TEACH Instructor Resource Manual

for

Torres and Ehrlich Modern Dental Assisting

Ninth Edition

TEACH Instructor Resource Manual

for

Torres and Ehrlich Modern Dental Assisting

Ninth Edition

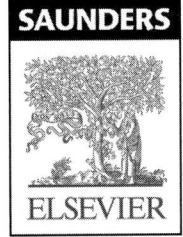

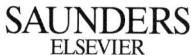

SAUNDERS
ELSEVIER

11830 Westline Industrial Drive
St. Louis, Missouri 63146

TEACH Instructor Resource Manual for
Torres and Ehrlich Modern Dental Assisting   ISBN: 978-1-4160-4263-1

Notice

Knowledge and best practice in this field are constantly changing. As new research and experience broaden our knowledge, changes in practice, treatment and drug therapy may become necessary or appropriate. Readers are advised to check the most current information provided (i) on procedures featured or (ii) by the manufacturer of each product to be administered, to verify the recommended dose or formula, the method and duration of administration, and contraindications. It is the responsibility of the practitioner, relying on their own experience and knowledge of the patient, to make diagnoses, to determine dosages and the best treatment for each individual patient, and to take all appropriate safety precautions. To the fullest extent of the law, neither the Publisher nor the Editors assumes any liability for any injury and/or damage to persons or property arising out of or related to any use of the material contained in this book.

The Publisher

International Standard Book Number 978-1-4160-4263-1

Senior Editor: John Dolan
Managing Editor: Jaime Pendill
Book Production Manager: Linda McKinley
Project Manager: Stephen Bancroft

Printed in United States of America

Last digit is the print number: 9 8 7 6 5 4 3 2 1

Working together to grow
libraries in developing countries

www.elsevier.com | www.bookaid.org | www.sabre.org

ELSEVIER   BOOK AID
            International   Sabre Foundation

How to Use This Instructor Resource Manual

Welcome to TEACH, your Total Curriculum Solution!

This Instructor Resource Manual is designed to help you prepare for classes using **Torres and Ehrlich Modern Dental Assisting**, by Doni Bird and Deborah Robinson. We hope it will reduce your lesson preparation time, give you new and creative ideas to promote student learning, and help you to make full use of the rich array of resources in the Bird/Robinson teaching package.

This Instructor Resource Manual is comprised of lesson plans, lecture outlines/slides with talking points, an appendix containing the answer keys for the workbook and textbook questions, and a test bank.

The lesson plans are designed to promote active student learning and get students involved in class discussions and activities. They include assessment tools to help you gauge your students' understanding of the course material and adapt lessons to their needs.

Each textbook chapter is divided into 50-minute lessons – building blocks that can be sequenced to fit your class schedule. The lesson plans are available in electronic format so that you can customize them to fit the requirements of your course.

Every lesson includes a wide variety of teaching resources. In many cases, our subject matter experts have provided more resources and activities than can be covered in a 50-minute lesson. We encourage you to choose activities that match the needs of your students and your curriculum, and the materials and resources available at your school.

Lesson plans can be a valuable tool for documenting how your curriculum covers and applies learning objectives. The Instructor Resource Manual helps you integrate learning resources into your program's curriculum to enhance students' learning experiences and may also help them achieve higher pass rates in the classroom and on the DANB certification exam. The activities in this Instructor Resource Manual will encourage your students to use learning resources such as the library or the Internet to complement their textbook.

Instructor Resource Manual Formats

This Instructor Resource Manual is available in 2 formats:

1. As a printed manual including a CD-ROM with Word files of the lesson plans and lecture outlines, PowerPoint slides of the lectures, and an electronic test bank in Exam View
2. Or online at http://TEACH.elsevier.com or http://evolve.elsevier.com/Bird/modern/. Access codes are available from your sales representative.

Instructor Resource Manual Organization

TEACH lesson plans complement Elsevier textbooks; there is a lesson plan chapter for each book chapter.

Each lesson plan chapter includes 3 sections:

1. **Preparation:** checklists to help you prepare classes based on the chapter

2. **Lessons:** Each chapter is divided into 50-minute lessons, to provide you with the building blocks for your curriculum
3. **Lecture Outlines:** teaching tips and questions for class discussion to accompany the PowerPoint slides

Preparation

The Preparation section ensures that you're well prepared for class. It includes the following checklists:

- *Teaching Focus* — identifies key student learning goals for the chapter

- *Materials and Resources* — lists materials needed for each lesson within the chapter

- *Lesson Checklist* — includes instructor preparation suggestions
- *Key Terms* — provides page references for each key term in the chapter
- *Additional Resources* — lists instructor resources available for this chapter
- *Key Terms* — provides page references for each key term in the chapter
- *Reference List* — lists instructor resources available for this chapter

Lessons

Each lesson includes the following sections:

Pretest and Background Assessment. The first lesson in each chapter includes a Pretest and two Background Assessment questions, designed to help you gauge your students' readiness for the lesson. Depending on students' responses, you may wish to modify your lesson. Students who are comfortable with the topic may need more challenging activities. Students who have difficulty with the topic may need to start by addressing more fundamental concepts.

Critical Thinking Question. Every lesson includes a Critical Thinking Question to motivate students by demonstrating real-world applications of the lesson content.

Lesson Roadmap. The heart of the TEACH lesson plan is the 3-column roadmap that links Objectives and Content from **Torres and Ehrlich Modern Dental Assisting** with its Teaching Resources. Teaching Resources reference all the elements of the ancillary package and include additional teaching tips such as Class Activities, discussion topics, and much more. This section correlates your textbook and its ancillary materials with the objectives upon which your course is based.

Homework/Assignments, Instructor's Notes/Student Feedback. These sections are provided for you to add your own notes for assignments, for recording student feedback, and for other notes relating to the lesson.

Lecture Outline

The Lecture Outlines include PowerPoint slides to provide a compelling visual presentation and summary of the main chapter points. Lecture notes for each slide highlight key topics and provide questions for discussion – to help create an interactive classroom environment.

We encourage you to select material from the Instructor Resource Manual that meets your students' needs, to integrate TEACH into your existing lesson plans, and to put your own teaching approach into the plans. We hope TEACH will be an invaluable tool in your classroom.

Answer Keys

This appendix includes answers to questions and exercises presented in other parts of the Modern Dental Assisting learning package. Answers to the Workbook exercises are included, divided by chapter. The Recall questions presented in the textbook are included with their answers, also divided by chapter. Answers are available only to instructors in the TEACH Instructor Resource Manual, or on the Evolve Web site.

Test Bank

A test bank with over 1,000 questions is available electronically on the accompanying CD-ROM or on the Evolve Web site. The test bank has been prepared in Exam View, a program that allows instructors to randomize test questions. Rationales for the correct and incorrect answer choices are included, as well as cross references to page numbers in the textbook.

Table of Contents
Torres and Ehrlich Modern Dental Assisting, 9th ed.

LESSON PLANS AND LECTURE OUTLINES

Chapter

Part One - The Dental Assisting Profession

Part Two - Sciences in Dentistry

Part Three - Oral Health and Prevention of Dental Disease

Part Four - Infection Control in Dentistry

Part Five - Occupational Health and Safety

PART THREE: ORAL HEALTH AND PREVENTION OF DENTAL DISEASE

PART FOUR: INFECTION CONTROL IN DENTISTRY

PART FIVE: OCCUPATIONAL HEALTH AND SAFETY

PART SIX: PATIENT INFORMATION AND ASSESSMENT

PART SEVEN: FOUNDATION OF CLINICAL DENTISTRY

Lesson Plan

1 History of Dentistry

TEACHING FOCUS

This chapter will give students the opportunity to learn about the history of dentistry. Early discoveries in dentistry, the educational and professional development of dentistry in the United States, as well as the history of dental assisting and dental hygiene will be discussed.

MATERIALS AND RESOURCES

☐ computer and PowerPoint projector (all Lessons)
☐ dry erase board and markers (all Lessons)
☐ index cards (Lesson 1.1)

LESSON CHECKLIST

Preparations for this lesson include:

- lecture
- guest speaker: dental professional, female dentist
- evaluation of student knowledge of the history of dentistry, including:
  - early history of dentistry
  - development of dentistry, including professional education, in the United States
  - history of dental assisting
  - history of dental hygienists

Bird/Robinson

KEY TERMS

Commission on Dental Accreditation of the
American Dental Association (p. 9)
dental treatise (p. 6)
forensic dentistry (p. 6)

periodontal disease (p. 3)
preceptorship (p. 6)
silver amalgam paste (p. 4)

ADDITIONAL RESOURCES

PowerPoint slides (Evolve): 1-38

Legend

CTQ
Critical
Thinking
Question

DVD
Multimedia
Procedures
Videos and
Animations

ESLR
EVOLVE
Student
Learning
Resources

IDO
Interactive
Dental
Office
CD-ROM

SW
Student
Workbook

TB
Test Bank
on the
TEACH
CD-ROM

PPT
PowerPoint
Slides

Class Activities are indicated in ***bold italic***.

ELSEVIER

Torres and Ehrlich Modern Dental Assisting, 9th ed.

Bird/Robinson

LESSON 1.1

PRETEST

1. What term signifies study under the guidance of a dentist or other professional without attending an institution of higher learning?
   a. accreditation
   b. preceptorship
   c. working unit
   d. curriculum

2. Who was the first African-American female dental graduate from a U.S. dental college?
   a. Malvina Cueria
   b. Ida Gray-Rollins
   c. Lucy B. Hobbs-Taylor
   d. Emeline Robert Jones

3. Who is the earliest dentist whose name is known and in what country or region did he reside?
   a. T'ing To-t'ung (China)
   b. Cornelius Celsus (Rome)
   c. Hesi-Re (Egypt)
   d. Diocles of Carystus (Greece)

4. Who is the "Grand Old Man of Dentistry"?
   a. Chapin A. Harris
   b. Horace H. Hayden
   c. Green Vardiman Black
   d. Wilhelm Conrad Roentgen

5. Who is credited with beginning forensic dentistry?
   a. Paul Revere
   b. Isaac Greenwood
   c. John Baker
   d. Horace Hayden

6. Who is Pierre Fauchard?
   a. originated the title of "surgeon dentist"
   b. George Washington's dentist
   c. showed the usefulness of nitrous oxide sedation
   d. "Father of Modern Surgery"

7. Who was the source of the famous oath—a solemn obligation to refrain from wrongdoing and to treat patients with confidentiality and to the best of one's ability?
   a. Aristotle
   b. Diocles
   c. Hippocrates
   d. Celsus

8. In which state did the first dental college start?
   a. Connecticut
   b. Virginia
   c. California
   d. Maryland

9. Who was the first to describe the difference between molars and premolars?
   a. Ambroise Paré
   b. Pierre Fauchard
   c. Joseph Warren
   d. Leonardo da Vinci

10. Who was the first dentist to employ a dental assistant?
    a. C. Edmund Kells
    b. Joseph Warren
    c. Emeline Robert Jones
    d. Green Vardiman Black

Answers

1. b	3. c	5. a	7. c	9. d
2. b	4. c	6. a	8. d	10. a

BACKGROUND ASSESSMENT

Question: What is the Hippocratic Oath and how does it apply to dentistry?
Answer: Hippocrates, a Greek physician who lived from 460 to 377 BC, brought his famous oath to both the medical and dental field alike. He believed it was the solemn obligation of any healthcare professional to refrain from wrongdoing and to treat patients with confidentiality and to the best of one's ability.

Bird/Robinson

Question: Who is the "Grand Old Man of Dentistry" and what were his contributions to the field of dentistry?

Answer: Dr. Green Vardiman Black (1836-1915), known worldwide as G.V. Black, earned the title of the "Grand Old Man of Dentistry" through his unmatched contributions to the profession. Two of his major contributions to dentistry were (1) the principle of extension for prevention, in which the margins of a filling were extended to be within reach of a toothbrush for cleaning the tooth, and (2) establishing standardized rules of cavity preparation and filling.

CRITICAL THINKING QUESTION

A male patient is offered nitrous oxide for pain control during a dental procedure. He is concerned about the use of this type of anesthesia and asks the dental assistant for more background information on this drug. He wants to know how long nitrous oxide has been in use for patient comfort. How should the dental assistant respond to the patient's questions?

Guidelines: The dental assistant should acknowledge the patient's concerns about receiving inhalation anesthesia and then share some history about the use of nitrous oxide. The dental assistant can explain to the patient that a dentist by the name of Horace Wells discovered inhalation anesthesia in the mid-nineteenth century (1844). The dental assistant can reassure the patient that since that time, patients are made to feel more comfortable by the controlled use of nitrous oxide during dental treatment. It is a procedure that complements local anesthesia and other forms of pain control.

OBJECTIVES	CONTENT	TEACHING RESOURCES
Pronounce, define, and spell the Key Terms.	■ Key terms (p. 2)	▣ TB question 11 ▣ SW Fill in the Blank questions 2-5 (p. 2) ▣ ESLR Electronic Flashcards ▸ Discuss each of the key terms in Chapter 1, focusing on the definition, pronunciation, and spelling of each term. *Class Activity Ask the students to get together in small groups. Have each group create flash cards for the key terms. On one side of the flash card, have the groups paraphrase the definition of the term. On the flip side of the flash card, have them correctly spell the key term and include a phonetic spelling of the term. Collect all the flash cards and present them to the class for review, sometimes reading the term and asking for the definition, sometimes reading the definition and asking for the term.*
Describe the role of Hippocrates in history.	■ Early times (p. 3) ☐ The Egyptians (p. 3) ☐ The Greeks (p. 3)	▣ PPT 6-7 ▣ TB question 2 ▣ SW Short-Answer Questions 1; Fill in the Blank question 4; Multiple Choice questions 1-3; Activity: Questions to Ask (pp. 1-3) Table 1-1 Highlights in the History of Dentistry (p. 4) Figure 1-1 Ancient Etruscan gold-banded bridge with built-in calf's tooth (p. 3) Recall questions 1-2 (p. 3) ▽ CTQ 1-2, 4 (p. 10)

OBJECTIVES	CONTENT	TEACHING RESOURCES
		▸ Discuss what medicine might have been like before Hippocrates. ▸ Discuss why Hippocrates believed dental health was important and how it factored into his concept of the human body. ***Class Activity** Have the students interview a dental professional and ask three questions about the Hippocratic Oath. Have them prepare a report on their findings to share with the class. (For students to prepare for this activity, see Homework/Assignments #1.)*
State the basic premise of the Hippocratic Oath.	☐ The Greeks (p. 3) ☐ The Chinese (pp. 3-4) ☐ The Romans (p. 4) ■ The Renaissance (p. 5) ■ Early America (pp. 5-6)	▣▤ PPT 7-14 ▥ TB questions 3-5 ▨ SW Short-Answer Questions 2; Fill in the Blank question 3; Multiple Choice questions 4-11 (pp. 1-3) Recall questions 3-12 (pp. 5-6) Figure 1-2 Pierre Fauchard (p. 5) Figure 1-3 John Greenwood (p. 6) ♡ CTQ 5 (p. 10) ▸ Discuss early American history with regard to dentistry and the development of the science of forensic medicine. ***Class Activity** The modern Hippocratic Oath in part states the obligation of physicians to prevent disease from occurring whenever they can. Choose one student to read that section out loud to the rest of the class. Then ask the students to give specific examples of how dental professionals can help prevent disease. List their responses on the board.*

1.1 Homework/Assignments:

1. Ask the students to interview a dental professional and ask three questions about the Hippocratic Oath. Have the students come to class prepared to share their findings.

1.1 Instructor's Notes/Student Feedback:

ELSEVIER

Torres and Ehrlich Modern Dental Assisting, 9th ed.

LESSON 1.2

CRITICAL THINKING QUESTION

A dental assistant is working with a young African-American girl who expresses an interest in becoming a dentist, although she admits she has never seen a woman dentist. The young girl's dentist (the dental assistant's employer) is male. She also wonders if being part of a minority group would affect her ability to pursue a career in dentistry. How should the dental assistant advise this young patient?

Guidelines: Having studied the history of dentistry, the dental assistant should share with this young woman that many women from various ethnicities have entered the dental field. The dental assistant should tell the young patient about Ida Gray, the very first African-American women dentist, who practiced in Chicago more than 50 years ago. The dental assistant should continue to explain that, currently, women represent almost 50 percent of students in some dental schools. It is projected that by the year 2020, 20% of all dental practitioners in the United States will be women. Today, women are active in dental associations, specialty organizations, public health, and the military. The dental assistant should encourage this young patient to follow her dreams and pursue her professional passion.

OBJECTIVES	CONTENT	TEACHING RESOURCES
Discuss the contributions of Horace H. Hayden and Chapin A. Harris.	■ Educational and professional development in the United States (p. 6)	PPT 18 SW Short-Answer Questions 6; Fill in the Blank question 2; Multiple Choice question 12 (pp. 1-3) Recall question 13 (p. 7) ▸ Discuss the impact of Hayden and Harris on modern dentistry. ▸ Discuss the various ways that students were trained in dentistry before the founding of a formal dental college. *Class Activity Divide the class into small groups. Have each group access the Internet and browse the website for the American Dental Association (ADA) at http://www.ada.org. Ask students to compare the first dental organization founded by Harris to the ADA as it now functions. What changes were necessary for the dental association to develop its new roles? (For students to prepare for this activity, see Homework/Assignments #1.)*
Describe two major contributions of G.V. Black.	■ Educational and professional development in the United States (p. 6)	PPT 19-21 TB question 6 SW Short-Answer Questions 7; Multiple Choice question 13 (pp. 1, 3) Recall question 14 (p. 7) Figure 1-4 G.V. Black (p. 6) Figure 1-5 Black's dental treatment room (p. 7) ▸ Discuss the two major contributions to modern dentistry of G.V. Black and describe his impact on modern dentistry.

Bird/Robinson

OBJECTIVES	CONTENT	TEACHING RESOURCES
		▸ Discuss the similarities and differences between Black's dental treatment room and modern dental treatment rooms.
		Class Activity Ask three students to prepare to play the game "Who's the real Dr. Black?" by becoming familiar with the contributions that G. V. Black made to the dental profession. Have the rest of the students try to stump the three panelists by asking them prepared questions. The panelist who is best prepared is given the title of "Grand Old Dental Assistant" for the day.
Name the scientist who discovered radiographs.	■ Educational and professional development in the United States (p. 6)	PPT 22-23 TB question 7 SW Short-Answer Questions 10; Fill in the Blank question 6 (pp. 1-2) Figure 1-6 Roentgen (p. 7) ▸ Discuss the impact of the discovery of radiographs to dentistry. *Class Activity Invite a dental professional to speak to the class about several standard dental practices, making sure to contrast how they were performed before and after the development of dental x-ray technology. Have students take part in a question-and-answer session based on the presentation.*
Name the physician who first used nitrous oxide for tooth extractions.	■ Educational and professional development in the United States. (p. 6)	PPT 24 TB question 8 SW Short-Answer Questions 11; Multiple Choice question 15 (pp. 1, 3) Recall question 15 (p. 7) ▸ Discuss what drugs were used before nitrous oxide and whether they would be considered reliable anesthetics. ▸ Discuss how nitrous oxide might have been discovered and recognized as useful in medicine and dentistry. *Class Activity Divide the class into small groups, and ask each to research and prepare a timeline on the history of pain control in dentistry. Have a volunteer from each group present the group's timeline to the rest of the class. (For students to prepare for this activity, see Homework/ Assignments #2.)*
Name the first woman to graduate from a college of dentistry.	☐ Women in dentistry (p. 7)	PPT 25 TB questions 1, 9 SW Short-Answer Questions 3; Multiple Choice

OBJECTIVES	CONTENT	TEACHING RESOURCES
		question 17 (pp. 1, 3)
		Figure 1-7 Dental instrument kit (p. 7)
		Figure 1-8 Lucy B. Hobbs-Taylor (p. 8)
		Table 1-2 Highlights of Women in Dentistry (p. 8)
		Recall question 19 (p. 10)
		CTQ 3 (p. 10)
		▸ Discuss how society in general viewed women going to medical school in the nineteenth century and how those views changed in the twentieth century.
		Class Activity Divide the class into small groups, and have each group develop an ad campaign aimed at women about joining the field of dentistry. Make sure the advertisement stresses the visibility of women in the dental profession. Have a volunteer from each group present the group's advertisement to the class for discussion.
Name the first African-American woman to receive a dental degree in the United States.	☐ Women in dentistry (p. 7)	PPT 26 SW Short-Answer Questions 5; Fill in the Blank question 7 (pp. 1-2) Recall question 20 (p. 10) ▸ Discuss how the experiences of an African-American woman in learning and practicing medicine would differ from those of a Caucasian woman. ▸ Discuss how African-American female dentists would affect dental care in the African-American communities of the United States. *Class Activity Before class, have the students obtain statistics from the National Dental Association on the ethnic diversity of the members of the dental community. Ask the students to share this information with the class. (For students to prepare for this activity, see Homework/Assignments #3.)*
Name the first woman to practice dentistry in the United States.	☐ Women in dentistry (p. 7)	PPT 27-29 SW Short-Answer Questions 4; Multiple Choice question 16 (pp. 1, 3) ▸ Discuss how a male patient might react to being treated by a female dentist. ▸ Discuss how a woman in the nineteenth century would balance a career in dentistry with a family life.

Torres and Ehrlich Modern Dental Assisting, 9ᵗʰ ed.
Bird/Robinson

OBJECTIVES	CONTENT	TEACHING RESOURCES
		Class Activity Invite a woman dentist to speak to the class about her decision to join the dental field. Ask her to address any gender-related challenges she may have faced in her profession and how she handled them. Have the students create brief interview questions in preparation for her visit.
Name the first dentist to employ a dental assistant.	☐ History of dental assisting (p. 8)	PPT 30 TB question 10 SW Short-Answer Questions 8; Multiple Choice question 14 (pp. 1, 3) Figure 1-9, C. Edmund Kells and his "working unit" (p. 9) Recall question 17 (p. 10) ▸ Discuss how C. Edmund Kells developed the idea of employing a dental assistant. ▸ Discuss what qualities a dentist in the nineteenth century might have looked for in a woman being hired as a dental assistant. *Class Activity Divide the class into two groups. Ask each group to create a collage of pictures and words depicting the development of accredited dental-assisting educational programs.*
Name the first female dental assistant.	☐ History of dental assisting (p. 8) ☐ History of dental hygiene (pp. 8-9) ☐ Dental accreditation (p. 9)	PPT 31-36 TB question 11 SW Short-Answer Question 9; Fill in the Blank questions 1, 5 (pp. 1-2) Figure 1-10 Dental hygienist during the 1960s working in a standing position (p. 9) Figure 1-11 Dental students at University of California San Francisco (p. 9) Figure 1-12 Modern dental-assisting students (p. 10) Recall question 18 (p. 10) ▸ Discuss how the role of dental assistants has changed from the nineteenth century to modern times. ▸ Discuss how the introduction of dental hygienists has changed the nature of dentistry. ▸ Discuss how dental accreditation changed dentistry and what elements were first included in that accreditation. *Class Activity Ask the class to create a hypothetical student award in honor of the first dental assistant. The award is to be presented to a worthy student upon graduation. Have the class make a list of the attributes*

Bird/Robinson

OBJECTIVES	CONTENT	TEACHING RESOURCES
		that a student must possess in order to be considered for such an award. Then have the class decide on a name for the award.
Discuss the purpose and activities of the National Museum of Dentistry.	☐ National Museum of Dentistry (pp. 9-10)	🖥️ PPT 37-38 💻 TB question 12 📖 SW Short-Answer Questions 12; Multiple Choice question 18 (pp. 1, 3) Figure 1-13 Dr. Samuel D. Harris National Museum of Dentistry (p. 10) Recall question 21 (p. 10) Legal and Ethical Implications (p. 10) Eye to the Future (p. 10) ▸ Discuss how a museum changes society's view of a profession. ▸ Discuss what would be the most important items to include in a museum of dentistry. *Class Activity Divide the class into three groups. Ask the groups to access the Internet and browse the website for the National Museum of Dentistry (NMD) at http://www.dentalmuseum.umaryland.edu/. Have each group report on one of the three ways to get involved in NMD:* *1. Ways to donate* *2. Ways to participate* *3. Opportunities to provide museum leadership* *(For students to prepare for this activity, see Homework/Assignments #4.)*
Performance Evaluation		💻 TB 📖 SW questions (pp. 1-3) 📀 ESLR Electronic Flashcards 📀 ESLR Practice Quiz Recall questions (pp. 5-7, 10)

Torres and Ehrlich Modern Dental Assisting, 9th ed.

Bird/Robinson

1.2 Homework/Assignments:

1. Have the students access the Internet and browse the website for the American Dental Association (ADA) at http://www.ada.org. Ask the students to compare the current ADA to the organization founded by Harris.

2. Ask students to research and prepare a time line with their group that concerns the history of pain control in dentistry.

3. Have the students obtain statistics from the National Dental Association on the ethnic diversity of the members of the dental community.

4. Divide the class into three groups. Ask the groups to access the Internet and browse the Web site for the National Museum of Dentistry (NMD) at http://www.dentalmuseum.umaryland.edu/. Have each group report on one of the three ways to get involved in NMD: (1) ways to donate, (2) ways to participate, (3) opportunities to provide museum leadership.

1.2 Instructor's Notes/Student Feedback:

Slide 1

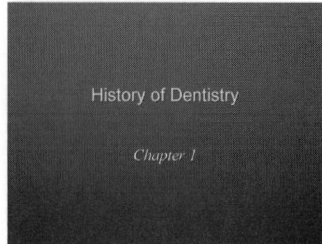

History of Dentistry

Chapter 1

Slide 2

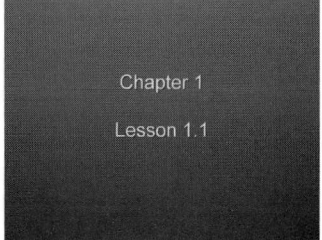

Chapter 1

Lesson 1.1

Slide 3

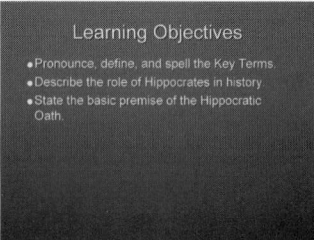

Learning Objectives
- Pronounce, define, and spell the Key Terms.
- Describe the role of Hippocrates in history.
- State the basic premise of the Hippocratic Oath.

Slide 4

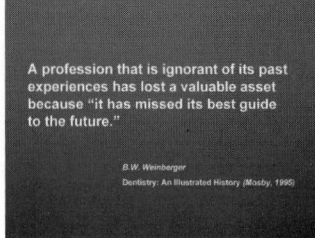

A profession that is ignorant of its past experiences has lost a valuable asset because "it has missed its best guide to the future."

B.W. Weinberger

Dentistry: An Illustrated History (Mosby, 1995)

Slide 5

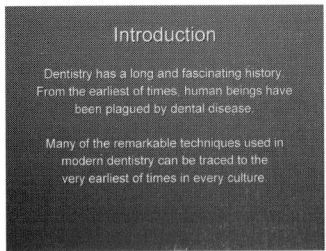

- What constitutes dental disease? *(Dental disease can include cavities or caries and gum disease or periodontal disease We now know that dental disease can lead to systemic, somatic disease.)*
- What is the earliest record of dentistry?

Slide 6

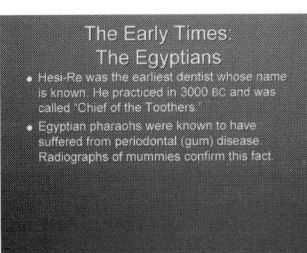

- Were teeth full of caries (cavities) in ancient times? *(The mummies of this time prove that teeth were not necessarily bad, as we had assumed, without modern dental information and techniques. The wear from a rougher, non-processed diet removed small cavities before they had a chance to get established, and also helped to clean out the space between teeth. This rougher diet also helped to keep teeth straighter. This changed and caries became more common as we moved to the more modern world of the Renaissance. Changes included the technology to produce softer food, sugar, and the use of the fork.)*

Slide 7

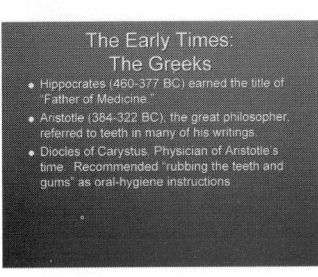

- Aristotle mistakenly stated that men had 32 teeth and women had only 30. From this came the use of the term "wisdom teeth," which only men supposedly had.
- Diocles advised rubbing teeth and gums with bare fingers using ground-up mint to remove particles of food, a forerunner of today's modern "minty" toothpastes.
- What is the history of toothpastes? *(Long ago, people used ground-up chalk or charcoal, lemon juice, ashes, or even a mixture of tobacco and honey to clean their teeth. It was only about 100 years ago that someone created a minty cream to clean teeth.)*

Slide 8

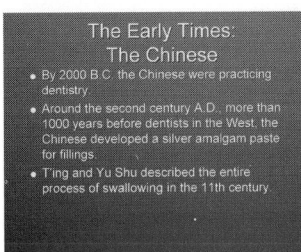

- China sets aside September 20th as a national holiday known as "Love Your Teeth Day." The ancient Chinese wrapped tiny pieces of parchment containing written prayers and incantations around painful teeth.
- How do we celebrate teeth in the U.S.? *(We have the annual observance of National Children's Dental Health Month. It began as a one-day event in Cleveland, Ohio on 2/3/1941. The American Dental Association held the first national observance of Children's Dental Health Day on 2/8/1949. This single-day observance became a week-long event in 1955, and in 1981 it was extended to a month-long celebration.)*

ELSEVIER

Torres and Ehrlich Modern Dental Assisting, 9th ed.

Bird/Robinson

Slide 9

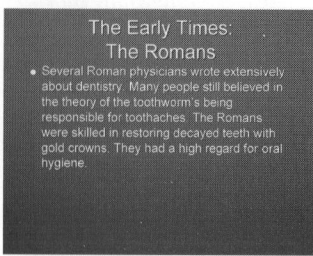

- What is a toothworm? *(People of ancient times believed that a toothworm caused toothaches. They thought the worm just appeared, or drilled its way into a tooth. If the tooth pain was severe, it meant that the worm was moving around. If the aching stopped, then the worm was resting. People smeared their aching teeth with honey and waited all night with tweezers in hand, ready to pull out the toothworm.)*

- Did the Romans have toothbrushes? *(They were called "chew sticks" and were actually small branches, with one frayed end. They were rubbed on teeth to scrape off any particles.)*

Slide 10

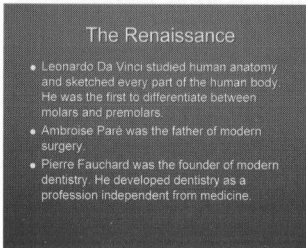

- Ambroise Paré was an apprentice to a barber surgeon.

- His writings include dental extraction methods and reimplantation of teeth.

- He is also credited with being the first to use artificial eyes, hands, and legs.

Slide 11

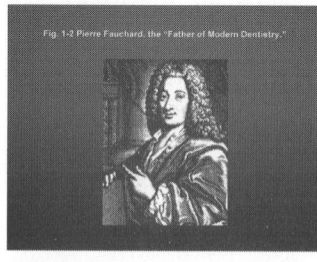

- Why is Pierre Fauchard regarded as the "Father of Modern Dentistry"? *(He developed dentistry as an independent profession and came up with the title of "surgeon dentist." In the United States, the degree conferred on dentists is Doctor of Dental Surgery [DDS].)*

Slide 12

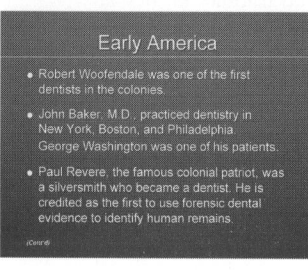

- How did Paul Revere become involved in forensic dentistry? *(He performed the first identification of a corpse based on dental history. The corpse was that of Dr. Joseph Warren, whom Revere identified by a two-unit bridge he had made for him years earlier.)*

- What does a forensic dentist do today? *(He performs dental identification of deceased individuals.)*

Slide 13

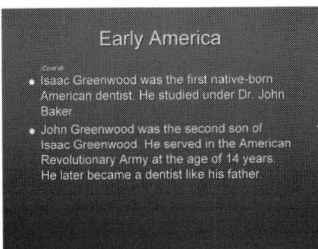

- What was John Greenwood's claim to fame? (*He was one of George Washington's dentists.*)

Slide 14

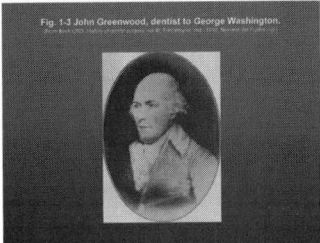

- What was George Washington's dental history? Did he really have wooden teeth? (*When George Washington was elected President, he had only one tooth—a lower left premolar. He never had wooden teeth. His dentures were manufactured from gold, hippopotamus tusk, elephant ivory, and human teeth.*)

- Where was the first dental college established?

Slide 15

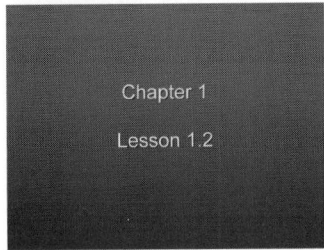

Slide 16

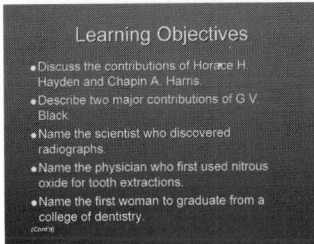

Bird/Robinson

Slide 17

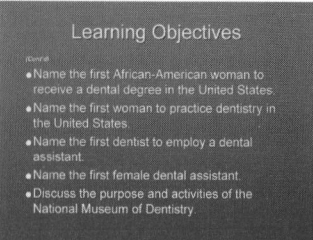

Slide 18

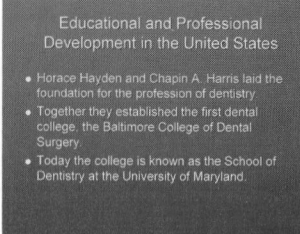

- How did dentists learn their profession before dental schools? *(They learned by preceptorship, where a practicing dentist trained another dentist on the job to perform dental duties.)*

Slide 19

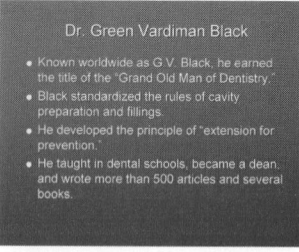

- Who is the "Grand Old Man of Dentistry"?

- What does "extension for prevention" mean? *(The margins of a filling or restoration were extended to within reach of a toothbrush for cleaning the tooth.)*

- Instead of "extension for prevention," today's cavity prevention is designed to preserve the health of the tooth over a lifetime. Minimally invasive dentistry is the adoption of detection, diagnosis, limited surgical intervention for excavation of decay, and restoration, with a view toward maximum preservation of tooth structure and adjunctive remineralization therapy.

Slide 20

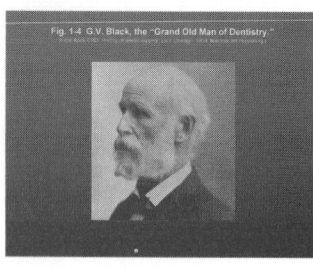

- Dr. Black studied with his brother, a doctor, before going into dentistry.

- Dr. Black believed that dentistry should stand as a profession independent from and equal to that of medicine.

- His first book was called *The Formation of Poisons by Microorganisms.*

- What did Dr. Black use to study microorganisms? *(A microscope; he later formed a Microscope Club for the same reason. He obtained one of the first microscopes in Illinois and became the de facto consulting pathologist for the region. He developed modem techniques for filling teeth based upon biological principles and microscopic evaluation.)*

Slide 21

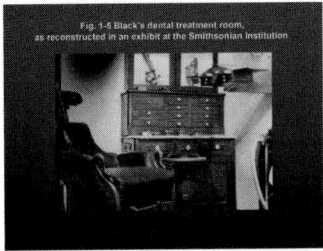

- Look carefully at Dr. Black's dental treatment room. Compare this dental treatment room to today's modern rooms.
  - Would the dental professional stand or sit? *(Stand.)*
  - Would the patient always be sitting or laying supine? *(Always sitting.)*
  - Would there be suction or just a spittoon? *(Spittoon only.)*
  - How would the patient's mouth be rinsed? *(Bulb with water.)*

Slide 22

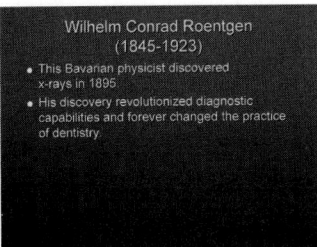

- How did the discovery of x-rays change dentistry forever?

Slide 23

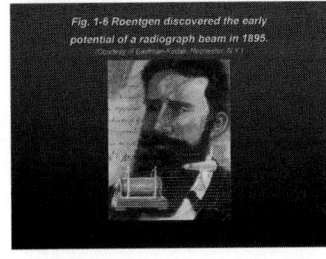

- The first x-rays were called "roentgenograms."
- Roentgen was awarded the Nobel Prize for his work in x-rays.
- *(Tie this slide in with Chapter 38: Foundations of Radiography, Radiographic Equipment, and Radiologic Safety.)*

Slide 24

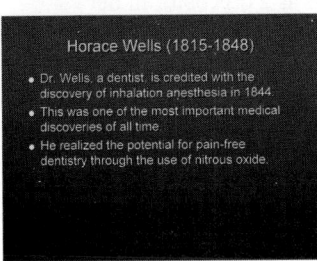

- What pain remedies were available for patients before there were pain control procedures such as nitrous oxide? *(Brute force, alcohol, and opium were used. Dosing of oral drugs was inaccurate, leaving patients either undermedicated or overmedicated. Patients could die of exhaustion or shock if an operation lasted more than 20 minutes.)*
- *(Tie this slide in with Chapter 37: Anesthesia and Pain Control.)*
- Was dentistry the first to use nitrous oxide? *(Yes, but after Dr. Wells' success, the medical community later modified and adopted inhalation anesthesia as a standard surgical management procedure.)*

Bird/Robinson

Slide 25

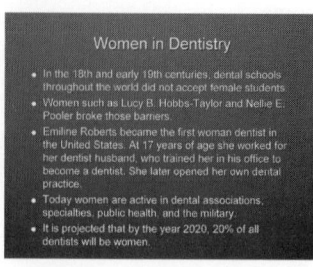

- During her preceptorship with her husband and another local dentist, Emiline Roberts saved several hundred extracted teeth and secretly placed restorations in them to practice.

- Dr. Roberts trained her son, David, in a preceptorship in dentistry. Then she sent him to Yale University and Harvard's School of Dental Medicine.

- Today, women represent almost 50% of students in some dental schools.

Slide 26

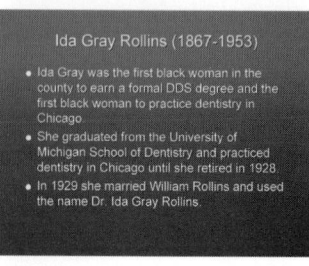

- Who was the first black male dentist? *(Dr. Robert Tanner Freeman)*

- Is there an association for the black dental professional today? *(The National Dental Association [NDA] is a national forum for minority dentists and a leader in advancing their rights within the dental profession.)*

- What is the relationship between the NDA and ADA? *(NDA received ADA's empathic support for its insistence on removal of racial discrimination in dentistry's predominant organization. In 1965, unprecedented action by the ADA House of Delegates nullified sanctioned racial discrimination within the dental profession.)*

Slide 27

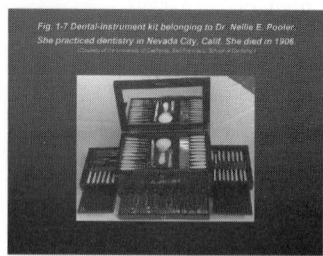

- Look closely at the instruments. Note the forceps in the bottom drawer.

- Forceps are one of the oldest of all dental instruments. Forceps were known by such names as parrot's beak, crow's bill, and stork's bill.

- Forceps were and still are the key instrument for extraction of teeth.

Slide 28

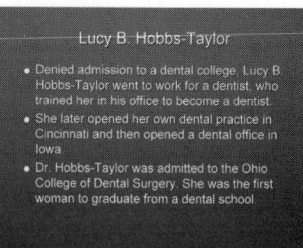

- Lucy Hobbs-Taylor received credit for time as a preceptor in her husband's practice.

Bird/Robinson

Slide 29

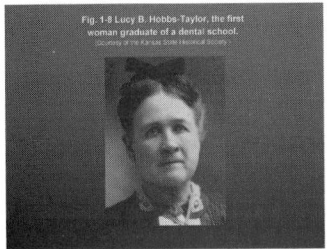

- Lucy's admission to dental school prompted a dentist to write in the *Dental Times* that "the very form and structure of a woman unfits her for its duties" and that "the female of the species (does not have) the necessary strength which the practice of dentistry requires."

- Does this prejudice (that women are not strong enough for dentistry) still exist today?

Slide 30

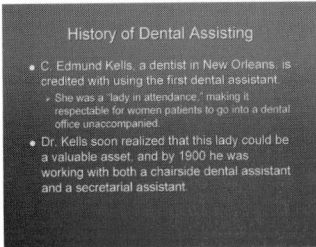

- What would it have been like to be the first dental assistant? *(The assistant's duties, as listed by the ADA in its dental history records, included chair-side assistance, instrument cleaning, inventory, appointments, bookkeeping, and reception—not unlike today.)*

- How did dental-assisting education start? *(Other dentists began training dental assistants in their own offices. In 1930, a committee was formed to draft training courses to be used as educational guides. In 1948, the Certifying Board of the American Dental Assistants Association was established, now the Dental Assisting National Board. By 1950, there were one- and two-year programs for dental-assisting education.)*

Slide 31

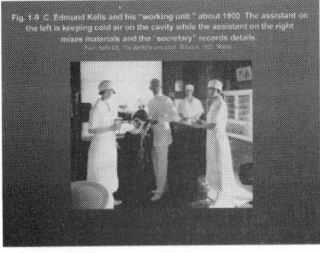

- Who was the first female dental assistant? *(Malvina Cueria.)*

- Dr. Kells was also the first to use radiographs in dental practice.

- When, at age 40, he first began his work with X-rays, Dr. Kells was unaware of the unseen danger of cumulative doses of radiation. He often held the films in place with his own fingers. By the time Kells reached 50, he had developed cancer in his right hand. Over the next 20 years, Kells endured 42 operations. He progressively lost his hand, his arm, and his shoulder.

Slide 32

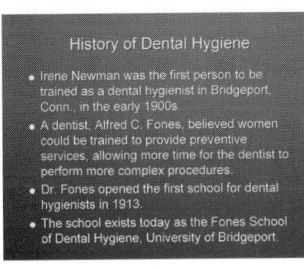

- What happened to the first dental hygiene graduates? *(Most of the 27 graduates of the first class were employed by the local Board of Education to clean the teeth of school children. The greatly reduced incidence of caries among these children gave strength to the dental hygienist movement.)*

Slide 33

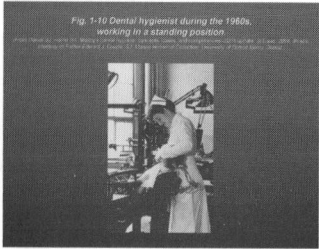

- Is standing all the time while working on a patient hard on a dental professional? *(Yes, today we recognize that it is important to practice the correct ergonomic standards to prevent work-related injury.)*

Slide 34

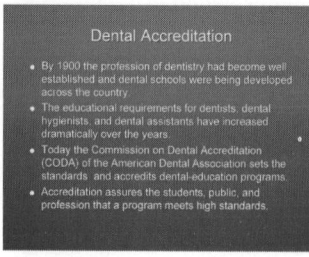

- What is the mission of the Commission on Dental Accreditation (CODA)? *(Its mission is to serve the public by establishing, maintaining, and applying standards that ensure the quality and continuous improvement of dental and dental-related education and reflect the evolving practice of dentistry.)*

- What dental professions does CODA regulate? *(The scope of CODA includes dental, advanced dental, and allied dental education programs.)*

Slide 35

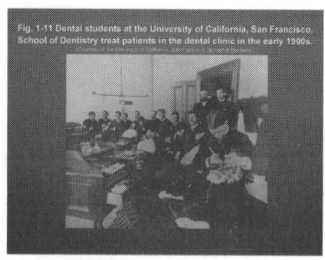

- What stands out about this picture? *(The dentists are wearing street clothes, and are not wearing masks, eyewear, or gloves. Now we practice dentistry with strict infection control standards.)*

- When was the first fully reclining dental chair introduced? *(1958.)*

- What does the seal for dentistry mean? *(The design uses a serpent entwined about an ancient Arabian cautery in the manner of the single serpent of Aesculapius, the Greek god of medicine, coiled about a rod. The Greek letter Δ for dentistry and the Greek letter Ο for odont (tooth) form the periphery of the design. In the background are 32 leaves and 20 berries, representing the permanent and temporary teeth.)*

Slide 36

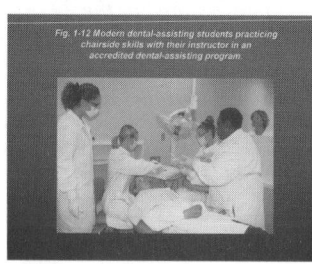

- Compare this dental treatment room to the one used by Dr. Black and the old dental school.

  - Does the dental professional stand or sit? *(Sit.)*

  - Is the patient sitting or lying supine? *(Lying supine.)*

  - Would there be suction or just a spittoon? *(Suction is available.)*

  - How would the patient's mouth be rinsed? *(Hand water spray.)*

  - What is the dental professional wearing to help with infection control standards? *(Lab coat, mask, eyewear, and gloves.)*

- How often are dental-assisting schools reviewed to maintain their accreditation status? *(Every seven years.)*

ELSEVIER

Torres and Ehrlich Modern Dental Assisting, 9th ed.

Bird/Robinson

Slide 37

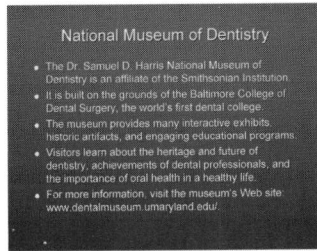

- What are the most recent advances in dentistry in the last 25 years?

  - *1980s—Per-Ingvar Branemark describes techniques for the osseointegration of dental implants.*

  - *1989—The first commercial home tooth-bleaching product is marketed.*

  - *1990s—New tooth-colored restorative materials plus increased usage of bleaching, veneers, and implants inaugurate an era of aesthetic dentistry.*

  - *1997—FDA approves the erbium YAG laser, the first for use on dentin, to treat tooth decay.*

Slide 38

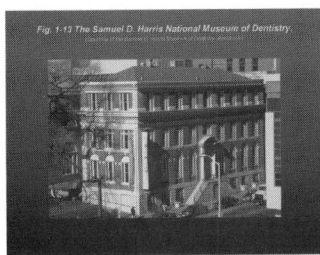

- Many of the remarkable techniques in modern dentistry can be traced to the earliest times in every culture.

- List what we still use today in dentistry? *(X-rays, local anesthesia, nitrous oxide, surgical instruments, amalgam, etc.)*

- Think of dentistry's past: first use of x-rays, first women dentist or dental assistant, first use of pain control. What will be the new "firsts" in the future of dentistry?

- Additional dental museums include the Pierre Fauchard Museum of Dental History at the Community College of Southern Nevada, United States, and the Pierre Fauchard Museum of Dentistry at Paris, France.

2 The Professional Dental Assistant

TEACHING FOCUS

This chapter will give the student the opportunity to learn about aspects of the career of the professional dental assistant. These include the different roles of the dental assistant, the importance of maintaining a professional appearance, the qualities needed to be a dental assistant, and the professional organizations for dental assistants.

MATERIALS AND RESOURCES

☐ computer and PowerPoint projector (Lesson 2.1)

LESSON CHECKLIST

Preparations for this lesson include:

- lecture
- guest speakers: representatives from ADAA and DANB; dental assistant
- evaluation of student knowledge and skills needed to perform all entry-level activities related to the profession of dental assistant, including:
  - confidentiality
  - knowledge and skills
  - personal qualities
  - professional appearance
  - professional organizations

KEY TERMS

American Dental Assistants Association
(ADAA) (p. 13)
certified dental assistant (CDA) (p. 15)

Dental Assisting National Board (DANB) (p. 15)
HIPAA (p. 13)
professional (p. 12)

ADDITIONAL RESOURCES

PowerPoint slides (Evolve): 1-29

Legend

CTQ
Critical
Thinking
Question

DVD
Multimedia
Procedures
Videos and
Animations

ESLR
EVOLVE
Student
Learning
Resources

IDO
Interactive
Dental
Office
CD-ROM

SW
Student
Workbook

TB
Test Bank
on the
TEACH
CD-ROM

PPT
PowerPoint
Slides

Class Activities are indicated in ***bold italic.***

Torres and Ehrlich Modern Dental Assisting, 9th ed.

Bird/Robinson

LESSON 2.1

PRETEST

1. What is the nationally recognized credential of the dental assistant who has passed the DANB certification examination and keeps up current practice through continuing education?
   a. CDA
   b. ADAA
   c. EFDA
   d. HIPAA

2. Which of the following roles of a dental assistant involves the delegation of the functions—such as placing a retraction cord—that vary among states, depending on the individual state's dental practice act,?
   a. chairside dental assistant
   b. expanded-functions dental assistant
   c. administrative assistant
   d. secretarial assistant

3. Which of the following is always considered part of professional attire for a dental assistant?
   a. appropriate undergarments
   b. excessive makeup
   c. excessive jewelry
   d. perfumes and scents

4. What do the letters in TEAM stand for?
   a. Time, Effort, Allowance, Majority
   b. Together, Everyone Accomplishes More
   c. Time Evolves And More
   d. Together, Effort Always Matters

5. When the dental assistant is working in the hospital, what should he or she always wear?
   a. surgical gowns
   b. scrubs with clean shoes
   c. street clothes
   d. full personal protective wear

6. What is the new set of federal privacy laws for healthcare patients?
   a. OSHA
   b. EFDA
   c. HIPAA
   d. DANB

7. Who is the founder of ADAA?
   a. Malvina Cueria
   b. Juliette A. Southard
   c. Edmund Kells
   d. Emeline Robert Jones

8. Which of the following are in the DANB examination?
   a. radiology, infection control, ethics and jurisprudence
   b. radiology, infection control, general chairside
   c. infection control, oral pathology, general chairside
   d. oral pathology, ethics and jurisprudence, tooth morphology

9. When a dental assistant becomes certified, which of the following does he or she obtain?
   a. expanded-function licensure
   b. pin and certificate
   c. registration in any state
   d. use of the ADAA credentials

10. Professionalism is what distinguishes people who only "pursue a job" from those who
    a. "have a business."
    b. "work overtime."
    c. "pursue a career."
    d. "work weekends."

Answers

1. a	3. a	5. a	7. b	9. b
2. b	4. b	6. c	8. b	10. c

ELSEVIER

Bird/Robinson

BACKGROUND ASSESSMENT

Question: What are three key elements of a dental assistant's professional appearance?

Answer: The key elements are good health, good grooming, and appropriate dress. To stay in good health, you must get an adequate amount of rest, eat well-balanced meals, and exercise enough to keep fit. Good grooming requires paying attention to the details of your personal appearance. Appropriate dress involves wearing clothing appropriate for the type of dental office in which the dental assistant is working. Regardless of the type of professional wear, it must be clean, wrinkle-free, and worn over appropriate undergarments.

Question: On your first position as a dental assistant, you are not sure how to talk to patients. Should you talk to them as if you are good friends, or is there another way to relate to patients that is more professional? Should you discuss your private life or keep the conversation pleasant but light? What should one do when patients seem upset when visiting the office?

Answer: The dental assistant must demonstrate sensitivity to the patient's needs, show empathy, say "the right thing at the right time," and be sincere. Again, avoid discussing aspects of your personal life with your patients. By learning to be a good listener, you will develop sensitivity for the opinions and concerns of others. It is nearly impossible to build rapport (good relations) with the patients in your office if they do not trust you.

CRITICAL THINKING QUESTION

Your first employer does not know there is a dental assisting association or anything about certification of dental assistants. You would like to join the association and eventually become certified; you want your employer to understand what this means and how it can add to your professional standing. What do you say to your dentist?

Guidelines: In a courteous and professional manner, inform the dentist about the Dental Assisting National Board (DANB), the national agency responsible for administering the certification examination and issuing the credential of certified dental assistant. This certification is the nationally recognized credential of the dental assistant who keeps up current practice through continuing education. Also tell the dentist about the American Dental Assistants Association (ADAA), the organization that represents the profession of dental assisting. Let your dentist know that by pursuing certification and professional standing, you hope to gain respect from your colleagues and patients, and increase your value as a member of the dental health care team.

OBJECTIVES	CONTENT	TEACHING RESOURCES
Pronounce, define, and spell the Key Terms.	■ Key terms (p. 11)	SW Short-Answer Questions 4, 6, 7 (p. 5) ESLR Electronic Flashcards ▶ Discuss each of the key terms in Chapter 2, focusing on the definition, pronunciation, and spelling of each term. ▶ Discuss what motivates someone to want to become a dental assistant. *Class Activity Invite local representatives from ADAA and DANB as guest speakers to discuss the profession of dental assisting.*
Discuss the concept of professionalism.	■ Characteristics of a professional dental assistant (p. 12)	PPT 6-8 TB question 1 SW Short-Answer Questions 1 (p. 5) ▶ Discuss the difference between a professional and a nonprofessional worker.

Bird/Robinson

OBJECTIVES	CONTENT	TEACHING RESOURCES
		▸ Discuss the concept of professionalism as an attitude that infuses aspects of how a professional conducts his or her work. *Class Activity **Divide the class into small groups, and have group members take turns role-playing professional behavior in dental assisting. Have the groups perform the role-plays in front of the class.***
Demonstrate the characteristics of a professional dental assistant.	☐ Professional appearance (p. 12) ☐ Knowledge and skills (p. 12) ☐ Teamwork (p. 13) ☐ Attitude (p. 13) ☐ Dedication (p. 13) ☐ Responsibility and initiative (p. 13) ☐ Confidentiality (p. 13)	PPT 9-14 TB questions 2-4 SW Short-Answer Questions 2; Multiple Choice questions 1-2; Activities 2 (pp. 5-6) Guidelines for a Professional Appearance (p. 12) Many Roles of Dental Assistants (p. 14) Recall questions 1-2 (pp. 12-13) Figure 2-1 The dental assistant is an important member of the dental healthcare team (p. 12) Figure 2-2 The professional dental assistant's attire may vary depending on the duties performed (p. 13) CTQ 1, 4-5 (p. 17) ▸ Discuss the concept of working as part of a team and why it is important in a dental office. ▸ Discuss the ways a dental assistant could demonstrate responsibility and initiative in a dental office. *Class Activity **Have students prepare a confidential self-evaluation of their particular characteristics, both good and bad, as they relate to professionalism. Ask the students to submit the self-evaluation to the instructor. Discuss some of the statements, keeping the writers' identities anonymous.***
Identify the purpose of the Health Insurance Portability and Accountability Act of 1996 (HIPAA).	☐ Confidentiality (p. 13)	PPT 14 TB question 5 SW Short-Answer Questions 7; Fill in the Blank question 4; Multiple Choice questions 5-6 (pp. 5-6) CTQ 3 (p. 17) ▸ Discuss the background of HIPAA and its impact on the dental profession. ▸ Discuss whether or not it is appropriate for a dental assistant to share information about an experience with a patient even if the patient was not identified by name.

OBJECTIVES	CONTENT	TEACHING RESOURCES
		Class Activity Before class, have students research HIPAA as it relates to dentistry. Divide the class into small groups, and have each group prepare educational materials on HIPAA. Then have the groups present their findings to the class. (For students to prepare for this activity, see Homework/Assignments #1.)
Demonstrate the personal qualities of a professional dental assistant.	☐ Personal qualities (p. 13)	PPT 15-16 TB question 6 SW Short-Answer Questions 3 (p. 5) Check Your Personal Qualities as a Dental Assistant (p. 14) ▸ Discuss the personal qualities that are most important for a dental assistant to possess. ▸ Discuss how someone would evaluate his or her own personal qualities to determine if he or she is suited to any profession. *Class Activity List on the board the personal qualities of a professional dental assistant. Then have the class discuss the qualities and why they are important for a professional.*
Describe the role and purpose of the American Dental Assistants Association (ADAA).	■ Professional organizations (p. 13) ☐ American Dental Assistants Association (p. 13)	PPT 17-19 TB question 7 SW Short-Answer Questions 4; Fill in the Blank question 1; Multiple Choice question 3 (pp. 5-6) Figure 2-3 Juliette A. Southard (p. 14) Figure 2-4 The ADAA seal (p. 15) ADAA Mission Statement (p. 15) Recall question 3 (p. 15) ▸ Discuss the concept of a tripartite organization and how that would benefit a dental assistant. *Class Activity Divide the class into small groups, and have each group discuss how the formation of a professional organization benefits members of that profession. Then have the groups present their findings to the class.*
Describe the benefits of membership in the ADAA.	– Benefits of membership (pp. 14-15)	TB question 8 SW Short-Answer Questions 5 (p. 5) Where to obtain more information: ADAA (p. 15) CTQ 2 (p. 17) ▸ Discuss how a dental assistant would benefit from membership in the ADAA and how to evaluate those benefits.

Bird/Robinson

OBJECTIVES	CONTENT	TEACHING RESOURCES
		▶ Discuss how participation in ADAA activities would benefit a dental assistant. *Class Activity Before class, have students visit the ADAA Web site and print one piece of information to share with the class. Then have the students discuss with the class what they learned about the ADAA. (For students to prepare for this activity, see Homework/Assignments #2.)*
Describe the role of the Dental Assisting National Board (DANB).	☐ Dental Assisting National Board (p. 15) – Certified dental assistant (p. 15) – Specialty certification (pp. 15-16)	🖳 PPT 20-29 🖥 TB questions 9-11 📖 SW Short-Answer Questions 6; Fill in the Blank questions 2-3; Multiple Choice question 4 (pp. 5-6) Recall questions 4-5 (p. 16) Figure 2-5 Official logo of the DANB (p. 15) Figure 2-6 Official certificate of CDA (p. 16) Box 2-1 Summary of Dental Assisting National Board Eligibility Pathways (p. 16) ▶ Discuss the specific benefits of being certified by the DANB. *Class Activity Divide the class into small groups, and have each group discuss the difference between a regular DANB certification and a specialty certification and whether it would benefit a dental assistant to have both types of certification. Then have each group present its findings to the class.*
Explain where to obtain information about the DANB.	– Specialty certification (pp. 15-16)	Recall question 5 (p. 16) Where to Obtain More Information (DANB) (p. 16) Eye to the Future (p. 16) *Class Activity Invite a local dental assistant who has taken the DANB and become a CDA as a guest speaker to discuss the certification process.*
Performance Evaluation		🖥 TB 📖 SW Questions (pp. 5-6) 🄴 ESLR Electronic Flashcards 🄴 ESLR Practice Quiz Recall questions (pp. 12-16) 💡 CTQ (p. 17)

ELSEVIER

Torres and Ehrlich Modern Dental Assisting, 9th ed.

Bird/Robinson

2.1 Homework/Assignments:
1. Have the students research HIPAA as it relates to dentistry. 2. Have the students visit the ADAA Web site and print one piece of information they want to share with the class.

2.1 Instructor's Notes/Student Feedback:

ELSEVIER

Slide 1

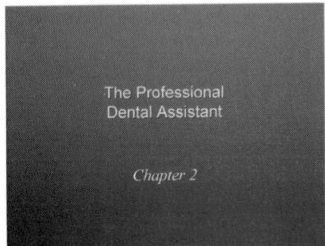

Slide 2

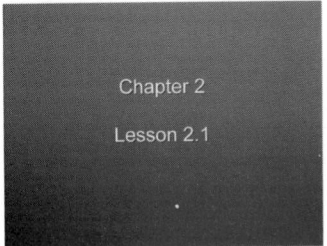

Slide 3

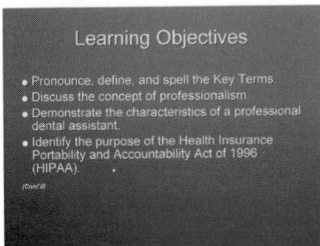

Slide 4

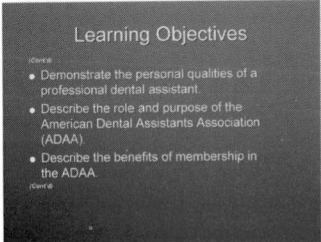

Slide 5

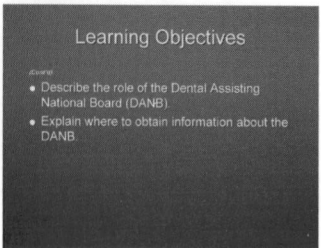

Slide 6

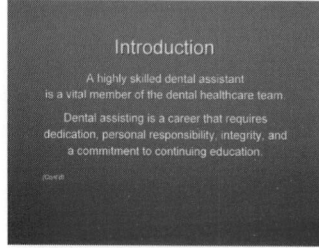

- What is a typical day for a dental assistant?
- Why do we need continuing education (CE)?
- What is professionalism, and what does it mean for the dental assisting profession?

Slide 7

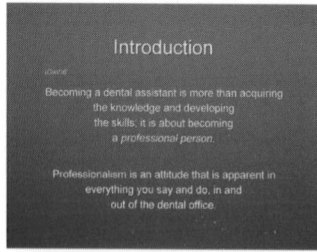

- Why is it important to be professional in dentistry?

Slide 8

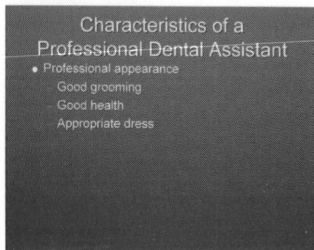

- How do you stay in good health?
- What does good grooming involve?

Slide 9

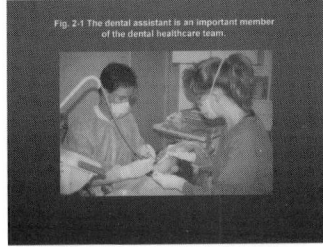

- Does this dental assistant have a professional appearance?
- Does she have good grooming?
- Does she appear to be in good health?
- And is she wearing appropriate dress for practice?
- Would she promote confidence in this dental office and improve the patient's dental experience?

Slide 10

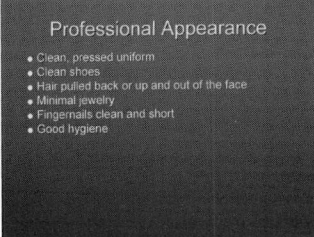

- What might a patient think when seeing a dental assistant with a messy uniform, hair in the face, dirty shoes, and dirty nails?

Slide 11

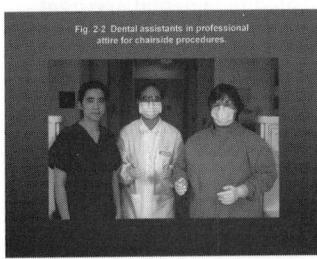

- What is appropriate attire for a dental assistant?
- Note that the first dental assistant (from the left) is in scrubs, which is basic acceptable wear at all times. The second one is in full personal protective wear, which is indicated for chairside procedures. The third assistant wears a surgical gown, which is indicated for surgery or hospital dentistry.

Slide 12

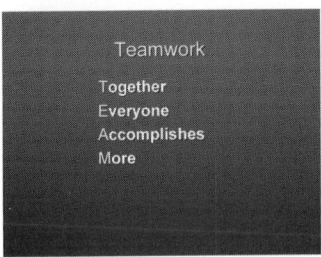

- What does teamwork mean?
- Should a dental assistant have both front-desk and chairside background?

Torres and Ehrlich Modern Dental Assisting, 9th ed.

Bird/Robinson

Slide 13

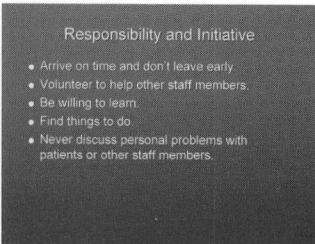

- How should a dental assistant act with patients?
- How do you maintain a relationship with your dentist employer?
- What does confidentiality mean in the dental office?

Slide 14

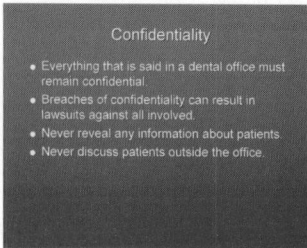

- There is federal legislation called HIPAA (Health Insurance Portability and Accountability Act) that affects all types of healthcare providers with regard to methods that must be taken to ensure that patient privacy is protected while health information is shared among healthcare providers.

Slide 15

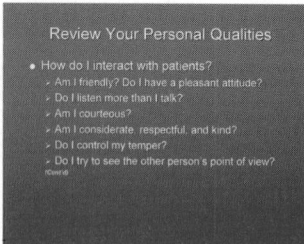

- Most people do not enjoy a visit to the dentist, and many are stressed or intimidated. How would you like to be treated by a dental assistant if you were stressed?

Slide 16

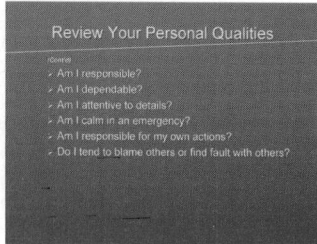

- Take time to answer each question and see what areas of professionalism you need to work on.
- Your conduct in a professional capacity ultimately establishes your status as a professional.
- By striving to be a professional, you can make a significant contribution to dentistry, society, and the patients you serve.

Torres and Ehrlich Modern Dental Assisting, 9th ed.

Bird/Robinson

Slide 17

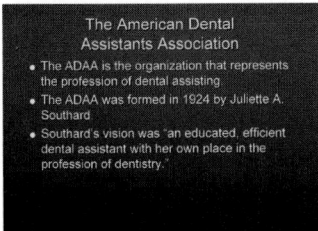

- Why would you join the ADAA?

Slide 18

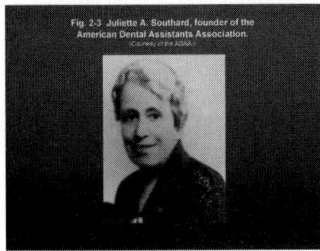

- There is an annual Juliette A. Southard/Oral-B Scholarship awarded to ten students enrolled in a dental assisting program or applicable courses aimed at furthering careers in dental assisting.

Slide 19

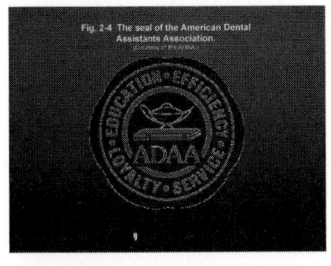

- When is Dental Assistant Recognition Week (DARW)? *(First full week in March.)*
- What are the advantages of a dental assisting career? *(Variety, flexibility, excellent working conditions, and personal satisfaction.)*
- Is there a national test for the certification of dental assistants?

Slide 20

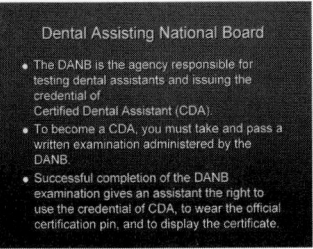

- Why would you want to become a CDA?

Slide 21

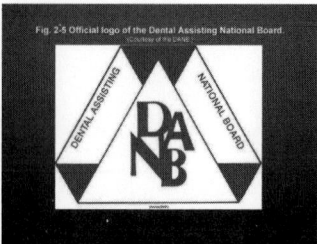

- How many states recognize DANB? *(Certification through DANB is recognized or required in more than 30 states.)*

Slide 22

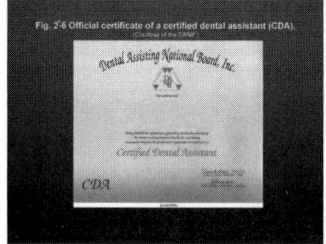

- What topics are covered on the national board examination? *(Three major categories: radiology, infection control, and general chairside.)*
- The applicant must pass all three categories in order to become a CDA.

Slide 23

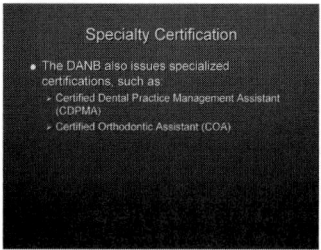

- How do the responsibilities of a CDPMA differ from those of a COA?

Slide 24

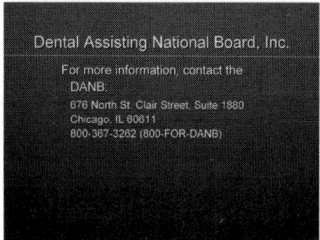

Bird/Robinson

Slide 25

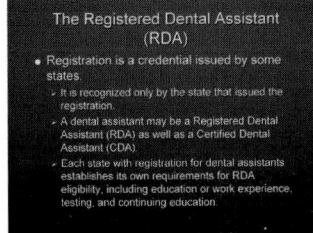

- What are the regulations imposed on dental assistants in our state? *(Instructor: check with the dental board/commission in your state; you will find this information on ADA's Web site, www.ada.org.)*

Slide 26

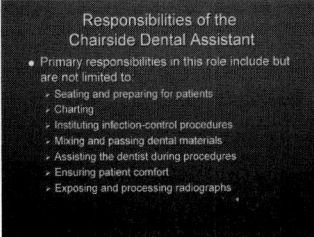

- What are the roles of the chairside dental assistant?

Slide 27

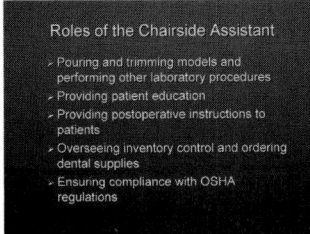

- What does OSHA stand for? *(Occupational Safety & Health Administration.)*

- What is OSHA's mission? *(To assure the safety and health of America's workers by setting and enforcing standards; providing training, outreach, and education; establishing partnerships; and encouraging continual improvement in workplace safety and health.)*

Slide 28

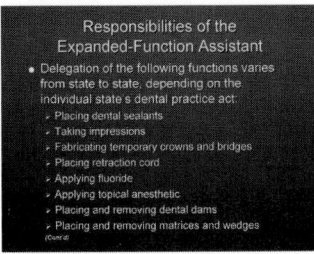

- Why do some states allow expanded functions for dental assisting? *(The program is designed to provide current dental assistants with advanced training, ,thereby increasing the dentist's overall productivity.)*

- What are the roles of the expanded-function assistant?

Bird/Robinson

Slide 29

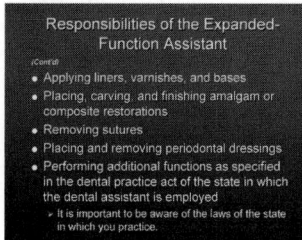

- *(Tie this in with Chapter 5: Dentistry and the Law and its discussion of state dental boards.)*

Torres and Ehrlich Modern Dental Assisting, 9th ed.

Bird/Robinson

TEACHING FOCUS

This chapter will introduce the student to the roles, responsibilities, and educational requirements of various members of the dental healthcare team, including the dentist, dental specialist, registered dental hygienist, dental assistant, and dental laboratory technician. The student will also have the opportunity to learn about the dental team's supporting services, legal and ethical issues, and future implications. The student will have the opportunity to put this information into context by participating in classroom activities and discussions.

MATERIALS AND RESOURCES

☐ computer and PowerPoint projector (Lesson 3.1)

LESSON CHECKLIST

Preparations for this lesson include:

- lecture
- guest speakers: dentist, dental specialist, registered dental hygienist, dental assistant, dental laboratory technician
- evaluation of student knowledge and skills needed to perform all entry-level activities related to understanding the dental healthcare team, including:
  - describing each of the recognized dental specialties
  - describing supportive services
  - identifying responsibilities of the dental assistant
  - identifying roles of the various members of the dental healthcare team
  - learning minimum educational requirements of each team member

Torres and Ehrlich Modern Dental Assisting, 9th ed.

KEY TERMS

certified dental technician (p. 23)
dental assistant (p. 21)
dental equipment technician (p. 24)
dental hygienist (p. 19)
dental laboratory technician (p. 19)
dental public health (p. 20)
dental spa (p. 24)
dental supply person (p. 23)
dentist (p. 19)

detail person (p. 24)
endodontics (p. 20)
oral and maxillofacial radiology (p. 20)
oral and maxillofacial surgery (p. 20)
oral pathology (p. 20)
orthodontics (p. 20)
pediatric dentistry (p. 20)
periodontics (p. 20)
prosthodontics (p. 20)

ADDITIONAL RESOURCES

PowerPoint slides (Evolve): 1-26

Legend

CTQ
Critical
Thinking
Question

DVD
Multimedia
Procedures
Videos and
Animations

ESLR
EVOLVE
Student
Learning
Resources

IDO
Interactive
Dental
Office
CD-ROM

SW
Student
Workbook

TB
Test Bank
on the
TEACH
CD-ROM

PPT
PowerPoint
Slides

Class Activities are indicated in ***bold italic.***

ELSEVIER

Torres and Ehrlich Modern Dental Assisting, 9th ed.

Bird/Robinson

LESSON 3.1

PRETEST

1. Which of the following performs services such as fabricating crowns, bridges, and dentures, as specified by the dentist's written prescription?
   a. certified dental assistant
   b. certified dental technician
   c. dental equipment technician
   d. dental supply person

2. Which dental specialist diagnoses and treats diseases of the pulp?
   a. prosthodontist
   b. periodontist
   c. oral surgeon
   d. endodontist

3. Which of the following members of the dental team is focused on tasks such as payroll?
   a. dental hygienist
   b. dental assistant
   c. business assistant
   d. dentist

4. When does the dentist usually refer a patient?
   a. when it is a more difficult case
   b. when less training is needed
   c. when the patient load is too great
   d. when there is less staff in the office

5. How many years does a dental hygienist have to attend college?
   a. at least 1
   b. at least 2
   c. at least 3
   d. at least 4

6. What type of dental assistant serves as an extra pair of hands where needed throughout the clinical areas of the practice?
   a. business assistant
   b. sterilization assistant
   c. circulating assistant
   d. chairside assistant

7. Who approves many of the dental professional schools?
   a. ADAA
   b. ADA
   c. CODA
   d. HIPAA

8. What dental specialty involves developing policies at county, state, and national levels for programs to control and prevent disease?
   a. dental laboratory technician
   b. prosthodontics
   c. pediatric dentistry
   d. dental public health

9. What is the minimum length of an accredited dental assisting program?
   a. at least 4 months
   b. at least 8 months
   c. at least 1 year
   d. at least 18 months

10. What is the term used when one chairside assistant works primarily with the dentist?
    a. one-handed dentistry
    b. two-handed dentistry
    c. four-handed dentistry
    d. six-handed dentistry

Answers

1. b	3. c	5. b	7. c	9. c
2. d	4. a	6. c	8. d	10. c

BACKGROUND ASSESSMENT

Question: Your patient wants to know why your dentist has a "DMD" after her name and not "DDS." What do you tell the patient? Does it make a difference to patient care?

Answer: The initials after the dentist's name indicate the degree awarded upon graduation from dental school to become a general dentist. DDS stands for doctor of dental surgery; DMD stands for doctor of dental medicine. There is no difference between the two degrees; dentists who have a DMD or DDS have the

Bird/Robinson

same education. Universities have the prerogative to determine what degree is awarded. Both degrees use the same curriculum requirements, which are set by the ADA Commission on Dental Accreditation.

Question: A friend of yours wants to go to an online dental assisting school that claims that it is accredited. The school lasts only four weeks. You doubt that the school is accredited. What information does your friend need to check before enrolling in the school if she wants to practice in her home state? How do you explain the need to attend an accredited school for your education as a dental assistant?

Answer: Although not all states require formal education for dental assistants, minimal standards for schools accredited by the Commission on Dental Accreditation (CODA) require a program of approximately one academic year in length, conducted in a post–high-school educational institution. The curriculum must include didactic, laboratory, and clinical content. Dental assistants may also receive training at vocational schools or proprietary schools accredited through the state's Board of Dentistry. So your friend would need to check whether the online school is accredited either through the state board or through CODA. You tell her that attending school to become a dental assistant was important to you because each dental practice is unique and has specific needs, and the educationally qualified dental assistant is quick to adapt to new situations as the needs arise.

CRITICAL THINKING QUESTION

Your parents do not understand why you want to become an expanded-functions dental assistant in a dental office, a profession allowed in your state. How do you explain about this role in patient care?

Guidelines: An expanded-functions dental assistant (EFDA) has received additional training and is legally permitted to provide certain intraoral patient-care procedures beyond the duties traditionally performed by a dental assistant. In some settings, the expanded-functions dental assistant is a key member in providing care to patients. The dentist and dental hygienist cannot provide all the care needed for a patient. The chairside and other dental assisting roles do not have the additional training needed. Many dental assistants want increased responsibilities in patient care to meet their professional needs. Duties delegated to the EFDA vary according to the dental practice act in each state. It is important that a dental assistant performs only functions trained for and allowed by state law so as to maintain personal and public professionalism.

OBJECTIVES	CONTENT	TEACHING RESOURCES
Pronounce, define, and spell the Key Terms.	■ Key terms (p. 18)	🅔 ESLR Electronic Flashcards *Class Activity **List the key terms related to dental specialties or dental team members on the board and ask the students to give a short description of those positions.***
Name the members of the dental healthcare team and describe their roles.	■ Introduction (p. 19)	PPT 5-6 Roles and Responsibilities of Dental Healthcare Team Members (p. 19) *Class Activity **List the members of the dental healthcare team on the board and call on students to describe the role of each one.***
Name and describe each of the recognized dental specialties.	■ Dentist (p. 19) ■ Dental specialists (p. 20)	PPT 6-10 TB questions 3, 13-15 SW Short-Answer Questions 4 (p. 7); Fill in the Blank questions 2-3, 7-13 (pp. 7-8) SW Case Study questions 1-2 (p. 8) Recall questions 1-2 (p. 20)

OBJECTIVES	CONTENT	TEACHING RESOURCES
		Dental Specialties Recognized by the American Dental Association (p. 20) CTQ 3 (p. 24) ▸ Discuss how a dentist is trained and legally permitted to perform all dental functions. Explain the circumstances under which a dentist might choose to refer a patient to a dental specialist. ▸ Discuss the difference between endodontics and periodontics. *Class Activity Invite members of the dental community from the different specialties to speak to the class. Have students prepare questions in advance.*

Name the members of the dental healthcare team and describe their roles.	■ Dentist (p. 19)
	
	■ Dental specialists (p. 20)
	
	■ Registered dental hygienist (p. 20)
	
	■ Dental assistant (p. 21)
	
	☐ Clinical dental assistant (p. 21)
	
	  – Chairside assistant (p. 21)
	
	  – Circulating assistant (p. 21)
	
	☐ Sterilization assistant (p. 22)
	
	☐ Expanded-functions dental assistant (p. 22)
	
	☐ Business assistant (p. 22)
	
	■ Dental laboratory technician (p. 23)
		PPT 11-12
		
		TB questions 1, 4, 6, 9
		
		SW Short-Answer Questions 1; Fill in the Blank questions 4-6; Multiple Choice questions 1, 5 (pp. 7-8)
		
		Recall question 3 (p. 21)
		
		Figure 3-1 Dental hygienist performing an oral prophylaxis (p. 21)
		
		Figure 3-3 Chairside dental assistant supported by a circulating dental assistant (p. 22)
		
		Figure 3-5 A sterilization assistant is an important member of the team (p. 22)
		
		Figure 3-6 EFDA removing excess cement (p. 22)
		
		Figure 3-7 A patient is greeted by a business assistant before meeting the dental hygienist (p. 23)
		
		Figure 3-8 Dental laboratory technicians working in a large commercial dental laboratory (p. 23)
		
		Figure 3-9 Laboratory dental cases are stored in work pans (p. 23)
		
		▸ Discuss the dentist's clinical, managerial, and business operational roles in a private dentistry practice.
		
		▸ Discuss the differences between the role of the dental hygienist and the role of the dental assistant.
		
		Class Activity Divide the class into small groups, and have each group discuss the roles of the dental assistant in four-handed dentistry and six-handed dentistry. Have the groups report their discussion to the class.

OBJECTIVES	CONTENT	TEACHING RESOURCES
Describe the various roles and responsibilities of a dental assistant.	■ Dentist (p. 19) ■ Dental specialists (p. 20) ■ Registered dental hygienist (p. 20) □ Clinical dental assistant (p. 21) – Chairside assistant (p. 21) – Circulating assistant (p. 21) □ Sterilization assistant (p. 22) □ Expanded-functions dental assistant (p. 22) □ Business assistant (p. 22) ■ Dental laboratory technician (p. 23)	⊠▤ PPT 13-23 ▣ TB questions 5, 8 ▨ SW Fill in the Blank question 1 (p. 7) ▨ SW Case Study questions 3-4 (p. 9) ♀ CTQ 2, 4-5 (p. 24) ▸ Discuss the role and responsibilities of the sterilization assistant. Note that this role is sometimes shared among dental assistants. ▸ Discuss how training as a chairside assistant can help an individual move into a position as a business assistant. *Class Activity Divide the class into small groups. Have each group create educational materials comparing the responsibilities of the chairside assistant, circulating assistant, sterilization assistant, and expanded-functions dental assistant. Have the groups share their materials with the class.*
Identify the minimal educational requirements for each member of the dental healthcare team.	■ Dentist (p. 19) ■ Dental specialists (p. 20) ■ Registered dental hygienist (p. 20) ■ Dental assistant (p. 21) □ Clinical dental assistant (p. 21) – Chairside assistant (p. 21) – Circulating assistant (p. 21) □ Sterilization assistant (p. 22) □ Expanded-functions dental assistant (p. 22) □ Business assistant (p. 22) ■ Dental laboratory technician (p. 23)	▣ TB questions 2, 7, 10-12 ▨ SW Short-Answer Questions 2; Multiple Choice questions 2-4 (pp. 7-8) Recall questions 4-6 (p. 23) ▸ Discuss the minimal educational requirements for dentists. Note the requirement that dentists pass both a written national board examination and a clinical state board examination before being allowed to practice. ▸ Discuss the minimal educational and training requirements for dental laboratory technicians and certified dental technicians. *Class Activity Divide the class into small groups, and have each group research one of the dental team members' educational requirements in your local community or state. They can use the Internet, but the students should make at least two phone calls to gather the information. Have each group present its findings to the class. (For students to prepare for this activity, see Homework/Assignments #1.)*

Bird/Robinson

OBJECTIVES	CONTENT	TEACHING RESOURCES
Describe the supportive services provided by other members of the dental healthcare team.	■ Supporting services (p. 23)	⊠▤ PPT 24-26 📕 SW Short-Answer Questions 3 (p. 7) 📕 SW Case Study question 5 (p. 9) Legal and Ethical Implications (p. 24) Eye to the Future (p. 24) 💡 CTQ 6 (p. 24) ▸ Discuss the roles of the dental supply person, detail person, and dental equipment technician. ▸ Discuss dental spas, describing the amenities offered in a dental spa. Ask the class to predict whether dental spas will turn out to be a fad or an emerging trend in dentistry. *Class Activity **On the board, list activities that are beyond the scope of practice and training of the dental assistant. As a class, discuss the legal and ethical implications of these activities.***
Performance Evaluation		🖥 TB 📕 SW questions (pp. 7-9) ⓔ ESLR Electronic Flashcards ⓔ ESLR Practice Quiz Recall questions (pp. 20-23) 💡 CTQ (p. 24)

3.1 Homework/Assignments:

1. Have each group research the educational requirements for one of the dental team members in your local community or state. They can use the Internet but need to make at least two phone calls to gather the information.

3.1 Instructor's Notes/Student Feedback:

ELSEVIER

Torres and Ehrlich Modern Dental Assisting, 9th ed.

Bird/Robinson

3

Slide 1

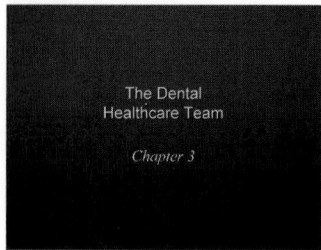

The Dental
Healthcare Team

Chapter 3

Slide 2

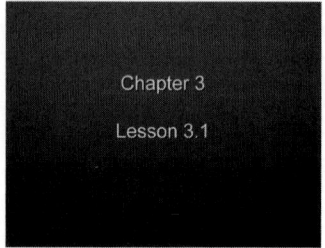

Chapter 3

Lesson 3.1

Slide 3

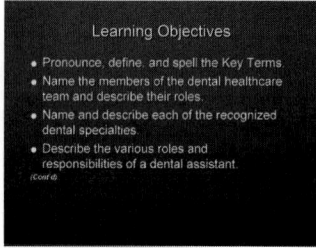

Learning Objectives

- Pronounce, define, and spell the Key Terms.
- Name the members of the dental healthcare team and describe their roles.
- Name and describe each of the recognized dental specialties.
- Describe the various roles and responsibilities of a dental assistant.

(Cont'd)

Slide 4

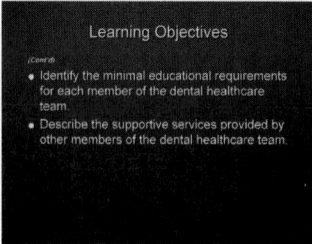

Learning Objectives

(Cont'd)

- Identify the minimal educational requirements for each member of the dental healthcare team.
- Describe the supportive services provided by other members of the dental healthcare team.

ELSEVIER

Torres and Ehrlich Modern Dental Assisting, 9th ed.

Bird/Robinson

Slide 5

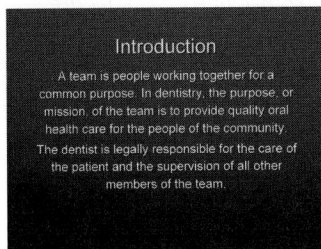

- What does a dentist do?

- How does one apply for dental school?

- Has anyone worked for a dentist before? Did that dentist act like he or she was the head of the dental team? What made the dentist head of the dental team?

- Who are the other members of the dental team besides the dentist?

Slide 6

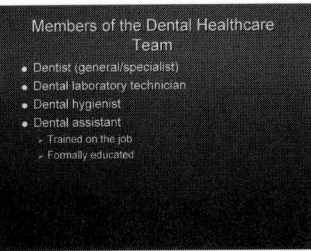

- What is the current job outlook for these careers?

Slide 7

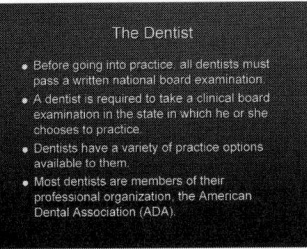

- What is the difference between a DDS - Doctor of Dental Surgery and a DMD - Doctor of Dental Medicine? *(There is no difference between the two degrees.)*

- Can a general dentist perform all treatments needed by a patient? *(Although a general dentist is trained and legally permitted to perform all dental functions, many dentists prefer to refer more difficult cases to specialists who have advanced training in certain areas.)*

- When did the ADA form? *(In 1859, 26 dentists met in Niagara Falls, New York.)*

- What is the national organization that most dentists belong to?

Slide 8

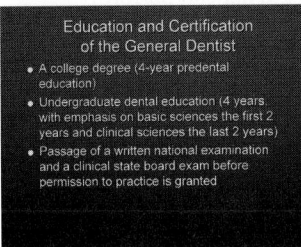

- What is the role of the general dentist?

- Where can a general dentist practice?

- How many are general dentists and how many are in the dental specialties? *(More than 80% are general practitioners, while about 20% are dental specialists.)*

- Are all general practices the same?

- How long does it take to become a dentist?

Torres and Ehrlich Modern Dental Assisting, 9th ed.
Bird/Robinson

Slide 9

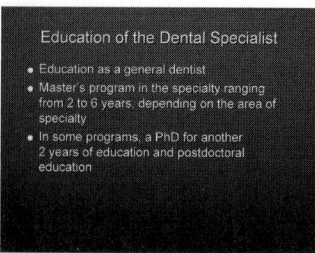

- How are the dental specialties determined? *(Specialties are recognized by the ADA in those areas where advanced knowledge and skills are essential to maintain or restore oral health.)*

- How many dental assistants work in the various types of dental practice? *(Endodontic 2%; oral surgery 5%; orthodontic 10%; pedodontic 3%; periodontic 3%; prosthodontic 2%; general dentistry 62%; from a DANB survey.)*

Slide 10

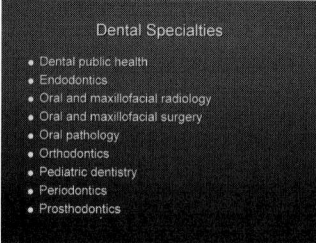

- What is endodontics? *(Diseases of the pulp.)*

- What is oral and maxillofacial radiology? *(Diagnosis of disease through various forms of imaging.)*

- What is oral and maxillofacial surgery? *(Conditions of the mouth, face, upper jaw, and associated areas.)*

- What is oral pathology? *(Diseases of the oral structures.)*

- What is prosthodontics? *(Restoration and replacement of natural teeth.)*

Slide 11

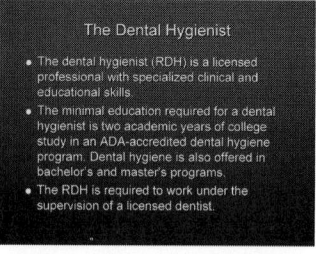

- What are the duties of the dental hygienist?

- Where can a dental hygienist practice?

- What are the main traits of dental hygiene?

Slide 12

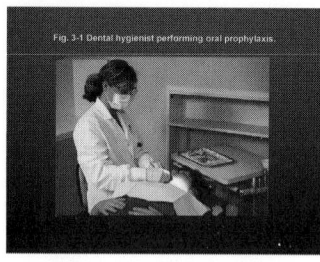

- What is an oral prophylaxis? *(Supragingival and subgingival [below the gumline] removal of plaque, calculus, and stain.)*

- How are the duties regulated that a dental hygienist can perform? *(Varies from state to state.)*

- What is the career outlook for a dental hygienist? *(Projected to be one of the 30 fastest-growing occupations.)*

Bird/Robinson

Slide 13

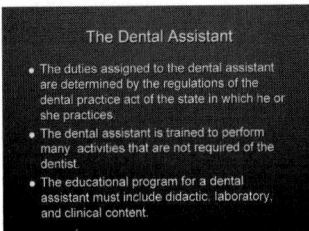

- What are the main traits noted in the profession of dental assisting? *(Variety, security, flexibility, personal satisfaction.)*

- Dentists look for people who are reliable, can work well with others, and have good manual dexterity.

- The American Dental Association's Commission on Dental Accreditation approved 265 dental-assisting training programs as of January 2005.

Slide 14

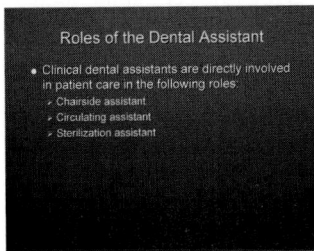

- In what settings do dental assistants work?

- What are the benefits offered by the job?

- What role in dental assisting would you like to be involved with that entails patient care? Do you think you would like to try all of them?

Slide 15

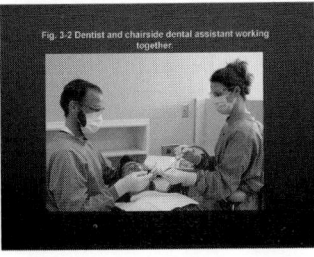

- The chairside assistant mixes dental materials, exchanges instruments, and provides oral evacuation during dental procedures.

- When did this type of dentistry become popular in the United States? *(Sit-down, four-handed dentistry became popular in the United States in the 1960s because this technique improves productivity and shortens treatment time.)*

- What personal protective wear is the assistant wearing?

- Notice her personal grooming.

Slide 16

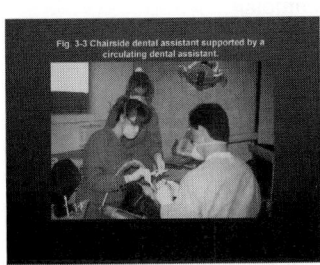

- In many practices, the circulating assistant is also responsible for seating and dismissing patients, as well as for preparing and caring for instruments and treatment rooms.

- What personal protective wear are they both wearing?

- Notice their personal grooming.

Slide 17

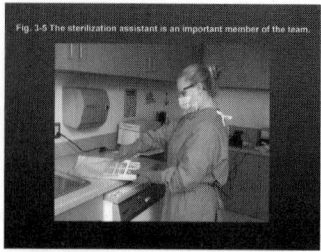

- In many offices the responsibility for sterilization procedures is delegated to a specific individual. In other offices all dental assistants share this important responsibility.

- The sterilization assistant efficiently and safely processes all instruments and manages biohazard waste. Other responsibilities include weekly monitoring of sterilizers and maintenance of sterilization monitoring reports.

- What special personal protective wear is she wearing?

Slide 18

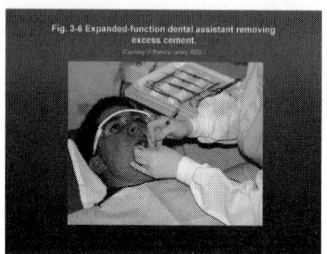

- An expanded-functions dental assistant (EFDA) has received additional training and is legally permitted to provide certain intraoral patient care procedures beyond the duties traditionally performed by a dental assistant.

- Duties delegated to the EFDA vary according to the dental practice act in each state. It is important that a dental assistant performs only functions allowed by state law.

- What if I am asked to perform procedures that I am not allowed to do?

- Are you interested in becoming an expanded-functions dental assistant?

Slide 19

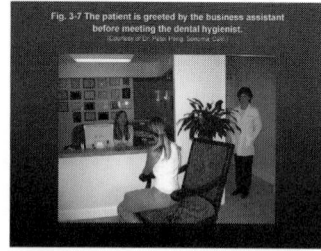

- What are business assistants?

- Who is the first person the patient meets from the dental office? Who is the first person from the dental office who talks to the patient on the phone? Are first impressions important?

- Do you think you may be interested in becoming a business assistant in the dental office?

Slide 20

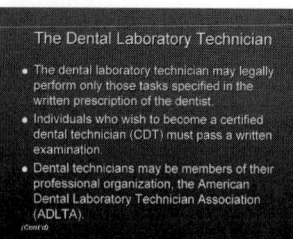

- What is the role of the dental laboratory technician?

- In some laboratories technicians perform all stages of the work, and in other labs each technician does only a few.

- Dental laboratory technicians can specialize in one of five areas: orthodontic appliances, crowns and bridges, complete dentures, partial dentures, or ceramics. Job titles can reflect specialization in these areas.

- About seven out of ten dental laboratory technician jobs are in medical equipment and supply manufacturing laboratories, which often are small, privately owned businesses.

Slide 21

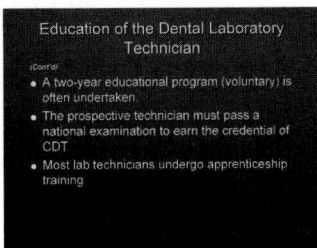

- What background does a technician need? *(Extensive knowledge of dental anatomy and materials as well as excellent manual dexterity.)*

- Most dental laboratory technicians learn their craft on the job, beginning with simple tasks, such as pouring plaster into an impression, and progressing to more complex procedures, such as making porcelain crowns and bridges.

- Becoming a fully trained technician requires an average of 3 to 4 years, depending upon the individual's aptitude and ambition, but it may take a few years more to become an accomplished technician.

Slide 22

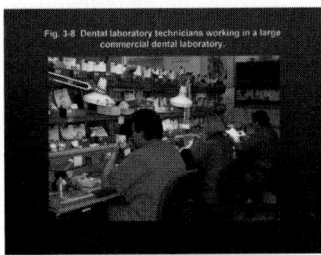

- The dental assistant often communicates with the dental laboratory technician regarding the length of time needed to return a case or to relay special instructions from the dentist about a case. It is important to have a good working relationship with the dental laboratory.

Slide 23

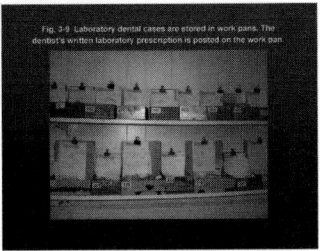

Slide 24

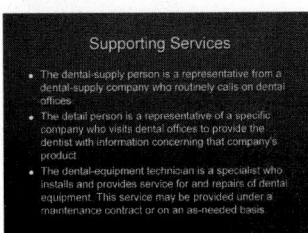

- Why are the supporting services important to the dental office?

- When visiting a dental office, have you noticed any people providing supporting services to the dental office? Do you think you would ever become involved in supporting services?

- Who is involved in the supporting services that are available in the dental office?

Torres and Ehrlich Modern Dental Assisting, 9th ed.

Bird/Robinson

Slide 25

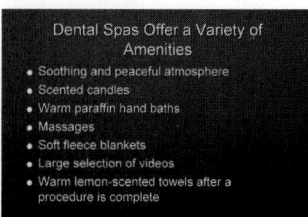

- Why offer dental spas?
- Have you been to a dental office that offered these extras?
- Would you like to work in an office that offered these extras?
- Do you think it helps to reduce the fear and tension that sometimes accompanies a visit to a dental office?

Slide 26

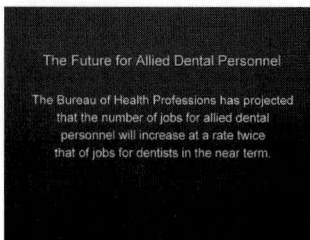

- What are the job prospects for the dental assistant in the future? *(Employment in this field is expected to grow much faster than the average for all occupations through the year 2012.)*
- Why is there such growth in this profession?

4 Lesson Plan
Dental Ethics

TEACHING FOCUS

This chapter will introduce the student to topics related to dental ethics. The student will have the opportunity to become acquainted with the basic principles of ethics, confidentiality, the American Dental Assistants Association professional code of ethics, applying ethical principles, and guidelines for solving ethical dilemmas.

MATERIALS AND RESOURCES

☐ computer and PowerPoint projector (all Lessons)

LESSON CHECKLIST

Preparations for this lesson include:

- lecture
- guest speakers: ADAA representative
- evaluation of student knowledge needed to perform all entry-level activities related to dental ethics, including:
  - explaining and giving examples of the basic principles of ethics
  - discussing the American Dental Assistants Association Code of Ethics
  - explaining the difference between being "legal" and being "ethical"
  - describing the steps in ethical decision making
  - giving examples of personal ethics and unethical behaviors
  - developing case studies involving ethical dilemmas

KEY TERMS

code of ethics (p. 28)
ethics (p. 26)

HIPAA (p. 27)
laws (p. 26)

ADDITIONAL RESOURCES

PowerPoint slides (Evolve): 1-20

Legend

CTQ
Critical
Thinking
Question

DVD
Multimedia
Procedures
Videos and
Animations

ESLR
EVOLVE
Student
Learning
Resources

IDO
Interactive
Dental
Office
CD-ROM

SW
Student
Workbook

TB
Test Bank
on the
TEACH
CD-ROM

PPT
PowerPoint
Slides

Class Activities are indicated in ***bold italic.***

ELSEVIER

Torres and Ehrlich Modern Dental Assisting, 9th ed.

Bird/Robinson

LESSON 4.1

PRETEST

1. What is the term used for a voluntary standards of behavior established by a profession?
   a. laws
   b. code of ethics
   c. practice acts
   d. licensure requirements

2. How is the principle of nonmaleficence easily described?
   a. beneficence
   b. "do no harm"
   c. autonomy
   d. "silence is golden"

3. What is the first step in solving an ethical dilemma?
   a. Determine the professional implications.
   b. Rank the alternatives.
   c. Choose a course of action.
   d. Identify the alternatives.

4. Which of the following is correct concerning ethics and the law?
   a. Ethical standards are always of a higher order than the law.
   b. The law is always of a higher order than ethical standards.
   c. The law refers to what you should do, not what you must do.
   d. Ethics deals with what you must do.

5. Ethical behavior is important to dental health care professionals because they
   a. provide dental care to their patients.
   b. must answer to the law.
   c. can have large patient flow.
   d. work with insurance companies.

6. Which of the following best describes the principle of autonomy?
   a. actions are ethical as long as they will benefit a person or community
   b. the right to privacy, freedom of choice, and the acceptance of responsibility for one's actions
   c. treating people fairly and giving people what they deserve and are entitled to receive
   d. the principle that comes from Hippocrates' oath for healthcare practitioners

7. Which of the following is related to the concept of ethics?
   a. Many absolutes exist.
   b. There are no gray areas to regard.
   c. Ethics is subject to individual interpretation.
   d. There is only the right or wrong of particular situations.

8. What would be an example of the principle of promotion of well-being?
   a. instituting a break in the mornings for those who come early
   b. making sure all dental assistants have the same level of salary
   c. not discussing patients and their health histories
   d. volunteering in dental health education programs

9. What concept is demonstrated in the philosophy that all patients should receive the same quality of dental care?
   a. justice
   b. beneficence
   c. autonomy
   d. confidentiality

10. Which of the following is an act signed into law that requires that the transactions of all patient health care information be formatted in a standardized electronic style?
    a. USDHHS
    b. HIPAA
    c. TOP
    d. PHI

Answers

1. b	3. d	5. a	7. c	9. a
2. b	4. a	6. b	8. d	10. b

ELSEVIER

Bird/Robinson

BACKGROUND ASSESSMENT

Question: What is ethics? Why do dental assistants need to consider ethics before working in a dental office?

Answer: Ethics with moral conduct (right and wrong behavior, "good" and "evil"). Ethics includes the values, high standards of conduct, and personal obligations in our interactions with other professionals and patients. Ethical behavior is important to dental health care professionals as they provide dental care to their patients.

Question: Why do we need ethics if the state board of dentistry outlines the legal standards for the practice of dentistry? Maybe we should just follow the letter of the law and then we do not have to worry about any ethical concerns. Do we not already know right from wrong?

Answer: As a general rule, ethical standards are of a higher order than the minimum legal standards established by the law. A behavior can be unethical and still be legal, but it cannot be illegal and still be ethical. There are very few absolutes and many gray areas regarding ethics. Ethical issues are subject to individual interpretation as to the right or wrong of particular situations.

CRITICAL THINKING QUESTION

You have been working for an older dentist whose care is becoming what you would consider substandard. You wonder if you should report him, since his treatment is bordering on being harmful to patients. However, the patients are older, too, and probably would not receive any care elsewhere because he charges very little for his treatments. What should you do? You like working for him and he cares greatly for his patients. Should you talk to him or his family? Should your report him to your state board of dentistry? Should you seek employment elsewhere?

Guidelines: A dental assistant is not legally obligated to report questionable actions of the dentist or to attempt to alter the circumstances. However, an ethical dental assistant would not wish to participate in substandard care or unlawful practices that may be harmful to patients. You may want to speak to him or his family carefully but seek employment elsewhere that meets your ethical standards of providing excellent care to patients. These decisions are difficult, especially if you like your employer and enjoy your job.

OBJECTIVES	CONTENT	TEACHING RESOURCES
Pronounce, define, and spell the Key Terms.	■ Key terms (p. 25)	*e* ESLR Electronic Flashcards *Class Activity Call out the definitions of key terms in the chapter and have students identify and properly pronounce the term.*
Explain the difference between being "legal" and being "ethical."	■ Introduction (p. 26) ■ Sources for ethics (p. 26)	PPT 5-7, 15-16 TB questions 1-3 SW Short-Answer Questions 3-4; Fill in the Blank questions 1, 4; Multiple Choice question 3 (pp. 11-12) Recall question 1 (p. 26) ▸ Discuss how ethical standards are of a higher order than the minimal legal standards established by the law. ▸ Discuss the various sources of ethics, including basic instinct, parents, teachers, religious teachings, and other people's behavior. *Class Activity Create two columns on the board labeled "Ethical" and "Legal." Have students identify characteristics of each and write them in the correct*

Bird/Robinson

OBJECTIVES	CONTENT	TEACHING RESOURCES
		column on the board. Next, as a class, discuss the similarities and distinguishing characteristics between activities that are ethical and those that are legal.
Explain and give examples of the basic principles of ethics.	■ Basic principles of ethics (p. 26) □ Regard for self-determinations (autonomy) (p. 26) □ To "do no harm" (nonmaleficence) (p. 26) – Promotion of well-being (beneficence) (p. 26) □ Regard for justice (p. 26) ■ Confidentiality (p. 27)	▣ PPT 8-12 ▣ TB questions 4-6, 8 ▣ SW Short-Answer Questions 1; Fill in the Blank questions 3, 5; Multiple Choice questions 1, 4 (pp. 11-12) ▣ SW Activity 1 (p. 12) Table 4-1 Basic Ethical Principles (p. 26) Figure 4-1 Patients have the right to expect confidentiality of their conversations in the dental office (p. 27) Recall question 2 (p. 27) ▢ CTQ 2 (p. 29) ▸ Discuss the four basic principles of ethics and relate each principle to the healthcare setting. Describe how a dental assistant will behave ethically in a dental practice. ▸ Discuss the basic requirements of HIPAA, including privacy standards, patient's rights, and administrative requirements. *Class Activity Divide the class into small groups. Have each group define and provide an example that illustrates each of the principles of ethics: autonomy, nonmaleficence, beneficence, and fairness. Then have each group share its results with the class for discussion.*
Discuss the American Dental Assistants Association Code of Ethics.	■ Professional code of ethics (pp. 27-28)	▣ PPT 13-14 ▣ TB question 7 ▣ SW Short-Answer Questions 2; Fill in the Blank question 2; Multiple Choice question 2 (pp. 11-12) ▣ SW Activity 2 (p. 12) Recall question 3 (p. 28) ADAA: Principles of Ethics and Code of Professional Conduct (p. 27) ▸ Discuss the professional code of ethics for dental assistants and review the principles of ethics and code of professional conduct established by the American Dental Assistants Association. *Class Activity Invite a representative of the ADAA to talk to the class about the association's Code of Ethics. Ask the representative to present situations in which a member violated the code of ethics, how the member should have acted in accordance with the code, and the consequences of the member's unethical act.*

Bird/Robinson

OBJECTIVES	CONTENT	TEACHING RESOURCES
Give examples of personal ethics and unethical behaviors.	■ Applying ethical principles (p. 28)	SW Short-Answer Questions 6 (p. 11) 💡 CTQ 3 (p. 29) ▸ Discuss examples of how people might apply ethical principles in their daily lives. ▸ Discuss examples of unethical behaviors and their repercussions. *Class Activity Ask students to write down one example of personal ethics and one example of unethical behavior they have witnessed or performed in their personal lives. Ask several students to volunteer their examples and discuss as a class how ethical principles should be applied in each example.*
Give examples of ethical dilemmas for each principle of ethics.	■ Ethical dilemmas (p. 28)	🖥 TB question 9 ▸ Discuss ethical dilemmas. Note that an ethical dilemma occurs when one or more ethical principles are in conflict. ▸ Discuss two examples of ethical dilemmas for each of the four principles of ethics. *Class Activity In small groups, have students identify the ethical principles involved in each of the following situations and discuss how the principles relate to the situation described:* *1. An HIV-positive dentist performs surgery without revealing his illness to the patient or his staff.* *2. A dentist performs unnecessarywork on a patient..* *3. A dental assistant notices that his or her employer is charging a patient's insurance company for work that has not been provided.* *4. A dentist volunteers to provide free dental work to children in poor communities.*
Develop case studies involving ethical dilemmas.	☐ Case study (p. 28)	▸ Discuss a case study of an ethical dilemma and ask students how they would resolve it. *Class Activity Have each student develop a case study from what he or she has learned so far in dentistry that he or she would consider an ethical dilemma. Share the case studies with the class. As a class, discuss the case studies, identifying the dilemma and the principles of ethics that apply.*
Describe the steps in ethical decision-making.	■ Steps for solving ethical dilemmas (pp. 28-29)	🖼 PPT 17-20 🖥 TB questions 10-11 📖 SW Short-Answer Questions 5 (p. 11)

Torres and Ehrlich Modern Dental Assisting, 9th ed.

Bird/Robinson

OBJECTIVES	CONTENT	TEACHING RESOURCES
		Legal and Ethical Implications (p. 29)
		Eye to the Future (p. 29)
		♀ CTQ 1 (p. 29)
		▶ Discuss steps for solving ethical dilemmas. Describe four steps, including identifying the alternatives, determining the professional implications, ranking the alternatives, and choosing a course of action.
		▶ Discuss what sources dental assistants can approach for help if they face an ethical dilemma.
		Class Activity ***Present the following situations to the class:***
		1. A patient can't pay for services. Should the patient be asked to leave the office even if the patient needs care?
		2. A dentist asks the staff to do unethical procedures to make a profit.
		As a class, go through the steps of ethical decision making with each situation,, asking students to identify the alternatives, determine the professional implications, rank the alternatives, and choose a course of action. Are students in agreement about the course of action? Discuss why or why not.
Performance Evaluation		🖥 TB
		📕 SW questions (pp. 11-12)
		🅔 ESLR Electronic Flashcards
		🅔 ESLR Practice Quiz
		Recall questions (pp. 26-28)
		♀ CTQ (p. 29)

4.1 Homework/Assignments:

4.1 Instructor's Notes/Student Feedback:

Torres and Ehrlich Modern Dental Assisting, 9th ed.

Bird/Robinson

Slide 1

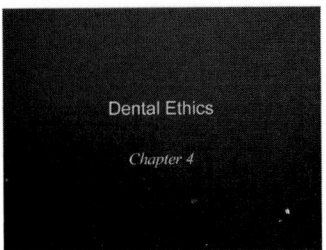

Dental Ethics

Chapter 4

Slide 2

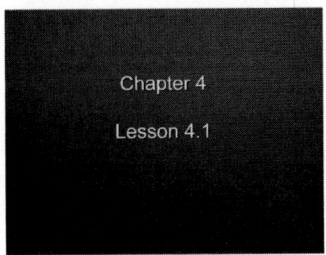

Chapter 4

Lesson 4.1

Slide 3

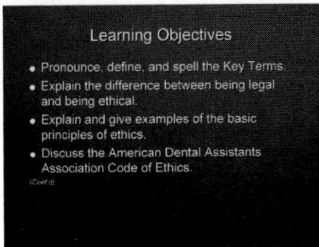

Learning Objectives

- Pronounce, define, and spell the Key Terms.
- Explain the difference between being legal and being ethical.
- Explain and give examples of the basic principles of ethics.
- Discuss the American Dental Assistants Association Code of Ethics.
(Cont'd)

Slide 4

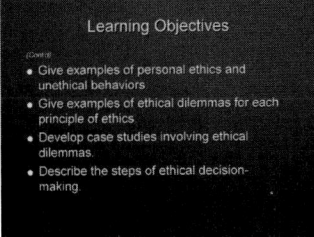

Learning Objectives

(Cont'd)
- Give examples of personal ethics and unethical behaviors.
- Give examples of ethical dilemmas for each principle of ethics.
- Develop case studies involving ethical dilemmas.
- Describe the steps of ethical decision-making.

ELSEVIER

Torres and Ehrlich Modern Dental Assisting, 9th ed.

Bird/Robinson

Slide 5

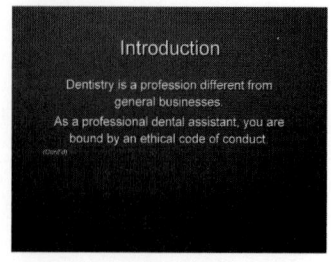

- What is ethics? *(Moral standards of conduct; rules or principles that govern proper conduct.)*
- An ethics curriculum is now required in all U.S. dental schools (although at present 80% of all dental schools offer courses in ethics, the emphasis in many is on jurisprudence).
- What is meant by conduct? *(To comport oneself or behave in a specified way.)*

Slide 6

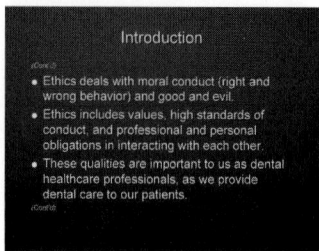

- How does ethics relate to dentistry?
- Sometimes a practitioner's recommendation may conflict with what the patient wants. Sometimes what the patient wants may sound foolish to the dentist. How the dentist responds to these problems and many others determines the character of a dentist's practice.
- What questions does ethics seek to answer for the professional person?

Slide 7

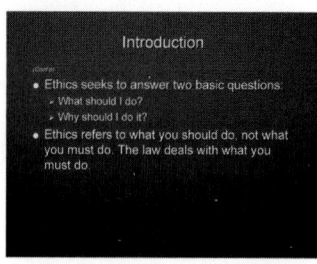

- Basic principles of ethics:
  - Do no harm (nonmaleficence): This principle comes from Hippocrates' dictate to "do no harm." It is the most basic element in morality.
  - Promotion of well-being (beneficence): This principle is based on the idea that actions are ethical as long as they will benefit a person or community.
  - What is justice?
  - What is self-determination?

Slide 8

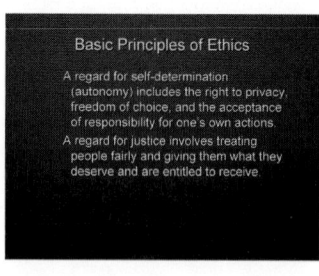

- What are principles? *(A basic generalization that is accepted as true and can be used as a basis for reasoning or conduct.)*
- Some define justice in terms of equality: each person should get or have the same amount, regardless of how hard he or she works.
- Others define justice in terms of equity: people should get benefits in proportion to what they contributed to producing those benefits.
- Still other people believe in equity with a bottom "safety-net" level which protects people who, because of misfortune or disability, are unable to work or even help themselves.

Bird/Robinson

Slide 9

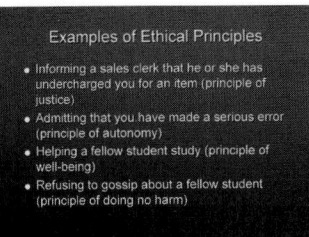

- Can you provide additional examples?

- We live in a constantly changing world. With technological advances come hard choices that may challenge existing moral standards.

- Our values are understood in the context of the life we live and the decisions of individuals and of society around us. We cannot separate our values from our experiences.

Slide 10

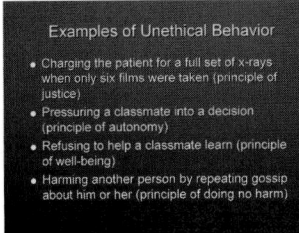

- Can you provide additional examples?

- Some situations occur so often that they may not even be recognized as having ethical content. Other times the circumstances are complex, and the answers are not readily apparent. In both situations a background in philosophical ethics can be helpful as support for making sound decisions.

Slide 11

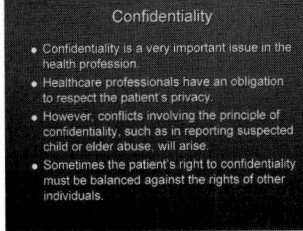

- What is confidentiality? *(A property by which information relating to an entity or party is not made available or disclosed to unauthorized individuals, entities, or processes.)*

- Reporting abuse and neglect: The ADA recognizes the responsibility of its members to report suspected cases of abuse and neglect of patients to appropriate authorities.

Slide 12

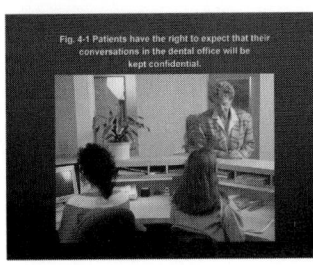

- Healthcare professionals have an obligation to respect a patient's privacy. In addition to moral and ethical principles for patient confidentiality, the HIPAA (Health Insurance Portability and Accountability Act) has very definite legal requirements for confidentiality of patients' health information.

- Why is it important that dental professionals adhere to HIPAA standards?

- Dentists will need to write privacy policies for their offices—documents for their patients that detail their particular office's practices.

- Would this conversation between the front desk personnel and the patient be private if another patient were present?

Torres and Ehrlich Modern Dental Assisting, 9th ed.

Bird/Robinson

Slide 13

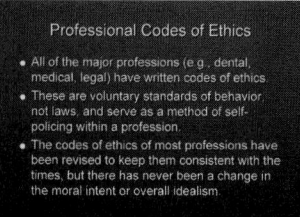

- Do you have a personal code of ethics?
- A code of ethics can provide a benchmark to use for self-evaluation.

Slide 14

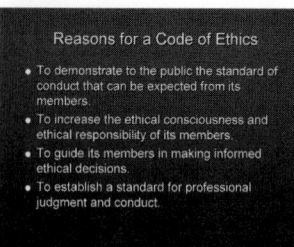

- What is the code of ethics for ADAA?
- How is the law related to ethics?

Slide 15

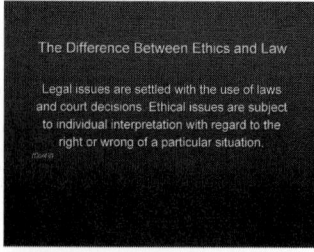

- Ethical obligations may, and often do, exceed legal duties. In resolving any ethical problem not explicitly covered by the ethical code, dental professionals should consider the ethical principles, the patient's needs and interests, and any applicable laws.

Slide 16

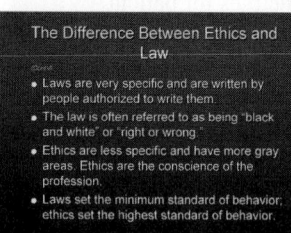

- The connection between law and ethics is very close.
- Discuss how laws set a minimum while ethics sets the highest standard of behavior.

Torres and Ehrlich Modern Dental Assisting, 9th ed.

Bird/Robinson

Slide 17

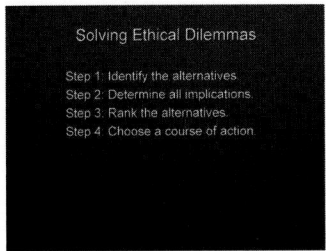

- How do you know if you are making the right decisions at each step?
- To whom can you go for help resolving ethical dilemmas arising in your professional environment?
- When you follow these steps and make a decision about what should and should not be done ethically and professionally, you will be more comfortable with your decision.

Slide 18

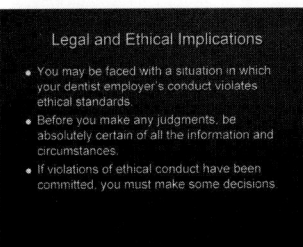

- What is a standard of care? *(A diagnostic and treatment process that a clinician should follow for a certain type of patient, illness, or clinical circumstance. In legal terms, the level at which the average, prudent provider in a given community would practice. It is how similarly qualified practitioners would have managed the patient's care under the same or similar circumstances.)*
- The healthcare malpractice plaintiff must establish the appropriate standard of care and demonstrate that the standard of care has been breached.

Slide 19

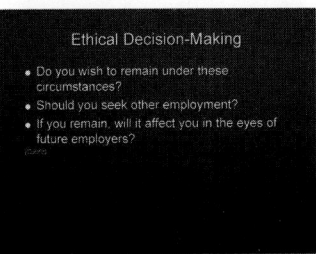

- Discuss ethical dilemmas a dental assistant might face that would cause him or her to ask these questions.

Slide 20

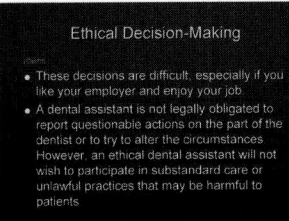

- More sources of information about dental ethics:
  - The ADA Code of Ethics.
  - The American College of Dentists has published an ethics handbook for dentists and now includes a section on dental ethics in each issue of its journal.
  - The United States-based Professional Ethics in Dentistry Network.
  - An international dental ethics association has been formed called IDEALS (the International Dental Ethics and Law Society).

Bird/Robinson

TEACHING FOCUS

This chapter gives the student an opportunity to learn about various types of laws and contracts that pertain to the dental profession. The legal ramifications of licensing, auxiliary supervision, abandonment, negligence, and malpractice suits are also discussed. Situations for which written consent or consent of a minor seeking care is necessary are highlighted. Since all health care providers are designated as mandated reporters, indications of child abuse and neglect are also discussed.

MATERIALS AND RESOURCES

- ☐ blank informed consent forms from professional organizations, insurance companies, and school dental clinic (Lesson 5.4)
- ☐ blank dental chart used to illustrate how documentation is performed (Lesson 5.4)

- ☐ computer and PowerPoint projector (all Lessons)
- ☐ copies of meeting minutes from state board of dentistry (Lessons 5.1 and 5.2)
- ☐ copies of state dental practice act (Lesson 5.1)
- ☐ poster board and markers (Lesson 5.4)

LESSON CHECKLIST

Preparations for this lesson include:

- lecture
- guest speakers: representative from state dental association child-abuse protection program or national program
- evaluation of student knowledge and skills needed to perform all entry-level activities related to dentistry and the law, including:
  - ○ types of laws and contracts
  - ○ what constitutes effective supervision, due care, abandonment
  - ○ means to avoid malpractice suits
  - ○ means and methods of informed consent
  - ○ proper documentation and correction of patients' records
  - ○ awareness of indicators of child abuse and neglect

ELSEVIER

Torres and Ehrlich Modern Dental Assisting, 9th ed.

Bird/Robinson

KEY TERMS

abandonment (p. 34)
administrative law (p. 32)
board of dentistry (p. 33)
civil law (p. 31)
contract law (p. 32)
criminal law (p. 31)
dental auxiliary (p. 33)
direct supervision (p. 33)
due care (p. 35)
expanded functions (p. 33)
expressed contract (p. 32)
felony (p. 32)
general supervision (p. 33)
implied consent (p. 36)
implied contract (p. 32)
informed consent (p. 36)

infraction (p. 32)
licensure (p. 33)
malpractice (p. 35)
mandated reporters (p. 38)
misdemeanor (p. 32)
patient of record (p. 33)
reciprocity (p. 33)
res gestae (p. 36)
res ipsa loquitur (p. 35)
respondeat superior (p. 33)
standard of care (p. 34)
state dental practice act (p. 32)
statutory law (p. 31)
tort law (p. 32)
written consent (p. 36)

ADDITIONAL RESOURCES

PowerPoint slides (Evolve): 1-44

Legend

CTQ
Critical
Thinking
Question

DVD
Multimedia
Procedures
Videos and
Animations

ESLR
EVOLVE
Student
Learning
Resources

IDO
Interactive
Dental
Office
CD-ROM

SW
Student
Workbook

TB
Test Bank
on the
TEACH
CD-ROM

PPT
PowerPoint
Slides

Class Activities are indicated in ***bold italic.***

ELSEVIER

Torres and Ehrlich Modern Dental Assisting, 9th ed.

Bird/Robinson

LESSON 5.1

PRETEST

1. What does abandonment mean in the dental office?
   a. a patient not paying his dental bill because it seems unfair to him or her
   b. termination by the dentist of a patient relationship without reasonable notice
   c. firing of a dental staff member because the person did not abide by privacy laws
   d. not taking into account general supervision of the dental staff

2. Which of the following is a felony?
   a. offense that usually results in only a fine
   b. offense that may result in imprisonment of six months to one year
   c. conviction that can result in imprisonment of one year or more
   d. conviction that results in a fine and probation

3. Which term allows individuals in one state to obtain a license in another state without retesting?
   a. reciprocity
   b. *respondeat superior*
   c. misdemeanor
   d. due care

4. What is it called when a dentist is negligent for not meeting the standard of care?
   a. due care
   b. derelict
   c. *res ipsa loquitur*
   d. informed consent

5. What does "Silence Is Golden" refer to?
   a. *respondeat superior*
   b. *res ipsa loquitur*
   c. *res gestae*
   d. tort law considerations

6. The main purpose of licensure is to protect the public from
   a. unqualified or incompetent practitioners.
   b. poor infection control.
   c. lesser levels of tort law.
   d. due care from practitioners.

7. What is malpractice?
   a. professional negligence
   b. using due care
   c. abiding by the practice act
   d. allowing informed refusal

8. Which of the following is an example of an expanded duty that may be delegated to a trained dental assistant?
   a. polishing coronal surfaces of teeth
   b. making chart entries correctly
   c. legally correcting chart entries
   d. rinsing the patient's mouth

9. Who interprets and implements state dental regulations?
   a. the state legislature
   b. the state Board of Dentistry
   c. the governor
   d. dental associations

10. Who technically owns a patient's dental chart?
    a. the patient
    b. the state dental board
    c. the dentist
    d. the insurance company

Answers

1. b	3. a	5. c	7. a	9. b
2. c	4. b	6. a	8. a	10. c

Bird/Robinson

BACKGROUND ASSESSMENT

Question: What are the legal duties of the patient to the dentist?
Answer: The patient is legally required to pay a reasonable and agreed-upon fee for the dentist's services. The patient also is expected to cooperate and follow instructions regarding treatment and home care.

Question: What items are included in the patient's dental chart?
Answer: Patients' dental charts are important legal documents that must be protected and handled with care. All examination records, diagnoses, radiographs, consent forms, updated medical histories, copies of medical and laboratory prescriptions, and correspondence to or about a patient are filed together in the patient chart. Financial information is not included in the patient chart. Original records and radiographs are not allowed to leave the dental practice without the dentist's permission. In most situations, duplicate radiographs will satisfy the patient's needs.

CRITICAL THINKING QUESTION

A chairside dental assistant works for a dentist whose business has increased in the last year. The dentist is often behind schedule. The dentist's wife has asked the dental assistant to perform procedures (dental sealants) that assistants are not allowed to perform according to the state's dental practice act. The wife tells the assistant that nobody will know that the assistant performs the procedures and that licensure is not really important. Is it illegal for the dental assistant to perform these procedures? Is it a criminal act or does it fall under a civil act? Is it a felony?
Guidelines: The dental practice act specifies the legal requirements for the practice of dentistry in every state. In every state, anyone who practices dentistry without a license is guilty of an illegal act. If the dental assistant performs procedures that the state practice act states can be performed only by a dentist, the assistant is guilty of an illegal act and can be held accountable. Ignorance of the dental practice act is no protection. A dental assistant who performs a procedure that is not legal is in violation of criminal law. Performing procedures that are not legal is the same as practicing dentistry without a license, which is a criminal act. Placing a sealant would possibly be considered a misdemeanor or an infraction and not a felony.

OBJECTIVES	CONTENT	TEACHING RESOURCES
Pronounce, define, and spell the Key Terms.	■ Key terms (pp. 30-31)	*ESLR* Electronic Flashcards ▸ Discuss each of the key terms in Chapter 5, focusing on the definition, pronunciation, and spelling of each term. *Class Activity Give the students copies of the state dental practice act with key terms underlined. Have them write out the definitions of the underlined terms.*
Describe the differences between civil and criminal law.	■ Statutory law (p. 31) ☐ Contract law (p. 32) ☐ Tort law (p. 32)	PPT 4, 21-23 TB questions 1-3 SW Short-Answer Questions 6; Fill in the Blank questions 9, 13, 17-18; Multiple Choice questions 9-10 (pp. 13-16) Recall questions 1-3 (p. 32) ▸ Discuss at least one example of criminal law and one example of civil law as they pertain to the field of dentistry. ▸ Discuss how tort and contract laws specifically apply to health care workers.

Torres and Ehrlich Modern Dental Assisting, 9th ed.

Bird/Robinson

OBJECTIVES	CONTENT	TEACHING RESOURCES
		Class Activity **Have each student write a short paragraph that describes the differences between civil and criminal law. Then have student volunteers read their work to the class for discussion.**
Explain the purpose of the state dental practice act.	■ State dental practice act (p. 32) □ Board of dentistry (p. 33)	▣ PPT 5-6 ▦ TB questions 4-5 ◪ SW Short-Answer Questions 1; Fill in the Blank questions 6-7; Multiple Choice question 2 (pp. 13-15) ▶ Discuss the specific features of your state's dental practice act and how these apply directly to various job descriptions within the practice. *Class Activity* **Give the students copies of the state dental practice act. Have the students highlight the provisions that concern the dental assistant.**
Explain the purpose for licensing dental health professionals.	■ State dental practice act (p. 32) □ Board of dentistry (p. 33)	▣ PPT 6-9 ▦ TB questions 6-7 ◪ SW Short-Answer Questions 2; Fill in the Blank questions 8, 10, 19; Multiple Choice question 1 (pp. 13-15) Recall questions 4-6 (p. 33) ▶ Discuss whether current state licensure requirements are adequate, too rigid, or need to be revised. Make suggestions for how licensure could better serve the purpose it was intended to perform. *Class Activity* **Give the students copies of the state dental practice act. Discuss the provisions that concern dental team members who must be licensed and how that license is to be obtained. Emphasize whether the dental assistant must be registered or licensed in the state.**

5.1 Homework/Assignments:

5.1 Instructor's Notes/Student Feedback:

Torres and Ehrlich Modern Dental Assisting, 9th ed.

Bird/Robinson

LESSON 5.2

CRITICAL THINKING QUESTION

A business assistant in a dental office notices that when the dentist is on vacation, the office manager asks other dental assistants to perform procedures on patients that the state dental practice act states must be performed under direct supervision. The dentist seems to be aware of this violation of the practice act. What is direct supervision? Who is responsible if something goes wrong while the dentist is on vacation? Is the dental assistant covered under the dentist's liability insurance?

Guidelines: Direct supervision generally means that the dentist has delegated a specific procedure to be performed for a patient of record by a legally qualified dental auxiliary (who meets the requirements of the state board of dentistry). The dentist must examine the patient before delegating the procedure and again when the procedure is complete. The dentist must be physically present in the office at the time the procedure is performed. Under the doctrine of *respondeat superior* ("Let the master answer"), the employer is responsible for any harm caused by its employee's actions while the employee is carrying out the employer's business. In a dental practice, this means that the patient may sue the dentist for an error committed by any of the dentist's employees. However, because an employee is also responsible for his or her own actions, the injured patient may also file suit against the dental assistant. The dentist's liability insurance cannot be relied upon to provide complete coverage for the dental assistant. Many dental assistants who provide direct patient care choose to carry their own liability insurance.

OBJECTIVES	CONTENT	TEACHING RESOURCES
Give an example of *respondeat superior*.	■ State dental practice act (p. 32) ☐ Board of dentistry (p. 33) ☐ Expanded functions and supervision (p. 33)	PPT 12-14 TB questions 8-9 SW Short-Answer Questions 14; Fill in the Blank questions 2-5; Multiple Choice questions 3-4 (pp. 13-15) Recall question 7 (p. 33) ▸ Discuss examples of how an employer might be held liable for errors committed by an employee. *Class Activity **Give the students copies of meeting minutes from the state board of dentistry that deal with dental violations encountered in your state. Have them discuss the violations as a group.***
Describe the types of dental auxiliary supervision.	☐ Expanded functions and supervision (p. 33) ☐ Unlicensed practice of dentistry (pp. 33-34)	PPT 15-17 TB question 10 SW Short-Answer Questions 3; Fill in the Blank questions 1, 14; Multiple Choice question 5 (pp. 13-15) Recall question 8 (p. 33) ▸ Discuss the pros and cons of delegating functions that a dentist usually performs to a dental assistant or hygienist. *Class Activity **Describe to the class several situations involving supervision issues, such as when the dentist is late for work, on vacation, out to lunch, etc. Have the students call out the type of supervision described.***

Torres and Ehrlich Modern Dental Assisting, 9th ed.

Bird/Robinson

OBJECTIVES	CONTENT	TEACHING RESOURCES
Explain the circumstances required for patient abandonment.	■ Dentist-patient relationship (p. 34) ☐ Duty of care/standard of care (p. 34) ☐ Abandonment (p. 34) ☐ Patient responsibilities (p. 35) ☐ Due care (p. 35)	PPT 18-20 TB questions 11-13 SW Short-Answer Questions 4; Fill in the Blank questions 11-12; Multiple Choice questions 6-8 (pp. 13-15) Recall questions 9-10 (p. 35) CTQ 1-3 (p. 41) ▸ Discuss ways a dentist could adequately address the choice to terminate treatment with a patient without concerns of liability. *Class Activity **Divide the class into small groups. Have the groups work up cases of abandonment, either done correctly or done negligently. Assign students to act as judges and juries and decide the cases.***
Describe ways to prevent malpractice suits.	■ Malpractice (p. 35) ☐ Acts of omission and commission (p. 35) ☐ Doctrine of *res ipsa loquitur* (p. 35) ■ Risk management (p. 35) ☐ Avoiding malpractice lawsuits (p. 35)	PPT 24-27 TB questions 14-16 SW Short-Answer Questions 7; Fill in the Blank questions 15, 23; Multiple Choice questions 11-12 (pp. 13-16) Recall questions 11-13 (p. 35) Figure 5-1 The role of good communication with patient (p. 36) Legal and Ethical Implications (p. 41) Eye to the Future (p. 41) ▸ Discuss ways a dentist can practice effective communication with patients in order to reduce the risk of lawsuits. *Class Activity **Have students research recent malpractice suits on the Internet and prepare a short report. Have student volunteers share their work with the class. (For students to prepare for this activity, see Homework/Assignments #1.)***

5.2 Homework/Assignments:

1. Have students research recent malpractice suits on the Internet and prepare a short report.

5.2 Instructor's Notes/Student Feedback:

Bird/Robinson

LESSON 5.3

CRITICAL THINKING QUESTION

A dentist has asked the office's business assistant to put together a manual for the office. The dentist wants the assistant to include procedures for informed refusal. What is informed refusal? How can it be obtained from a patient?

Guidelines: If a patient refuses a proposed treatment, the dentist must inform the patient about the likely consequences and obtain the patient's informed refusal. Obtaining the patient's informed refusal does not, however, release the dentist from the responsibility of providing the standard of care. A patient may not consent to substandard care, and the dentist may not legally or ethically agree to provide such care. The dentist may request that the patient sign a written and dated informed refusal for treatment. The form should also be signed by the dentist and a witness, and the patient should receive a copy of the form. The informed refusal should then be filed with the patient's record.

OBJECTIVES	CONTENT	TEACHING RESOURCES
Give an example of *res gestae*.	■ Risk management (p. 35) ☐ Avoiding malpractice lawsuits (p. 35) ☐ Silence is golden (pp. 35-36)	PPT 30 TB question 17 SW Short-Answer Questions 15; Multiple Choice question 13 (pp. 13, 16) Recall question 14 (p. 36) ▸ Discuss common slips of the tongue in the course of dental treatment that could be used as evidence against the practice in the court of law. How could these slips be avoided? *Class Activity Have each student write a short paragraph that gives an example of* **res gestae.** *Have student volunteers share their work with the class for discussion.*
Describe the difference between written and implied consent.	☐ Guidelines for informed consent (p. 36) – Informed patient consent (p. 36)	PPT 31-32 TB questions 18-19 SW Short-Answer Questions 8; Fill in the Blank question 16; Multiple Choice question 14 (pp. 13, 15-16) Recall question 15 (p. 37) ▸ Discuss the steps that must occur between a patient's implied consent and obtaining written consent. *Class Activity Lead a class discussion on written consent and implied consent. Ask students to come up with examples of each.*
Explain when it is necessary to obtain an informed refusal.	– Informed refusal (p. 36) – Exceptions to disclosure (p. 36)	PPT 33 SW Short-Answer Questions 11; Fill in the Blank question 20 (pp. 13, 15) ▸ Discuss the consequences of a dentist not performing the standard of care necessary even when that patient has given informed refusal.

OBJECTIVES	CONTENT	TEACHING RESOURCES
		Class Activity Divide the class into small groups. Have the groups work on a statement for an office manual on how to obtain informed refusal, using the textbook and ADA Web site as resources. Have each group present its work to the class for discussion.
Describe the exceptions for disclosure.	– Exceptions to disclosure (p. 36)	SW Short-Answer Questions 12 (p. 13) ▸ Discuss examples where disclosure is not clear-cut and judgment must be used. Discuss decision-making criteria for these types of situations. *Class Activity Divide the class into small groups. Have each group create a list of exceptions for disclosure. See which group can list the most exceptions in a 5- or 10-minute period.*

5.3 Homework/Assignments:

5.3 Instructor's Notes/Student Feedback:

Torres and Ehrlich Modern Dental Assisting, 9th ed.

Bird/Robinson

LESSON 5.4

CRITICAL THINKING QUESTION

A dental assistant did not overhear the dentist's chart entry correctly because the patient was talking at the same time as the dentist. This resulted in an error in the patient's dental chart. Why must the chart be corrected?

Guidelines: The purpose of correcting the chart is to ensure that the original entry is still readable and the change is permanent. Dental charts, also called patient records, are important legal documents that must be protected and handled with care. Every entry in a chart should be made as if the chart will be seen in a court of law. The dental assistant should never use white correction fluid or attempt to cover up the original entry.

OBJECTIVES	CONTENT	TEACHING RESOURCES
Describe the procedure for obtaining consent for minor patients.	– Informed consent for minors (p. 36)	📊 PPT 35-36 💻 TB question 20 📕 SW Short-Answer Questions 9 (p. 13) ▸ Discuss the proper procedure for obtaining parental consent when the parents are living separately. *Class Activity **Divide the class into small group,s and have students take turns role-playing a dental assistant obtaining consent for minor patients. Have various students act as a parent, guardian, or child patient. Have selected groups present their role-plays to the class for discussion.***
Describe the procedure for documenting informed consent.	– Documenting informed consent (p. 37) – Content of informed consent forms (p. 37)	💻 TB question 21 📕 SW Short-Answer Questions 10 (p. 13) ▸ Discuss the essential components that should be documented when obtaining informed consent. *Class Activity **Give the students a variety of informed consent forms. Divide the class into small groups and have them develop their own forms that include all the pertinent information and signature areas.***
Explain the principle of contributory negligence.	☐ Patient referral (p. 37) – Failure to refer (p. 37) ☐ Guarantees (p. 37) ☐ Contributory negligence (p. 37)	📊 PPT 37-38 💻 TB question 22 📕 SW Short-Answer Questions 5 (p. 13) Recall question 16 (p. 37) ▸ Discuss how broken appointments or last-minute cancellations can be interpreted as contributory negligence. *Class Activity **Give the students directions, and then have them practice recording a missed appointment in the progress notes of a dental chart.***

ELSEVIER

Bird/Robinson

OBJECTIVES	CONTENT	TEACHING RESOURCES
Discuss the indications of child abuse and neglect.	☐ Ownership of dental records and radiographs (p. 38) ■ Reporting child abuse and neglect (p. 38) ☐ Immunity (p. 40)	PPT 40-44 TB questions 25-26 SW Short-Answer Questions 16; Fill in the Blank questions 21-22; Multiple Choice questions 16-17 (pp. 14-16) Figure 5-3 Victim of child abuse (p. 39) Recall questions 17-18 (p. 41) ▸ Discuss the most prominent indicators of child abuse and neglect and how these can be distinguished from accidents. *Class Activity* **Divide the class into groups, and have them create posters that show the importance of reporting child abuse and neglect as well as information on the procedure for doing so in the state. Post the best posters in the school's dental clinic.**
Performance Evaluation		TB SW questions (pp. 13-16) ESLR Electronic Flashcards ESLR Practice Quiz Recall questions (pp. 32-41) CTQ

5.4 Homework/Assignments:

5.4 Instructor's Notes/Student Feedback:

Torres and Ehrlich Modern Dental Assisting, 9th ed.

Bird/Robinson

Slide 1

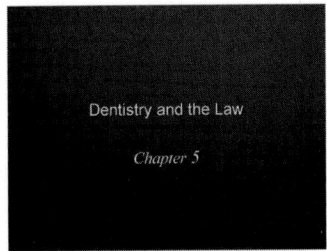

Slide 2

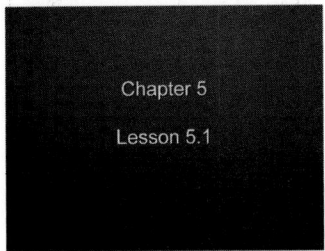

Slide 3

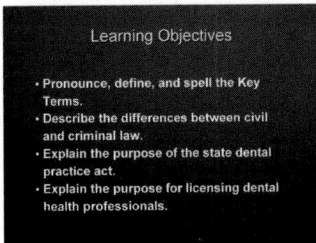

Slide 4

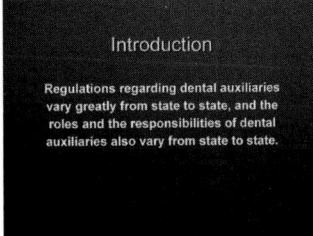

- Why do we have regulations in each state? *(To protect the public from incompetent dental healthcare providers.)*

Slide 5

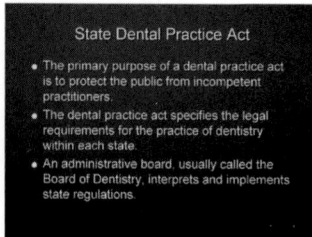

- Each state's dental practice act is now accessible on the Internet at http://www.ada.org.

Slide 6

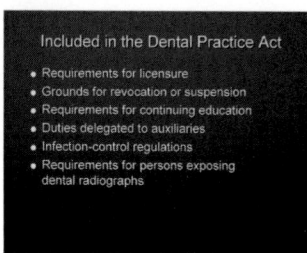

- What state was the first to enact laws to regulate dentistry? *(In 1841 Alabama enacted the first dental practice act, regulating dentistry in the United States.)*

Slide 7

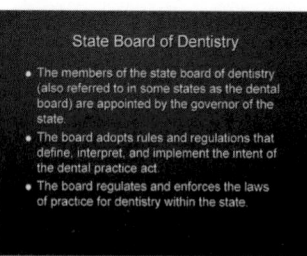

- How does the ADA relate to these state boards? *(The ADA believes states should have the power to decide who is qualified to practice dentistry and who is not.)*

- Are there only dentists on the boards? *(Some states have dental hygienists, dental assistants, and consumers as members of the board.)*

Slide 8

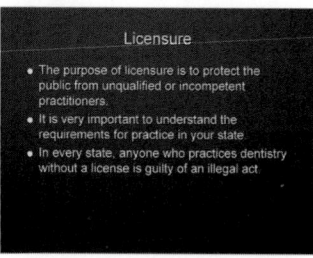

- The dentist and dental hygienist are usually licensed in their state to practice their profession. Many states now have licensure for differing levels of dental-assisting skill sets.

- Licensure can vary from state to state.

- What is meant by reciprocity?

Slide 9

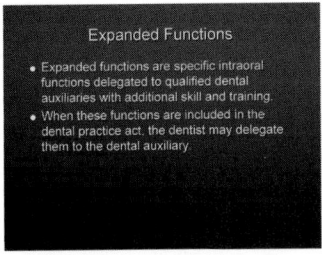

- Example of a state (California) that has expanded functions for qualified dental auxiliaries:
  - **Vocations Requiring License**: Hygienist and Registered Dental Assistant.
  - **Examination Frequency**: Two times per year.
  - **Experience Requirement**: Must be a licensed dental hygienist or registered dental assistant and have successfully completed the board-approved program in extended functions.

Slide 10

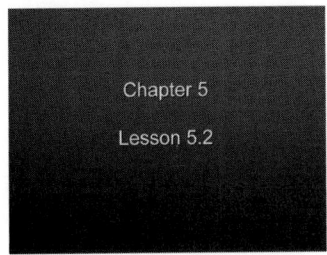

Slide 11

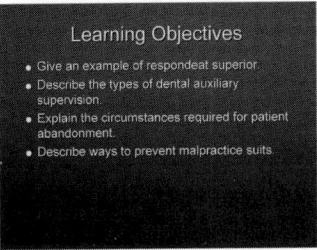

Slide 12

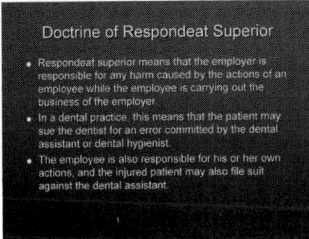

- Why would dental professionals need malpractice insurance for themselves?

Slide 13

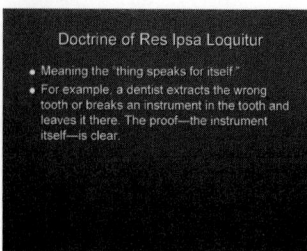

- If the evidence is clear, sometimes an expert witness is not necessary in a malpractice suit.

Slide 14

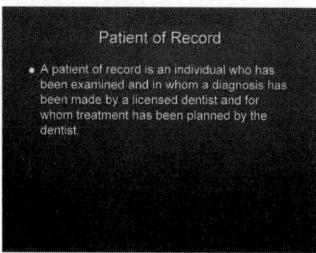

- Are you a patient of record for a dentist to whom you regularly go?

Slide 15

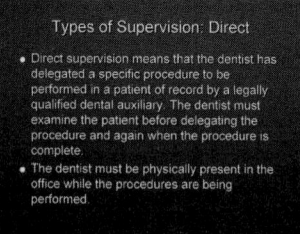

- What type of supervision is performed by the dentist in regard to his staff and their functions?
- How does direct supervision compare with general supervision?

Slide 16

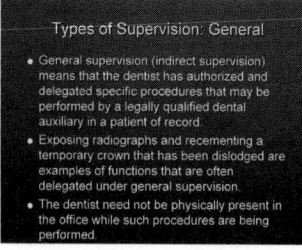

- In what situations may a dental office be open if the dentist is not physically present?

Torres and Ehrlich Modern Dental Assisting, 9th ed.

Bird/Robinson

Slide 17

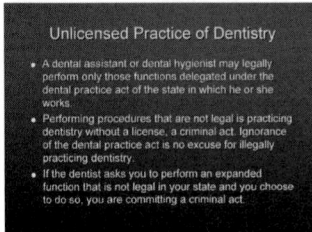

- What should you do if a dentist asks you to perform any duties the state does not legally allow an assistant to perform?

Slide 18

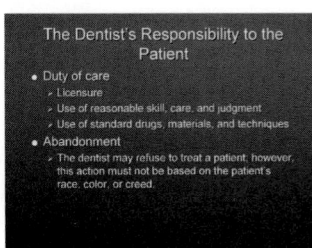

- What are dentists responsible for in regard to their patients?

- Can a dentist refuse to treat a patient because he or she has HIV infection?

- Abandonment refers to discontinuation of care after treatment has begun, but before it has been completed. The dentist may be liable for abandonment if the dentist ends the dentist-patient relationship without giving the patient reasonable notice.

Slide 19

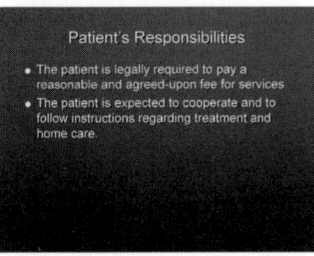

- Sometimes dental professionals forget that patients have some responsibility for their oral health, and we need to gently remind them of this fact.

Slide 20

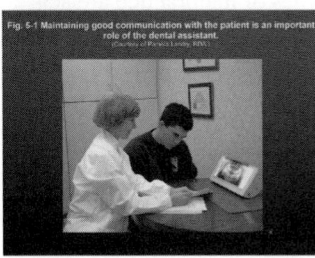

- Prevention and good communication with the patient are the best defenses against malpractice. Patients are less likely to initiate a lawsuit when they have a clear understanding of the following:

  - The planned treatment

  - Reasonable treatment results

  - Potential treatment complications

  - Their financial obligations

Slide 21

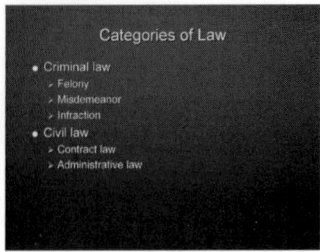

- What is a felony? *(A major crime, such as fraud or drug abuse; conviction can result in imprisonment of one year or more.)*

- What is a misdemeanor? *(A lesser offense that may result in a variety of penalties, including fines, loss or suspension of the license to practice dentistry, mandatory continuing education, counseling, or community service.)*

- What is an infraction? *(A minor offense that usually results in only a fine.)*

Slide 22

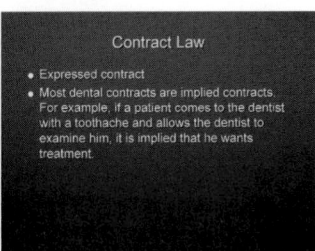

- What is the difference between an expressed contract and an implied contract?

Slide 23

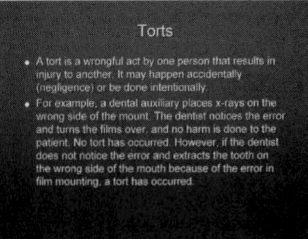

- What is a tort and how does it occur?

Slide 24

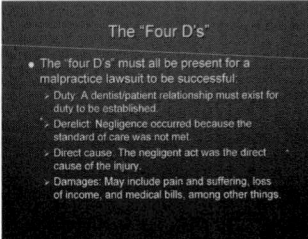

- Malpractice is professional negligence, or the failure to use due care or the lack of due care. In dentistry, the two types of malpractice are acts of omission and acts of commission.

- What is the typical insurance policy carried by a general dentist? *($1 million per occurrence to a maximum of $3 million.)*

Torres and Ehrlich Modern Dental Assisting, 9th ed.

Bird/Robinson

Slide 25

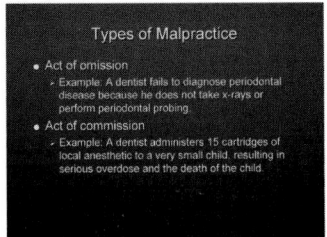

- What is the difference between an act of omission and an act of commission?

Slide 26

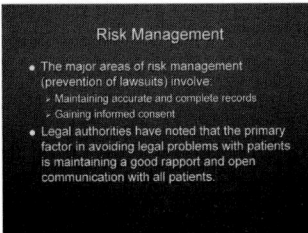

- How great are malpractice claims in dentistry today?
  (Dental malpractice claims are inherently smaller than in other medical fields. The average claim is between $12,000 and $15,000. The frequency and severity of the claims have remained fairly steady over the last 10 years.)

Slide 27

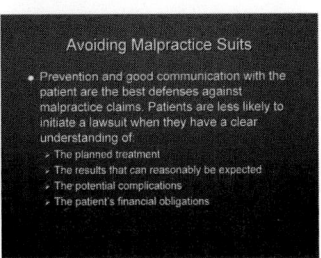

- The number of lawsuits in dentistry increases each year. Remember that a dental assistant may be involved in a malpractice suit or may be called to testify even if no longer employed in the practice.

Slide 28

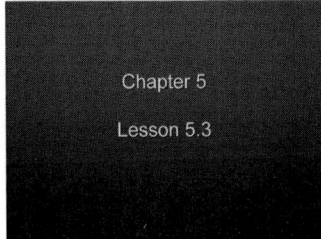

Torres and Ehrlich Modern Dental Assisting, 9th ed.
Bird/Robinson

Slide 29

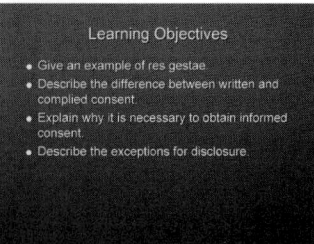

Slide 30

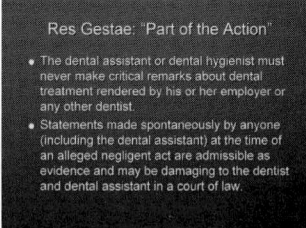

- Comments such as "woops" or "uh-oh" may unnecessarily frighten the patient and should be avoided.

Slide 31

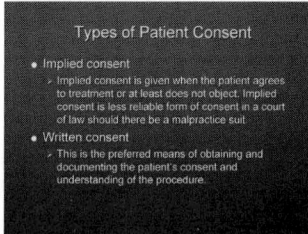

- How do these two types of consent compare with each other?

- What is the more reliable of the two in a legal situation?

- Have you been asked for written consent in a dentist's office?

Slide 32

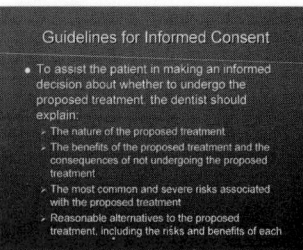

- What does "informed consent" mean? *(The patient must be given enough information about his or her condition and the available treatment options to make a decision.)*

Slide 33

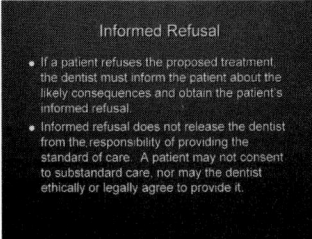

- What must be included in the patient's chart concerning informed refusal?

Slide 34

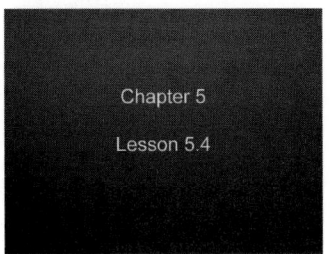

Slide 35

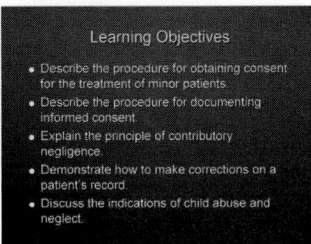

Slide 36

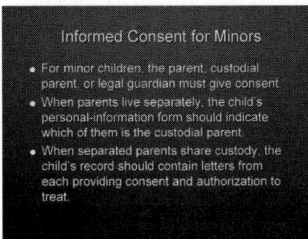

- What is a minor? *(A person under age 18, the age of legal majority.)*
- What is legal custody? *(The relationship with a child created by court order which gives a person legal responsibility for the physical possession of a minor and the duty to protect, care for, and discipline the child.)*

Slide 37

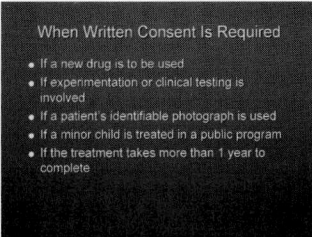

- Someone participating in a clinical trial will have many forms that concern written consent.

Slide 38

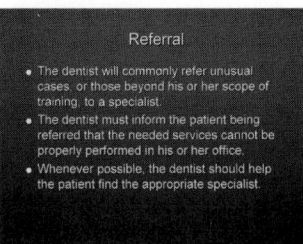

- As a patient what types of referrals have you encountered from your family dentist?

Slide 39

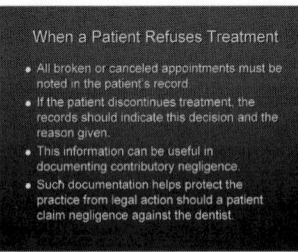

- What happens if there is a disagreement with a patient over a clinic record? *(The dental assistant should not attempt to make a decision but should immediately refer the matter to the dentist.)*

Slide 40

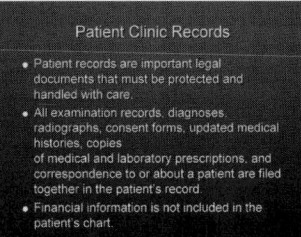

- The patient record is also called a dental chart.

Slide 41

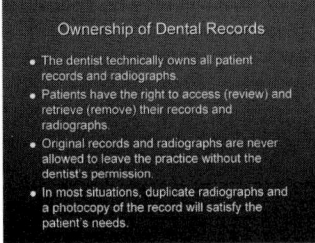

- Are patient records acceptable in court? *(Yes. Clearly show the date and the details of services rendered for each patient. Nothing should be left to memory. Incomplete or unclear records are damaging evidence in a malpractice case. Every entry in a chart should be made as if the chart will be seen in a court of law.)*

Slide 42

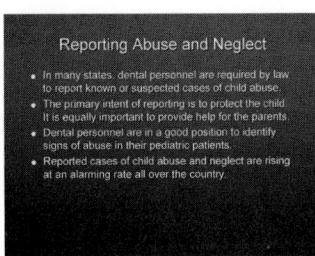

- Why are dental professionals involved in child abuse cases? *(Dental personnel are appropriate health care providers to identify signs of abuse in their pediatric patients.)*

Slide 43

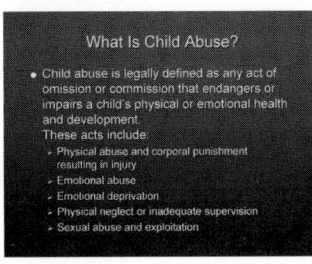

- What are the behaviors associated with child abuse?
  - *Child is frightened of parents or wary of adult contacts.*
  - *Child is apprehensive when other children cry.*
  - *Child is afraid to go home.*
  - *Child exhibits overly compliant, passive, and undemanding behaviors to avoid confrontation with abuser.*
  - *Child lags in development of motor skills, toilet training, socialization, or language.*

Slide 44

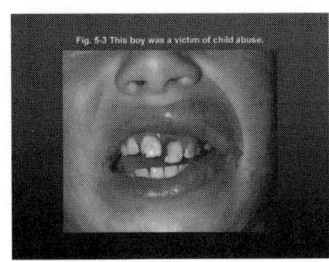

- What are the signs noted in dentistry of neglect or abuse?
  - *Untreated rampant caries that are easily detectable by a layperson.*
  - *Untreated pain, infection, bleeding, or trauma affecting orofacial region (as shown).*
  - *Injuries or tears to labial frenum, indicating forced feedings.*
  - *Cuts, bleeding, cigarette burns, bite or finger marks on ears, or "cauliflower ear."*
  - *Bald or sparse spots on scalp, indicating malnutrition or hair pulling.*

Slide 45

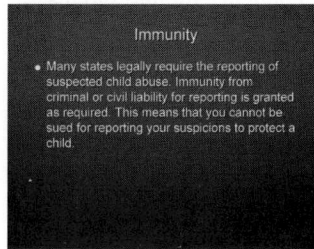

- What is legal immunity? *(Immunity confers a status on a person or body that makes that person or body free from otherwise legal obligations.)*

Torres and Ehrlich Modern Dental Assisting, 9th ed.

Bird/Robinson

TEACHING FOCUS

This chapter will give students an opportunity to learn about general anatomy of the human body with an emphasis on planes and body direction. Structural units of cells, tissues, organs, and body systems will also be discussed, along with the major body cavities and regions.

MATERIALS AND RESOURCES

☐ computer and PowerPoint projector (all Lessons)

LESSON CHECKLIST

Preparations for this lesson include:

- lecture
- guest speakers: dentist, dental hygienist, anatomy or physiology instructor
- evaluation of student knowledge and skills needed to perform all entry-level activities related to general anatomy, including:
  - the difference between anatomy and physiology
  - various planes and directions of the body
  - structural units of cells, tissues, organs, and body systems
  - major body cavities and regions

KEY TERMS

abdominal cavity (p. 51)
abdominopelvic (p. 51)
anatomical position (p. 45)
anatomy (p. 45)
anterior (p. 47)
apendicular (p. 51)
axial (p. 51)
connective tissue (p. 50)
cranial cavity (p. 51)
cytoplasm (p. 48)
differentiation (p. 47)
distal (p. 47)
dorsal cavity (p. 51)
epithelial tissue (p. 48)
frontal plane (p. 45)
horizontal plane (p. 45)
medial (p. 47)

midsaggital plane (p. 45)
muscle tissue (p. 50)
nerve tissue (p. 50)
nucleus (p. 48)
organelle (p. 48)
parietal (p. 51)
pelvic cavity (p. 51)
physiology (p. 45)
planes (p. 45)
posterior (p. 47)
proximal (p. 47)
spinal cavity (p. 51)
superior (p. 47)
thoracic cavity (p. 51)
ventral cavity (p. 51)
visceral (p. 49)

ADDITIONAL RESOURCES

PowerPoint slides (Evolve): 1-24

Legend

CTQ	DVD	ESLR	IDO	SW	TB	PPT
Critical Thinking Question	Multimedia Procedures Videos and Animations	EVOLVE Student Learning Resources	Interactive Dental Office CD-ROM	Student Workbook	Test Bank on the TEACH CD-ROM	PowerPoint Slides

Class Activities are indicated in **bold italic**.

Torres and Ehrlich Modern Dental Assisting, 9th ed.

Bird/Robinson

LESSON 6.1

PRETEST

1. Which body cavity contains the stomach, liver, gallbladder, spleen, and most of the intestines?
   a. cranial
   b. dorsal
   c. abdominal
   d. pelvic

2. A specialized part of a cell that performs a specialized function is a(n)
   a. cell membrane.
   b. organelle.
   c. cytoplasm.
   d. flagella.

3. Which body designation is farther away from the trunk of the body?
   a. proximal
   b. medial
   c. distal
   d. axial

4. The body's major support material is
   a. fat tissue.
   b. epithelial tissue.
   c. nerve tissue.
   d. connective tissue.

5. Which of the following describes cytoplasm?
   a. gel-like fluid inside the cell
   b. tissue that forms the covering of all body surfaces
   c. "control center" of the cell
   d. space in the body that houses the brain

6. Which of the following body designations means toward the front?
   a. axial
   b. anatomical
   c. anterior
   d. appendicular

7. Which body plane divides the body into right and left sides?
   a. horizontal
   b. frontal
   c. midsagittal
   d. coronal

8. Study of the functions of the human body is known as
   a. anatomy.
   b. histology.
   c. embryology.
   d. physiology.

9. Several types of tissues that group together to perform a single function form
   a. cells.
   b. tissues.
   c. organs.
   d. systems.

10. Which type of tissue secretes digestive juices, hormones, milk, perspiration, and mucus?
    a. connective
    b. nerve
    c. muscle
    d. epithelial

Answers

1. c	3. c	5. a	7. c	9. c
2. b	4. d	6. c	8. d	10. d

BACKGROUND ASSESSMENT

Question: How can one describe the human body so that everyone understands the same concepts?
Answer: When describing the human body, it is assumed that the body is in "anatomical position." Anatomical (or anatomic) position is the body standing erect with face forward, feet together, arms hanging at the sides, and palms forward.

ELSEVIER

Torres and Ehrlich Modern Dental Assisting, 9th ed.
Bird/Robinson

Question: How would you describe the function of the cell nucleus?

Answer: The nucleus is the "control center" of the cell and directs the cell's metabolic activities. All cells have at least one nucleus at some time during their existence. Some cells (e.g., red blood cells) lose their nucleus as they mature. Other cells (e.g., skeletal muscle cells) have more than one nucleus. The nucleus of every cell contains a complete set of the body's chromosomes, which contain DNA (deoxyribonucleic acid) and RNA (ribonucleic acid), two chemicals that carry all genetic information.

CRITICAL THINKING QUESTION

What is the study of anatomy, and why is it important for dental assistants to learn about anatomy?

Guidelines: Anatomy is the study of the human body's shape and structure. Sciences form the foundation of a dental assistant's caree; therefore, it is important for the dental assistant to understand the body's basic shape and structure. Dental assisting students will use their knowledge of anatomy as they progress through their studies, as well as every day in their careers. Because anatomy and physiology are closely related, an understanding of anatomy will also help students understand the physiology of the body. This understanding will help students with their study of oral pathology and considerations of the patient's health history, because the body and the mouth influence one another.

OBJECTIVES	CONTENT	TEACHING RESOURCES
Pronounce, define, and spell the Key Terms.	■ Key terms (p. 44)	SW Short-Answer Questions 1 (p. 17) *e* ESLR Electronic Flashcards ***Class Activity Have each student use one of the key terms in a clinically relevant sentence in order to define the term. Continue until all terms have been used. If a student becomes stuck, have the rest of the class offer suggestions.***
Explain the difference between anatomy and physiology.	■ Introduction (p. 45)	PPT 4 TB questions 1-2 SW Short-Answer Questions 2; Fill in the Blank questions 1-2; Multiple Choice questions 1-2 (pp. 17-18) Recall question 1 (p. 45) CTQ 1 (p. 51) ▶ Discuss why it is important for a dental assistant to be familiar with the anatomy and physiology of the human body. ***Class Activity Divide the class into groups. Ask each group to develop an explanation of the difference between anatomy and physiology. Have them give examples of each type of study. Have each group present its explanation to the class for discussion.***
Identify the planes and associated body directions used to divide the body into	■ Planes and body directions (p. 45)	PPT 5-8 TB questions 3-5, 12 SW Short-Answer Questions 3; Fill in the Blank questions 3-5, 11-16; Multiple Choice questions 3-4

Torres and Ehrlich Modern Dental Assisting, 9th ed.

Bird/Robinson

OBJECTIVES	CONTENT	TEACHING RESOURCES
sections.		(pp. 17-18)
		Table 6-1 Directional Terms for the Human Body (p. 47)
		Figure 6-1 Body in anatomical (anatomic) position (p. 46)
		Recall question 2 (p. 45)
		▶ Discuss mnemonic devices that could be used to help learn the body's directional terms.
		Class Activity Divide the class into groups. Have one student from each group stand in anatomical position while the remaining students use a meterstick to demonstrate the different planes of the body. Then have students use correct anatomical nomenclature to describe the parts of the body.
Identify the four levels of organization in the human body.	■ Structural units (p. 45)	⊠▤ PPT 9-11 ▦ TB question 8 ▰ SW Short-Answer Questions 4; Multiple Choice question 7 (pp. 17, 19) Figure 6-2 Organizational levels of the body (p. 47) ▶ Discuss various ways that knowing the four levels of organization in the body can aid one's understanding of bodily processes. *Class Activity Lead a class discussion about body systems. Ask students to identify the different body systems and to list their included organs. Then, have students explain the basic functions of each system. Record student responses on the board for comparison.*

6.1 Homework/Assignments:

6.1 Instructor's Notes/Student Feedback:

Torres and Ehrlich Modern Dental Assisting, 9th ed.

Bird/Robinson

LESSON 6.2

CRITICAL THINKING QUESTION

How can the complex subject of anatomy be broken down to make it easier to study and learn?
Guidelines: The human body is incredibly complex. However, anatomy is not difficult to study when it is broken down into smaller units. The study of the human body begins with the smallest units and builds systematically to larger and larger units. The human body has four organizational levels. Beginning with the simplest and proceeding to the most complex, the organizational levels are as follows: cells, tissues, organs, and body systems. Cells are the basic units of structure of the human body.

OBJECTIVES	CONTENT	TEACHING RESOURCES
Describe the components of a cell.	■ Structural units (p. 45) ☐ Cells (pp. 45, 47) – Cell membrane (p. 47) – Cytoplasm (p. 48) – Nucleus (p. 48)	PPT 14-16, 18 TB questions 6-7 SW Short-Answer Questions 5; Fill in the Blank questions 6-8; Multiple Choice questions 5, 8 (pp. 17-19) Figure 6-3 Basic human cell (p. 48) Visualizing the Semipermeable Function of the Cell (p. 48) Recall question 3 (p. 48) CTQ 3 (p. 51) ▸ Discuss the type of metabolic activities the cell nucleus performs. *Class Activity Divide the class into groups and assign each group one of the following parts of a cell: cell membrane, cytoplasm, or nucleus. Have each group diagram its assigned cell part and explain its functions in detail. Have each group present its findings to the class.*
Identify and describe the four types of tissues in the human body.	☐ Tissues (pp. 48-50) ☐ Organs (p. 50) ☐ Body systems (p. 50)	PPT 17, 19-21 TB question 9 SW Short-Answer Questions 6; Fill in the Blank questions 10, 17; Multiple Choice question 6 (pp. 17-19) Box 6-1 Types of Tissues and Functions in the Human Body (pp. 49-50) Recall questions 4-5 (p. 50) CTQ 2 (p. 51) ▸ Discuss the unique function of each of the four types of tissues and their locations in the body. *Class Activity Lead a class discussion about body tissues. Ask students to identify three examples of each type of tissue and explain where each is found in the body and its function. Record student responses on the board for comparison.*

Torres and Ehrlich Modern Dental Assisting, 9th ed.

Bird/Robinson

OBJECTIVES	CONTENT	TEACHING RESOURCES
Name and locate the two major body cavities and their components.	■ Body cavities (pp. 50-51)	⊠▤ PPT 22-23 💻 TB question 10 📘 SW Short-Answer Questions 7; Fill in the Blank questions 9, 17-19; Multiple Choice question 8 (pp. 17-19) Recall question 6 (p. 51) Figure 6-4 Spaces within the body (p. 51) ▸ Discuss the various sub-cavities contained in each of the two major cavities and the function of each. *Class Activity Divide the class into groups, and assign each group one or more different body cavities. Have each group outline the basics of its systems and present its findings to the class.*
Name and locate the two reference regions of the body.	■ Body regions (p. 51)	⊠▤ PPT 24 💻 TB question 11 📘 SW Short-Answer Questions 8; Fill in the Blank question 20; Multiple Choice questions 9-10 (pp. 17-19) Recall question 7 (p. 51) Legal and Ethical Implications (p. 51) ▸ Discuss both reference regions of the body and assess the usefulness of categorizing the body into these realms. What practical benefits do these distinctions provide healthcare workers? *Class Activity Divide the class into groups. Have each group list 10 movements that use only the axial region and 10 movements that use only the appendicular region. Have each group present its lists to the class and demonstrate its movements.*
Performance Evaluation		💻 TB 📘 SW questions (pp. 17-19) 🅔 ESLR Electronic Flashcards 🅔 ESLR Practice Quiz 🅔 ELSR Labeling Exercise 1: Identify the planes of the body Recall questions (pp. 45-51) 💡 CTQ (p. 51)

ELSEVIER

Torres and Ehrlich Modern Dental Assisting, 9th ed.

Bird/Robinson

6.2 Homework/Assignments:

6.2 Instructor's Notes/Student Feedback:

Torres and Ehrlich Modern Dental Assisting, 9th ed.

Bird/Robinson

Slide 1

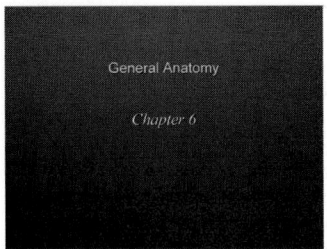

Slide 2

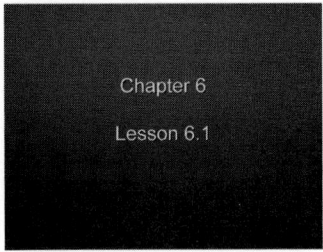

Slide 3

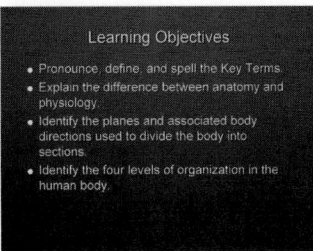

Slide 4

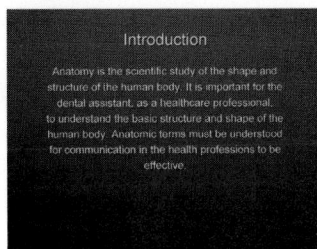

- How does physiology relate to anatomy?
- Why is it important for dental assistants to have an understanding of anatomy and physiology?

Slide 5

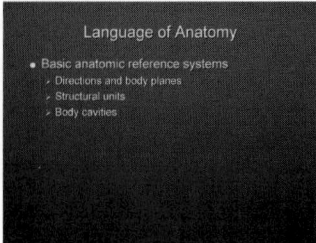

- What is the purpose of having anatomic reference systems?

Slide 6

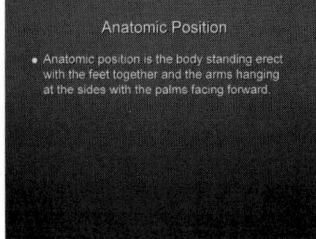

- How is anatomic position different from how you normally stand?

Slide 7

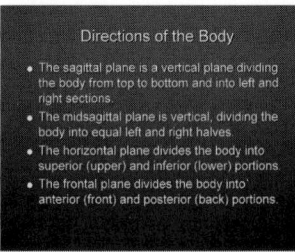

- What are planes in the study of anatomy? *(Planes are three imaginary lines used to divide the body into sections.)*

Slide 8

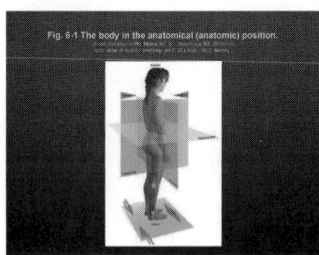

- When describing the human body, it is assumed that the body is in "anatomical position."

Bird/Robinson

Slide 9

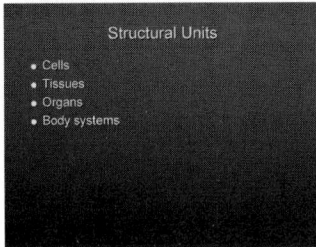

- Breaking the structures of the human body down into smaller parts makes it easier to study.

Slide 10

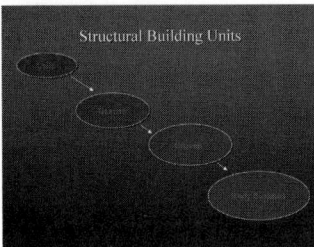

- Cells are the most basic units of structure in the body, and body systems are the most complex.

Slide 11

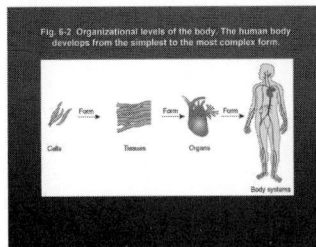

- What are examples of each unit of the body?
- *Cell (Epithelial cell, neuron, myyofiber, chondrocyte, fibroblast, erythrocyte, macrophage, sperm)*
- *Tissue (Epithelium, nervous tissue, muscle, cartilage, bone, blood)*
- *Organ (Skin, brain, heart, liver)*
- *System (Central nervous system, respiratory system, immune system, cardiovascular system)*

Slide 12

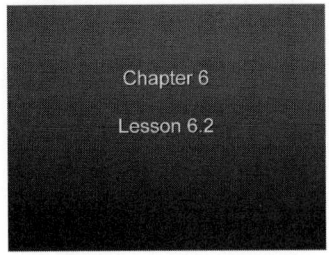

Slide 13

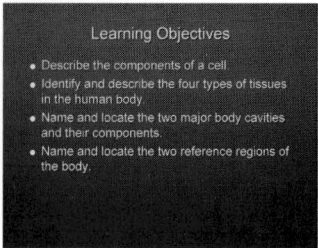

Slide 14

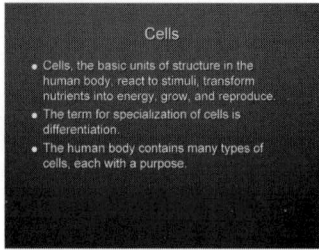

- How do cells differ?

- How are cells joined to one another? *(Some cells in tissues are joined by intercellular junctions. These are mechanical attachments between cells and possibly between cells and nearby noncellular surfaces.)*

Slide 15

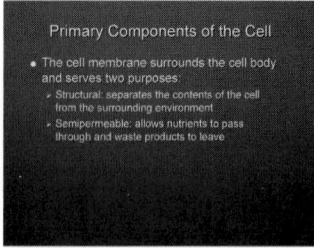

- What is the cell membrane structural mechanism like?

- What is the semipermable function of the cell membrane like?

Slide 16

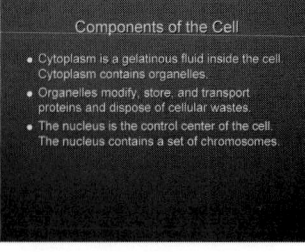

- What makes up most of the cytoplasm? *(It consists primarily of water; about two thirds of the body's water is found in the cytoplasm of cells.)*

- What are the components of the nucleus?

Bird/Robinson

Slide 17

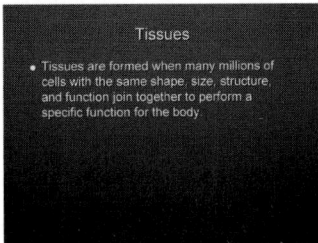

- What is histology? *(The study of the microscopic structure and function of cells and their tissues.)*

Slide 18

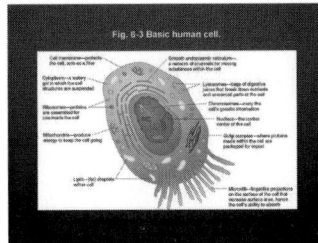

- What are some organelles located in the cell?

  - *Smooth endoplasmic reticulum: a network of channels for moving substances within the cell.*

  - *Golgi complex: where proteins made within the cell are packaged for export.*

  - *Lysosomes: bags of digestive juices that break down nutrients and unwanted parts of the cell.*

  - *Mitochondria: produce energy to keep the cell going.*

Slide 19

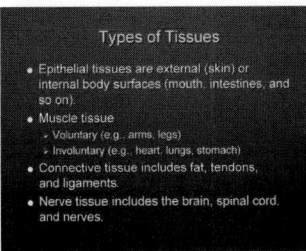

- Tissues form when millions of the same type of cell come together to perform a specific function.

Slide 20

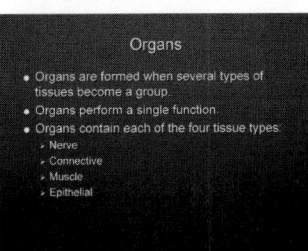

- What are examples of organs?
- How do organs communicate with the body systems?

Bird/Robinson

Slide 21

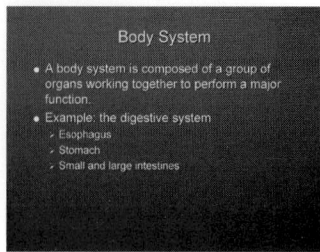

- What are the different body systems?
- How does disease affect the anatomy of the body systems?

Slide 22

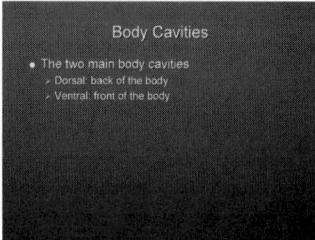

- A body cavity is a space in the body that is internally lined by a membrane and contains structures such as organs.

- Body surfaces not only separate the outside from the inside, they also keep structures and substances in their proper places so that they can function properly.

Slide 23

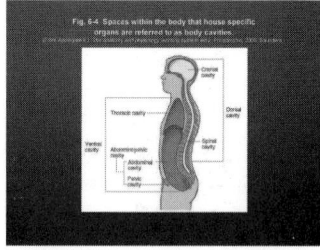

- Which organs are contained in each of the cavities?

Slide 24

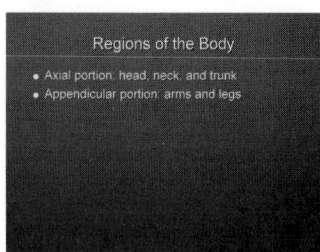

- Because of the relationship between disease and anatomy, methods of seeing into the body have become a mainstay of the diagnosis and treatment of disease.

TEACHING FOCUS

This chapter will give students the opportunity to learn about each of the 10 body systems. The location, purpose, and components of each system will be discussed, along with how each body system functions. Students will also have the opportunity to understand the signs and symptoms of common diseases and disorders related to each of the body systems. Conditions that affect more than one body system will be discussed.

MATERIALS AND RESOURCES

- ☐ chart of the human body with body systems illustrated
- ☐ computer and PowerPoint projector (all Lessons)

LESSON CHECKLIST

Preparations for this lesson include:

- lecture
- guest speaker: dentist or physician
- evaluation of student knowledge and skills needed to perform all entry-level activities related to general physiology, including:
  - ○ the cardiovascular system
  - ○ the digestive system
  - ○ the endocrine system
  - ○ the integumentary system
  - ○ the muscular system
  - ○ the nervous system
  - ○ the reproductive system
  - ○ the respiratory system
  - ○ the skeletal system
  - ○ the urinary system

KEY TERMS

apocrine sweat glands (p. 73)
appendicular skeleton (p. 53)
arteries (p. 62)
articulation (p. 56)
axial skeleton (p. 53)
bone marrow (p. 54)
cancellous bone (p. 54)
capillaries (p. 62)
cartilage (p. 55)
central nervous system (CNS) (p. 65)
compact bone (p. 54)
integumentary system (p. 71)
involuntary muscles (p. 58)
joints (p. 56)
muscle insertion (p. 59)

muscle origin (p. 59)
neurons (p. 66)
osteoblasts (p. 54)
pericardium (p. 60)
periosteum (p. 53)
peripheral nervous system (PNS) (p. 65)
peristalsis (p. 69)
plasma (p. 62)
red blood cells (p. 62)
sebaceous glands (p. 73)
Sharpey's fibers (p. 54)
sudoriferous glands (p. 73)
veins (p. 62)
white blood cells (p. 62)

ADDITIONAL RESOURCES

PowerPoint slides (Evolve): 1-66

Legend

CTQ
Critical
Thinking
Question

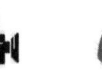

DVD
Multimedia
Procedures
Videos and
Animations

ESLR
EVOLVE
Student
Learning
Resources

IDO
Interactive
Dental
Office
CD-ROM

SW
Student
Workbook

TB
Test Bank
on the
TEACH
CD-ROM

PPT
PowerPoint
Slides

Class Activities are indicated in ***bold italic.***

ELSEVIER

Bird/Robinson

LESSON 7.1

PRETEST

1. What is the chemical messenger used by the endocrine system?
   - a. seminal fluid
   - b. hormone
   - c. saliva
   - d. lymph

2. The urinary system is also known as the
   - a. circulatory system.
   - b. digestive system.
   - c. endocrine system.
   - d. excretory system.

3. What is diabetes mellitus?
   - a. excess salivary production
   - b. increased sucrose uptake by the blood
   - c. impaired glucose uptake by the cells
   - d. decreased liver enzyme production

4. Which of the following is an appendage of the skin?
   - a. nares
   - b. nail
   - c. node
   - d. nephron

5. What is the first line of defense against disease?
   - a. kidneys
   - b. liver
   - c. skin
   - d. blood system

6. What connective tissue covers all bones?
   - a. periosteum
   - b. cartilage
   - c. synovial fluid
   - d. bursae

7. What is produced by the red bone marrow?
   - a. lymphocytes
   - b. erythyrocytes
   - c. plasma cells
   - d. macrophages

8. What is considered a mass of lymphoid tissue?
   - a. thyroid
   - b. tonsils
   - c. kidneys
   - d. liver

9. The central nervous system consists of the brain and the
   - a. cranial nerves.
   - b. peripheral nerves.
   - c. autonomic nerves.
   - d. spinal cord.

10. What is another name for a cerebrovascular accident?
    - a. heart attack
    - b. diabetic coma
    - c. kidney stone
    - d. stroke

Answers

1. b	3. c	5. c	7. b	9. d
2. d	4. b	6. a	8. b	10. d

BACKGROUND ASSESSMENT

Question: What are tonsils, where are they located, and how are they involved in both health and disease in the body?

Answer: The tonsils are masses of lymphatic tissue located in the upper portions of the nose and throat, where they form a protective ring. The nasopharyngeal tonsils, also known as adenoids, are found in the nasopharynx. The palatine tonsils are located in the oropharynx between the anterior and posterior pillars of fauces (throat) and are visible through the mouth. The lingual tonsils are located on the back of the tongue. Tonsils place lymphocytes into lymph to destroy invading microorganisms and may become infected in the process. This can cause tonsillitis, or inflammation of the tonsils. If the tonsils become a site of chronic infection, a physician may recommend their removal (tonsillectomy).

Question: What neurological condition can involve a cranial nerve and facial pain? What is another name for this condition? Where does the pain occur on the face and how is the pain described?

Answer: Trigeminal neuralgia is a neurologic condition of the trigeminal facial nerve. It is also known as tic douloureux. It triggers severe pain caused by inflammation of the trigeminal (fifth cranial) nerve. Depending on which of the three nerve branches is affected, the pain could occur around the eyes and over the forehead; in the upper lip, nose, and cheek; or in the tongue and lower lip. This pain, which has been described as excruciating, stabbing, and searing, may last for a few seconds; however, the initial incident is usually followed by other episodes, often of increasing severity.

CRITICAL THINKING QUESTION

One of the patients who will be coming to your dental office has had a heart transplant. Should the office be ready for an emergency? What are the emergency signs of heart failure? What happens if the patient's heart fails, and is the rest of the body affected?

Guidelines: The office should be prepared for an emergency with this patient and may want to have a physician's consult before treatment. If the patient experiences breathlessness, weakness, fatigue, dizziness, confusion, and hypotension, it is likely due to decreased blood pressure and thus the loss of oxygen to the body systems. During heart failure, the heart can no longer pump an adequate supply of blood. Red blood cells in the blood contain the blood protein hemoglobin, which plays an essential role in oxygen transport. Inadequate supplies of oxygen can quickly affect all body systems including that of the heart itself, the brain, and muscles.

OBJECTIVES	CONTENT	TEACHING RESOURCES
Pronounce, define, and spell the Key Terms.	■ Key terms (p. 52)	⊘ ESLR Electronic Flashcards ▸ Discuss each of the key terms, focusing on the definition, pronunciation, and spelling of each term. *Class Activity Have student pairs make flash cards of the key terms with the terms on one side and the definitions on the reverse. Then have the students quiz each other on the terms; correct their pronunciation as needed.*
Name and locate each of the 10 body systems.	■ Introduction (p. 53)	🖳 PPT 4-6 🖳 TB question 1 📖 SW Short-Answer Questions 1 (p. 21) Table 7-1 Major Body Systems (p. 54) ▸ Discuss the 10 body systems by locating where each one is in the body. *Class Activity Divide the class into small groups, and have each group create a list of the 10 body systems and where they are located in the body. Ask the group with the most complete list to share its work with the class.*
Describe the components of each body system.	■ Skeletal system (p. 53) ☐ Bone (p. 53) ☐ Cartilage (p. 55) ☐ Joints (p. 56) ■ Muscular system (p. 56)	🖳 PPT 9-66 🖳 TB questions 2, 4-8, 10-12, 17-18 📖 SW Short-Answer Questions 3; Fill in the Blank questions 1-10, 12-14, 17-19, 21; Multiple Choice questions 1-7, 10, 13-16, 22-23 (pp. 21-24)

Torres and Ehrlich Modern Dental Assisting, 9th ed.

Bird/Robinson

OBJECTIVES	CONTENT	TEACHING RESOURCES
	☐ Striated muscle (p. 56)	Figure 7-1 The skeletal system (p. 55)
	☐ Smooth muscle (p. 56)	Figure 7-2 The structure of bone (p. 55)
	☐ Cardiac muscle (p. 58)	Figure 7-3 Cortical bone and cancellous bone (p. 56)
	☐ Muscle function (p. 59)	Figure 7-4 Types of joints (p. 57)
	■ Cardiovascular system (p. 59)	Recall questions 1-7 (pp. 55-56, 58)
	☐ Circulatory system (p. 60)	Figure 7-5 Muscles of the body, anterior view (p. 58)
		Figure 7-6 Muscles of the body, posterior view (p. 59)
	☐ Heart (p. 60)	Figure 7-7 The heart and great vessels (p. 61)
	– Heart chambers (p. 60)	Figure 7-8 Coronary vessels (p. 61)
		Recall question 10 (p. 61)
	– Heart valves (p. 60)	Figure 7-9 Arteries carry blood from the heart to the body (p. 63)
	– Blood flow through the heart (p. 61)	
	– Blood vessels (p. 62)	Figure 7-10 Hematocrit (p. 64)
	– Blood and blood cells (p. 62)	Figure 7-11 Lymphatic system (p. 64)
		Figure 7-12 The tonsils (p. 65)
	– Blood typing and Rh factor (p. 62)	Figure 7-13 The central nervous system (p. 65)
		Figure 7-14 Structure of the respiratory system (p. 68)
	☐ Lymphatic system (p. 62)	Figure 7-15 Major structures of the digestive system (p. 70)
	– Lymph vessels (p. 62)	Figure 7-16 Endocrine glands (p. 71)
	– Lymph nodes (p. 64)	Figure 7-17 The urinary system (p. 71)
	– Lymph fluid (p. 64)	Figure 7-18 Three most common forms of skin cancer (p. 73)
	– Lymphoid organs (p. 65)	Recall questions 13-15, 23 (pp. 65, 73)
	■ Nervous system (p. 65)	▸ Discuss the components and structures of each body system.
	☐ Neurons (p. 66)	***Class Activity** List the components of the 10 body systems on the board in random order. As you read each item aloud, ask the students to identify its system.*
	☐ Central nervous system (p. 66)	
	– Brain (p. 66)	
	– Spinal cord (p. 67)	
	☐ Peripheral nervous system (p. 67)	
	■ Respiratory system (p. 67)	
	☐ Structures (p. 67)	

ELSEVIER

Torres and Ehrlich Modern Dental Assisting, 9th ed.

Bird/Robinson

OBJECTIVES	CONTENT	TEACHING RESOURCES
	– Nose (p. 67)	
	– Pharynx (p. 67)	
	– Epiglottis (p. 67)	
	– Larynx (p. 68)	
	– Trachea (p. 68)	
	– Lungs (p. 68)	
	■ Digestive system (p. 69)	
	☐ Digestive process (p. 69)	
	☐ Structures (p. 69)	
	– Mouth (p. 69)	
	– Pharynx (p. 69)	
	– Esophagus (p. 69)	
	– Stomach (p. 69)	
	– Small intestine (p. 70)	
	– Large intestine (p. 70)	
	– Liver, gallbladder, and pancreas (p. 70)	
	■ Endocrine system (p. 70)	
	■ Urinary system (p. 70)	
	■ Integumentary system (p. 71)	
	☐ Skin structures (p. 71)	
	– Epidermis (p. 71)	
	– Dermis (p. 71)	
	– Subcutaneous fat (p. 72)	
	☐ Skin appendages (p. 72)	
	– Hair (p. 72)	
	– Nails (p. 72)	
	– Glands (p. 73)	
	■ Reproductive system (p. 73)	
	☐ Female (p. 73)	
	☐ Male (p. 73)	

Torres and Ehrlich Modern Dental Assisting, 9th ed.

Bird/Robinson

OBJECTIVES	CONTENT	TEACHING RESOURCES
Explain the purpose of each body system.	All chapter content supports this learning objective.	⊠ PPT 9-66 🖥 TB 📄 SW Short-Answer Questions 2 (p. 21) Recall question 18 (p. 70) ▸ Discuss the purpose or function that each body system serves. ***Class Activity** Divide the class into small groups, and assign each group several of the body systems. Have each group discuss the purpose of their assigned body systems and have the groups present their findings to the class.*

7.1 Homework/Assignments:

7.1 Instructor's Notes/Student Feedback:

Bird/Robinson

LESSON 7.2

CRITICAL THINKING QUESTION

A diabetic patient from your office needs to be referred to an oral surgeon. The patient is not on insulin and feels fine with no symptoms. The referring office needs to know if the diabetes is type 1 or type 2. What is diabetes? Will anything be compromised by oral surgery because of the patient's diabetes?

Guidelines: Diabetes mellitus is an impairment of glucose uptake by the cells because of not having insulin (type 1) or having poor insulin metabolism (type 2). The endocrine system is the system involved by way of the endocrine gland, the pancreas. The patient probably is a type 2 diabetic because he is not on insulin and has no symptoms. There is a recognized association between periodontal disease and diabetes; thus the patient has an increased risk of periodontal disease that must be considered before oral surgery. He also may need to have a physician's consult to rule out any complications postsurgery.

OBJECTIVES	CONTENT	TEACHING RESOURCES
Explain how each body system functions.	All chapter content supports this learning objective.	PPT 9-66 TB questions 9, 13-16, 19 SW Short-Answer Questions 4; Fill in the Blank questions 11, 15-16, 20; Multiple Choice questions 9, 11-12, 17-21 (pp. 21-23) Recall questions 9, 11, 12, 16, 17, 19-22 (pp. 61-62, 65-66, 69, 70-71, 73) CTQ 3 (p. 75) ▸ Discuss how each of the 10 body systems functions. *Class Activity Divide the class into small groups, and assign a body system to each group. Ask each group to create and act out a short presentation about how its body system functions for an imaginary audience of elementary school children. Encourage the use of sound effects, physical gestures, and colorful descriptions. Discourage the use of jargon and technical language.*
Describe the signs and symptoms of common disorders related to each body system.	All chapter content supports this learning objective.	TB questions 20-25 SW Short-Answer Questions 5; Multiple Choice question 8 (pp. 21, 23) Box 7-1 Disorders of the Skeletal System (p. 54) Box 7-2 Disorders of the Muscular System (p. 57) Recall question 8 (p. 59) Box 7-3 Disorders of the Heart (p. 60) Box 7-4 Disorders of the Lymphatic System (p. 60) Box 7-5 Disorders of the Nervous System (p. 66) Box 7-6 Disorders of the Respiratory System (p. 67) Box 7-7 Disorders of the Digestive System (p. 69)

ELSEVIER

Torres and Ehrlich Modern Dental Assisting, 9th ed.

Bird/Robinson

OBJECTIVES	CONTENT	TEACHING RESOURCES
		Box 7-8 Disorders of the Endocrine System (p. 72)
		Box 7-9 Disorders of the Urinary System (p. 72)
		Box 7-10 Disorders of the Integumentary System (p. 72)
		Box 7-11 Disorders of the Female Reproductive System (p. 74)
		Box 7-12 Disorders of the Male Reproductive System (p. 74)
		💡 CTQ 1, 2, 4 (pp. 74-75)
		▸ Discuss common disorders of each of the 10 body systems. Be sure to discuss the signs and symptoms of each disorder.
		Class Activity Have each student choose a common disorder of one of the systems of the body, research it on the Internet, and prepare a report to deliver to the rest of the class. (For students to prepare for this activity, see Homework/Assignments #1.)
Give examples of conditions that require interaction of the body systems.	■ The interaction of the ten body systems (p. 73)	📘 SW Short-Answer Questions 6 (p. 21)
		📘 SW Activity (p. 24)
		Legal and Ethical Implications (p. 74)
		Eye to the Future (p. 74)
		▸ Discuss how the body systems interact with one another.
		▸ Discuss conditions that involve more than one body system.
		Class Activity Invite a dentist or a physician to speak to the class about the connections between dental health and the overall health of the body. Have students prepare questions beforehand. (For students to prepare for this activity, see Homework/Assignments #2.)
Performance Evaluation		💻 TB
		📘 SW questions (pp. 21-24)
		🅔 ESLR Electronic Flashcards
		🅔 ESLR Practice Quiz
		Recall questions (pp. 55-73)
		💡 CTQ (pp. 74-75)

Bird/Robinson

7.2 Homework/Assignments:

1. Have each student choose a common disorder of one of the systems of the body, research it on the Internet, and prepare a report to deliver to the rest of the class.

2. Have students prepare questions for a guest speaker—a dentist or a physician—who can discuss the connection between dental health and the overall health of the body.

7.2 Instructor's Notes/Student Feedback:

Slide 1

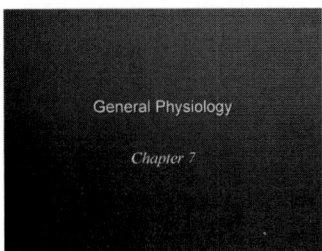

Slide 2

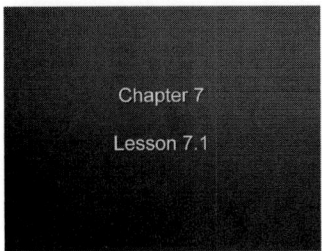

Slide 3

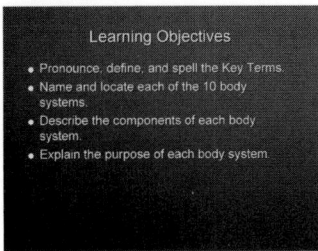

Slide 4

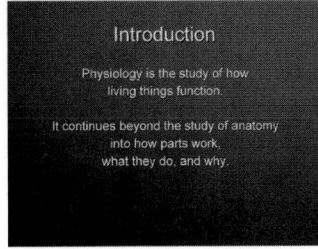

- What is human anatomy? *(Anatomy is the study of the shape and structure of the human body.)*
- How many body systems does the body have?

Torres and Ehrlich Modern Dental Assisting, 9th ed.

Bird/Robinson

Slide 5

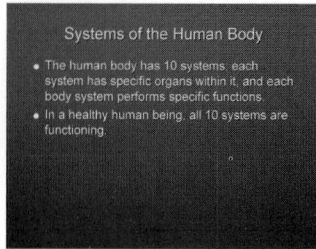

- Body systems do not operate independently; they exert important effects on each other.

- For example, when you exercise hard, your muscular system needs extra oxygen, so your respiratory system works harder than usual to supply it.

- The ovaries and testes clearly belong to the reproductive system. However, since one of their functions is to produce hormones, they are also components of the endocrine system.

- When something happens in one system, it can often affect another system. For example, if your nervous system reacts to upsetting information while you are eating, your digestive system may not function as well as usual.

Slide 6

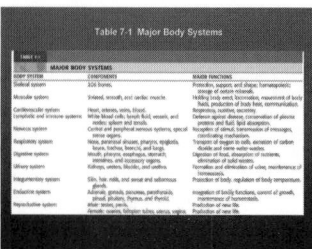

- The human body has 10 systems: (1) skeletal, (2) muscular, (3) cardiovascular (including lymphatic and immune systems), (4) nervous, (5) respiratory, (6) digestive, (7) endocrine, (8) urinary, (9) integumentary (skin), and (10) reproductive.

- Each system has specific organs within it, and each body system performs specific functions. When all 10 systems are functioning well, the person is healthy.

Slide 7

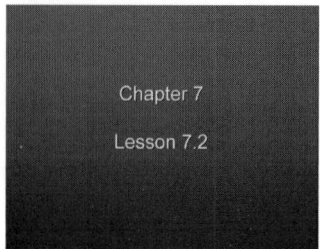

Slide 8

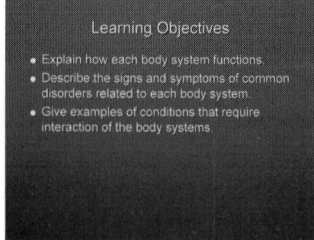

Torres and Ehrlich Modern Dental Assisting, 9th ed.

Bird/Robinson

Slide 9

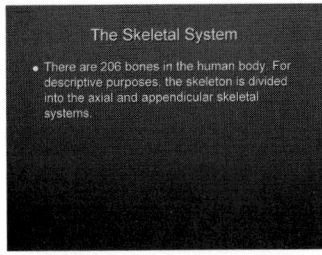

- The major functions of the skeletal system are protection, support, and shape; hematopoietic (makes blood cells); and storage of certain minerals.
- Remember that "axial" pertains to the body region that is made up of the head, neck, and trunk, and "appendicular" pertains to the body region that consists of the arms and legs.

Slide 10

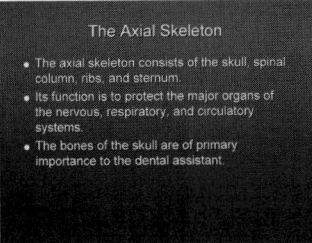

- What is the skull? *(It is the skeletal structure of the head, composed of the facial and cranial bones. The skull houses and protects the brain and most of the chief sense organs; i.e., the eyes, ears, nose, and tongue. Among humans, some 14 bones shape the face, most occurring in symmetrical pairs.)*
- Why is the skull of primary importance to the dental assistant?

Slide 11

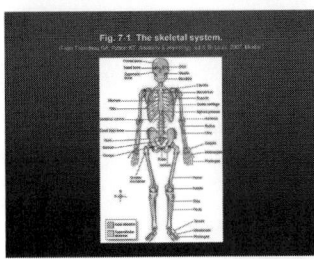

- The skull, spine, and rib cage form the axial skeleton and account for 80 of the 206 bones in the human body.
- What are the two divisions of the skeleton?

Slide 12

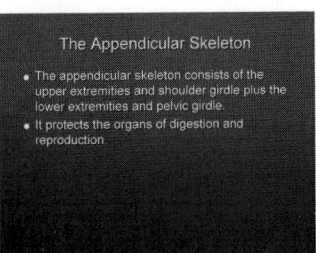

- What tissue makes up most of the human skeleton?

Slide 13

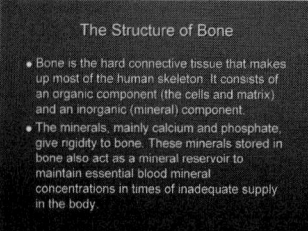

- Why is it important that we have calcium in our diets when we are growing?

Slide 14

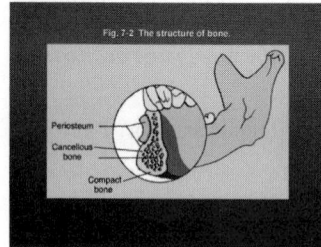

- The three layers of bone are (1) periosteum, (2) compact bone, and (3) cancellous bone and bone marrow.

- The periosteum is the first layer of the bone. It is a thin layer of whitish connective tissue and contains nerves and blood vessels. It supplies the cells from which the hard bone below the periosteum is built up. It is necessary for bone growth and repair, nutrition, and carrying away waste.

- Compact bone, also known as cortical bone, is hard, dense, and very strong. It forms the outer layer of the bones.

- Cancellous bone, also known as spongy bone, is found inside the bone.

Slide 15

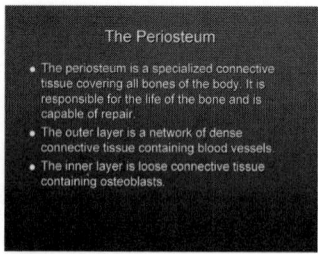

- During dental surgery, care is taken not to traumatize the periosteum of the jaws.

- What are osteoblasts? *(The cells that produce bone tissue.)*

- How many kinds of bone are found in the body?

Slide 16

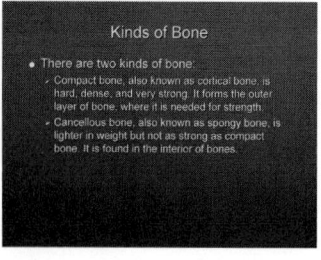

- What is osteoporosis? *(Osteoporosis, or "porous bone," is a disease characterized by low bone mass and structural deterioration of bone tissue, leading to bone fragility and an increased susceptibility to fractures of the hip, spine, and wrist. Men as well as women suffer from osteoporosis, a disease that can be prevented and treated.)*

- How are these two types of bone different?

Slide 17

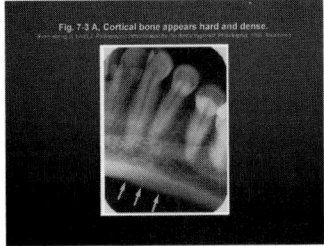

- View of the mandible on a periapical radiograph.

- Compact bone, also known as cortical bone, is hard, dense, and very strong. It forms the outer layer of the bones (where the arrows are), where it is needed for strength. Cancellous bone, also known as spongy bone, is lighter in weight but not as strong as compact bone and is found in the interior of bones.

- Where is the cancellous bone on this radiograph?

Slide 18

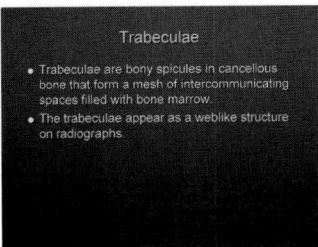

- What are spicules? *(Small pieces of bone.)*

Slide 19

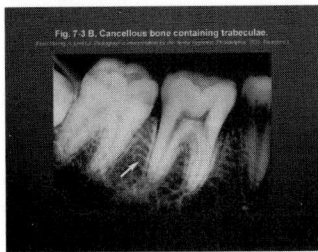

- Periapical radiograph shows the alveolar bone.

- The trabeculae in cancellous bone appear as a weblike structure in a radiograph (arrow).

- Where is the compact bone in this radiograph?

- What is bone marrow and how does it function?

Slide 20

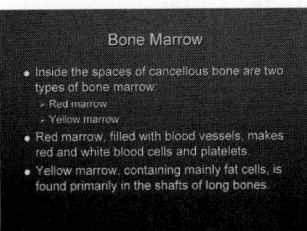

- People are born with only red bone marrow. As a person matures, the red marrow in many of the bones is replaced by yellow marrow. By adulthood, only about half of the bone marrow is red. Red bone marrow is found mostly in the ribs, breastbone, shoulder blades, collarbones, hip bones, skull, and spine.

- This means that the elderly are more prone to infections and cancers because fewer lymphocytes are being produced, since the red bone marrow is decreasing.

Slide 21

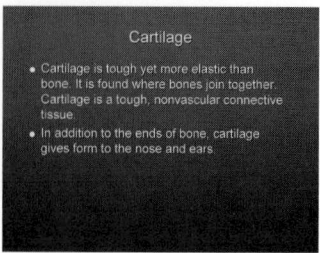

- How many types of cartilage are there? *(There are three basic forms of cartilage; hyaline cartilage serves as the "type" and the other two forms are described with reference to it. Elastic cartilage and fibrous cartilage are the other two. Many authorities regard the last as a transitional form between cartilage and connective tissue proper.)*

Slide 22

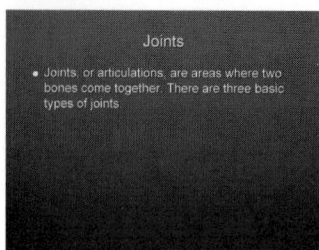

- What are the three basic types of joints?

Slide 23

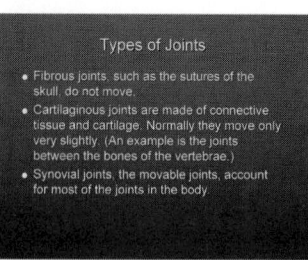

- What is arthritis? *(Arthritis is a painful condition resulting from inflammation of the joints. Tens of millions of Americans experience chronic or acute pain and physical limitations because of more than 100 forms of arthritis.)*
- Unlike osteoarthritis, which results from wear and tear on your joints, rheumatoid arthritis is an inflammatory condition. The exact cause is unknown, but it is believed to be the body's immune system attacking the synovium — the tissue that lines the joints.

Slide 24

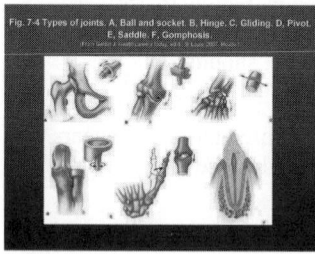

- What are the features of synovial joints? *(They consist of two bones whose articular surfaces are covered with hyaline cartilage.)*
- The joint space is enclosed by a fibrous capsule. Thickened and organized areas of this capsule consists of the named ligaments.
- The synovial membrane lines the joint space. This membrane secretes synovial fluid, which fills the joint space and provides lubrication and nourishment to the articular cartilage.
- Is the temporomandibular joint a synovial joint?

Bird/Robinson

Slide 25

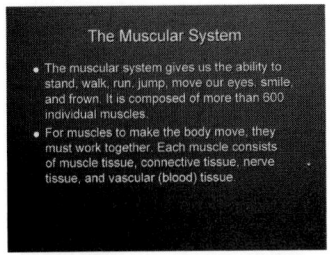

- The major functions of the muscles are holding the body erect, locomotion, movement of body fluids, production of body heat, and communication.

- What are the three types of muscle tissue?

- What distinguishes the appearance of each muscle type?

Slide 26

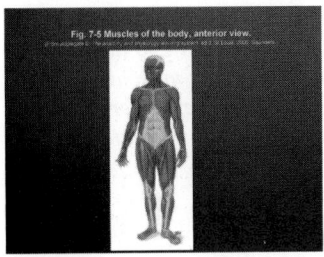

- Muscles are the primary means by which we communicate and interact with the environment. Speech is dependent on the muscles of the larynx, mouth and tongue (spoken words); verbal communication can also be accomplished with the muscles of your fingers (written words or sign language).

- What other activities are dependent on the skeletal muscles?
  (Body language, dancing, running, playing, eating, building, or fighting.)

Slide 27

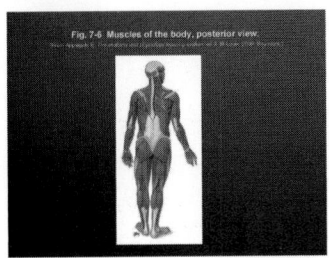

- Because muscles are so crucial to any animal, they are incredibly sophisticated. They are efficient at turning fuel into motion; they are long-lasting; they are self-healing, and they are able to grow stronger with practice. They do everything from allowing you to walk to keeping your blood flowing.

Slide 28

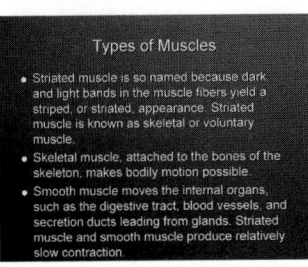

- Which muscle has the striations?

- Which muscle type is attached to the skeleton?

- Which muscles help digestion and move blood?

Torres and Ehrlich Modern Dental Assisting, 9th ed.

Bird/Robinson

Slide 29

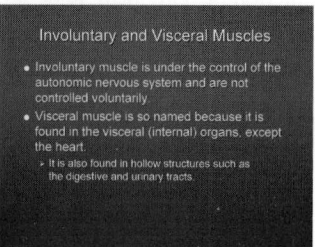

Slide 30

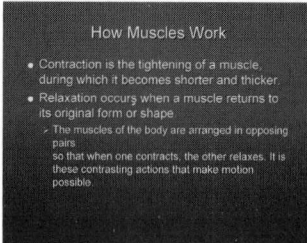

- Try contracting a facial muscle, then let it relax.

- What is muscular dystrophy? *(A group of rare inherited muscle diseases in which muscle fibers are unusually susceptible to damage and become progressively weaker. In the late stages of muscular dystrophy, fat and connective tissue often replace muscle fibers. In some types of muscular dystrophy, heart muscle, other involuntary muscles and other organs are affected.)*

Slide 31

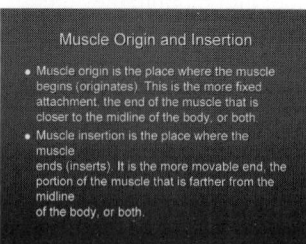

- Where is the midline of the body?

- What is the difference between the origin and the insertion of a muscle?

Slide 32

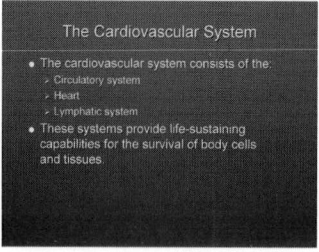

- The main functions of the cardiovascular system are respiratory, nutritive, and excretory.

- Studies now show a relationship between periodontal disease and cardiovascular disease. People who have cardiovascular disease and periodontal disease are at increased risk because of bacterial products that can migrate into the pleural cavity and infect the heart.

- What are the main functions of the circulatory system?

Torres and Ehrlich Modern Dental Assisting, 9th ed.

Bird/Robinson

Slide 33

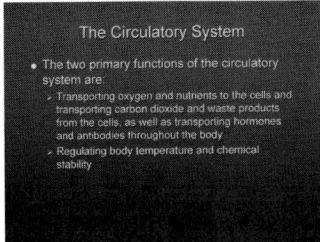

- What is carbon dioxide? *(A colorless, odorless gas, CO$_2$, which is a by-product of respiration. Plants require CO$_2$ to photosynthesize, which generates molecular oxygen.)*

Slide 34

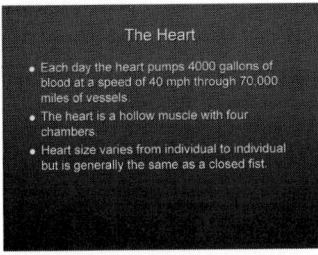

- What are the symptoms of a heart attack (myocardial infarction)? *(Some heart attacks are sudden and intense—the "movie heart attack," where no one doubts what's happening. But most heart attacks start slowly, with mild pain or discomfort. Often people affected aren't sure what's wrong and wait too long to get help.)*

- What is high blood pressure, how does it occur in the body, and how do we record it?

Slide 35

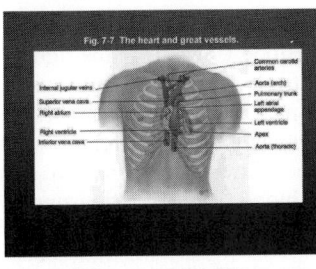

- The right atrium receives blood from the superior and inferior venae cavae, the largest veins that enter the heart. Blood flows from the right atrium into the right ventricle. The right ventricle receives blood from the right atrium and pumps it into the pulmonary artery, which carries it to the lungs.

- The left atrium receives oxygenated blood from the lungs through the four pulmonary veins. Blood flows from here into the left ventricle. The left ventricle receives blood from the left atrium. Blood then goes into the aorta, the largest of the arteries, and is pumped to all parts of the body, except the lungs.

Slide 36

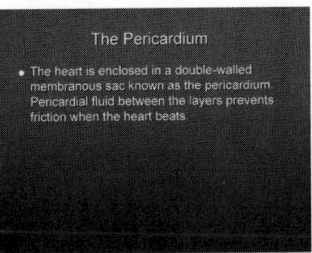

- What are the upper and lower chambers of the heart?

Slide 37

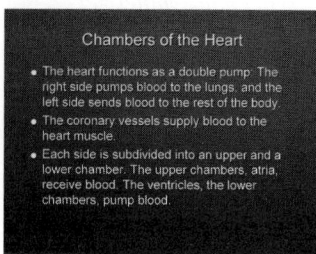

- The "coronary arteries" are the vessels that bring the blood to the heart muscle. Blockages of these vessels are the number one cause of death in the United States.

- Why does the blood go to the lungs?

- What are the names and functions of the three main types of blood vessels?

Slide 38

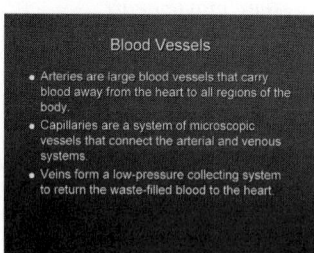

- Which way do arteries go in relationship to the heart?

- Which way do veins go in relationship to the heart?

- Where are capillaries located in relationship to the arteries and veins?

Slide 39

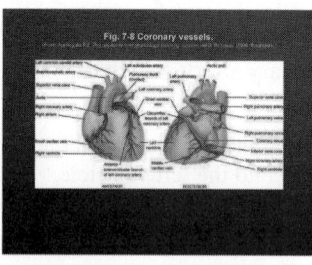

- The heart functions as a double pump; the right side pumps blood to the lungs, and the left side sends blood to the rest of the body.

- The right atrium receives blood from the superior and inferior venae cavae, the largest veins that enter the heart. Blood flows from the right atrium into the right ventricle. The right ventricle receives blood from the right atrium and pumps it into the pulmonary artery, which carries it to the lungs. The left atrium receives oxygenated blood from the lungs through the four pulmonary veins. Blood flows from here into the left ventricle. The left ventricle receives blood from the left atrium. Blood then goes into the aorta.

Slide 40

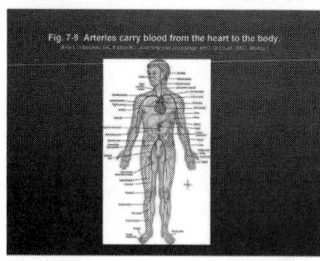

- The arteries are the large blood vessels that carry blood away from the heart to all regions of the body. The walls of the arteries are made up of three layers. This structure makes arteries both muscular and elastic so that they can expand and contract with the pumping beat of the heart.

- The capillaries are a system of microscopic vessels that connect the arterial and venous system.

- The veins form a low-pressure collecting system to return the waste-filled blood to the heart.

Bird/Robinson

Slide 41

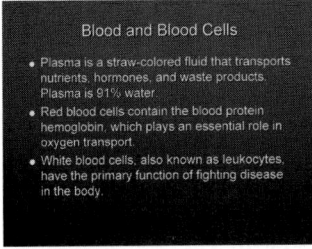

- One drop of blood contains 5 million red blood cells, 7500 white blood cells, and 300,000 platelets. The remaining 9% of plasma consists mainly of plasma proteins, including albumin and globulin.
- White blood cells, also known as leukocytes, have the primary function of fighting disease in the body. The five major groups of leukocytes are as follows:

  1. Basophils have imprecisely understood functions.
  2. Eosinophils increase in number in allergic conditions.
  3. Lymphocytes are important in the immune process to protect the body.
  4. Monocytes act as macrophages and dispose of dead and dying cells and other debris.
  5. Neutrophils fight disease by engulfing germs.

Slide 42

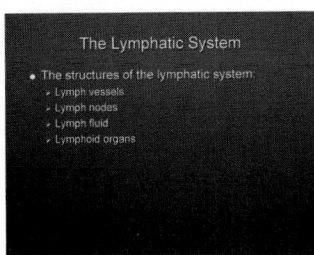

- The main functions of the lymphatic system are defense against disease, conservation of plasma proteins and fluid, systems and nodes, and spleen and tonsils lipid absorption.

Slide 43

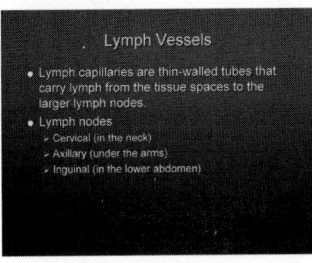

- The bean-shaped lymph nodes of the lymphatic system are connected by vessels. Lymph nodes are usually present in clusters in the armpits, on either side of the neck, and in the groin.
- The lymph nodes contain lymphocytes (white blood cells), which help destroy foreign bacteria or other harmful cells. The lymph nodes may become enlarged or swollen when they fight an infection, since they must produce additional white blood cells. The lymph nodes may feel tender or inflamed as they are actively fighting a foreign body.

Slide 44

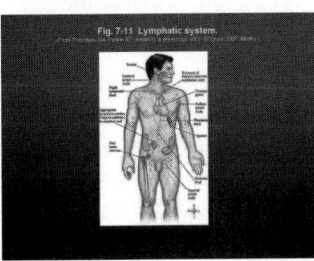

- The structures of the lymphatic system include the lymph vessels, lymph nodes, lymph fluid, and lymphoid organs. Fluid leaves circulatory capillaries to bathe tissues and cells to keep them moist. This same clear, light yellow fluid, called lymph, is reabsorbed by the lymphatic system and returned to the blood through the veins.
- Lymph nodes are small round or oval structures located in lymph vessels.
- The spleen is the largest of the lymphoid organs. The spleen produces lymphocytes and monocytes, which are important components of the immune system. It also filters microorganisms and other debris not destroyed by the lymphatic system.

ELSEVIER

Torres and Ehrlich Modern Dental Assisting, 9th ed.

Bird/Robinson

Slide 45

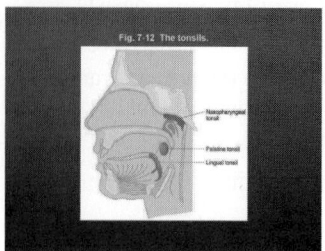

- The tonsils are masses of lymphatic tissue located in the upper portions of the nose and throat, where they form a protective ring of lymphatic tissue.

- The nasopharyngeal tonsils, also known as adenoids, are found in the nasopharynx.

- The palatine tonsils are located in the oropharynx between the anterior and posterior pillars of fauces (throat) and are visible through the mouth.

- The lingual tonsils are located on the back of the tongue.

Slide 46

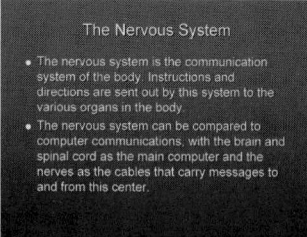

- The main functions of the nervous system are reception of stimuli, transmission of messages, coordination of mechanism systems, and special sense organs.

- What are the two divisions of the autonomic nervous system?

Slide 47

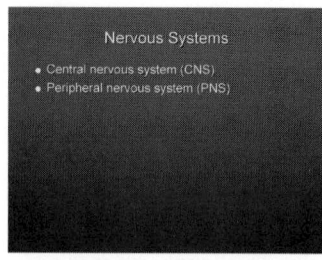

- The nervous system is made up of the central and the peripheral nervous systems.

- The central nervous system (CNS) consists of the brain and spinal cord.

- The peripheral nervous system (PNS) consists of the cranial nerves and the spinal nerves. The PNS also includes the autonomic nervous system, which is divided into the sympathetic and parasympathetic nervous systems.

Slide 48

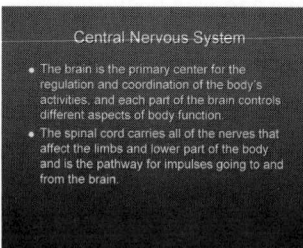

- Injury to the brain:

  - Head injury can be caused by a blunt trauma to the head or a break in the skull.

  - Brain tumors can be benign (noncancerous) or malignant (cancerous); a tumor's effect on brain and bodily functions depends on its location and whether it is exerting pressure on surrounding tissues.

  - Migraine headache results from vasodilation and increased blood flow to the head.

  - Cerebrovascular accident—commonly called a stroke—is the interruption of blood flow to the brain. It results in numbness, altered mental status, vertigo, and loss of muscle coordination. It can be caused by a hemorrhage or a blood clot.

Bird/Robinson

Slide 49

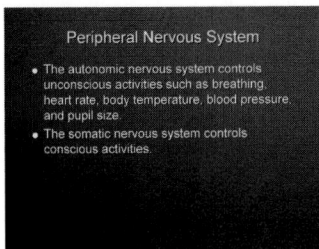

- What system controls breathing?
- What system controls walking?
- What system controls whether or not you sweat?
- What system controls speaking?

Slide 50

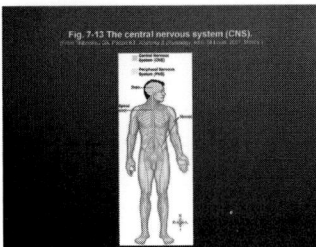

- The nervous system is the communication system of the body. Instructions and directions are sent out by this system to the various organs in the body.
- The central nervous system (CNS) consists of the brain and spinal cord.
- The peripheral nervous system (PNS) consists of the cranial nerves and the spinal nerves.
- The PNS also includes the autonomic nervous system, which is divided into the sympathetic and parasympathetic nervous systems.

Slide 51

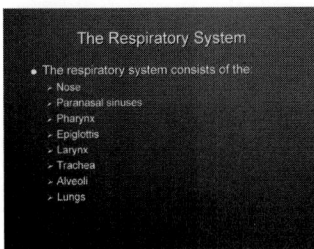

- The main functions of the respiratory system are transport of oxygen to cells, and excretion of carbon dioxide and some water and waste.
- The larynx, also known as the voice box, contains the vocal bands, which make speech possible.
- Air passes from the larynx to the trachea. The trachea extends from the neck into the chest, directly in front of the esophagus.
- The trachea divides into two branches called bronchi. Each bronchus leads to a lung, where it divides and subdivides into increasingly smaller branches; bronchioles are the smallest of these branches. Alveoli are the tiny grape-like clusters found at the end of each bronchiole. During respiration, the exchange of gases between the lungs and the blood takes place in the alveoli.

Slide 52

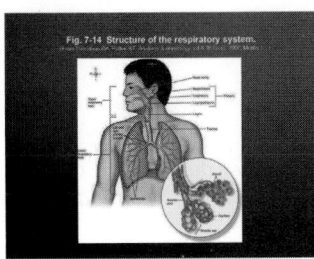

- Air enters the body through the nostrils (nares) of the nose and passes through the nasal cavity. The nose is divided by a wall of cartilage called the nasal septum. The nose and respiratory system are lined with mucous membrane, which is a specialized form of epithelial tissue.
- The incoming air is filtered by the cilia, thin hairs attached to the mucous membrane just inside the nostrils. Mucus secreted by the mucous membranes helps to moisten and warm the air as it enters the nose.

Torres and Ehrlich Modern Dental Assisting, 9th ed.

Bird/Robinson

Slide 53

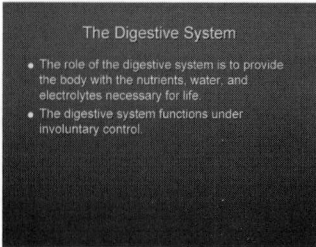

- The main functions of the digestive system are digestion of food, absorption of nutrients, and elimination of solid wastes.
- What are the five actions of the digestive system?

Slide 54

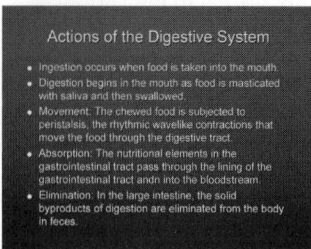

Slide 55

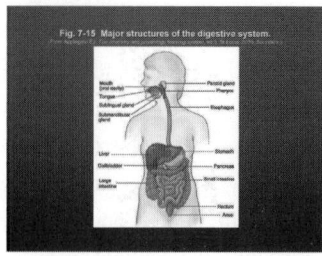

- The major structures of the digestive system are the mouth, pharynx, esophagus, stomach, small intestine, large intestine, liver, gallbladder, and pancreas.
- The digestive system works like an assembly line in reverse. It takes in whole foods and breaks them down into their chemical components. Food that has been eaten is broken down by digestive juices into small absorbable nutrients that generate energy and provide the body with the nutrients, water, and electrolytes necessary for life. The digestive system functions under involuntary control.

Slide 56

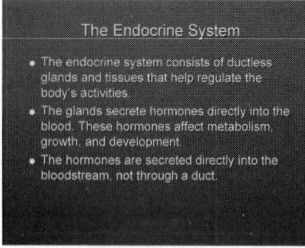

- Studies now show that there is a relationship between periodontal disease and diabetes, an endocrine disease, and its control.

  - What is diabetes? *(Diabetes mellitus is a chronic disease involving abnormalities in the body's ability to use sugar. Diabetes is characterized by:*

  - *Elevated blood sugars for months to years.*

  - *Both hereditary and environmental factors leading to its development and progression.*

  - *A relative or absolute deficiency of effective circulating insulin. Insulin is a substance made by the pancreas; it lowers blood sugar in conjunction with meals.)*

Slide 57

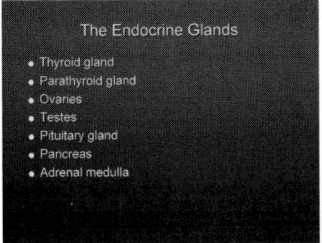

Slide 58

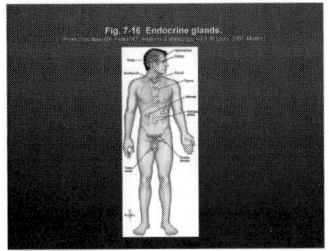

- Endocrine glands include the thyroid gland, the parathyroid gland, the ovaries, the testes, the pituitary gland, the pancreas, and the adrenal medulla.

- The endocrine system uses chemical messengers called hormones that move through the bloodstream and can reach every cell in the body. Hormones help maintain a constant environment inside the body (homeostasis), adjusting the amount of salt and water in the tissues and sugar in the blood to suit the particular conditions that exist. Hormones produce both long-term changes, such as a child's growth and sexual maturation, and rhythmic ones, such as the menstrual cycle.

Slide 59

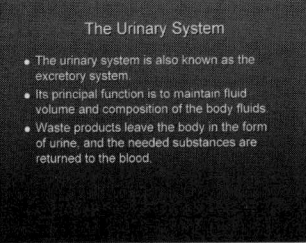

- Why is it important that we get enough fluids in our bodies during the day?

Slide 60

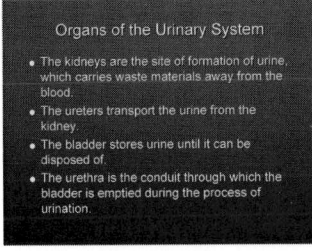

- Kidney disease results from damage to the nephrons, the tiny structures inside your kidneys that filter blood. Usually the damage—which happens in both kidneys—occurs very gradually over years. Kidney disease is often asymptomatic.

  - Common causes of kidney disease:

  - Diabetes mellitus: The glucose stays in your blood and acts like a poison.

  - High blood pressure, which can damage the small blood vessels in the kidneys. When this happens, the kidneys cannot effectively filter wastes from the blood..

  - Heredity: Some kidney diseases result from hereditary factors, and can run in families. If your family has a history of any kind of kidney problems, you may be at risk for kidney disease and should talk to your doctor.

Torres and Ehrlich Modern Dental Assisting, 9th ed.
Bird/Robinson

Slide 61

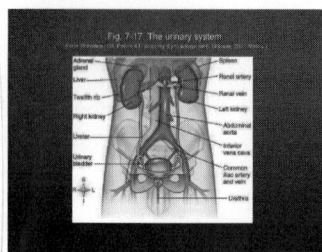

- The urinary system consists of
  - the kidneys, where urine is formed to carry away waste materials from the blood;
  - the ureters, which transport the urine from the kidneys;
  - the bladder, where the urine is stored until it can be eliminated; and
  - the urethra, through which the bladder is emptied to the outside through the process of urination.

Slide 62

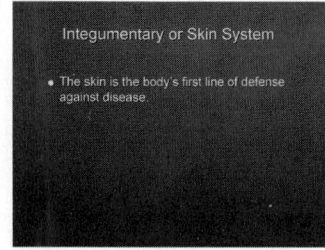

- What are the functions of the skin?
- What are the appendages of the skin?

Slide 63

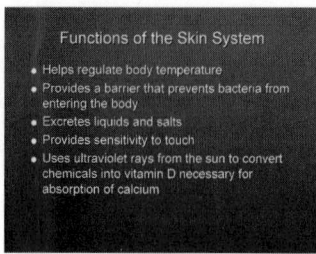

- What is calcium used for in the body? *(Calcium is essential to the formation and maintenance of strong bones and teeth. In the human adult, the bone calcium is chiefly in the form of the phosphate and carbonate salts. A sufficient store of vitamin D in the body is necessary for the proper utilization of calcium. Calcium also functions in the regulation of the heartbeat and in the conversion of prothrombin to thrombin, a necessary step in the clotting of blood.)*
- What is skin cancer? *(Skin cancer is the uncontrolled growth of skin cells. If left unchecked, these cancer cells can spread from the skin into other tissues and organs.)*

Slide 64

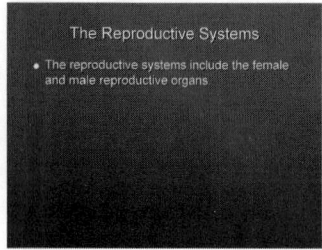

Torres and Ehrlich Modern Dental Assisting, 9th ed.

Bird/Robinson

Slide 65

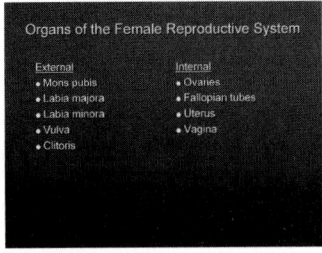

- The female reproductive system consists of the external and internal genitalia. The external genitalia consist of the mons pubis, labia majora and labia minora, vulva, and clitoris. The internal genitalia consist of the ovaries, fallopian tubes, uterus, and vagina.

- Fertility, the normal functioning of the reproductive system, begins at puberty (the onset of menstruation) and ceases at menopause. Many disorders can affect the female reproductive system.

- What is the uterus? *(It is the womb--a pear-shaped organ in women—that holds and nourishes the growing embryo and fetus. The uterus has three areas: the body or upper part; the isthmus or the narrowed central area; and the cervix, the lower portion.)*

Slide 66

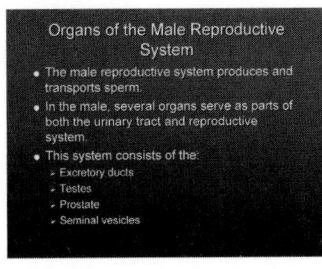

- The male reproductive system consists of the testes, excretory ducts, and accessory organs. The accessory organs include the prostate and seminal vesicles. In the male, several organs serve as parts of both the urinary tract and the reproductive system.

- A disorder may interfere with the function of either system or both systems.

- What is the prostate? *(A gland in the male that surrounds the neck of the bladder and urethra. The prostate contributes to the seminal fluid.)*

ELSEVIER

8 Oral Embryology and Histology

TEACHING FOCUS

This chapter will give students an opportunity to understand oral embryology, especially embryonic development of the face and oral cavity. The chapter also includes information on developmental disturbances. Furthermore, students will have an opportunity to learn about facial development after birth and the life cycle of a tooth. Finally, the chapter provides information on oral histology, including the crown, root, enamel, dentin, cementum, pulp, and periodontium.

MATERIALS AND RESOURCES

☐ computer and PowerPoint projector (all Lessons)
☐ unlabeled copies of Figure 8-15 (Lesson 8.2)
☐ unlabeled copies of Figure 8-19 (Lesson 8.3)

LESSON CHECKLIST

Preparations for this lesson include:

- lecture
- evaluation of student knowledge and skills needed to perform all entry-level activities related to oral embryology and histology, including:
  - prenatal development
  - embryonic development of the face and oral cavity
  - development disturbances
  - facial development after birth
  - life cycle of a tooth
  - oral histology

ELSEVIER

Torres and Ehrlich Modern Dental Assisting, 9th ed.

Bird/Robinson

KEY TERMS

alveolar crest (p. 95)
alveolar socket (p. 95)
ameloblasts (p. 87)
anatomic crown (p. 89)
apex (p. 87)
apical foramen (p. 94)
cementoblasts (p. 87)
cementoclasts (p. 97)
cementum (p. 90)
clinical crown (p. 89)
conception (p. 78)
coronal pulp (p. 94)
cortical plate (p. 95)
dental lamina (p. 86)
dental papilla (p. 86)
dental sac (p. 84)
dentin (p. 93)
dentinal fiber (p. 93)
dentinal tubules (p. 93)
deposition (p. 83)
embryo (p. 78)
embryology (p. 78)
embryonic period (p. 78)
enamel lamellae (p. 93)
enamel organ (p. 86)
enamel spindles (p. 93)
enamel tufts (p. 92)
exfoliation (p. 87)
fetal period (p. 79)
fibroblasts (p. 94)
gestation (p. 78)
histology (p. 78)
Hunter-Schreger bands (p. 92)
hydroxyapatite (p. 92)

hyoid arch (p. 81)
lamina dura (p. 95)
lining mucosa (p. 98)
mandibular arch (p. 81)
masticatory mucosa (p. 98)
meiosis (p. 78)
modeling (p. 83)
odontoblasts (p. 87)
odontogenesis (p. 86)
osteoblasts (p. 83)
osteoclasts (p. 83)
periodontium (p. 91)
preimplantation period (p. 78)
prenatal development (p. 78)
primary cementum (p. 94)
primary dentin (p. 93)
primary palate (p. 82)
prisms (p. 92)
pulp chamber (p. 94)
radicular pulp (p. 94)
remodeling (p. 86)
resorption (p. 83)
secondary cementum (p. 94)
secondary dentin (p. 93)
secondary palate (p. 82)
specialized mucosa (p. 98)
stomodeum (p. 79)
stratified squamous epithelium (p. 98)
striae of Retzius (p. 92)
succedaneous teeth (p. 86)
tertiary dentin (p. 94)
tooth buds (p. 86)
zygote (p. 78)

ADDITIONAL RESOURCES

PowerPoint slides (Evolve): 1-66

Legend

CTQ
Critical
Thinking
Question

DVD
Multimedia
Procedures
Videos and
Animations

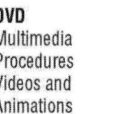

ESLR
EVOLVE
Student
Learning
Resources

IDO
Interactive
Dental
Office
CD-ROM

SW
Student
Workbook

TB
Test Bank
on the
TEACH
CD-ROM

PPT
PowerPoint
Slides

Class Activities are indicated in ***bold italic***.

Torres and Ehrlich Modern Dental Assisting, 9th ed.

Bird/Robinson

LESSON 8.1

PRETEST

1. Which cells form the enamel?
   - a. odontoblasts
   - b. osteoblasts
   - c. ameloblasts
   - d. cementoblasts

2. Which portion of the healthy tooth is visible in the oral cavity?
   - a. anatomic root
   - b. clinical root
   - c. anatomic crown
   - d. clinical crown

3. In which stage of tooth development do the cells of the tooth grow and increase in number?
   - a. cap stage
   - b. bud stage
   - c. bell stage
   - d. maturation stage

4. What is the hardest substance in the body?
   - a. dentin
   - b. bone
   - c. cementum
   - d. enamel

5. What is the stomodeum in a developing human embryo?
   - a. primitive eye
   - b. primitive tooth
   - c. primitive mouth
   - d. primitive ear

6. When the embryo is 5 to 6 weeks old, the first signs of tooth development are found in the
   - a. upper posterior.
   - b. lower posterior.
   - c. upper anterior.
   - d. lower anterior.

7. How many teeth are in development at birth?
   - a. 16
   - b. 20
   - c. 36
   - d. 44

8. Which cells form new bone?
   - a. odontoblasts
   - b. osteoblasts
   - c. ameloblasts
   - d. cementoblasts

9. From what embryonic layer does the cementum form?
   - a. neural crest cells
   - b. endoderm
   - c. mesoderm
   - d. ectoderm

10. What portion of the tooth germ is directly responsible for dentin formation?
    - a. dental sac
    - b. dental lamina
    - c. dental papilla
    - d. dental cuticle

Answers

1. c	3. a	5. c	7. d	9. c
2. d	4. d	6. d	8. b	10. c

BACKGROUND ASSESSMENT

Question: Of what mineral are the hard tissues of the teeth and alveolar bone composed? Of the hard tissues of the tooth, what is the most mineralized tissue of the tooth and what is the least mineralized?

Answer: Hydroxyapatite, which consists primarily of calcium, is the most abundant mineral component in the hard tissues of the tooth. Enamel is the most mineralized, followed by dentin. The cementum and alveolar bone are less mineralized than either enamel or dentin.

ELSEVIER

Question: What are the tissues of the tooth germ and during what stage does it form? From what embryonic layers do they come? What tissues will they form in the future and what is the cell involved?

Answer: The tooth germ is composed of the enamel organ, dental papilla, and dental sac that forms during the cap stage. The enamel organ is derived from the ectoderm by way of the dental lamina. The dental papilla and dental sac are derived from the mesoderm. The enamel organ will produce enamel from the ameloblasts. The dental papilla will produce dentin from the odontoblasts, and pulp will be derived from the central cells of dental papilla. The dental sac will produce the periodontal ligament from the fibroblasts, cementum from the cementoblasts, and alveolar bone from the osteoblasts.

CRITICAL THINKING QUESTION

A patient who has Down syndrome is coming to the office. You want to investigate this syndrome before the patient comes in so you can understand the patient's needs. What is this syndrome, and what are its signs and symptoms? Why did it occur, and what process was involved?

Guidelines: With conception, the union of the egg and sperm subsequently forms a fertilized egg, or zygote. In the zygote, the 23 chromosomes in the sperm unite with the 23 chromosomes in the egg, providing a new life with a full complement of 46 chromosomes. These chromosomes will determine its inherited characteristics and direct its growth and development. The process of joining each parent's chromosomes is called meiosis. Meiosis ensures that the future embryo will have the correct number of chromosomes. An extra chromosome that results from a disturbance in meiosis during fertilization causes Down syndrome. A child with this syndrome has a flat, broad face with wide-set eyes, a flat-bridged nose, oblique eyelid fissures, and other defects. An affected child can have various levels of mental retardation. Children with Down syndrome have increased levels of periodontal (gum) disease and abnormally shaped teeth.

OBJECTIVES	CONTENT	TEACHING RESOURCES
Pronounce, define, and spell the Key Terms.	■ Key terms (pp. 76-77)	ⓔ ESLR Electronic Flashcards ▸ Discuss each of the key terms, focusing on the definition, pronunciation, and spelling of each term. *Class Activity Divide the class into two teams. Have one team call out the definition of a key term and a member of the other team answer with the term, using correct pronunciation and spelling. Have each team alternate providing the definition until all the key terms from the chapter have been used.*
Define embryology and histology.	■ Introduction (p. 78)	⊠ PPT 4-5, 40 TB questions 1-2 SW Short-Answer Questions 1; Fill in the Blank questions 1-2 (p. 25) ▸ Discuss and define embryology and histology. *Class Activity Divide the class into groups, and have them develop definitions of embryology and histology and give examples of each. Have each group present its explanation to the class, and then have the class vote on which explanation was the most thorough.*
Describe the three periods of prenatal development.	■ Oral embryology (p. 78) ☐ Prenatal development (p. 78)	⊠ PPT 6-13 TB question 3 SW Short-Answer Questions 2; Fill in the Blank questions 3-5; Multiple Choice questions 1-3 (pp. 25-27)

ELSEVIER

Torres and Ehrlich Modern Dental Assisting, 9th ed.
Bird/Robinson

OBJECTIVES	CONTENT	TEACHING RESOURCES
		SW Topics for Discussion questions 1, 3-5 (p. 28)
		Recall questions 1, 2 (p. 79)
		Figure 8-1 Periods and structure in prenatal development (p. 78)
		Figure 8-2 Sperm fertilizes the ovum and unites with it to form the zygote (p. 79)
		Figure 8-3 A fetus at various weeks of development (p. 79)
		Figure 8-4 Scanning electron micrograph of the head and neck of an embryo at four weeks (p. 81)
		Figure 8-5 A human embryo during the fifth week of development (p. 81)
		Box 8-1 Developmental Disturbances (p. 80)
		Legal and Ethical Implications (p. 99)
		Eye to the Future (p. 99)
		CTQ 2 (p. 99)
		▸ Discuss the three distinct periods of prenatal development.
		▸ Discuss the most critical period of prenatal development and the reasons why.
		Class Activity Divide the class into small groups, and have them prepare charts contrasting the three periods of prenatal development. Students may use figures from the text to illustrate their charts. Have each group present its chart to the class and discuss its contents.
Discuss prenatal influences on dental development.	☐ Embryonic development of the face and oral cavity (p. 79) – Primary embryonic layers (p. 79) – Early development of the mouth (p. 81) – Branchial arches (p. 81) – Hard and soft palates (p. 82) – Facial development (p. 82) – Tooth development (p. 83)	PPT 14-15, 18-19 SW Short-Answer Questions 3; Multiple Choice questions 5, 7 (pp. 25, 27) Recall questions 3-5, 7 (pp. 79, 82-83) ▸ Discuss the time period in prenatal development when the face and its related tissues begin to form. ▸ Discuss the early development of the mouth. *Class Activity Assign each student a disorder of the teeth that occurs in prenatal development. Have each student research the disorder and present a brief synopsis of it to the class, using photos or drawings if possible.*

Torres and Ehrlich Modern Dental Assisting, 9th ed.

Bird/Robinson

OBJECTIVES	CONTENT	TEACHING RESOURCES
Describe the steps in the formation of the palate.	– Hard and soft palates (p. 82) – Facial development (p. 82) – Tooth development (p. 83)	PPT 16-17 SW Short-Answer Questions 5; Multiple Choice question 6 (pp. 25, 27) Recall question 6 (p. 82) Figure 8-6 Adult palate and developmental divisions (p. 82) Figure 8-7 (A) An infant with a left unilateral complete cleft lip and palate; (B) The infant after corrective surgeries are performed (p. 82) ▶ Discuss the process of the formation of the soft and hard palates. ▶ Discuss the time period in which palate formation occurs. ***Class Activity** As a class, discuss the formation of the palate, including identification of the steps in the process and when each occurs. Create a time line of the process on the board. Identify and discuss the aberration in the process that forms a cleft palate.*

8.1 Homework/Assignments:

8.1 Instructor's Notes/Student Feedback:

Torres and Ehrlich Modern Dental Assisting, 9th ed.

Bird/Robinson

LESSON 8.2

CRITICAL THINKING QUESTION

During what period of prenatal development is the child more vulnerable to malformations from environmental factors? What are these factors called, and why is the embryo so susceptible to environmental influences? Is the mother's dental health also affected?

Guidelines: Because all of the organ systems are formed during the embryonic period, the fetus is less vulnerable than the embryo to malformations caused by radiation, viruses, and drugs. The embryonic period is the stage of human development that occurs from the beginning of the second week to the end of the eighth week. Adverse environmental influences are called teratogens and include infections, drugs, and exposure to radiation. Drugs taken during pregnancy may cause birth defects, including prescribed medication, over-the-counter remedies such as aspirin and cold tablets, and abused drugs including alcohol. Antibiotics, particularly tetracycline, taken during pregnancy may result in a stain on the primary teeth. Women of childbearing age should avoid teratogens from the time of their first menstrual period. Specifically, the teratogens can include rubella virus that causes German measles, alcohol that causes fetal alcohol syndrome, and high levels of radiation that causes cell death and retardation of mental development and physical growth (dental radiation is not implicated, but care must be taken to avoid unnecessary radiation at this time). The mother's dental health is also of concern. Toxins from a dental infection may be dangerous to both mother and child (e.g., toxins from periodontal disease in the mother are linked to low birth weight in the infant). Fever in the mother during pregnancy will leave marks in the developing teeth of the fetus.

OBJECTIVES	CONTENT	TEACHING RESOURCES

Describe the stages in development of a tooth.	– Tooth development (p. 83)	🖥 TB question 7
		
		SW Short-Answer Questions 6 (p. 25)
		
		Recall question 8 (p. 83)
		
		Table 8-1 Stages of Tooth Development (p. 84)
		
		💡 CTQ 3 (p. 99)
		
		▸ Discuss the tooth development in an embryo.
		
		***Class Activity** Present the following stages of tooth development to students:*
		
		   – Bell stage
		
		   – Initiation stage
		
		   – Cap stage
		
		   – Bud stage
		
		   – Maturation stage
		
		   – Apposition stage
		
		Have groups work as quickly as possible to place the stages in the correct order and correctly identify the characteristics of each stage.

Discuss genetic and environmental factors that can affect dental development.	☐ Developmental disturbances (p. 83) – Genetic factors (p. 83) – Environmental factors (p. 83)	🖻 PPT 22-24, 39 🖥 TB question 5 SW Short-Answer Questions 7; Multiple Choice question 9 (pp. 25, 27)

Torres and Ehrlich Modern Dental Assisting, 9th ed.

Bird/Robinson

OBJECTIVES	CONTENT	TEACHING RESOURCES
		Recall question 9 (p. 83)
		▸ Discuss genetic factors that can affect prenatal dental development.
		▸ Discuss environmental factors that can affect prenatal dental development.
		Class Activity Write the following genetic and environmental factors in columns on the board.
		– Jaw and Tooth Size
		– Infections
		– Drugs
		– Exposure to Radiation
		Have students identify the dental disorders that can result from these factors and write them in the correct column. Then, discuss ways in which these factors can be avoided or treated.
Describe the function of osteoclasts and osteoblasts.	☐ Facial development after birth (p. 83) – Tooth movement (p. 86)	🖥 PPT 27-28 💻 TB question 8 📑 SW Short-Answer Questions 4; Fill in the Blank questions 11-12 (pp. 25-26) Recall questions 10-11 (p. 86) Figure 8-8 Changes in facial contours from birth to adulthood (p. 85) Figure 8-9 The mandible grows by displacement, resorption, and deposition (p. 86) Figure 8-10 Process of orthodontic tooth movement (p. 86) Recall question 25 (p. 95) *Class Activity As a class discuss and define osteoclasts and osteoblasts. Have students identify their functions and discuss and answer the following questions: What is the benefit of resorption and how does it occur? Is resorption always beneficial? When is new bone required?*
Discuss the life cycle of a tooth.	☐ Life cycle of a tooth (p. 86) – Growth periods (p. 86) – Calcification (p. 87) – Eruption of primary teeth (p. 87)	🖥 PPT 29-38 💻 TB questions 7-10 📑 SW Fill in the Blank questions 6, 13; Multiple Choice questions 8, 12-13, 15, 17 (pp. 26-27) 📑 SW Topics for Discussion question 2 (p. 28) Recall questions 12-15 (p. 87)

ELSEVIER

Torres and Ehrlich Modern Dental Assisting, 9th ed.

Bird/Robinson

OBJECTIVES	CONTENT	TEACHING RESOURCES
	– Shedding of primary teeth (p. 87) – Eruption of permanent teeth (p. 87)	Figure 8-11 (A) Chronologic order of primary dentition (p. 90); (B) Permanent dentition (pp. 88-89) Figure 8-12 Stages in the process of tooth eruption (p. 90) Figure 8-13 Radiograph showing normal resorption of the roots (p. 90) Figure 8-14 Examples of mixed dentition with the primary and permanent teeth erupting (p. 91) ▸ Discuss the three growth periods in the process of tooth formation: bud stage, cap stage, and bell stage. ▸ Discuss the calcification process. *Class Activity **Divide the class into five groups, and assign each group one of the stages of the tooth life cycle: growth periods, calcification, eruption of primary teeth, shedding of primary teeth, or eruption of permanent teeth. Have each group discuss its assigned stage. Meanwhile, create a time line of the life cycle of a tooth on the board with each stage identified. Then have group representatives summarize their discussions to the class.***
Explain the difference between the clinical and anatomic crowns.	■ Oral histology (pp. 87-88) □ Crown (pp. 88-89)	⊠▤ PPT 39-40, 44-46 ▧ SW Short-Answer Questions 8; Multiple Choice questions 14, 16 (pp. 25, 27) Recall questions 16-17 (p. 90) Figure 8-16 (A) The anatomic crown; (B) The clinical crown (p. 92) ▸ Discuss the attributes of the anatomic crown. ▸ Discuss the attributes of the clinical crown. *Class Activity **Create two columns on the board: Clinical Crowns and Anatomic Crowns. Then have students identify as many characteristics of each as they can and write them on the board in the correct column. Next, have class discuss the similarities and distinguishing characteristics of the two types of crowns.***

Torres and Ehrlich Modern Dental Assisting, 9th ed.

Bird/Robinson

8.2 Homework/Assignments:

8.2 Instructor's Note/Student Feedback::

LESSON 8.3

CRITICAL THINKING QUESTION

You want to work for an endodontist. However, when he asks you about pulp testing, you are not certain what he is talking about. What is the pulp, where is it located in the tooth, and how does it form? Why does the pulp feeling pain from the pulp tester mean that the pulp is healthy?

Guidelines: The pulp is inside the dentin of the tooth, which is then covered by enamel. Thus the pulp is in both the crown and root of the tooth. The pulp is made up of blood vessels and nerves that enter the pulp chamber through the apical foramen. The blood supply is derived from branches of the dental arteries and from the periodontal ligament. The pulp also contains connective tissue, which consists of cells, intercellular substance, and tissue fluid. Fibroblasts, one type of cell in connective tissue, are responsible for the formation of the intercellular substance of the pulp. The pulp forms from dental papilla's cells as the dentin forms around the pulp chamber and root canal areas. The nerve supply of the pulp receives and transmits pain stimuli. When the stimulus is weak (tapping on tooth, chewing), the response by the pulpal system is weak, and the interaction goes unnoticed. When the stimulus is great (pulp tester or infection), the reaction is stronger, and pain quickly calls attention to the threatened condition of the tooth. If the tooth's pulp is no longer viable, the tooth will not react to stimuli.

OBJECTIVES	CONTENT	TEACHING RESOURCES
Name and describe the tissues of the teeth.	☐ Root (p. 90) ☐ Enamel (pp. 90-93) ☐ Dentin (p. 93) ☐ Cementum (p. 94) ☐ Pulp (p. 94) ☐ Periodontium (p. 95) – Attachment apparatus (p. 95) – Gingival unit (p. 98)	PPT 43-44, 47-49, 52-53, 55 TB questions 11-13 SW Short-Answer Questions 9; Fill in the Blank question 10 (pp. 25-26) Figure 8-15 Anterior (top or front) tooth and posterior (bottom or back) tooth showing the dental tissues (p. 92) CTQ 2 (p. 99) ▸ Discuss and describe the various tissues of the teeth: root, enamel, dentin, cementum, pulp, and periodontium. ***Class Activity Provide unlabeled copies of Figure 8-15 (p. 94) to the class, face down. Have students turn over their copies of the diagram and label the tissues of the teeth as quickly as they can. The first student to correctly label all tissues wins. Next, call on students to describe each of the tissues and have the class provide feedback.***
Name and describe the three types of dentin.	☐ Dentin (p. 93) ☐ Cementum (p. 94) ☐ Pulp (p. 94) ☐ Periodontium (p. 95) – Attachment apparatus (p. 95) – Gingival unit (p. 98)	PPT 49-51 SW Fill in the Blank questions 8-9; Multiple Choice questions 18-21 (pp. 26-28) Recall questions 18-21 (pp. 93-94) Figure 8-17 Enamel rod, the basic unit of enamel (p. 93) Figure 8-18 Scanning electron micrograph of dentinal tubules (p. 93) ▸ Discuss primary, secondary, and tertiary dentin.

ELSEVIER

Bird/Robinson

OBJECTIVES	CONTENT	TEACHING RESOURCES
		Class Activity, Have students create three columns on a sheet of paper: Primary, Secondary, and Tertiary. Next, call out the following characteristics of dentin and have the students identify in which column the characteristic appears. The first student to place the characteristics in the correct columns wins. – *Narrows the pulp chamber as the person ages* – *Forms the bulk of the tooth* – *Begins formation after eruption* – *Known as reparative dentin* – *Continues formation at a slow rate throughout the life of the tooth* – *Formed before eruption* – *Forms in response to irritation* – *Appears as a localized deposit on the wall of the pulp chamber*
Describe the structure and location of the dental pulp.	☐ Pulp (p. 94) ☐ Periodontium (p. 95) – Attachment apparatus (p. 95) – Gingival unit (p. 98)	PPT 53-54 TB questions 14-15 SW Short-Answer Questions 11; Multiple Choice questions 22-23 (pp. 25, 28) Recall questions 23-24 (p. 95) Figure 8-19 The dental pulp (p. 94) ▸ Discuss the structure and location of dental pulp. ▸ Discuss the differences between coronal pulp and radicular pulp. *Class Activity Provide unlabeled copies of Figure 8-19 (p. 97) to the class, face down. Have students turn over their copies of the diagram and label the pulp structures as quickly as they can. The first student to correctly label all pulp structures wins.*
Name and describe the components of the periodontium.	☐ Periodontium (p. 95) – Attachment apparatus (p. 95) – Gingival unit (p. 98)	PPT 55-61 TB questions 16-17 SW Short-Answer Questions 12; Fill in the Blank question 7 (pp. 25-26) Figure 8-20 Periodontium of the tooth with its components identified (p. 95) Figure 8-21 Anatomy of the alveolar bone (p. 96) Figure 8-22 The alveolar crest as it appears in a radiograph (p. 97)

Torres and Ehrlich Modern Dental Assisting, 9th ed.

Bird/Robinson

OBJECTIVES	CONTENT	TEACHING RESOURCES
		▸ Discuss the function of periodontium.
		***Class Activity** As a class, discuss the two major units of periodontium: attachment apparatus and gingival unit and their components. Call out specific components and have students volunteer a description of the component.*
Describe the functions of periodontal ligaments.	☐ Periodontium (p. 95) – Attachment apparatus (p. 95) – Gingival unit (p. 98)	PPT 62-63 TB question 18 SW Short-Answer Questions 13; Multiple Choice question 24 (pp. 25, 28) Recall questions 26-27 (p. 98) Figure 8-23 Periodontal fiber groups (p. 97) Figure 8-24 Some of the fiber subgroups of the gingival fiber group (p. 98) ▸ Discuss the functions of the various periodontal ligaments. ▸ Discuss the various types of periodontal ligaments. ***Class Activity** Divide the class into four groups and assign each group one of the following functions of periodontal ligaments.* – *Supportive and protective* – *Sensory* – *Nutritive* – *Formative and resorptive* *Have groups develop patient teaching materials about the functions of periodontal ligaments and present them to the class for feedback.*
Describe the types of oral mucosa and give an example of each.	– Gingival unit (p. 98)	PPT 64-66 TB questions 19-21 SW Short-Answer Questions 14; Fill in the Blank questions 14-15; Multiple Choice question 25 (pp. 25-26, 28) Recall question 28 (p. 99) Figure 8-25 (A) A dense masticatory type of mucosa makes up the gingiva; (B) The delicate lining type of mucosa covers the vestibule (p. 98) ▸ Discuss the three types of oral mucosa: lining mucosa, masticatory mucosa, and specialized mucosa.

ELSEVIER

Torres and Ehrlich Modern Dental Assisting, 9th ed.

Bird/Robinson

OBJECTIVES	CONTENT	TEACHING RESOURCES
		Class Activity, Have students create three columns on a sheet of paper: Lining Mucosa, Masticatory Mucosa, and Specialized Mucosa. Without using their texts, have students identify as many characteristics of oral mucosa as they can in 5 minutes and list them in the proper column. Have students share their answers and the student with the most correct answers wins.
Performance Evaluation		TB. TB SW questions (pp. 25-28) *e* ESLR Electronic Flashcards *e* ESLR Practice Quiz *e* ESLR Labeling Exercise 2: Identify the dental tissues of an anterior tooth *e* ESLR Labeling Exercise 3: Identify the dental tissues of a posterior tooth Recall questions (pp. 79-99) CTQ (p. 99)

8.3 Homework/Assignments:

8.3 Instructor's Notes/Student Feedback:

Torres and Ehrlich Modern Dental Assisting, 9ᵗʰ ed.

Bird/Robinson

Slide 1

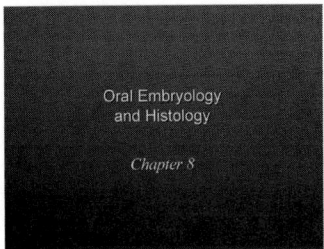

Slide 2

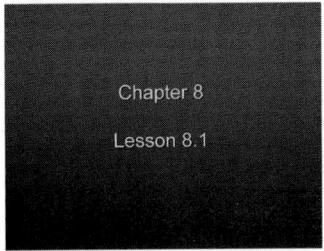

Slide 3

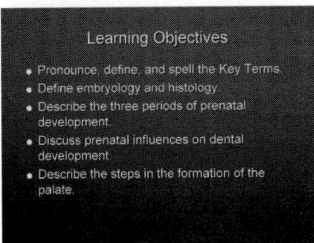

Slide 4

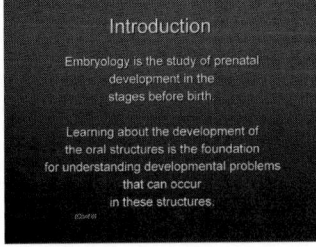

- Why does a dental assistant need to know about embryology?

- What is histology?

- How does embryology compare with histology?

Bird/Robinson

Slide 5

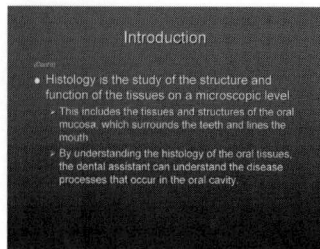

- Why does a dental assistant need to know about histology?
- When does pregnancy occur and what happens during conception?

Slide 6

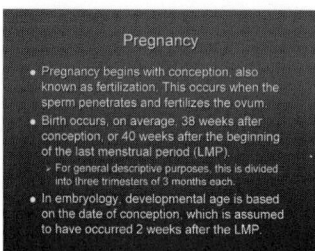

- What are the three periods of prenatal development?
- What can happen with the chromosomes after fertilization, such as happens with Down syndrome?
- Which period of prenatal development is the most critical and why?

Slide 7

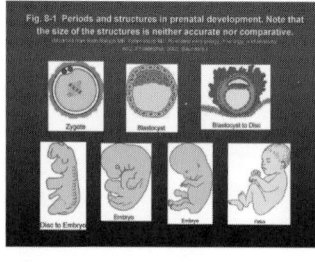

- Prenatal development consists of three distinct periods: preimplantation, embryonic, and fetal.
- Discuss what occurs in each period.

Slide 8

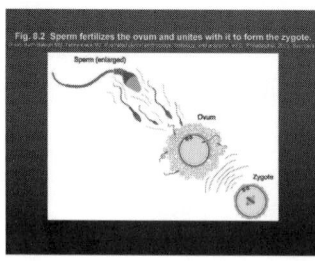

- Pregnancy begins with conception, also known as fertilization. This occurs when the sperm penetrates and fertilizes the ovum.
- The penetration of the egg by a sperm cell has an immediate effect on the surface of the egg: the outer coating of the egg changes, so that no other sperm cell can enter.
- The union of the egg and sperm subsequently forms a fertilized egg, or zygote.
- In the zygote, the 23 chromosomes in the sperm unite with the 23 chromosomes in the egg, providing a new life with a full complement of 46 chromosomes.

Torres and Ehrlich Modern Dental Assisting, 9th ed.

Bird/Robinson

Slide 9

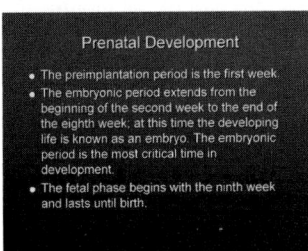

- What is the timeline in prenatal development? What period is first, what period is second, and what period is third? How many days or months is each period?

- Because all the organ systems are formed during the embryonic period, the fetus is less vulnerable than the embryo to malformations caused by radiation, viruses, and drugs.

Slide 10

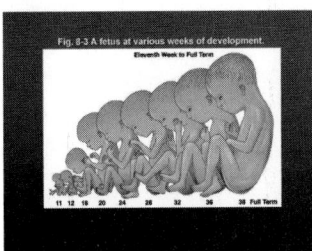

- What is the fetus and when does it form? *(The fetal period is the stage of human development that starts at the beginning of the ninth week and ends at birth; it involves the fetus. The fetus forms from the embryo.)*

- What is meant by full term (how many weeks)?

- Look at the size of the brain over time, as compared to the mandible.

- What are the three primary embryonic layers?

Slide 11

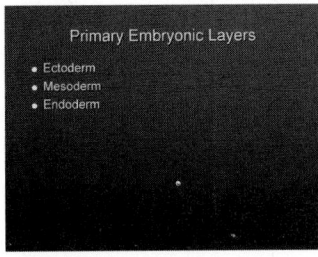

- During the third week of development, the cells of the embryo form the three primary embryonic layers: the ectoderm, mesoderm, and endoderm.

- The cells within each layer multiply and differentiate into the specialized cells needed to form the organs and tissues of the body.

- What are the outer, middle, and inner layers of the embryo?

Slide 12

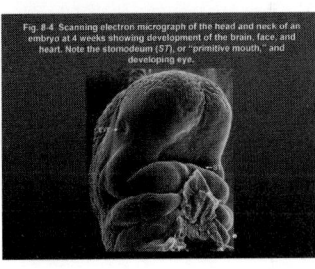

- The embryonic period extends from the beginning of the second week to the end of the eighth week, and the new individual is known as an embryo.

- The cells begin to proliferate (increase in number), differentiate (change into tissues and organs), and integrate (form systems).

- At about the end of the eighth week of pregnancy, a baby graduates from embryo to fetus. This name change signifies a change in the baby's level of development.

- Why is the eye on the lateral surface of the embryo?

- What are the folds of tissue below the stomodeum?

Torres and Ehrlich Modern Dental Assisting, 9th ed.

Bird/Robinson

Slide 13

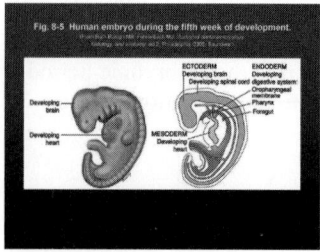

- In the fourth week, the stomodeum (primitive mouth) and the primitive pharynx merge, and the stomodeum develops into part of the mouth.
- Where is the beginning of the primitive mouth or stomodeum on the cross section of the embryo?
- Looking at the three embryonic tissues, what is the primitive brain developing mainly from?
- What is the digestive system mainly developing from?
- What is the heart mainly developing from?

Slide 14

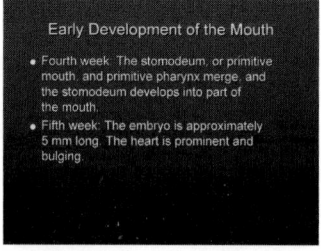

Slide 15

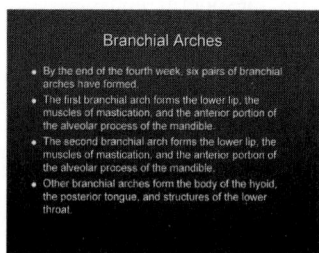

- What are the branchial arches and what do they form on the head and neck?
- Which branchial arch forms the bones, muscles, nerves of the face, and lower lip?
- Which branchial arch forms the side and front of the neck?

Slide 16

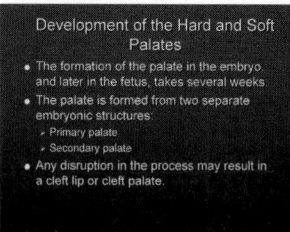

- Note that the palate is formed over both the embryonic and fetal periods.
- Has anyone seen a cleft lip or palate before surgical correction?
- Note that the branchial arches are forming structures in the lower face and neck area in order of their placement.
- What are the three stages of palate formation?

ELSEVIER

Torres and Ehrlich Modern Dental Assisting, 9th ed.

Bird/Robinson

Slide 17

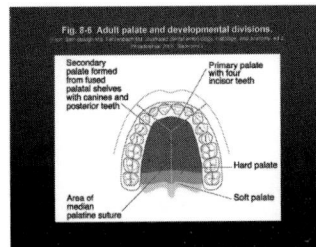

- The formation of the palate takes several weeks to occur.
- Discuss the formation of the palate.
- Can you feel the midline on your hard palate where the suture fused? What is it called? *(Median palatine suture.)*
- Fusion usually begins from the anterior during the ninth week. The palate is then completed during the twelfth week within the fetal period.
- When does the development of the human face occur?

Slide 18

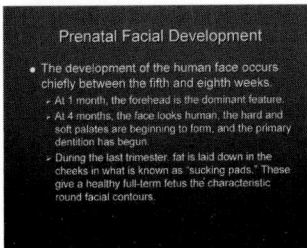

- At what time does the embryo have a dominant forehead?
- When does the face look human?
- When does the face become rounded?
- At birth, how many teeth are in various stages of development?

Slide 19

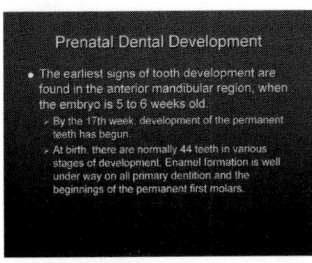

- What are the two major categories of factors that can adversely influence dental development?

Slide 20

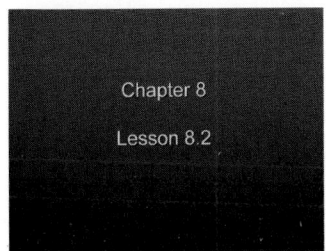

Torres and Ehrlich Modern Dental Assisting, 9th ed.
Bird/Robinson

Slide 21

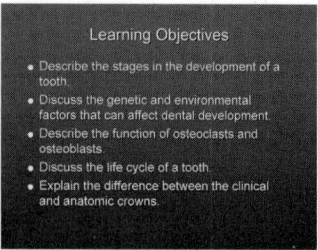

Slide 22

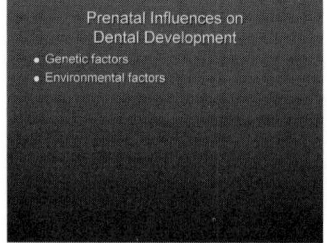

- In prenatal tooth development, the genetic factor that is most often a concern is tooth size and jaw size. Why?
- Do your teeth fit your jaw, or do you have a size discrepancy?
- How many have had tooth extraction, orthodontics, or other means to help regulate their teeth and jaws?

Slide 23

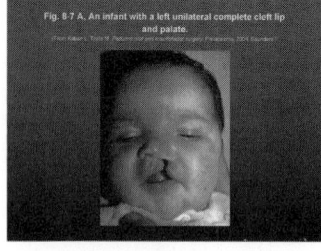

- Any disruption in the process of the formation of the lip and palate may result in a cleft lip or cleft palate.
- Note that this child has both cleft lip and palate.
- Would feeding be difficult for this infant?

Slide 24

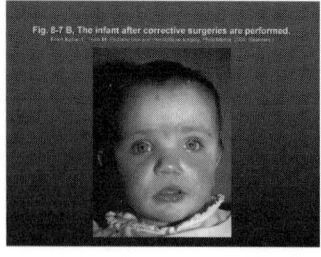

- What does cleft surgery involve?
- Do you notice any scar from the infant's surgery?
- Can the infant more easily eat? Will speech be easier in the future?

Torres and Ehrlich Modern Dental Assisting, 9th ed.

Bird/Robinson

Slide 25

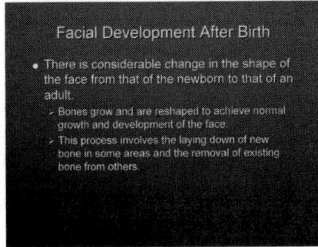

- As you were growing up, did you notice that your face and jaws changed over time?

Slide 26

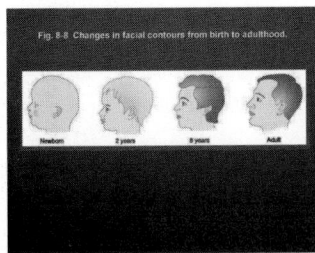

- If you look at photos of yourself as you grew, you will notice the same changes in facial contour as this slide shows. Look closely at the forehead, maxilla, and mandible as they make the facial contours change.
- The development of the human face occurs primarily between the fifth and eighth weeks.
- What is the process of adding bone?
- What is the process of bone loss or removal?

Slide 27

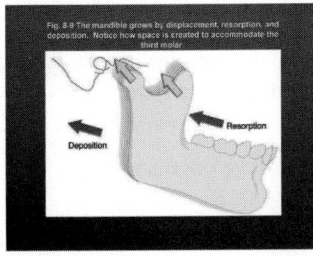

- Facial bones grow and are reshaped to achieve normal growth and development. This process involves the deposition of new bone in some areas and resorption of existing bone from other areas.
- What is deposition?
- What is resorption?
- Do you have your third molars? Was there enough room for them?

Slide 28

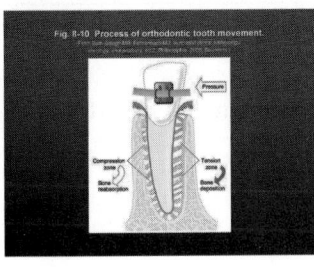

- Deposition is the process of "laying down" or adding new bone. Osteoblasts are the cells responsible for new bone formation.
- Resorption occurs when the body removes bone. Osteoclasts are the cells responsible for this process, in which bone cells are resorbed (taken away) by the body.
- Remodeling occurs in response to forces placed on the tooth within its socket.

ELSEVIER

Bird/Robinson

Slide 29

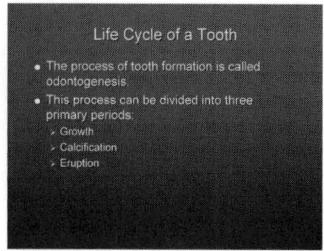

- What is the process of tooth formation called?
- What are the three stages in the growth period?
- What are the three primary periods in tooth formation?

Slide 30

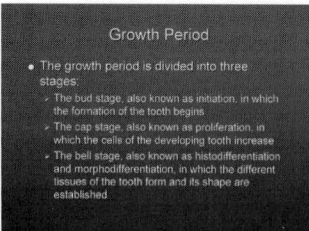

- Note that these stages are based on the shape of the tooth germ over time.

Slide 31

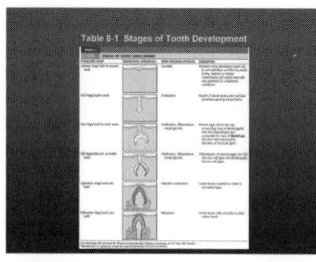

- When the embryo is 5 to 6 weeks old, the first signs of tooth development are found in the anterior mandibular region.
- Shortly after the mandibular anteriors develop, the anterior maxillary teeth begin to develop, and the process of tooth development progresses toward the posterior in both jaws.
- By the seventeenth week, all primary teeth are developed and the development of the permanent teeth has begun.
- At birth, there are normally 44 teeth in various stages of development. Enamel formation is well under way on all primary dentition and may be just beginning on the permanent first molars.

Slide 32

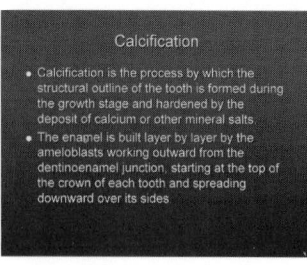

- What produces enamel? Where does enamel formation start and move on to?
- Ameloblasts are very sensitive cells and can be disturbed by birth, fevers, and drug usage.

Bird/Robinson

Slide 33

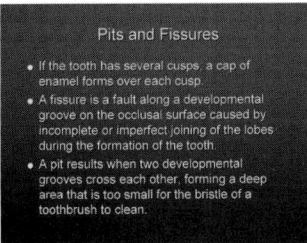

- The enamel may be particularly thin, and these areas are often inaccessible for cleaning and are thus sites where decay frequently begins. This can be prevented by the placement of an enamel sealant.
- When a tooth has several cusps, what structures are formed when the cusps join?

Slide 34

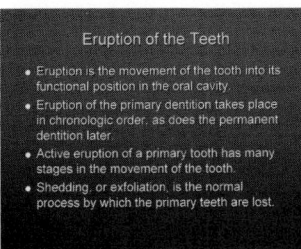

- What is Nasmyth's membrane? *(When the teeth are forming in the jaws, they are surrounded by a soft tissue membrane called Nasmyth's membrane, named after Alexander Nasmyth, a Scottish dental surgeon in London who died in 1847.)*
- What is the name of the process by which teeth move into the oral cavity?

Slide 35

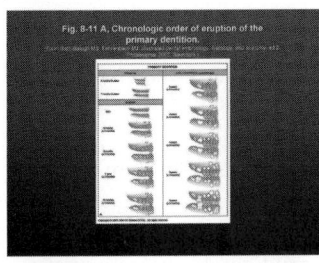

- What is the primary dentition period?
- Look closely at these diagrams to get an overall feel for tooth eruption and then shedding of the primary dentition.
- Which teeth are first to arrive in the infant and which are first to be shed?
- Which are the first permanent teeth to erupt?

Slide 36

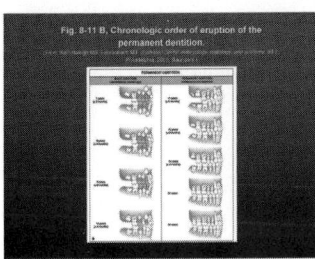

- What is the mixed dentition period?
- What problems would the young patient encounter having a mixed dentition? How does their mouth look? Is oral hygiene easy?
- What is the permanent dentition period?
- Look closely at this eruption of the permanent teeth and the shedding of the primary teeth. What are the last teeth to be shed from the primary dentition? What are the last teeth to enter the permanent dentition?

Bird/Robinson

Slide 37

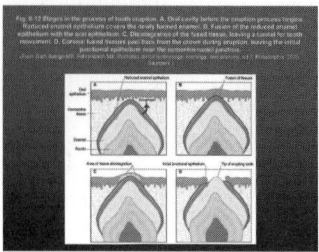

- Active eruption of a primary tooth has many stages in the movement of the tooth. The period of tissue disintegration causes an inflammatory response known as "teething," which may be accompanied by tenderness and swelling of the local tissues.

- The process of eruption for a succedaneous tooth is the same as for the primary tooth.

- When a permanent tooth starts to erupt before the primary tooth is fully shed, problems in spacing can occu.

- What are the functions of osteoblasts and osteoclasts?

- What is passive eruption?

Slide 38

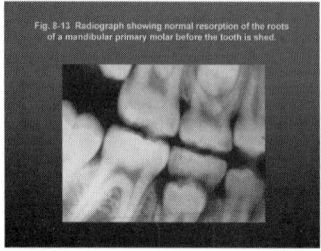

- Shedding, or exfoliation, is the normal process by which the primary teeth are lost as the succedaneous (permanent) teeth develop.

- When it is time for a primary tooth to be lost, osteoclasts cause the resorption of the root, beginning at the apex and continuing in the direction of the crown.

- Eventually the crown of the tooth is lost because of lack of support.

- The process of shedding is intermittent because at the same time that osteoblasts replace resorbed bone, odontoblasts and cementoblasts are replacing resorbed portions of the root.

Slide 39

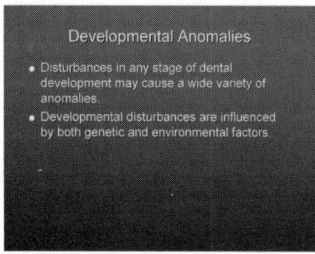

- The mother's dental health is also of concern.
  - Toxins from a dental infection may be dangerous to both mother and child (e.g., toxins from periodontal disease in the mother are linked to low birth weight in the infant).
  - Fever in the mother during pregnancy will leave marks in the developing teeth of the fetus.
- When pregnant women take the systemic antibiotic tetracycline during the fetal period, permanent staining of the child's primary teeth may result.

Slide 40

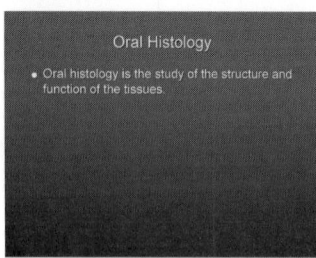

- This section discusses anatomic parts and histology of the teeth, the supporting structures, and the oral mucosa, which surrounds the teeth and lines the mouth.

Slide 41

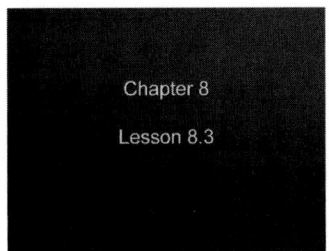

Slide 42

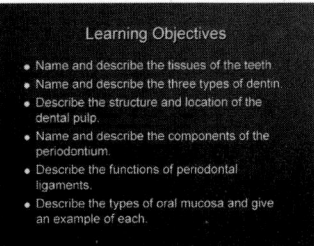

Slide 43

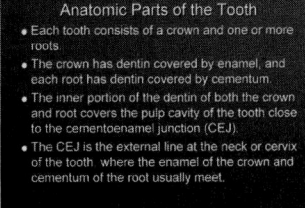

- Enamel is translucent (allows some light to pass through it) and ranges in color from yellow to grayish white.

- These variations in shade are caused by differences in the thickness and translucency of the enamel and in the color of the dentin beneath it.

- Enamel is the whiter tissue; the dentin is more yellow..

- Any exposed cementum is quickly abraded off the root, leaving exposed dentin.

- Cementum is light yellow and is easily distinguishable from enamel by its lack of luster and its darker hue. It is somewhat lighter in color than dentin.

Slide 44

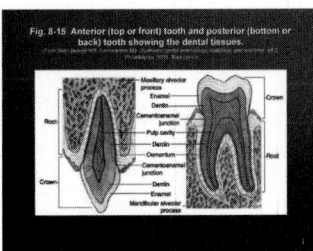

- Anatomic Parts of the Tooth:

  - Each tooth consists of a crown and one or more roots.

  - The crown has dentin covered by enamel, and each root has dentin covered by cementum.

  - The inner portion of the dentin of both the crown and root covers the pulp cavity of the tooth close to the cementoenamel junction (CEJ).

  - The CEJ is the external line at the neck or cervix of the tooth where the enamel of the crown and cementum of the root usually meet.

- What is the difference between the anatomic crown and the clinical crown?

Slide 45

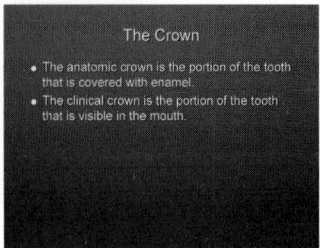

Slide 46

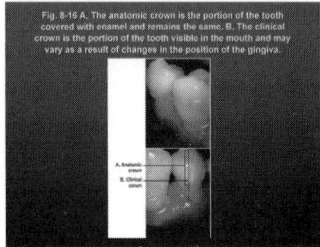

- What is the difference between the anatomic crown and the clinical crown?

Slide 47

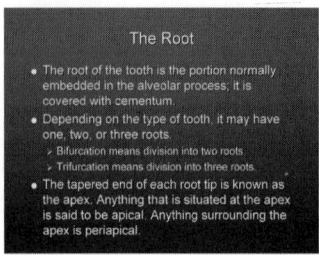

- Which teeth have two or three roots? *(In the permanent dentition, all the maxillary molars are trifurcated and the mandibular molars are bifurcated. The maxillary first premolar is bifurcated also. Many times, the third molars have fused roots; so it is hard to see how many roots they have.)*

Slide 48

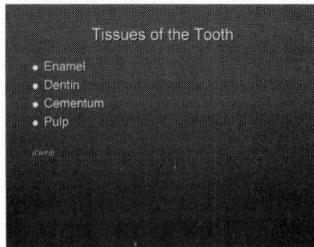

- What is the hardest substance in the human body?
- Where are enamel, dentin, and cementum located on the tooth?
- How does dentin transmit sensations of pain?
- What are the three types of dentin?
- What are the two types of cementum?

Torres and Ehrlich Modern Dental Assisting, 9th ed.

Bird/Robinson

Slide 49

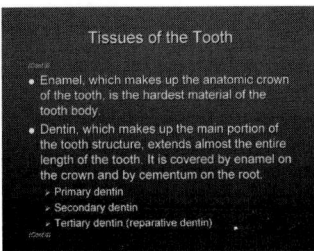

- Because it is capable of continued growth and repair, dentin consists of the following three major types:

  - Primary dentin, which is formed before eruption, forms most of the tooth.

  - Secondary dentin begins formation after eruption and continues at a very slow rate throughout the life of the tooth.

  - Tertiary dentin, also known as reparative dentin, is formed in response to irritation and appears as a localized deposit on the wall of the pulp chamber.

- Where does enamel form from embryologically?

Slide 50

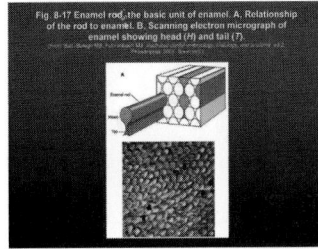

- Discuss the structure of enamel.

- What is the most abundant mineral component in enamel?

- What happens during tooth whitening? *(The staining components that are found between the enamel rods whiten and become more opaque, so that the tooth appears whiter and brighter.)*

Slide 51

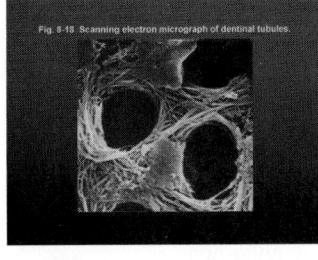

- Discuss the formation, structure, and function of dentin.

- Where is the border of the dentinal tubule? Where is the dentinal fiber located?

Slide 52

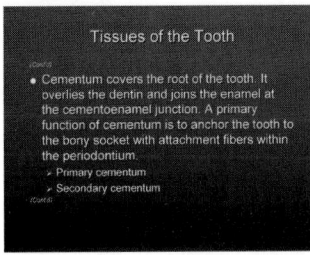

- As the root develops, primary cementum, also known as acellular cementum, is formed outward from the cementodentinal junction for the full length of the root.

- After the tooth has reached functional occlusion, secondary cementum continues to form on the apical half of the root.

- As a result, the cervical half of the root is covered with a thin layer of primary cementum, and the apical half of the root has a thickened cementum covering.

Slide 53

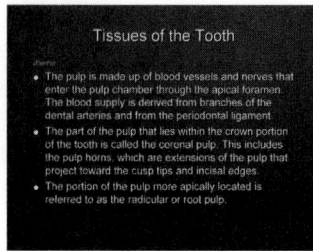

- What happens with a toothache?
- What is the only sensation that the pulp feels, no matter if it is traumatized, burned, or dried out? *(Pain.)*

Slide 54

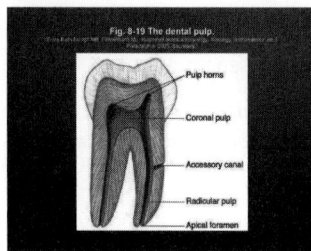

- What type of tissue makes up the pulp?
- What cells form the intercellular substance of the pulp?

Slide 55

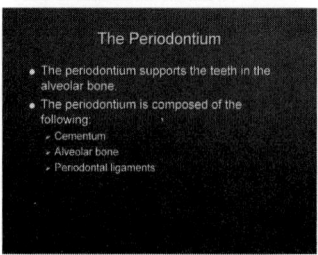

- The periodontium also protect and nourish the teeth by way of the blood vessels and the immune response.
- What is the primary function of the periodontal ligaments?
- To which structures are the periodontal ligaments attached?

Slide 56

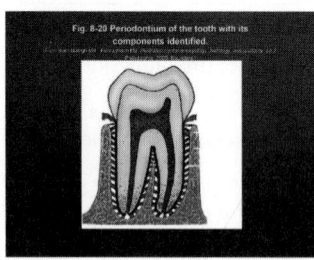

- The periodontium supports the teeth in the alveolar bone.
- The periodontium consists of cementum, alveolar bone, and the periodontal ligaments. These tissues also protect and nourish the teeth.
- The periodontium is divided into two major units: the attachment apparatus and the gingival unit.
- What tissues embryonically helped form the tissues of the periodontium?

Bird/Robinson

Slide 57

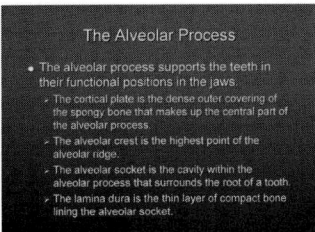

- What type of bone forms the cortical plate and the lamina dura?
- What does the lamina dura look like on a radiograph?

Slide 58

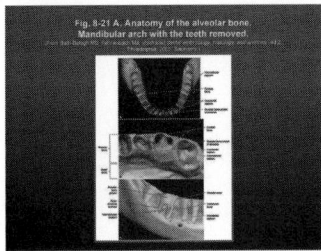

- The alveolar processes are the extensions of the bone from the body of the mandible and the maxilla that support the teeth in their functional positions in the jaws.
- The cortical plate is the dense outer covering of the spongy bone that makes up the central part of the alveolar process.
- The alveolar socket is the cavity within the alveolar process that surrounds the root of a tooth.

Slide 59

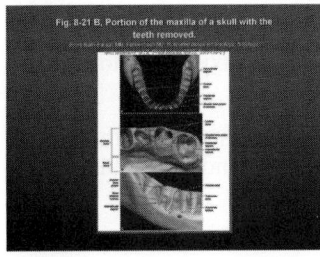

- Note that the bone is formed to accommodate multirooted teeth and single rooted teeth.
- What is the name of the bone between the roots of the teeth?
- What type of bone is between the cortical plates and the alveolar process or lamina dura?

Slide 60

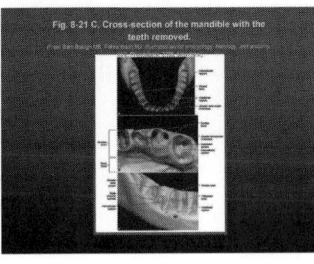

- The alveolar process develops in response to the growth of the developing teeth.
- After teeth have been lost, bone from the alveolar process is resorbed, and the ridge decreases in size and changes shape.

Slide 61

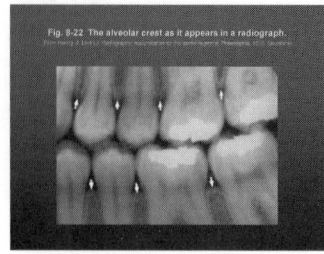

Fig. 8-22 The alveolar crest as it appears in a radiograph.

- The cortical plate is the dense outer covering of the spongy bone that makes up the central part of the alveolar process.

- The alveolar crest is the highest point of the alveolar ridge.

- The alveolar socket is the cavity within the alveolar process that surrounds the root of a tooth.

- The lamina dura, also known as the cribriform plate, is thin, compact bone that lines the alveolar socket.

- How is the alveolar crest on your radiographs? Is it healthy and pointed, or is it blunt like the ones above that show bone loss?

Slide 62

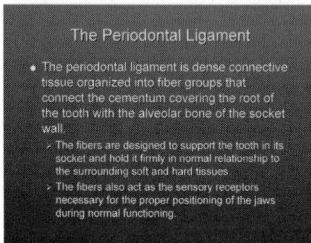

The Periodontal Ligament
- The periodontal ligament is dense connective tissue organized into fiber groups that connect the cementum covering the root of the tooth with the alveolar bone of the socket wall.
  - The fibers are designed to support the tooth in its socket and hold it firmly in normal relationship to the surrounding soft and hard tissues.
  - The fibers also act as the sensory receptors necessary for the proper positioning of the jaws during normal functioning.

- What does periodontal ligament connect?

- What does the periodontal ligament consist of?

Slide 63

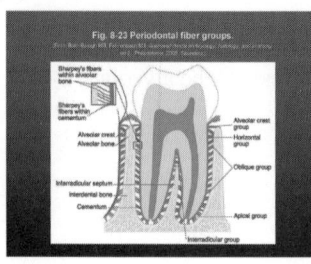

Fig. 8-23 Periodontal fiber groups.

- Alveolar crest fibers run from the crest of the alveolar bone to the cementum in the region of the CEJ.

- Horizontal fibers course at right angles to the long axis of the tooth, from the cementum to the bone.

- Oblique fibers run in an upward direction, from cementum to the bone. These fiber bundles are the most numerous fibers and constitute the main attachment of the tooth.

- Discuss and describe apical and transseptal fibers.

Slide 64

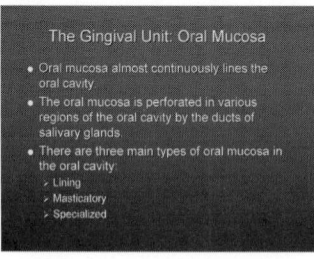

The Gingival Unit: Oral Mucosa
- Oral mucosa almost continuously lines the oral cavity.
- The oral mucosa is perforated in various regions of the oral cavity by the ducts of salivary glands.
- There are three main types of oral mucosa in the oral cavity:
  - Lining
  - Masticatory
  - Specialized

- Oral mucosa is composed of stratified squamous epithelium overlying connective tissue. Although oral mucosa is present throughout the mouth, different types of mucosal tissues are present in different regions of the mouth. The three main types of oral mucosa in the oral cavity are lining, masticatory, and specialized mucosa.

Slide 65

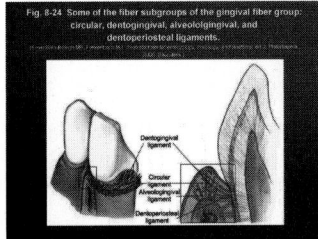

Fig. 8-24 Some of the fiber subgroups of the gingival fiber group: circular, dentogingival, alveologingival, and dentoperiosteal ligaments.

- The gingival fibers are divided into the following four groups:
    - Dentogingival fibers extend from the cervical cementum outward and upward into the lamina propria.
    - Alveologingival fibers extend upward from the alveolar crest into the lamina propria.
    - Circular fibers form a band around the neck of the tooth and are interlaced by other groups of fibers in the unattached gingiva.
    - Dentoperiosteal fibers extend facially and lingually from the cementum, pass over the crest of the alveolar bone, and insert into the periosteum of the alveolar process.

Slide 66

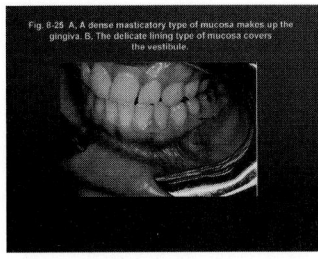

Fig. 8-25 A, A dense masticatory type of mucosa makes up the gingiva. B, The delicate lining type of mucosa covers the vestibule.

- Although oral mucosa is present throughout the mouth, different types of mucosal tissues are present in different regions of the mouth. The three main types of oral mucosa in the oral cavity are lining, masticatory, and specialized mucosa.

- What are the characteristics and functions of each type of mucosa?

TEACHING FOCUS

This chapter focuses on the specific regions of the head, with an emphasis on the bones, muscles, blood vessels, nerves, the temporomandibular joint, and salivary glands. Students will have an opportunity to identify the regions of the head and the bones of the cranium and face; the muscles, nerves and blood routes of the head and neck; and the components and actions of the termporomandibular joint. In addition, students will have the opportunity to identify and locate the salivary glands and major lymph node sites and discuss the divisions of the trigeminal nerve. Finally, this chapter discusses how to integrate knowledge of the head and neck into clinical practice.

MATERIALS AND RESOURCES

- ☐ computer and PowerPoint projector (all Lessons)
- ☐ model of a human skull (all Lessons)
- ☐ unlabeled copies of Figures 9-1 and 9-11 (Lesson 9.1)
- ☐ unlabeled copies of Figures 9-25 and 9-26 (Lesson 9.2)

LESSON CHECKLIST

Preparations for this lesson include:

- lecture
- evaluation of student knowledge and skills needed to perform all entry-level activities related to head and neck anatomy, including:
  - ○ the bones of the cranium and face
  - ○ the actions and the location of the temporomandibular joint
  - ○ the major and minor salivary glands, parasinuses, and lymph nodes
  - ○ the division of the trigeminal nerve
  - ○ integrating knowledge about head and neck anatomy into clinical practice

KEY TERMS

alveolar process (p. 104)
articular disc (p. 111)
articular eminence (p. 110)
articular space (p. 111)
buccal (p. 102)
circumvallate lingual papillae (p. 117)
condyloid process (p. 110)
coronal suture (p. 102)
cranium (p. 102)
external auditory meatus (p. 102)
foramen (p. 102)
foramen magnum (p. 102)
fossa (p. 103)
frontal (p. 102)
frontal process (p. 104)
glenoid fossa (p. 103)
greater palatine nerve (p. 120)
hamulus (p. 103)
infraorbital (p. 102)
lacrimal bones (p. 106)
lambdoid suture (p. 102)
lateral pterygoid plate (p. 103)
lymphadenopathy (p. 123)
masseter (p. 115)
mastoid process (p. 103)
maxillary tuberosity (p. 104)
meatus (p. 102)

medial pterygoid plate (p. 103)
mental (p. 102)
mental protuberance (p. 108)
nasal (p. 102)
nasal conchae (p. 106)
occipital (p. 102)
oral (p. 102)
orbital (p. 102)
ossicles (p. 103)
parietal (p. 102)
parotid duct (p. 117)
process (p. 103)
pterygoid process (p. 103)
sagittal suture (p. 102)
sphenoid sinuses (p. 103)
sternocleidomastoid (p. 114)
styloid process (p. 103)
symphysis menti (p. 109)
temporal (p. 102)
temporal process (p. 104)
temporomandibular joint (p. 109)
trapezius (p. 114)
trigeminal nerve (p. 120)
zygomatic (p. 102)
zygomatic arch (p. 104)
zygomatic process (p. 104)

ADDITIONAL RESOURCES

PowerPoint slides (Evolve): 1-75

Legend

CTQ
Critical
Thinking
Question

DVD
Multimedia
Procedures
Videos and
Animations

ESLR
EVOLVE
Student
Learning
Resources

IDO
Interactive
Dental
Office
CD-ROM

SW
Student
Workbook

TB
Test Bank
on the
TEACH
CD-ROM

PPT
PowerPoint
Slides

Class Activities are indicated in ***bold italic***.

Torres and Ehrlich Modern Dental Assisting, 9th ed.

Bird/Robinson

LESSON 9.1

PRETEST

1. Which part of the temporomandibular joint is the raised portion of the temporal bone just anterior to the glenoid fossa?
   a. eminence
   b. space
   c. fossa
   d. notch

2. What bony process creates the cheekbone?
   a. zygomatic arch
   b. maxillary tuberosity
   c. mandibular notch
   d. coronoid process

3. How many bones form the cranium?
   a. two
   b. four
   c. six
   d. eight

4. What bone forms the sides of the cranium?
   a. occipital
   b. parietal
   c. frontal
   d. temporal

5. The mastoid process is located
   a. in front of the ear.
   b. behind the ear.
   c. at the base of the nose.
   d. at the top of the nose.

6. Which bone forms the joint with the mandible?
   a. temporal
   b. occipital
   c. frontal
   d. zygomatic

7. Which of the following salivary glands is the largest?
   a. submandibular
   b. von Ebner's
   c. sublingual
   d. parotid

8. The aorta ascends from the
   a. left ventricle.
   b. right ventricle.
   c. left atrium.
   d. right atrium.

9. Another name for the parotid duct is
   a. Bartholin's.
   b. Stensen's.
   c. von Ebner's.
   d. Wharton's.

10. Which artery is the larger of the two terminal branches of the external carotid?
    a. mandibular
    b. maxillary
    c. inferior alveolar
    d. lingual

Answers

1. a	3. d	5. b	7. d	9. a
2. a	4. d	6. a	8. a	10. b

BACKGROUND ASSESSMENT

Question: What is the zygomatic arch?
Answer: The zygomatic arch is formed from the articulation of the temporal process of the zygomatic bone and the zygomatic process of the temporal bone. The zygomatic arch creates the prominence of the cheek.

Question: How does the inferior alveolar nerve subdivide, and what tissues are served? Where does this nerve originally branch off from?
Answer: The inferior alveolar nerve subdivides to serve the following tissues: the mylohyoid nerve supplies the mylohyoid muscles and the anterior belly of the digastric muscle; small dental nerves supply the molar

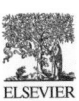

and premolar teeth, alveolar process, and periosteum; the mental nerve moves outward and anteriorly through the mental foramen and supplies the chin and mucous membrane of the lower lip; the incisive nerve continues anteriorly within the bone and gives off small branches to supply the incisor teeth. The inferior alveolar nerve branches off of the mandibular division of the trigeminal nerve (cranial nerve V).

CRITICAL THINKING QUESTION

A patient has headaches caused by joint problems. What is this joint and how does it move? How does it cause headaches?

Guidelines: The patient is suffering from temporomandibular disorder (TMD) which results from problems with the temporomandibular joint (TMJ). The TMJ is the joint on either side of the head that allows for movement of the mandible (chewing and speech). The TMJ receives its name from the two bones that enter into its formation, the temporal bone and the mandible. The mandible is attached to the cranium by the ligaments of the TMJ. The mandible is held in position by the muscles of mastication. The TMJ performs two basic types of movement, a hinge action and a gliding movement. With these two types of movement, the jaws can open and close and shift from side to side. TMD is a complex disorder that involves many factors, such as stress. The diagnosis and treatment of TMD can be difficult. Frequently, the diagnosis of TMD requires a multidisciplinary approach. For a complete analysis of the patient's condition, some cases require involvement of psychiatrists and others. Patients with TMD may report a wide range of pains, including headaches.

OBJECTIVES	CONTENT	TEACHING RESOURCES
Pronounce, define, and spell the Key Terms.	■ Key terms (pp. 100-101)	SW Fill in the Blank questions 1-18 (p. 30) ESLR Electronic Flashcards ▸ Discuss each of the key terms, focusing on the definition, pronunciation, and spelling of each term. *Class Activity Go around the room and have each student use one of the key terms in a clinically relevant sentence in order to define the term. Continue until all terms have been used; if students become stuck, have the rest of the class offer suggestions.*
Identify the regions of the head.	■ Regions of the head (p. 102)	PPT 4-6 SW Short-Answer Questions 1; Fill in the Blank questions 4, 6, 9; Multiple Choice question 1 (pp. 29-31) Recall question 1 (p. 102) Figure 9-1 Regions of the head (p. 102) ▸ Discuss the regions of the head and their locations. *Class Activity Provide students with unlabeled copies of Figure 9-1 (p. 105). In groups, have students fill in the missing labels without using their textbooks. Have groups share their answers with the class.*
Locate and identify the bones of the cranium and face.	■ Bones of the skull (p. 102) ☐ Bones of the cranium (p. 102) – Parietal bones (p. 102)	PPT 7-22 TB questions 1-6, 20 SW Short-Answer Questions 2; Fill in the Blank questions 2, 7; Multiple Choice questions 2-6, 11 (pp. 29-31)

OBJECTIVES	CONTENT	TEACHING RESOURCES
	– Frontal bone (p. 102)	Table 9-1 Bones of the Skull (p. 103)
	– Occipital bone (p. 102)	Table 9-2 Terminology of Anatomic Landmarks of Bones (p. 103)
	– Temporal bones (p. 102)	Figure 9-2 Lateral view of the skull (p. 104)
	– Sphenoid bone (p. 103)	Figure 9-3 Frontal view of the skull (p. 105)
	– Ethmoid bone (p. 103)	Figure 9-4 Posterior view of the skull (p. 106)
	– Auditory ossicles (p. 103)	Recall questions 2-5 (pp. 103, 106)
	☐ Bones of the face (p. 103)	Figure 9-5 View of external base of the skull (p. 107)
	– Zygomatic bones (p. 104)	Figure 9-6 Anterior view of the facial bones and overlying facial tissue (p. 108)
	– Maxillary bones (p. 104)	Figure 9-7 Bones and landmarks of the hard palate (p. 108)
	– Palatine bones (p. 105)	Recall questions 6-7 (p. 108)
	– Nasal bones (p. 105)	Figure 9-8 The mandible (p. 109)
	– Lacrimal bones (p. 106)	Figure 9-9 The fetal skull (p. 110)
	– Vomer (p. 106)	Recall question 8 (p. 109)
	– Nasal Conchae (p. 106)	Figure 9-10 Stages of postnatal development of the human skull (p. 111)
	– Mandible (p. 106)	⚲ CTQ 2 (p. 124)
	☐ Hyoid bone (p. 108)	▸ Discuss the function of the hyoid bone. What is its shape, and why is it unique?
	☐ Postnatal Development (p. 108)	▸ Discuss and identify the two sections of the skull. Which section protects the brain?
	– Fusion of bones (p. 108)	*Class Activity Lead a class discussion about the differences between an infant's skull and that of an adult. Why does an infant lack vertical dimensions, and what spurs vertical growth? Record student responses on the board for comparison.*
	– Development of the facial bones (p. 108)	
	☐ Differences between male and female skulls (p. 109)	

ELSEVIER

Torres and Ehrlich Modern Dental Assisting, 9th ed.
Bird/Robinson

OBJECTIVES	CONTENT	TEACHING RESOURCES
Identify the components of the temporomandibular joint.	■ Temporomandibular joints (p. 109) □ Capsular ligament (p. 110) □ Articular space (p. 111)	PPT 23-26 SW Short-Answer Questions 5; Fill in the Blank question 12 (pp. 29-30) Figure 9-11 Lateral view of the joint capsule of the temporomandibular joint (p. 111) ▸ Discuss the three parts that make up the temporomandibular joint. ▸ Discuss how the temporomandibular joint received its name. ***Class Activity Provide students with unlabeled copies of Figure 9-11 (p. 115). In groups, have students fill in the missing labels without using their textbooks. Have groups share their answers with the class.***
Describe the action of the temporomandibular joint.	□ Jaw movements (p. 111) – Hinge action (p. 112) – Gliding movement (p. 112)	PPT 27-28 TB questions 7-9, 11 SW Short-Answer Questions 6; Fill in the Blank questions 14-15; Multiple Choice question 8 (pp. 29-31) Figure 9-12 Hinge and gliding actions of the temporomandibular joint (p. 112) Recall question 9 (p. 113) ▸ Discuss the different types of gliding movements performed by the temporomandibular joint. ***Class Activity Lead a class discussion about the actions of the temporomandibular joint. Ask students to identify how the anatomy of the joint enables its movements, and how the joint can lead to headaches and other health problems. Record student responses on the board for comparison.***
Integrate the knowledge about head and neck anatomy into clinical practice.	□ Temporomandibular disorders (p. 112) – Symptoms (p. 113) – Causes (p. 113)	PPT 29-31 SW Short-Answer Questions 11; Multiple Choice question 9 (pp. 29, 31) Table 9-3 Categories of Temporomandibular Disorders (p. 113) Figure 9-13 Palpation of the patient (p. 113) Figure 9-14 Palpation of the sternocleidomastoid muscle (p. 114) Recall question 10 (p. 113) ▸ Discuss possible known causes of TMD. ▸ Discuss the symptoms of temporomandibular disorder. Why is treatment and diagnosis of TMD difficult?

Bird/Robinson

OBJECTIVES	CONTENT	TEACHING RESOURCES
		Class Activity Have students research the pathophysiology of TMD and its treatments and present their findings to the class. (For students to prepare for this activity, see Homework/Assignments #1.)

9.1 Homework/Assignments:

1. Have students research the pathophysiology of TMD and its treatments and present their findings to the class.

9.1 Instructor's Notes/Student Feedback:

Torres and Ehrlich Modern Dental Assisting, 9th ed.

Bird/Robinson

LESSON 9.2

CRITICAL THINKING QUESTION
How is saliva produced, and what is its function?
Guidelines: Saliva is produced by the salivary glands. The salivary glands include major glands (the parotid, submandibular, and sublingual) as well as minor glands (von Ebner's). Saliva lubricates and cleanses the oral cavity and aids in digestion of food by an enzymatic process. Saliva also helps maintain the integrity of tooth surfaces through a process of remineralization. Saliva also contributes to plaque formation, and it supplies the minerals for supragingival calculus formation. Changes in salivary flow and function are extremely sensitive to subtle changes in general health.

OBJECTIVES	CONTENT	TEACHING RESOURCES
Locate and identify the muscles of the head and neck.	■ Muscles of the head and neck (p. 113) ☐ Major muscles of the neck (p. 114) ☐ Major muscles of facial expression (p. 114) ☐ Major muscles of mastication (p. 114) ☐ Muscles of the floor of the mouth (p. 114) ☐ Muscles of the tongue (p. 116) ☐ Muscles of the soft palate (p. 116)	PPT 34-46 TB questions 10-11 SW Short-Answer Questions 3; Fill in the Blank questions 8, 11, 16 (pp. 29-30) Table 9-4 Major Muscles of the Neck (p. 114) Table 9-5 Major Muscles of Facial Expression (p. 115) Figure 9-15 Major muscles of mastication (p. 114) Table 9-6 Major Muscles of Mastication (p. 115) Figure 9-16 The origin and insertion of the geniohyoid muscle (p. 115) Figure 9-17 Extrinsic muscles of the tongue (p. 116) Recall questions 11-12 (p. 116) Table 9-7 Muscles of the Floor of the Mouth (p. 116) Table 9-8 Extrinsic Muscles of the Tongue (p. 116) Table 9-9 Major Muscles of the Soft Palate (p. 117) ▸ Discuss why it is important for a dentist to know the location and actions of the neck muscles. ***Class Activity** Divide the class into small groups and assign each group one of the following muscle groups: neck, facial expression, mastication, floor of the mouth, extrinsic muscles of the tongue, soft palate. Have each group make paper cutouts in the shape of the major muscles in the group's assigned muscle group. Then, one at a time, have each group correctly place its cutouts over a model of a human skull.*
Identify the location of major and minor salivary glands and associated ducts.	■ Salivary Glands (p. 116) ☐ Minor salivary glands (p. 117) ☐ Major salivary glands (p. 117)	PPT 47-54 TB question 12 SW Short-Answer Questions 7, 11; Fill in the Blank questions 5, 10, 17-18; Multiple Choice questions 12-13 (pp. 29-31)

ELSEVIER

Torres and Ehrlich Modern Dental Assisting, 9th ed.

Bird/Robinson

OBJECTIVES	CONTENT	TEACHING RESOURCES
		Figure 9-18 The salivary glands (p. 117)
		Recall questions 13-14 (p. 118)
		Figure 9-19 Sialoliths (p. 118)
		▸ Discuss how a sialolith may prevent saliva from flowing into the mouth. What is the treatment?
		▸ Discuss the roles of the three major paired salivary glands.
		Class Activity Divide the class into groups. Have each group list the major and minor salivary glands, identify their associated ducts, and explain where the minor salivary glands seem to be located by their inspection of the oral cavity. Have each groups share its findings with the class for discussion.
Identify and trace the routes of the blood vessels of the head and neck.	■ Blood supply to the head and neck (p. 118) ☐ Major arteries of the face and oral cavity (p. 118) – External carotid artery (p. 118) – Facial artery (p. 119) – Lingual artery (p. 119) – Maxillary artery (p. 119) – Mandibular artery (p. 119) ☐ Major veins of the face and mouth (p. 119)	▦ PPT 55-57 ▤ TB questions 13-14 ▨ SW Short-Answer Questions 4; Fill in the Blank question 1; Multiple Choice questions 14-15 (pp. 29-31) Figure 9-20 Major arteries and veins of the face and oral cavity (p. 118) Table 9-10 Major Arteries to the Face and Mouth (p. 119) Recall questions 15-16 (p. 119) ▸ Discuss and name the artery behind the ramus. Name its five branches. ***Class Activity Divide the class into groups. Have each group create a diagram that illustrates the routes of the major veins and arteries from the heart to the head and neck. Have groups share their diagrams with the class for discussion.***
Describe and locate the divisions of the trigeminal nerve.	■ Nerves of the head and neck (p. 120) ☐ Cranial nerves (p. 120) ☐ Innervation of the oral cavity (p. 120) – Maxillary division of trigeminal nerve (p. 120) – Mandibular division of trigeminal nerve (p. 120)	▦ PPT 58-65 ▤ TB questions 15-17 ▨ SW Short-Answer Questions 8, 11; Fill in the Blank questions 3, 13; Multiple Choice questions 7, 10, 16-17 (pp. 29-31) Figure 9-21 Facial paralysis resulting from damage to lower motor neurons of the facial nerve (cranial nerve VII) (p. 120) Figure 9-22 The 12 cranial nerves (p. 121) Figure 9-23 Maxillary and mandibular innervation (p. 122)

Bird/Robinson

OBJECTIVES	CONTENT	TEACHING RESOURCES
		Figure 9-24 Palatal, lingual, and buccal innervation (p. 122)
		Clinical Considerations: Facial Paralysis (p. 120)
		Recall questions 17-18 (p. 120)
		▸ Discuss why removing an impacted third molar could be complicated. What injury could result?
		▸ Discuss the three main divisions of the trigeminal nerve. What is the primary function of the trigeminal nerve?
		***Class Activity** Have students label a simplified diagram showing the routes of the two important divisions of the trigeminal nerve. Make sure the diagrams include the portions that the nerves innervate such as teeth, tongue, and other soft tissues. Have students share their diagrams with the class.*
Identify the location of major lymph node sites of the body.	■ Lymph nodes of the head and neck (p. 122) □ Structure and function (p. 122) □ Superficial lymph nodes of the head (p. 123) □ Deep cervical lymph nodes (p. 123) □ Lymphadenopathy (p. 123)	PPT 66-72 TB question 18 SW Short-Answer Questions 9; Multiple Choice questions 18-19 (pp. 29, 31) Figure 9-25 (A) Superficial lymph nodes of the head and associated structures; (B) Deep cervical lymph nodes and associated structures (p. 123) Recall questions 19-20 (p. 124) CTQ 1 (p. 124) ▸ Discuss why a dental professional must be careful when examining and palpating the lymph nodes of the head and neck. ▸ Discuss what happens when a patient has an infection or cancer in the lymph nodes. ***Class Activity** Divide the class into pairs and have students palpate their partners to look for any palpable lymph nodes, using a checklist. Then have students share their observations with the class and describe lymph node pathology and locations.*
Identify and locate the paranasal sinuses of the skull.	■ Paranasal sinuses (p. 124)	PPT 73-75 TB question 19 SW Short-Answer Questions 10 (p. 29) Clinical C9.2 Instructor's Notes/Student Feedback:onsiderations: Toothaches and Sinus Pain (p. 124)

OBJECTIVES	CONTENT	TEACHING RESOURCES
		Figure 9-26 The paranasal sinuses (p. 124) ▸ Discuss the three functions of the sinuses. What are they named and where are they located? ▸ Discuss the relationship between toothaches and sinus pain. *Class Activity Provide students with unlabeled copies of Figure 9-26 (p. 129). In groups, have students fill in the missing labels and share their answers with the class.*
Performance Evaluation		▣ TB ▤ SW questions (pp. 29-32) ⤷ ESLR Electronic Flashcards ⤷ ESLR Practice Quiz ⤷ ESLR Labeling Exercises 4-12 Recall questions (pp. 102-124) ♁ CTQ (p. 124)

9.2 Homework/Assignments:

9.2 Instructor's Notes/Student Feedback:

Torres and Ehrlich Modern Dental Assisting, 9th ed.

Bird/Robinson

Slide 1

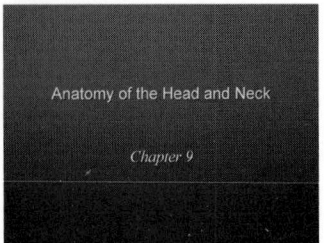

Slide 2

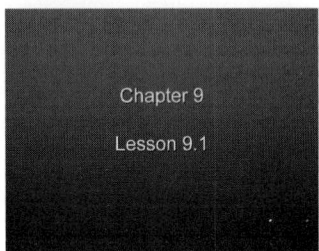

Slide 3

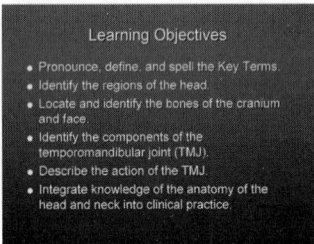

Slide 4

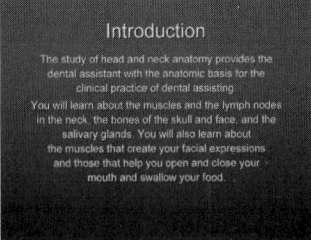

Torres and Ehrlich Modern Dental Assisting, 9th ed.

Bird/Robinson

Slide 5

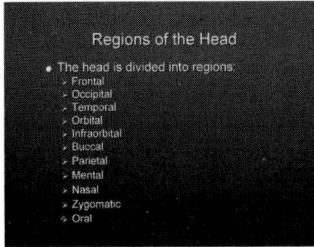

- As you can see, many of the regions are based on the bony surfaces underneath the skin and other surface structures.
- Why should a dental assistant study the anatomy of the head and neck?

Slide 6

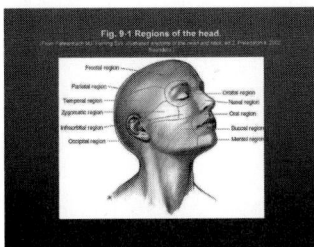

- In a newborn the anterior *fontanelle* is the soft spot where the sutures between the frontal and parietal bones have not yet closed.

Slide 7

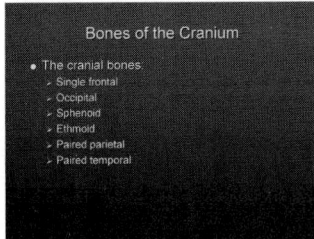

- What organ does the cranium protect? *(Brain.)*
- What passes through the "foramen magnum" of the occipital bone? *(Blood vessels, nerves, and ligaments, through the spinal cord.)*
- Which bone encloses the ear? *(Temporal.)*

Slide 8

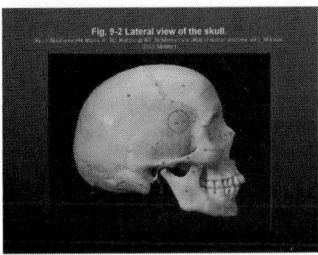

- What is a lateral view?
- What bone forms the forehead?
- What bone forms the back and base of the cranium?
- What bone forms the sides of the cranium?

ELSEVIER

Torres and Ehrlich Modern Dental Assisting, 9th ed.
Bird/Robinson

Slide 9

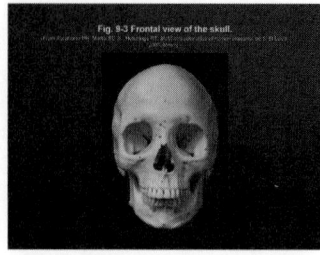

- What is a frontal view?
- Review the cranium bones numbered in the photo by accessing Fig. 9-3 on p. 105 of the book.

Slide 10

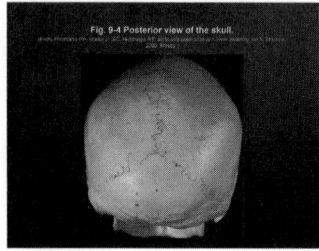

- What is a posterior view? How is this different from a frontal view?
- Quiz students on the bones numbered in the photo by going to Fig. 9-4 on p. 106.

Slide 11

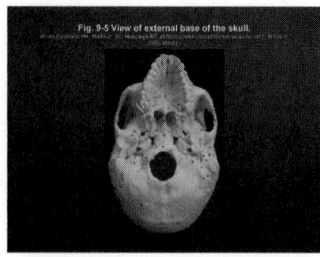

- What is the large opening in the base of the skull? *(The foramen magnum.)*
- What are the bones of the face?
- Review the bones numbered in the photo by going to Fig. 9-5 on p. 107 in the book.

Slide 12

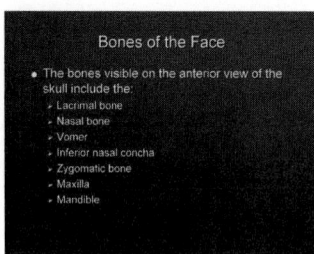

- What bones form the cheek?
- What bones form the upper jaw and hard palate?
- What bone develops prenatally as two parts, then hardens into a single bone during childhood? *(The mandible. It is also the strongest and longest bone in the face.)*

Torres and Ehrlich Modern Dental Assisting, 9th ed.

Bird/Robinson

Slide 13

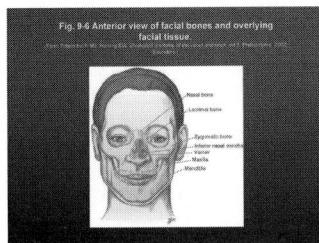

- The bones visible on the anterior view of the skull include the:
  - Lacrimal bone
  - Nasal bone
  - Vomer
  - Inferior nasal concha
  - Zygomatic bone
  - Maxilla
  - Mandible

Slide 14

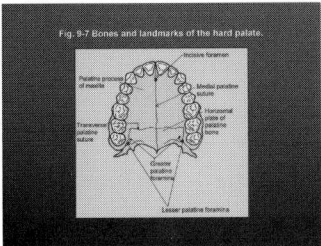

- The two maxillary bones, also known as the *maxillae* (singular *maxilla*), form the upper jaw and part of the hard palate.
- The two palatine bones are not strictly considered facial bones but are considered here for ease of learning.
- The horizontal plates of the palatine bones form the posterior part of the hard palate of the mouth and the floor of the nose.
- The vertical plates form part of the lateral walls of the nasal cavity. Anteriorly, they articulate (join) with the maxillary bone.

Slide 15

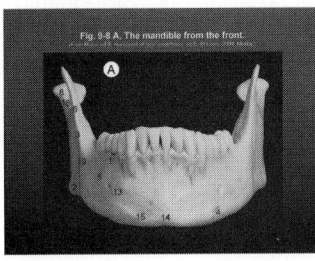

- The mandible forms the lower jaw and is the movable bone of the skull.
- The alveolar process of the mandible supports the teeth of the mandibular arch.
- The mental protuberance, or chin, reaches full development in puberty.
- Can you feel your mental protuberance?
- What is the only movable bone in the skull?
- Where is the mental foramen located?

Slide 16

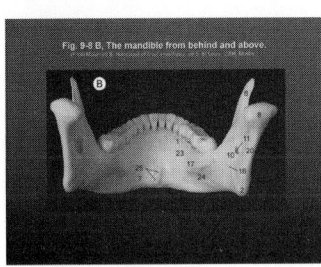

- Can you feel the angle of your mandible?
- Where do the two salivary glands fit into the area of the mandible?

ELSEVIER

Torres and Ehrlich Modern Dental Assisting, 9th ed.

Bird/Robinson

Slide 17

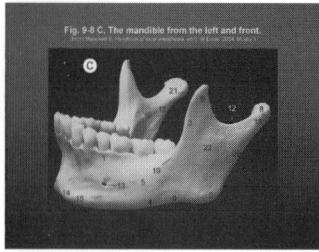

- The mandibular foramen is a landmark for the dentist when giving a mandibular block for the lower teeth.

Slide 18

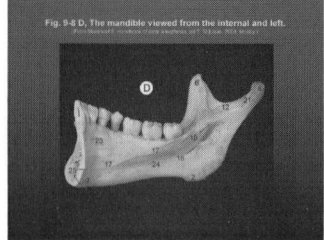

- What parts of the mandible are involved in the temporomandibular joint?
- What types of bone make up the mandible as shown by cross section?

Slide 19

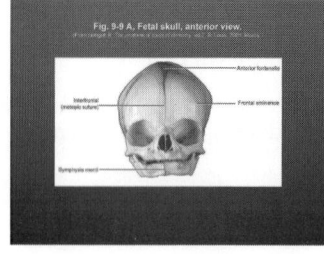

- At birth:
  - The cranial vault is large, and the cranial base and face are small.
  - The face lacks vertical dimension because the teeth have not yet erupted.
  - The mandible is in two halves separated by the symphysis menti.
  - The maxilla is entirely filled with the developing tooth buds.
- During the first year of life:
  - The symphysis menti fuses.

Slide 20

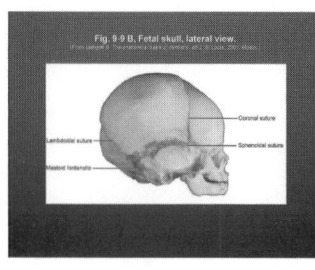

- Several bones of the skull have not fused as single bones at the time of birth.
- Various components of the temporal, occipital, sphenoid, and ethmoid will fuse during infancy and early childhood.
- What is the difference between the skulls and teeth of males and females? (*The female skull tends to be smaller and lighter, with thinner walls; male skulls are larger and heavier, with larger frontal sinuses.*)

Slide 21

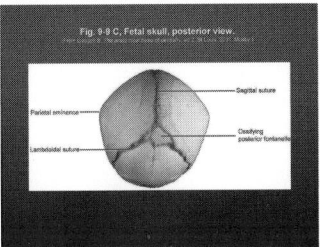

- Can you see the open sutures that have not fused?

Slide 22

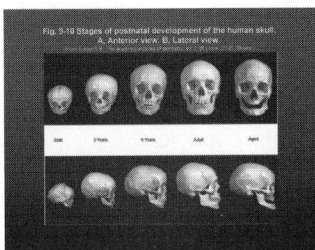

- Look over the growth pattern of the human skull from a frontal view and then from a lateral view. The oldest skull has lost its teeth so it has lost some of its alveolar bone. However, the base of the jaws remains.

Slide 23

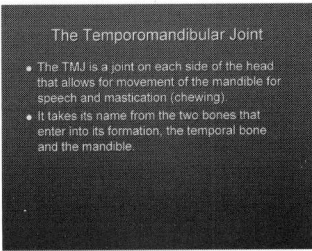

- Put your finger gently in your outer ear and then open and close your jaws to feel the temporomandibular joint. You can also feel it when you clench your teeth.

Slide 24

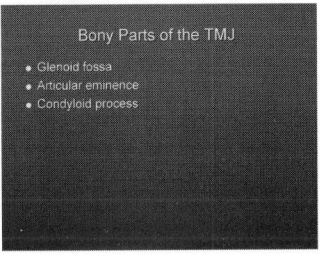

- What structure completely encloses the joint? *(A fibrous joint capsule.)*

- The glenoid fossa is an oval depression in the temporal bone just anterior to the external auditory meatus.

- The articular eminence is a raised portion of the temporal bone just anterior to the glenoid fossa.

- The condyloid process of the mandible lies in the glenoid fossa.

Slide 25

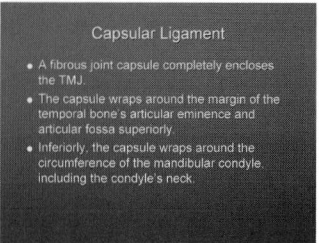

Slide 26

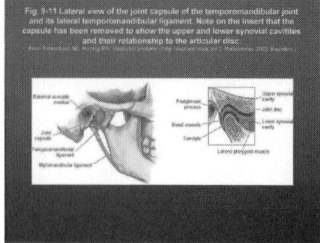

- The capsule wraps around the margin of the temporal bone's articular eminence and articular fossa superiorly.

- Inferiorly, the capsule wraps around the circumference of the mandibular condyle, including the condyle's neck.

- The articular space is the area between the capsular ligament and between the surfaces of the glenoid fossa and the condyle.

- What are the two basic types of movement by the TMJ? (*A hinge action and a gliding movement.*)

Slide 27

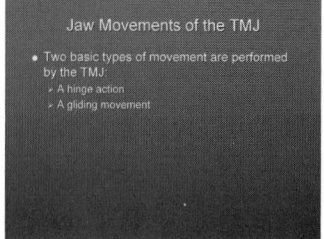

Slide 28

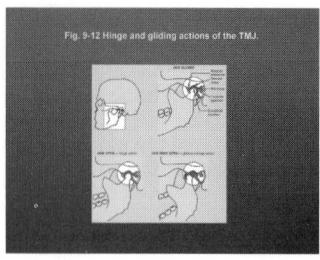

- The hinge action occurs when the mouth is opened.

- The gliding movement occurs during protrusion and in combination with the hinge action during the wider opening of the mouth.

Torres and Ehrlich Modern Dental Assisting, 9th ed.

Bird/Robinson

Slide 29

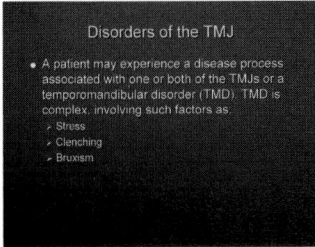

- Clenching is holding the teeth tightly together for prolonged periods. The muscle of the jaws (masseter) becomes enlarged.

- Bruxism is the habitual grinding of the teeth, especially at night. The chewing surfaces of the teeth can be worn down.

Slide 30

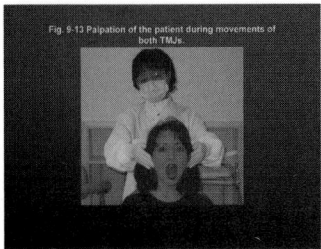

- The dental professional is having the patient open and close her mouth to check for pain, sounds, and other symptoms that may be related to TMD.

- TMD can also be caused by trauma to the jaw, systemic diseases such as osteoarthritis, or wear from aging.

- The diagnosis and treatment of TMD can be difficult. Frequently, the diagnosis of TMD requires a multidisciplinary approach. For a complete analysis of the patient's condition, some cases require involvement of dentists, physicians, psychiatrists, psychologists, neurologists, neurosurgeons, and others.

Slide 31

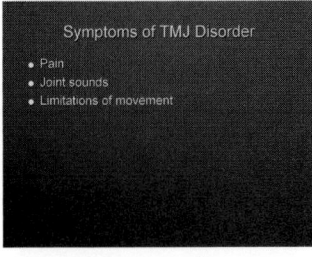

- Symptoms include headaches, pain in and around the ear, pain while chewing, muscle spasms, and clicking or popping sounds in the jaw.

- *Crepitus* is a term used to describe the cracking sound that may be heard in a joint.

- Limitations of movement lead to difficulty and pain during actions such as chewing and yawning.

- *Trismus* is a term used to describe a spasm of the muscles of mastication.

Slide 32

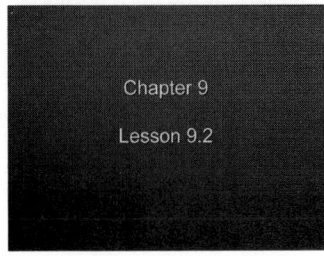

Slide 33

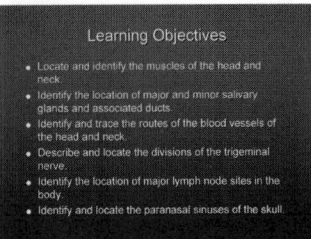

Slide 34

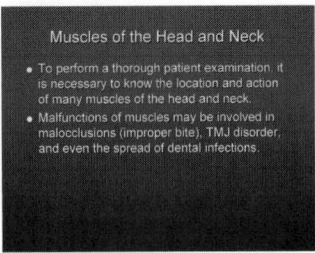

Slide 35

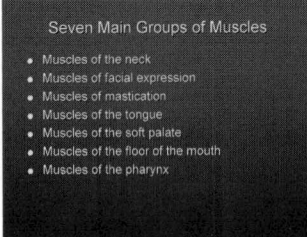

- What are the two major muscles of the neck? *(Sternocleidomastoid and trapezius.)*

- Have students locate their own sternocleidomastoid and trapezius muscles.

- Discuss how each muscle has a point of origin that is fixed (nonmovable) and a point of insertion (movable).

Slide 36

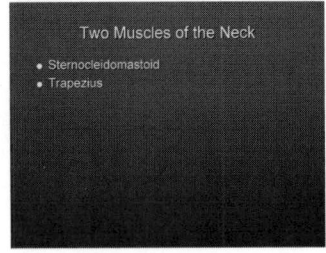

- Sternocleidomastoid divides the neck region into anterior and lateral posterior cervical triangles; it serves as a landmark of the neck during extraoral examination.

- Trapezius lifts the clavicle and scapula (shoulder blade), as when the shoulders are shrugged.

Torres and Ehrlich Modern Dental Assisting, 9th ed.

Bird/Robinson

Slide 37

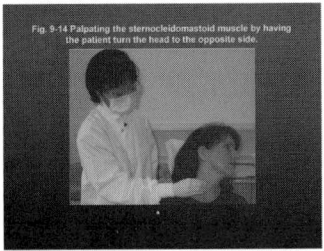

- Notice that the dental professional has the patient move her head to one side. This helps make the sternocleidomastoid muscle stand out more. The deep cervical lymph nodes are found around and deep in this muscle.

- Move your head to the left and then the right and see if your large strap muscle stands out more.

Slide 38

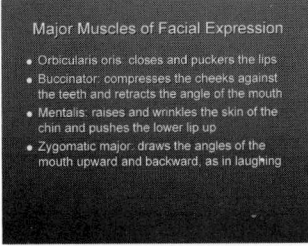

- The muscles of facial expression are paired muscles (left and right) and originate from the bone and insert on skin tissue.

- The seventh cranial (facial) nerve innervates all the muscles of facial expression.

Slide 39

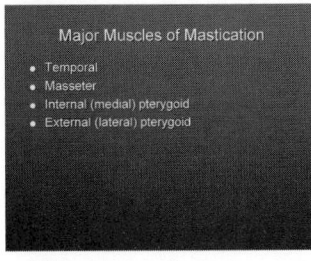

- These muscles are attached to the mandible.

- Which cranial nerve innervates all muscles of mastication? *(Fifth, or trigeminal.)*

Slide 40

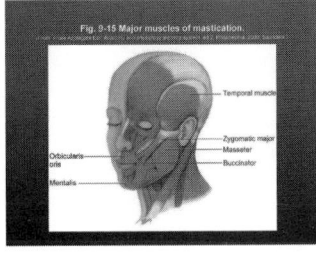

Bird/Robinson

Slide 41

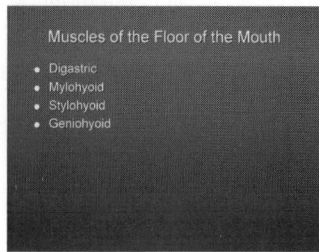

- These muscles are located between the mandible and the hyoid bone.
- These muscles work with the TMJ to make all movements of the mandible possible.

Slide 42

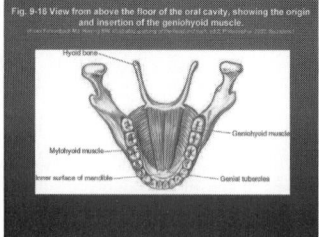

- The geniohyoid muscle is attached to the inner surface of the mandible at the genial tubercles and also the hyoid bone.
- The mylohyoid muscle forms the floor of the mouth.
- The hyoid bone functions as a primary support for the tongue and other muscles.

Slide 43

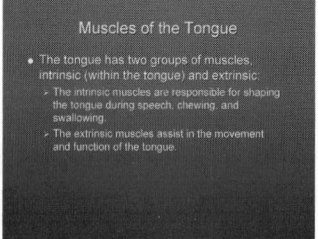

Slide 44

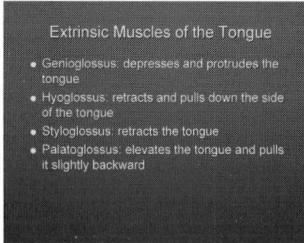

- Have students go through the actions of the tongue (depress, protrude, retract, pull down the sides, elevate, pull the tongue slightly backwards) and name the muscles involved (perhaps not at the same time).

ELSEVIER

Bird/Robinson

Slide 45

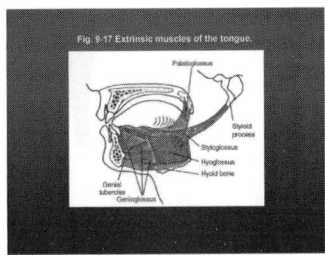

- Functions of the extrinsic muscles of the tongue:
    - Genioglossus muscle: depresses and protrudes the tongue.
    - Hyoglossus muscle: retracts and pulls down the side of the tongue.
    - Styloglossus muscle: retracts the tongue.
    - Palatoglossus muscle: elevates the tongue and pulls it slightly backward.

Slide 46

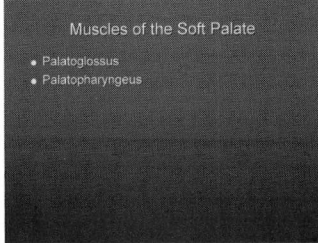

- The pharyngeal plexus innervates both of these muscles.

Slide 47

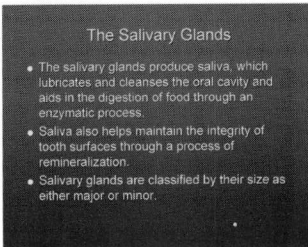

- What is a term used for dry mouth? *(Xerostomia.)*
- What causes most cases of dry mouth? *(Prescription drug use.)*

Slide 48

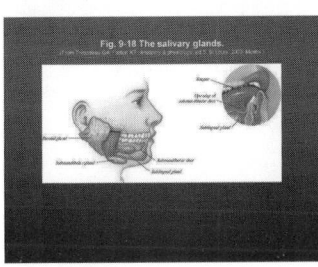

- The three major salivary glands are:
    - Parotid salivary gland. It is located in an area just below and in front of the ear.
    - Submandibular salivary gland. It lies beneath the mandible in the submandibular fossa, posterior to the sublingual salivary gland.
    - Sublingual salivary gland.

Slide 49

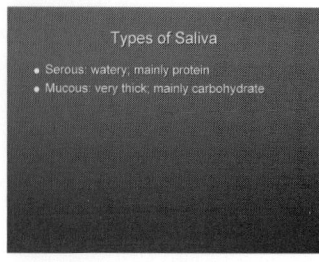

- Serous is produced by the parotid.

- Both the submandibular and sublingual produce a combination of serous and mucous salivary product.

Slide 50

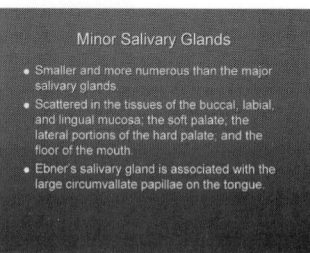

Slide 51

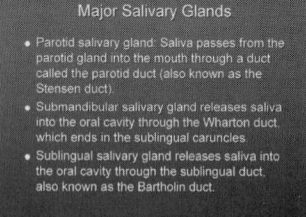

- The parotid salivary gland is the largest but provides only 25% of the total volume of saliva.

- The submandibular salivary gland provides 60% to 65% of the total volume of saliva

- The sublingual salivary gland is the smallest of the three major salivary glands. It provides only 10% of total salivary volume.

- What is the opening landmark on the buccal mucosa for Stensen's duct?

Slide 52

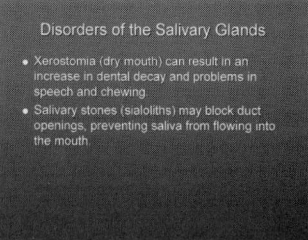

Slide 53

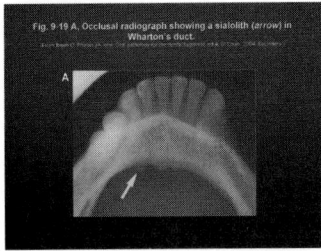

Fig. 9-19 A, Occlusal radiograph showing a sialolith (arrow) in Wharton's duct.

- The most common salivary gland that has them is the submandibular gland, since its duct is prone to them (as shown here).
- Why is the stone "whitish"?
- Where does the stone come from?

Slide 54

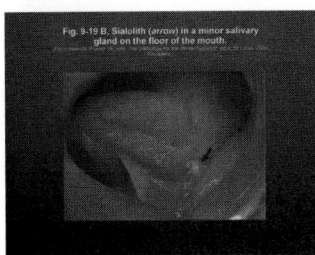

Fig. 9-19 B, Sialolith (arrow) in a minor salivary gland on the floor of the mouth.

- Sometimes the stone or sialolith can actually be seen, as it is here, on the floor of the mouth. Minor surgery can remove it, but it tends to recur.

Slide 55

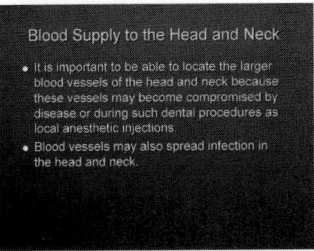

Blood Supply to the Head and Neck

- It is important to be able to locate the larger blood vessels of the head and neck because these vessels may become compromised by disease or during such dental procedures as local anesthetic injections.
- Blood vessels may also spread infection in the head and neck.

Slide 56

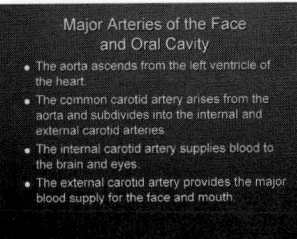

Major Arteries of the Face and Oral Cavity

- The aorta ascends from the left ventricle of the heart.
- The common carotid artery arises from the aorta and subdivides into the internal and external carotid arteries.
- The internal carotid artery supplies blood to the brain and eyes.
- The external carotid artery provides the major blood supply for the face and mouth.

- When you take your pulse in your neck, you are checking your carotid pulse of the carotid artery.

ELSEVIER

Torres and Ehrlich Modern Dental Assisting, 9th ed.

Bird/Robinson

Slide 57

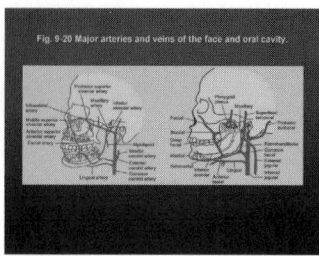

- Common carotid arises from the aorta and subdivides into the internal and external carotid.
- To what does the internal carotid artery supply blood? *(The brain and eyes.)*
- To what does the external carotid provide blood? *(The face and mouth.)*
- How does an artery travel from the heart?
- What artery is behind the ramus and branches into five arteries?
- What artery supplies the maxillary molars and premolars and gingivae?

Slide 58

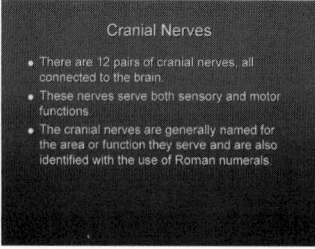

- These nerves come through the cranium, which protects the brain.

Slide 59

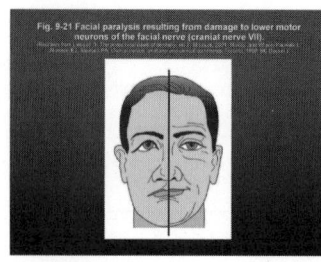

- The facial nerve serves the muscles of facial expression. Damage to this nerve means that the facial muscles on one side are unusable. Which side is the damaged side?

Slide 60

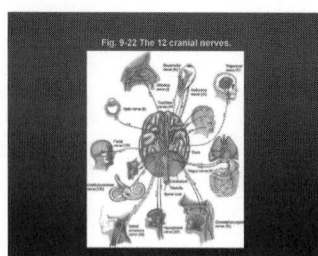

- The 12 cranial nerves serve both sensory and motor functions.
- The cranial nerves are generally named for the area or function they serve and are identified with Roman numerals.
- The trigeminal nerve is the primary source of innervation for the oral cavity. It subdivides into three main branches:
  - Maxillary
  - Mandibular
  - Ophthalmic (not discussed in this chapter)

Slide 61

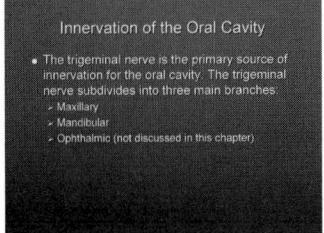

- What Roman numeral stands for the trigeminal nerve? *(V.)*

Slide 62

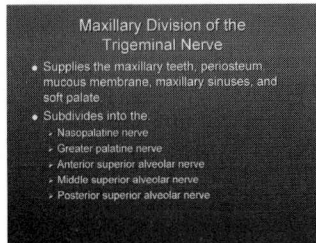

- Dental personnel sometimes use short names for these nerves when discussing local anesthetic injections. What are they?

Slide 63

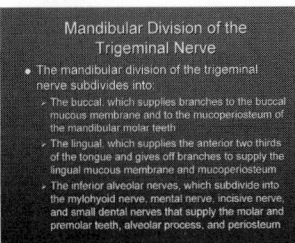

- Which branch of the mandibular division supplies the tongue?

- Which branch of the mandibular division supplies the teeth?

- Which branch of the mandibular division does not supply either the tongue or the teeth?

Slide 64

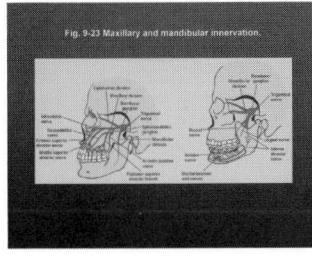

- The maxillary division of the trigeminal nerve supplies the maxillary teeth, periosteum, mucous membrane, maxillary sinuses, and soft palate.

- The mandibular division of the trigeminal nerve subdivides into:
  - Buccal nerve
  - Lingual nerve
  - Inferior alveolar nerve

Torres and Ehrlich Modern Dental Assisting, 9th ed.

Bird/Robinson

Slide 65

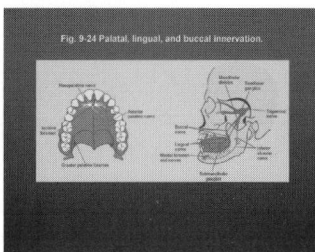

- What does each of these nerves supply?
  - The nasopalatine nerve?
  - The greater palatine nerve?
  - The buccal nerve?
  - The lingual nerve?
  - The inferior alveolar nerve?

Slide 66

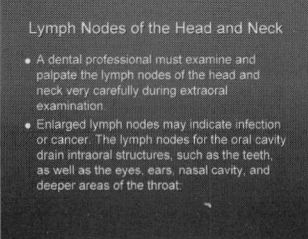

- What is the term for enlarged or palpable lymph nodes? *(Lymphadenopathy.)*
- Why does enlargement occur to the lymph node? *(Infection or cancer results in an increase in size and count of lymphocytes in the area.)*

Slide 67

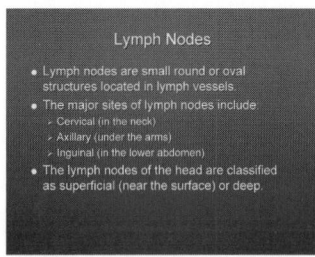

- All the nodes of the head drain either the right or the left tissues in the area, depending on their location.
- What is one cause of swollen axillary nodes? *(Underarm deodorant draining into lymph nodes.)*

Slide 68

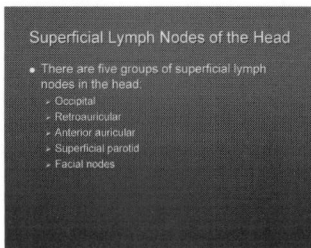

Bird/Robinson

Slide 69

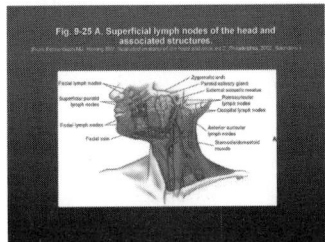

• Can you feel any of your facial lymph nodes?

Slide 70

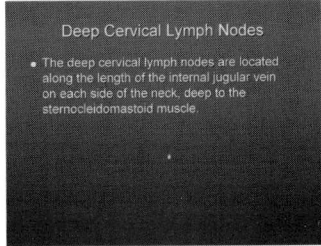

• The dental professional needs to palpate deep around the sternocleidomastoid muscle in order to palpate the deep cervical lymph nodes.

• Explain why the dental professional needs to be careful when palpating this muscle.

Slide 71

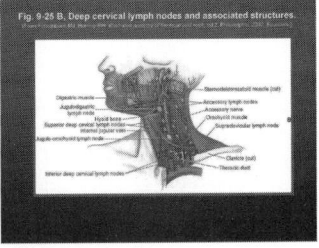

Slide 72

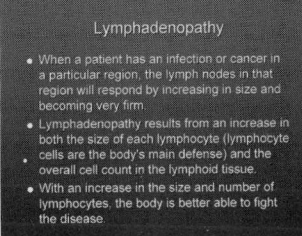

• The dentist will make an appropriate referral to a physician when any enlarged lymph nodes are found during an examination.

Bird/Robinson

Slide 73

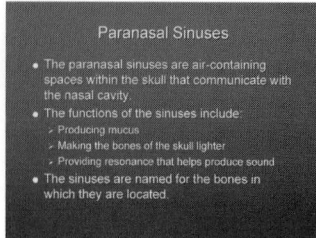

- Explain to students why a patient with an infected sinus might complain of a toothache. *(The roots of the maxillary teeth lie close to the sinus floor. Because the teeth and the maxillary sinus share a common nerve supply, inflammation of the sinus may cause a generalized aching of the maxillary teeth.)*

Slide 74

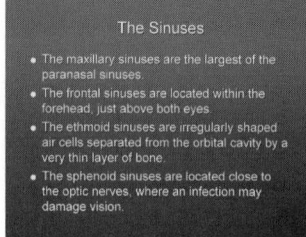

- When people say they have a sinus headache, the headache may involve one or more of these sinuses.

- Have your sinuses ever felt congested when you have a cold or are in an airplane?

Slide 75

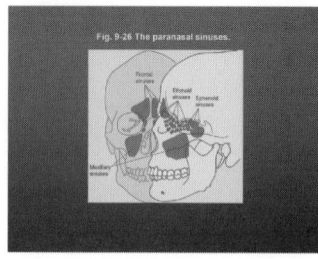

- Have students point to each of the sinuses on their own faces: frontal and maxillary.

Torres and Ehrlich Modern Dental Assisting, 9th ed.

Bird/Robinson

TEACHING FOCUS

This chapter gives students an opportunity to learn about the normal characteristics of the oral cavity. The landmarks of the face and oral cavity will be discussed, with an emphasis on the proper identification and pronunciation of the name of each landmark. Students will have the opportunity to learn about the structure and function of the oral cavity, the characteristics of the gingival tissue, and the function and location of the taste buds.

MATERIALS AND RESOURCES

- ☐ computer and PowerPoint projector (all Lessons)
- ☐ cotton tip applicators (all Lessons)
- ☐ model of a human skull (all Lessons)
- ☐ unlabeled copies of Figures 10-4 and 10-5 (Lesson 10.1)

LESSON CHECKLIST

Preparations for this lesson include:

- lecture
- evaluation of student knowledge and skills needed to perform all entry-level activities related to landmarks of the face and oral cavity, including:
  - structures found in the vestibular region of the oral cavity
  - the area of the oral cavity proper
  - the characteristics of normal gingival tissue
  - the function of the taste buds

ELSEVIER

Bird/Robinson

KEY TERMS

ala (p. 126)
angle of the mandible (p. 127)
angular cheilosis (p. 128)
anterior faucial pillar (p. 131)
anterior naris (p. 126)
buccal vestibule (p. 129)
canthus (p. 126)
filiform papillae (p. 133)
fordyce's spots (p. 129)
frenum (p. 130)
fungiform papillae (p. 133)
gingiva (p. 130)
glabella (p. 126)
incisive papilla (p. 131)
isthmus of fauces (p. 131)
labia (p. 127)
labial commissure (p. 127)
labial frenum (p. 130)
linea alba (p. 129)

lingual frenum (p. 130)
mental protuberance (p. 127)
mucobuccal fold (p. 128)
mucogingival junction (p. 129)
nasion (p. 126)
nasolabial sulcus (p. 127)
oral cavity proper (p. 128)
parotid papilla (p. 129)
philtrum (p. 126)
posterior faucial pillar (p. 131)
root (p. 126)
septum (p. 126)
tragus (p. 126)
uvula (p. 131)
vallate papillae (p. 133)
vermilion border (p. 127)
vestibule (p. 128)
zygomatic arch (p. 127)

ADDITIONAL RESOURCES

PowerPoint slides (Evolve): 1-37

Legend

CTQ
Critical
Thinking
Question

DVD
Multimedia
Procedures
Videos and
Animations

ESLR
EVOLVE
Student
Learning
Resources

IDO
Interactive
Dental
Office
CD-ROM

SW
Student
Workbook

TB
Test Bank
on the
TEACH
CD-ROM

PPT
PowerPoint
Slides

Class Activities are indicated in ***bold italic.***

ELSEVIER

Torres and Ehrlich Modern Dental Assisting, 9th ed.

Bird/Robinson

LESSON 10.1

PRETEST

1. The winglike tip of the outer side of each nostril is called the
   a. ala.
   b. nares.
   c. septum.
   d. glabella.

2. The thin fold of mucous membrane that extends from the floor of the mouth to the underside of the tongue is the
   a. labial frenum.
   b. incisive papilla.
   c. lingual frenum.
   d. parotid papilla.

3. For the purpose of identifying landmarks, how many regions can the face be divided into?
   a. three
   b. five
   c. seven
   d. nine

4. The distinct line of color change in the tissue where the alveolar membrane meets with attached gingivae is called the
   a. lingual fold.
   b. mucobuccal fold.
   c. linea alba.
   d. mucogingival junction.

5. The darker-colored border around the lips is called the
   a. vermilion zone.
   b. vermilion border.
   c. lingual frenum.
   d. lingual fold.

6. What type of gingival tissue extends from the base of the sulcus to the mucogingival junction?
   a. free gingiva
   b. marginal gingiva
   c. attached gingiva
   d. sulcular gingiva

7. The posterior part of the roof of the mouth is called the
   a. soft palate.
   b. hard palate.
   c. maxillary tuberosity.
   d. posterior vestibule.

8. The opening between the two arches is called the isthmus of
   a. fauces.
   b. pillars.
   c. vestibules.
   d. tonsils.

9. The anterior two thirds of the tongue is the
   a. ventral surface.
   b. lateral surface.
   c. body.
   d. root.

10. The taste buds are located on the
    a. root of the tongue.
    b. dorsum of the tongue.
    c. surface of the salivary glands.
    d. ducts of the salivary glands.

Answers

| 1. a | 3. d | 5. b | 7. a | 9. c |
| 2. c | 4. d | 6. c | 8. a | 10. b |

BACKGROUND ASSESSMENT

Question: What is the vermilion border? What changes in the vermilion border may be associated with oral cancer?

Answer: Normally there is a distinct darker-colored border between the lips and the surrounding skin of the face; this is called the vermilion border. Color change in or disappearance of the vermilion border may be associated with oral cancer. A biopsy is the only way to determine if the cells are cancerous.

Question: What is the mucobuccal fold, and where is it located?

Answer: The mucobuccal fold is located at the base of the vestibule where the buccal mucosa meets the alveolar mucosa, in the space between the teeth and the inner mucosal lining of the lips and cheeks. The vestibules are lined with mucosal tissue. The vestibular mucosa is thin, red, and loosely bound to the underlying alveolar bone.

CRITICAL THINKING QUESTION

A patient who is scheduled for nitrous oxide next week says that he cannot breathe out of his left nostril because bridge of his nose was recently hit by a football. How should the dental assistant describe this situation to the dentist?

Guidelines: Because this patient has breathing problems that could complicate the use of nitrous oxide, the dental assistant must accurately describe the situation to the dentist. Using the landmarks of the face, the dental assistant should explain to the dentist that the patient has a deviated nasal septum and that he cannot breathe out of the left anterior nares because of a trauma to the root of the nose. With the help of the dentist the dental assistant should also write up the progress notes for the day, using this same terminology.

OBJECTIVES	CONTENT	TEACHING RESOURCES
Pronounce, define, and spell the Key Terms.	■ Key terms (p. 125)	SW Fill in the Blank questions 1-15 (pp. 33-34) ESLR Electronic Flashcards ▶ Discuss each of the key terms, focusing on the definition, pronunciation, and spelling of each term. *Class Activity Have each student use one of the key terms in a clinically relevant sentence. Continue until all terms have been used and defined. If students become stuck, have the rest of the class offer suggestions.*
Name and identify the landmarks of the face.	■ Landmarks of the face (p. 126) ☐ Regions of the face (p. 126) ☐ Features of the face (p. 126) ☐ Skin (p. 127) ☐ Lips (p. 127)	PPT 4-10 TB questions 1-3 SW Short-Answer Questions 1; Multiple Choice questions 1-2 (pp. 33-34) SW Activities questions 1 and 3 (pp. 35-36) Figure 10-1 Regions of the face (A) At rest; (B) Smiling (p. 127) Figure 10-2 Landmarks of the face (p. 127) Recall questions 1-2 (pp. 127-128) Clinical Considerations with the Lips (p. 128) Figure 10-3 Frontal view of the lips (p. 127) ▶ Discuss why a dental professional should examine the lips before examining the oral cavity. ▶ Discuss other facial landmarks that a dental assistant should be able to identify. *Class Activity Divide the class into pairs. Have each pair create an examination list that includes the regions and features of the face. Then have each student use the list to examine his or her partner's face and note the findings. Have students share their observations with the class.*

OBJECTIVES	CONTENT	TEACHING RESOURCES
Name and identify the landmarks of the oral cavity.	■ The oral cavity (p. 128)	▣▤ PPT 11 ▣ TB questions 4-7 ▣ SW Short-Answer Questions 2; Multiple Choice questions 3, 5 (pp. 33-34) ▣ SW Activities question 2 (p. 35) Recall questions 3-5 (p. 130) ▸ Discuss the two areas that make up the oral cavity. ***Class Activity** Provide students with unlabeled copies of Figures 10-4 and 10-5 (p. 134). In groups, have students fill in the missing labels without using their textbooks and share their answers with the class.*
Describe the structures found in the vestibular region of the oral cavity.	☐ Vestibules (pp. 128-129) ☐ Labial and other frenula (p. 130)	▣▤ PPT 12-14, 20 ▣ SW Short-Answer Questions 3; Multiple Choice question 4 (pp. 33-34) Figure 10-4 Vestibule and vestibular tissue of the oral cavity (p. 128) Figure 10-5 Buccal vestibule and buccal mucosa of the cheek (p. 129) ▸ Discuss the components of the vestibular region of the oral cavity. Where does the intraoral vestibule begin? ▸ Discuss normal variations that might appear on the buccal mucosa. ***Class Activity** Divide the class into groups and assign each group one of the following vestibular structures: mucobuccal fold, mucogingival junction, buccal vestibule, parotid papilla, Fordyce's spots, linea alba. Have each group describe its structure in detail, explain its structure's functions in the oral cavity, and present its findings to the class for discussion.*

Bird/Robinson

10.1 Homework/Assignments:

10.1 Instructor's Notes/Student Feedback:

Torres and Ehrlich Modern Dental Assisting, 9th ed.

Bird/Robinson

LESSON 10.2

CRITICAL THINKING QUESTION

A patient says that she has been experiencing a burning sensation in the front part of the roof of her mouth, the top of the front part of the tongue, and in the corners of the mouth. How should the dental assistant relate this information to the dentist?

Guidelines: The dental assistant should be familiar with the landmarks of the oral cavity in order to accurately relate the information to the dentist. The dental assistant should explain that the patient has been experiencing a burning sensation on the hard palate, the dorsum of the body of the tongue, and on the labial commissures. With the help of the dentist, the dental assistant should also write up the progress notes for the day, using this terminology.

OBJECTIVES	CONTENT	TEACHING RESOURCES
Describe the characteristics of normal gingival tissue.	☐ Gingiva (p. 130) – Unattached gingiva (p. 130) – Interdental gingiva (p. 130) – Gingival groove (p. 130) – Attached gingiva (p. 130)	⊠▤ PPT 17-19, 21-24 ▤ TB questions 8-9 ▤ SW Short-Answer Questions 5; Multiple Choice questions 6-8 (pp. 33-34) Figure 10-6 View of gingivae and associated anatomic landmarks (p. 129) Figure 10-7 Linea alba (p. 129) Figure 10-8 It is normal for the color of the gingiva to vary according to the pigmentation of the individual (p. 130) Figure 10-9 Close-up view of gingivae and associated anatomic landmarks (p. 130) Recall questions 6-8 (p. 130) ▸ Discuss the normal characteristics of the gingival tissue. ▸ Discuss the various levels of severity for gingivitis and periodontitis. *Class Activity Present the class with several pictures of gingiva. Have students determine which pictures depict healthy gingiva and which depict unhealthy gingiva, and hae them identify which type of gingiva each picture represents. Have students share and discuss their answers with the class.*
Describe the area of the oral cavity proper.	■ The oral cavity proper (p. 131) ☐ Hard palate (p. 131) ☐ Soft palate (p. 131) ☐ Tongue (p. 132)	⊠▤ PPT 25-36 ▤ TB questions 10-13, 15 ▤ SW Short-Answer Questions 4; Multiple Choice questions 9-12 (pp. 33-35) Recall questions 9-10 (p. 132) Figure 10-10 (A) Surface features of the hard palate; (B) Surface features of the soft palate (p. 131)

ELSEVIER

OBJECTIVES	CONTENT	TEACHING RESOURCES
		Clinical Considerations with the Gag Reflex (p. 133)
		Figure 10-11 Dorsum of the tongue (p. 132)
		Figure 10-12 Sublingual aspect of the tongue (p. 132)
		Clinical Considerations with the Lingual Frenula (p. 133)
		🔅 CTQ 1-2 (p. 133)
		▶ Discuss the components of the oral cavity proper. Where does the oral cavity proper link with the vestibule?
		▶ Discuss where on the hard palate an injection of anesthesia would be administered to the nasopalatine nerve.
		***Class Activity** In class, have students practice the following: Have each hold his or her teeth together, and with the tongue feel the areas of the oral cavity proper and the hard palate. Then have students use mouth mirrors to examine their fungiform papillae. Have students discuss their observations with the class.*
Locate and describe the functions of the taste buds.	☐ Taste buds (p. 133) ☐ Teeth (p. 133)	🖼️ PPT 37 💻 TB question 13 📖 SW Short-Answer Questions 6 (p. 33) Recall questions 11-12 (p. 133) 🔅 CTQ 3 (p. 133) ▶ Discuss where the teeth are situated in the oral cavity. Name the parts that are visible. ▶ Discuss the location and function of the taste buds. What else is necessary to stimulate the taste buds? ***Class Activity** Have students research taste bud histology, taste sensations, or loss of taste and present their findings to the class. (For students to prepare for this activity, see Homework/Assignments #1.)*
Performance Evaluation		💻 TB 📖 SW questions (pp. 33-36) 💶 ESLR Electronic Flashcards 💶 ESLR Practice Quiz 💶 ESLR Labeling Exercise 13: Identify the orofacial structures of the face Recall questions 1-12 (pp. 127-133) 🔅 CTQ (p. 133)

| **10.2 Homework/Assignments:** |
| 1. Have student research taste-bud histology, taste sensations, or loss of taste and present their findings to the class. |

| **10.2 Instructor's Notes/Student Feedback:** |
| |

Slide 1

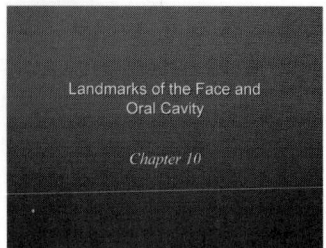

Slide 2

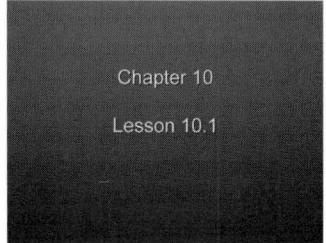

Slide 3

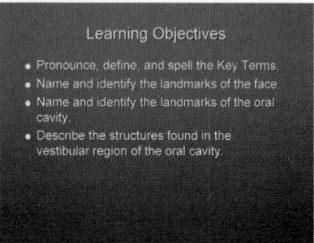

Slide 4

- What deeper structures do facial features help to pinpoint?

Torres and Ehrlich Modern Dental Assisting, 9th ed.
Bird/Robinson

Slide 5

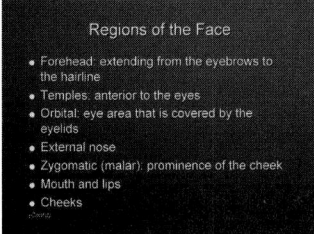

- The face is defined as the part of the head that is visible in a frontal view. It includes everything that lies between the hairline and the chin.

Slide 6

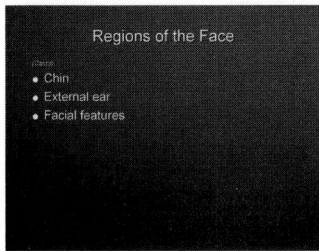

- What is the mandibular protuberance? *(The part of the mandible that forms the chin.)*
- Name and point out the parts of the external ear, such as the external canal, tragus, antitragus, and helix.

Slide 7

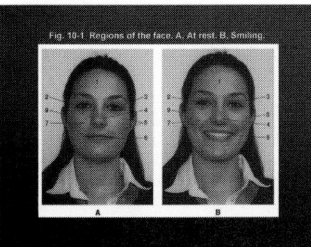

- How does facial skin differ from skin on the rest of the body?

Slide 8

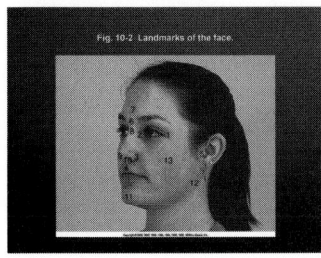

- Identify the 13 landmarks of the face, numbered in the picture. *(1) the outer canthus of the eye, (2)the inner canthus of the eye, (3) the ala of the nose, (4) the philtrum, (5) the tragus of the ea,r, (6) the nasion' (7) the glabella, (8) the root of the nose, (9) the septum (10) the anterior naris, (11) the mental protuberance, (12) the angle of the mandible, and (13) the zygomatic arch.)*

Slide 9

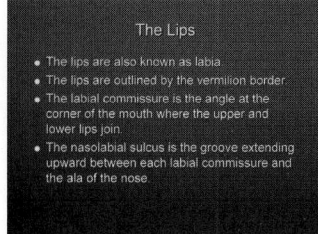

- What is the philtrum? *(A rectangular area that extends from just under the nose to the midline of the upper lip.)*
- Where are lip ointments applied? *(In the vermilion zone.)*
- What is the area of color change around the border of the lips?

Slide 10

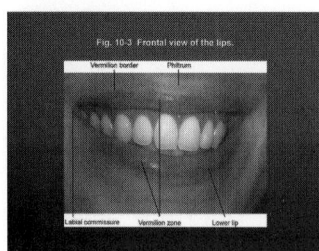

- Grasp your lip between your thumb and forefinger to feel the pulsations of the labial branches of the facial artery. The upper and lower lips are continuous at the angles of the mouth and blend with the cheeks.

Slide 11

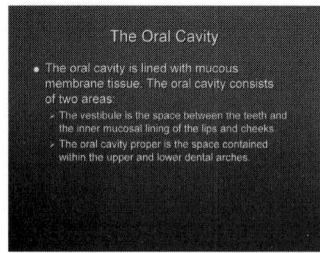

- How many vestibules does a person have?
- What is the difference between the vestibules and the oral cavity proper?

Slide 12

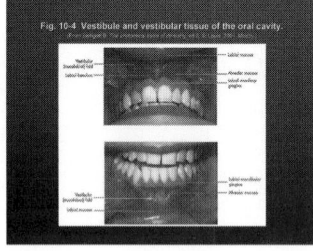

- The muccobuccal fold is where the dentist will inject the local anesthetic on the maxillary arch.
- What type of tissues cover the oral cavity?
- What are the two regions of the oral cavity?
- What is the name of the structure that passes from the oral mucosa to the facial midline of the mandibular arch?

Torres and Ehrlich Modern Dental Assisting, 9th ed.

Bird/Robinson

Slide 13

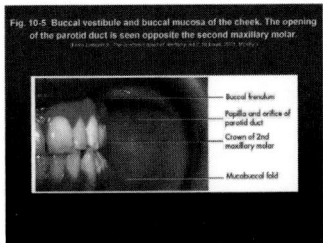

- Have you ever seen Fordyce's spots in the oral cavity? What do these spots consist of? *(Enlarged ectopic sebaceous glands in the mucosa of the mouth.)*

- What product does the parotid produce in the oral cavity? *(Saliva.)*

- Can you feel your parotid papillae with your tongue? Where in the mouth are they located?

Slide 14

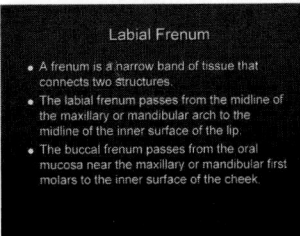

- Some members of the dental community feel that the labial frenum may exert force on the teeth and believe that it may need to be surgically corrected if it presents a problem for a patient.

Slide 15

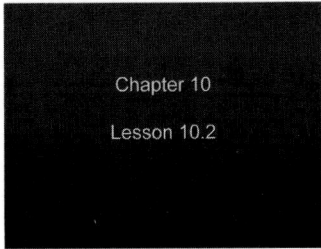

Slide 16

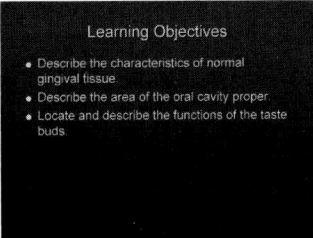

Slide 17

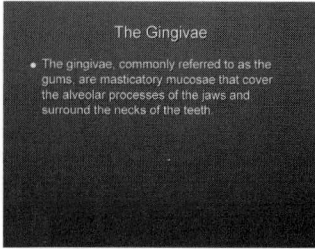

- What role do the gums play in oral health?

Slide 18

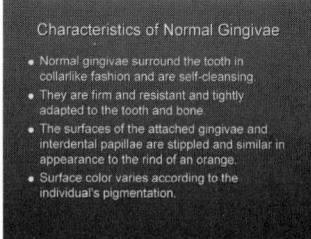

- Sometimes the gingiva does not completely cover the roots of the teeth and the roots become exposed. This condition, called gingival recession, can lead to sensitivity and root cavities (caries).

Slide 19

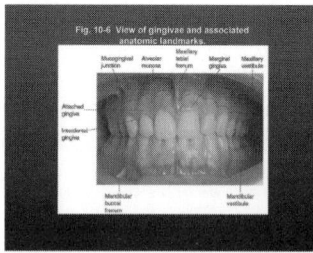

- The distinct line of color change where the alveolar membrane meets the attached gingivae is the mucogingival junction.
- What are the characteristics of normal gingival tissue?

Slide 20

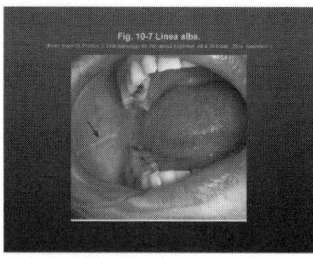

- Do you have a wide or extensive linea alba?
- Is it the same on both sides?
- Do you ever chew your buccal mucosa?
- Do you bite your buccal mucosa?

Torres and Ehrlich Modern Dental Assisting, 9th ed.

Bird/Robinson

Slide 21

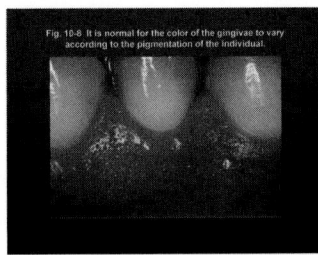

- In dark-skinned people, the gingiva may contain melanin pigment to a greater extent than the nearby alveolar mucosa. This melanin pigment is synthesized in specialized cells and is produced as granules that are stored within the cells that produce melanin.

Slide 22

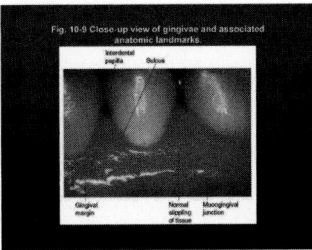

- When you floss, where does the floss fit?

Slide 23

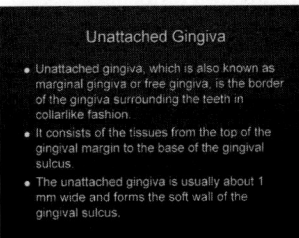

- Unattached gingiva is the first tissue to become inflamed.

Slide 24

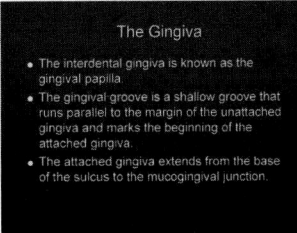

- Can you feel with your tongue the firmness of the attached gingiva compared with the softer alveolar mucosa of the vestibules?

- How does the attached gingiva look in a healthy mouth? Can you see the groove when you look at your gingiva?

- How does the interdental gingiva look in a healthy mouth? Does it fill in the spaces between the teeth or is it blunted or enlarged?

Torres and Ehrlich Modern Dental Assisting, 9th ed.

Bird/Robinson

Slide 25

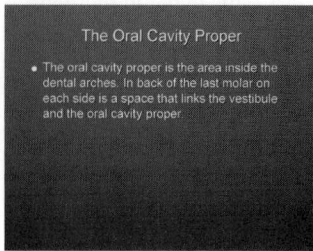

- What is the difference between the oral cavity proper and the vestibules?

Slide 26

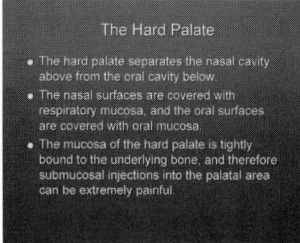

- What is another term used to refer to the hard palate? *(The roof of the mouth.)*

Slide 27

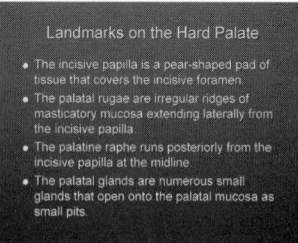

- The incisive papilla can easily be burned with hot food and drinks. It is the landmark for the dentist to give a palatal injection of local anesthesia to numb the soft tissue of the hard palate.

Slide 28

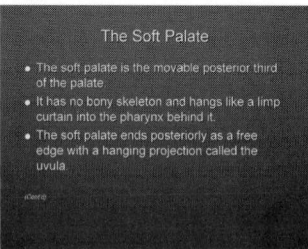

- Does the tissue feel soft to your tongue when you gently touch it? Does it feel muscular?
- Try to swallow and notice that the soft palate, unlike the hard palate, is movable.

Bird/Robinson

Slide 29

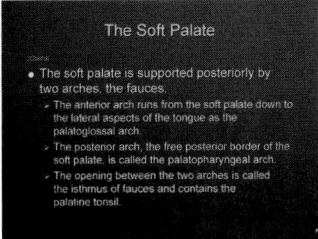

- What is the palatine tonsil?

Slide 30

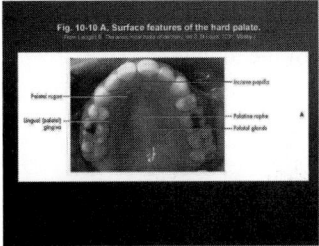

- What are the landmarks of the hard palate?

Slide 31

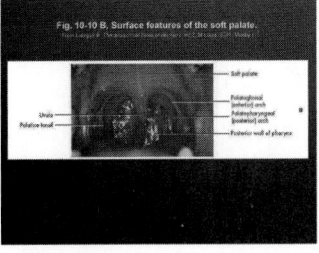

- How does the soft palate differ from the hard palate?

Slide 32

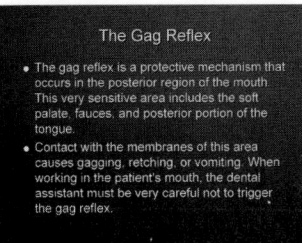

- Use of nitrous oxide can help to curb the gag reflex. The gag reflex may occur when radiographs and impressions of patients' mouths are taken. Exciting the gag reflex could trigger vomiting.

Slide 33

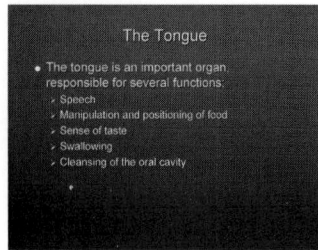

- What is the term for the upper surface of the tongue?
- What is the thin fold of mucous membrane that extends from the floor of the mouth to the underside of the tongue?

Slide 34

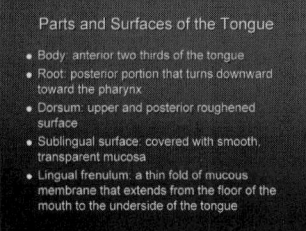

- What are the implications of tongue piercing?
- What is a common region for oral cancer? *(The root of the tongue.)*
- What is another name for the undersurface of the tongue? *(Ventral surface.)*

Slide 35

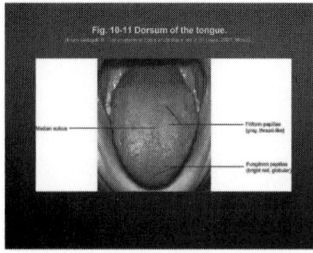

- Why does the dorsum of the tongue feel rough?
- Look at the fungiform lingual papillae and notice how they look like red dots.
  - Microscopically, they look like little red mushrooms, thus the name.
  - The taste buds are located on the sides of the mushroom in the epithelial tissues.

Slide 36

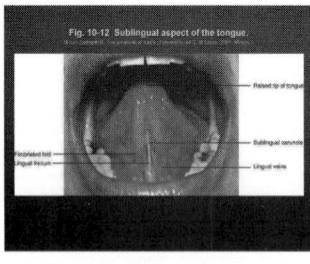

- The submandibular ducts are located at either side of the lingual frenulum.
- This is one of the places where saliva enters the mouth.

Bird/Robinson

Slide 37

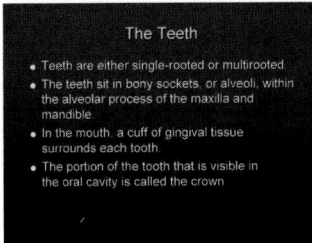

- Which teeth are usually multirooted? *(Molars and maxillary first premolars.)*

- Which teeth are usually single rooted? *(All other teeth.)*

- When people talk about getting their teeth "capped," what part of a tooth is being restored?

- What part of the tooth is found within the jaw bones in a healthy person?

11 Overview of the Dentitions

TEACHING FOCUS

This chapter,will introduce students to dentitions. Students will have the opportunity to learn to identify how tooth function is determined by size and shape, locations of each tooth surface, landmarks of the teeth, types of occlusions, and the three primary systems of tooth numbering.

MATERIALS AND RESOURCES

- ☐ computer and PowerPoint projector (all Lessons)
- ☐ typodonts (all Lessons)

LESSON CHECKLIST

Preparations for this lesson include:

- lecture
- evaluation of student knowledge and skills surrounding dentitions, including:
  - ○ size and shape of teeth
  - ○ tooth landmarks
  - ○ tooth-numbering systems
  - ○ tooth surfaces
  - ○ types of occlusions

ELSEVIER

Bird/Robinson

KEY TERMS

Angle's classification (p. 144)
anterior (p. 139)
apical third (p. 143)
buccal surface (p. 141)
buccolingual division (p. 143)
centric occlusion (p. 143)
cervical third (p. 143)
concave (p. 145)
contact area (p. 142)
convex (p. 145)
curve of Spee (p. 145)
curve of Wilson (p. 145)
deciduous (p. 136)
dentition (p. 135)
distal surface (p. 141)
distoclusion (p. 145)
embrasure (p. 142)
facial surface (p. 141)
functional occlusion (p. 143)
incisal surface (p. 141)
interproximal space (p. 141)
labial surface (p. 141)
labioversion (p. 145)
line angle (p. 142)

lingual surface (p. 141)
linguoversion (p. 145)
malocclusion (p. 143)
mandibular arch (p. 137)
masticatory surface (p. 141)
maxillary arch (p. 137)
mesial surface (p. 141)
mesioclusion (p. 145)
mesiodistal division (p. 143)
middle third (p. 143)
mixed dentition (p. 136)
neutroclusion (p. 144)
occlusal surface (p. 141)
occulsion (p. 143)
occlusocervical division (p. 143)
palatal surface (p. 141)
point angle (p. 142)
posterior (p. 139)
primary dentition (p. 136)
proximal surfaces (p. 141)
quadrant (p. 137)
sextant (p. 139)
succedaneous teeth (p. 136)

ADDITIONAL RESOURCES

PowerPoint slides (Evolve): 1-52

Legend

CTQ
Critical
Thinking
Question

DVD
Multimedia
Procedures
Videos and
Animations

ESLR
EVOLVE
Student
Learning
Resources

IDO
Interactive
Dental
Office
CD-ROM

SW
Student
Workbook

TB
Test Bank
on the
TEACH
CD-ROM

PPT
PowerPoint
Slides

Class Activities are indicated in ***bold italic***.

LESSON 11.1

PRETEST

1. What is the maximum contact between the occluding surfaces of the maxillary and mandibular teeth?
   a. functional occlusion
   b. malocclusion
   c. centric occlusion
   d. distoclusion

2. When is the estimated time for the eruption of the permanent mandibular second molar?
   a. 9 to 11 years
   b. 10 to 12 years
   c. 11 to 13 years
   d. 12 to 14 years

3. Which permanent tooth has a lingual surface like a shovel?
   a. molars
   b. premolars
   c. canines
   d. incisors

4. How many teeth are present in the primary dentition?
   a. 12
   b. 16
   c. 18
   d. 20

5. What is a name given in the past to the premolars?
   a. eye tooth
   b. bicuspid
   c. wisdom tooth
   d. cuspid

6. Which tooth type is present in the permanent dentition but not in the primary dentition?
   a. molars
   b. premolars
   c. canines
   d. incisors

7. What is the term for the junction of two surfaces and derives its name from the combination of the two surfaces that join?
   a. point angle
   b. embrasure
   c. height of contour
   d. line angle

8. Which of Angle's classifications is also considered neutroclusion?
   a. Class I
   b. Class II, division 1
   c. Class II, division 2
   d. Class III

9. Which of the following numbering systems uses capital letters for the primary dentition?
   a. Angle's
   b. Palmer
   c. Universal
   d. FDI

10. Which dentition period has some teeth of both dentitions present?
    a. deciduous
    b. primary
    c. mixed
    d. permanent

Answers

1. c	3. d	5. b	7. d	9. c
2. c	4. d	6. b	8. a	10. c

BACKGROUND ASSESSMENT

Question: When might a patient have both primary and permanent teeth present in the mouth? How does this happen?

Answer: A patient in the mixed dentition period, usually between the ages of 6 and 12, will have both primary and permanent teeth. Until a child is about the age of 6, the primary dentition is in place. At about that same age, the first permanent teeth begin to emerge in the mouth. This begins a period in which there is a mixture of permanent teeth and primary teeth until about age 12, when all the primary teeth have been lost.

ELSEVIER

Question: What is malocclusion? What is the method by which malocclusion can be assessed initially? What is the basis for this method? What types of malocclusion does this system involve?

Answer: Malocclusion refers to abnormal or malpositioned relationships of the maxillary teeth to mandibular teeth when they are in centric occlusion. Centric occlusion widely distributes the occlusal forces and provides the greatest comfort and stability. Angle's classification system is the initial method used for assessing a malocclusion. The basis of this system is that the permanent maxillary first molar is the key to occlusion. Angle's system assumes that a patient is occluding in a centric position. This system involves three main classifications: Class I, Class II, and Class III.

CRITICAL THINKING QUESTION

An 11-year-old patient is very upset. Her teeth seem very crooked and of different sizes and her gums are bleeding. She asks if her teeth will be this way forever. She wants her teeth to be nice and straight. What should the dental assistant tell her to help her understand her dental situation? What will be important to stress for her to maintain her oral health?

Guidelines: The patient is in a mixed dentition period that occurs usually between the ages of 6 and 12 years, until all the primary teeth have been lost. The mixed dentition period is often a difficult time for children because color differences between the primary and permanent teeth become apparent (primary teeth are whiter than permanent teeth), and they may notice the difference in the crown size between the larger permanent teeth and the smaller primary teeth. Some children may notice crowding of the teeth as they shift positions during eruption. This crowding makes oral hygiene difficult, and gingivitis may occur. The dental assistant should assure the patient that, with care, her mouth will change for the better. The dental assistant should stress to the patient that she will need to spend extra time with her oral hygiene to help fight the gingivitis that is causing her gingiva to bleed.

OBJECTIVES	CONTENT	TEACHING RESOURCES
Pronounce, define, and spell the key terms.	■ Key terms (p. 134) ■ Introduction (p. 135)	PPT 4 ESLR Electronic Flashcards ▶ Discuss the challenges of learning dentitions for a dental assistant. *Class Activity Have students make flash cards for the key terms with the terms on one side and the definitions on the reverse. Then have the students quiz each other with the flash cards. Correct their pronunciation as needed.*
Explain the differences between primary, mixed, and permanent dentitions.	■ Dentition periods (pp. 135-136) □ Primary dentition (p. 136) □ Mixed dentition (p. 136) □ Permanent dentition (p. 137) ■ Dental arches (p. 137) □ Quadrants (p. 137) □ Sextants (p. 139) □ Anterior and posterior teeth (p. 139)	PPT 5-18 TB questions 1-7 SW Short-Answer Questions 5; Fill in the Blank questions 1-3, 6-9; Multiple Choice questions 1-3 (pp. 37-38) Table 11-1 Dentition Periods and Clinical Considerations (p. 136) Table 11-2 Primary Dentition in Order of Eruption (p. 136) Table 11-3 Permanent Dentition in Order of Eruption (p. 137) Figure 11-1 Example of the primary dentition (p. 136) Figure 11-2 Example of the oral cavity during the mixed dentition period (p. 137)

ELSEVIER

Torres and Ehrlich Modern Dental Assisting, 9th ed.

Bird/Robinson

OBJECTIVES	CONTENT	TEACHING RESOURCES
		Figure 11-3 Facial and buccal view of a permanent dentition (p. 137)
		Figure 11-4 Primary and permanent dentition separated into quadrants (p. 138)
		Figure 11-5 Permanent dentition separated into sextants (p. 139)
		Figure 11-6 Occlusal view of the permanent and primary dentition (p. 140)
		Recall questions 1-4 (p. 139)
		⚲ CTQ 1-2 (p. 148)
		▸ Discuss the common terms used for the different periods of dentition.
		▸ Discuss the different types of dental arches and the common terms used to describe them.
		***Class Activity** Draw on the board a table with the following column headings: Primary, Mixed, and Permanent. Have students call out characteristics for each dentition period and write them in the correct column on the board. Next, have class, discuss the similarities and differences among the dentition periods.*
Explain how the size and shape of teeth determine the functions of different types of teeth.	■ Types and functions of teeth (pp. 139-140) ☐ Incisors (p. 140) ☐ Canines (p. 140) ☐ Premolars (p. 140) ☐ Molars (p. 140)	⊠▤ PPT 19-26 ⌨ TB questions 8-10 ✎ SW Short-Answer Questions 1-2, 4; Fill in the Blank questions 4-5; Multiple Choice questions 4-6 (pp. 37-38) Recall questions 5-6 (p. 141) ▸ Discuss how each type of tooth works in the chewing and mastication of food. ▸ Discuss what the effects might be on a patient who is absent one or more of the different types of teeth. ***Class Activity** Divide the class into four groups. Assign each group one of the following tooth types: incisors, canines, premolars, and molars. Next, using typodonts, have each group explain how the size and shape of its assigned tooth type helps contribute to the function of the tooth. Have the class provide feedback.*
Name and identify the location of each tooth surface.	■ Tooth surfaces (p. 141)	⊠▤ PPT 27-28 ⌨ TB questions 11-12 ✎ SW Short-Answer Questions 3; Fill in the Blank questions 10-12; Multiple Choice question 7 (pp. 37-39)

Torres and Ehrlich Modern Dental Assisting, 9th ed.

Bird/Robinson

OBJECTIVES	CONTENT	TEACHING RESOURCES
		Figure 11-7 Surfaces of the teeth (p. 141)
		Recall question 7 (p. 142)
		▸ Discuss how the surface of a tooth can be compared to a box with sides.
		▸ Discuss how to describe the tooth surfaces when they are adjacent to each other.
		***Class Activity** Using typodonts for each type of tooth, point to different areas on each typodont and have the students call out the tooth surface. Next, call out a tooth surface and have student volunteers identify the surface on a typodont.*

Utilize terminology to identify landmarks of the teeth.	■ Anatomic features of teeth (p. 141)
	
	☐ Contours (p. 141)
	
	  – Facial and lingual contours (p. 141)
	
	  – Mesial and distal contours (p. 141)
	
	☐ Contacts (p. 142)
	
	☐ Height of contour (p. 142)
	
	☐ Embrasures (p. 142)
		PPT 29-33
		
		TB question 13
		
		SW Fill in the Blank questions 13; Multiple Choice questions 8-10 (pp. 38-39)
		
		Figure 11-8 Tooth contours (p. 141)
		
		Figure 11-9 Example of a permanent anterior tooth with the contact area and height of contour identified (p. 142)
		
		Figure 11-10 Embrasures may diverge facially, lingually, occlusally, or apically (p. 142)
		
		Recall questions 8-10 (p. 142)
		
		▸ Discuss how learning about the anatomic features of the teeth can help the dental assistant locate specific areas of the teeth.
		
		▸ Discuss how abnormal tooth contours might affect a patient's dental health.
		
		***Class Activity** Place numbered labels on the surfaces of typodonts at laboratory stations. Divide the class into small groups, and have students name each site on a prepared form, using terms such as height of contour, embrasure, or contact area.*

11.1 Homework/Assignments:

11.1 Instructor's Notes/Student Feedback:

Bird/Robinson

LESSON 11.2

CRITICAL THINKING QUESTION

A dental assistant has started working for an orthodontist. The office uses a different system of numbering the teeth than the Universal/National system—one that uses a bracket and quadrant numbers. What is this numbering system? Give examples of the use of the system.

Guidelines: The orthodontist's office is using the Palmer Notation system. In this system, each of the four quadrants is given its own tooth bracket made up of a vertical line and a horizontal line. It uses a shorthand diagram of the teeth as if viewing the patient's teeth from the outside. The teeth in the right quadrant would have the vertical midline bracket to the right of the tooth numbers or letters—just as when looking at the patient. The midline is to the right of the teeth in the right quadrant. For example, if the tooth is a maxillary tooth, the number or letter should be written above the horizontal line of the bracket, thus indicating an upper tooth. Conversely, a mandibular tooth symbol should be placed below the line, indicating a lower tooth. The number or letter assigned to each tooth depends on its position relative to the midline. For example, central incisors, the teeth closest to the midline, have the lowest number, 1, for permanent teeth, and the letter A for primary teeth. All central incisors, maxillary and mandibular, are given the number 1. All lateral incisors are given the number 2, all canines are given the number 3, premolars are numbers 4 and 5, molars are 6 and 7, and the third molars are assigned number 8.

OBJECTIVES	CONTENT	TEACHING RESOURCES
Utilize terminology to identify landmarks of the teeth.	■ Angles and divisions of teeth (p. 142) □ Line and point angles (p. 142) □ Divisions into thirds (p. 143)	PPT 36-39 SW Fill in the Blank question 14; Multiple Choice question 11 (pp. 38-39) Figure 11-11 Line and point angles (p. 143) Figure 11-12 An anterior tooth and a posterior tooth (p. 143) Recall questions 11-12 (p. 143) ▸ Discuss how identifying the angles of the teeth can help identify specific areas of the teeth. ▸ Discuss how angles and divisions of the teeth relate to the surfaces of the teeth in identifying specific areas of the teeth. ***Class Activity** Place numbered labels on the surfaces of typodonts at laboratory stations. Then divide the class into small groups, and have the students name each site on a prepared form, using identifying terminology such as line angle, point angle, or third of the tooth.*
Explain the terms *occlusion*, *centric occlusion*, and *malocclusion*.	■ Occlusion and malocclusion (p. 143)	PPT 40-43 TB questions 14-15 SW Short-Answer Questions 6; Fill in the Blank questions 15-18; Multiple Choice questions 12-14 (pp. 37-39) Recall questions 13-14 (p. 144) Figure 11-13 Lingual view of the teeth in centric occlusion (p. 144)

OBJECTIVES	CONTENT	TEACHING RESOURCES
		▶ Discuss the concept of occlusion and its importance to dental health.
		***Class Activity** Have class discuss and define the terms occlusion, centric occlusion, and malocclusion. Why is centric occlusion considered normal? How might malocclusion affect a patient's health?*
Explain Angle's classification of malocclusion.	☐ Angle's classification (p. 144) – Class I (p. 144) – Class II (p. 145) – Class III (p. 145) ■ Stabilization of the arches (p. 145) ☐ Closure (p. 145) ☐ Curve of Spee (p. 145) ☐ Curve of Wilson (p. 145)	PPT 44-47 TB question 16 SW Short-Answer Questions 7; Multiple Choice questions 15-17 (pp. 37, 39) Recall questions 15-16 (p. 145) Table 11-4 Angle's Classifications of Malocclusion (p. 144) Recall question 17 (p. 146) Figure 11-14 Radiograph showing the mesial drift of the mandibular second molar (p. 145) Figure 11-15 Curves noted in the dental arch (p. 146) ▶ Discuss how Angle's classification can aid in identifying different types of occlusions. ▶ Discuss the importance of stable and efficient arches to a patient's dental health. ***Class Activity** Divide the class into small groups. Present the following situations to the groups, and have them classify each situation according to Angle's classification system, providing a rationale for each. Have each group share its results with the class.* *1. The mandibular dental arch is in a distal relationship to the maxillary arch. The lower lip is tucked behind the upper incisors.* *2. The mesiobuccal cusp of the permanent maxillary first molar occludes with the mesiobuccal groove of the mandibular first molar. Anterior teeth are malaligned.* *3. The mandible appears to protrude.*
Name and describe the three primary systems of tooth numbering.	■ Tooth-numbering systems (p. 146) ☐ Universal/National System (p. 146) ☐ International Standards Organization System (p. 146)	PPT 48-52 TB question 17 SW Short-Answer Questions 8 (p. 37) ▶ Discuss how tooth-numbering systems might have been developed and their importance in dentistry.

OBJECTIVES	CONTENT	TEACHING RESOURCES
	☐ Palmer Notation System (p. 147)	▸ Discuss how a dentist's assistant might choose one particular numbering system to identify teeth.
		*Class Activity **In a class discussion compare and contrast the Universal/National System, the International Standards Organization System, and the Palmer Notation System. Have students identify and discuss benefits and shortcomings of each system.***
Identify teeth using the Universal/ National system, the Palmer Notation System, and the ISO/FDI system.	■ Tooth-numbering systems (p. 146) ☐ Universal/National System (p. 146) ☐ International Standards Organization System (p. 146) ☐ Palmer Notation System (p. 147)	⊠ PPT 48-52 TB questions 18-20 SW Activity (pp. 39-40) Table 11-5 Tooth Designation Systems (p. 147) Example of Palmer Notation System (p. 146) Figure 11-16 Palmer Notation System (p. 148) Legal and Ethical Implications (p. 148) Eye to the Future (p. 148) CTQ 3-4 (p. 148) ▸ Discuss the advantages and disadvantages of the three systems of tooth numbering. ▸ Discuss how a dental assistant can memorize the different types of tooth-numbering systems for later use in the profession. *Class Activity **Divide the class into three groups. Assign each group one of the primary tooth-numbering systems. Using its assigned system, have each group identify and number each tooth in a blank figure of the mouth. Have each group share its results with the class.***
Performance Evaluation		TB SW questions (pp. 37-40) ESLR Electronic Flashcards ESLR Practice Quiz ESLR Labeling Exercise 14: Identify the surfaces of the teeth Recall questions (pp. 139-146) CTQ (p. 148)

11.2 Homework/Assignments:

11.2 Instructor's Notes/Student Feedback:

Slide 1

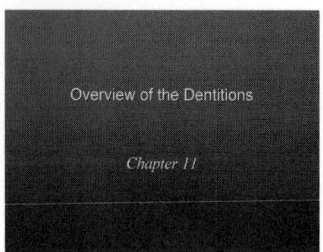

Slide 2

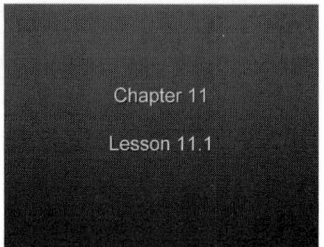

Slide 3

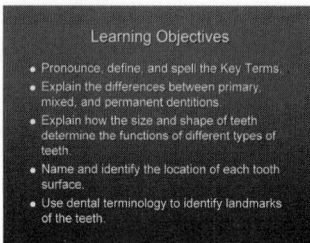

Slide 4

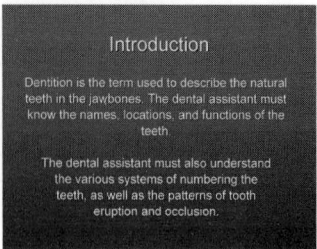

- Why do we number the teeth in each dentition?

- What occurs during tooth eruption?

- What does occlusion mean?

- How many teeth are in each dentition?

- What is the term for the four sections of the divided dental arches?

- What are the terms for the front teeth and for the back teeth?

Torres and Ehrlich Modern Dental Assisting, 9th ed.

Bird/Robinson

Slide 5

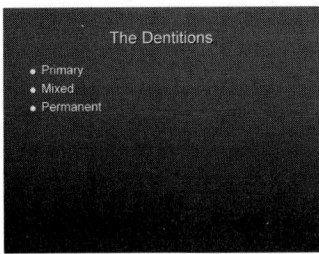

- Decisions regarding dental treatment are often based on the dentition period.
- Ask students to define each dentition.
- What are the four types of teeth?
- Which tooth is referred to as the "cornerstone" of the dental arch?

Slide 6

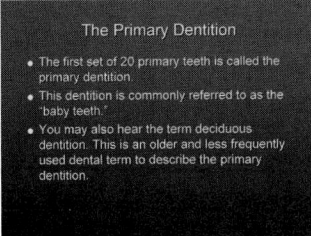

- Do you still have any of your shed primary teeth?
- Why were the primary teeth called deciduous?

Slide 7

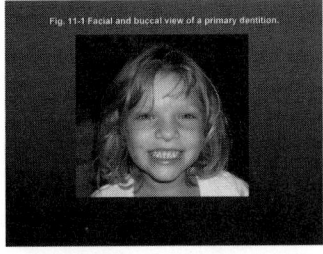

- Are baby teeth important or should parents just let them decay and fall out?
- Do you notice how white these teeth are? Why are they whiter?

Slide 8

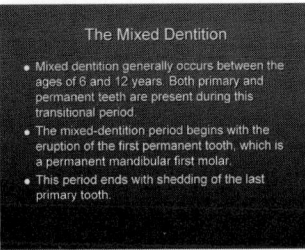

- Why can the mixed dentition period be difficult for the child? *(The mixed dentition period is often a difficult time for children because color differences between the primary and permanent teeth become apparent, and they may notice the difference in the crown size between the larger permanent teeth and the smaller primary teeth. Some children may notice crowding of the teeth as they shift positions during eruption.)*

Slide 9

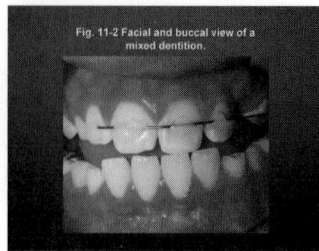

- Why is this the mixed dentition? Which teeth are primary teeth and which are permanent teeth?
- Why during this time do orthodontists start therapy as shown here?

Slide 10

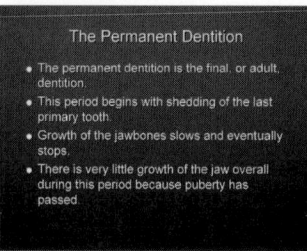

- After eruption of the permanent canines and premolars and the second permanent molars, the permanent dentition is complete at about age 14 to age 15, except for the third molars, which are not completed until about age 18 to 25.
- It includes eruption of all the permanent teeth, except for teeth that are congenitally (from the time of birth) missing or impacted and cannot erupt (usually the third molars).

Slide 11

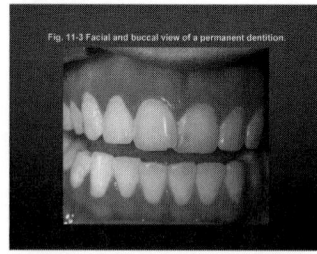

- The *permanent dentition* is the final or adult dentition.
- Why is this called the permanent dentition?
- Why are these teeth more yellow than the primary teeth?

Slide 12

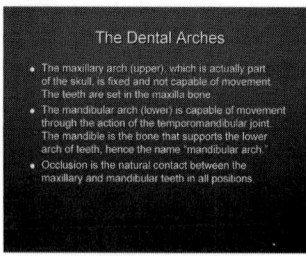

- How is each arch divided for treatment in the dental office?
- How is occlusion assessed?

Slide 13

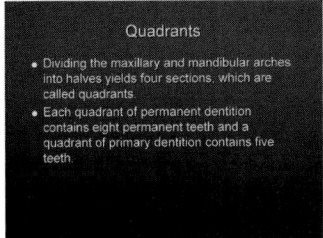

- Remember that as one looks into the patient's oral cavity, the directions are reversed.

Slide 14

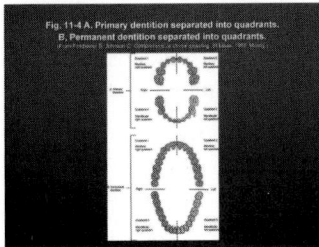

- Which ones are the maxillary arches and which are the mandibular arches?
- How are the arches divided?

Slide 15

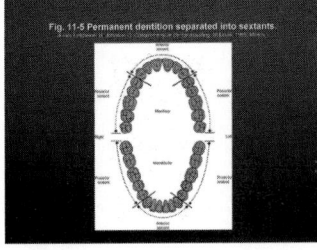

- How is a sextant different from a quadrant in the mouth?
- Would it take longer to polish a sextant or quadrant?

Slide 16

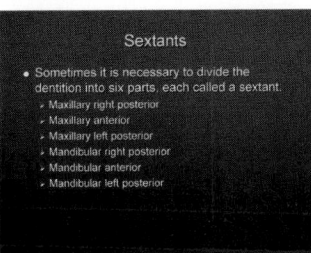

- How many teeth are in each sextant of the mouth?

ELSEVIER

Torres and Ehrlich Modern Dental Assisting, 9th ed.

Bird/Robinson

Slide 17

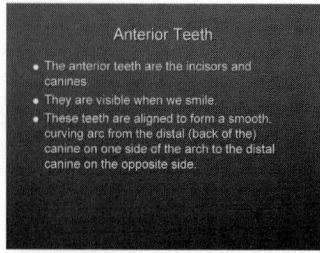

- To help in describing their location and functions, the teeth are classified as being anterior (toward the front) or posterior (toward the back).
- How many incisors are in the primary dentition?
- How many incisors are in the permanent dentition?
- How many canines are in either the primary or permanent dentition?

Slide 18

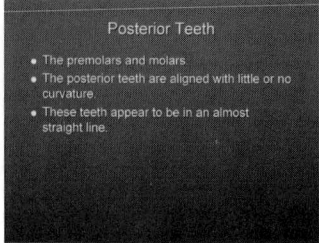

- What is the other name for premolars?
- How many premolars are in the permanent dentition? How many molars?
- How are the posterior teeth aligned in contrast to the anterior teeth?

Slide 19

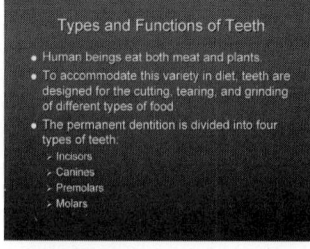

- How do the teeth help during mastication (chewing food)?

Slide 20

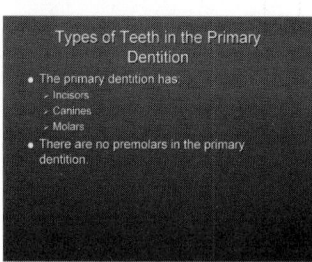

- What tooth type is absent in the primary dentition?
- What teeth types are the same for the permanent and primary dentition?

Torres and Ehrlich Modern Dental Assisting, 9th ed.

Bird/Robinson

Slide 21

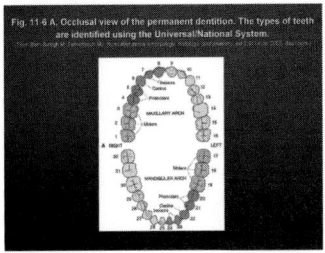

- The permanent teeth are numbered from 1 to 32 with the Universal/National Numbering System.
- Numbering begins with the upper right third molar, works around to the upper left third molar, drops to the lower left third molar, and works around to the lower right third molar.
- What teeth are usually extracted from the permanent dentition?
- What tooth is the first one to erupt into the permanent dentition?

Slide 22

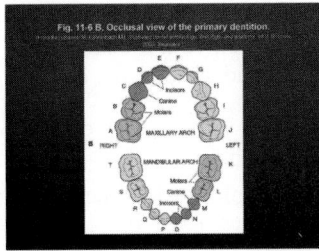

- In the Universal/National System, the primary teeth are lettered with capital letters from A to T.
- How many molars does the primary dentition have as compared to the permanent dentition?

Slide 23

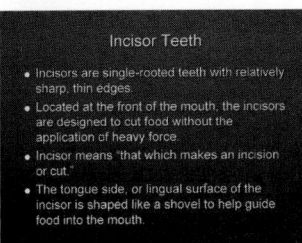

- Ask students to feel their incisors with their tongues and note the sharp and thin edges these teeth have.

Slide 24

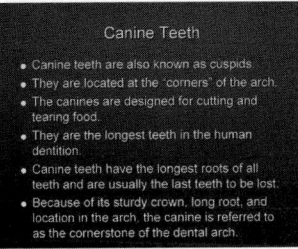

- Why are canines called "canines"?

Slide 25

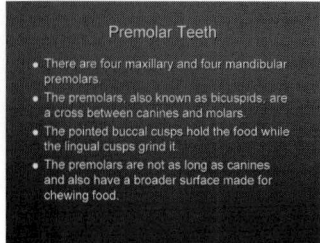

- With your tongue, feel the cusps of your premolars.
- Ask students if they have all of their premolars. Many times for spacing requirements in orthodontic therapy, the first premolar is extracted.

Slide 26

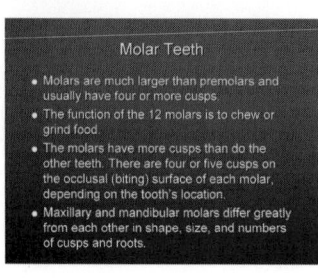

- How many types of molars does the permanent dentition have as compared to the primary dentition?
- Ask students the following question: Do you have all your molars? Many times because of impaction or spacing considerations, the third molar is extracted.
- What is the name for the space between adjacent teeth?
- What is the name of the area where adjacent teeth physically touch?
- What is the name of the triangular space toward the gingiva between adjacent teeth?

Slide 27

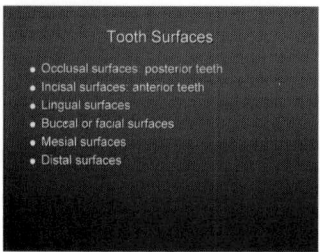

- The facial surface is the surface closest to the face.
- The lingual surface is the surface of mandibular and maxillary teeth that is closest to the tongue.
- The masticatory surface is the chewing surface. On anterior teeth, it is the incisal surface (or incisal edge), and on posterior teeth it is the occlusal surface.
- The mesial surface is the surface of the tooth toward the midline.
- The distal surface is the surface of the tooth distant from the midline.

Slide 28

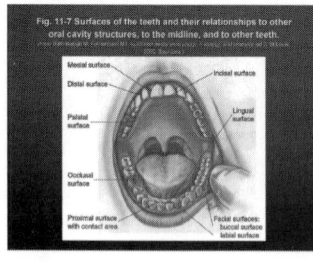

- What tooth surfaces usually get the most wear?
- What surfaces usually have the most caries?
- Which surfaces need a mirror to retract the tongue to see the gingival tissue?
- What surfaces are hard to see without a mirror?
- Which surfaces may need reflected light off the mirror to see them?

Slide 29

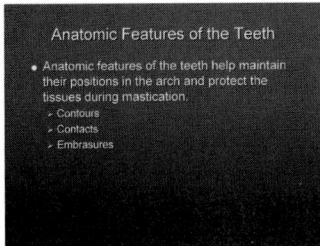

- Why do teeth have anatomic features?

Slide 30

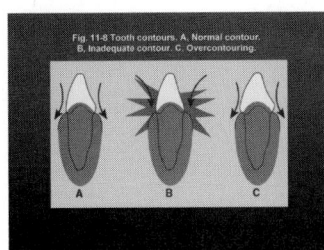

- All teeth have a curved surface except when the tooth is fractured or worn. Some surfaces are convex (curved outward); others are concave (curved inward).

- Although the general contours vary, the general principle that the crown of the tooth narrows toward the cervical line is true for all types of teeth.

- What is the term for the junction of two tooth surfaces?

Slide 31

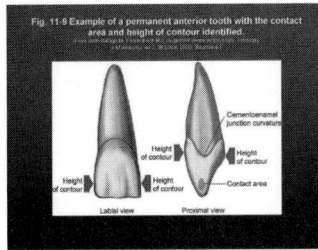

- A proper contact relationship between adjacent teeth:

  - Prevents food from being trapped between the teeth

  - Stabilizes the dental arches by holding the teeth in either arch in positive contact with each other

  - Protects the interproximal gingival tissue from trauma during mastication

- Where is the contact area on this maxillary central incisor on its labial view? Is this the same as its height of contour on its proximal surfaces?

- Note that the height of contour on this tooth on its buccal and lingual surface is not the same.

Slide 32

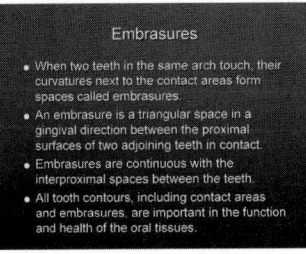

- Ask the students the following question: Can you feel the embrasures of your teeth with your tongue?

Slide 33

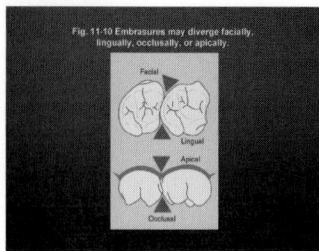

- Curvatures adjacent to the contact areas form spaces called embrasures.

Slide 34

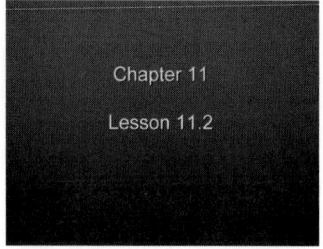

Slide 35

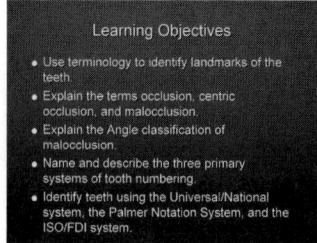

Slide 36

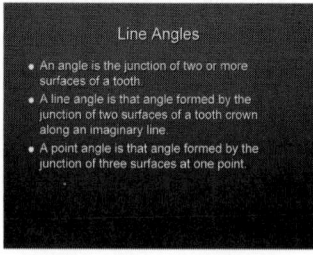

- In order to better describe the teeth, the crowns and roots of the teeth have been divided into thirds, and junctions of the crown surfaces are described as line angles and point angles.

- Actually, there are no angles or points on the teeth. Line and point angles are used only as descriptive terms to indicate specific locations.

Slide 37

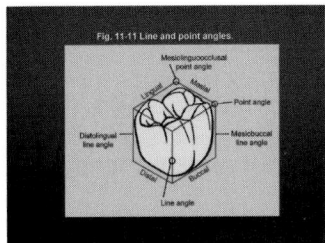

- Why is it important to have terms to indicate specific locations in dentistry?

Slide 38

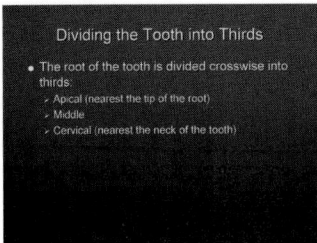

- Why is each tooth divided into thirds?

Slide 39

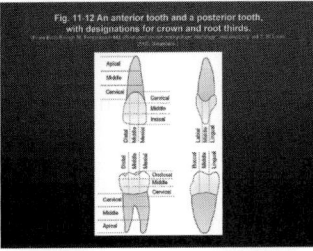

- To help identify a specific area of the tooth, each surface is divided into imaginary thirds.
- The crown of the tooth is divided into thirds in three divisions:
  - Occlusocervical division
  - Mesiodistal division
  - Buccolingual division
- Which third of the molar's crown usually decays first?

Slide 40

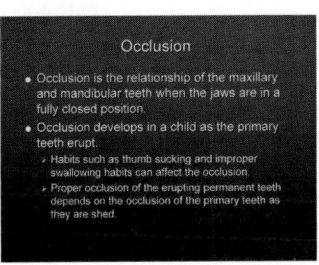

- Why is occlusion important in the overall health of a patient? *(Occlusion-related problems could affect the teeth, joints, and muscles of the head and neck and cause periodontal trauma.)*
- What is the name for the position of the teeth in chewing movements?
- What is the term for teeth that are in poor occlusion?

Torres and Ehrlich Modern Dental Assisting, 9th ed.
Bird/Robinson

Slide 41

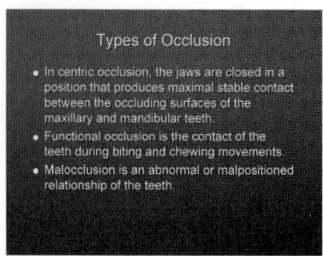

Types of Occlusion

- In centric occlusion, the jaws are closed in a position that produces maximal stable contact between the occluding surfaces of the maxillary and mandibular teeth.
- Functional occlusion is the contact of the teeth during biting and chewing movements.
- Malocclusion is an abnormal or malpositioned relationship of the teeth.

- What is the difference between centric and functional occlusion?

- Is appearance the important thing when teeth are in a malocclusion, or does the malocclsion affect the health of the mouth?

- Is it harder to keep a malocclusion clean during oral hygiene procedures?

- Which teeth will have more caries and periodontal concerns: an aligned dentition or a malocclusion?

Slide 42

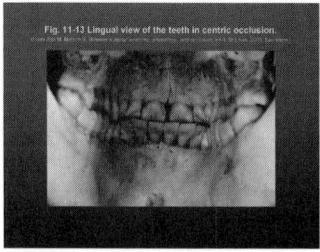

Fig. 11-13 Lingual view of the teeth in centric occlusion.

Slide 43

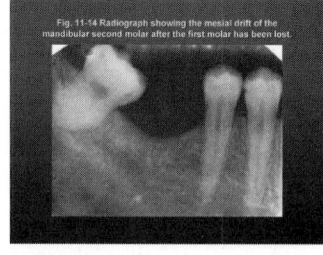

Fig. 11-14 Radiograph showing the mesial drift of the mandibular second molar after the first molar has been lost.

- Permanent posterior teeth exhibit physiological mesial drift—the tendency to drift mesially when space is available. If the primary second molars are lost prematurely, the first permanent molars drift anteriorly and block out the second premolars.

- If a primary second molar is extracted prematurely, a space maintainer can be fabricated by the dentist.

- Why does the bone undergo resorption when a tooth is lost?

- Does mesial drift help increase the crowding of the mandibular anteriors over time?

Slide 44

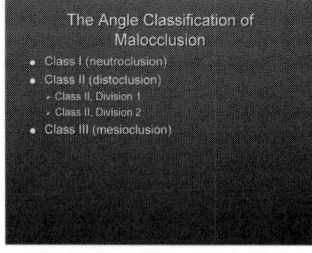

The Angle Classification of Malocclusion
- Class I (neutroclusion)
- Class II (distoclusion)
  - Class II, Division 1
  - Class II, Division 2
- Class III (mesioclusion)

- What is malocclusion?

- Why does malocclusion occur?

- Dr. Edward H. Angle developed this classification system to describe and classify occlusion and malocclusion.

- Describe each class in Angle's classification system.

- What classification is neutroclusion?

Bird/Robinson

Slide 45

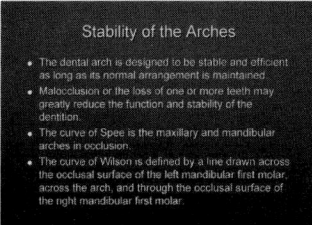

- Once the teeth erupt into the oral cavity, the position of teeth is affected by other teeth, both in the same dental arch and in the opposing dental arch.
- Tooth loss leaves one or more teeth without an antagonist. Also, teeth drift, tip, and rotate when other teeth in the arch are extracted.

Slide 46

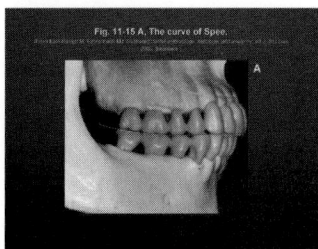

- The curve of Spee is described by the maxillary and mandibular arches in occlusion.
- On a radiograph, the occlusal line of the teeth appears to be smiling (as it does here).

Slide 47

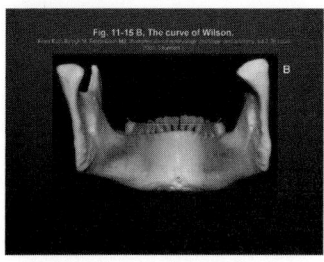

- The curve of Wilson is defined by a line drawn across the occlusal surface of the left mandibular first molar, across the arch, and through the occlusal surface of the right mandibular first molar.
- The curve of Wilson is flatter than the curve of Spee.

Slide 48

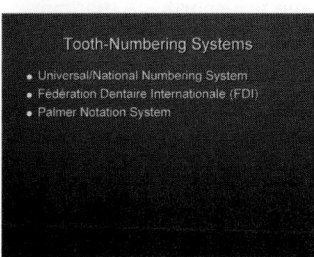

- Numbering systems are used as a simplified means of identifying the teeth for charting and descriptive purposes.
- Three basic numbering systems are used, and the dental assistant must be familiar with each system.

Slide 49

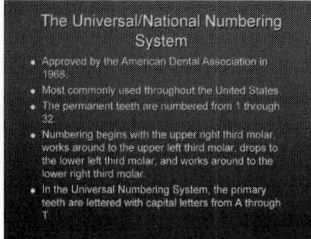

- Does the numbering of the teeth for the Universal or National System proceed in a clockwise fashion or counter-clockwise fashion?

- Extreme care must be taken when entering tooth numbers on records or carrying out verbal instructions regarding a specific tooth. Errors have resulted in the extraction of the wrong tooth.

- Remember that all dental records are legal documents. Learn the charting systems, and make charting entries accurately. They may have to be explained in a court of law.

Slide 50

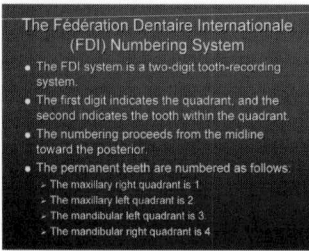

- The FDI system is used in Canada and around the world. It is simpler to use on a computer.

- To avoid miscommunication internationally, the ISO/FDI system also designates areas in the oral cavity. A two-digit number designates these, and at least one of the two digits is zero (0).

- In this system, for example, "00" designates the whole oral cavity, and "01" indicates the maxillary area only.

Slide 51

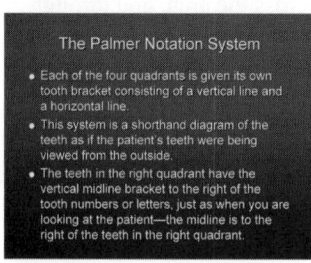

- When is the Palmer system used? Can you make up the tooth bracket needed to use the Palmer system?

Slide 52

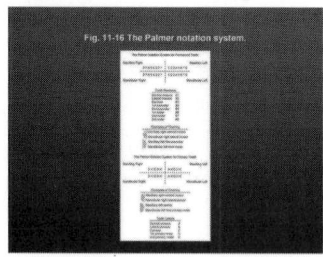

- Each of the four quadrants is given its own tooth bracket made up of a vertical line and a horizontal line. This system is a shorthand diagram of the teeth as if the patient's teeth were being viewed from the outside.

12 Lesson Plan
Tooth Morphology

TEACHING FOCUS

This chapter will introduce the student to topics related to tooth morphology. The student will have the opportunity to learn the location, features, and clinical considerations of each permanent tooth, as well as the features and clinical considerations of the primary dentition.

MATERIALS AND RESOURCES

- ☐ ADA/dental clinic form for charting teeth (Lesson 12.1)
- ☐ computer and PowerPoint projector (all Lessons)
- ☐ dental mirrors (Lesson 12.2)
- ☐ sets of teeth for identification (all Lessons)
- ☐ tooth chart (Lesson 12.1)

LESSON CHECKLIST

Preparations for this lesson include:

- lecture
- evaluation of student knowledge and skills needed to understand tooth morphology, including:
  - ○ clinical considerations of permanent teeth and primary dentition
  - ○ features of permanent teeth and primary dentition
  - ○ location of permanent teeth

ELSEVIER

KEY TERMS

bicanineate (p. 157)
bifurcated (p. 156)
bifurcation (p. 159)
canine eminence (p. 153)
central groove (p. 155)
cingulum (p. 150)
cusp (p. 153)
cusp of Carabelli (p. 158)
diastema (p. 152)
fossa (p. 150)
furcation (p. 156)
imbrication lines (p. 152)
incisal edge (p. 151)

inclined cuspal planes (p. 155)
mamelon (p. 151)
marginal groove (p. 155)
marginal ridge (p. 150)
molars (p. 154)
morphology (p. 150)
nonsuccedaneous (p. 158)
pegged laterals (p. 152)
succedaneous (p. 150)
triangular groove (p. 155)
tricanineate (p. 157)
trifurcated (p. 158)
trifurcation (p. 158)

ADDITIONAL RESOURCES

PowerPoint slides (Evolve): 1-98

Legend

CTQ
Critical
Thinking
Question

DVD
Multimedia
Procedures
Videos and
Animations

ESLR
EVOLVE
Student
Learning
Resources

IDO
Interactive
Dental
Office
CD-ROM

SW
Student
Workbook

TB
Test Bank
on the
TEACH
CD-ROM

PPT
PowerPoint
Slides

Class Activities are indicated in **_bold italic._**

ELSEVIER

Torres and Ehrlich Modern Dental Assisting, 9th ed.

Bird/Robinson

LESSON 12.1

PRETEST

1. What is a bicanineate?
   a. a two-cusp type of tooth
   b. a tooth with two roots
   c. two ridges on the occlusal table
   d. an area in which two roots divide

2. Where is the cusp of Carabelli located on the maxillary first molar?
   a. buccal to the distolingual cusp
   b. lingual to the mesiolingual cusp
   c. facial to the mesiobuccal cusp
   d. palatal to the distobuccal cusp

3. What is the term for a space between two teeth?
   a. primate space
   b. diastema
   c. fossa
   d. furcation

4. Which of the following do all mature anterior teeth have?
   a. lingual pit
   b. lingual fossa
   c. cingulum
   d. mamelons

5. What are the Universal System numbers for the maxillary central incisor teeth?
   a. #6 and #11
   b. #8 and #9
   c. #2 and #14
   d. #5 and #12

6. Which of the following is a common developmental anomaly for lateral incisors?
   a. pegged laterals
   b. fused root
   c. furcated root
   d. shovel-shaped

7. Which tooth is the "cornerstone of the dentition"?
   a. molar
   b. premolar
   c. canine
   d. incisor

8. Which tooth is usually the first permanent tooth to erupt in the oral cavity?
   a. mandibular incisors
   b. mandibular canines
   c. mandibular premolars
   d. mandibular first molars

9. Which of the following is correct concerning the primary teeth in contrast with the permanent teeth?
   a. whiter due to increased enamel opacity
   b. longer crowns than overall length
   c. wider roots than crown
   d. shorter roots than crown

10. For how many years are primary teeth needed for chewing, appearance, and speech?
    a. 2 to 4 years
    b. 4 to 6 years
    c. 5 to 11 years
    d. 7 to 16 years

Answers

1. a	3. b	5. b	7. c	9. a
2. b	4. c	6. a	8. d	10. c

BACKGROUND ASSESSMENT

Question: Which teeth are the last to be lost? Why do they last so long?
Answer: The permanent canines are the longest teeth in the dentition. The canine has a particularly long, thick root. The root is usually the same length as, or twice the length of, the crown. The crown of the canine is shaped in a manner that promotes cleanliness. Because of the self-cleansing shape and the sturdy anchorage in the jaws, the canines are usually the last teeth to be lost.

Question: How many molars are in the permanent dentition? What do their names indicate and what is their function? How many types are found in the permanent dentition? What is their eruption pattern? How many cusps and roots do they have?

Answer: There are 12 molars in the permanent dentition, 3 in each quadrant. The permanent molars are the largest teeth in the dentition. The name molar comes from the Latin word for "grinding," one of the functions of the molar teeth. There are three types of molars: the first molar, second molar, and third molar. The first and second molars are also called the 6-year and 12-year molars, respectively, because of the approximate ages at eruption. Many times the third molar does not erupt because of impaction. The molar crowns have four or five short, blunt cusps, and each molar has two or three roots that help to support the larger crown.

CRITICAL THINKING QUESTION
The mother of your child patient is concerned that her child's new teeth have unsightly bumps on them. She points them out to you and wants to know why something is not being done to make her daughter have a better smile. She wants the dentist to grind down the teeth so they look straight. What can you say to her?
Guidelines: You need to let her know that when newly erupted, the central and lateral incisors have three mamelons, or rounded enamel extensions on the incisal ridge, or edge. The mamelons usually undergo attrition (wearing away of a tooth surface) shortly after eruption. Then the incisal ridge appears flattened and becomes the incisal edge. There is no need to have these small extensions removed by the dentist.

OBJECTIVES	CONTENT	TEACHING RESOURCES
Pronounce, define, and spell the Key Terms.	■ Key terms (p. 149)	SW Fill in the Blank questions 1-13 (pp. 41-42) ESLR Electronic Flashcards *Class Activity Have student pairs make flash cards of the key terms with the terms on one side and the definitions on the other. Then, have the students quiz each other on the terms. Correct their pronunciation as needed.*
Use the correct terminology when discussing features of the permanent dentition.	■ Introduction (p. 150)	PPT 5-7 TB question 1 SW Short-Answer Questions 3; Fill in the Blank questions 6, 9; Multiple Choice questions 1-3 (pp. 41-42) SW Activity 5 (p. 44) Figure 12-1 Stainless steel crowns are available in a variety of sizes for each tooth (p. 150) CTQ 1 (p. 166) ▶ Discuss the various clinical applications that would use tooth morphology. *Class Activity Discuss as a class how tooth morphology may vary from patient to patient and how a dental assistant can still identify the tooth.*
Identify each tooth using the correct terms and Universal/ National System code numbers.	■ Anterior permanent dentition (p. 150)	PPT 8-10 SW Short-Answer Questions 1; Multiple Choice question 18 (pp. 41, 43) Figure 12-2 Attractive teeth are important for a nice smile (p. 150) Recall questions 1-3 (p. 152)

Torres and Ehrlich Modern Dental Assisting, 9th ed.

Bird/Robinson

OBJECTIVES	CONTENT	TEACHING RESOURCES
		♀ CTQ 3 (p. 166)
		▸ Discuss how the Universal Numbering System for permanent teeth can aid in tooth morphology.
		▸ Discuss the importance of the anterior teeth in a person's appearance.
		*Class Activity **Have pairs of students chart each other's permanent dentition using the standard ADA form or school dental clinic form by coloring the teeth present and crossing out teeth not present. Have them note any anomalies in form or numbers.***
Identify the location of each permanent tooth.	☐ Permanent incisors (p. 151)	PPT 11
		SW Short-Answer Questions 2 (p. 41)
		Figure 12-3 Various views of a newly erupted permanent maxillary incisor showing its features (p. 151)
		Recall question 4 (p. 152)
		▸ Discuss the differences between maxillary and mandibular incisors.
		▸ Discuss the clinical considerations of the permanent incisors.
		*Class Activity **Have students fill in the numbers of the permanent incisors on a tooth chart, just showing the outlines.***
Describe the general and specific features of each tooth in the permanent dentition.	– Maxillary central incisors (p. 151) – Maxillary lateral incisors (pp. 151-152) – Mandibular incisors (p. 152)	PPT 12-24
		TB questions 2-4
		SW Short-Answer Questions 4; Fill in the Blank questions 7-8, 10; Multiple Choice questions 4-5, 7 (pp. 41-42)
		Figure 12-4 Various views of a permanent maxillary right central incisor (p. 151)
		Figure 12-5 Mamelons are the rounded portions of the incisal edge of the lower central incisors (p. 151)
		Figure 12-6 Various views of a permanent maxillary right lateral incisor (p. 152)
		Figure 12-7 Pegged maxillary lateral incisor (p. 152)
		Figure 12-8 Various views of a permanent mandibular right central incisor (p. 153)
		Figure 12-9 Various views of a permanent mandibular right lateral incisor (p. 153)
		Recall questions 5-7 (p. 154)

OBJECTIVES	CONTENT	TEACHING RESOURCES
		▸ Discuss the importance of mamelons on newly erupted teeth and how they change over time. *Class Activity* **Divide the class into small groups, and have each group discuss the unique anatomic features of the maxillary central incisors. Then have each group present its findings to the class.**
Discuss clinical considerations of each tooth in the permanent dentition.	– Maxillary central incisors (p. 151) – Maxillary lateral incisors (pp. 151-152) – Mandibular incisors (p. 152)	SW Short-Answer Questions 5 (p. 41) Clinical Considerations: Incisors (p. 153) ▸ Discuss how the maxillary and mandibular incisors function together. *Class Activity* **Divide the class into small groups, and have each group discuss the reasons a dental assistant must know the location of grooves and ridges in incisor teeth. Then have each group present its findings to the class.**
Identify the location of each permanent tooth.	☐ Permanent canines (p. 153)	TB question 5 SW Short-Answer Questions 2; Fill in the Blank questions 1, 4 (pp. 41-42) ▸ Discuss the derivation of the term "canine" and why that term was used to describe these types of teeth. *Class Activity* **Place a set of canines on a classroom table, and have the students identify surfaces and landmarks of the teeth. Then lead a class discussion on the importance of knowing the surfaces and landmarks.**
Describe the general and specific features of each tooth in the permanent dentition.	– Maxillary canines (p. 153) – Mandibular canines (p. 154)	PPT 25-28 TB question 6 SW Short-Answer Questions 4; Fill in the Blank question 4 (pp. 41-42) Recall questions 5-7 (p. 154) Figure 12-10 Views of permanent mandibular and maxillary canines (p. 154) Figure 12-11 Various views of a permanent mandibular right canine (p. 154) ▸ Discuss the difference between the canine and the incisor. ▸ Discuss how the cusp slopes can change with attrition. *Class Activity* **Divide the class into small groups, and have each group prepare a list of the challenges presented to the dental assistant by the similarities in appearance of the maxillary and mandibular canines. Write each list on the board, and lead a class discussion.**

Bird/Robinson

OBJECTIVES	CONTENT	TEACHING RESOURCES
Discuss clinical considerations of each tooth in the permanent dentition.	– Maxillary canines (p. 153) – Mandibular canines (p. 154)	PPT 29-31 SW Short-Answer Questions 5 (p. 41) Clinical Considerations: Canines (p. 154) ▶ Discuss why permanent canines are called the cornerstone of the dental arches. ▶ Discuss why the canines are the last teeth a person might lose with age. *Class Activity Divide the class into small groups, and have each group discuss the differences in appearance between a mandibular canine and maxillary canine. Have each group draw the teeth with indications of the differences. Then have each group present its drawings to the class for discussion.*

12.1 Homework/Assignments:

12.1 Instructor's Note/Student Feedback:

LESSON 12.2

CRITICAL THINKING QUESTION

You have a young pediatric patient with a mixed dentition in the chair. He has had many caries in his primary dentition. He has a poor diet and does not have parental supervision for dental care at home. What can be done by the dental office for the child's emerging dentition, and what teeth and surfaces would it involve?

Guidelines: You can support the recommendation by the dentist to place sealants. These would be placed on the permanent molars (and possibly the premolars) as soon as they erupt. The natural pits and grooves between the cusps on these teeth make them very susceptible to tooth decay. The dental sealants will fill the pits and fissures, thus preventing tooth decay.

OBJECTIVES	CONTENT	TEACHING RESOURCES
Identify the location of each permanent tooth.	■ Posterior permanent dentition (pp. 154-155) □ Permanent premolars (p. 155)	PPT 34-39 TB question 7 SW Short-Answer Questions 2; Fill in the Blank questions 2, 5, 11; Multiple Choice questions 8-9 (pp. 41-43) Figure 12-12 Occlusal surface on a permanent posterior tooth and its features (p. 155) Figure 12-13 Other features of the occlusal table on a permanent posterior tooth (p. 155) ▸ Discuss what constitutes the posterior permanent teeth. ▸ Discuss what features are unique to the posterior permanent teeth. *Class Activity Give the students dental mirrors; have each student look at his or her permanent posterior teeth and identify the three types and two arches.*
Describe the general and specific features of each tooth in the permanent dentition.	– Maxillary first premolars (p. 155) – Maxillary second premolars (p. 156) – Mandibular first premolars (p. 156) – Mandibular second premolars (p. 157)	PPT 40-50 TB questions 8-10 SW Short-Answer Questions 4; Fill in the Blank question 3; Multiple Choice questions 6, 10-11 (pp. 41-43) SW Activities 1-3 (p. 43) Figure 12-14 Various views of a permanent maxillary first premolar (p. 156) Figure 12-15 Various views of a permanent mandibular right first premolar (p. 156) Recall questions 8-11 (p. 157) Figure 12-16 Various views of a permanent mandibular second premolar (p. 157) Figure 12-17 Occlusal views of a permanent mandibular second premolar (p. 157)

OBJECTIVES	CONTENT	TEACHING RESOURCES
		▸ Discuss how to identify a first premolar and a second premolar.
		▸ Discuss the differences between tricanineate and bicanineate teeth.
		*Class Activity **Have each student write a short paragraph on the clinical considerations of the permanent posterior teeth. Select students at random to read their paragraphs, and then lead a class discussion.***
Discuss clinical considerations of each tooth in the permanent dentition.	– Maxillary first premolars (p. 155) – Maxillary second premolars (p. 156) – Mandibular first premolars (p. 156) – Mandibular second premolars (p. 157)	SW Short-Answer Questions 5 (p. 41) Clinical Considerations: Posterior Teeth (p. 155) Clinical Considerations: Premolars (p. 155) ▸ Discuss why dental sealants are sometimes applied to posterior teeth as soon as they erupt. ▸ Discuss the effect on a person's appearance when they lose their molars. *Class Activity **Divide the class into small groups, and have each group prepare educational materials for an elementary school class on how the premolars work with the other teeth in chewing food. Have each group share its materials with the class.***
Identify the location of each permanent tooth.	☐ Permanent molars (p. 157)	PPT 51-52 TB question 11 SW Short-Answer Questions 2; Fill in the Blank question 12; Multiple Choice questions 12-16 (pp. 41-43) SW Activity 4 (p. 43) *Class Activity **Place a set of molars on a classroom table, and have the students identify surfaces and landmarks of the teeth. Then lead a class discussion on the importance of knowing the surfaces and landmarks.***
Describe the general and specific features of each tooth in the permanent dentition.	– Maxillary molars (p. 157) – Mandibular molars (p. 159)	PPT 53-59 TB questions 12-16, 20 SW Short-Answer Questions 4 (p. 41) Figure 12-18 (A) Maxillary first molar; (B) Mandibular first molar (p. 158) Figure 12-19 Various views of a permanent maxillary right first molar (p. 158) Figure 12-20 Various views of a permanent maxillary right second molar (p. 159) Recall questions 12-14 (p. 159)

OBJECTIVES	CONTENT	TEACHING RESOURCES
		Figure 12-21 Buccal views of permanent maxillary right molars (p. 159)
		Figure 12-22 Various views of permanent maxillary right third molars (p. 159)
		Figure 12-23 Various views of a permanent mandibular right first molar (p. 160)
		Figure 12-24 Various views of a permanent mandibular right second molar (p. 160)
		Recall questions 15-16 (p. 160)
		Figure 12-25 Various views of the permanent mandibular right third molar (p. 161)
		Figure 12-26 Buccal views of permanent mandibular right molars (p. 161)
		▸ Discuss the unique features of the permanent molars.
		▸ Discuss the differences between the mandibular first, second, and third molars.
		Class Activity Divide the class into small groups, and have the groups discuss the concept of bifurcation in the mandibular teeth and how the roots are identified. Then have each group present its findings to the class.
Discuss clinical considerations of each tooth in the permanent dentition.	– Maxillary molars (p. 157) – Mandibular molars (p. 159)	PPT 60-73 SW Short-Answer Questions 5 (p. 41) Clinical Considerations: Maxillary Molars (p. 158) Clinical Considerations: Mandibular Molars (p. 159) ▸ Discuss how patients can confuse pain caused by a sinus infection with pain caused by their maxillary teeth. ▸ Discuss why the mandibular molars can present difficulty in positioning the oral evacuator. *Class Activity Have pairs of students take turns role-playing a dental assistant teaching a patient about the difficulties and importance of oral hygiene with mandibular molars.*

12.2 Homework/Assignments:

12.2 Instructor's Notes/Student Feedback:

ELSEVIER

Torres and Ehrlich Modern Dental Assisting, 9th ed.

Bird/Robinson

LESSON 12.3

CRITICAL THINKING QUESTION

The father of a child with extensive decay of the primary molars wants the dentist just to pull the molars out. He does not see the need to restore "baby teeth" if they are just going to fall out anyway. You notice that there is already a loss of space on the maxillary arch caused by past tooth loss due to decay because the permanent teeth are not erupting in the proper sequence. How can you convince the father that the primary teeth are important? What do you need to stress with the father to help prevent further primary tooth loss?

Guidelines: You will need to tell him that although the "baby teeth" are only temporary, if they are lost prematurely, there may be serious problems with tooth alignment, spacing, and occlusion for the child later on. The primary teeth play an important role in "saving" space for the permanent teeth. In addition to providing for chewing, appearance, and speech for about 5 to 11 years, primary teeth support the cheeks and lips and a normal facial appearance. You can point out the loss of space that has already occurred, showing him on the radiographs the teeth that are having difficulty erupting in proper sequence. You can also ask the dentist to provide a referral to an orthodontist so that the general office can work with the specialist to restore the needed space for the permanent teeth in the maxillary arch. You must stress to the father that early dental health education and dental care are essential for keeping the primary dentition healthy because the enamel and dentin are thinner in primary teeth and this allows decay to travel quickly through the enamel to the pulp, possibly causing loss of the tooth and further space problems for the child.

OBJECTIVES	CONTENT	TEACHING RESOURCES
Compare and contrast the features of the primary and permanent dentitions.	■ Primary dentition (pp. 160-161)	PPT 76-78 TB questions 17-19 SW Short-Answer Questions 6; Multiple Choice question 17 (pp. 41, 43) CTQ 2, 4 (p. 166) Figure 12-27 (A) Primary mandibular molar; (B) Permanent mandibular molar (p. 161) ▶ Discuss the differences between the primary teeth and permanent teeth. ▶ Discuss how the primary teeth are identified in the Universal Numbering System. *Class Activity Place permanent teeth and primary teeth at stations in the classroom, and have students fill out a checklist to identify iwhether the teeth are permanent or primary.*
Describe the general and specific features of the primary dentition.	☐ Primary incisors (p. 161) – Maxillary central incisors (p. 161) – Maxillary lateral incisors (p. 162) – Mandibular central incisors (p. 162) – Mandibular lateral incisors (p. 162)	PPT 79-98 SW Short-Answer Questions 7; Multiple Choice questions 19-20 (pp. 41, 43) Figure 12-28 Various views of a primary maxillary right central incisor (p. 162) Figure 12-29 Various views of a primary maxillary lateral incisor (p. 162) Figure 12-30 Various views of a primary mandibular central incisor (p. 163)

Torres and Ehrlich Modern Dental Assisting, 9th ed.

Bird/Robinson

OBJECTIVES	CONTENT	TEACHING RESOURCES

	☐ Primary canines (p. 162)
	  – Maxillary canines (p. 162)
	  – Mandibular canines (p. 164)
	☐ Primary molars (p. 164)
	  – Maxillary first molars (p. 164)
	  – Maxillary second molars (p. 165)
	  – Mandibular first molars (p. 165)
	  – Mandibular second molars (p. 165)
		Figure 12-31 Various views of a primary mandibular lateral incisor (p. 163)
		Figure 12-32 Various views of a primary maxillary canine (p. 163)
		Figure 12-33 Various views of a primary mandibular canine (p. 164)
		Figure 12-34 Various views of a primary maxillary first molar (p. 164)
		Recall questions 17-18 (p. 164)
		Figure 12-35 Various views of a primary maxillary second molar (p. 165)
		Figure 12-36 Various views of a primary mandibular first molar (p. 165)
		Figure 12-37 Various views of a primary mandibular second molar (p. 165)
		Recall questions 19-21 (p. 166)
		Eye to the Future (p. 166)
		▸ Discuss the differences between the maxillary canines and mandibular canines.
		▸ Discuss what aspects of the teeth can most easily identify them as primary maxillary and mandibular teeth.
		Class Activity Divide the class into small groups, and have the groups prepare a patient education brochure on the importance of the primary dentition. Then have each group present its brochure to the class.

Discuss clinical considerations of each tooth in the permanent dentition.	☐ Primary incisors (p. 161)
	  – Maxillary central incisors (p. 161)
	  – Maxillary lateral incisors (p. 162)
	  – Mandibular central incisors (p. 162)
	  – Mandibular lateral incisors (p. 162)
	☐ Primary canines (p. 162)
	  – Maxillary canines (p. 162)
	  – Mandibular canines (p. 164)
	☐ Primary molars (p. 164)
		SW Short-Answer Questions 8 (p. 41)
		Clinical Considerations: Primary Teeth (p. 161)
		▸ Discuss why decay can become more rampant in primary teeth.
		Class Activity Have the class discuss why "baby teeth" are important to a person's long-term dental health.

Bird/Robinson

OBJECTIVES	CONTENT	TEACHING RESOURCES
	– Maxillary first molars (p. 164)	
	– Maxillary second molars (p. 165)	
	– Mandibular first molars (p. 165)	
	– Mandibular second molars (p. 165)	
Performance Evaluation		TB SW questions (pp. 41-43) SW Activities (pp. 43-44) ESLR Electronic Flashcards ESLR Practice Quiz Recall questions (pp. 152-166) CTQ (p. 166)

12.3 Homework/Assignments:

12.3 Instructor's Notes/Student Feedback:

Slide 1

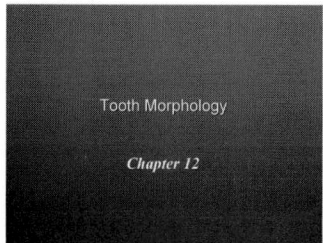

Slide 2

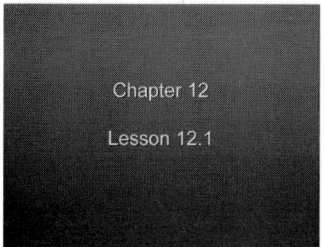

Slide 3

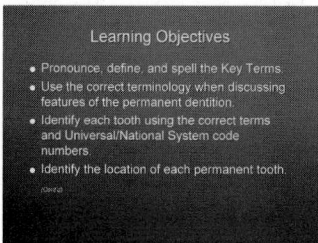

Slide 4

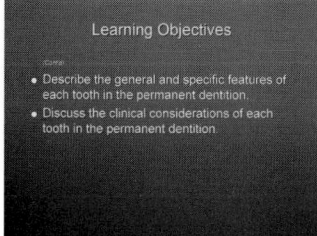

Slide 5

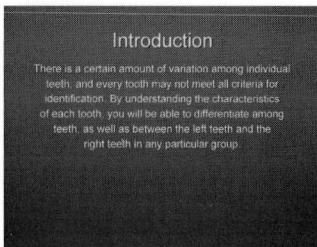

- What does "morphology" mean?

Slide 6

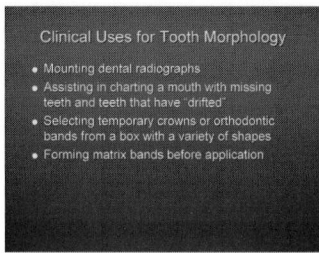

- Although morphology provides useful guidelines for the shape and positioning of teeth, there is always a certain amount of individual variation.

- Understanding the general characteristics of teeth allows for identification and differentiation of an individual's teeth.

Slide 7

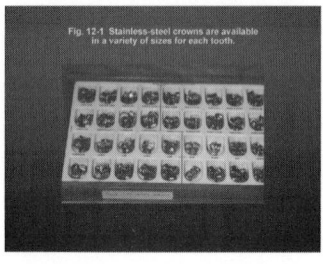

- A thorough understanding of tooth morphology is useful in selecting appropriate appliances.

Slide 8

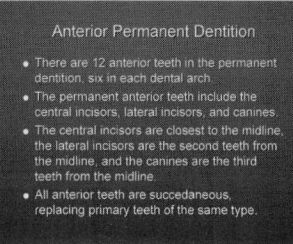

- Permanent anterior teeth tend to be the first to erupt and replace primary teeth.

Torres and Ehrlich Modern Dental Assisting, 9th ed.

Bird/Robinson

Slide 9

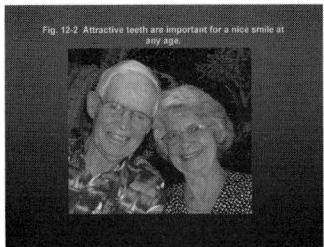

- People can be extremely self-conscious about the appearance of their front teeth and may take better care of a nice smile than one they are not proud of.

- The size, shape, color, and position of the anterior teeth may affect a person's appearance and self-esteem.

Slide 10

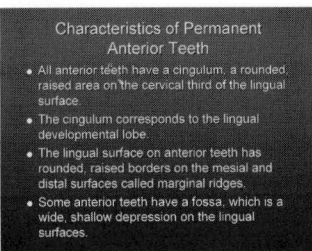

- Do these lingual surfaces make a difference when brushing the anterior teeth?

Slide 11

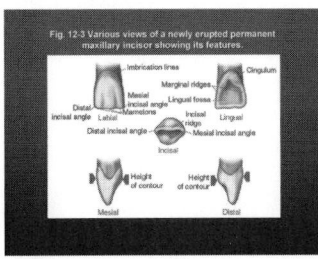

- What features do all anterior teeth have?

- Note the thin crown on the incisor, which is an adaptation for tearing food.

Slide 12

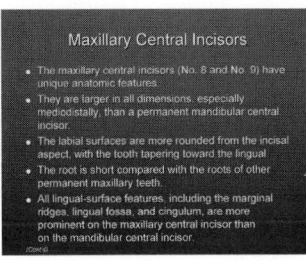

- What is the meaning of "mesiodistally"?

- The maxillary central incisors are the most prominent teeth in the mouth.

ELSEVIER

Torres and Ehrlich Modern Dental Assisting, 9th ed.

Bird/Robinson

Slide 13

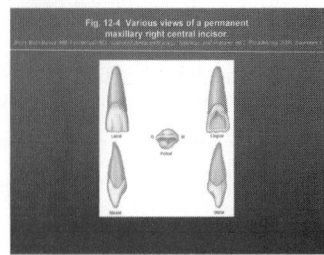

- The incisors present a triangular outline.
- Note the virtually straight incisal edge and curve in the cervical line.

Slide 14

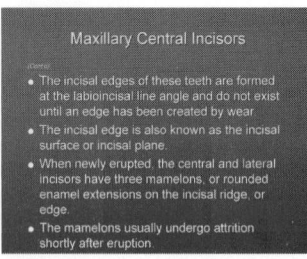

- What feature do newly erupted central and lateral incisors have on the incisal ridge?
- Some incisors may present with a distinctive shovel-shaped appearance on the lingual aspect. This feature appears more frequently in persons of Asian origin, and in many Native Americans.

Slide 15

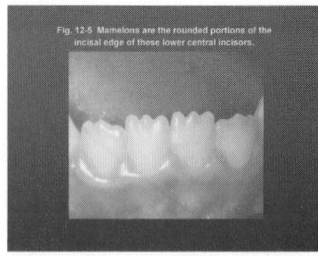

- What is meant by attrition? *(Mechanical wear of teeth during use.)*

Slide 16

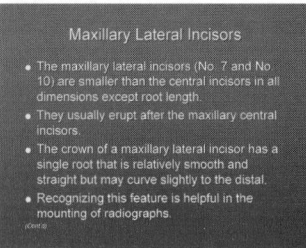

- When a lingual pit is present, the tooth is more susceptible to caries.

Bird/Robinson

Slide 17

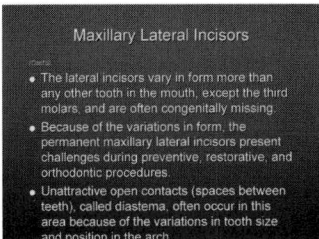

- Treatment for diastemas can include orthodontic treatment, crowns, or veneers.

Slide 18

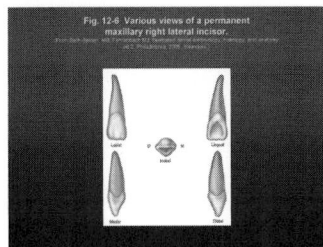

- Note the narrow, cone-shaped appearance of the incisor.

- These teeth are among the most likely to be missing congenitally or because of heredity.

Slide 19

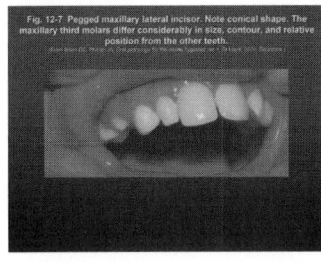

- What are pegged laterals? *(Maxillary lateral incisors with a pointed or tapered shape.)*

Slide 20

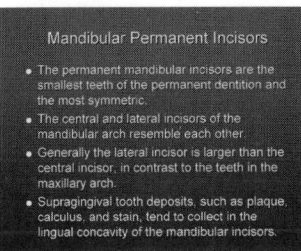

- In general, the mandibular central incisor is the smallest tooth in the human mouth.

- Supernumerary teeth often form among the upper incisors.

Bird/Robinson

Slide 21

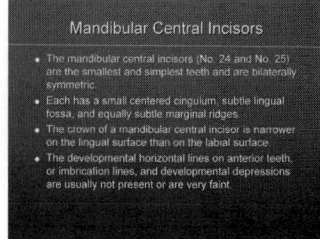

- The mandibular central incisors present with a strong degree of bilateral symmetry.

Slide 22

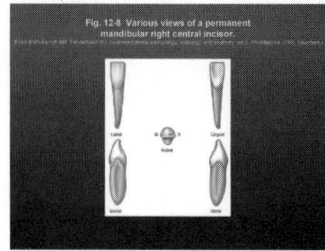

- Note the symmetrical nature of the tooth.
- The lingual surface is concave, with slight fossa and cingulum.

Slide 23

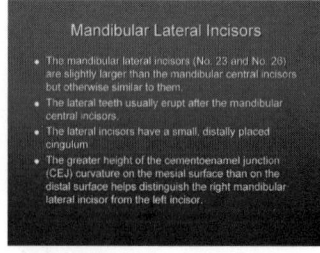

- There is less symmetry than in the mandibular central incisors.
- The mandibular lateral incisors have slightly larger roots than the central incisors.

Slide 24

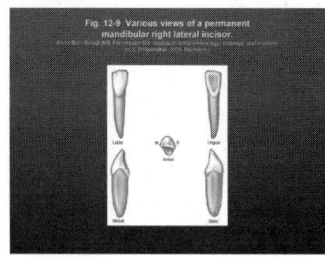

- Note the "twist" in the incisal edge.
- The distal surface tends to have a more pronounced curve than that on the central incisors.

Bird/Robinson

Slide 25

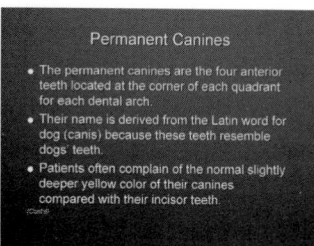

- "Cuspid" is an older term that has been used in place of "canine."
- A cusp is a major elevation on a chewing surface.

Slide 26

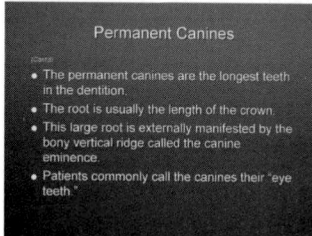

- Canines are considered the "cornerstones" of the dentition.

Slide 27

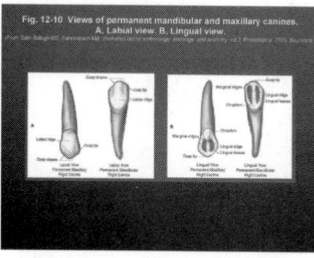

- Canines are the only teeth with one cusp.
- Note the single root and canine eminence.

Slide 28

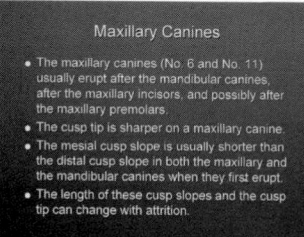

- The maxillary canine is narrower than the central incisor.

Slide 29

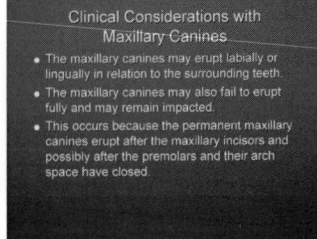

- What makes the canine teeth self-cleaning? *(Their location and shape.)*
- Why are the canines frequently the last teeth to be lost?
- The canines are very important in establishing a natural facial contour.

Slide 30

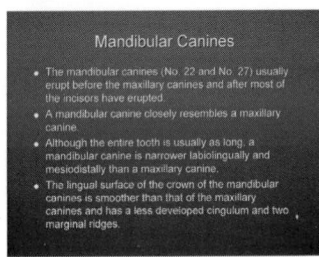

- Lower permanent canines on occasion have a bifurcation near the apex, resulting in two short roots.

Slide 31

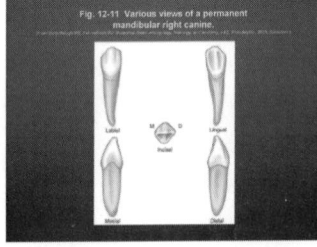

- Note the lack of symmetry common to all canines.

Slide 32

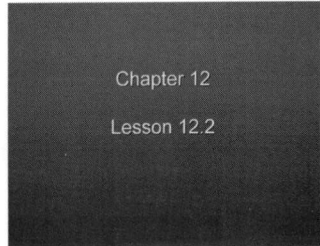

Torres and Ehrlich Modern Dental Assisting, 9th ed.

Bird/Robinson

Slide 33

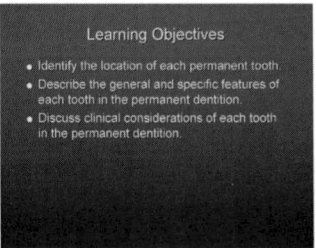

Slide 34

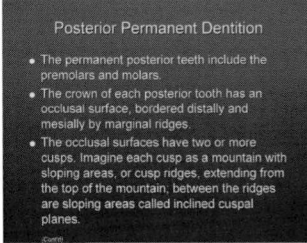

- The posterior dentition is important for grinding and chewing food and for maintaining the shape of the face.

Slide 35

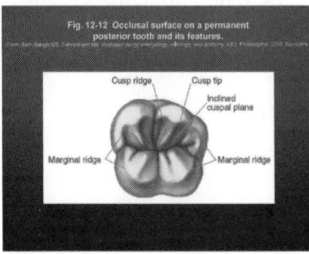

- The premolars are also known as bicuspids because of the two large prominences.

Slide 36

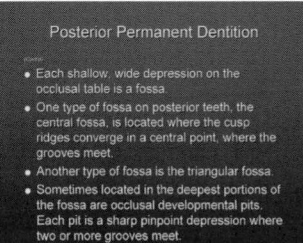

- How do occlusal pits relate to the fossa on the tooth?
- How might dental sealants help with grooves, pits, etc.?

Slide 37

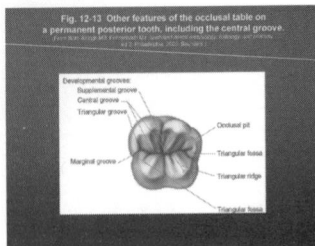

- What are developmental grooves?
- Note the occlusal pit formed by the junction of grooves.
- Pits are more common in teeth with three cusps.

Slide 38

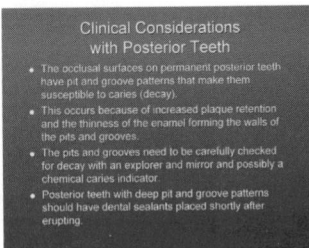

- Would the morphology and position of the posterior teeth make identification of caries more difficult? Why?

Slide 39

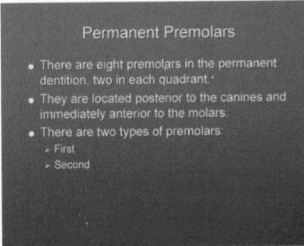

- Primitive mammals had four premolars per quadrant. The most mesial two have been lost in New World monkeys, apes, and humans.

Slide 40

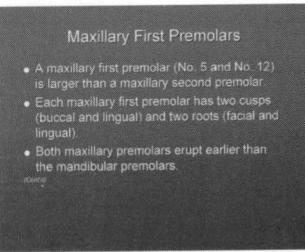

- The buccal cusp is the larger of the two cusps.
- The lower second premolar may, at times, present with two lingual cusps.

Slide 41

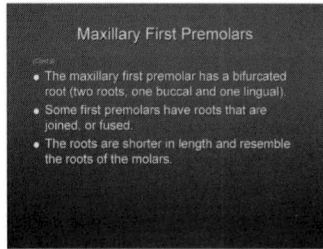

- In contrast to the roots, the crown of the first premolars may closely resemble the canines.
- Most upper premolars have two roots; less than one fifth present with a single root.

Slide 42

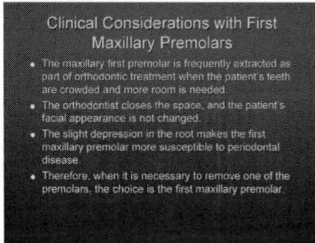

Slide 43

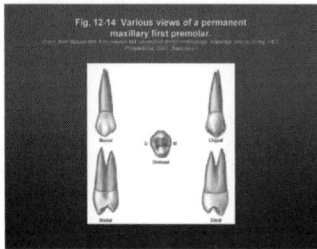

- Note the larger buccal cusps and the well-defined occlusal groove.
- The concave depression near the root line is known as the canine fossa. Why might this term be misleading?
- Why is the buccal cusp large and sharp?

Slide 44

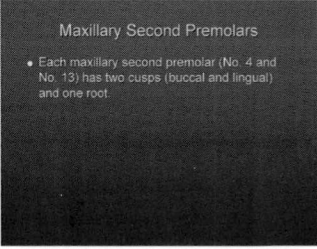

- The buccal cusp is shorter, less pointed, and more rounded than the first.

Bird/Robinson

Slide 45

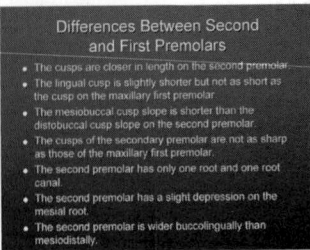

- In most facets, second premolars are similar to first premolars but less defined.
- Many features tend to be more rounded in second premolars.

Slide 46

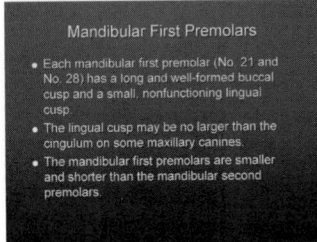

- The lingual cusp on this tooth is the smallest of any tooth.

Slide 47

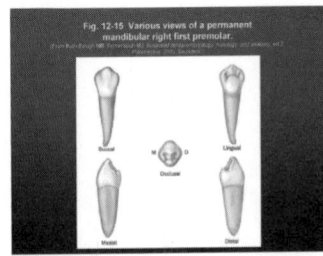

- Note the bilateral symmetry.
- Note the large buccal cusp and the diamond shape of the occlusal outline.

Slide 48

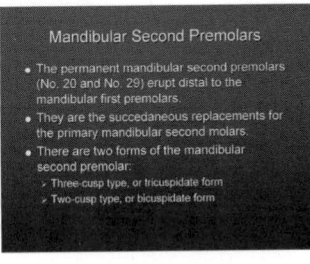

- Mandibular second premolars tend to be larger than the first, but the buccal cusp is less pronounced.
- This tooth is among the most frequently missing because of heredity or congenital factors.

Bird/Robinson

Slide 49

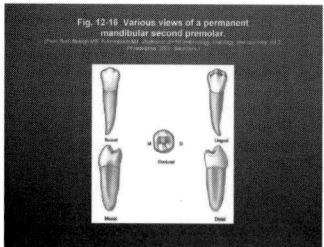

Slide 50

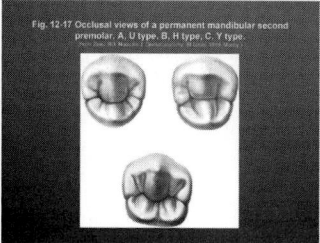

- Note the single deep groove in the two-cusp teeth, compared to the distinctive Y pattern of the three-cusp tooth.

Slide 51

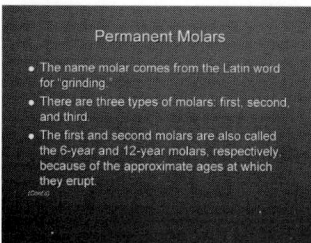

- The permanent molars are the largest teeth in the dentition.

- Molar teeth are not preceded by primary teeth.

Slide 52

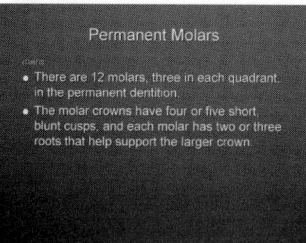

- In most individuals, lower molars have two lingual cusps while upper permanent molars present with two buccal cusps.

- Lower molars generally have two roots whereas upper molars generally have three roots.

Torres and Ehrlich Modern Dental Assisting, 9th ed.

Bird/Robinson

Slide 53

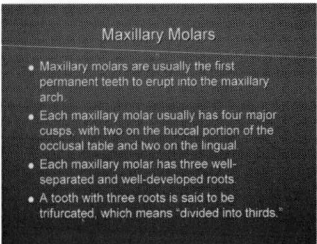

Slide 54

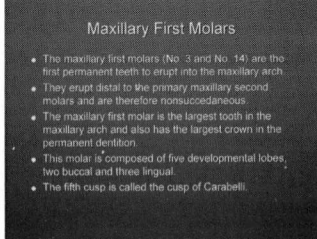

- The cusp of Carabelli is much less pronounced than the other cusps and has little practical use.

- Because of the typical age at eruption, children and parents may need to be educated that the maxillary and mandibular first molars are permanent dentition.

Slide 55

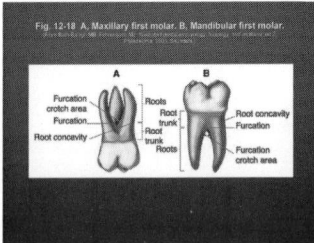

- Note the three roots on the maxillary molar, compared to two roots on the mandibular.

- Note that mandibular molars tend to be wider than maxillary, with larger cusps.

Slide 56

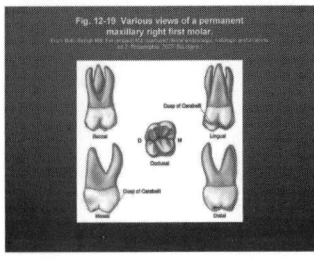

- Note that the size of the roots parallels the buccal and two lingual cusps.

- According to anthropologists, the fourth and fifth cusps are more recent in human development. The cusps are used to trace population movements in prehistory

- Note that the size of the roots tends to parallel the size of the cusps.

Torres and Ehrlich Modern Dental Assisting, 9th ed.

Bird/Robinson

Slide 57

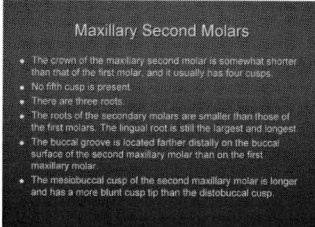

- Differences in cusp size are more noticeable on the maxillary second molars than on the first.
- Roots in the second molars are close together and sometimes fuse.

Slide 58

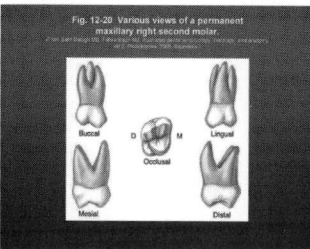

- The distolingual cusp may vary in size from fairly prominent to very small.
- Note the proximity of the three roots.

Slide 59

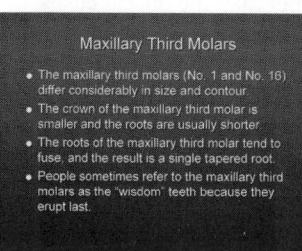

- Maxillary third molars show more variation in morphology than other teeth.
- These teeth are the most likely to be missing because of heredity or congenital causes.

Slide 60

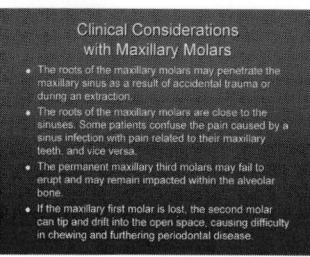

- Diagnostic tests can rule out maxillary teeth involvement when a patient may have a sinus problem.
- What advice would you give a patient having difficulty brushing the maxillary molars?
- Impacted third molars can irritate the surrounding tissue, leading to pain and swelling.

Bird/Robinson

Slide 61

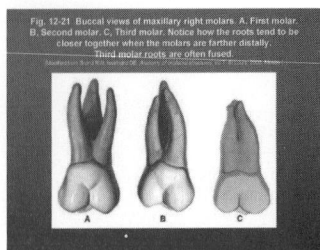

- Note the pattern of increasing proximity of the roots from first to third molar.
- Note how both cusp size and root length diminish in parallel.

Slide 62

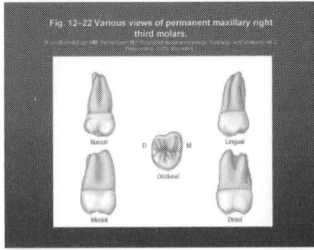

- Note the closely proximate or fused roots and the less pronounced cusps compared to the first or second molars.

Slide 63

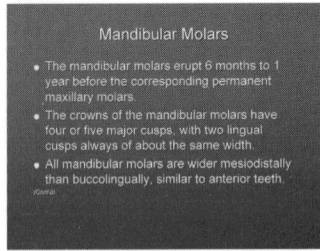

- The lingual cusps tend to be longer and sharper than the buccal cusps.

Slide 64

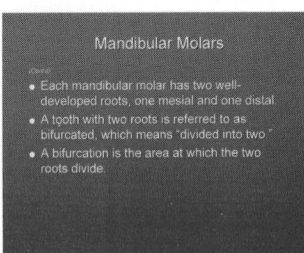

- The mesial root is wider than the distal.
- Both roots are generally the same length.

Bird/Robinson

Slide 65

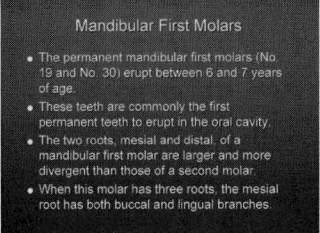

- A third root presents in rare cases, often among Native Americans.

Slide 66

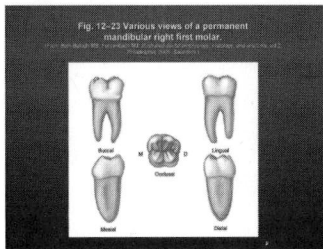

- Note that the buccal cups are the largest (and widest) of the cusps.
- In general, the distal cusp is poorly developed. In some cases, the molar may have four cusps.
- Rare cases present with a sixth cusp.

Slide 67

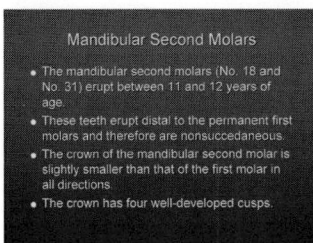

- Roots on the second molars tend to be shorter than on the first.
- A fifth cusp is seen in rare cases.

Slide 68

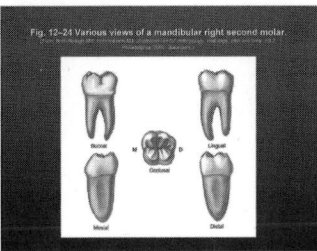

- Note the prominent buccal cusps and the bifurcated roots.

Slide 69

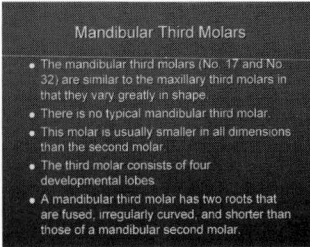

- The crown of the mandibular third molar tends to be more rounded than the first or second molars.
- Four or five cusps may be present.

Slide 70

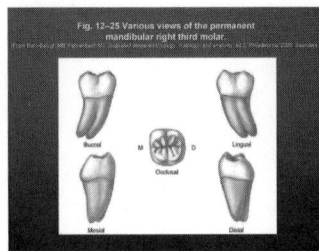

- Note the rounded shape of the cusps, and the nearly fused appearance of the roots.

Slide 71

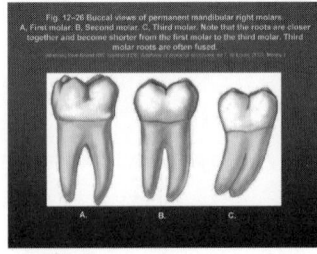

- Note the diminishing prominence of the cusps and the increasingly rounded appearance of the crowns.

Slide 72

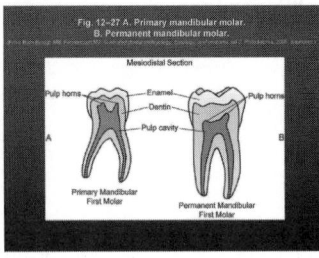

- How do the pulp chambers and pulp horns in primary teeth differ from those in permanent teeth?

ELSEVIER

Bird/Robinson

Slide 73

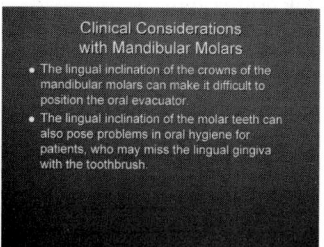

- What advice would you give a patient having difficulty with oral hygiene for the mandibular molars?

Slide 74

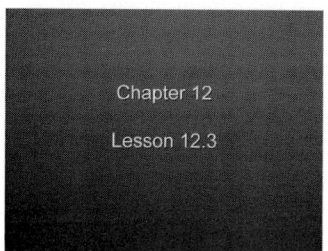

Slide 75

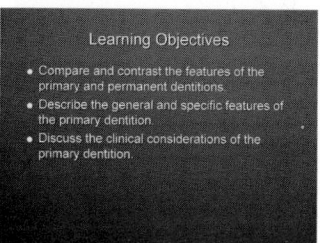

Slide 76

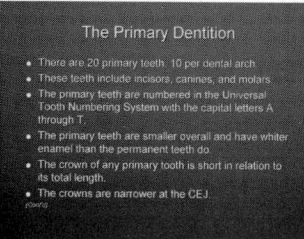

- The primary teeth are commonly known as "primary," "baby," or "milk" teeth.
- They are also known clinically as the deciduous dentition.

Bird/Robinson

Slide 77

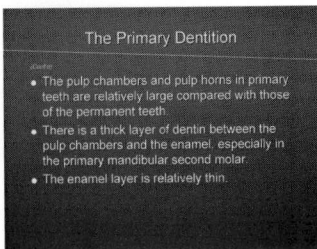

The Primary Dentition

- The pulp chambers and pulp horns in primary teeth are relatively large compared with those of the permanent teeth.
- There is a thick layer of dentin between the pulp chambers and the enamel, especially in the primary mandibular second molar.
- The enamel layer is relatively thin.

- In addition to normal tooth function, the key role of the primary dentition is to maintain proper spacing for the eruption of the permanent dentition.
- It is for this reason, more than others, that proper care of the primary dentition is so important.

Slide 78

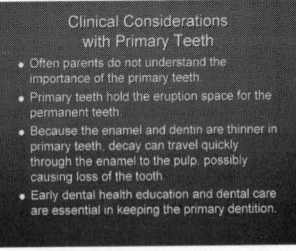

Clinical Considerations with Primary Teeth

- Often parents do not understand the importance of the primary teeth.
- Primary teeth hold the eruption space for the permanent teeth.
- Because the enamel and dentin are thinner in primary teeth, decay can travel quickly through the enamel to the pulp, possibly causing loss of the tooth.
- Early dental health education and dental care are essential in keeping the primary dentition.

- Among the primary teeth, it is particularly important to retain the second molars. If these teeth are lost, the first permanent molars are likely to drift out of position.

Slide 79

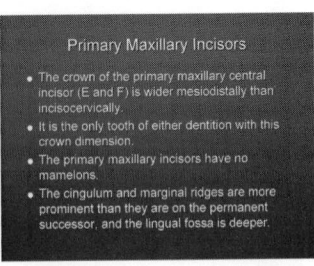

Primary Maxillary Incisors

- The crown of the primary maxillary central incisor (E and F) is wider mesiodistally than incisocervically.
- It is the only tooth of either dentition with this crown dimension.
- The primary maxillary incisors have no mamelons.
- The cingulum and marginal ridges are more prominent than they are on the permanent successor, and the lingual fossa is deeper.

- The incisors are the first teeth to erupt, beginning at 6 ½ months to about 8 months after birth.
- Primary incisor teeth are functional for 5 to 6 years.

Slide 80

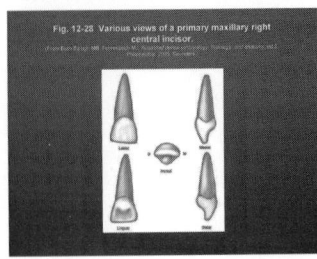

Fig. 12-28 Various views of a primary maxillary right central incisor.

- Note the narrow root and the short crown length relative to the root length.
- Note the relatively large cingulum.

Slide 81

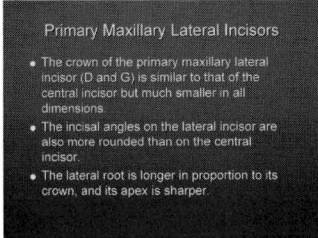

- The maxillary lateral incisor is more rounded than a central incisor, and is longer than it is wide.

Slide 82

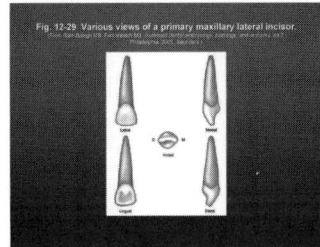

- Note the similarity, except for size, to the central incisors.
- Note the sharp apex and long root.

Slide 83

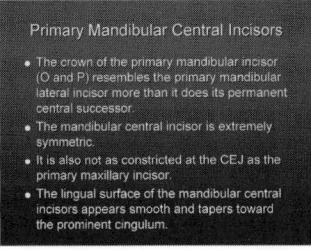

- The crown of the mandibular central incisor is slightly bigger than the permanent lateral incisor.

Slide 84

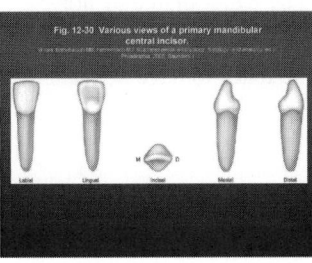

- The root is slender and rather long.
- How would you compare the morphology of this tooth with the permanent lateral incisor? What are the similarities?

Bird/Robinson

Slide 85

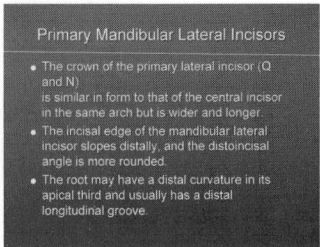

Primary Mandibular Lateral Incisors

- The crown of the primary lateral incisor (Q and N) is similar in form to that of the central incisor in the same arch but is wider and longer.
- The incisal edge of the mandibular lateral incisor slopes distally, and the distoincisal angle is more rounded.
- The root may have a distal curvature in its apical third and usually has a distal longitudinal groove.

Slide 86

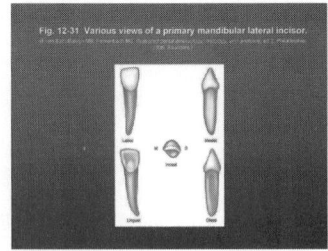

Fig. 12-31 Various views of a primary mandibular lateral incisor.

- Note that the cingulum is more noticeable, and the fossa is deeper than in the central incisor.

Slide 87

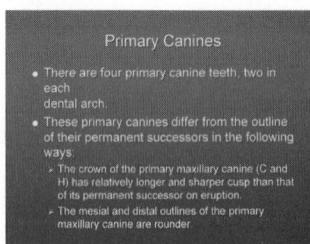

Primary Canines

- There are four primary canine teeth, two in each dental arch.
- These primary canines differ from the outline of their permanent successors in the following ways:
  - The crown of the primary maxillary canine (C and H) has relatively longer and sharper cusp than that of its permanent successor on eruption.
  - The mesial and distal outlines of the primary maxillary canine are rounder.

- The canines erupt between 16 months and 20 months after birth.
- The primary canines are sometimes removed to allow other teeth to align properly.

Slide 88

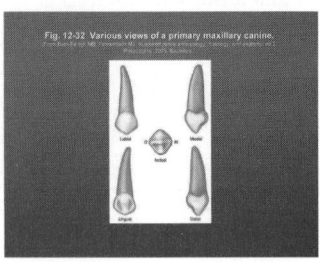

Fig. 12-32 Various views of a primary maxillary canine.

- Note that the primary canines may appear to be wider than they are long. This is an optical illusion
- This tooth has a well-developed cingulum and tends to have noticeable ridges on the mesial slope.

Slide 89

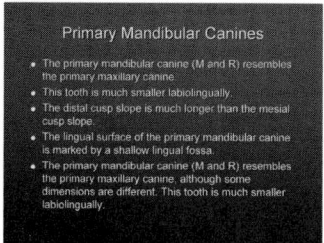

Slide 90

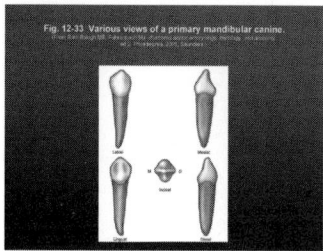

- Note the thin root, and the less-obvious cingulum compared to the maxillary canine.

Slide 91

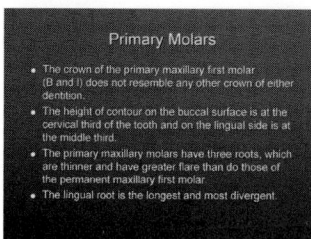

- The crown of the first maxillary molar is the smallest found in the primary molars.

Slide 92

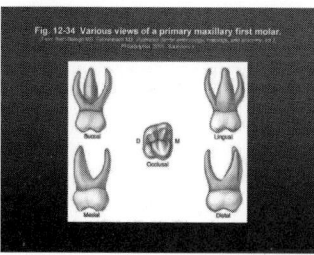

- The first molars erupt between 12 months and 16 months after birth.

Slide 93

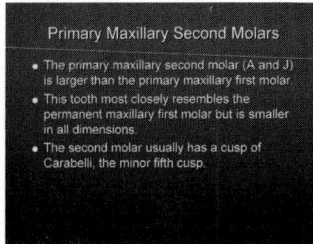

- How many pronounced cusps will a primary maxillary second molar have? *(Four.)*

Slide 94

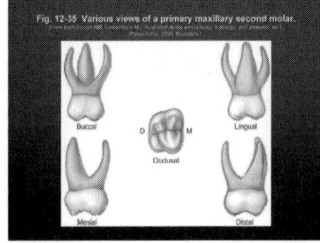

- The first permanent first maxillary molar may resemble the primary second molar.

- Primary maxillary molars have three roots, while mandibular molars have two roots.

Slide 95

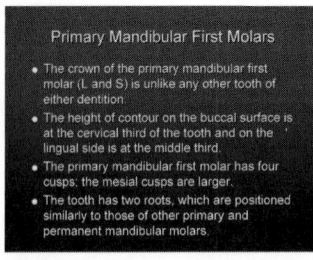

- The mesial cusps are the highest and largest to be found on any tooth.

Slide 96

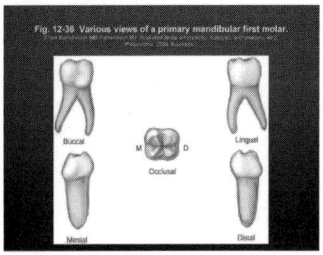

- What makes this tooth's morphology unique?

Bird/Robinson

Slide 97

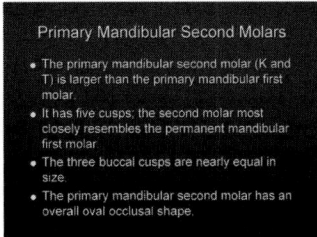

Primary Mandibular Second Molars

- The primary mandibular second molar (K and T) is larger than the primary mandibular first molar.
- It has five cusps; the second molar most closely resembles the permanent mandibular first molar.
- The three buccal cusps are nearly equal in size.
- The primary mandibular second molar has an overall oval occlusal shape.

Slide 98

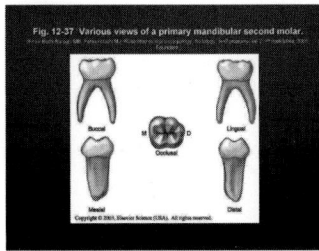

Fig. 12-37 Various views of a primary mandibular second molar.

- Note the five cusps and the equal size of the buccal cusps.
- The distal root tends to be smaller and narrower than the mesial root.

TEACHING FOCUS

This chapter will give students the opportunity study and to recognize dental caries as an infectious disease. The process of dental caries, the role of infective agents in the caries process, and the modes of transmission will be discussed. Students will have the opportunity to learn about caries diagnosis. Risk assessment and methods of caries intervention will be described.

MATERIALS AND RESOURCES

- ☐ agar carrier (Lesson 13.2)
- ☐ blank cards for flash cards (Lesson 13.1)
- ☐ caries activity test (Lesson 13.2)
- ☐ computer and PowerPoint projector (all Lessons)
- ☐ CRT kit (Lesson 13.2)
- ☐ culture incubator (Lesson 13.2)
- ☐ cup, china (Lesson 13.1)
- ☐ cups, paper (all Lessons)
- ☐ disclosing agent tablets (Lesson 13.1)
- ☐ disinfected extracted teeth (Lesson 13.2)
- ☐ eggs (Lesson 13.1)
- ☐ evaluation chart (Lesson 13.2)
- ☐ explorer (Lesson 13.2)

- ☐ fluoride toothpaste (Lesson 13.2)
- ☐ $NaHCO_3$ tablet (sodium, hydrogen, carbonate) (Lesson 13.2)
- ☐ overhead projector
- ☐ plastic overviews (Lesson 13.2)
- ☐ paraffin pellet (Lesson 13.2)
- ☐ pen with waterproof ink (Lesson 13.2)
- ☐ pipette (Lesson 13.2)
- ☐ plastic wrap (Lesson 13.1)
- ☐ Quigley Hein Plaque Index and student chart (Lesson 13.1)
- ☐ radiographs (Lesson 13.2)
- ☐ test vial (Lesson 13.2)
- ☐ vinegar (Lesson 13.1)

LESSON CHECKLIST

Preparations for this lesson include:

- lecture
- guest speakers: dentist, dental hygienist
- evaluation of student knowledge and skills needed to perform all entry-level activities related to dental caries, including:
  - ○ causes and stages of caries development
  - ○ the differences among secondary (recurrent), rampant, and root caries
  - ○ means and methods of diagnosis
  - ○ the importance of saliva diagnosis of caries
  - ○ methods of caries intervention

ELSEVIER

Bird/Robinson

KEY TERMS

caries (p. 169)
cavitation (p. 171)
demineralization (p. 171)
early childhood caries (p. 172)
fermentable carbohydrates (p. 170)
fluoride (p. 171)
incipient caries (p. 171)
lactobacilli (p. 169)

mutans streptococci (p. 169)
pellicle (p. 170)
plaque (p. 169)
rampant caries (p. 172)
remineralization (p. 171)
saliva flow rate test (p. 175)
xerostomia (p. 172)
xylitol (p. 175)

ADDITIONAL RESOURCES

PowerPoint slides (Evolve): 1-39

Legend

CTQ
Critical
Thinking
Question

DVD
Multimedia
Procedures
Videos and
Animations

ESLR
EVOLVE
Student
Learning
Resources

IDO
Interactive
Dental
Office
CD-ROM

SW
Student
Workbook

TB
Test Bank
on the
TEACH
CD-ROM

PPT
PowerPoint
Slides

Class Activities are indicated in ***bold italic.***

ELSEVIER

Torres and Ehrlich Modern Dental Assisting, 9th ed.

Bird/Robinson

LESSON 13.1

PRETEST

1. What term refers to tooth decay?
   a. remineralization
   b. xerostomia
   c. caries
   d. fluorosis

2. What term refers to the film from saliva that adheres to the teeth?
   a. pellicle
   b. immunoglobulins
   c. hydroxyapatite
   d. plaque

3. What term indicates an exposed root?
   a. rampant
   b. recession
   c. recurrent
   d. cavitation

4. What dental instrument is usually used to check for decay?
   a. pliers
   b. chisel
   c. explorer
   d. spatula

5. What term refers to minerals that are redeposited in the tooth?
   a. demineralization
   b. carbonization
   c. remineralization
   d. cavitation

6. What is the main cause of tooth decay?
   a. presence of saliva
   b. size of tooth
   c. presence of plaque
   d. position of tooth

7. What is the most mineralized tissue in the body?
   a. bone
   b. enamel
   c. cartilage
   d. dentin

8. What is the earliest sign of tooth decay?
   a. dark stained tooth
   b. white spot
   c. hole or cavity
   d. pain in area

9. Where does pit-and-fissure decay first occur?
   a. smooth surfaces
   b. interproximally
   c. occlusal surface
   d. root surfaces

10. What term indicates multiple decayed areas throughout the mouth?
    a. rampant caries
    b. incipient caries
    c. frank caries
    d. overt caries

Answers

1. c	3. b	5. c	7. b	9. c
2. a	4. c	6. c	8. b	10. a

BACKGROUND ASSESSMENT

Question: What is dental plaque? What is plaque's relationship to saliva?

Answer: Dental plaque is a colorless, soft, sticky coating that adheres to the teeth. Plaque forms on the pellicle—the thin coating of saliva that clings to the teeth. Acids from bacteria in the plaque are ultimately responsible for tooth decay.

Question: What are the methods of reducing the risk of caries for patients? Who would be a candidate for risk assessment tests and why?

Answer: The carious process can be interrupted or prevented by fluoride, antibacterial therapy, dietary changes, and increasing salivary flow. New patients with signs of caries and those experiencing a sudden

Bird/Robinson

increase in incidence are candidates for testing because they are at risk for further caries. Pregnant patients are candidates because this will reduce the transmission of caries-causing bacteria to the infant. Because saliva protects against caries, patients taking medications that reduce the flow of saliva, those with xerostomia, and those with autoimmune diseases are candidates for caries risk assessment. Patients with upcoming chemotherapy are at increased risk of caries because of the likelihood of frequent vomiting. Patients who frequently consume fermentable carbohydrates are candidates because these are key to the carious process.

CRITICAL THINKING QUESTION

A young pregnant woman wonders how she can make certain that her child never has caries. The young woman has a mouth full of fillings and remembers all the pain and discomfort she had as a child, as well as the missed schooldays and activities. She plans on bottle feeding her child. What issues can the dental team discuss with her so she can plan ahead for feeding her child? What can the dentist recommend to help her preserve her child's teeth?

Guidelines: The dental team can inform the mother that after the child is born, the bacteria that cause caries, mutans streptococcus and lactobacillus, can be transmitted from parent to child by means of saliva. The mother can reduce the amount of bacteria in her mouth by keeping her mouth as clean as possible; the dentist may recommend that she rinse for two weeks with chlorhexidine, an oral antiseptic, after she receives a professional prophylaxis. As soon as the child's teeth erupt, the mother should clean the teeth with fluoridated toothpaste. She can also make sure that the baby is not put to bed with a bottle of juice or milk. All these caries prevention strategies will reduce the risk of her child having caries, thus avoiding future dental pain and missed school or activities.

OBJECTIVES	CONTENT	TEACHING RESOURCES
Pronounce, define, and spell the Key Terms.	■ Key terms (p. 168)	SW Fill in the Blank question 1 (p. 46) ESLR Electronic Flashcards ▸ Discuss each of the key terms in Chapter 13, focusing on the definition, pronunciation, and spelling of each term. *Class Activity Have students make flash cards of the key terms with the terms on one side and the definitions on the reverse. Then have the students quiz one another with the flash cards Correct their pronunciation as needed.*
Name the most common chronic disease in children.	■ Introduction (p. 169)	SW Short-Answer Questions 12 (p. 45) SW Case Study (p. 47) ▸ Discuss the prevalence of dental caries in children, and compare it to the prevalence of other disorders. Discuss how the prevalence of dental caries affects children, such as in the number of school hours children miss each year because of dental caries. ▸ Discuss how the approach used to fight dental caries has shifted in recent years from restoring teeth to reducing dental caries. *Class Activity Have the students write a one-page essay of their dental experiences as children. Using the knowledge they have gained from this chapter, ask students to summarize caries prevention strategies they could have used as children. Have students report their conclusions to the class.*

ELSEVIER

Torres and Ehrlich Modern Dental Assisting, 9th ed.

Bird/Robinson

OBJECTIVES	CONTENT	TEACHING RESOURCES
Recognize dental caries as an infectious disease.	■ Introduction (p. 169)	PPT 9 SW Short-Answer Questions 1 (p. 45) ▸ Discuss the process of tooth decay as an infectious bacterial disease, including the role of diet and dental plaque. ▸ Discuss how the structure of the enamel is affected by acids in plaque and saliva. *Class Activity **Have students conduct Internet research on mutans streptococci (MS) and write a two-paragraph report on the subject.** (For students to prepare for this activity, see Homework/Assignments #1.)*

Describe the modes of transmission of dental caries.	■ Bacterial infection (p. 169)	PPT 9-10
		
		TB question 2
		
		SW Short-Answer Questions 5; Multiple Choice questions 1, 2 (pp. 45-46)
		
		Recall questions 1, 2 (p. 169)
		
		▸ Discuss how mothers can transmit disease-causing mutans streptococci (MS) to their infants.
		
		*Class Activity **Refer to the Critical Thinking Question for Lesson 13.1. Divide the class into small groups, and assign each group one of the discussion points below. After 15 minutes, have the groups share their findings with the class.***
		
		   — *Group 1: How does the mother transmit the bacteria to the child, and how does this affect the child?*
		
		   — *Group 2: How can the mother reduce the amount of bacteria in her mouth?*
		
		   — *Group 3: How can the dentist help the mother reduce the bacteria in her mouth?*
		
		   — *Group 4: After her child has teeth, what can the mother do for the child to reduce the risk of caries?*

Identify the infective agent in the caries process.	■ Bacterial infection (p. 169) ☐ Dental plaque (p. 169)	PPT 9-12 TB question 1 SW Short-Answer Questions 6; Fill in the Blank questions 4, 5; Multiple Choice questions 3, 4 (pp. 45-46) Figure 13-1 Dental plaque made visible with disclosing agent (p. 170) Recall question 3 (p. 170)

OBJECTIVES	CONTENT	TEACHING RESOURCES
		▶ Discuss the two specific groups of bacteria in the mouth that are responsible for dental caries. How are MS bacteria transmitted to an infant?
		Class Activity After chewing disclosing- agent tablets, the students can go to the clinic after oral hygiene, estimate the amount of plaque using an index (Quigley Hein Plaque Index), and record it on a chart. Be sure that students with any tooth-colored restorations protect them with petroleum jelly before chewing the tablets. This index evaluates the plaque revealed on both the buccal side and the lingual side of the teeth on a scale from 0 to 5 where:
		0 = no plaque
		1 = isolated flecks of plaque near the gingival (gum) margin
		2 = a 1 mm band of plaque at the gingival margin
		3 = up to one third of the surface covered with plaque
		4 = disclosed plaque from one third to two thirds of the surface
		5 = disclosed plaque on more than two thirds of the surface
Explain the process of dental caries.	☐ Enamel structure (p. 170) ■ The caries process (p. 170) ☐ Stages of caries development (p. 171) ☐ Root caries (p. 172) ☐ Secondary (recurrent) caries (p. 172)	PPT 13-15, 17-23 TB questions 3, 10 SW Short-Answer Questions 2; Fill in the Blank questions 6-8 (pp. 45-46) SW Case Study (p. 47) Recall questions 4, 5, 7 (pp. 170-172) Figure 13-2 Factors involved in the formation of carious defects (p. 170) Figure 13-3 Demineralization and remineralization of the tooth (p. 171) Figure 13-4 (A) Early carious lesion or white spot of demineralization; (B) Overt carious lesion; (C) Rampant caries (p. 171) Figure 13-5 Severely decayed molar on a child (p. 172) Figure 13-6 Decay on the lingual surface of a maxillary lateral incisor (p. 172) ▶ Discuss the three factors that must occur at the same time for caries to develop. ▶ Discuss the process that enables caries to develop.

OBJECTIVES	CONTENT	TEACHING RESOURCES
		Class Activity Have the students work in small groups to prepare a patient education pamphlet, with graphics, that explains how the caries process occurs (similar to that shown in Figure 13-2). Students can add the factors of diet and bacteria to fully illustrate the process.
		Class Activity Have the students perform an experiment using eggs to represent the enamel and how the carious process and acid affects it. Pour enough vinegar into a china cup to cover the egg, and then carefully place the egg into the vinegar with the spoon. Rest the spoon on top of the egg to keep it under the vinegar, and cover the cup with plastic wrap. Leave the egg in vinegar until the egg softens (7 to 13 hours).
Describe the relationship between diet and dental caries.	■ The caries process (p. 170) ☐ Stages of caries development (p. 171) ☐ Root caries (p. 172) ☐ Secondary (recurrent) caries (p. 172)	SW Short-Answer Questions 8 (p. 45); Fill in the Blank question 12 (pp. 45-46) CTQ 2 (p. 179) ▸ Discuss how a diet rich in fermentable carbohydrates can contribute to dental caries. *Class Activity Have each student prepare a one-day journal of all the food eaten the day before and rate each food according to its caries risk level (slight, moderate, high).*

13.1 Homework/Assignments:

1. Have the students conduct Internet research on mutans streptococci and write a two-paragraph report on the subject.

13.1 Instructor's Notes/Student Feedback:

LESSON 13.2

CRITICAL THINKING QUESTION

An older woman patient will soon be undergoing chemotherapy for her recently diagnosed breast cancer. She already has areas of recession, and she experiences dry mouth because of the medicine she takes for high blood pressure. She wonders what she should do to preserve her dental health because her physician says her cancer therapy may cause vomiting. What issues can the dental assistant discuss with this patient regarding her risk of tooth decay? What preventive interventions can be implemented to reduce the risk of dental decay?

Guidelines: Vomit contains acid that can increase the patient's risk of dental caries by causing demineralization of her teeth. She can undergo a risk assessment test before her chemotherapy to determine her overall risk of caries. She already has an increased risk because she has xerostomia from her medicine and from recession. Saliva is protective against caries. Her recession has exposed the root surface and the roots are especially prone to caries because the surface is not as mineralized. Many methods of intervention could reduce her risk of caries. She can increase her use of fluoride to strengthen her teeth, possibly by using prescription methods recommended by the dentist. The dentist may want to use oral antibacterial therapy to reduce the bacteria that cause caries. Her diet should be discussed by the dental team so as to decrease the amount and frequency of fermentable carbohydrates. Methods to increase her saliva, such as chewing gum and drinking water, should be discussed, and she should be told how to rinse out her mouth should vomiting occur.

OBJECTIVES	CONTENT	TEACHING RESOURCES
Explain the remineralization process.	■ The caries process (p. 170) 　□ Stages of caries development (p. 171) 　□ Root caries (p. 172) 　□ Secondary (recurrent) caries (p. 172)	PPT 14, 17-18 TB questions 4, 8 SW Short-Answer Questions 9; Fill in the Blank questions 2, 3; Multiple Choice question 5 (pp. 45-46) Recall question 6 (p. 172) ▶ Discuss the ongoing caries process characterized by alternating periods of demineralization and remineralization. Describe both demineralization and remineralization. ***Class Activity** Have the students use eggs to represent tooth enamel and demonstrate how fluoride can prevent caries. First, place a full tube of fluoridated toothpaste completely over the egg. Next, place the egg in a cup, cover it tightly with plastic wrap, and leave it at room temperature for at least 4 full days (96 hours). After the treatment, with clean hands, rinse all the paste off the egg with warm tap water and let the egg dry overnight. The next day add the vinegar as in the earlier Class Activity (Lesson 13.1), and see whether the egg retains its softness. This exercise demonstrates how the egg is protected from the acid by the fluoride, which is similar to the remineralization of enamel.* ***Class Activity** Have students research fluoride use on the Internet. Then, divide the class into two groups and have a panel discussion on the pros and cons of fluoride use. (For students to prepare for this activity, see Homework/Assignments #1.)*

OBJECTIVES	CONTENT	TEACHING RESOURCES
Distinguish between root caries and smooth surface caries.	■ The caries process (p. 170) ☐ Stages of caries development (p. 171) ☐ Root caries (p. 172) ☐ Secondary (recurrent) caries (p. 172)	PPT 17, 26-29 TB question 5 SW Short-Answer Questions 10; Fill in the Blank question 9; Multiple Choice questions 6, 7 (pp. 45-47) Recall question 8 (p. 172) Figure 13-7 Root surface caries (p. 172) Figure 13-8 Radiograph showing recurrent decay under an amalgam restoration (p. 172) CTQ 1 (p. 178) ▶ Discuss the definitions for smooth surface caries and root caries. ▶ Discuss why root caries are a concern for elderly persons. ***Class Activity** Have students use an explorer to check the surfaces of disinfected extracted teeth. Have them point out areas of root caries and smooth-surface caries, marking them for other students to see.*
Explain the role of saliva in oral health.	■ The importance of saliva (p. 173)	PPT 30 TB question 6 SW Short-Answer Questions 7; Fill in the Blank questions 10, 11; Multiple Choice questions 8 (pp. 45-47) Recall question 9 (p. 173) ▶ Discuss the physical, chemical, and antibacterial protective measures that saliva provides for the teeth. ***Class Activity** Refer to the Critical Thinking Question for Lesson 13.2. Divide the class into small groups. Ask one group to address each of the discussion points below. After 15 minutes, have the groups share their findings with the class, making use of the front board to illustrate their findings graphically.* *– Group 1: What is the role of saliva in the formation of plaque?* *– Group 2: How does saliva protect the tooth against caries?* *– Group 3: Why does this woman have a dry mouth?* *– Group 4: What can the woman and the dentist do to help reduce her risk of caries?* ***Class Activity** Have the students conduct Internet research to discover how many drugs cause dry mouth. Insert the following criterion into an Internet search engine: "dry mouth drug side effect." Have students make a list of the drugs with this side effect.*

ELSEVIER

Torres and Ehrlich Modern Dental Assisting, 9th ed.
Bird/Robinson

OBJECTIVES	CONTENT	TEACHING RESOURCES
Explain the purpose of caries activity tests.	■ Diagnoses of caries (p. 174) ☐ Dental explorer (p. 174) ☐ Radiographs (p. 174) ☐ Visual appearance (p. 174) ☐ Indicator dyes (p. 174) ☐ Laser caries detector (p. 174)	☒ PPT 31 TB question 7 SW Short-Answer Questions 4 (p. 45) ▸ Discuss the following methods of detecting dental caries, including how each one works and its limitations: dental explorer, radiographs, visual appearance, indicator dyes, laser caries detector. *Class Activity Provide the students with radiographs to examine in small groups. Direct the students to see whether they can visualize radiographic evidence of caries. Students can mark the areas of concern on a plastic overview sheet.*
Describe the advantages and disadvantages of the laser caries detection device.	☐ Laser caries detector (p. 174)	☒ PPT 32-34 SW Short-Answer Questions 11 (p. 45) Figure 13-11 The DIAGNOdent directs a laser beam into the occlusal surface (p. 174) Figure 13-12 Visual and radiographic appearance of seemingly intact molar (p. 174) Figure 13-13 Cross section of molar showing decay (p. 174) ▸ Discuss how a laser caries detector works. ▸ Discuss the advantages and disadvantages of using a laser caries detector. *Class Activity Have each student conduct Internet research on the pros, cons, and costs of buying a laser caries detector for a dental office where they work. Have them write a three-paragraph report on their findings to discuss in class. (For students to prepare for this activity, see Homework/Assignments #2.)*
Identify the risk factors for dental caries.	■ Methods of caries intervention (p. 175) ■ Risk assessment for caries (p. 175) Procedure 13-1 Performing Caries Risk Assessment (pp. 176-178) (SW/ESLR Competency 13-1, pp. 49-50)	☒ PPT 35-39 TB question 9, 11 SW Short-Answer Questions 3 (p. 45) SW/ESLR Competency 13-1 Performing Caries Risk Assessment (pp. 49-50) CTQ 3 (p. 179) ▸ Discuss risk factors for dental caries. What patients are at highest risk for developing dental caries? ▸ Discuss what a high bacterial count indicates as the result of a caries risk-assessment test. *Class Activity Have each student create a chart listing the risk factors for caries in their mouths and the mouths of two family members. Have students describe how each factor is involved in caries activity.* *Class Activity In groups, have the students perform the caries activity test on each other using Competency 13-1 (SW pp. 47-48).*

OBJECTIVES	CONTENT	TEACHING RESOURCES
Performance Evaluation		📺 TB
		📖 SW questions (pp. 45-47)
		📖 SW Case Study (p. 47)
		📖 *e* SW/ESLR Competency 13-1 Performing Caries Risk Assessment (pp. 49-50)
		e ESLR Electronic Flashcards
		e ESLR Practice Quiz
		Recall questions (pp. 169-173)
		💡 CTQ (p. 178-179)

13.2 Homework/Assignments:

1. Have students research fluoride use on the Internet. Then, divide the class into two groups, and have a panel discussion with the students on the pros and cons of fluoride.

2. Have each student conduct Internet research on the pros, cons, and costs of buying a laser caries detector for a dental office where they work. Have them write a three-paragraph report on their findings to discuss in class.

13.2 Instructor's Notes/Student Feedback:

ELSEVIER

Bird/Robinson

Slide 1

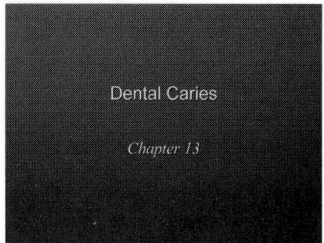

Dental Caries

Chapter 13

Slide 2

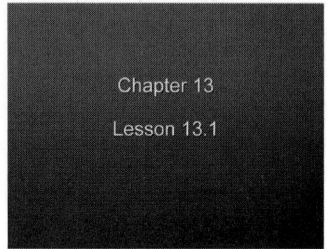

Chapter 13

Lesson 13.1

Slide 3

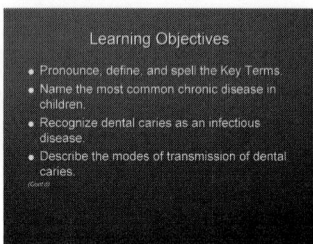

Learning Objectives

- Pronounce, define, and spell the Key Terms.
- Name the most common chronic disease in children.
- Recognize dental caries as an infectious disease.
- Describe the modes of transmission of dental caries.

Slide 4

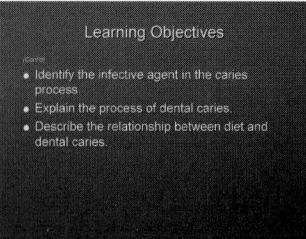

Learning Objectives

- Identify the infective agent in the caries process.
- Explain the process of dental caries.
- Describe the relationship between diet and dental caries.

Torres and Ehrlich Modern Dental Assisting, 9th ed.

Bird/Robinson

Slide 5

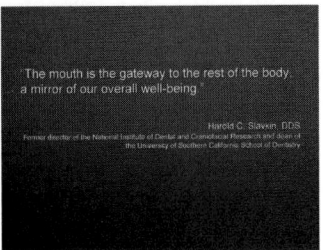

Slide 6

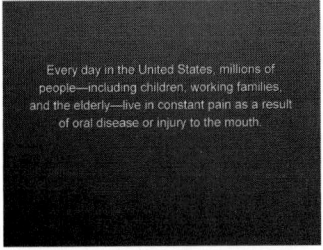

- The development of dental caries is a complex, multistage process. Even though many younger patients do not exhibit caries, tooth decay still affects a large portion of patients (20% of patients have 80% of the tooth decay), regardless of gender, age, and ethnicity. However, caries tend to affect low-income individuals more frequently than other demographic groups.

- What are the signs and symptoms of the disease? *(In most cases there is tooth sensitivity to sweet foods and to hot and cold food or drinks. If a tooth is sensitive to heat, it frequently requires a root canal. There may be no symptoms until a cavity becomes very large or a tooth abscess forms. An abscess can cause pain, swelling, and fever.)*

Slide 7

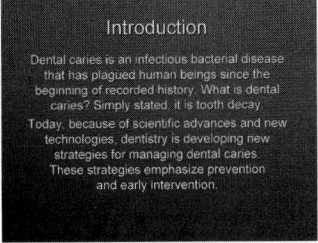

Slide 8

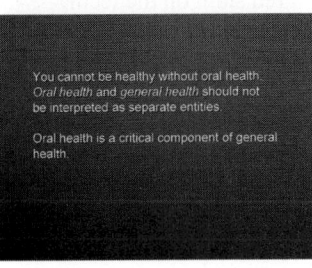

- Many patients do not understand this concept because oral health is usually not viewed as being connected to the general health of the body.

- It is important for the dental health care team to believe this concept and to reinforce it with patients.

- Thus it is important that dental healthcare professionals try to see the "whole" patient and not think that only the mouth is being treated.

- Many important factors involved in the patient's oral health and disease are lost when only a narrow focus on oral health is considered.

Slide 9

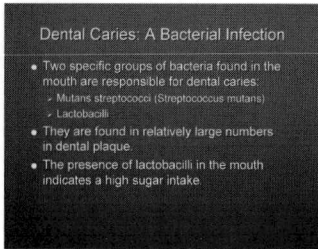

- The earliest recorded reference to oral disease is from an ancient Sumerian text (c. 5000 BC) that describes "tooth worms" as a cause of dental decay.
- Skulls of Cro-Magnon peoples, who inhabited the earth 25,000 years ago, show evidence of tooth decay.

Slide 10

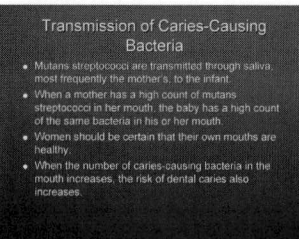

- How could a mother transmit her saliva with its bacteria to her infant? *(It could be transmitted by kissing and touching the child after the mother's hands have picked up bacteria from her mouth. Remember: no one advocates not kissing or touching babies, but rather keeping the mother's mouth healthy. This may include dietary counseling, professional cleanings, oral hygiene instruction, topical fluoride application, and removal of any caries. If necessary, an antibacterial, such as chlorhexidine, may be prescribed and placed in the mouth daily for about two weeks.)*

Slide 11

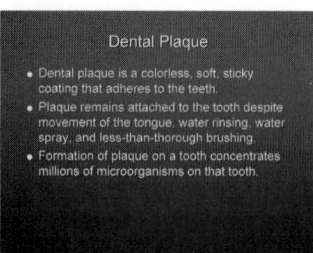

- Many healthcare professionals are now stressing that plaque is a biofilm.
- What is a biofilm? *(Biofilms are made up of microbial communities that are attached to an environmental surface. These microorganisms usually encase themselves in an extracellular polysaccharide or slime matrix. Therefore, plaque is an outstanding biofilm.)*

Slide 12

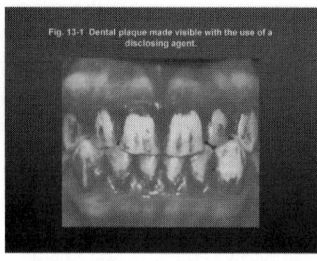

- Usually the patient rinses with, or chews tablets of, the nontoxic disclosing agent, and plaque is revealed as a red stain on the teeth. This stain is subsequently removed by brushing and flossing. This is an easy aid to help patients look for areas they are missing in their daily oral care.
- Care must be taken to cover areas of tooth-colored fillings with petroleum jelly to protect them. Areas of hardened plaque or tartar (calculus) will remain stained until the stain is removed professionally or wears off. The tongue will also appear stained, but plaque forms on it, too, and needs to be gently brushed off.

Slide 13

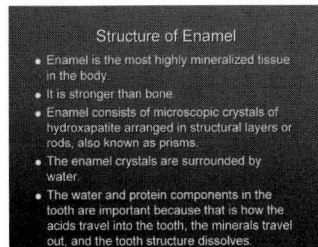

- How mineralized is enamel? *(Enamel is composed of 95% calcium minerals.)*

Slide 14

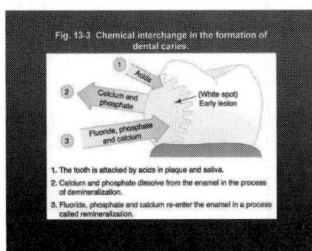

- How can fluoride be provided to the patient to aid in remineralization? *(It can be contained in water, toothpastes, or oral rinses. It can also be applied as a treatment at a dental office or used at home on recommendation of the dentist.)*

Slide 15

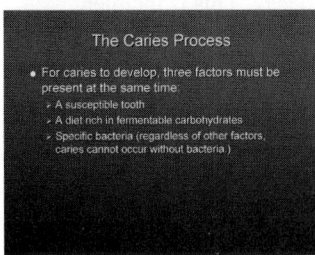

- Caries can also develop as a result of the constant intake of acidic foods. This is called erosion.

- What types of food or drink could be considered risky to the tooth because of their acid content? *(This could include soft drinks or lemon cough drops.)*

- If a patient drinks only diet soda rather than regular soda, does this positively affect tooth health? *(It does not. Acid breakdown of the tooth can occur with bacteria in the caries process or it can occur with acidic foods. Diet soda is more acidic than nondiet soda.)*

Slide 16

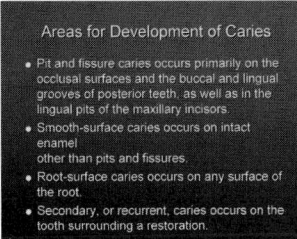

- No surface is really safe from decay. Many patients believe that once they restore a tooth it cannot become decayed again. What type of decay can occur in these teeth? *(Secondary or recurrent caries.)*

Slide 17

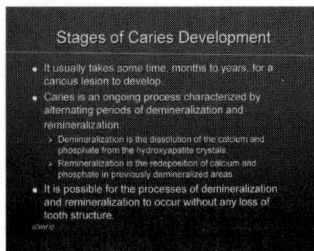

- Minerals that are replaced during remineralization actually make the tooth *stronger* against acid attack than the original.
- It is important to note that newly erupted teeth are especially vulnerable to acid attack because they have fewer minerals present at the surface (hypomineralization); this is similar to the exposure of roots with their layers of less mineralized tissue.
- What can be done in the dental office to help promote remineralization of newly erupted teeth.?

Slide 18

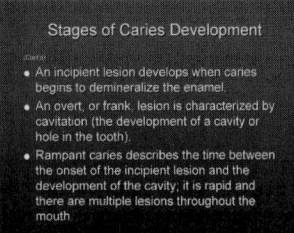

- At what stage of caries development should the teeth be protected from demineralization? *(Incipient lesion.)*
- At what stage does the patient usually first notice the lesion? *(Overt or frank lesion.)*
- At what stage is it most difficult for the dentist to restore good health to the mouth? *(Rampant caries.)*

Slide 19

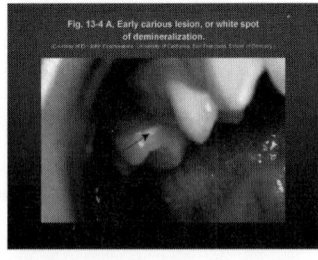

- The chalky white area in the photo is called the "white spot." It is an area of decalcification, the earliest sign of decay. This is incipient caries.
- How would it feel to a dental assistant who went over this area with a dental instrument such as an explorer? *(It would feel rough, which indicates that the enamel structure has broken down.)*
- Is this lesion very painful to the patient? *(There generally is no pain with this lesion other than sensitivity to sweet foods, and hot and cold food or drinks.)*

Slide 20

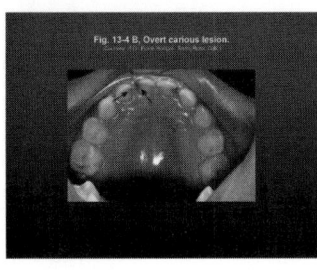

- Where are the dental caries located in this patient's mouth? *(They appear as dark-stained areas between the anterior teeth and the areas in the pits and fissures of the posterior teeth that do not polish or scale off. Thus, visual appearance is not always an exact way to diagnose caries.)*
- Are these early signs of decay?
- The occlusal surface that is decayed will "stick" when the dentist presses into the pits and fissures with a dental explorer in order to diagnose decay. But this method of using the explorer is not as effective once the teeth have been exposed to fluoride.

Bird/Robinson

Slide 21

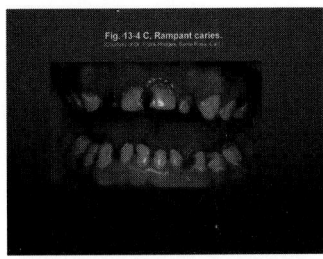

- What type of decay is in this patient's mouth? *(This is rampant decay. Multiple lesions are always present with this type of caries.)*

- Note that some of the carious lesions look as if they were prepared for restorations at one time. These lesions could also be considered secondary or recurrent caries.

- How could this happen to the patient? *(Poor diet, poor dental care, or xerostomia [dry mouth].)*

Slide 22

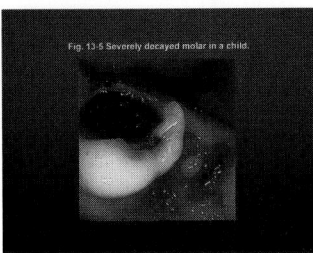

- This might be an example of "baby bottle" tooth decay, which is caused by frequent exposure of a child's teeth for long periods of time to liquid that contains sugars. It can occur when the baby falls asleep with a bottle containing formula, milk, or juice, with use of a pacifier dipped in honey, or even while breast feeding.

- Primary teeth have thinner layers of tooth tissue overlying the pulp, so they easily decay when compared to thicker-layered permanent teeth.

- The teeth most likely to be damaged are the maxillary anterior teeth. They are some of the first teeth to erupt and thus have the longest exposure time to the sugars in the bottle.

Slide 23

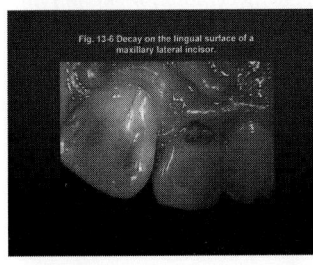

- Why caused this lesion to occur? *(It could be due to the patient having a natural pit in this area of the tooth that was susceptible to the carious process.)*

- The dentist will use an explorer to visually check for any natural pits and fissures in the teeth; or the dentist may use a laser device.

- How can the patient protect the natural pits and fissures from decay? *(The patient can perform good oral hygiene, watch his or her diet, use fluoride products, and have the pits and fissures sealed in the dental office.)*

Slide 24

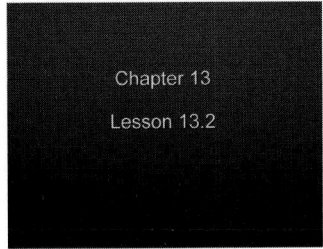

Chapter 13

Lesson 13.2

Torres and Ehrlich Modern Dental Assisting, 9th ed.

Bird/Robinson

Slide 25

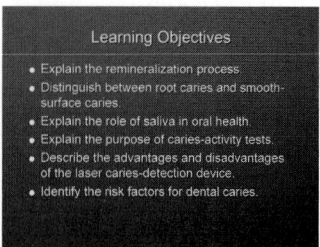

Slide 26

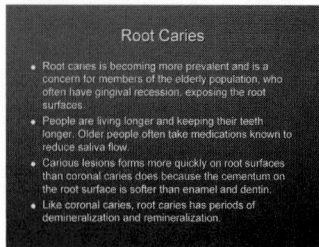

- Recession may be seen on an older person's front teeth.

- Why does the root surface become exposed? *(Many factors are involved. Two of them are age and periodontal disease; others include hard brushing and tooth placement.)*

- One factor that may be involved in recession is "abfraction," which occurs when the enamel structure breaks down and chips off, causing recession and deep cervical cuts. This happens with oral habits such as grinding or clenching of the teeth.

Slide 27

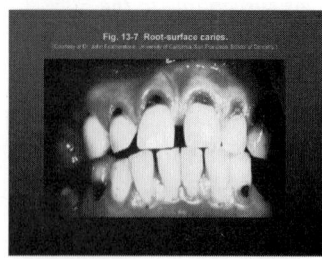

- Would these root carious lesions cause as much pain as other types of lesions already reviewed? *(Usually root caries are slow to form and do not cause much pain until most of the tooth's neck or cervix is undermined. However, rampant decay can lead to extensive pain and suffering.)*

Slide 28

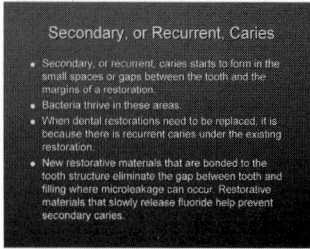

- Today there are many choices in sealant surface protection.

- The old standby is the unfilled resin systems that have been available for years.

- One of the relatively new types is the glass ionomer sealant. It releases high levels of fluoride to assist in remineralization of the surrounding area.

- Another new sealant uses the latest system of amorphous calcium phosphate to release these important minerals to assist in remineralization.

Slide 29

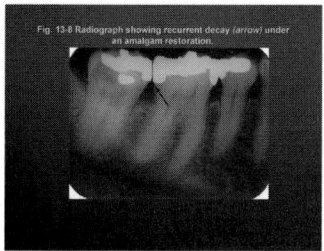

- What indicates to the dentist that decay is present on this radiograph? *(It is a dark area located interproximally, as indicated by the arrow. You can see that the radiograph must have good contrast to allow the dentist to see any carious lesions.)*

- Note that decay is often two times deeper and more widespread than it appears on radiographs. So using a radiograph alone is not the best way to diagnose decay. But a visual exam using an explorer would not show this lesion.

- Would it be possible to see early decay on the occlusal surface on a radiograph? *(No, only extensive decay of the occlusal surface on a radiograph would be seen.)*

Slide 30

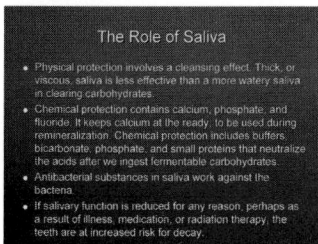

- Fluoride varnishes currently exist that are safer and easier to use than gels or foams because there is less systemic intake for the patient for remineralization. New toothpastes, candies, and rinses are available that incorporate this type of remineralization; however, they need to be studied further in relationship to the overall processes occurring in the mouth.

- New antibacterials are also expected to become available in the form of rinses, gels, and varnishes.

- What is another name for dry mouth? *(Xerostomia.)* What types of medications cause dry mouth? *(Prescribed medications for high blood pressure, allergies, and mental anxiety.)* How will you know if your patient has dry mouth?

Slide 31

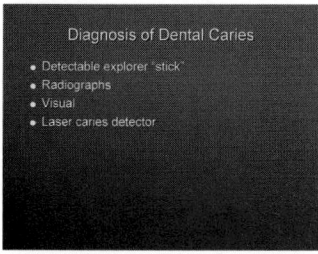

- Which is the best method for the dentist to use to diagnose caries? What are the pros and cons to each method of caries detection?

- Even the latest approach, the laser caries detector, has limitations. At the current level of technology, it cannot detect caries interproximally, or under sealants or restorations. But it is useful in nonrestored areas and around margins of restorations.

Slide 32

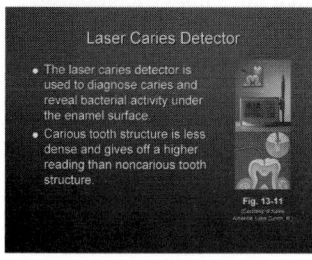

- One other method that may soon move from the lab to the office is the Quantitative Light-Induced Fluorescence method that uses the autofluorescence of teeth.

- When teeth are illuminated with high-intensity, harmless blue light, they will start to emit light in the green part of the spectrum, with the data going to a computer.

- The fluorescence of the dental material is directly related to the mineral content of the enamel. A loss due to caries would be easily detected on any exposed tooth surface, including the root.

Torres and Ehrlich Modern Dental Assisting, 9th ed.
Bird/Robinson

Slide 33

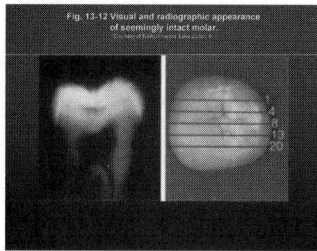

- As you can see, the molar appears intact but the readings from the laser tell another story. The readings indicate to the dentist that decalcification is occurring on the occlusal surface of this tooth.

- The laser comes with a chart that helps the dentist determine what treatment needs to be performed on the tooth surface.

Slide 34

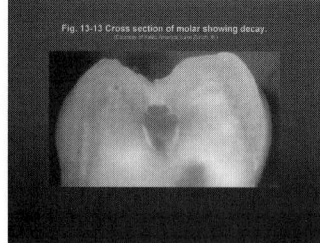

- It is important that the tooth be clean to obtain consistent readings with the laser.

- At the specific wavelength at which the laser operates, clean, healthy tooth structure exhibits little or no fluorescence, resulting in very low-scale readings on the display.

- However, carious tooth structure will exhibit fluorescence that is proportionate to the degree of caries, resulting in elevated scale readings on the display.

Slide 35

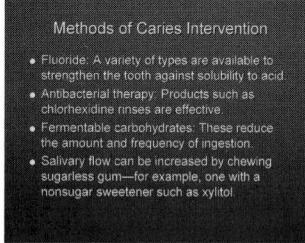

- How can the dental office help a patient with caries intervention?

- Looking at caries prevention using protection and remineralization, there are some possible risk interventions that patients can consider.

- It is important to note that preventive strategies are more effective when two or more are combined.

Slide 36

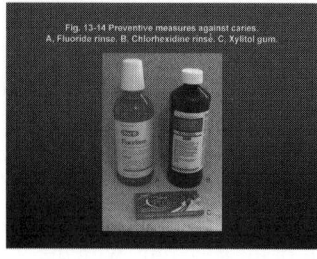

- Which of these preventive measures would be the easiest for the patient to use on a daily basis? *(Sugar-free gum.)*

- What is compliance? *(The extent to which a patient follows the recommendations of a doctor or health care professional, particularly with respect to medication or other treatments.)*

- Compliance may be poor with a procedure that does not taste good, so manufacturers attempt to provide rinses that have a pleasant taste.

Bird/Robinson

Slide 37

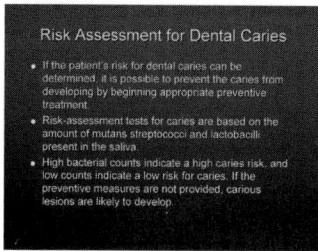

- There has been an important shift in the strategy concerning caries control because we are now able to promote remineralization and protection of the tooth surface.

- Today, the emphasis is on a prevention model and moving away from a repair model.

- Restoring the teeth did nothing to control caries.

Slide 38

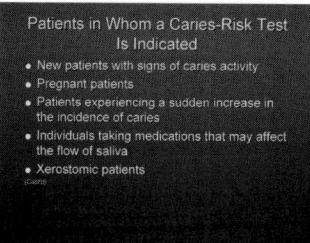

- What is your caries risk level? What factors can promote or even reduce the incidence of decay? *(A dental professional should seek ways to take care of his or her own mouth as an example to the patients. Consider taking the caries risk test.)*

Slide 39

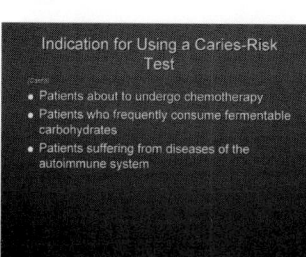

- What is chemotherapy, and why does it indicate a risk for caries? *(Treatment using anticancer drugs. The teeth should be protected before this treatment is undertaken because the patient may vomit as a result of using these drugs, which will cause acid contact with the teeth.)*

- What are fermentable carbohydrates? *(There is a considerable range in the ease by which different carbohydrates can be attacked by microorganisms. The most vulnerable are sugars and cooked starches.)*

- Why do autoimmune diseases indicate a risk for caries? *(Many diseases of the autoimmune system have a side effect of xerostomia or dry mouth.)*

Bird/Robinson

14 Lesson Plan
Periodontal Disease

TEACHING FOCUS

This chapter,will introduce the student to topics related to periodontal disease. The student will become acquainted with the various systemic conditions linked to periodontal disease, the types of periodontal disease, and signs and symptoms of periodontal disease.

MATERIALS AND RESOURCES

- ☐ computer and Powerpoint projector (Lesson 14.1)
- ☐ unlabeled copies of Figure 14-1 (Lesson 14.1)

LESSON CHECKLIST

Preparations for this lesson include:

- lecture
- guest speaker: dental assistant
- evaluation of student knowledge and skills needed to perform all entry-level activities related to periodontal disease, including:
  - ○ the tissues and structures of the periodontium
  - ○ systemic factors that influence periodontal disease
  - ○ the two main types of periodontal disease and their associated risk factors
  - ○ the significance of plaque and calculus in periodontal disease
  - ○ the progression of periodontal disease

Bird/Robinson

KEY TERMS

calculus (p. 182)
gingivitis (p. 184)
periodontal (p. 181)
periodontitis (p. 185)
periodontium (p. 181)

perioscopy (p. 188)
plaque (p. 182)
subgingival (p. 182)
supragingival (p. 182)

ADDITIONAL RESOURCES

PowerPoint slides (Evolve): 1-23
The Interactive Dental Office CD-ROM: Louisa Van Doren

Legend

CTQ
Critical
Thinking
Question

DVD
Multimedia
Procedures
Videos and
Animations

ESLR
EVOLVE
Student
Learning
Resources

IDO
Interactive
Dental
Office
CD-ROM

SW
Student
Workbook

TB
Test Bank
on the
TEACH
CD-ROM

PPT
PowerPoint
Slides

Class Activities are indicated in ***bold italic.***

ELSEVIER

Torres and Ehrlich Modern Dental Assisting, 9th ed.

Bird/Robinson

LESSON 14.1

PRETEST

1. A soft deposit on teeth that consists of bacteria and bacterial byproducts is
   a. plaque.
   b. acquired pellicle.
   c. calculus.
   d. material alba.

2. What percentage of Americans have some form of periodontal disease?
   a. 35%
   b. 40%
   c. 60%
   d. 75%

3. How many more times is a diabetic likely to have periodontal support loss?
   a. twice
   b. three
   c. four
   d. five

4. Which of the following has been linked to alveolar bone loss?
   a. testosterone loss
   b. estrogen loss
   c. calcium supplementation
   d. vitamin D supplementation

5. How many drugs cause the side effect of xerostomia?
   a. fewer than 25
   b. about 50
   c. around 200
   d. more than 400

6. The use of phenytoin, cyclosporine, and calcium channel blockers such as nifedipine and verapamil results in
   a. gingival ulceration.
   b. plaque-induced gingivitis.
   c. gingival enlargement.
   d. hematologic gingival disease.

7. Which of the following is associated with necrotizing ulcerative periodontitis?
   a. leukemia
   b. HIV/AIDS
   c. NSAIDs
   d. diabetes mellitus

8. Directly between the tooth and the free gingiva is the
   a. interdental papilla.
   b. marginal gingiva.
   c. gingival sulcus.
   d. attached gingiva.

9. Most cases of periodontal disease start in the
   a. interdental papilla.
   b. marginal gingiva.
   c. gingival sulcus.
   d. attached gingiva.

10. The portion of the tooth that anchors the tooth to the bony socket with the attachments of the periodontal ligaments is the
    a. cementum.
    b. enamel.
    c. dentin.
    d. pulp.

Answers

1. a	3. b	5. d	7. b	9. c
2. d	4. b	6. c	8. c	10. a

BACKGROUND ASSESSMENT

Question: How do medications react with the periodontium?

Answer: Medications such as tetracycline and NSAIDs have a beneficial effect on the periodontium. Other medications such as diuretics, antihistamines, antipsychotics, antihypertension agents, and analgesics have a harmful effect on the periodontium by decreasing salivary flow (xerostomia), which results in dry tissue, increases levels of plaque growth, and harms the periodontium. Antiseizure drugs and hormones such as estrogen and progesterone can also cause gingival enlargement, which harms the periodontium by making oral hygiene difficult.

Question: How should home care instructions be documented?
Answer: It is important to observe and chart the patient's oral hygiene status at every visit and to document all home-care instructions. Conversations about oral hygiene and the risks for developing periodontal disease should also be documented in the patient chart; documentation should include that the patient has been clearly informed about the potential for future periodontal disease if the home care does not improve and that the patient understands the risks.

CRITICAL THINKING QUESTION

A 38-year-old woman with severe periodontitis is in her tenth week of pregnancy. When the dental assistant tries to discuss oral hygiene and future appointments for scaling, the patient becomes angry and says that she can live with bleeding gums and brown teeth from her smoking. She also says that she is not interested in learning about hygiene because her teeth will eventually fall out anyway. How could the dental assistant convince this patient of the importance of oral hygiene?

Guidelines: The dental assistant should explain to the patient that periodontal disease may actually increase her susceptibility to certain systemic conditions. Individuals with periodontal disease have a higher incidence of coronary heart disease, which results in a greater occurrence of strokes and heart attacks. Individuals with severe periodontal disease have 3 times the risk of stroke and 3.6 times the risk of coronary heart disease when compared with individuals without periodontal disease, and they are at greater risk for developing respiratory infections. Studies show that oral bacteria can easily spread into the bloodstream, attach to fatty plaques in the coronary arteries, and contribute to clot formation and heart attacks. Women with severe periodontal disease also have 7 times the risk for delivering preterm and low-birth-weight babies as women with little or no periodontal disease. Preterm birth and low birth weight are the two most significant predictors of the health and survival of an infant.

OBJECTIVES	CONTENT	TEACHING RESOURCES
Pronounce, define, and spell the Key Terms.	■ Key terms (p. 180)	SW Fill in the Blank questions 1-8 (pp. 51-52) ESLR Electronic Flashcards *Class Activity Have each student use one of the key terms in a clinically relevant sentence in order to define the term. Continue until all terms have been used; if students become stuck, have the rest of the class offer suggestions.*
Name and describe the tissues of the periodontium.	■ Prevalence (p. 181)	TB question 1 SW Short-Answer Questions 1; Fill in the Blank question 4 (pp. 51-52) ▸ Discuss periodontal disease. Explain that periodontal disease is an infectious process that involves inflammation of the periodontium. Note that the periodontium is made up of the structures that surround, support, and are attached to the teeth. ▸ Discuss the tissues of the periodontium. Describe the location of the gingivae and the epithelial attachment. *Class Activity Have each student draw a simplified diagram of how periodontal disease influences overall health and how health and lifestyle factors can influence the progression of periodontal disease. Have students share their diagrams with the class for discussion.*

ELSEVIER

Torres and Ehrlich Modern Dental Assisting, 9th ed.

Bird/Robinson

OBJECTIVES	CONTENT	TEACHING RESOURCES
Name the structures that make up the periodontium.	■ Prevalence (p. 181)	🖵 PPT 9 💻 TB question 1 📘 SW Short-Answer Questions 3; Fill in the Blank question 3 (pp. 51-52) Table 14-1 Structures of the Periodontium (p. 181) Figure 14-1 Structures of the periodontium: junctional epithelium, gingival sulcus, periodontal ligaments, and cementum (p. 181) ▸ Discuss periodontal disease. State that periodontal disease causes a breakdown of the periodontium, resulting in loss of tissue attachment and destruction of the alveolar bone. ▸ Discuss the structures of the periodontium. Note the locations of the periodontal ligaments, the cementum, and the alveolar bone. ***Class Activity Provide students with unlabeled copies of Figure 14-1 (p. 189). In small groups, have students fill in the missing labels without using their textbooks. Have groups share their answers with the class.***
Describe the prevalence of periodontal disease.	■ Prevalence (p. 181)	🖵 PPT 7 💻 TB question 2 📘 SW Short-Answer Questions 2 (p. 51) ▸ Discuss the prevalence of periodontal disease among adults. Why are most people unaware of the condition? ▸ Discuss the role of early detection and treatment in preventing tooth loss. ***Class Activity Have students research the latest statistics for periodontal disease in their region and present their findings to the class. (For students to prepare for this activity, see Homework/Assignments #1.)***
Describe the systemic conditions that are linked to periodontal disease.	■ Periodontal disease and systemic health (p. 181) ☐ Cardiovascular disease (p. 181) ☐ Preterm low birth weight (p. 182) ☐ Respiratory disease (p. 182) ■ Causes of periodontal disease (p. 182)	🖵 PPT 8 💻 TB question 3 📘 SW Short-Answer Questions 8; Multiple Choice question 5 (pp. 51-52) ▸ Discuss how periodontal disease can lead to other systemic conditions. ***Class Activity Divide the class into groups, and assign each group one of the following systemic conditions: cardiovascular disease, preterm low birth weight, respiratory disease, dental plaque, calculus. Have each***

OBJECTIVES	CONTENT	TEACHING RESOURCES

	☐ Dental plaque (p. 182)
	
	☐ Calculus (p. 182)
	
	  – Supragingival calculus (p. 182)
	
	  – Subgingival calculus (p. 183)
		group outline how periodontal disease is linked to its assigned condition and explain its treatments and short- and long-term implications. Have each group present its findings to the class.

Identify systemic factors influencing periodontal disease.	■ Periodontal disease and systemic health (p. 181)
	
	☐ Cardiovascular disease (p. 181)
	
	☐ Preterm low birth weight (p. 182)
	
	☐ Respiratory disease (p. 182)
	
	■ Causes of periodontal disease (p. 182)
	
	☐ Dental plaque (p. 182)
	
	☐ Calculus (p. 182)
	
	  – Supragingival calculus (p. 182)
	
	  – Subgingival calculus (p. 183)
		⊞ PPT 8
		
		SW Short-Answer Questions 4 (p. 51)
		
		▸ Discuss systemic factors influencing periodontal disease. Note that while the vast majority of periodontal disease cases are caused by plaque, some cases are caused by factors such as malocclusions, certain medications, and serious nutritional deficits.
		
		▸ Discuss systemic factors influencing periodontal disease. Explain that systemic factors include the body's response to the bacteria present in the mouth as well as the individual's particular number and mix of risk factors.
		
		Class Activity Lead a class discussion about periodontal disease. Ask students to identify systemic factors that influence periodontal disease. Record student responses on the board for comparison.

Explain the significance of plaque and calculus in periodontal disease.	■ Causes of periodontal disease (p. 182)
	
	☐ Dental plaque (p. 182)
	
	☐ Calculus (p. 182)
	
	  – Supragingival calculus (p. 182)
	
	  – Subgingival calculus (p. 183)
		⊞ PPT 10-13
		
		TB questions 4-6
		
		SW Short-Answer Questions 6 (p. 51)
		
		SW Fill in the Blank questions 1-2 (pp. 51-52)
		
		Figure 14-2 10-day-old supragingival plaque. The first symptoms of gingival inflammation are becoming visible (p. 182)
		
		Figure 14-3 Heavy calculus deposits on the lingual surfaces of the lower anterior teeth (p. 182)
		
		Tooth Deposits (p. 183)
		
		▸ Discuss the link between periodontal disease and plaque.
		
		Class Activity Divide the class into groups. Have each group outline the significance of plaque and calculus in periodontal disease and describe how supragingival calculus and subgingival calculus cause disease. Then have groups share their findings with the class.

Bird/Robinson

OBJECTIVES	CONTENT	TEACHING RESOURCES
Identify the risk factors that contribute to periodontal disease.	□ Other risk factors (p. 183)	SW Short-Answer Questions 7 (p. 51) SW/IDO Patient Case Exercise questions 1-2 (p. 53) (The Interactive Dental Office CD-ROM) Table 14-2 Common Risk Factors for Periodontal Disease (p. 183) CTQ 1-3 (p. 188) ▸ Discuss medications that can increase a person's risk of developing periodontal disease. ***Class Activity Lead a class discussion about periodontal disease. Ask students to identify risk factors for developing the disease and discuss the dental assistant's role communicating those risks to patients. Record student responses on the board for comparison.***
Identify and describe the two main types of periodontal diseases.	■ Types of periodontal disease (p. 183)	PPT 14 TB question 7 SW Short-Answer Questions 5 (p. 51) Figure 14-4 Gingivitis type I (p. 184) Table 14-3 Terminology Used to Describe Observations Associated with Clinical Assessment of Gingiva (p. 184) Recall questions 1-3 (p. 184) ▸ Discuss the different forms of periodontal disease. ▸ Discuss the characteristics of periodontal disease. ***Class Activity Present slides of the two main types of periodontal disease to the class and have students identify which type each slide represents.***
Describe the clinical characteristics of gingivitis.	□ Gingivitis (p. 184)	PPT 15-18 TB question 8 SW Short-Answer Questions 9; Fill in the Blank questions 5-7; Multiple Choice questions 1-3 (pp. 51-52) SW Case Study questions 1-5 (p. 52) Figure 14-5 Medication-induced gingivitis (p. 185) Figure 14-6 Gingival inflammation and enlargement associated with orthodontic appliance and poor oral hygiene (p. 185) Box 14-1 Characteristics of Plaque-Induced Gingival Diseases (p. 185)

ELSEVIER

Bird/Robinson

OBJECTIVES	CONTENT	TEACHING RESOURCES
		▸ Discuss gingivitis. Note that some types of gingivitis are associated with puberty, pregnancy, and use of birth control medications.
		▸ Discuss gingivitis. Compare plaque-induced gingivitis with plaque-induced gingival diseases modified by systemic factors.
		Class Activity Divide the class into groups, and assign each group one of the following gingival characteristics: color, contour, consistency, surface texture. Have each group outline its characteristic's location, distribution, and severity in both a healthy mouth and with the presence of gingivitis. Have groups present their findings to the class for discussion.
Describe the progression of periodontitis.	☐ Periodontitis (p. 185) ■ Description of periodontal disease (pp. 185, 187) ■ Signs and symptoms (p. 187)	PPT 19-23 TB questions 9-11 SW Short-Answer Questions 10; Fill in the Blank question 8; Multiple Choice question 4 (pp. 51-52) SW/IDO CD-ROM Patient Case Exercise questions 1-2 (p. 53) (The Interactive Dental Office CD-ROM) Figure 14-7 Cross-section of a tooth and associated anatomical structures (p. 186) Figure 14-8 The arrows indicate varying amounts of bone loss because of periodontal disease (p. 186) Figure 14-9 Generalized chronic periodontitis in a woman with 20-year smoking habit. A. The clinical view shows minimal place and inflammation. B. The radiographs show severe, generalized, horizontal pattern of bone loss. (p. 186) Box 14-2 Characteristics of Periodontitis (p. 187) Recall questions 4-6 (p. 187) ▸ Discuss the characteristics of periodontitis. Note that as the disease progresses, connective tissues attachments at the base of periodontal pockets are destroyed. ▸ Discuss the different types of periodontal disease defined by the American Academy of Periodontology. ▸ Discuss signs and symptoms of periodontal disease. List the signs and symptoms most often found in patients with periodontal disease. *Class Activity Choose two student volunteers to role-play a dental assistant informing a patient with early periodontal disease about the progression of the disease. Encourage the rest of the class to offer comments and suggestions.*

Torres and Ehrlich Modern Dental Assisting, 9th ed.

Bird/Robinson

OBJECTIVES	CONTENT	TEACHING RESOURCES
Performance Evaluation		TB questions
		SW questions (pp. 51-52)
		SW Case Study questions (pp. 52-53)
		SW/IDO Patient Case Exercise (p. 53) (The Interactive Dental Office CD-ROM)
		ESLR Electronic Flashcards
		ESLR Practice Quiz
		ESLR Labeling Exercise 15: Anatomical Structures of a Tooth and Surrounding Area
		Recall questions (pp. 184, 187)
		CTQ (p. 188)

14.1 Homework/Assignments:

1. Have students research the latest statistics for periodontal disease in their region and present their findings to the class.

14.2 Instructor's Notes/Student Feedback:

Slide 1

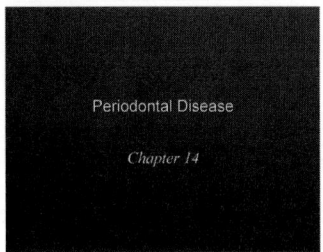

Periodontal Disease

Chapter 14

Slide 2

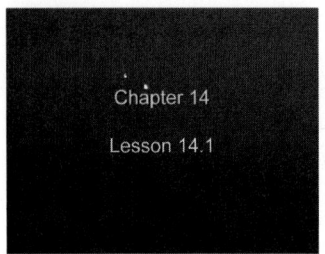

Chapter 14

Lesson 14.1

Slide 3

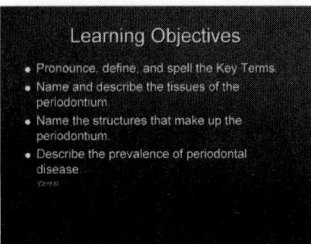

Learning Objectives

- Pronounce, define, and spell the Key Terms.
- Name and describe the tissues of the periodontium.
- Name the structures that make up the periodontium.
- Describe the prevalence of periodontal disease.

Slide 4

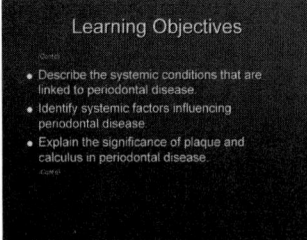

Learning Objectives

- Describe the systemic conditions that are linked to periodontal disease.
- Identify systemic factors influencing periodontal disease.
- Explain the significance of plaque and calculus in periodontal disease.

Bird/Robinson

Slide 5

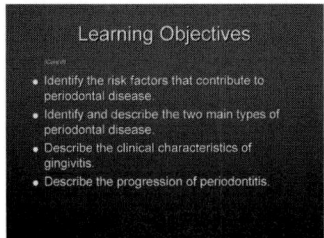

Slide 6

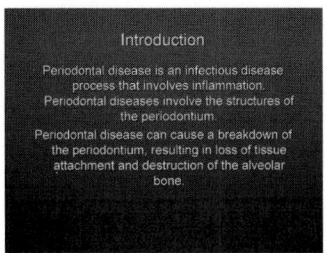

- What is the periodontium? *(Structures that surround, support, and are attached to the teeth.)*

- Failure to recognize periodontal disease and refer patients to a periodontist is a very common cause for a malpractice suit.

- Periodontal disease is a silent disease. Patients rarely experience pain and are often unaware that a problem exists.

Slide 7

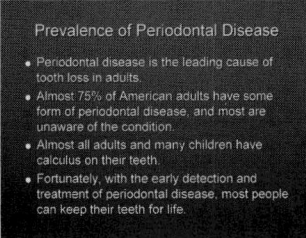

- What is calculus and how is it removed from the teeth? *(Calcium and phosphate salts in saliva that become mineralized and adhere to tooth surfaces; it is scaled off the teeth by hand or by ultrasonic instrumentation.)*

Slide 8

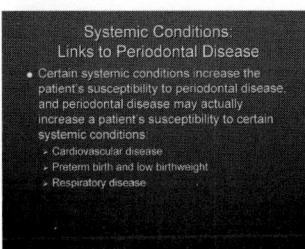

- Oral bacteria can spread into the bloodstream, attach to fatty plaques in the coronary arteries, and contribute to clot formation and heart attacks.

Bird/Robinson

Slide 9

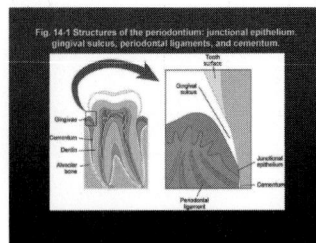

- Periodontal disease:
  - Involves inflammation
  - Involves the structures of the periodontium
- Can cause a breakdown of the periodontium resulting in:
  - loss of tissue attachment
  - destruction of the alveolar bone

Slide 10

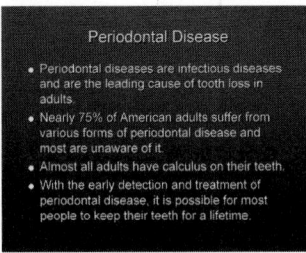

- The American Dental Association (ADA) and the American Academy of Periodontology (AAP) have developed systems for classifying periodontal diseases. What are the two main types of periodontal disease?
- Peri-implantitis is a new category established by the AAP. Patients in this category have implants that exhibit a "periodontitis-like-process" similar to natural teeth.

Slide 11

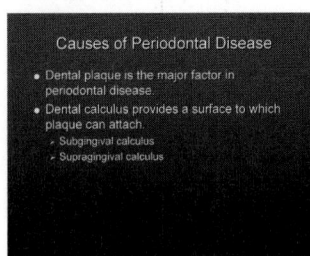

- What is dental plaque? *(It is a soft deposit of bacteria and bacterial by-products.)*
- How is most plaque removed? *(Plaque is removed by brushing and flossing.)*
- What is calculus? *(Calculus is calcium and phosphate salts that adhere to tooth surfaces.)*
- What is the difference between subgingival and supragingival calculus? Which is more harmful for the periodontium?

Slide 12

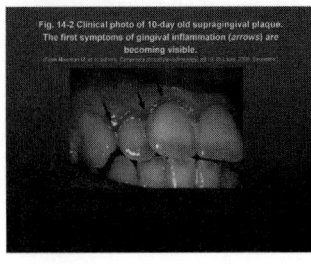

- Plaque cannot be removed by rinsing.
- Bacteria produce enzymes and toxins that destroy the periodontal tissues and lower defenses.
- The dental team must explain the need for improved home care to a patient and must document the instructions.
- If the patient's home care remains unimproved, that is contributory negligence leading to the development of periodontal disease.

Slide 13

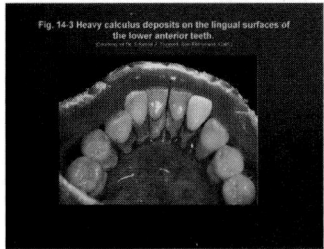

- How are the tissues in the figure responding to the calculus?
- What structures does this infection involve?
- What would the symptoms be?
- What would the radiographs look like?

Slide 14

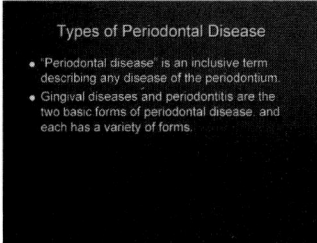

- What are the differences between gingival disease and periodontitis?

Slide 15

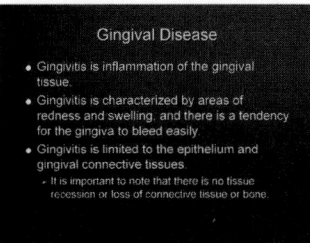

- How does gingivitis compare to periodontitis?

Slide 16

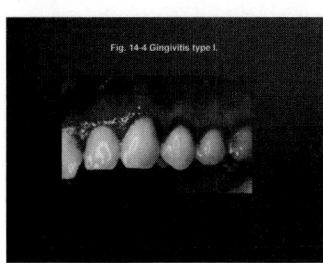

- Gingivitis is limited to the epithelium and gingival connective tissues.
- When would these gums bleed?

Bird/Robinson

Slide 17

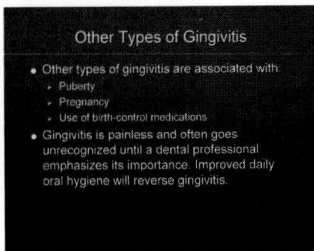

- Necrotizing ulcerative gingivitis (NUG) is characterized by sudden onset of pain, necrosis of the tips of the gingival papillae, and bleeding.

Slide 18

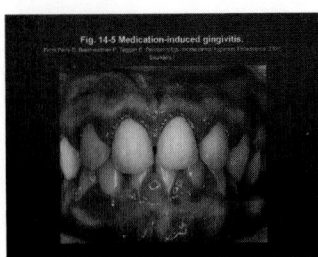

- Antiseizure drugs and hormones such as estrogen and progesterone can cause gingival enlargement.

Slide 19

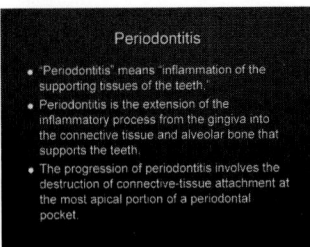

- What is periodontitis?

- How is severity determined?

Slide 20

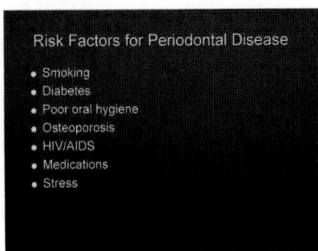

- Smokers have greater (1) loss of attachment, (2) bone loss, (3) periodontal pocket depths, (4) calculus formation, and (5) tooth loss.

- Periodontal treatments are less effective in smokers than in nonsmokers.

Slide 21

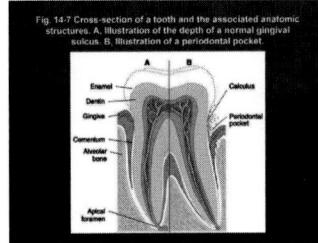

- The main area involved in periodontal disease is the gingival sulcus, a pocket between the teeth and the gums.

- What is a periodontal pocket? *(It is a pathologically deepened gingival sulcus--a feature of periodontal disease.)*

- How is this pocket measured? *(The dentist or dental hygienist can measure these pockets with a small probe to determine the extent of the disease.)*

Slide 22

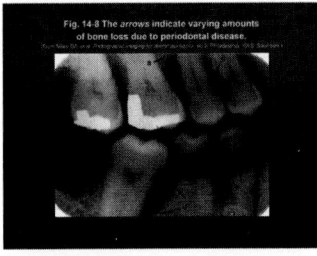

- The resulting bone loss is irreversible; the bone will not usually grow back.

- If the bone loss continues and the tooth support is compromised, the teeth become mobile and eventually are lost.

- Bone loss is also a major problem for dental patients who have had teeth extracted.

Slide 23

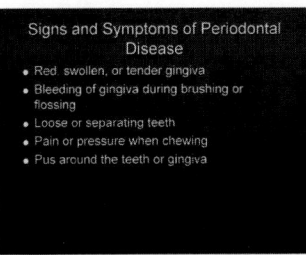

- Periodontal disease is described in terms of the severity of the disease and how much of the mouth is affected.

Bird/Robinson

TEACHING FOCUS

This chapter will give the student an opportunity to learn about preventive dentistry and the role of the dental assistant. Preventive dental care requires effective patient education, correct assessment and use of fluorides, a plaque control program, and nutritional considerations. Types of toothbrushes and brushing techniques will also be discussed along with procedures for assisting patients with dental floss, mouthrinses, oral irrigation devices, and proper cleaning of dentures.

MATERIALS AND RESOURCES

- ☐ blank food diary (Lesson 15.4)
- ☐ computer and PowerPoint projector (all Lessons)
- ☐ examples of topical forms of fluoride (Lesson 15.1)
- ☐ fluoride needs assessment form (Lesson 15.3)
- ☐ model of a set of teeth to illustrate proper flossing method (Lesson 15.4)
- ☐ model of dentures to show proper cleaning method (Lesson 15.4)
- ☐ photo of periodontal disease (Lesson 15.1)
- ☐ samples of mouthrinses available to consumers (Lesson 15.4)

- ☐ samples of sugar substitutes (Lesson 15.4)
- ☐ samples of various styles of toothbrushes (Lesson 15.4)
- ☐ typodont (Lessons 15.1 and 15.3)
- ☐ various chemotherapeutic products available to consumers (Lesson 15.3)
- ☐ video showing flossing techniques (Lesson 15.4)
- ☐ video showing the application of topical fluoride gel or foam (Lesson 5.3)
- ☐ video showing toothbrushing methods (Lesson 15.4)

LESSON CHECKLIST

Preparations for this lesson include:

- lecture
- guest speakers: dentist, dental hygienist
- evaluation of student knowledge and skills needed to perform all entry-level activities related to preventive dentistry, including:
  - ○ correct citing of the components of a comprehensive preventive dentistry program
  - ○ patient education on removal of plaque, proper toothbrushing method, and selection of home-care aids
  - ○ accurate fluoride needs assessment
  - ○ proper analysis of a food diary
  - ○ applying topical fluoride gel or foam
  - ○ assisting patients with dental floss

ELSEVIER

Torres and Ehrlich Modern Dental Assisting, 9th ed.

Bird/Robinson

KEY TERMS

dental sealant (p. 192)
disclosing agent (p. 191)
pontic (p. 207)

preventive dentistry (p. 190)
systemic fluoride (p. 192)
topical fluoride (p. 192)

ADDITIONAL RESOURCES

PowerPoint slides (Evolve): 1-64
Multimedia Procedures DVD:
    Applying Topical Fluoride Gel or Foam
    Flossing Techniques
    Toothbrushing Methods

Legend

	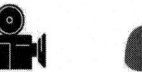					
CTQ Critical Thinking Question	**DVD** Multimedia Procedures Videos and Animations	**ESLR** EVOLVE Student Learning Resources	**IDO** Interactive Dental Office CD-ROM	**SW** Student Workbook	**TB** Test Bank on the TEACH CD-ROM	**PPT** PowerPoint Slides

Class Activities are indicated in ***bold italic***.

LESSON 15.1

PRETEST

1. What is the term used to describe a program that combines patient education, fluorides, sealants, nutrition, and plaque control?
   - a. restorative dentistry
   - b. preventive dentistry
   - c. periodontal dentistry
   - d. general dentistry

2. What is the goal of preventive dentistry?
   - a. prevent new and recurring disease
   - b. restore diseased teeth to proper function
   - c. replace missing teeth
   - d. to extract teeth

3. Systemic fluoride is ingested by which means?
   - a. toothpaste
   - b. mouthwash
   - c. floss
   - d. water

4. Topical fluoride is applied by which means?
   - a. water
   - b. toothpaste
   - c. food
   - d. tablets

5. Chronic overexposure to fluoride can result in which of the following?
   - a. fluorosis
   - b. cavities
   - c. premature loss of teeth
   - d. xerostomia

6. Prescription fluoride rinses generally contain
   - a. 0.10% stannous fluoride.
   - b. 0.63% stannous fluoride.
   - c. 1.00% stannous fluoride.
   - d. 1.40% stannous fluoride.

7. What is the term used to describe "caries causing"?
   - a. carcinogenic
   - b. preventive
   - c. restorative
   - d. cariogenic

8. What measurement or analysis is performed to determine if food intake is contributing to carious activity?
   - a. weigh-in
   - b. fat analysis
   - c. dietary analysis
   - d. hereditary analysis

9. What is the goal of a plaque control program?
   - a. to remove plaque once daily
   - b. to remove plaque once a week
   - c. to remove plaque at a patient's recall appointments
   - d. to remove plaque only when problems occur

10. What is the most frequently recommended toothbrushing method?
    - a. Charters
    - b. Modified Stillman
    - c. Fones
    - d. Modified Bass

Answers

1. b	3. d	5. a	7. d	9. a
2. a	4. b	6. b	8. c	10. d

BACKGROUND ASSESSMENT

Question: What is a dental sealant?

Answer: A dental sealant is a plastic-like coating that is applied over the occlusal pits and fissures of the teeth. Sealants are used to protect those areas because they are more difficult to clean on a regular basis. Dental sealants may be used on primary or permanent teeth.

ELSEVIER

Bird/Robinson

Question: What is the importance of patient education in preventive dentistry?

Answer: Patient education plays an important role in the success of preventive dentistry. In order for preventive dentistry to be successful, dental team members must educate patients through repetitive instructions about their home care. They must first listen carefully to the patient to understand how a patient perceives his or her dental health care needs. The dental team should instruct patients on how to remove plaque with the use of disclosing agents to show the patients the areas they are missing during their toothbrushing sessions. However, to receive the full cooperation of the patient, the dental team must recognize the patient's level of motivation and work with the patient according to the patient's needs. It is also very important to instruct the patient in the use of home-care aids. Finally, home care should be reinforced so the patients can meet their needs for good oral health.

CRITICAL THINKING QUESTION

How can dental team members identify patients who are in need of a therapeutic fluoride program?

Guidelines: Dental team members can determine an individual's need for a fluoride program by obtaining a "fluoride needs assessment." This assessment asks the patient a series of questions about such topics as current fluoride use, multiple restorations, candy consumption, snacking, soda consumption, and toothbrushing habits. This assessment will help the dental team and the patient by helping the patient identify areas that can be improved. It also allows the dentist to correctly identify the appropriate therapeutic program for the individual.

OBJECTIVES	CONTENT	TEACHING RESOURCES
Pronounce, define, and spell the Key Terms.	■ Key terms (p. 189)	*e* ESLR Electronic Flashcards ▸ Discuss each of the key terms in Chapter 15, focusing on the definition, pronunciation, and spelling of each term. *Class Activity **Have students use the key terms in an appropriate sentence.***
Explain the goal of preventive dentistry.	■ Introduction (p. 190)	PPT 4 TB question 1 SW Short-Answer Questions 1; Multiple Choice questions 1-2 (pp. 55-56) Recall questions 1-2 (p. 190) ▸ Discuss the challenges associated with preventive care as it pertains to patient habits and self-care patterns. *Class Activity **Show students examples of materials that are used to educate patients, including:*** *– videos* *– pamphlets* *– toothbrushes, floss, mouthrinses*
Describe the components of a preventive dentistry program.	■ Partners in prevention (p. 190)	PPT 5 TB questions 2-3, 22 SW Short-Answer Questions 3; Fill in the Blank question 1 (p. 55) Figure 15-1 Mother looks for early signs of decay (p. 190)

OBJECTIVES	CONTENT	TEACHING RESOURCES
		Table 15-1 Comprehensive Preventive Dentistry Care (p. 190) ▸ Discuss the most prominent nutritional deficiencies or needs of patients and how these affect good oral health. *Class Activity **Demonstrate the sealant procedure on a typodont. Ask students to identify other components that should be part of a preventive dentistry program and how these components might be influenced by patient characteristics. Discuss specific patient education points for a preventive dentistry program.***
Assist patients in understanding the benefits of preventive dentistry.	■ Patient education (p. 191)	PPT 6-8 SW Short-Answer Questions 2 (p. 55) Figure 15-2 Dental assistant uses intraoral camera to assist with patient education (p. 191) Recall question 3 (p. 191) ▸ Discuss ways to motivate patients to consistently practice better oral hygiene.. *Class Activity **Have students break into small groups. Each group must create a plan of action for the following situation. Discuss each plan when completed.*** *A patient comes in with concern about a recent diagnosis of high carious activity. The patient has been cavity-free for 10 years, drinks 10 sodas per day, does not floss, consumes well water, and is very motivated to find out what can be done to change the current situation.*

15.1 Homework/Assignments:

15.1 Instructor's Notes/Student Feedback:

Bird/Robinson

LESSON 15.2

CRITICAL THINKING QUESTION

A 7-year-old girl has just had a prophylaxis completed. During the dental examination the dentist informs the patient's mother that she will need sealants on her 6-year molars. The patient's mother feels that sealants are not necessary since her daughter is already 7 years old and hasn't had any cavities yet. What information can the dental assistant provide to the patient's mother about the benefits of having sealants placed?

Guidelines: The first thing the dental assistant should do is to compliment the young girl on her brushing habits since she has not had any cavities thus far. It is important to give all patients positive reinforcement on their oral health practices. In this patient's case, prevention is the goal of placing sealants. Sealants will prevent cavities from forming in the occlusal surfaces of her first molars, and although she doesn't have cavities now, it doesn't necessarily mean she won't develop them at a later date. The assistant should also explain to the patient's mother that sealants are a noninvasive procedure that will protect the chewing surfaces of the teeth from bacteria that could attack the hard-to-clean areas of these molars.

OBJECTIVES	CONTENT	TEACHING RESOURCES
Discuss techniques for educating patients in preventive care.	■ Patient education (p. 191) ■ Dental sealants (p. 192)	PPT 11-12 SW Short-Answer Questions 5; Fill in the Blank question 3; Multiple Choice questions 3-5 (pp. 55-56) Patient education guidelines (p. 191) Recall questions 4-5 (pp. 191-192) ▸ Discuss criteria for assessing and selecting the appropriate home care aids for patients. *Class Activity Conduct a group discussion on how to appropriately instruct the patient using the patient education guidelines. Use the following situations:* *1. A 30-year-old woman comes to the office with questions regarding manual toothbrushing versus automatic toothbrushing.* *2. An 8-year-old girl lives in the country (well water); the mother is concerned about inefficient fluoride in the water system. The girl's first molars have fully erupted.* *3. A 33-year-old man has had several bridges placed, was never shown how to properly clean around bridges, and is concerned that the lack of instruction will affect the success of the bridges.*
Describe the effect of water fluoridation on the teeth.	■ Fluoride (p. 192) ☐ How fluoride works (p. 193) – Preeruptive development (p. 193) – Posteruptive development (p. 193)	PPT 13-17 TB questions 4-6 SW Multiple Choice question 6 (p. 56) Figure 15-5 Topical forms of fluoride (p. 193) Recall questions 6-7 (p. 193) ▸ Discuss the pros and cons of commercial and professional uses of fluoride.

ELSEVIER

OBJECTIVES	CONTENT	TEACHING RESOURCES
		***Class Activity** Have students research the fluoridated water process and the level of fluoridation for the area in which they live. (For students to prepare for this activity, see Homework/Assignments #1.)*
Describe the effects of excessive amounts of fluoride.	☐ Safe and toxic levels (p. 193) ☐ Precautions (p. 193)	⊠▤ PPT 18 🖥 TB questions 7 📄 SW Short-Answer Questions 7; Fill in the Blank question 4; Multiple Choice questions 8-9 (pp. 55-56) 📄 SW Discussion question 3 (p. 57) Figure 15-6 Mild and moderate fluorosis (p. 193) Recall questions 8-9 (p. 193) ▸ Discuss the guidelines for safe use of fluoride in a young child. ***Class Activity** Discuss as a class the effects of fluorosis. Identify ways in which someone may develop fluorosis. Are children more susceptible to fluorosis?*

15.2 Homework/Assignments:
1. Have students research the fluoridated water process and the level of fluoridation for the area in which they live.

15.2 Instructor's Notes/Student Feedback:

LESSON 15.3

CRITICAL THINKING QUESTION

A 43-year-old man is concerned that his children are not getting the appropriate levels of fluoride because the area where they live does not supply fluoridated water. How can the patient ensure that his children are receiving the appropriate amounts of fluoride?

Guidelines: The patient's children are probably receiving some fluoride through the foods they eat, but there are other ways for the children to receive fluoride supplements. Topical fluoride is available in many home-care products such as fluoridated toothpastes and mouthrinses. However, depending on the age of his children, they may not be good candidates for these topical applications. In coordination with the dentist, the patient's children may be good candidates for a prescribed fluoride supplement that is dispensed in tablets, drops, or lozenges. This type of supplementation is recommended only for those under the age of 16.

OBJECTIVES	CONTENT	TEACHING RESOURCES
Describe the purpose of a fluoride needs assessment.	■ Fluoride needs assessment (p. 194) □ Fluoride needs assessment (checklist) (p. 194) □ Sources of fluoride (p. 194)	PPT 21-26 TB questions 8-9 SW Short-Answer Questions 8 (p. 55) ▶ Discuss the benefits of sharing the results of a fluoride needs assessment with a patient. Which aspects should be emphasized the most? *Class Activity **Have the students complete a fluoride needs assessment for another student, then have students assess their own need for fluoride.***
Identify sources of systemic fluoride.	□ Sources of systemic fluoride (p. 194) – Foods and beverages (p. 194) – Prescribed dietary supplements (p. 194)	PPT 27-28 TB question 10 SW Short-Answer Questions 4 (p. 55) ▶ Discuss best and worst sources of systemic fluoride in foods, beverages and dietary supplements. *Class Activity **Have students find five examples of systemic fluoride. Discuss the factors the dentist will consider before prescribing a dietary fluoride supplement.***
Discuss three methods of fluoride therapy.	□ Sources of topical fluoride (p. 195) – Toothpastes (p. 195) – Mouthrinses (p. 197) – Gels (p. 197) – Professional applications (p. 197) [Procedure] 15-1 Applying topical fluoride gel or foam (pp. 198-199) (SW/ESLR Competency 15-1, p. 59)	PPT 29-32 Multimedia Procedures DVD: Applying a Topical Fluoride Gel or Foam TB question 11 SW Short-Answer Questions 6; Fill in the Blank question 5; Multiple Choice question 7 (pp. 55-56) SW/ESLR Competency 15-1 Applying Topical Fluoride Gel or Foam (p. 59) Figure 15-7 Fluoride dispensed in tablet form (p. 195) Figure 15-8 Prescription-strength mouthrinse and dentrifice to prevent dental decay (p. 195) Table 15-2 Types of Professionally Applied Fluorides (p. 195)

OBJECTIVES	CONTENT	TEACHING RESOURCES
		Table 15-3 Fluoride Therapies for Home Use (p. 196) Figure 15-9 The dental assistant is applying a fluoride varnish to this child's teeth (p. 195)
		Figure 15-10 Training toothpaste for young children (p. 197)
		Figure 15-11 Various chemotherapeutic products available to consumers (p. 197)
		▶ Discuss the advantages or disadvantages of home-use fluoride treatments versus professionally applied treatments.
		Class Activity **Have students demonstrate the three methods of fluoride therapy on a typodont. Ask students to compare and contrast the three methods and identify the specific benefits of each method.**

15.3 Homework/Assignments:

15.3 Instructor's Notes/Student Feedback:

LESSON 15.4

CRITICAL THINKING QUESTION

A 72-year-old woman comes to the office with questions regarding toothbrushes. Currently, she is using a large-headed, hard-bristled toothbrush that is approximately 15 months old. She states that her gums have been quite tender lately and she has been scrubbing those areas more aggressively, because she fears there may be cavities there. She also states that her arthritis has been acting up lately, and she is having difficulties holding the floss. The patient also states she is using herbal toothpaste that does not contain fluoride. What advice should be given to the patient about her home care?

Guidelines: After listening to the patient's concerns, it is important to acknowledge the efforts of her oral home care. She should then be informed that there are several options for toothbrushes, but a hard-bristled toothbrush may not be the best option for her at this time. Soft-bristled toothbrushes adapt to the contours of the tooth, and are less traumatic to the gum tissue. It should also be explained that toothbrushes should be replaced when the bristles have shown signs of wear and tear—generally around 8 to 12 weeks. It is important to discuss the toothbrushing method that the patient is using, and encourage her to use the Modified Bass method. This method requires the bristles to be in the sulcus at a 45° angle. Short, gentle strokes are followed by a "rolling stroke" that is repeated approximately five times for each area. The importance of using fluoride toothpaste should also be explained, but if the patient is opposed to changing brands, she could be encouraged to use a fluoride supplement such as a brush-on gel, dental rinse, or a prescription rinse to help ward off decay. Since the patient has mentioned that her arthritis is affecting her flossing abilities, she can try using an automatic flosser. Once the floss has been placed interproximally, the automatic flosser is turned to the 'on' position and will vibrate to help remove plaque from those areas.

OBJECTIVES	CONTENT	TEACHING RESOURCES
Explain the steps in analyzing a food diary.	■ Nutrition and dental caries (p. 197) □ Sugar substitutes (p. 197) – Xylitol (p. 199) □ Dietary analysis (p. 199) – Steps for analyzing a food diary (p. 200)	PPT 35-39 TB questions 13-14 SW Multiple Choice questions 10-12 (p. 56) SW Discussion question 1 (p. 57) Figure 15-12 Ford Xtreme Xylitol gum and Sugar Free Dental Care gum containing xylitol and sorbitol (p. 200) Hard facts about soft drinks (p. 200) Recall questions 10-12 (p. 200) CTQ 1 (p. 210) ▸ Discuss when a food diary is necessary and the best ways to help patients maintain consistency in recording their dietary intake. *Class Activity Have students keep a food diary for themselves for three days; have students assess whether their dietary intake is affecting their oral health.*
Compare and contrast the methods of toothbrushing techniques.	■ Plaque control program (p. 200) □ Toothbrushes and toothbrushing (p. 201) – Manual toothbrushes (p. 201)	PPT 40-56 Multimedia Procedures DVD: Flossing Techniques; Toothbrushing Methods TB questions 15-19 SW Short-Answer Questions 9; Fill in the Blank question 2; Multiple Choice questions 13-17, 19 (pp. 55-56)

ELSEVIER

Torres and Ehrlich Modern Dental Assisting, 9th ed.

OBJECTIVES	CONTENT	TEACHING RESOURCES
	– Automatic toothbrushes (p. 201) – Toothbrushing methods (p. 201) – Toothbrushing precautions (p. 204) – Toothbrushing for unusual conditions (p. 204) ☐ Dental floss or tape (p. 205) – When to floss (p. 205) ☐ Interdental aids (p. 205) – End tuft brushes (p. 207) – Bridge threaders (p. 207) – Automatic flossers (p. 207) – Perio-aid (p. 207) **Procedure** 15-2 Assisting the patient with dental floss (p. 206) (SW/ESLR Competency 15-2, p. 61)	▱ SW Discussion questions 2, 4 (p. 57) ▱ *e* SW/ESLR Competency 15-2 Assisting the Patient with Dental Floss (p. 61) Figure 15-14 Examples of manual toothbrushes (p. 201) Figure 15-15 Proper positioning of a powered toothbrush head and bristle tips is critical to achieving effective cleaning results (p. 202) Table 15-4 Examples of Powered Toothbrushes (p. 202) Table 15-5 Toothbrushing Methods (p. 203) Figure 15-16. Bass method (p. 204) Figure 15-17 Observing toothbrushing technique (p. 204) Figure 15-18 Improper brushing techniques resulting in abrasions of the tooth surface causing gingival recession (p. 204) Figure 15-19 The dental assistant helping with patient flossing (p. 205) Figure 15-20 Interproximal cleaning devices (p. 205) Figure 15-21 An interdental hygienic aid (p. 205) Figure 15-22 A bridge threader used as an aid to clean under a fixed bridge (p. 207) Figure 15-23 Powered flossing devices (p. 207) Figure 15-24 Perio-aid (p. 208) ♀ CTQ 2-3 (p. 210) Recall questions 13-17; 19-20 (pp. 204-205; 209) ▸ Discuss ways to assess and correct a patient's ineffective or harmful toothbrushing method. *Class Activity Have students demonstrate how they brush their teeth now; identify changes that should be implemented, and discuss how they will adapt to the recommended changes.*
Describe the process for cleaning a denture.	☐ Dentures (p. 207) ☐ Toothpaste (p. 207) ☐ Mouthrinses (p. 209) ☐ Oral irrigation devices (p. 209) ☐ General guidelines for home care products (p. 209)	⊠ PPT 57-64 ▱ TB questions 19-21 ▱ SW Short-Answer Questions 10; Multiple Choice question 18 (pp. 55, 56) ▱ SW Discussion question 5 (p. 57) Figure 15-25 Denture and denture brush (p. 208) Figure 15-26 Toothpaste for children (p. 208) Table 15-6 Types of Toothpastes (p. 208) Figure 15-27 Mouthrinses (p. 209)

OBJECTIVES	CONTENT	TEACHING RESOURCES
		Figure 15-28 Irrigator (p. 209)
		Figure 15-29 The American Dental Association's Seal of Acceptance (p. 209)
		Recall question 18 (p. 209)
		▸ Discuss the particular aspects of cleaning dentures that are different from regular brushing of natural teeth.
		***Class Activity** Demonstrateon a denture the procedure for cleaning a denture or partial denture. Discuss the types of cleaners and brush strokes that should be used when cleaning dentures.*
Performance Evaluation		🖥 TB
		📘 SW questions (pp. 55-57)
		📘 *e* SW/ESLR Competency 15-1 Applying Topical Fluoride Gel or Foam (p. 59)
		📘 *e* SW/ESLR Competency 15-2 Assisting the Patient with Dental Floss (p. 61)
		e ESLR Electronic Flashcards
		e ESLR Practice Quiz
		Recall questions (pp. 190-193, 200, 204-205, 209)

15.4 Homework/Assignments:

15.4 Instructor's Notes/Student Feedback:

Torres and Ehrlich Modern Dental Assisting, 9th ed.

Bird/Robinson

Slide 1

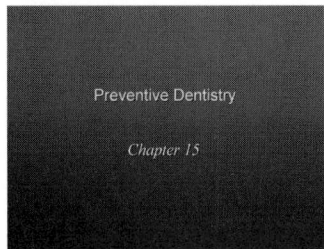

Slide 2

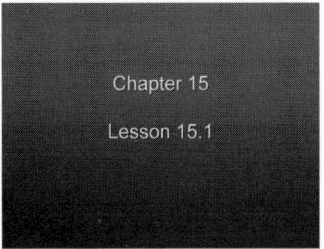

Slide 3

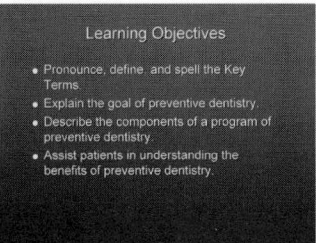

Slide 4

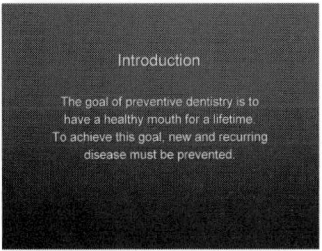

- What are the two most common types of dental diseases?
- Preventive dentistry:
    - Used to achieve optimal oral health for a lifetime
    - An ongoing process

Torres and Ehrlich Modern Dental Assisting, 9th ed.
Bird/Robinson

Slide 5

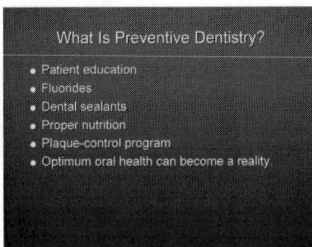

What Is Preventive Dentistry?

- Patient education
- Fluorides
- Dental sealants
- Proper nutrition
- Plaque-control program
- Optimum oral health can become a reality.

- If the patient is unwilling to cooperate or is unmotivated, has "preventive dentistry" been accomplished?

Slide 6

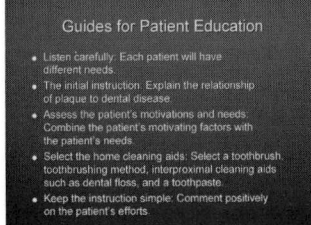

Guides for Patient Education

- Listen carefully: Each patient will have different needs.
- The initial instruction: Explain the relationship of plaque to dental disease.
- Assess the patient's motivations and needs: Combine the patient's motivating factors with the patient's needs.
- Select the home cleaning aids: Select a toothbrush, toothbrushing method, interproximal cleaning aids such as dental floss, and a toothpaste.
- Keep the instruction simple: Comment positively on the patient's efforts.

- Patient education:
  - It requires a partnership between the patient and the dental team.
  - It is used to develop and maintain good oral habits.
- How often do we need to educate the patient on his or her oral habits?

Slide 7

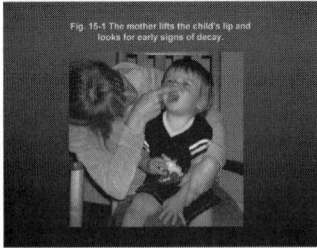

Fig. 15-1 The mother lifts the child's lip and looks for early signs of decay.

Slide 8

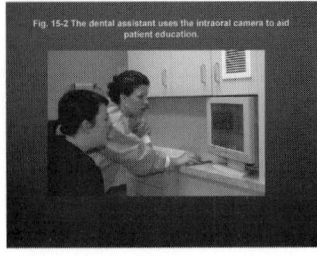

Fig. 15-2 The dental assistant uses the intraoral camera to aid patient education.

- What is the benefit of using an intraoral camera? *(To show patients a close-up view of their teeth.)*

Slide 9

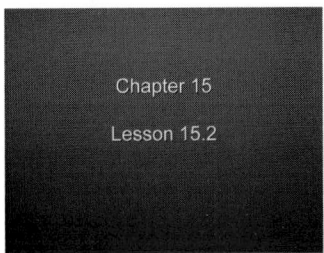

Slide 10

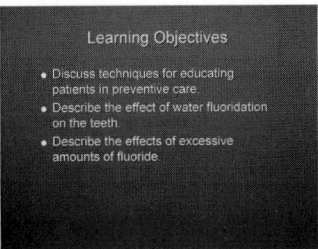

Slide 11

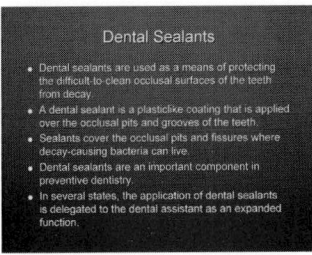

- Sealants are generally placed on permanent teeth, but if a child is susceptible to decay, sealants can be placed on primary teeth.

- Can sealants be placed on anterior teeth? *(Yes, on lingual pits of anterior teeth.)*

Slide 12

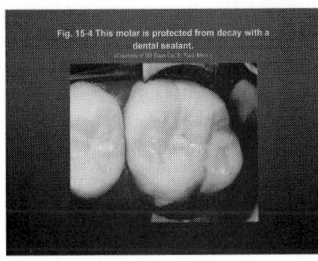

- Sealants are white or clear. White sealants are used to visualize placement and retention.

Slide 13

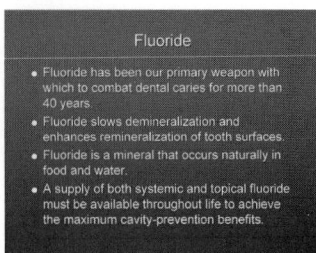

- What is demineralization? *(The removal of mineral components from mineralized tissues.)*
- What is remineralization? *(The process of restoring minerals to a mineralized tissue that has been demineralized.)*

Slide 14

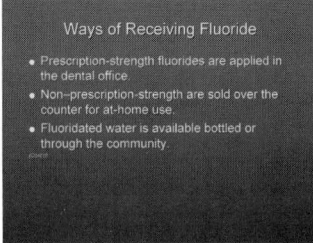

- How the patient receives fluoride is based on the patient's needs.
- Needs will vary from patient to patient.

Slide 15

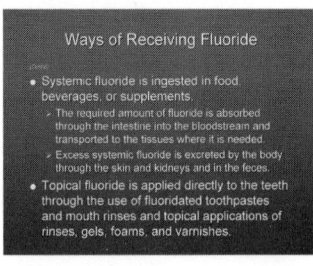

- Systemic fluroide is available in bottled water, meat, vegetables, cereals, citrus fruits, tea, and fish.
- Topical fluoride is included in in-office application of fluoride, fluoride rinses, and fluoride toothpastes.

Slide 16

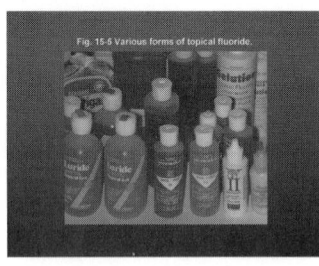

- In-office fluoride comes in gel, foam, rinse, or liquid form.
- It is flavored for patient comfort; patient chooses flavor.
- Each has different contact time; check manufacturer's directions.
- It is used with disposable trays after a prophylaxis has been completed.
- Patients are instructed not to eat or drink anything for 30 minutes after placement of topical fluoride.

Bird/Robinson

Slide 17

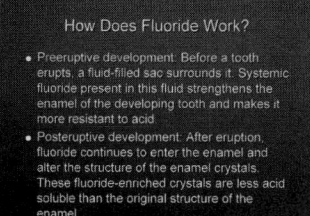

- Before birth, fluoride comes from the expectant mother's diet.
- Posteruptive development requires systemic and topical fluoride for the remineralization process.

Slide 18

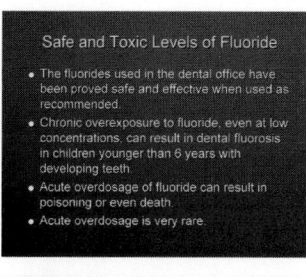

- What is fluorosis? *(Mottled enamel caused by excessive fluoride intake.)*
- What is mottled enamel? *(Discoloration of enamel; mostly white)*
- Lethal dose of fluoride varies from 2.5 to 10 g in adults to as low as 0.25 g in infants.
- When a fluoride overdose is suspected, instruct patient to drink milk.
- Milk will soothe irritated mucous membranes.
- Patient should seek medical attention immediately.

Slide 19

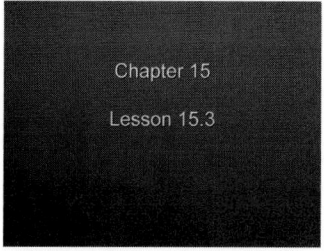

Slide 20

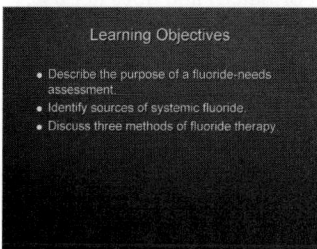

Bird/Robinson

Slide 21

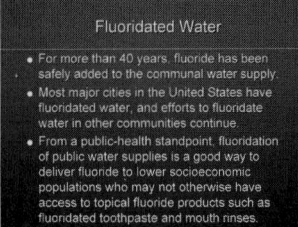

- Very controversial issue; many people are opposed to fluoridated water.
- Does your area supply fluoridated water?
- Do you know the levels in your area?
- Dental team members need to stay up-to-date with fluoride controversy.

Slide 22

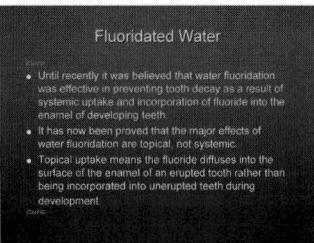

- Fluoridated water is a source of which fluoride? *(Systemic.)*

Slide 23

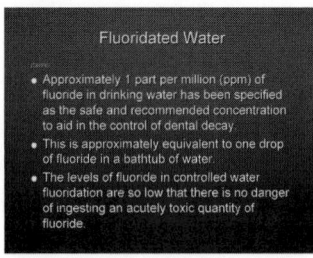

- Some states have water that naturally contains more than twice the optimum levels of fluoride.

Slide 24

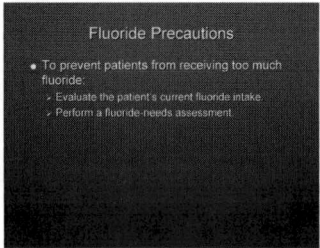

- If a patient has well water (generally not fluoridated) and does not use fluoride toothpaste, should the dentist prescribe a fluoride supplement?
- Needs assessment determines the patient's need for a fluoride program.

Bird/Robinson

Slide 25

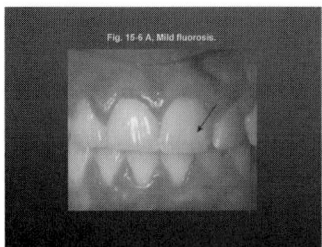

- White "spots" on teeth indicate mild fluorosis.

Slide 26

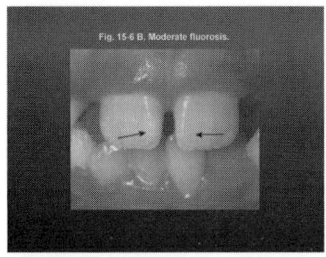

- Discoloration due to moderate fluorosis.
- Do any of the students have fluorosis?

Slide 27

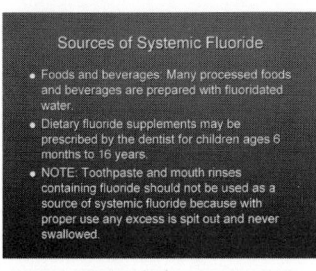

- Food: meat, vegetables, cereals, and citrus fruits naturally contain small amounts of fluoride; tea and fish have slightly higher levels of fluoride.
- Not all bottled water contains fluoride; check labels.
- Prescribed fluoride treatments would include tablets, drops, and rinses.

Slide 28

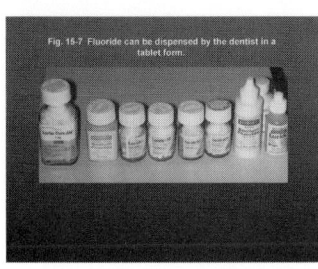

- Examples of tablets that are dispensed by the dentist
- What is the recommended age group for prescribed fluoride supplements? *(Six months to 16 years of age.)*

Slide 29

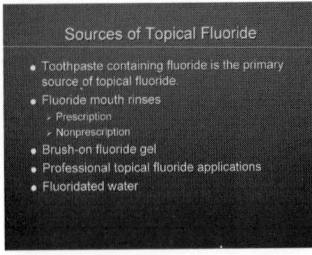

- Applied to make teeth more resistant to demineralization and to assist in the remineralization of decalcified areas
- Can reduce caries by 40% to 50%.
- OTC rinses contain 0.05% sodium fluoride.
- Rx rinses contain 0.63% stannous fluoride or 0.2% sodium fluoride.
- OTC gels contain 1.1% sodium fluoride.
- Rx gels contain 2% sodium fluoride.

Slide 30

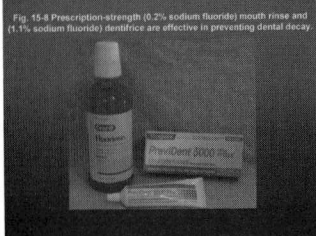

- Examples of fluoride rinses and fluoride toothpastes.
- How many of the students use a fluoride toothpaste?
- Of those who do not, how many use another type of fluoride supplement?

Slide 31

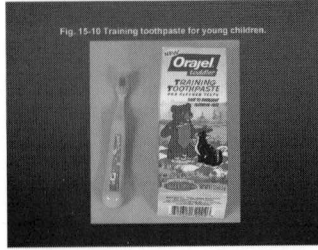

- Training toothpastes do not contain fluoride.
- Length of toothbrushing should not change.
- Small amount of toothpaste should be used.

Slide 32

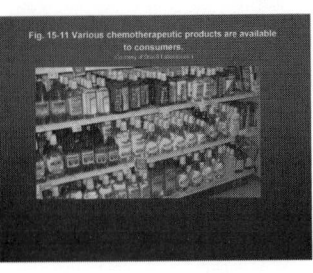

- Examples of rinses that are available.

Slide 33

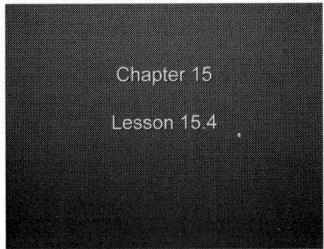

Slide 34

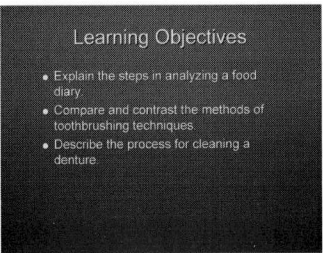

Slide 35

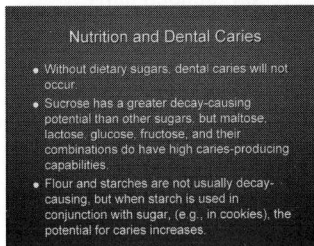

- What is another term for "decay-causing?" *(Cariogenic.)*

- Patients should be asked about their dietary intake when assessing their fluoride needs.

Slide 36

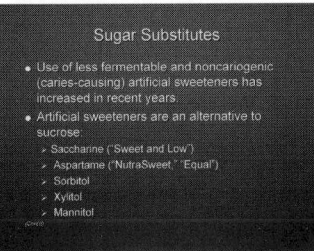

- Artificial sweeteners were initially developed for diabetics and those who struggled with obesity.

Torres and Ehrlich Modern Dental Assisting, 9th ed.
Bird/Robinson

Slide 37

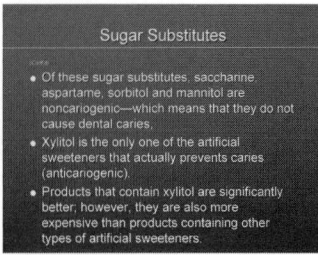

- Xylitol is derived from birch trees, corn cobs, oats, bananas, and certain mushrooms.

- Studies are constantly conducted to find reasons why Xylitol prevents tooth decay.

Slide 38

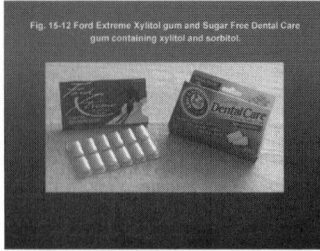

- Xylitol is approximately 10 times more expensive than sucrose.

- Xylitol gum is more expensive than Arm & Hammer gum.

Slide 39

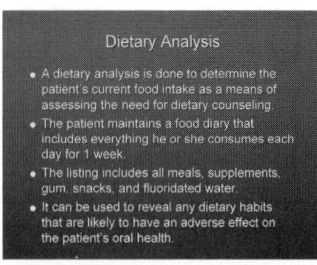

- Food diary includes: times food/snacks were eaten; foods sweetened with added sugars; fresh fruit vs. dried fruit; recommended daily allowance vs. actual daily consumption.

- Diary should also include any fluoride supplements that have been used.

Slide 40

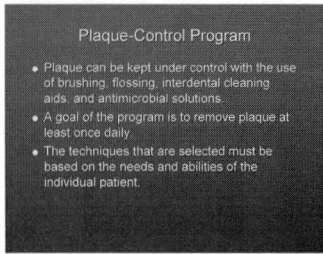

- What is plaque? *(A soft deposit on the teeth consisting of bacteria and bacteria products.)*

- How is plaque removed from the teeth?

- Once removed, it takes plaque 24 hours to accumulate.

Bird/Robinson

Slide 41

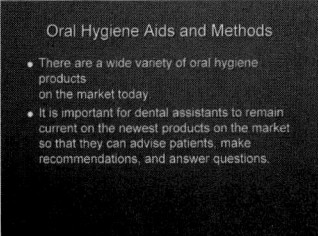

- Should be part of the patient education program.
- Dental team members should be aware of different products.
- Which products do the students use?

Slide 42

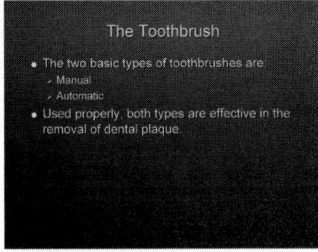

- Toothbrush:
  - When used with a fluoridated toothpaste, can be very effective.
  - Many sizes are available (infant, child/teen, adult, appliances).
- What types of toothbrushes do the students use?

Slide 43

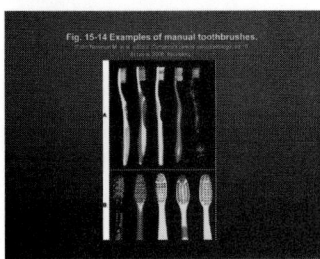

- Soft bristled brushes are recommended; they are gentler on the gum tissue.
- Nylon bristles are preferred; the ends are rounded.
- The brush should be replaced every 8 to 12 weeks or when bristles are worn.
- Different-sized handles are available.

Slide 44

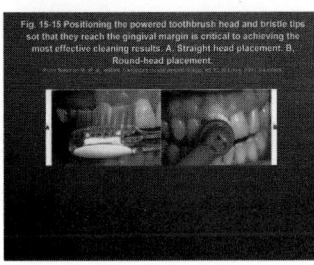

- Many automatic toothbrushes available on the market.
- How many students use an automatic toothbrush?
- Powered toothbrush:
  - It can have built-in timers.
  - It can have pulsating or ultrasonic action.
  - Heads are interchangeable, so that many people may use one unit.
  - Larger handles are especially good for children and the elderly.

Bird/Robinson

Slide 45

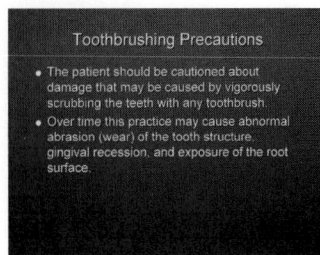

- The dental team can observe the toothbrushing techniques of patients to ensure they are using their toothbrushes properly.

- Toothbrushes should be sized and shaped correctly to allow for sufficient cleaning and easy management (i.e., an adult should not use a child-size toothbrush).

Slide 46

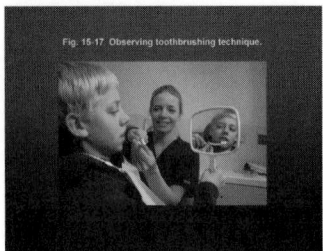

- As part of the patient education program, the dental team should have the patient brush his or her teeth and give instruction on how to correct bad habits.

- A disclosing agent could be used after this procedure to show the patient where he or she is missing during toothbrushing sessions.

Slide 47

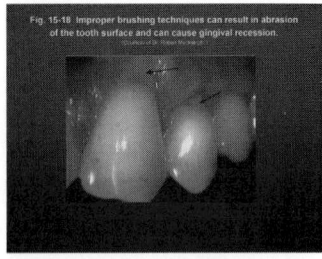

- Which teeth are involved?

- What instruction should be given to this patient to improve toothbrushing technique?

Slide 48

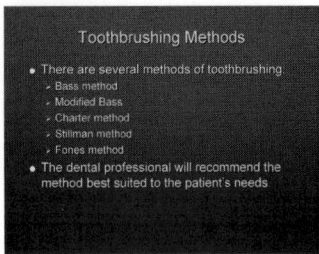

- The most common is the Modified Bass.

- What method do the students use?

- What is the recommended length a patient should brush his or her teeth? *(3 minutes.)*

- Patients who have good plaque control due to good brushing habits should be commended—but continue to coach them.

Slide 49

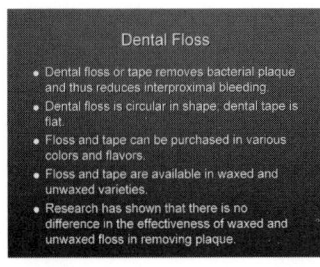

Dental Floss

- Dental floss or tape removes bacterial plaque and thus reduces interproximal bleeding.
- Dental floss is circular in shape; dental tape is flat.
- Floss and tape can be purchased in various colors and flavors.
- Floss and tape are available in waxed and unwaxed varieties.
- Research has shown that there is no difference in the effectiveness of waxed and unwaxed floss in removing plaque.

- How many students floss their teeth on a regular basis?
- What type of floss do they use?
- Flossing has been shown to be the most effective way of removing plaque from the interproximal areas.
- Flossing should be done *before* brushing teeth.
- Patients should use approximately 18 inches of floss.

Slide 50

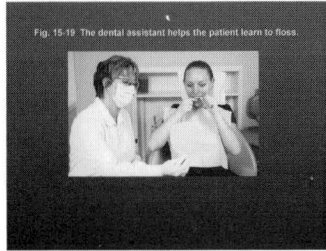

Fig. 15-19 The dental assistant helps the patient learn to floss.

- Patients should be instructed to "wrap" the floss around the tooth and move in an "up and down" direction.
- Patients should be instructed never to floss using a "sawing" motion.
- Flossing aids are available to help during the procedure.

Slide 51

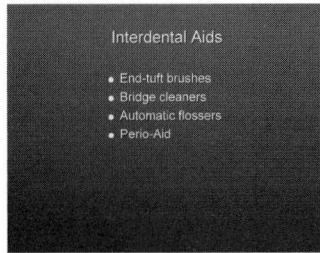

Interdental Aids

- End-tuft brushes
- Bridge cleaners
- Automatic flossers
- Perio-Aid

- Many different aids are available depending on the patient's needs.
- Interdental aids are used for cleaning under fixed bridges, orthodontic work, or cleaning in open spaces.

Slide 52

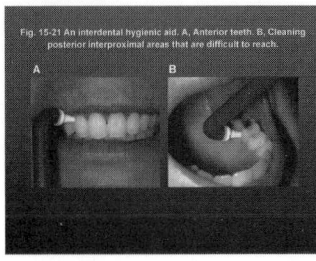

Fig. 15-21 An interdental hygienic aid. A, Anterior teeth. B, Cleaning posterior interproximal areas that are difficult to reach.

- End-tuft toothbrush:
  - It is made much like a regular toothbrush, but has a much smaller head
  - Soft, nylon bristles are used.
  - It is used to clean hard-to-reach areas.
  - It can be used to clean around orthodontic brackets.

Torres and Ehrlich Modern Dental Assisting, 9th ed.

Bird/Robinson

Slide 53

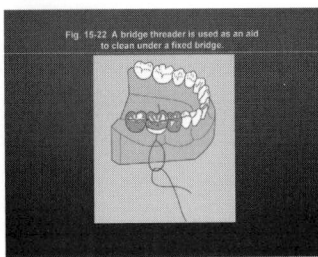

Fig. 15-22 A bridge threader is used as an aid to clean under a fixed bridge.

- Regular cleaning under a bridge is important for the success of the bridge.
- Patients should be instructed on the appropriate technique for using a floss threader.
- Bridge cleaner is made of flexible plastic and looks like a large needle.
- Floss is "threaded" through the bridge cleaner; floss threader is then "threaded" under the pontic.
- Floss threaders may also be used on patients who have fixed orthodontics (brackets).

Slide 54

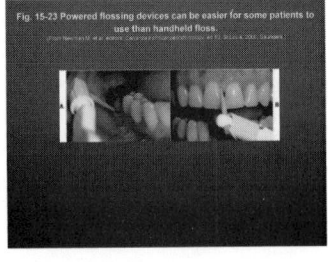

Fig. 15-23 Powered flossing devices can be easier for some patients to use than handheld floss.
(From Newman et al. editors: Carranza's clinical periodontology, ed 10, St Louis, 2006, Saunders.)

- Automatic flosser:
  - Designed to help those that have difficulty using the traditional flossing technique
  - Good for patients who have arthritis
  - Inserted interproximally and turned "on"
  - Uses vibrations to remove plaque interproximally
  - Disposable heads
  - Replacement heads available

Slide 55

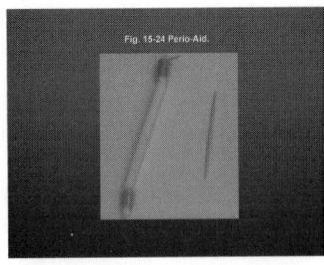

Fig. 15-24 Perio-Aid.

- PerioAid:
  - Designed to hold toothpicks
  - Used to clean hard-to-reach areas
  - Can be used to stimulate gingival tissue

Slide 56

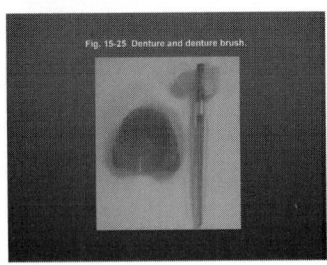

Fig. 15-25 Denture and denture brush.

- Specific brushes are available to clean dentures, partial dentures, and orthodontic appliances.
- Brushes can be used with toothpaste, denture cleaner, mild soap, or dishwashing liquid.
- Unlike a toothbrush, this brush has stiffer bristles.
- Dentures, partial dentures, and orthodontic appliances should be cleaned daily.

Slide 57

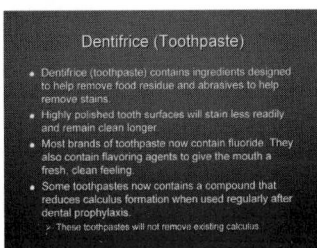

- Use only toothpastes that have been tested and approved by the ADA.
- What is the ADA? *(American Dental Association.)*
- Many different types of toothpastes are available.
- A small, pea-sized amount should be used.
- What type of toothpaste do the students use? Why?

Slide 58

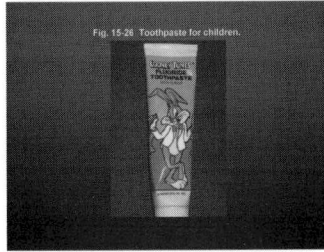

- Toothpastes for children have "kid-oriented" flavors, such as bubble gum.
- Cartoons on packaging are a good motivating factor for children.

Slide 59

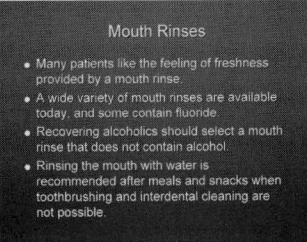

- Mouth rinses should be used in conjunction with other plaque removal techniques.

Slide 60

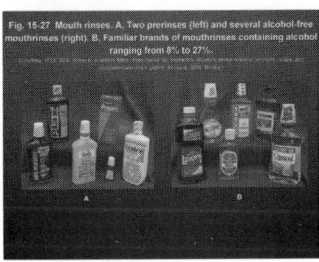

- Mouth rinses are used for cosmetic or therapeutic purposes.
- Rinsing can loosen debris from the oral cavity but does not remove it completely.
- Rinsing can give patients fresh breath.
- Some mouth rinses do contain alcohol.
- What type of mouth rinse should be avoided by a recovering alcoholic?
- Dental team members should be up-to-date on new products that are available.

Bird/Robinson

Slide 61

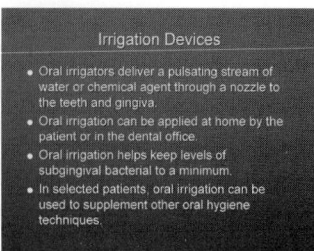

Irrigation Devices

- Oral irrigators deliver a pulsating stream of water or chemical agent through a nozzle to the teeth and gingiva.
- Oral irrigation can be applied at home by the patient or in the dental office.
- Oral irrigation helps keep levels of subgingival bacterial to a minimum.
- In selected patients, oral irrigation can be used to supplement other oral hygiene techniques.

Slide 62

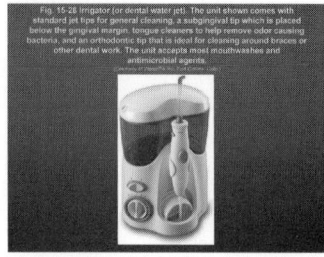

Fig. 15-28 Irrigator (or dental water jet). The unit shown comes with standard jet tips for general cleaning, a subgingival tip which is placed below the gingival margin, tongue cleaners to help remove odor causing bacteria, and an orthodontic tip that is ideal for cleaning around braces or other dental work. The unit accepts most mouthwashes and antimicrobial agents.

- An oral irrigator is used to reduce levels of bacteria subgingivally.
- An oral irrigator should be used in conjunction with other oral hygiene techniques.

Slide 63

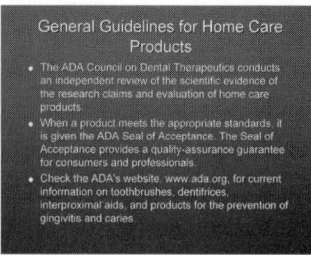

General Guidelines for Home Care Products

- The ADA Council on Dental Therapeutics conducts an independent review of the scientific evidence of the research claims and evaluation of home care products.
- When a product meets the appropriate standards, it is given the ADA Seal of Acceptance. The Seal of Acceptance provides a quality-assurance guarantee for consumers and professionals.
- Check the ADA's website, www.ada.org, for current information on toothbrushes, dentifrices, interproximal aids, and products for the prevention of gingivitis and caries.

- Dental team members should be up-to-date on new oral health care products.

Slide 64

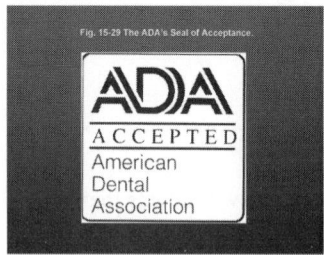

Fig. 15-29 The ADA's Seal of Acceptance.

Bird/Robinson

TEACHING FOCUS

This chapter will give students an opportunity to learn about the importance of nutrition in the context of overall oral health care. The primary nutrients will be emphasized along with dietary guidelines for intake; the role of antioxidants, how to read food labels, and proper eating habits will also be discussed. Students will also have the opportunity to learn about the effect of eating disorders on oral health.

MATERIALS AND RESOURCES

- ☐ computer and PowerPoint projector (all Lessons)
- ☐ food products with complicated labels (Lesson 16.2)
- ☐ samples of complex carbohydrates and simple sugars (Lesson 16.1)
- ☐ sample dietary analysis form (Lesson 16.2)

LESSON CHECKLIST

Preparations for this lesson include:

- lecture
- evaluation of student knowledge and skills needed to perform all entry-level activities related to nutrition, including:
  - o the role of nutrition in oral health
  - o the primary nutrients and their role in overall oral health
  - o correctly interpreting nutrition label facts and claims made about "organic" foods
  - o characteristics of anorexia and bulimia
  - o guidelines for healthy eating habits and the Food Guide Pyramid

Bird/Robinson

KEY TERMS

amino acids (p. 215)   fats (p. 215)
anorexia nervosa (p. 222)   nutrients (p. 212)
bulimia (p. 222)   organic (p. 221)
cariogenic (p. 214)   triglycerides (p. 215)

ADDITIONAL RESOURCES

PowerPoint slides (Evolve): 1-44

Legend

CTQ
Critical
Thinking
Question

DVD
Multimedia
Procedures
Videos and
Animations

ESLR
EVOLVE
Student
Learning
Resources

IDO
Interactive
Dental
Office
CD-ROM

SW
Student
Workbook

TB
Test Bank
on the
TEACH
CD-ROM

PPT
PowerPoint
Slides

Class Activities are indicated in ***bold italic***.

ELSEVIER

Torres and Ehrlich Modern Dental Assisting, 9th ed.

Bird/Robinson

LESSON 16.1

PRETEST

1. The components in food that are needed by the body to supply energy are called
   a. antioxidants.
   b. nutrients.
   c. triglycerides.
   d. multivitamins.

2. How many sections are in the Food Guide Pyramid?
   a. three
   b. four
   c. five
   d. six

3. Which section of the Food Guide Pyramid has the most recommended servings?
   a. vegetables
   b. fats, oils, and sweets
   c. bread, cereal, rice, and pasta
   d. fruits

4. Compounds in proteins used by the body to build and repair tissue are
   a. cariogenic.
   b. organic.
   c. reconstructive acids.
   d. amino acids.

5. In an average American, what percentage of calories comes from fat?
   a. 20%
   b. 40%
   c. 60%
   d. 80%

6. Proper bone and tooth formation is reliant on adequate supplies of
   a. vitamin A.
   b. vitamin B.
   c. vitamin D.
   d. vitamin K.

7. Which government agency requires that all food products contain a nutrition fact label?
   a. USDA
   b. FDA
   c. EPA
   d. OSHA

8. Foods that have been grown without the use of chemical pesticides, herbicides, or fertilizers are
   a. organic.
   b. minerals.
   c. inorganic.
   d. carbohydrates.

9. Which diet-related disorder is strongly correlated to obesity and high salt intake?
   a. anemia
   b. anorexia nervosa
   c. cirrhosis
   d. hypertension

10. Which diet-related disorder deals with an altered self-image?
    a. anemia
    b. anorexia nervosa
    c. bulimia
    d. hypertension

Answers

1. b	3. c	5. c	7. a	9. d
2. d	4. d	6. c	8. a	10. b

BACKGROUND ASSESSMENT

Question: What is good nutrition?

Answer: Nutrition is the science of the way the body uses food for development, repair, growth, and maintenance. Nutrients are needed by our bodies and are organized into six categories: carbohydrates, proteins, fats, water, vitamins, and minerals. Good nutrition is recommended for all age groups, but is extremely important in the elderly, young children, and pregnant women. Good nutrition can be obtained by following the recommended dietary (daily) allowances, and by limiting fermentable carbohydrate and sugar intake.

ELSEVIER

Bird/Robinson

Question: What are proteins?

Answer: Proteins are the only nutrients that have the ability to repair and build body tissues. Proteins build amino acids, which are used in the building and repairing process. There are 20 amino acids in an adult body; 8 of them are essential for normal growth and tissue maintenance. There are 3 types of proteins: complete, partially complete, and incomplete. Complete proteins include meat, fish, and poultry and are a balance of all 8 essential amino acids. Partially complete proteins include grains and vegetables; these maintain life, but do not support normal growth. Incomplete proteins include corn and gelatin; they support neither life nor normal growth.

CRITICAL THINKING QUESTION

When asked about his diet, a patient states that he has gained approximately 30 lbs in the last few months and expresses concern about his overall health and appearance. He also says that he has been eating a lot of fast food because he doesn't have time to cook, but that he is thinking of beginning an all-organic diet in order to lose weight. How should the dental assistant respond, and what other suggestions could be made?

Guidelines: Although eating organic foods may be healthier because pesticides, herbicides, or fertilizers haven't been used, it is important to educate the patient about other options. The first step should be to obtain an analysis of the patient's dietary consumption in order to identify the areas that require changes. It is crucial that the patient understand the recommended dietary (daily) allowance for individuals. Eating a healthier diet will help the patient to look and feel better as well as have more energy. This information may help the patient understand how to achieve overall healthy eating habits, rather than just switching to an all-organic diet.

OBJECTIVES	CONTENT	TEACHING RESOURCES
Pronounce, define, and spell the Key Terms.	■ Key terms (p. 211)	*e* ESLR Electronic Flashcards ▸ Discuss each of the key terms in Chapter 16, focusing on the definition, pronunciation, and spelling of each term. *Class Activity Have each student use one of the key terms in a clinically relevant sentence in order to define the term. Continue until all terms have been used; if students become stuck, have the rest of the class offer suggestions.*
Explain how diet and nutrition can affect oral conditions.	■ Introduction (p. 212)	🖳 PPT 5-6 📖 SW Short-Answer Questions 1 (p. 63) ▸ Discuss specific ways that diet and nutrition affect oral health and care. *Class Activity Have students research oral conditions that are affected by diet and nutrition and present their findings to the class. (For students to prepare for this activity, see Homework/Assignments #1.)*
Explain why the study of nutrition is important to the dental assistant.	■ Introduction (p. 212)	🖳 PPT 7-8 🖳 TB questions 1-2 📖 SW Short-Answer Questions 2; Fill in the Blank question 4; Multiple Choice question 1 (pp. 63-64) 📖 SW Topics for Discussion questions 4-5 (p. 65) Figure 16-1 Dental assistant discusses dental health with a patient (p. 212)

Bird/Robinson

OBJECTIVES	CONTENT	TEACHING RESOURCES
		Box 16-1 Functions of Five Major Nutrients (p. 212)
		Recall question 1 (p. 215)
		▸ Discuss the role of the dental assistant in educating patients about diet and nutrition.
		Class Activity Lead a class discussion about how to counsel patients on their dietary habits after the following procedures:
		– Surgical procedures
		– General dental procedures
		– Orthodontic procedures
		Record student responses on the board for comparison.
Explain the meaning of "recommended dietary (daily) allowance."	■ Recommended dietary allowances (RDAs) (p. 212)	PPT 9
		TB question 3
		SW Short-Answer Questions 5 (p. 63)
		SW Topics for Discussion questions 1-3 (p. 65)
		▸ Discuss the pros and cons of the recommended dietary allowance. When is it appropriate for a given nutrient to exceed the RDA?
		Class Activity Have each student make a chart that lists the types and amounts of foods that he or she consumed the previous day. Then have the students compare their intake with the recommended dietary (daily) allowance and share their findings with the class.
List the six areas of the Food Guide Pyramid.	■ MyPyramid (p. 212)	PPT 10-12
		TB questions 4, 17-18
		SW Short-Answer Questions 4 (p. 63)
		Six Key Nutrients (p. 212)
		Figure 16-2 MyPyramid (p. 213)
		CTQ 1-2 (p. 225)
		▸ Discuss the specific types of foods that the food pyramid encourages and the number of servings for each group.
		Class Activity Lead a class discussion about the six areas of the Food Guide Pyramid. Ask students to compare and contrast the RDAs for adults, children, pregnant women, and the elderly. Record student responses on the board for comparison.

OBJECTIVES	CONTENT	TEACHING RESOURCES
Describe the role of carbohydrates in the daily diet.	■ Carbohydrates (p. 213)	⊠▣ PPT 13-14 ▣ TB questions 5-6 ▐ SW Short-Answer Questions 7; Multiple Choice questions 2-3 (pp. 63-64) Recall questions 1-2 (p. 215) Table 16-1 Dietary Fiber in Some Common Foods (p. 214) ▸ Discuss the different types of carbohydrates. *Class Activity **Divide the class into groups. Have each group choose a carbohydrate-restricting diet and outline its philosophy, its guidelines, and its pros and cons. Then have each group present its findings to the class for discussion.***

Explain the relationship between frequency and amount of cariogenic foods in causing tooth decay.	☐ Foods that cause tooth decay (p. 214)	⊠▣ PPT 15-16
		
		▣ TB question 7
		
		Sources of Carbohydrates (p. 214)
		
		Recall question 3 (p. 215)
		
		▸ Discuss how certain foods promote tooth decay; identiry particularly problematic foods.
		
		*Class Activity **Present the following situations to the class, and lead a class discussion about the relationship between cariogenic foods and tooth decay:***
		
		   – *Drinking cola products all day long*
		
		   – *Drinking water all day long*
		
		   – *Frequent snacking on crackers*
		
		   – *Frequent snacking on fruits and vegetables*
		
		Record student responses on the board for comparison.

Describe the three types of proteins.	■ Proteins (p. 215) ■ Fats (lipids) (p. 215) ☐ Cholesterol (p. 215) ☐ Antioxidants (p. 216)	⊠▣ PPT 17-21 ▣ TB questions 8-10 ▐ SW Short-Answer Questions 3; Fill in the Blank question 1; Multiple Choice questions 4-8 (pp. 63-64) Sources of Protein (p. 215) Sources of Antioxidants (p. 217) Recall questions 4-8 (p. 215) Table 16-2 Common Sources of Fat and Cholesterol (p. 216) ▸ Discuss the distinctions among the three types of proteins and provide examples of each.

Torres and Ehrlich Modern Dental Assisting, 9th ed.

Bird/Robinson

OBJECTIVES	CONTENT	TEACHING RESOURCES
		Class Activity **Divide the class into groups, and assign each group one of the eight essential amino acids. Have each group do research and create a list of foods in which its assigned amino acid can be found and present its findings to the class.** *(For students to prepare for this activity, see Homework/Assignments #2.)*

16.1 Homework/Assignments

1. Have students research oral conditions that are affected by diet and nutrition and present their findings to the class.
2. Divide the class into groups and assign each group one of the eight essential amino acids. Have each group do research and create a list of foods in which its assigned amino acid can be found and present its findings to the class.

16.1 Instructor's Notes/Student Feedback:

Bird/Robinson

LESSON 16.2

CRITICAL THINKING QUESTION

A patient comes to the office for full-mouth extractions and delivery of immediate full-upper and full-lower dentures. What postoperative instructions must be given to the patient regarding his diet?
Guidelines: Multiple extractions and the placement of dentures will require this patient to alter his diet. Any patient who is receiving any type of dentures should be encouraged to chew certain foods by starting on the most posterior teeth. Because there is always a period of adjustment for the patient, it helps to begin by chewing on the molar teeth, with gradual movement toward the anterior teeth. Food should be cut into small pieces, and hard, crunchy foods should be avoided during this stage. Because the patient also had multiple extractions, he should be advised to stay away from hot, spicy food as it can irritate the healing gum tissues. Soft, cool foods such as yogurt, pasta, oatmeal, and pudding are encouraged because they maintain good nutrient levels and promote proper healing of the extraction sites.

OBJECTIVES	CONTENT	TEACHING RESOURCES
Describe the difference between vitamins and minerals.	■ Vitamins (p. 216) ■ Minerals (p. 218)	PPT 24 TB question 11 SW Short-Answer Questions 6; Multiple Choice questions 9-12 (pp. 63-64) Table 16-3 Vitamins: Best Sources, Primary Functions, Deficiency Symptoms, and Toxicity (pp. 217-218) Recall questions 9-11 (p. 216) ▸ Discuss the different roles vitamins play in the body as opposed to the role of minerals. *Class Activity Lead a class discussion about vitamins and minerals. Ask students to describe how each functions in the body and to compare and contrast their sources and actions. Record student responses on the board so students can evaluate the responses for completeness.*
Explain the need for minerals in the diet.	■ Minerals (p. 218) ■ Water (p. 218) ■ Diet modification (p. 218) ■ Dietary analysis (pp. 218, 220)	PPT 25-30 TB question 12 SW Short-Answer Questions 8; Multiple Choice question 13 (pp. 63-64) Table 16-4 Minerals: Best Sources, Primary Functions, Deficiency Symptoms, and Toxicity (pp. 219-220) Diet Recommendations in Dentistry (p. 221) Recall questions 12-13 (p. 218) Figure 16-3 Sample dietary analysis form (p. 222) ▸ Discuss what is meant by "essential" minerals. Why are some minerals more necessary than others? *Class Activity Lead a class discussion about daily mineral requirements. Ask students to identify which minerals are required in large amounts, and which require only trace amounts. What are the effects of consuming too many minerals?*

OBJECTIVES	CONTENT	TEACHING RESOURCES
Explain how to interpret food labels.	■ Reading food labels (p. 220) □ Product label information (p. 220) □ Labeling ingredients (p. 221) □ Label claims (p. 221)	⊠ PPT 31-34 TB question 13 SW Short-Answer Questions 10-11; Multiple Choice question 14 (pp. 63-64) Figure 16-4 Nutrition facts label (p. 223) Figure 16-5 Comparative versus absolute nutrient claims (p. 224) Recall question 14 (p. 223) CTQ 4 (p. 225) ▸ Discuss the aspects of reading food labels that seem most problematic for patients. What do they find most confusing? How could dental assistants bring clarity to these issues? *Class Activity **Have each student bring two food labels to class to practice reading and interpreting the nutritional information. (For students to prepare for this activity, see Homework/Assignments #1.)***
Explain the criteria for a food to be considered "organic."	□ Organic foods (p. 221)	⊠ PPT 35 TB question 14 SW Short-Answer Questions 12; Fill in the Blank question 5; Multiple Choice question 15 (pp. 63-64) Recall question 15 (p. 223) ▸ Discuss the criteria used to determine whether a product may legitimately be considered organic.. *Class Activity **Lead a class discussion about organic foods. Ask students to identify the advantages and disadvantages of consuming organic foods over non-organic foods and identify local markets that carry organic food.***
Discuss the health and oral implications of eating disorders.	■ Eating disorders (p. 221) □ Bulimia (p. 222) □ Anorexia nervosa (p. 222) □ Female athlete triad (p. 223) □ Management of eating disorders (p. 223) ■ Healthy habits (p. 223)	⊠ PPT 36-44 TB questions 15-16 SW Short-Answer Questions 9; Fill in the Blank question 2-3; Multiple Choice question 16 (pp. 63-64) Table 16-5 Common Diet-Related Disorders (p. 224) Recall question 16 (p. 223) CTQ 3 (p. 225) ▸ Discuss the steps a dental assistant might take if a patient was known to have an eating disorder. *Class Activity **Present the following situations to the class and lead a class discussion about how a dental assistant could recognize eating disorders in patients:***

ELSEVIER

Bird/Robinson

OBJECTIVES	CONTENT	TEACHING RESOURCES
		1. A 16-year-old girl comes in to the office with severe lingual erosion on the anterior teeth and seems to have lost a lot of weight since her last visit. *2. An 18-year-old boy comes in with advanced periodontal disease and comments several times that he feels fat even though he appears very thin for his large frame.*
Performance Evaluation		📺 TB 📖 SW questions (pp. 63-65) *e* ESLR Electronic Flashcards *e* ESLR Practice Quiz *e* ESLR Labeling Exercise 16: MyPyramid Recall questions (pp. 215-223) 💡 CTQ (p. 225)

16.2 Homework/Assignments:

1. Have each student bring two food labels to class to practice reading and interpreting the nutritional information.

16.2 Instructor's Notes/Student Feedback:

Torres and Ehrlich Modern Dental Assisting, 9th ed.

Bird/Robinson

Slide 1

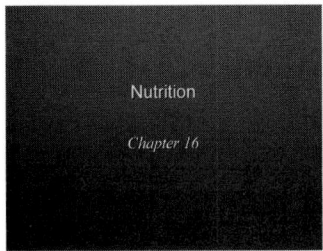

Nutrition

Chapter 16

Slide 2

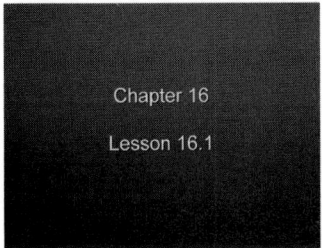

Chapter 16

Lesson 16.1

Slide 3

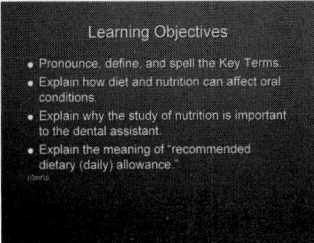

Learning Objectives

- Pronounce, define, and spell the Key Terms.
- Explain how diet and nutrition can affect oral conditions.
- Explain why the study of nutrition is important to the dental assistant.
- Explain the meaning of "recommended dietary (daily) allowance."

Slide 4

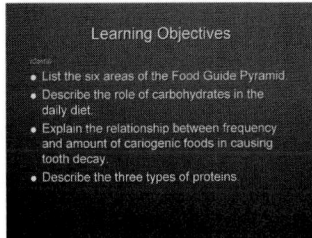

Learning Objectives

- List the six areas of the Food Guide Pyramid.
- Describe the role of carbohydrates in the daily diet.
- Explain the relationship between frequency and amount of cariogenic foods in causing tooth decay.
- Describe the three types of proteins.

Torres and Ehrlich Modern Dental Assisting, 9th ed.

Bird/Robinson

Slide 5

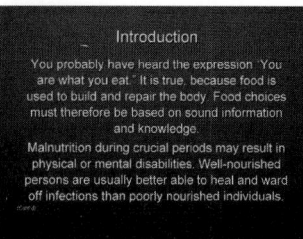

- Good nutrition is critical in pregnant women, young children, and the elderly.

Slide 6

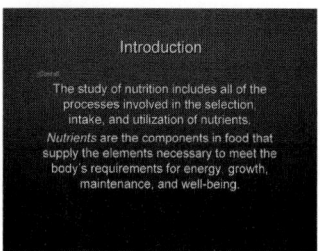

- Foods are used to meet the body's needs.

Slide 7

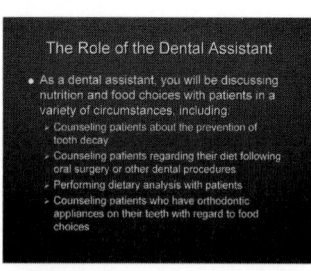

- Many people confuse diet with weight loss.

- Dental assistants are often given the responsibility of giving postoperative instructions following certain dental procedures.

Slide 8

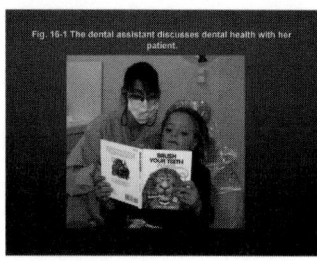

- The dental team must always listen to the patients' needs and assess their motivation levels regarding diet.

- Use terminology that is appropriate for a patient's age and understanding.

Slide 9

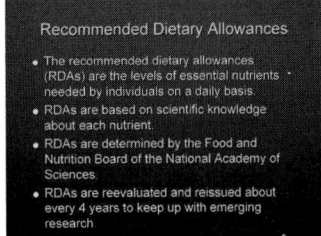

- Also known as the "recommended *daily* allowances."

Slide 10

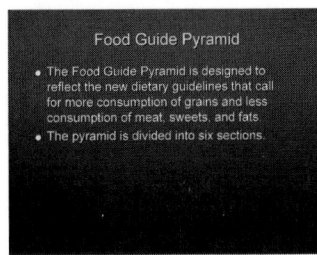

- The Pyramid is a guide meant to allow individuals to make healthful and varied food choices.

Slide 11

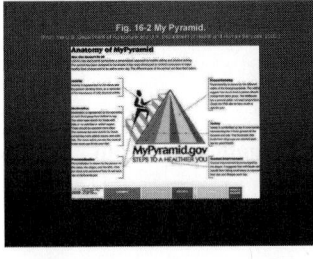

- Proportionality is shown by the different widths of the food group bands.

Slide 12

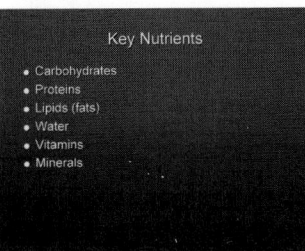

- What are nutrients? *(Components needed by the body.)*

Bird/Robinson

Slide 13

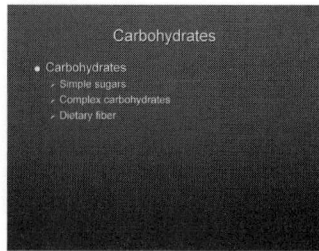

- Carbohydrates are the body's chief source of energy.
- Simple sugars are absorbed first; they are found in processed foods.
- Complex carbohydrates (starches) are found mainly in grains and must be processed before they can be absorbed.
- Dietary fiber is indigestible. It is commonly called roughage.

Slide 14

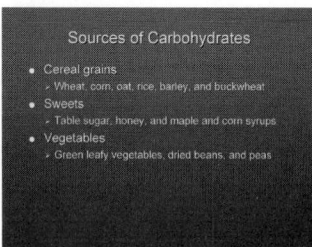

- Of the foods listed above, which are simple sugars, which are complex sugars, and which are dietary fibers?

Slide 15

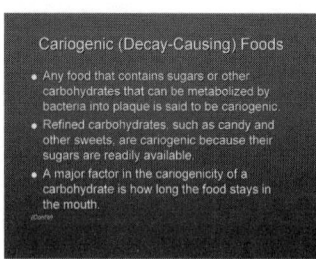

- Liquid sugars can be washed away from tooth surfaces, whereas sticky sugars can adhere to the tooth structure and cause decay.
- Salivary flow is important in washing away sugars. It has two functions:
  - To speed clearance of food from the mouth.
  - To provide dietary fluoride in order to strengthen the tooth.

Slide 16

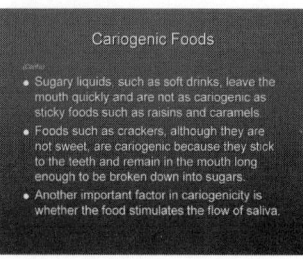

- Which foods stimulate saliva flow?

Torres and Ehrlich Modern Dental Assisting, 9th ed.

Bird/Robinson

Slide 17

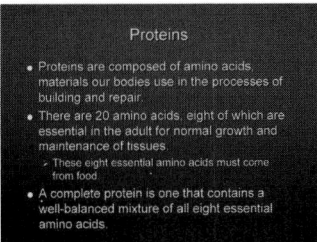

- Proteins provide structure, regulate body processes, and provide the body with energy.

Slide 18

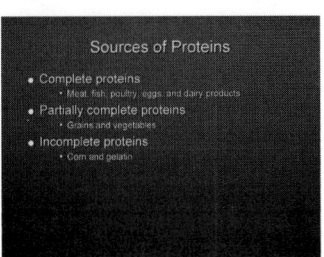

- Complete proteins are a well-balanced mix of all eight essential amino acids.

- Partially complete proteins are an unbalanced mix of eight essential amino acids.

- Incomplete proteins support neither life nor normal growth; they cannot be used as a sole source of protein.

- Each gram of protein supplies four calories.

- Where are proteins found on the MyPyramid?

Slide 19

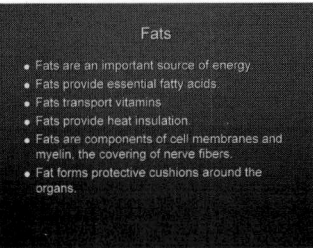

- Fats are also known as lipids.

- Consuming excessive amounts of fat is discouraged.

- In average Americans' diets, 40% of calories come from fat.

- Overconsumption of fat can lead to cardiovascular disease, obesity, diabetes, and some cancers.

Slide 20

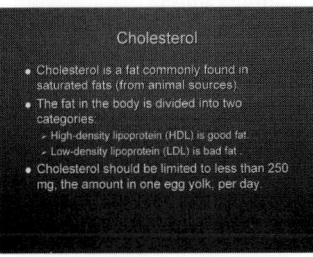

- Many foods that are high in fat are also high in cholesterol.

- What are examples of foods that are high in saturated fat?

Bird/Robinson

Slide 21

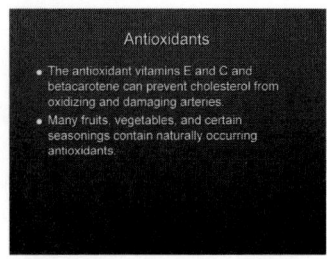

- Vitamin E: soy beans, almonds, oatmeal, chick peas, wheat germ, sunflower seeds

- Vitamin C: peppers, oranges, strawberries, tangerines, broccoli, lemons, raspberries, cabbage, grapefruit, black currants

- Beta-carotene: carrots, sweet potatoes, pumpkin, kale, winter squash, spinach, cantaloupe, apricots

- Seasonings: nutmeg, thyme, rosemary, sesame, cloves, green tea, pepper

Slide 22

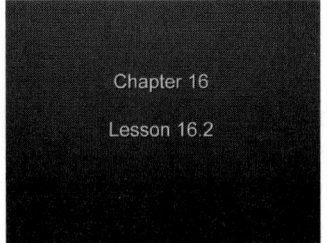

Slide 23

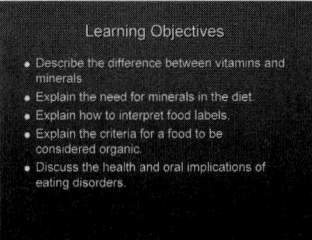

Slide 24

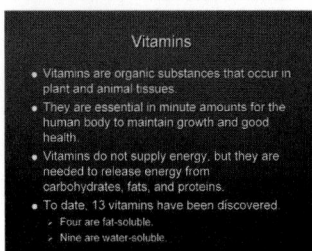

- Fat-soluble vitamins include vitamins A, D, E, and K.

- Water-soluble vitamins include vitamins B complex and C.

Slide 25

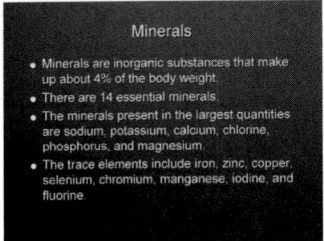

- Minerals are needed by the body in small amounts to maintain health and function.
- Minerals are supplied by diet alone.
- Minerals are components of the bones and teeth; they make bones and teeth rigid and strong.

Slide 26

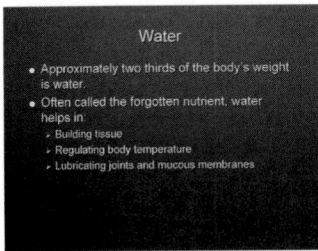

- Adults should consume at least 64 ounces of water each day.
- Humans can survive for longer without food than they can without water.
  - Water can come from some foods. For example:
  - Fruits and vegetables contain 80% water.
  - Meats contain 40% to 60% water.

Slide 27

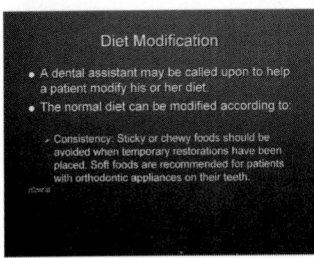

- The word "diet" is commonly confused with "weight loss."
- Postoperative instructions are given after orthodontic appliances are applied.
- What foods should an orthodontic patient avoid?

Slide 28

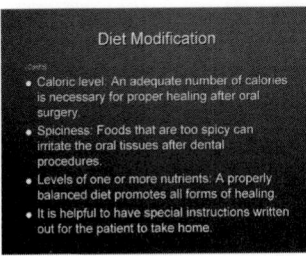

- Always give positive reinforcement when reviewing a patient's diet.
- First review diet modification orally, then provide the patient with written instructions.

Slide 29

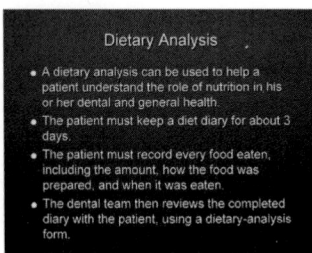

- Why is it necessary to obtain a dietary analysis of a patient?

Slide 30

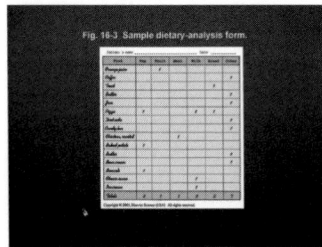

- Patients should be encouraged to complete a dietary analysis form openly and honestly.

- It is important that the dental assistant avoid making judgments; the purpose of the dietary analysis form is to provide education and instruction.

Slide 31

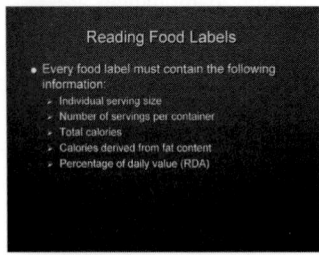

- How many students read food labels on a daily basis?

- Why?

Slide 32

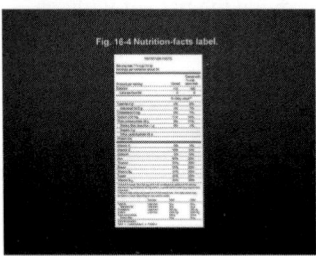

- What does the "percent daily value" mean?

Slide 33

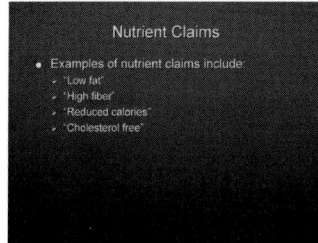

- Nutrient claims can be very confusing for consumers.

- What are comparison claims? *(For example, items that claim to be reduced fat must have at least 25% less fat than the regular items.)*

Slide 34

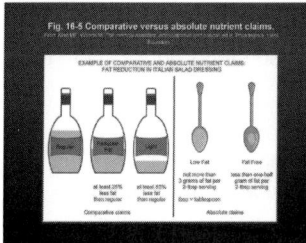

- The government has set strict conditions under which statements such as "low fat" can be used as part of the front label on a product.

Slide 35

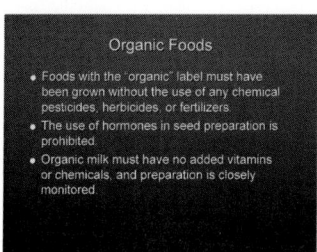

- USDA regulations protect consumers by ensuring that products are truly organic.

- What is the USDA? What regulations has it set forth?

Slide 36

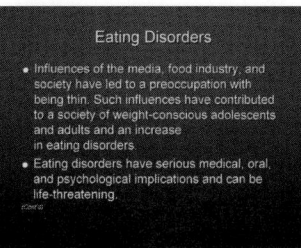

- Give some examples of negative media influences on body image. Are there any positive influences?

Slide 37

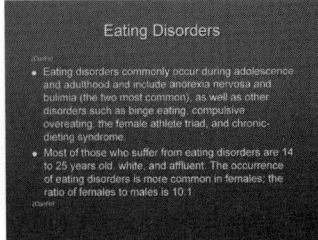

- What are the treatments of eating disorders? Are they successful?

Slide 38

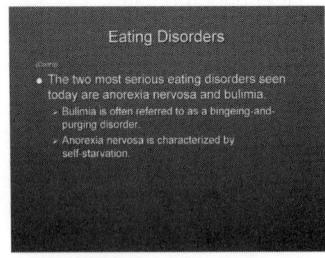

- Binging involves eating large amounts of food (as many as 5000 calories) in a short period of time. A person with bulimia often finds comfort in food.
- Purging is vomiting following a binge; the person feels guilty about the binge.
- Use of laxatives is another form of purging.
- Bulimics may have excessive wear of the lingual surfaces of the anterior teeth because of the acid that is produced from vomiting.
- Anorexia nervosa can be deadly because the body is deprived of essential nutrients.

Slide 39

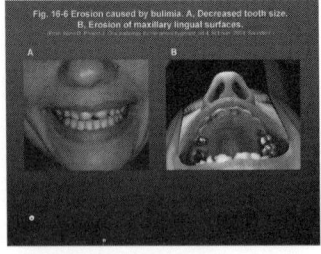

- Why would erosion be a consequence of bulimia?

Slide 40

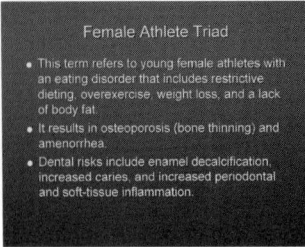

- What is amenorrhea? *(Missed menstrual periods.)*

Slide 41

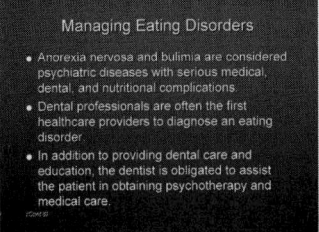

- How is it that dental professionals become aware of an eating disorder before other professionals?

- Therapy for such disorders can be lengthy and costly. It may also require inpatient care.

- Dental team members must always be empathetic and understanding.

Slide 42

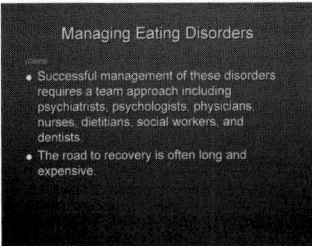

- What is the dentist's role in management and recovery of eating disorders?

Slide 43

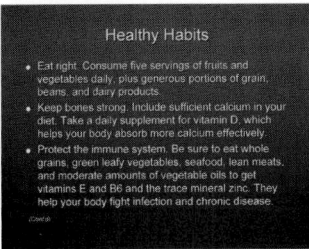

- What constitutes five servings of fruits and vegetables? Is it easy or difficult to consume the recommended amount?

Slide 44

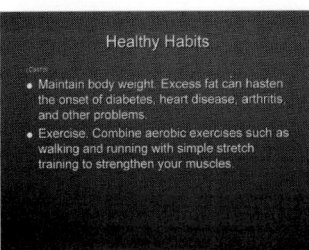

- How often should adults participate in physical exercise?

- Brochures on healthy habits are good educational tools to use with patients.

TEACHING FOCUS

This chapter will give students the opportunity to learn about pathologic conditions of the oral cavity. Students will become acquainted with the categories of diagnostic information, oral lesions, diseases of the oral soft tissues, conditions of the tongue, oral cancer, and the oral manifestations of HIV and AIDS. Development disorders along with other disorders, including abrasion, attrition, bruxism, bulimia, and orofacial piercings, will be discussed.

MATERIALS AND RESOURCES

☐ computer and PowerPoint projector (all Lessons)

LESSON CHECKLIST

Preparations for this lesson include:

- lecture
- guest speakers: oral surgeon, dentist, representative from AIDS clinic
- evaluation of student knowledge and skills needed to perform all entry-level activities related to oral pathology, including:
  - conditions of the tongue
  - developmental disorders
  - diseases of the oral soft tissues
  - making a diagnosis
  - oral cancer
  - oral lesions
  - oral manifestations of HIV and AIDS

KEY TERMS

abscess (p. 231)
acute inflammation (p. 230)
biopsy (p. 229)
candidiasis (p. 232)
carcinoma (p. 235)
cellulitis (p. 233)
chronic inflammation (p. 230)
congenital disorders (p. 241)
cyst (p. 231)
ecchymosis (p. 231)
erosion (p. 231)
inflammation (p. 230)
glossitis (p. 234)
granuloma (p. 231)

hematoma (p. 231)
lesion (p. 230)
leukemia (p. 236)
leukoplakia (p. 232)
lichen planus (p. 232)
lymphadenopathy (p. 238)
lymphoma (p. 238)
meth mouth (p. 247)
metastasize (p. 235)
pathology (p. 227)
petechia (p. 238)
sarcoma (p. 235)
xerostomia (p. 236)

ADDITIONAL RESOURCES

PowerPoint slides (Evolve): 1-106

Legend

CTQ
Critical
Thinking
Question

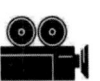
DVD
Multimedia
Procedures
Videos and
Animations

ESLR
EVOLVE
Student
Learning
Resources

IDO
Interactive
Dental
Office
CD-ROM

SW
Student
Workbook

TB
Test Bank
on the
TEACH
CD-ROM

PPT
PowerPoint
Slides

Class Activities are indicated in ***bold italic.***

ELSEVIER

Torres and Ehrlich Modern Dental Assisting, 9th ed.

Bird/Robinson

LESSON 17.1

PRETEST

1. What is the term used for a localized area of pus originating from an infection?
   a. ulcer
   b. abscess
   c. cyst
   d. hematoma

2. How would you describe the condition of cellulitis?
   a. superficial infection caused by a yeast-like fungus
   b. inflammation of cellular or connective tissue
   c. swelling or mass of blood collected in one area or organ
   d. formation of white spots or patches on the oral mucosa

3. Which of the following is considered a tumor of connective tissue?
   a. sarcoma
   b. carcinoma
   c. leukoplakia
   d. leukemia

4. What is xerostomia?
   a. ulcerated tongue
   b. enlarged lymph node
   c. dry mouth
   d. infected sinus

5. Which of the following is characterized by a bright red line along the border of the free gingival margin?
   a. leukemia
   b. HIV
   c. herpes zoster
   d. cytomegalovirus

6. What is the location of hairy leukoplakia?
   a. upper lip
   b. tongue dorsum
   c. hard palate
   d. soft palate

7. What diagnostic tool would be useful in diagnosing both periapical pathology and impacted teeth?
   a. pulp tester
   b. radiographs
   c. saliva tests
   d. periodontal probe

8. What procedure is done with soft tissue lesions in the mouth so they can be microscopically examined?
   a. radiograph
   b. biopsy
   c. disinfection
   d. ultrasonic

9. What type of diagnosis is made by providing a treatment and seeing how the condition responds?
   a. clinical
   b. radiographic
   c. culture
   d. therapeutic

10. Which of the following, if taken during pregnancy, may result in a yellow-gray-brown stain on the teeth of the fetus?
    a. laxatives
    b. stool softeners
    c. antibiotics
    d. high blood pressure medicines

Answers

1. b	3. a	5. b	7. b	9. d
2. b	4. c	6. b	8. b	10. c

BACKGROUND ASSESSMENT

Question: What is used by a dentist to help in the diagnosis of an oral pathological lesion?

Answer: Personal history, family history, medical and dental histories, and history of the lesion are often useful in making a diagnosis. Family histories are important because of genetic disorders. Medical histories can give information about medication the patient may be taking that could affect the oral tissues. In addition, the clinical appearance of the lesion, including the color, size, shape, and location, is often useful.

ELSEVIER

Bird/Robinson

Question: Which infection is seen as purplish lesions on the skin or oral mucosa of patients with HIV/AIDS? What type of infection is it?

Answer: Kaposi's sarcoma is one of the opportunistic infections that occur in patients with HIV infection. Oral lesions of Kaposi's sarcoma may appear as multiple bluish, blackish, or reddish blotches that are usually flat in the early stages. At present, no effective treatment exists for Kaposi's sarcoma. Surgical excision to decrease the size of the lesion is sometimes attempted, as well as radiation treatment and chemotherapy. Kaposi's sarcoma is one of the intraoral lesions used to diagnose AIDS. Because the immune system of a patient with AIDs is severely damaged, death is usually caused by an opportunistic infection. An opportunistic infection is one that normally would be controlled by the immune system but which cannot be controlled because the immune system is not functioning properly because of HIV/AIDS or other causes.

CRITICAL THINKING QUESTION

An experienced dental assistant does not understand why a dental assisting student must study oral pathology because the dentist is the only one who can legally and correctly identify diseases in the mouth. Why does a dental assistant need to know about oral pathology? How does oral pathology relate to patient care?

Guidelines: While it is true only a dentist may legally diagnose pathologic (disease) conditions, it is important for the dental assistant to be able to recognize the differences between normal and abnormal conditions that appear in the mouth. The dental assistant might notice a lesion in the patient's mouth that appears abnormal. Then the dentist would be informed so that a diagnosis could be made. In addition, many systemic diseases as well as infectious diseases have oral manifestations (signs and symptoms). The dental assistant should also understand how oral abnormalities affect the patient's general health and planned dental treatment. Finally, this information enables the dental assistant to communicate effectively with other professionals.

OBJECTIVES	CONTENT	TEACHING RESOURCES
Pronounce, define, and spell the Key Terms.	■ Key terms (pp. 226-227)	SW Fill in the Blank questions 3-8, 10-11, 19-20 (pp. 68) ESLR Electronic Flashcards ***Class Activity** As a class, discuss each of the key terms, focusing on the definition, pronunciation, and spelling of each term.*
Explain why oral pathology is important for the dental assistant.	■ Introduction (p. 227)	PPT 4-7 TB question 1 SW Short-Answer Questions 1; Fill in the Blank question 1 (pp. 67-68) ▸ Discuss the definition of the term "oral pathology." ***Class Activity** Divide the class into small groups and have each group discuss why it is important for dental assistants to be able to recognize the difference between normal and abnormal conditions that appear in the mouth. Have each group report its findings to the class.*
Explain why categories of diagnostic information are necessary.	■ Making a diagnosis (p. 227) ☐ Historical diagnosis (p. 228) ☐ Clinical diagnosis (p. 228)	PPT 8-27 TB question 2 SW Short-Answer Questions 2; Fill in the Blank question 19 (pp. 67-68)

ELSEVIER

OBJECTIVES	CONTENT	TEACHING RESOURCES
	☐ Radiographic diagnosis (p. 228)	Figure 17-1 Dentinogenesis imperfecta (p. 228)
		Figure 17-2 Melanin pigmentation (p. 228)
	☐ Microscopic diagnosis (p. 229)	Figure 17-3 Fissured tongue (p. 228)
	☐ Laboratory diagnosis (p. 229)	Figure 17-4 (A) Clinical appearance of bilateral mandibular tori; (B) Clinical appearance of lobulated torus palatinus (p. 228)
	☐ Therapeutic diagnosis (p. 229)	Figure 17-5 Median rhomboid glossitis (p. 229)
		Figure 17-6 Periapical pathology (p. 229)
	☐ Surgical diagnosis (p. 220)	Figure 17-7 Internal resorption (p. 229)
	☐ Differential diagnosis (p. 220)	Figure 17-8 Horizontal impaction of the third molar (p. 230)
		Figure 17-9 A white lesion is seen on the anterior floor and ventral surface of the tongue (p. 230)
		Figure 17-10 Angular cheilitis (p. 230)
		Figure 17-11 Traumatic bone cyst (p. 230)
		Figure 17-12 Static bone cyst (p. 230)
		▸ Discuss the eight sources of information that can be used to make a final diagnosis. Define and explain each.
		Class Activity Invite an oral surgeon to speak to the class about cases in oral pathology and how he or she diagnosed and treated each case.
Describe the classic signs of inflammation.	☐ Acute/chronic inflammation (p. 230)	Classic Signs of Inflammation (p. 231) ▸ Discuss the classic signs of inflammation. *Class Activity Divide the class into small groups and have each group develop a table that lists the classic signs of inflammation. Have each group present its table to the class for comparison and further discussion.*
Differentiate between chronic and acute inflammation.	☐ Acute/chronic inflammation (p. 230)	SW Short-Answer Questions 7 (p. 67) ▸ Discuss the definition of inflammation. *Class Activity Divide the class into small groups and have each group create educational materials on the differences between chronic and acute inflammation. Then have the groups present their materials to the class.*

17.1 Homework/Assignments:

17.1 Instructor's Notes/Student Feedback:

Torres and Ehrlich Modern Dental Assisting, 9th ed.

Bird/Robinson

LESSON 17.2

CRITICAL THINKING QUESTION

A teenage patient admits that he just started to chew tobacco when playing baseball. He says all the good baseball players chew tobacco. How can the dental assistant alert this patient to the dangers of chewing tobacco?

Guidelines: The dental assistant should let the patient know that smokeless tobacco, in the form of chewing tobacco or snuff, presents a serious health hazard. It is an addictive substance that may be hard for him to quit using as he grows older. This is a major concern because of the high rates of precancerous leukoplakia and oral cancer occurring among users of smokeless tobacco, even in young adults. Leukoplakia is a white patch that cannot be wiped off and may be associated with chemical agents or tobacco. In addition, cancers of the pharynx, larynx, and esophagus occur 400 to 500 times more frequently among users than among nonusers. Smokeless tobacco is also linked to serious irritation of the oral mucosa and an increased incidence of tooth loss from periodontal disease. By chewing tobacco, the patient is risking his oral health and his overall health.

OBJECTIVES	CONTENT	TEACHING RESOURCES
Describe the types of oral lesions.	■ Oral lesions (p. 230) □ Lesions extending below mucosal surface (p. 231) □ Lesions extending above mucosal surface (p. 231) □ Lesions even with mucosal surface (p. 231) □ Raised or flat lesions (p. 231)	PPT 30-31 TB questions 3-5 SW Short-Answer Questions 4; Fill in the Blank questions 3-8, 10; Multiple Choice questions 1-3 (pp. 67-69) Figure 17-13 Radiographs of dentigerous cysts (p. 231) Recall questions 1-3 (p. 231) ▸ Discuss the five categories of oral lesions. Define and explain each category. ▸ Discuss the causes of lesions. ***Class Activity Divide the class into five groups, and assign each group one of the general categories of lesions. Have each group research causes and treatment of the lesions and report its findings to the class. (For students to prepare for this activity, see Homework/Assignments #1.)***
Identify two oral conditions related to nutritional factors.	■ Diseases of the oral soft tissues (p. 242) □ Leukoplakia (p. 232) □ Lichen planus (p. 232) □ Candidiasis (p. 232) – Pseudomembranous candidiasis (p. 232) – Hyperplastic candidiasis (p. 233) – Atrophic candidiasis (p. 233) □ Aphthous ulcers (p. 233)	PPT 32-43 TB questions 6-7 SW Short-Answer Questions 8; Fill in the Blank questions 9, 11-12; Multiple Choice questions 4-7 (pp. 67-69) Figure 17-14 Leukoplakia (p. 232) Figure 17-15 Lichen planus on the buccal mucosa (p. 232) Figure 17-16 Pseudomembranous candidiasis (p. 232) Figure 17-17 Chronic hyperplastic candidiasis (p. 233) Figure 17-18 Minor aphthous ulcer (p. 233) Figure 17-19 Cellulitis (p. 234)

ELSEVIER

Torres and Ehrlich Modern Dental Assisting, 9th ed.

Bird/Robinson

OBJECTIVES	CONTENT	TEACHING RESOURCES
	☐ Cellulitis (p. 233)	Recall questions 4-7 (p. 234)
		💡 CTQ 3 (p. 248)
		▸ Discuss the definition of leukoplakia.
		▸ Discuss the fact that leukoplakia often appears before the development of a malignant lesion.
		Class Activity Divide the class into small groups and have each group prepare a brochure on smokeless tobacco, using Internet resources for descriptions and photographs. Then have each group present its materials so that the class can select the most effective brochure and discuss why it was selected. Display all the brochures in the classroom. (For students to prepare for this activity, see Homework/Assignments #2.)
Describe three conditions associated with the tongue.	■ Conditions of the tongue (p. 234)	🖥 PPT 44-51
		💻 TB question 8
		📖 SW Fill in the Blank question 13; Multiple Choice questions 8-9 (pp. 68-69)
		Figure 17-20 Black hairy tongue (p. 234)
		Figure 17-21 Geographic tongue (p. 234)
		Recall questions 8-10 (p. 235)
		Figure 17-22 Fissured tongue and attrition (p. 234)
		Figure 17-23 Angular cheilitis and depapillation of the tongue in a patient with pernicious anemia (p. 235)
		▸ Discuss the term "glossitis."
		Class Activity Divide the class into small groups, and have each group discuss the causes of and treatments for the following conditions:
		– Geographic tongue
		– Fissured tongue
		– Pernicious anemia
		Have each group present its findings to the class.

Bird/Robinson

17.2 Homework/Assignments:

1. Divide the class into five groups, and assign each group one of the general categories of lesions. Have each group research causes and treatment of the lesions and report its findings to the class.

2. Have each group prepare a brochure on smokeless tobacco, using Internet resources for descriptions and photographs.

17.2 Instructor's Notes/Student Feedback:

LESSON 17.3

CRITICAL THINKING QUESTION

A young adult man has come into the dental office right after being diagnosed with AIDS. He tells the dental assistant that he has only the initial symptoms of AIDS at this time and asks what he can expect to see in his mouth now or in the future. What will the assistant need to know about his overall state of health in order to gauge his oral health?

Guidelines: The dental assistant should let the patient know that oral lesions are prominent features of AIDS. AIDS is the end-stage disease for an individual infected with HIV. Initially, this patient may have a bright red line along the border of the free gingival margin that characterizes HIV gingivitis, also known as atypical gingivitis. He may also have candidiasis, which is often the initial oral sign of the progression from HIV-positive status to AIDS. In addition, hairy leukoplakia is an early sign of the change to AIDS status. Hairy leukoplakia is a white plaque usually found on one side or sometimes on both sides on the lateral borders of the tongue. Kaposi's sarcoma is another opportunistic infection that occurs in patients with HIV infection. Oral lesions of Kaposi's sarcoma may appear as multiple bluish, blackish, or reddish blotches that are usually flat in the early stages. Herpes simplex lesions might also be seen in this patient. In immunocompromised patients, such as those with AIDS, the herpes lesions may occur throughout the mouth, causing an ulcer-like lesion that may persist for longer than a month with the presence of AIDS. The dental assistant can tell him that lesions develop because the immune system is compromised when the T-helper cells become depleted as a result of the disease. Causes of oral lesions include opportunistic infections, tumors, and autoimmune-like diseases. Thus, the dental assistant will need to know the level of the patient's T-helper cells to gauge his oral health. These cells are indicators of how much his immune system is compromised.

OBJECTIVES	CONTENT	TEACHING RESOURCES
Describe the warning symptoms of oral cancer.	■ Oral cancer (p. 235) ☐ Leukemia (p. 236)	⊠▤ PPT 54-59 ▥ TB question 9 ▨ SW Short-Answer Questions 3; Fill in the Blank questions 14-17, 20; Multiple Choice questions 11, 13 (pp. 67-69) Table 17-1 Appearance of Early Cancer (p. 235) Figure 17-24 Clinical appearance of squamous cell carcinoma of the lower lip (p. 235) Oral Cancer Warning Signs (p. 236) Figure 17-25 Destruction of the mandible by squamous cell carcinoma (p. 236) Figure 17-26 Leukemia (p. 236) ▸ Discuss the types of lesions that signal the early appearance of cancer. Discuss the clinical appearance of each type. ▸ Discuss the early warning signs of oral cancer. *Class Activity **Divide the class into small groups, and have each group create a one-page flier concerning oral cancer to be placed on the school's Web site. The fliert can contain photographs and descriptions from the Internet or other sources. Have the class decide on the best flier to be placed on the Web site to increase public awareness of oral cancer.***

OBJECTIVES	CONTENT	TEACHING RESOURCES
Describe the appearance of lesions associated with the use of smokeless tobacco.	☐ Smokeless tobacco (p. 236)	⊠▣ PPT 60-61 ▣ TB question 10 ▣ SW Short-Answer Questions 6; Multiple Choice question 12 (pp. 67, 69) Figure 17-27 Tobacco chewer's white lesion (p. 236) Recall questions 11-15 (pp. 236-237) ***Class Activity** Have student pairs take turns role-playing a dental assistant discussing the dangers of chewing tobacco with a high school student who chews tobacco. Have the students research the long-term health effects of smokeless tobacco. (For students to prepare for this activity, see Homework/Assignments #1.)*
Describe the warning symptoms of oral cancer.	☐ Therapy for oral cancer (p. 237) ☐ Dental implications of radiation therapy (p. 236) – Xerostomia (p. 237) – Radiation caries (p. 237) – Osteoradionecrosis (p. 237) ☐ Dental implications of chemotherapy (p. 237)	⊠▣ PPT 62-63 ▣ SW Multiple Choice question 14 (p. 69) Figure 17-28 (A) and (B) Radiation mucositis; (C) Postradiation xerostomia (p. 237) Table 17-2 Dental Implications of Chemotherapy (p. 237) ▸ Discuss the dental implications of radiation therapy and chemotherapy. ***Class Activity** Invite a dentist to speak to the class about dental treatment for patients with oral cancer. Have the speaker address some of the related dental problems he or she has encountered in his or her practice and the interventions taken and outcomes achieve. Have students prepare questions for the speaker in advance.*
Name five lesions that are associated with HIV/AIDS.	■ Human immunodeficiency virus (HIV) and acquired immunodeficiency syndrome (AIDS) (p. 238) ☐ Oral manifestations (p. 238) – HIV gingivitis (p. 238) – HIV periodontitis (p. 238) – Cervical lymphadenopathy (p. 239) – Candidiasis (p. 238)	⊠▣ PPT 64-80 ▣ TB question 11 ▣ SW Short-Answer Questions 5; Multiple Choice questions 15-17 (pp. 67, 69) Oral Lesions Associated with HIV Infection (p. 238) Figure 17-29 Atypical periodontal disease in a patient with HIV infection (p. 238) Figure 17-30 Lymphadenopathy (p. 239) Figure 17-31 Candidiasis in a patient with HIV infection (p. 239) Figure 17-32 Intraoral lymphoma in a patient with AIDS (p. 239) Figure 17-33 Hairy leukoplakia on the lateral borders of the tongue (p. 239)

OBJECTIVES	CONTENT	TEACHING RESOURCES
	– Lymphoma (p. 238) ☐ Hairy leukoplakia (p. 239) ☐ Kaposi's sarcoma (p. 239) ☐ Herpes simplex (p. 240) ☐ Herpes zoster (p. 240) ☐ Human papillomavirus (p. 240)	Figure 17-34 Kaposi's sarcoma in a patient with AIDS (p. 240) Figure 17-35 Herpes simplex ulceration of the hard palate in a patient with HIV infection (p. 240) Figure 17-36 Papillary lesion of the upper lip caused by human papillomavirus in a patient with HIV infection (p. 241) Recall questions 16-18 (p. 240) 💡 CTQ 1 (p. 248) ▸ Discuss the lesions associated with HIV/AIDS. ▸ Discuss the oral manifestations of HIV/AIDS. **Class Activity** *Invite a representative from a local AIDS clinic to speak to the class about the disease.*

17.3 Homework/Assignments:

1. Have the students research the long-term health effects of smokeless tobacco.

17.3 Instructor's Notes/Student Feedback:

LESSON 17.4

CRITICAL THINKING QUESTION

While exposing radiographs or making impressions, the dental assistant may notice that the anatomy of the lingual surfaces of the patient's maxillary anterior teeth has an unusually smooth, glassy appearance. The dental assistant may see few, if any, stains or lines on the teeth and may notice a slight loss of occlusal anatomy on a patient's posterior teeth. What is this disorder and how does it affect the teeth? What can be done to lessen its effects? Should the dental assistant tell the patient to stop vomiting? If the dental assistant tells the patient anything, how should it be done?

Guidelines: These are common oral manifestations associated with bulimia. The erosion is caused by the acidic gastric fluids from chronic vomiting and movement of the tongue. Bulimia is an eating disorder characterized by food binges and followed by self-induced vomiting. The dental professional is often the first healthcare professional to diagnose a patient with bulimia. Generally, the person with bulimia maintains a normal body weight but is secretive about eating habits. Dental management of the patient with bulimia requires minimizing the effects of the stomach acids on tooth enamel by encouraging the daily use of a fluoride rinse and fluoridated toothpaste. Rinsing the mouth with water and thoroughly cleaning the teeth immediately after vomiting also lessen the effect of the acid, instead of immediately brushing the teeth. However, the patient should be told that there is erosion on the teeth and that it usually indicates an eating disorder. If the patient is then open to discussing her disorder, she should be encouraged to seek professional treatment to end the eating disorder.

OBJECTIVES	CONTENT	TEACHING RESOURCES
Define, describe, and identify the developmental anomalies discussed in this chapter.	■ Developmental disorders (pp. 240-241) ☐ Genetic factors (p. 241) ☐ Environmental factors (p. 241) ☐ Disturbances in jaw development (p. 242) ☐ Disturbances in lip, palate, and tongue development (p. 243) ☐ Disturbances in tooth development and eruption (p. 243) ☐ Disturbances in enamel formation (p. 245) ☐ Disturbances in dentin formation (p. 245) ☐ Abnormal eruption of the teeth (p. 245) – Premature eruption (p. 245) – Ankylosis (p. 245) – Impaction (p. 245)	⊠▤ PPT 84-97 ▥ TB questions 12-13, 19 ▨ SW Short-Answer Questions 12; Fill in the Blank question 18; Multiple Choice questions 18-20 (pp. 67-68, 70) Table 17-3 Dental Developmental Disturbances (p. 242) Known Teratogens Involved in Congenital Malformations (p. 241) Recall questions 19-20 (p. 241) Figure 17-37 Discoloration of teeth caused by tetracycline ingestion (p. 241) Figure 17-38 A newborn with bilateral complete cleft lip and palate (p. 243) Figure 17-39 Ankyloglossia (p. 243) Recall questions 21-23 (p. 243) ▶ Discuss genetic and environmental factors that can influence oral developmental disorders. ▶ Discuss disturbances in jaw development. ***Class Activity** Present the class with photographs and radiographs of developmental anomalies. Have the students identify the different anomalies and discuss the causes and clinical ramifications of each.*

ELSEVIER

Torres and Ehrlich Modern Dental Assisting, 9th ed.

Bird/Robinson

OBJECTIVES	CONTENT	TEACHING RESOURCES

List and define three anomalies that affect the number of teeth.	☐ Disturbances in tooth development and eruption (p. 243)
	
	☐ Disturbances in enamel formation (p. 245)
	
	☐ Disturbances in dentin formation (p. 245)
	
	☐ Abnormal eruption of the teeth (p. 245)
	
	   – Premature eruption (p. 245)
	
	   – Ankylosis (p. 245)
	
	   – Impaction (p. 245)
		⊠ PPT 98
		
		TB question 14
		
		SW Short-Answer Questions 10; Multiple Choice question 23 (pp. 67, 70)
		
		SW Case Study questions 1-4 (p. 70)
		
		Figure 17-40 Partial anodontia (p. 243)
		
		Figure 17-41 Radiograph showing unerupted supernumerary teeth (p. 244)
		
		Figure 17-42 Dens in dente (p. 244)
		
		▸ Discuss disorders that affect the number of teeth. Be sure to discuss disorders that cause a person to have too many teeth and those disorders that cause a person to have too few teeth.
		
		Class Activity Divide the class into small groups, and have each group discuss disorders that affect the number of teeth. Have the students identify the different disorders and discuss the causes and clinical ramifications of each. Then have the groups present a summary of their discussion to the class for feedback on completeness and accuracy.

List and define five anomalies related to the shape of the teeth.	☐ Disturbances in tooth development and eruption (p. 243)
	
	☐ Disturbances in enamel formation (p. 245)
	
	☐ Disturbances in dentin formation (p. 245)
	
	☐ Abnormal eruption of the teeth (p. 245)
	
	   – Premature eruption (p. 245)
	
	   – Ankylosis (p. 245)
	
	   – Impaction (p. 245)
		SW Short-Answer Questions 11; Multiple Choice questions 21-22 (pp. 67, 70)
		
		Figure 17-43 Hutchinson's incisors (p. 244)
		
		Figure 17-44 (A) Clinical picture of fusion involving a permanent lateral incisor; (B) Fusion of mandibular molars (p. 244)
		
		Recall questions 24-26 (p. 245)
		
		▸ Discuss disorders that affect the shape of the teeth.
		
		Class Activity Present the class with photographs and radiographs of disorders that affect the shape of teeth. Have the students identify the different disorders and discuss the causes and clinical ramifications of each.

Recognize developmental disorders of the dentition.	☐ Disturbances in enamel formation (p. 245) ☐ Disturbances in dentin formation (p. 245) ☐ Abnormal eruption of the teeth (p. 245)	TB questions 15-16 SW Short-Answer Questions 9; Multiple Choice question 24 (pp. 67, 70) Figure 17-45 Note loss of enamel in these teeth in a patient with hypocalcified amelogenesis imperfecta (p. 245) Figure 17-46 A radiograph of ankylosis of a deciduous

Torres and Ehrlich Modern Dental Assisting, 9th ed.

Bird/Robinson

OBJECTIVES	CONTENT	TEACHING RESOURCES
	– Premature eruption (p. 245) – Ankylosis (p. 245) – Impaction (p. 245)	molar (p. 245) Figure 17-47 Impactions in mixed dentition visible on a dental radiograph (p. 245) Recall questions 27-28 (p. 246) ▶ Discuss development disorders that affect the dentition. *Class Activity Divide the class into small groups, and have the groups research the causes and effects of developmental disorders. Have each group present a short report to the class on its findings. (For student to prepare for this activity, see Homework/Assignments #1.)*
Describe the oral conditions of a patient with bulimia.	■ Miscellaneous disorders (p. 246) ☐ Abrasion (p. 246) ☐ Attrition (p. 246) ☐ Bruxism (p. 246) ☐ Bulimia (p. 246) ☐ Orofacial piercings (p. 247) ☐ Meth mouth (p. 247)	⊠ PPT 99-106 TB questions 17-18 SW Short-Answer Questions 13; Multiple Choice question 25 (pp. 67, 70) Figure 17-48 Abrasion at the cervical area of mandibular premolars caused by toothbrushing (p. 246) Figure 17-49 (A) Attrition of adult dentition; (B) Attrition of adult dentition (in incisal view) (p. 246) Figure 17-50 Attrition of the mandibular anterior teeth resulting from bruxism (p. 246) Recall questions 29-31 (p. 247) Figure 17-51 Pierced tongue with jewelry (p. 247) Patient Education (p. 247) Legal and Ethical Implications (p. 247) Eye to the Future (p. 247) ▶ Discuss the oral disorders found in patients with bulimia. *Class Activity Divide the class into small groups. Have each group discuss ways that a dental assistant can help a patient with bulimia to minimize the effects of the disease on the patient's mouth. Have each group report its findings to the class.*
Performance Evaluation		TB SW questions (pp. 67-70) SW Case Study (p. 70) ℰ ESLR Electronic Flashcards ℰ ESLR Practice Quiz Recall questions (pp. 231-247) CTA (p. 248)

Torres and Ehrlich Modern Dental Assisting, 9th ed.

Bird/Robinson

17.4 Homework/Assignments:

1. Divide the class into small groups, and have the groups research the causes and effects of developmental disorders.

17.4 Instructor's Notes/Student Feedback:

Slide 1

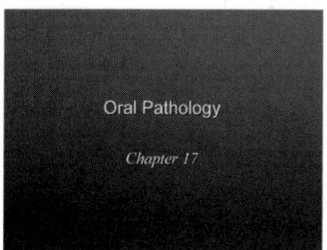

Slide 2

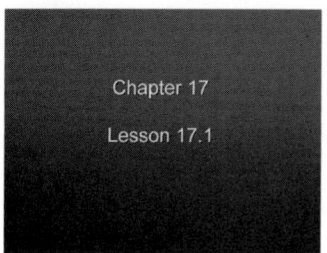

Slide 3

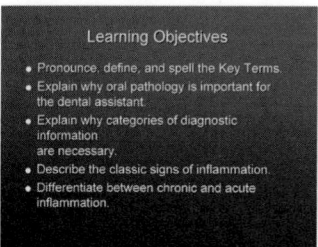

Slide 4

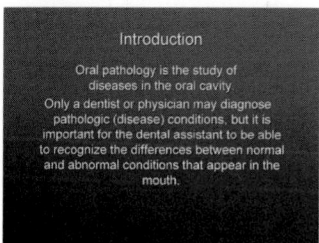

- Why is it important for a dental assistant to recognize normal and abnormal conditions in the oral cavity?

Slide 5

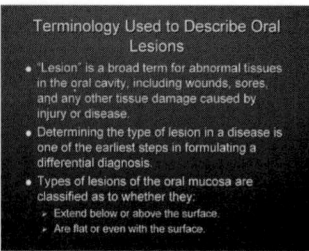

- Is recognizing a lesion the same as diagnosing it? Why or why not?

Slide 6

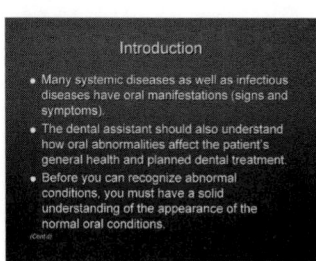

- What are some ways oral abnormalities may affect a patient's health?
- What terms could be used to describe normal oral conditions?

Slide 7

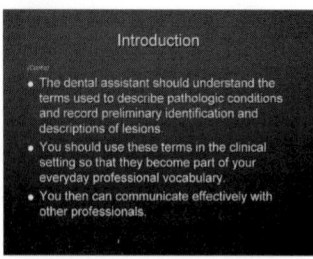

- What are examples of terms that might be used to describe lesions?
- Why is it important to have a shared vocabulary with other professionals?

Slide 8

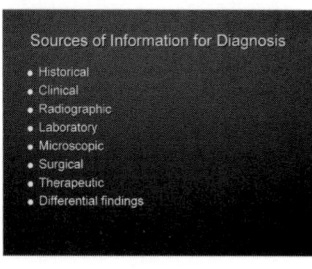

- Why is it useful to have more than one source of information for a diagnosis?
- How can the dental assistant be helpful in the formation of a diagnosis? (*By collecting family history, asking patients about symptoms, and reporting any lesions or other abnormalities to the dentist.*)

Torres and Ehrlich Modern Dental Assisting, 9th ed.

Bird/Robinson

Slide 9

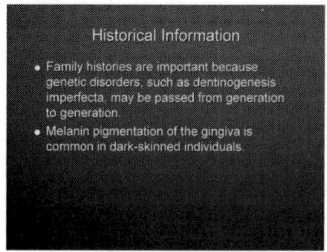

- Family history is also referred to as heredity.
- What are some other examples of genetic disorders?

Slide 10

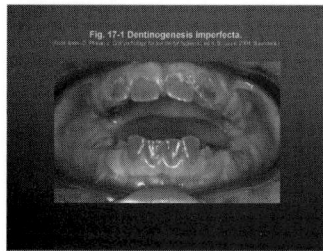

- Dentinogenesis imperfecta is a hereditary condition that affects the formation of dentin.
- Teeth having dentinogenesis imperfecta are opalescent and have an almost amber color.
- The enamel tends to chip away from the dentin, and the weakened teeth become worn down.

Slide 11

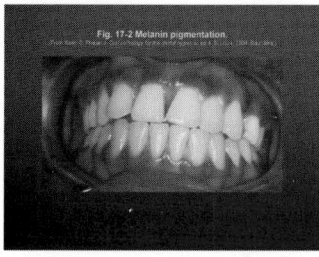

- This condition is not considered clinically harmful.
- It is more commonly found in African-Americans and Native Americans.

Slide 12

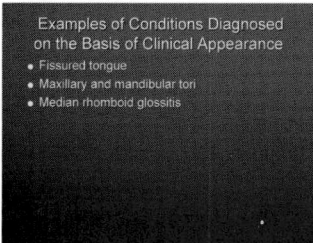

ELSEVIER

Torres and Ehrlich Modern Dental Assisting, 9th ed.
Bird/Robinson

Slide 13

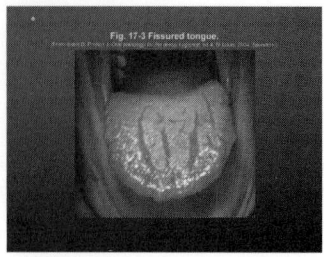

- The cause of fissured tongue is unknown. Theories include a vitamin deficiency or chronic trauma.

- The top of the tongue appears to have deep fissures or grooves that become irritated if food debris collects in them.

- The patient with a fissured tongue is advised to brush the tongue gently with a soft toothbrush to keep the fissures clean of debris and irritants.

- No treatment is indicated for this condition.

Slide 14

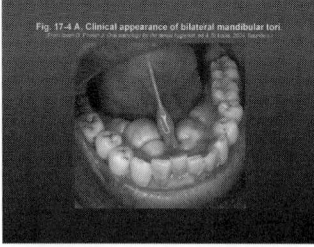

- A torus is a benign bony growth projecting outward from the surface of a bone.

- The slide shows a torus mandibularis, a bony overgrowth.

Slide 15

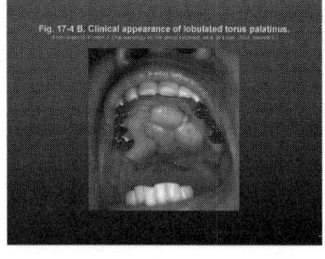

- A torus palatinus is a bony overgrowth in the midline of the hard palate.

Slide 16

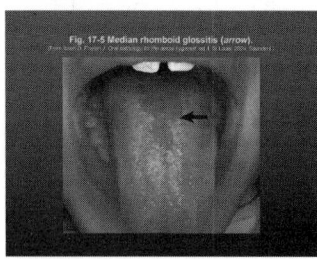

- Median rhomboid glossitis (posterior midline atrophic candidiasis) presents in the back of the tongue.

- Lesions are typically less than 2 cm.

- Most lesions, but not all, show a smooth, flat surface.

Bird/Robinson

Slide 17

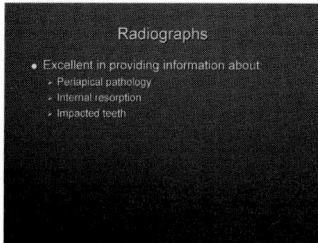

- What's the most familiar form of radiography? (*X-rays.*)

Slide 18

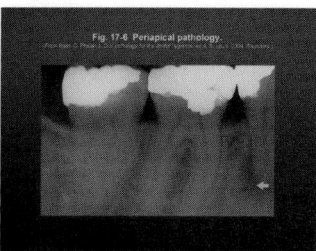

- Why is this radiograph important for patient care? (*Note the change in the bone of the mandible because of an infection. The pulp became infected because of caries and the infection caused bone resorption.*)

Slide 19

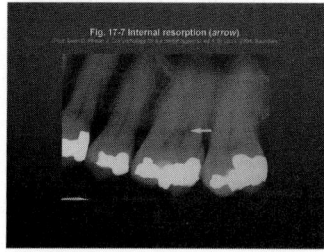

- The arrow is pointing to an area of internal resorption.
- The tooth often has a history of trauma or pulp cap.
- Discoloration may or may not be present.

Slide 20

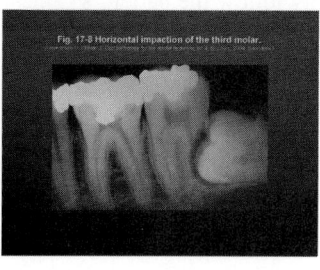

- An impacted tooth occurs when a tooth fails to fully emerge through the gingiva.
- The most common teeth to become impacted are the wisdom teeth, which normally emerge between the ages of 17 and 21.

Bird/Robinson

Slide 21

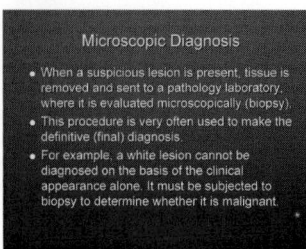

- It is essential that any suspicious malignancies be checked to see if they are malignant.

Slide 22

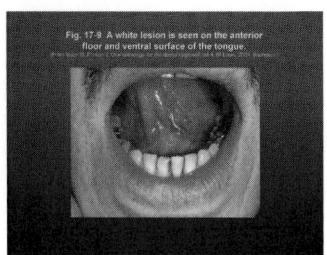

- How would you explain to a concerned patient the process of microscopic analysis of a lesion?

Slide 23

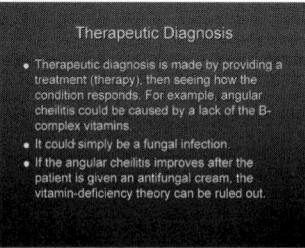

- Therapeutic diagnosis is also defined as an assessment of the objectives and available methods of treatment for an individual patient, considering the specific existing conditions.

Slide 24

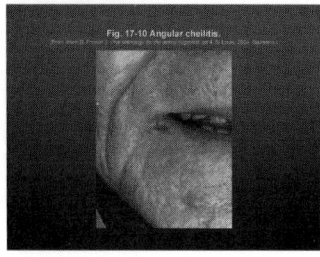

- The key to therapeutic diagnosis is to closely follow the patient's progress and monitor improvement or lack of improvement in the underlying condition.

Bird/Robinson

Slide 25

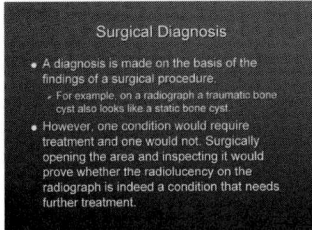

- Surgical diagnosis helps to distinguish between benign and potentially harmful conditions.

Slide 26

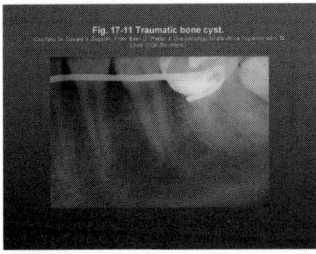

- Would surgical diagnosis more likely be used after other methods have not yielded a firm diagnosis?

Slide 27

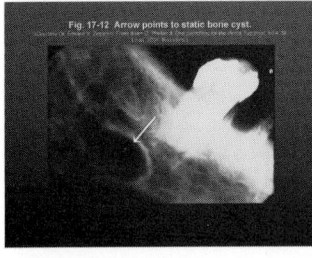

- The expertise of the dentist is the primary determining factor in making a differential diagnosis.

Slide 28

Slide 29

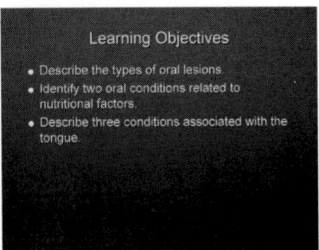

Slide 30

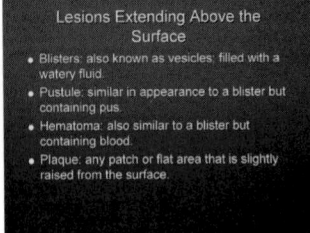

- Where would you expect to find a cyst? An abscess?
- Is erosion a symptom of disease or injury?

Slide 31

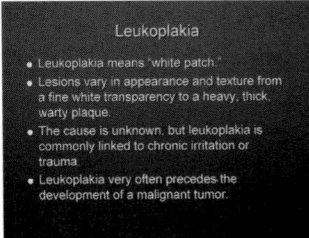

Slide 32

- What is a plaque? *(Any patch or flat area that is slightly raised from the surface.)*

Torres and Ehrlich Modern Dental Assisting, 9th ed.

Bird/Robinson

Slide 33

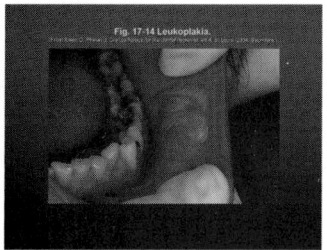

- How would you describe a leukoplakia lesion? *(Lesions vary in appearance and texture, from a fine white transparency to a heavy, thick, warty plaque.)*

- What is commonly linked to cases of leukoplakia? *(Chronic irritation or trauma.)*

- Why is early diagnosis of leukoplakia important?

Slide 34

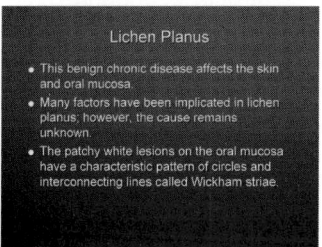

- Some forms of lichen planus can cause erosive lesions.

Slide 35

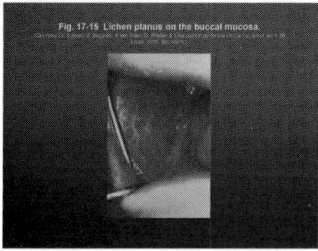

- Erosive lesions associated with lichen planus are made worse by stress.

Slide 36

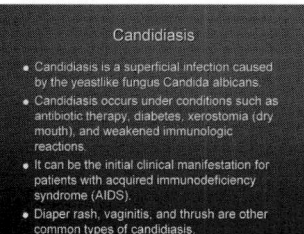

- What are some of the symptoms that can accompany candidiasis? *(Discomfort or pain, halitosis, and dysgeusis.)*

- Candidiasis is a common oral fungal infection; but actual incidence rates are low in healthy people.

Bird/Robinson

Slide 37

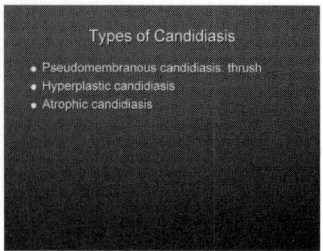

Slide 38

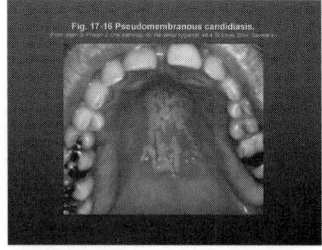

- Common patient complaints include feeling a burning sensation, having a bad tase in the mouth, or feeling that blisters are forming.

- The plaques can be scraped off and rarely bleed.

Slide 39

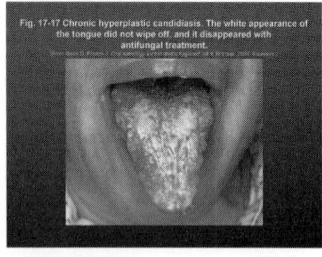

- Common treatment can take 10 days to 2 weeks.

- Like all forms of candidiasis, complications or lack of response to treatment may indicate more serious underlying disorders.

Slide 40

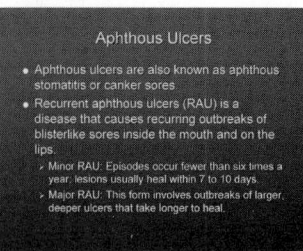

- Early signs are burning sensations and blister formation. The ulcers form when the blisters break.

Slide 41

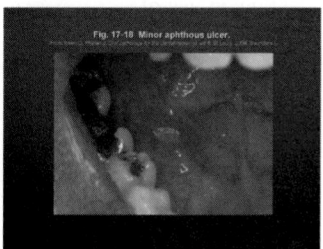

Slide 42

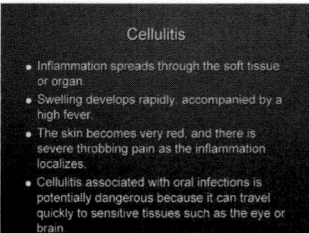

- What would be the keys to managing a case of cellulitis? *(Controlling inflammation and treating the underlying infection.)*

Slide 43

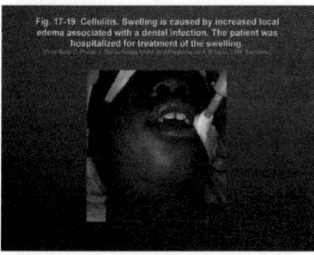

- What are common symptoms of cellulitis? *(The skin becomes very red, and there is severe throbbing pain as the inflammation localizes.)*

Slide 44

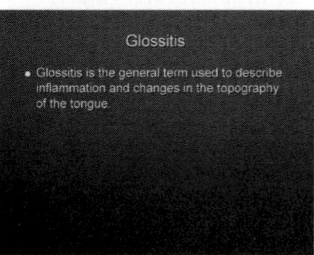

- Inflammation and pain in the tongue area can be disfiguring and also lead to difficulties in obtaining sufficient nutrition.

Slide 45

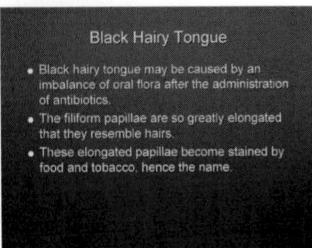

- What would you expect to learn about a patient's history if he or she presented with a case of black hairy tongue? (*Recent use of antibiotics.*)

Slide 46

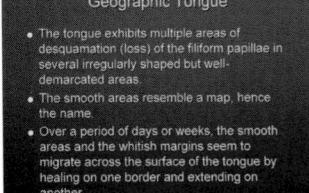

- What may cause black hairy tongue? (*Oral flora imbalance after the administration of antibiotics.*)
- What actually causes the hairlike appearance? (*The filiform papillae are so greatly elongated that they resemble hairs.*)

Slide 47

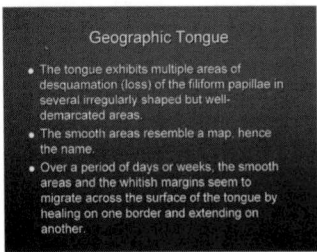

- What percentage of the population is affected by geographic tongue
- Which population is more often affected, women or men?

Slide 48

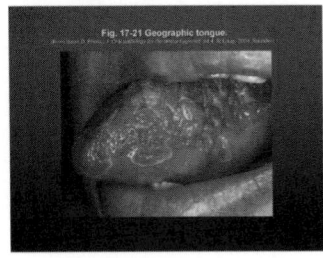

- What are the symptoms of geographic tongue evident in the slide? (*Multiple areas of loss of the filiform papillae in several irregularly shaped but well-demarcated areas.*)

Bird/Robinson

Slide 49

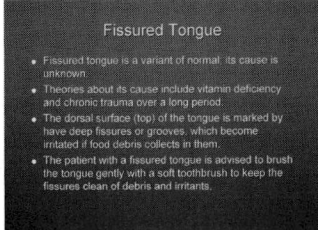

- Fissured tongue does not require medical treatment.

Slide 50

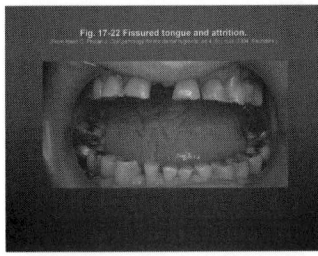

- What is the recommended self-care for a fissured tongue? *(The patient with a fissured tongue is advised to brush the tongue gently with a soft toothbrush to keep the fissures clean of debris and irritants.)*

Slide 51

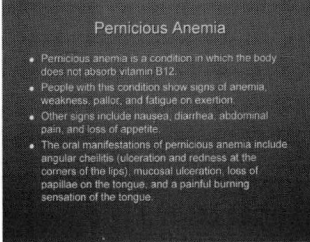

- Pernicious anemia is caused by a lack of intrinsic factor, a substance needed to absorb vitamin B12 from the gastrointestinal tract.
- Vitamin B12, in turn, is necessary for the formation of red blood cells.

Slide 52

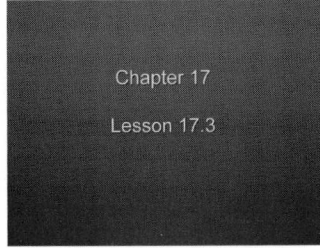

Slide 53

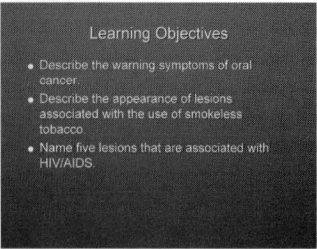

Slide 54

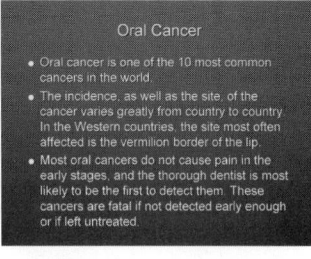

- Signs of oral cancer include:
  - A sore that bleeds easily or does not heal
  - A color change of the oral tissues
  - A lump, thickening, rough spot, crust, or small eroded area
  - Pain, tenderness, or numbness anywhere in the mouth or on the lips
  - Difficulty chewing, swallowing, speaking, or moving the jaw or tongue
  - A change in the way the teeth fit together

Slide 55

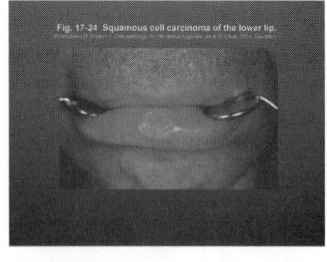

- Oral cancers may quickly metastasize (spread) to other regions of the body, usually the neck and cervical lymph nodes.

Slide 56

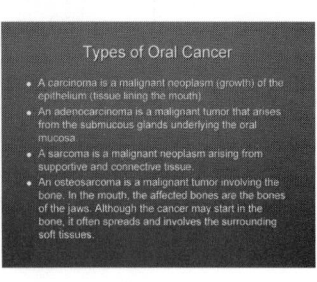

- Oral cancer most often occurs in those who use tobacco in any form.
- Alcohol use and poor diet also increase risk.
- Prolonged exposure to the sun increases the risk of lip cancer.
- More than 25% of oral cancers occur in people who do not smoke and have no other risk factors.

Slide 57

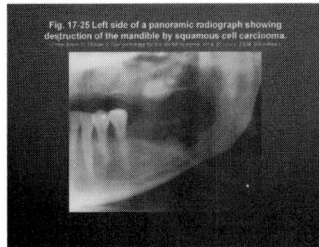

Fig. 17-25 Left side of a panoramic radiograph showing destruction of the mandible by squamous cell carcinoma.

- More than 90% of oral cancers are squamous cell carcinomas.

- Squamous cell cancer typically begins in the outer lining layer of cells in the oral cavity.

Slide 58

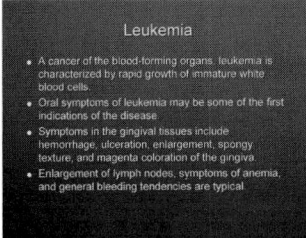

- Some 20% of chronic leukemia patients show no symptoms at diagnosis.

Slide 59

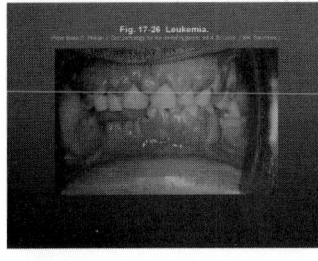

- Swollen, painful, and bleeding gums are common symptoms of acute leukemia.

Slide 60

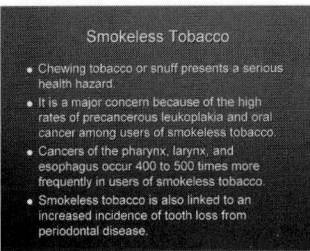

Slide 61

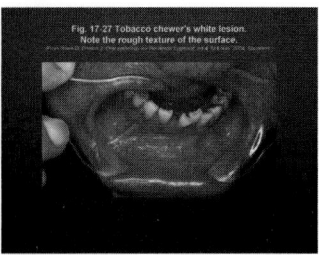

Slide 62

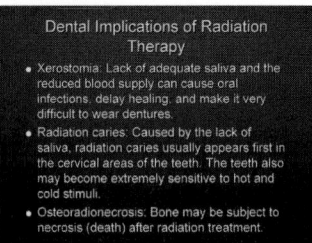

- It is strongly recommended that cancer patients visit the dentist before beginning radiation therapy.

- During treatment, the dentist can work with the patient to monitor complications such as dry mouth, increased cavities, or painful mouth sores.

Slide 63

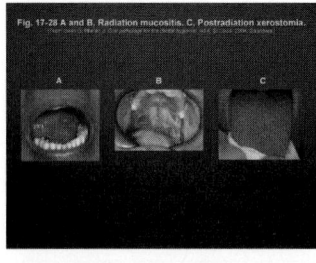

- Osteoradionecrosis is more common in cases of head and neck cancer, where the bone lies within the radiation field.

- Radiation technology now uses sophisticated computer algorithms to target beams so as to avoid healthy tissue and bone.

Slide 64

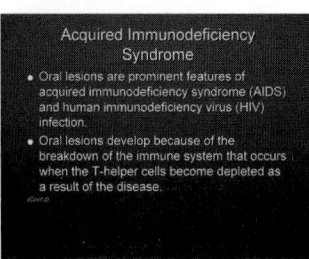

- The Americans with Disabilities Act requires that a patient with HIV cannot be refused treatment simply because of the disease.

- The only exception would be the HIV patient who has a special condition (e.g., severe periodontal disease) that requires the care of a specialist.

Bird/Robinson

Slide 65

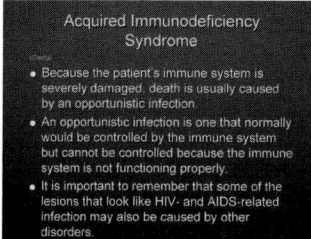

- More than a third of all people living with HIV have oral conditions related to a weakened immune system.
- Combination antiretroviral therapy has made some oral health problems less common, but has also involved side effects, such as xerostomia.

Slide 66

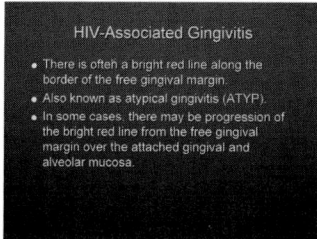

- HIV gingivitis progresses to HIV periodontitis.

Slide 67

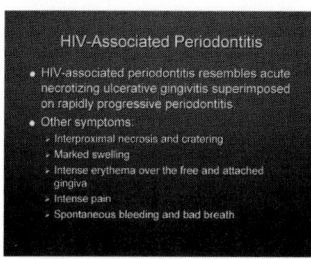

- HIV-associated periodontitis is much more aggressive than other forms.
- HIV-associated periodontitis may involve pain and spontaneous bleeding.

Slide 68

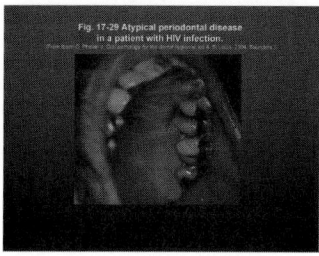

- A small percentage of cases does not respond to conventional treatment.

Bird/Robinson

Slide 69

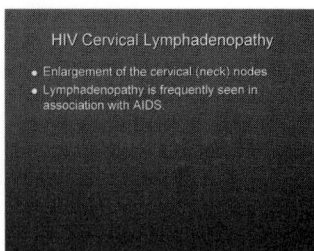

- Many infections are associated with lymphadenopathy. Care should be taken to avoid alarming a presenting patient without cause.

Slide 70

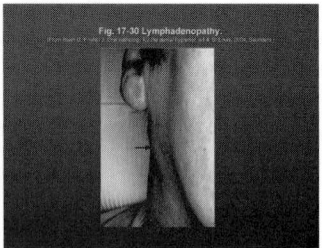

Slide 71

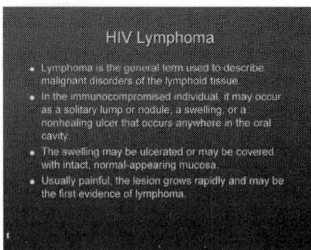

- Treatment involves radiation therapy for localized conditions and chemotherapy if the cancer has spread.

Slide 72

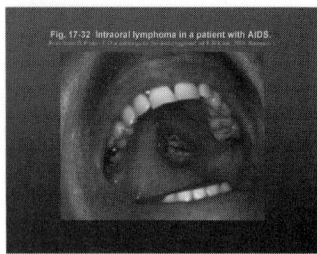

- Lymphoma lesions include firm masses and persistent ulcers.

- These lesions are difficult to distinguish from other forms of ulceration. Biopsy is usually required for firm diagnosis.

Bird/Robinson

Slide 73

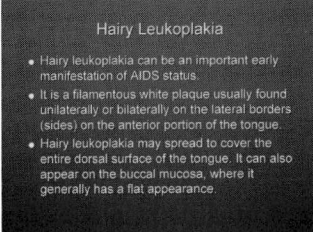

- In severe cases prescription medicines and pain relievers may be used to treat the symptoms.

Slide 74

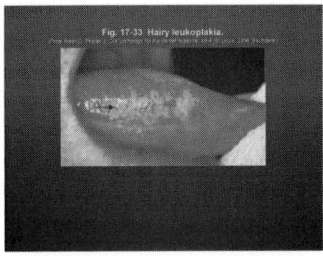

- Can the plaque associated with hairy leukopenia be brushed off?

Slide 75

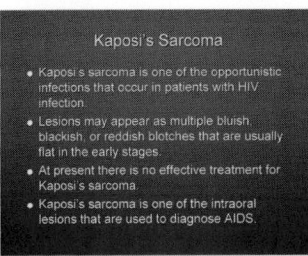

- What is an opportunistic infection? Why does the term apply to Kaposi's sarcoma?

Slide 76

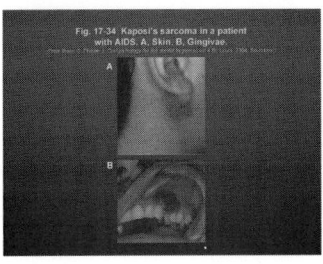

- The oral lesions associated with Kaposi's sarcoma appear as flat patches or swellings.
- Lesions may occur on the palate, gingiva, and tongue.
- Kaposi's sarcoma can become painful due to ulceration or infection.

Bird/Robinson

Slide 77

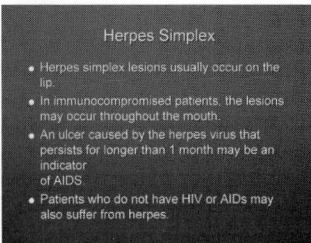

- Treatment includes prescription medications to promote healing and to control outbreaks.

Slide 78

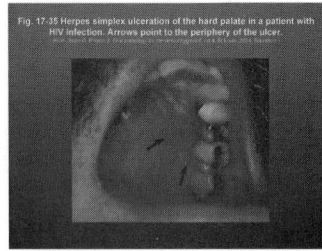

- In immunocompromised patients, lesions most commonly occur on the roof of the mouth.

Slide 79

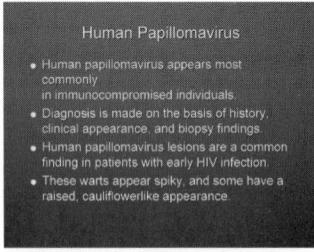

- A doctor can prescribe topical medications, excise warts surgically, or freeze the warts (cryosurgery).

Slide 80

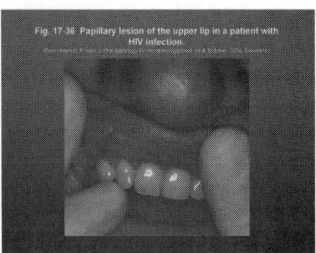

- Warts can return after treatment.

Slide 81

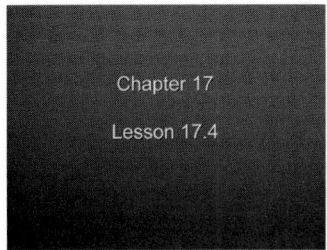

Slide 82

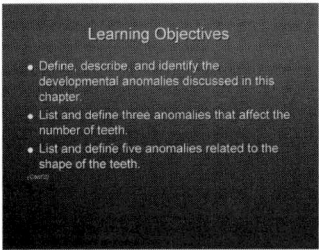

Slide 83

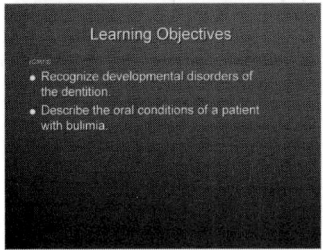

Slide 84

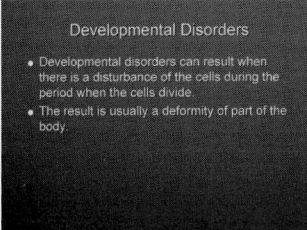

- What advice might you share with a patient who tells you she is pregnant?

Slide 85

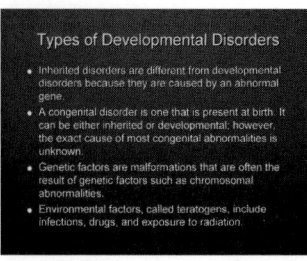

- Why would it be important for a dentist to know that a patient is pregnant?
- What teratogens might you find in a dental practice?

Slide 86

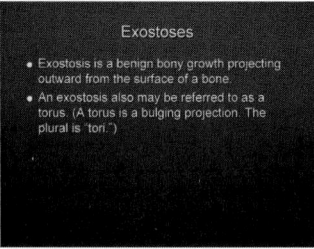

Slide 87

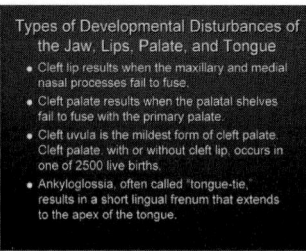

- Infants with clefts often routinely lose permanent teeth in the course of treatment and development.
- Modern dental techniques make it possible to preserve original dentition through careful monitoring and a treatment plan.

Slide 88

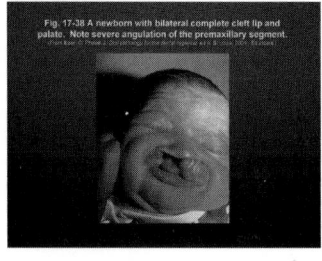

- With a cleft lip, an infant's dentition may be affected if the cleft involves the gum; otherwise, it is likely that dentition will be normal.
- A cleft of the palate and gum (alveolus) can produce a number of dental problems, including missing teeth, misshapen or misplaced teeth, and teeth that are slow to erupt.

Slide 89

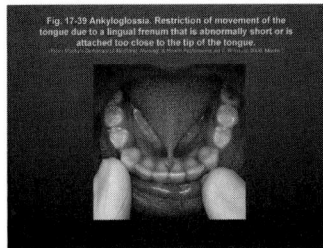

- Being "tongue-tied" does not affect speech development.

- In rare cases, an infant may have difficulty feeding due to ankyloglossia. This may indicate a need for treatment.

Slide 90

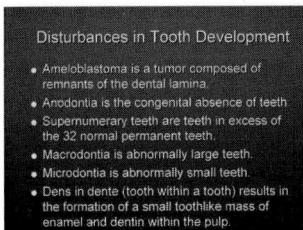

- Disturbances in tooth development may be linked to congenital diseases, but most are not.

Slide 91

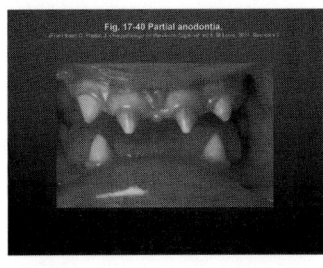

- Anodontia in the primary teeth does not necessarily indicate a similar prognosis for the permanent dentition.

Slide 92

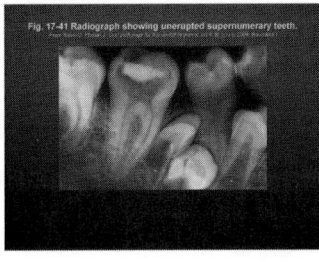

- Supernumerary teeth are classified according to their form and location. Their presence may give rise to a variety of clinical problems.

Slide 93

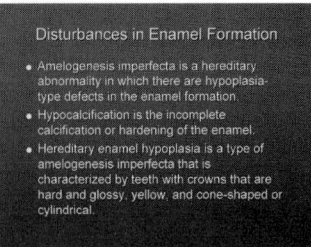

Disturbances in Enamel Formation

- Amelogenesis imperfecta is a hereditary abnormality in which there are hypoplasia-type defects in the enamel formation.
- Hypocalcification is the incomplete calcification or hardening of the enamel.
- Hereditary enamel hypoplasia is a type of amelogenesis imperfecta that is characterized by teeth with crowns that are hard and glossy, yellow, and cone-shaped or cylindrical.

Slide 94

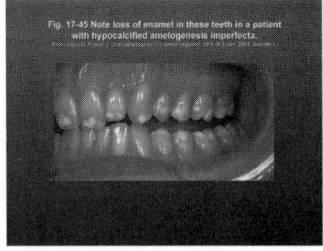

Fig. 17-45 Note loss of enamel in these teeth in a patient with hypocalcified amelogenesis imperfecta.

- As a result of amelogenesis imperfecta, a person's teeth are covered with thin, malformed enamel.
- Amelogenesis imperfecta is an inherited condition that is transmitted as a dominant trait.

Slide 95

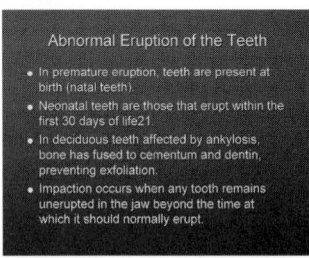

Abnormal Eruption of the Teeth

- In premature eruption, teeth are present at birth (natal teeth).
- Neonatal teeth are those that erupt within the first 30 days of life21.
- In deciduous teeth affected by ankylosis, bone has fused to cementum and dentin, preventing exfoliation.
- Impaction occurs when any tooth remains unerupted in the jaw beyond the time at which it should normally erupt.

- What is eruption? *(When a tooth comes through the gingiva, it is known as [active] tooth eruption and is a normal process of the body.)*

Slide 96

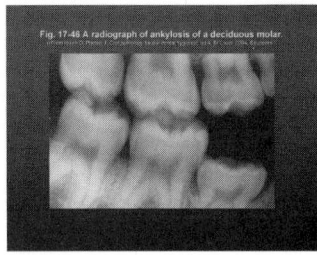

Fig. 17-48 A radiograph of ankylosis of a deciduous molar.

- Ankylosis can occur at any time during the course of eruption.

Bird/Robinson

Slide 97

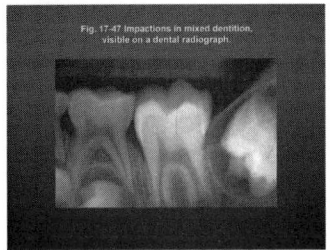

- Remember the processes that can lead to impaction:
  - Premature loss of baby teeth
  - Shifting of tooth into a horizontal position
  - Tooth crowding

Slide 98

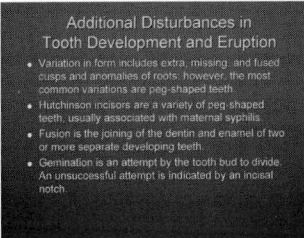

- Developmental dental disturbances may be hereditary.

Slide 99

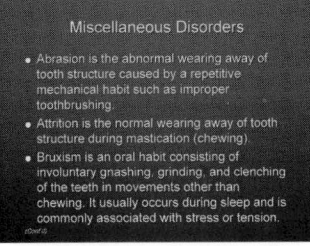

- These disorders are often caused by bad habits or lifestyle factors rather than disease or infection.

Slide 100

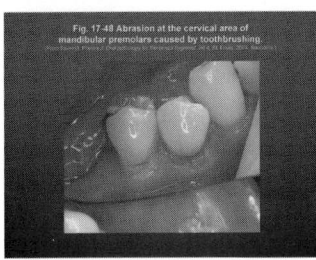

- What would be common advice for a patient presenting with abrasion?
- How might a patient's choice of toothbrush affect abrasion?

Slide 101

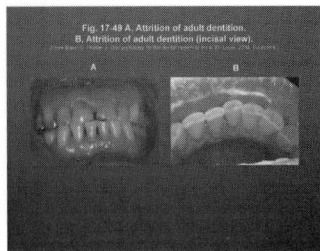

- How does attrition compare with abrasion or erosion?

Slide 102

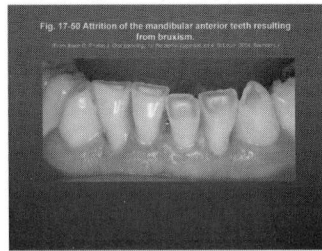

- Many cases of bruxism are mild and require no treatment. For more severe cases, relaxation therapy, protective devices, and sleep position changes may be recommended.

Slide 103

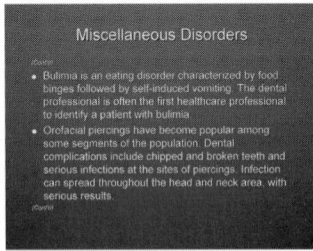

- Bulimia has also been linked to an increased rate of cavities.

- Piercing can also cause uncontrollable bleeding or nerve damage.

Slide 104

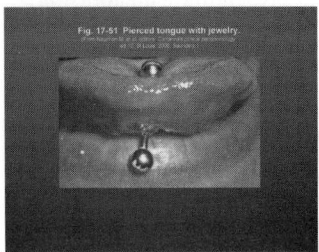

Bird/Robinson

Slide 105

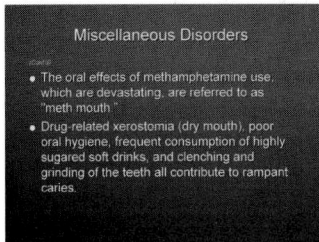

Miscellaneous Disorders

- The oral effects of methamphetamine use, which are devastating, are referred to as "meth mouth."
- Drug-related xerostomia (dry mouth), poor oral hygiene, frequent consumption of highly sugared soft drinks, and clenching and grinding of the teeth all contribute to rampant caries.

- Methamphetamine is a potent central nervous system stimulant that can cause brain damage, and severe oral health effects.

- Street names for methamphetamine include: *meth, speed, ice, chalk, crank, fire*, and *glass*.

Slide 106

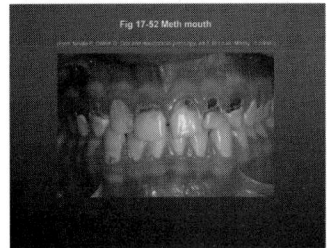

Fig 17-52 Meth mouth

TEACHING FOCUS

This chapter will give the student the opportunity to learn the basics of microbiology. The major groups of microorganisms, including bacteria, algae, protozoa, fungi, prions, and viruses, will be discussed. The student will also be introduced to viral and bacterial diseases and methods to prevent transmission of disease in the dental office.

MATERIALS AND RESOURCES

- ☐ computer and PowerPoint projector (all Lessons)
- ☐ index cards (Lessons 18.1-18.2)
- ☐ materials for students to create charts, lists, and tables (all Lessons)

LESSON CHECKLIST

Preparations for this lesson include:

- lecture
- guest speaker: dentist
- evaluation of student knowledge and skills needed to perform all entry-level activities related to microbiology, including:
  - ○ contributions of the pioneers in microbiology
  - ○ the importance of microbiology
  - ○ the major groups of microorganisms
  - ○ types of viral diseases
  - ○ types of bacterial diseases
  - ○ methods to prevent transmission of disease in the dental office

Bird/Robinson

KEY TERMS

aerobes (p. 255)
anaerobes (p. 255)
bacilli (p. 253)
candida (p. 256)
chancre (p. 262)
cocci (p. 253)
Creutzfeldt-Jakob disease (p. 256)
endospore (p. 252)
facultative anaerobes (p. 255)
fungi (p. 256)
Gram's stain (p. 253)
gram-negative (p. 255)
gram-positive (p. 253)
gram-variable (p. 255)
H5N1 (p. 261)
herpesvirus (p. 259)
latent (p. 257)

microbiology (p. 251)
nonpathogenic (p. 251)
oral candidiasis (p. 256)
pandemic (p. 261)
pathogens (p. 251)
percutaneous (p. 258)
Petri plate (p. 252)
prions (p. 253)
protozoa (p. 255)
provirus (p. 257)
spirochetes (p. 253)
staphylococci (p. 253)
streptococci (p. 253)
tyndallization (p. 252)
virulent (p. 255)
viruses (p. 253)

ADDITIONAL RESOURCES

PowerPoint slides (Evolve): 1-67

Legend

CTQ
Critical
Thinking
Question

DVD
Multimedia
Procedures
Videos and
Animations

ESLR
EVOLVE
Student
Learning
Resources

IDO
Interactive
Dental
Office
CD-ROM

SW
Student
Workbook

TB
Test Bank
on the
TEACH
CD-ROM

PPT
PowerPoint
Slides

Class Activities are indicated in ***bold italic***.

ELSEVIER

Torres and Ehrlich Modern Dental Assisting, 9th ed.

Bird/Robinson

LESSON 18.1

PRETEST

1. Who introduced the earliest belief that life was "spontaneously generated" from nonliving matter?
   - a. Aristotle
   - b. Leeuwenhoek
   - c. Tyndall
   - d. Lister

2. Which microorganism is known as the "perfect parasite" because of its ability to live inside cells of the host and produce 10,000 offspring in as quickly as 7 hours?
   - a. bacteria
   - b. algae
   - c. fungi
   - d. viruses

3. Gram's stain technique requires the sequential use of a crystal violet dye, iodine solution, alcohol solution, and
   - a. spore.
   - b. safranin dye.
   - c. capsule.
   - d. gram-positive bacteria.

4. Bacteria with a spherical shape are called
   - a. cocci.
   - b. bacilli.
   - c. spirochetes.
   - d. gram-negative.

5. What type of microorganism is the most resistant form of life?
   - a. bacteria
   - b. virus
   - c. spore
   - d. fungi

6. What is the main preventive measure a dental care worker can take to avoid contracting the virus hepatitis B?
   - a. blood donor screening
   - b. immunization
   - c. modifing risky behavior
   - d. ensuring safe drinking water

7. What does the term *percutaneous* mean?
   - a. a resistant, dormant structure
   - b. microorganisms that do not produce disease
   - c. performed through the skin
   - d. disease-producing microorganism

8. What does Epstein-Barr virus cause?
   - a. oral lesions
   - b. genital lesions
   - c. shingles and chicken pox
   - d. mononucleosis

9. What does HIV affect once it enters the body?
   - a. T-cells
   - b. C-cells
   - c. red blood cells
   - d. platelets

10. The first stage of syphilis is the presentation of a painless, ulcerating sore known as a
    - a. cold sore.
    - b. fever blister.
    - c. rash
    - d. chancre.

Answers

1. a	3. b	5. c	7. c	9. a
2. d	4. a	6. b	8. d	10. d

BACKGROUND ASSESSMENT

Question: What is microbiology? How does microbiology relate to the dental environment and the role of the dental assistant?

Answer: Microbiology is the study of microorganisms. The dental assistant needs a foundation in microbiology in order to understand the nature of pathogens or microorganisms that produce disease. The

Torres and Ehrlich Modern Dental Assisting, 9th ed.

Bird/Robinson

dental assistant's role is to prevent the transmission of disease in the dental office and dental treatment areas. Knowledge of microbiology helps the dental assistant to make important decisions regarding infection-control products and procedures.

Question: What are herpesviruses, and why do they pose a danger to dental care workers? What are the four major categories of herpesviruses, and what illnesses are associated with each?

Answer: Herpesvirus is a double-stranded DNA virus that causes infections in humans. It poses a danger to dental care workers because the virus may be dormant for years before becoming active and causing disease. There are four major herpesviruses that affect humans: (1) herpes simplex virus (HSV), (2) herpes zoster (HZV), (3) cytomegalovirus (CMV), and (4) Epstein-Barr virus (EBV). The herpes simplex virus is divided into two categories: HSV-1 and HSV-2. HSV-1 causes oral lesions commonly called fever blisters or cold sores, while HSV-2 causes genital lesions. Herpes zoster causes chicken pox and shingles. Cytomegalovirus does not cause disease but can affect a fetus during pregnancy, causing the infant to be born deaf or severely retarded. Epstein-Barr is associated with infectious mononucleosis, nasopharyngeal cancer, lymphoma, and oral hairy leukoplakia.

CRITICAL THINKING QUESTION

A dental assistant has been hired in a dental office setting where no infection-control protocol is in place. The dentist has asked the dental assistant to develop an infection-control program for the office and a training program for the staff. What resources or guidelines should the dental assistant consult? What aspects of microbiology should the dental assistant include in the training program and why?

Guidelines: A primary source to consult when developing infection control policy and procedures is the Centers for Disease Control and Prevention (CDC). The CDC is one of the 13 major operating components of the Department of Health and Human Services (HHS), which is the principal United States governmental agency responsible for protecting the health and safety of all Americans. Since it was founded in 1946 to help control malaria, the CDC has remained at the forefront of public health efforts to prevent and control infectious and chronic diseases, injuries, workplace hazards, disabilities, and environmental health threats. The training program must include discussion of the major groups of microorganisms, how microorganisms are identified, how microorganisms reproduce and cause disease, how various microorganisms are killed and destroyed, what results when cross contamination occurs, and what diseases can affect patients and dental-care workers. Including microbiology in the training program will provide dental staff the necessary foundation to understand organisms that cause disease.

OBJECTIVES	CONTENT	TEACHING RESOURCES
Pronounce, define, and spell the Key Terms.	■ Key terms (pp. 250-251)	⊕ ESLR Electronic Flashcards ▸ Discuss each of the key terms, focusing on the definition, pronunciation, and spelling of each term. *Class Activity Have students make flash cards for each key term by writing the key term on one side of an index card and the definition on the other side. Then have the students quiz each other with the flash cards.*
Explain why the study of microbiology is important for the dental assistant.	■ Introduction (pp. 251)	⊠ PPT 4 TB questions 1-2 SW Short-Answer Questions 2; Fill in the Blank questions 1-4; Multiple Choice question 1 (pp. 71-73) Recall question 1 (p. 252) Legal and Ethical Implications (p. 263) CTQ 2 (p. 263)

Torres and Ehrlich Modern Dental Assisting, 9th ed.

Bird/Robinson

OBJECTIVES	CONTENT	TEACHING RESOURCES
		▸ Discuss the reasons that a dental assistant needs a foundation in microbiology.
		▸ Discuss the meaning of *pathogens, microbiology,* and *nonpathogenic.*
		***Class Activity** Before reading Chapter 18, have each student write a paragraph on the importance of dental assistants having knowledge of microbiology. After reading the chapter, have each student write a second paragraph on the importance of dental assistants having knowledge of microbiology. Call on students to share how their opinions changed after reading the chapter.*
Discuss the contributions of early pioneers in microbiology.	▪ Pioneers in microbiology (p. 251)	⊠▤ PPT 5-9
		📖 SW Short-Answer Questions 1; Multiple Choice questions 2-4 (pp. 71, 73)
		Recall questions 2-4 (p. 252)
		Figure 18-1 Colonies of bacteria (p. 252)
		Figure 18-2 Discovery of rabies vaccine by Louis Pasteur, 1885 (p. 252)
		Figure 18-3 Louis Pasteur (p. 253)
		💡 CTQ 1 (p. 263)
		▸ Discuss Louis Pasteur's contribution to microbiology.
		▸ Discuss the roles that Aristotle, Leeuwenhoek, Tyndall, Cohn, Lister, and Koch played in microbiology.
		***Class Activity** Have each student research one pioneer of microbiology on the Internet and prepare a brief report of the pioneer's contributions to microbiology and how those contributions are still used today. Then have the students present their reports to the class. (For students to prepare for this Activity, see Homework/Assignments #1)*
Identify the types of bacteria according to their shape.	▪ Major groups of microorganisms (p. 252) ☐ Bacteria (p. 253) – Shape (p. 253)	⊠▤ PPT 10-13
		🖥 TB question 4
		📖 SW Short-Answer Questions 3; Fill in the Blank question 11; Multiple Choice questions 4, 6, 13 (pp. 71-73)
		Figure 18-4 Three basic shapes of bacteria (p. 254)
		Figure 18-5 Colonies of streptococci growing on agar medium are diagnostic for strep throat (p. 254)
		Figure 18-6 Golden-yellow colonies of staphylococci (p. 254)
		Recall question 5 (p. 255)

ELSEVIER

Torres and Ehrlich Modern Dental Assisting, 9th ed.

Bird/Robinson

OBJECTIVES	CONTENT	TEACHING RESOURCES
		▸ Discuss the three shapes of bacteria and the characteristics of each. *Class Activity* **Have each student create a chart or table describing and depicting the types and shapes of each bacteria. Then have each student share his or her chart with a classmate.**
List the major groups of microorganisms.	■ Major groups of microorganisms (p. 252) ☐ Bacteria (p. 253) – Shape (p. 253) – Gram-positive and gram-negative bacteria (p. 253) – Need for oxygen (p. 255) – Capsules (p. 255) – Spores (p. 255) – Rickettsiae (p. 255) ☐ Algae (p. 255) ☐ Protozoa (p. 255) ☐ Fungi (p. 256) ☐ Prions (p. 256) – Prion diseases (p. 256) – Future research (p. 256) ☐ Viruses (p. 257)	⊠▤ PPT 10, 14-18 ▤ TB questions 3, 7-8 ▤ SW Short-Answer Questions 4; Fill in the Blank questions 8-10, 13 (pp. 71-72) Recall questions 6-7 (p. 255) Figure 18-7 Gram-positive stain (p. 255) Figure 18-8 Gram-negative stain (p. 255) Figure 18-9 (A) Multiple white plaques of pseudomembranous candidiasis (thrush) in an HIV-infected individual; (B) Candida-associated denture stomatitis showing the edentulous maxillary arch (p. 256) ▤ CTQ 3 (p. 263) ▸ Discuss the five major groups of organisms: bacteria, algae, protozoa, fungi, and viruses. Discuss the characteristics of each. *Class Activity* **Divide the class into small groups, and assign each group one of the major groups of microorganisms (bacteria, algae, protozoa, fungi, and viruses). Have each group discuss the characteristics of its assigned microorganism. Then have the groups share their findings with the class.**

ELSEVIER

18.1 Homework/Assignments:

1. Have each student research one pioneer of microbiology on the Internet and prepare a brief report of the pioneer's contributions to microbiology and how those contributions are still used today. Then have the students present their reports to the class.

18.1 Instructor's Notes/Student Feedback:

LESSON 18.2

CRITICAL THINKING QUESTION

A dentist has asked a dental assistant to develop a chart to hang on the wall in the lab to inform the dental staff of the different types of microorganisms and their characteristics. What information should the dental assistant include?

Guidelines: The dental assistant should include the following information. The five major microorganisms are bacteria, algae, protozoa, fungi, and viruses. Members of the first four groups are easily recognized using a microscope. However, viruses are very small, and specialized equipment is required to view them. Bacteria are further identified by their shape: spherical (cocci), rod (bacilli), and spiral (spirochetes). Microorganisms are transmitted from host to host by different routes of entry: through the skin, into the respiratory tract, or into the gastrointestinal tract. Some microorganisms need oxygen to survive (aerobic) while others do not (anaerobic). Some bacteria have capsules that act as a protective layer. Bacteria also have the ability to change into spores. Spores represent the most resistant form of life known. Viruses are smaller than bacteria and invade a host cell, replicate themselves, then destroy the host cell.

OBJECTIVES	CONTENT	TEACHING RESOURCES
Describe the differences among aerobes, anaerobes, and facultative anaerobes.	■ Major groups of microorganisms (p. 252) □ Bacteria (p. 253) – Shape (p. 253) – Gram-positive and gram-negative bacteria (p. 253) – Need for oxygen (p. 255) – Capsules (p. 255) – Spores (p. 255) – Rickettsiae (p. 255) □ Algae (p. 255) □ Protozoa (p. 255) □ Fungi (p. 256) □ Prions (p. 256) – Prion diseases (p. 256) – Future research (p. 256) □ Viruses (p. 257)	PPT 21 TB question 5 SW Short-Answer Questions 5; Fill in the Blank questions 6-7; Multiple Choice question 7 (pp. 71-73) ▸ Discuss how aerobes, anaerobes, and facultative anaerobes grow. *Class Activity Have each student create a list containing three columns: Aerobes, Anaerobes, and Facultative Anaerobes. Have each student research names of microbes that fit into each column. Then have each student present his or her list to the class. Additional microbes should be added to each list as the students present the information.*
Compare viruses with bacteria, and name diseases caused by each.	■ Major groups of microorganisms (p. 252) □ Bacteria (p. 253) – Shape (p. 253)	PPT 22-27 TB questions 11-15 SW Short-Answer Questions 9; Multiple Choice question 10; Topics for Discussion questions 1-4 (pp. 71, 73-74)

ELSEVIER

OBJECTIVES	CONTENT	TEACHING RESOURCES
	– Gram-positive and gram-negative bacteria (p. 253) – Need for oxygen (p. 255) – Capsules (p. 255) – Spores (p. 255) – Rickettsiae (p. 255) ☐ Algae (p. 255) ☐ Protozoa (p. 255) ☐ Fungi (p. 256) ☐ Prions (p. 256) – Prion diseases (p. 256) – Future research (p. 256) ☐ Viruses (p. 257)	CTQ 4 (p. 263) ▸ Discuss the differences between bacteria and viruses. ▸ Discuss examples of bacteria and viruses. ***Class Activity** Have each student create a table comparing viruses to bacteria. The table should include shape, size, and what inactivates the microorganism. Have each student share his or her table with a classmate. Begin a class discussion by asking students whether they have any questions about the tables.*
Identify the most resistant form of life known, and explain how it survives.	■ Major groups of microorganisms (p. 252) ☐ Bacteria (p. 253) – Shape (p. 253) – Gram-positive and gram-negative bacteria (p. 253) – Need for oxygen (p. 255) – Capsules (p. 255) – Spores (p. 255) – Rickettsiae (p. 255) ☐ Algae (p. 255) ☐ Protozoa (p. 255) ☐ Fungi (p. 256) ☐ Prions (p. 256) – Prion diseases (p. 256) – Future research (p. 256) ☐ Viruses (p. 257)	PPT 23-27 TB question 6 SW Short-Answer Questions 7; Multiple Choice question 8 (pp. 71, 73) Recall question 8 (p. 255) ▸ Discuss the characteristics of spores. ▸ Discuss the differences between spores and the usual form of bacteria. ***Class Activity** Divide the class into small groups, and have each group design a presentation depicting the structure of a spore and how it defends itself. Then have each group give its presentation to the class.*

OBJECTIVES	CONTENT	TEACHING RESOURCES
Identify diseases caused by chlamydiae.	☐ Fungi (p. 256) ☐ Prions (p. 256) – Prion diseases (p. 256) – Future research (p. 256) ☐ Viruses (p. 257)	PPT 28-31 SW Short-Answer Questions 7 (p. 71) *Class Activity Have each student search the Internet for one disease caused by chlamydia. The student should identify the disease, its signs and symptoms, the route of transmission, and the incubation period. Then have each student present his or her findings to the class. (For students to prepare for this Activity, see Homework/Assignments #1.)*
Describe how prions differ from viruses and bacteria.	☐ Prions (p. 256) – Prion diseases (p. 256) – Future research (p. 256) ☐ Viruses (p. 257)	PPT 32 SW Short-Answer Questions 10; Multiple Choice question 9 (pp. 71, 73) Recall question 9 (p. 256) ▸ Discuss the definition of prions and their composition. ▸ Discuss how prions differ from bacteria and viruses. *Class Activity Divide the class into three groups. Have one group make flash cards by writing questions describing the characteristics of prions on one side of an index card and the answers to the questions on the other. Have the second group do the same for the characteristics of viruses. Have the third group do the same for the characteristics of bacteria. Then have each group quiz the other groups using the flash cards it created. The instructor should keep score of which group answers the most questions correctly.*
Name two diseases caused by prions.	☐ Prions (p. 256) – Prion diseases (p. 256) – Future research (p. 256) ☐ Viruses (p. 257)	PPT 33 TB questions 9-10 SW Short-Answer Questions 11; Fill in the Blank question 12 (pp. 71-72) ▸ Discuss diseases caused by prions. ▸ Discuss how prion diseases are transmitted. *Class Activity Have each student conduct Internet research for diseases caused by prions. Each student should write a brief paragraph about each disease. Then have the students present one of their paragraphs to the class. (For students to prepare for this Activity, see Homework/Assignments #2.)*
Explain why specificity in viruses is important.	☐ Viruses (p. 257) – Specificity (p. 257) – Latency (p. 257)	PPT 34-36 SW Short-Answer Questions 8 (p. 71) ▸ Discuss the meaning of specificity in relation to viruses.

OBJECTIVES	CONTENT	TEACHING RESOURCES
	– Treatment of viral diseases (p. 257) – Transmission of viral diseases (p. 257) – Viruses in the environment (p. 257)	▶ Discuss viral diseases that have a high degree of specificity. *Class Activity Divide the class into small groups, and assign each group a viral disease. Have each group discuss how specificity of the virus affects the disease cycle, disease treatment, and disease transmission from host to host. Then have each group present its findings to the class.*

18.2 Homework/Assignments:

1. Have each student search the Internet for one disease caused by chlamydia. The student should identify the disease, its signs and symptoms, the route of transmission, and the incubation period. Then have each student present his or her findings to the class.
2. Have each student conduct Internet research for diseases caused by prions. Each student should write a brief paragraph about each disease. Then have the students present one of their paragraphs to the class.

18.2 Instructor's Notes/Student Feedback:

LESSON 18.3

CRITICAL THINKING QUESTION

A dental assistant is reviewing a patient chart for a patient who is scheduled for an extraction. The dental assistant notices that the chart notes indicate the patient has a history of hepatitis B. What concerns would the dental assistant have for the safety of the patient as well as for the other members of the dental team? What are the precautionary measures that the dental assistant and the other team members can take for the future when a patient with hepatitis is scheduled for treatments?

Guidelines: Hepatitis B can cause a very serious disease that may result in prolonged illness, liver cancer, cirrhosis of the liver, liver failure, and even death. A medical consult with the patient's physician may be in order. Once the physician has approved the extraction, the extraction procedure should begin with the administration of local anesthetics that are not metabolized in the liver. The safety of the dental team is of concern as well, since the hepatitis B virus is transmitted percutaneously and through mucosal tissues. Precautionary measures to take to avoid transmission of hepatitis B from the patient to the dental care workers include the use of universal precautions, immunization, and infection-control practices. All healthcare providers should receive the hepatitis vaccine. The vaccine is considered safe even for women who are pregnant.

OBJECTIVES	CONTENT	TEACHING RESOURCES
Explain how each type of hepatitis is transmitted.	☐ Viral hepatitis (p. 257) – Hepatitis A (p. 257) – Hepatitis B (p. 257) – Hepatitis C (p. 258) – Hepatitis D (p. 259) – Hepatitis E (p. 259)	PPT 43-49 TB question 15,17 SW Short-Answer Questions 14-15; Fill in the Blank questions 14-15; Multiple Choice question 11 (pp. 71-73) Table 18-1 Primary Types of Hepatitis (p. 258) ▸ Discuss the five primary types of hepatitis, including the source of the virus, the route of transmission, and prevention. *Class Activity Ask students to call out the various types of hepatitis and write them on the blackboard. Then ask for student volunteers to come to the board and write how each type of hepatitis can be transmitted from host to host.*
Describe the effect of HIV on the immune system.	☐ Human immunodeficiency virus (p. 259)	PPT 50 SW Short-Answer Questions 16 (p. 71) ▸ Discuss how HIV affects the immune system. *Class Activity Divide the class into groups, and assign each group an immune response of a person infected with HIV. Have each group discuss the assigned immune response and then share its findings with the class.*
Identify methods of HIV transmission.	☐ Human immunodeficiency virus (p. 259)	PPT 51 TB question 19 SW Short-Answer Questions 17 (p. 71) Recall question 11 (p. 261)

Bird/Robinson

OBJECTIVES	CONTENT	TEACHING RESOURCES
		▸ Discuss ways that HIV can be transmitted.
		Class Activity Have the students conduct Internet research to determine how HIV is transmitted from one person to another. Have each student develop a table comparing the ways by which HIV can be transmitted and review his or her table with a classmate. (For students to prepare for this Activity, see Homework/Assignments #1.)
Describe the symptoms of West Nile virus.	☐ West Nile virus (p. 261)	🖼️ PPT 59

📘 SW Fill in the Blank question 17 (p. 71)

Recall question 12 (p. 261)

▸ Discuss the symptoms of West Nile virus.

Class Activity Have each student design a simple pamphlet describing the symptoms of West Nile virus. Pick the best pamphlets and share them with the class. |
| **Explain how West Nile virus is spread.** | ☐ West Nile virus (p. 261) | 🖼️ PPT 59

📘 SW Short-Answer Questions 14; Fill in the Blank question 16 (pp. 71-72)

▸ Discuss how West Nile virus is spread.

Class Activity Divide the class into small groups. Have each group discuss how West Nile virus is spread. Have each group present its findings to the class. |
| **Explain how the H5N1 virus is spread.** | ☐ Avian influenza viruses (p. 261) | 📘 SW Short-Answer Questions 13 (p. 71)

Recall question 13 (p. 261)

▸ Discuss how H5N1 is transmitted.

Class Activity As a class discuss the various routes of transmission of the H5N1 virus. Divide the class into small groups. Ask each group to make a list of the measures that can be employed in the dental setting to avoid transmission. Have each group share its list with the class. |
| **Name the bloodborne pathogens of concern in dentistry.** | ■ Viral diseases (p. 257)
☐ Viral hepatitis (p. 257)
– Hepatitis A (p. 257)
– Hepatitis B (p. 257)
– Hepatitis C (p. 258)
– Hepatitis D (p. 259)
– Hepatitis E (p. 259) | 🖼️ PPT 40-42, 52-58

💻 TB questions 16-17, 19-20

📘 SW Multiple Choice questions 14-15 (p. 73)

Table 18-1 Primary Types of Hepatitis (p. 258)

Recall questions 10, 14-16 (pp. 259, 263)

Figure 18-12 (A) Chancre on tongue seen in primary syphilis; (B) Chancre on lip (p. 262) |

OBJECTIVES	CONTENT	TEACHING RESOURCES
	☐ Human immunodeficiency virus (p. 259) ☐ Herpesvirus (p. 259) – Herpes simplex virus type 1 (p. 260) – Primary herpes (p. 260) – Recurrent herpes labialis (p. 260) – Herpes simplex virus type 2 (p. 260) – Herpes zoster virus (p. 260) – Cytomegalovirus (p. 260) – Epstein-Barr virus (p. 260) – Herpes transmission (p. 260) ☐ West Nile virus (p. 261) ☐ Avian influenza viruses (p. 261) ■ Bacterial diseases (p. 261) – Tuberculosis (p. 261) – Legionnaires' disease (p. 261) – Tetanus (p. 262) – Syphilis (p. 262)	Eye to the Future (p. 263) ▶ Discuss bloodborne pathogens that cause concern in dentistry. ▶ Discuss preventative measures to avoid occupational exposure to diseases. *Class Activity **Invite a dentist to speak to the class about bloodborne pathogens that may cause risk to dental care workers. Have the dentist explain how exposure to the pathogen can be avoided. Have the students prepare questions for the dentist beforehand.***
Performance Evaluation		▣ TB ▣ SW questions (pp. 71-74) *e* ESLR Electronic Flashcards *e* ESLR Practice Quiz Recall questions (pp. 252- 263) ♀ CTQ (p. 263)

18.3 Homework/Assignments:

1. Have the students conduct Internet research to determine how HIV is transmitted from one person to another. Have each student develop a table comparing how HIV can be transmitted and review his or her table with a classmate.

18.3 Instructor's Notes/Student Feedback:

Slide 1

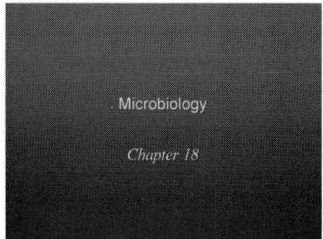

Slide 2

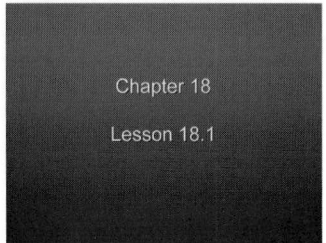

Slide 3

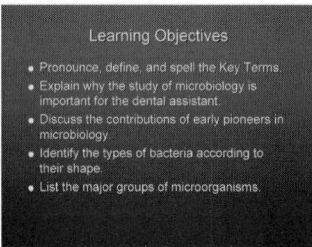

Slide 4

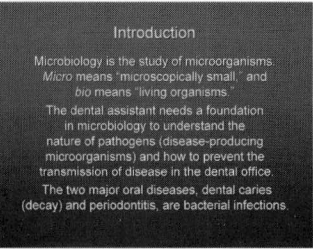

- Are all microorganisms bad? (*No. Most microorganisms are nonpathogenic— they do not produce human illness— and some are helpful.*)

- Can you think of ways microorganisms are helpful? (*Microorganisms are used in the production of flavorful cheeses and yogurt, in the disposal of waste products, in fertilization of soil, and in production of lifesaving drugs.*)

Slide 5

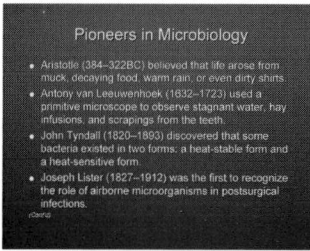

- Aristotle believed that life was "spontaneously generated." His theory remained unchallenged for more than 2000 years.

- Leeuwenhoek used a simple microscope with a 300 magnification lens. Who did he report his findings to? (*The Royal Society of London.*)

- Tyndall was an English physicist who explained the need for prolonged heating to destroy microorganisms.

- How did Lister lower the risk of infection after surgery? (*He applied carbolic acid to dressing.*)

Slide 6

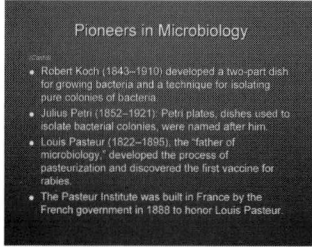

- Koch was a German physician who was a forerunner in providing the techniques and discipline that guided future microbiologists.

- The dishes Petri designed are still used in microbiology labs today.

- Which longtime theory was Pasteur responsible for disproving? (*The theory of spontaneous generation of life.*)

- Pasteur also designed S-shaped flasks with swanlike necks to prevent dust particles from contaminating microorganisms.

Slide 7

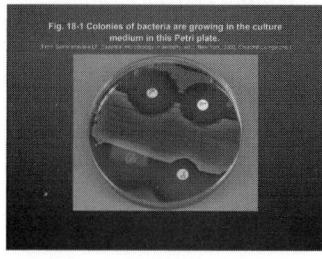

- This slide shows the two-part dish designed by Koch that makes the technique of isolating pure colonies of bacteria possible in microbiology labs.

- Who is the two-part dish named after? (*Julius Petri [1852-1921], a German bacteriologist.*)

Slide 8

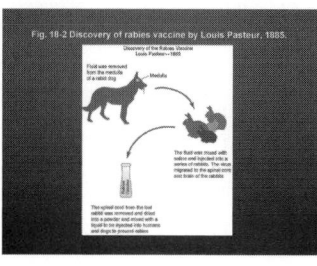

- Pasteur prepared the first vaccine for the fatal animal disease rabies.

- What is the medulla? (*A portion of the brainstem and spinal cord.*)

Slide 9

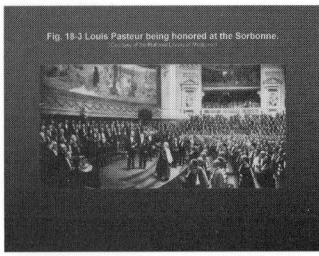

- The French government built the Pasteur Institute in 1888 to honor Pasteur.
- What were Pasteur's last words? (*"There is still a great deal to do."*)

Slide 10

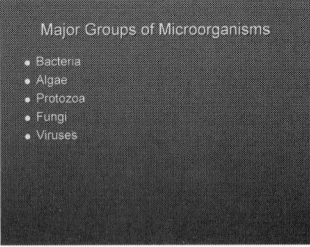

- Members of the first four groups are easily recognized with the aid of a microscope.
- Viruses can be viewed only under a powerful electron microscope.

Slide 11

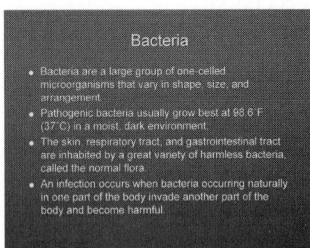

- What is the function or purpose of normal flora? (*They protect the human host by aiding in metabolism and preventing entrance of harmful bacteria.*)
- What are normal flora considered when normal bacteria invade another part of the body? (*Opportunistic bacteria that cause infection.*)
- What is an example of an opportunistic bacteria? (*Escherichia coli, which causes cystitis.*)

Slide 12

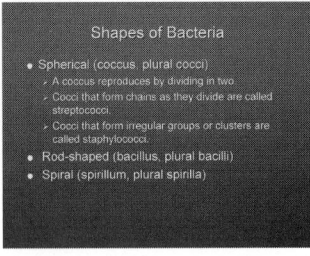

- The shapes of bacteria can be viewed under a microscope.
- What are examples of illnesses caused by cocci-shaped microorganisms? (*Strep throat, tonsillitis, pneumonia, and endocarditis.*)
- What is an example of an illness caused by rod-shaped microorganisms? (*Tuberculosis.*)
- What are examples of illnesses caused by spiral-shaped bacteria? (*Syphilis and Lyme disease.*)

Bird/Robinson

Slide 13

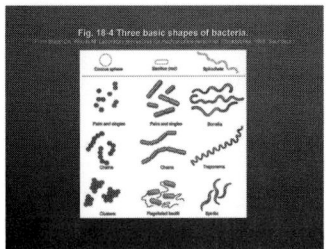

- Three shapes of bacteria are pictured: cocci (round or spherical), bacilli (rod-shaped), and spirochetes (helical-shaped).
- Even through the bacteria are classified in three different shapes, the individual classifications of shapes can vary. Cocci and rods can be single or paired, or actually form a chain. Rods can also appear to grow what looks like a tail, which acts as a propeller to guide the bacteria through their environment.
- The spiral-shaped bacteria can take on variations of waves and spirals.

Slide 14

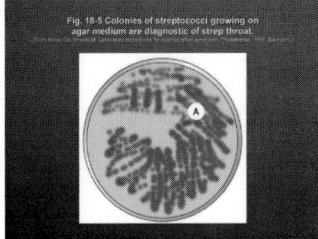

- Pictured on the slide are bacteria that cause infections such as pneumonia.
- Are there single, paired, or chainlike cocci? (*Mostly chainlike, but also single and paired cocci.*)

Slide 15

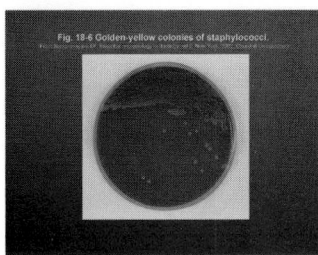

- Note the irregular groups or clusters that are formed by the cocci microorganisms.
- What are irregular clusters of cocci microorganisms called? (*Staphylococci.*)

Slide 16

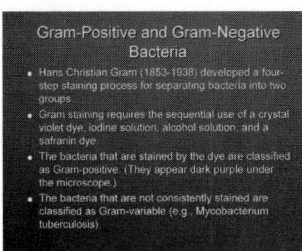

- How is gram staining used today? (*A physician can make a diagnosis on the basis of Gram's stain and begin appropriate antimicrobial therapy.*)

Slide 17

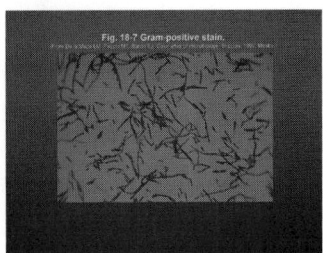

- Gram-positive bacteria are stained during the Gram stain process, making them appear darker in color or purple under microscopic examination.

- To what drugs or medications are most Gram-positive bacteria susceptible? (*Penicillins.*)

Slide 18

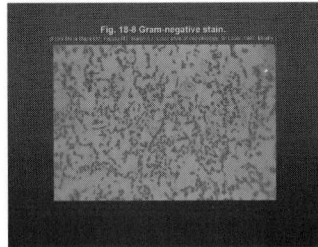

- Gram-negative bacteria are almost colorless or a light pink in color under microscopic examination.

- What are bacteria that are inconsistently stained called? (*Gram-variable.*)

Slide 19

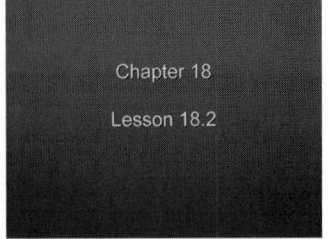

Chapter 18

Lesson 18.2

Slide 20

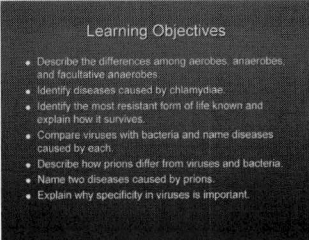

Learning Objectives

- Describe the differences among aerobes, anaerobes, and facultative anaerobes.
- Identify diseases caused by chlamydiae.
- Identify the most resistant form of life known and explain how it survives.
- Compare viruses with bacteria and name diseases caused by each.
- Describe how prions differ from viruses and bacteria.
- Name two diseases caused by prions.
- Explain why specificity in viruses is important.

ELSEVIER

Bird/Robinson

Slide 21

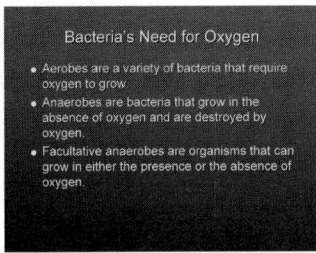

- A good supply of oxygen enhances the metabolism and the growth of many bacteria. Obligate or strict aerobes require oxygen to grow. Example: *Mycobacterium tuberculosis.*

- Obligate or strict anaerobes cannot grow in the presence of oxygen. An example is *Porphyromanas gingivalis.* However, microaerophiles also classified as anaerobic bacteria can survive when low levels of oxygen are present. Example: *Campylobacter fetus.*

- Facultative anaerobes use oxygen—if it is present—to generate energy by respiration. Examples: *Mutans streptococci* and *Escherichia coli.*

Slide 22

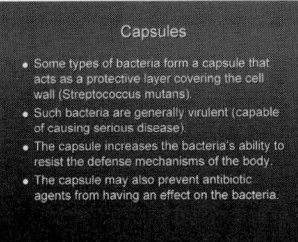

- The capsule is an amorphous, gelatin-like layer that surrounds the entire bacteria.

- Besides providing protection to the bacteria, what other role does the capsule play? (*It mediates adhesion of the bacteria to human tissues, which enhances the bacteria's ability to colonize and begin the infectious process.*)

Slide 23

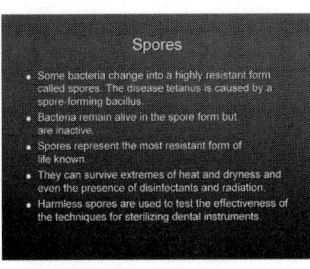

- When the bacteria are inactive in the spore form, they cannot reproduce or cause disease.

- Spore tests are performed with the use of biological monitors. Biological monitors are designed to prove sterilization.

- If the biological monitor claims that the spores were killed during the sterilization process, is it safe to assume that less-resistant bacteria have been destroyed? (*Yes.*)

Slide 24

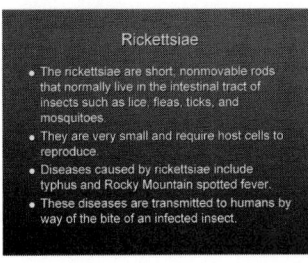

- Rickettsiae are smaller than bacteria but resemble them structurally and metabolically.

- The disease typhus is commonly seen in poor and malnourished individuals.

- These bacteria have a round or cocci shape with a multilayered outer cell wall resembling Gram-negative bacteria.

ELSEVIER

Torres and Ehrlich Modern Dental Assisting, 9th ed.

Bird/Robinson

Slide 25

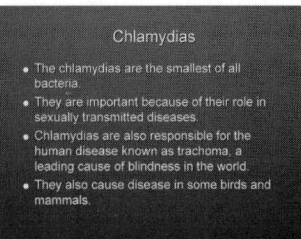

- *Chlamydia tachomatis* cause a spectrum of diseases, including ocular infections, genital infections, and pneumonia.
- Which is the most effective antibiotic against the chlamydia microorganisms? (*Tetracycline.*)

Slide 26

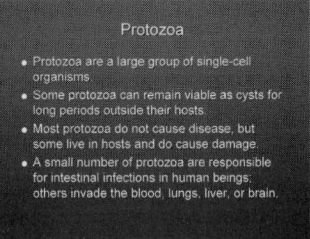

- Which common dental material is made from algae? (*Alginate.*)

Slide 27

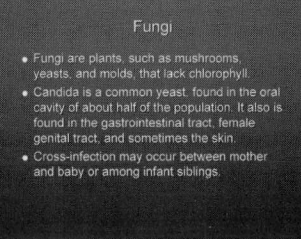

- Protozoa can live in the oral cavity as large, motile amoebae. The main species is *Entamoeba gingivalis*.
- Oral protozoa are often found in the periodontal tissues of patients who have just finished radiation therapy.

Slide 28

- The study of fungi is called mycology.
- Fungi are eukaryotic microorganisms, as opposed to bacteria, which are known as prokaryotic.
- Fungi exhibit two basic structural forms: yeast form and mould form.
- What is the difference between the two fungi forms? (*Yeast is unicellular and mould is multicellular.*)

ELSEVIER

Torres and Ehrlich Modern Dental Assisting, 9th ed.
Bird/Robinson

Slide 29

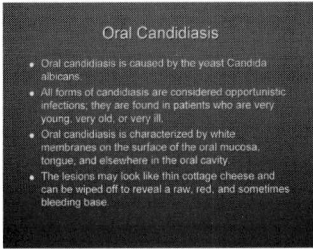

- *Candida albicans* can also be found in the gastrointestinal tract, female genital tract, and sometimes the skin.
- What is the common term for an oral candida infection? *(Thrush.)*

Slide 30

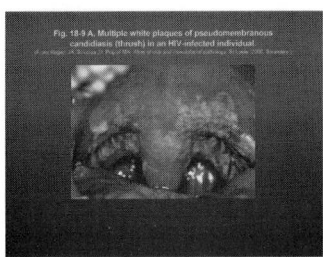

- In HIV-infected patients, candidiasis is virtually always mucocutaneous, involving the oropharynx, the esophagus, and the vagina.
- HIV infection by itself is not associated with the syndrome of disseminated candidiasis, which is characterized by candidemia, endophthalmitis, and multiple organ involvement.
- The precise immunologic processes that control candidal infection in HIV-infected patients are not known. However, mucocutaneous candidiasis is clearly related to the development of clinical cellular immunodeficiency. In fact, oropharyngeal candidiasis is an independent predictor of immunodeficiency in patients with AIDS.

Slide 31

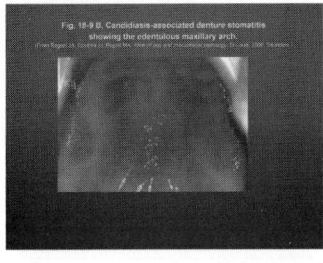

- Edentulous patients should have regular soft tissue checks with a dentist to avoid an outbreak of candidiasis-associated denture stomatitis.
- Proper fitting dentures and proper daily brushing of appliances and oral tissues will decrease the chance of an outbreak.

Slide 32

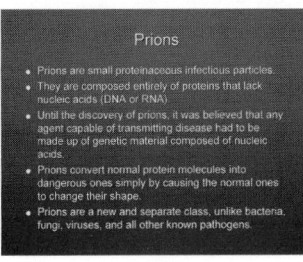

- Who discovered prions? *(Dr. Stanley Prusiner.)*
- Major characteristics of prions:
  - Neither viruses nor viroids
  - Do not contain DNA or RNA.
  - Can self-replicate.
  - Have a long incubation period.

ELSEVIER

Bird/Robinson

Slide 33

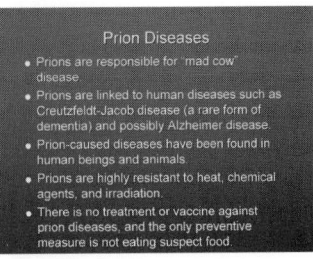

- The prion agent can be transmitted to cows, minks, cats, and mice when fed infected materials.
- Prions first appear in the lymphoid tissue and then in brain cells.

Slide 34

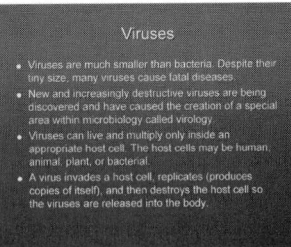

- Common characteristics of viruses:
  - Not visible with a light microscope
  - Not capable of free growth
  - DNA and RNA not present together
  - Do not have a rigid cell wall
  - Not susceptible to penicillin or tetracycline
  - Metabolically inactive outside the cells of susceptible hosts

Slide 35

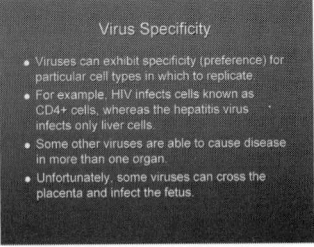

- Viruses can cause severe acute oral and orafacial disease, may produce oral signs of systemic infection, and may be transmitted to patients and dental staff.

Slide 36

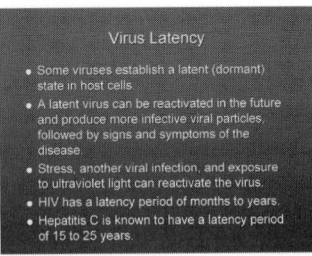

- What is another word for latent or dormant? (*Suppressed.*)
- Why are lengthy latent periods of concern to the dental team? (*A patient may be infected but have no signs, symptoms, or knowledge that he or she has an infection.*)

Torres and Ehrlich Modern Dental Assisting, 9th ed.

Bird/Robinson

Slide 37

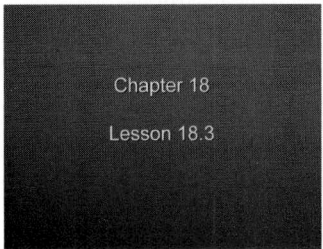

Slide 38

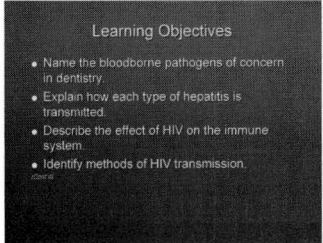

Slide 39

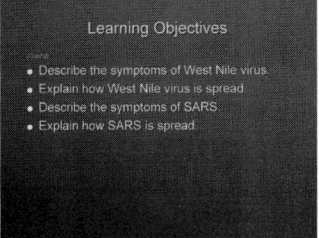

Slide 40

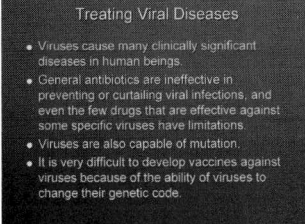

- Most viral diseases are treated symptomatically. What does the term "symptomatically" mean in this context? (*Treat the symptoms, not the infective cause.*)

- Why are general antibiotics ineffective against fighting viruses? (*Antibiotics either kill or interfere with the metabolic processes of bacteria. Because viruses do not function the same way as bacteria do, antibiotics are not effective against them.*)

- Why is having the capability to mutate such a powerful defense for viruses? (*Changing makes the viruses better suited to survive current conditions and resist efforts being made to kill them.*)

Bird/Robinson

Slide 41

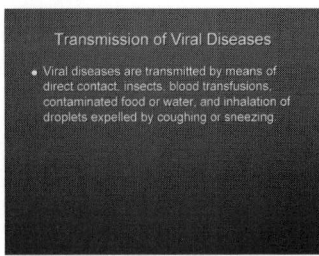

- Viruses are transmitted from one host to another via: inhalation through the respiratory tract, ingestion through the gastrointestinal tract, or inoculation through the skin and mucosa.

- The ability of organisms to adhere to host surfaces is a prerequisite for initiating infection.

- Viruses are completely devoid of organelles of transport, and are easily spread throughout the body by numerous routes.

Slide 42

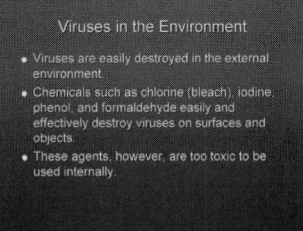

- How long do viruses live on surface areas such as countertops in a dental treatment room? (*Some viruses can live on countertops for up to 6 hours. Most viruses cannot live outside the human body for long periods of time.*)

Slide 43

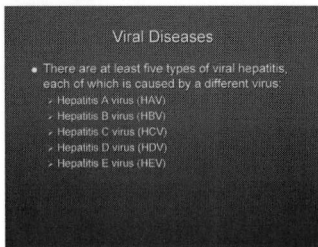

- What is viral hepatitis? (*Hepatitis is an inflammation of the liver caused by a virus.*)

- In the United States, hepatitis A, hepatitis B, and hepatitis C are the most common types.

Slide 44

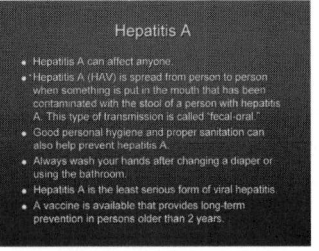

- Hepatitis A virus (HAV) is a small virus belonging to the picornavirus group (also includes poliovirus and coxsackievirus).

- HAV is inactivated by ultraviolet light, exposure to water at 100° C for 5 minutes, and by exposure to 2% glutaraldehyde for 15 minutes.

- What is the incubation period of HAV? (*It is 2 to 7 weeks.*)

Slide 45

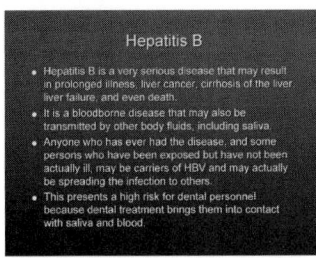

- What is the incubation period of HBV? (*It is 1 to 6 months.*)
- There are types of carriers of HBV:
  - Chronic persistent hepatitis or "healthy carriers": These patients usually have no liver damage and are generally in good health.
  - Chronic active hepatitis: Extremely infectious as these patients harbor infectious particles in their blood.
- Can people infected with HBV ever recover?
- What are the two best ways dental professionals can protect themselves from becoming infected with HBV?

Slide 46

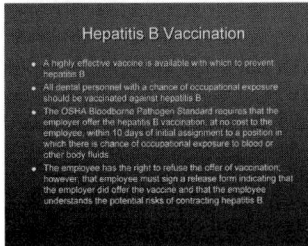

- Who is at greater risk of contracting HBV in a dental setting, the dental staff or the patient? (*The usual mode of transmission is from the patient to the dental operator.*)
- Where is the greatest concentration of HBV located intraorally? (*In the gingival sulcus due to continuous serum exudate.*)

Slide 47

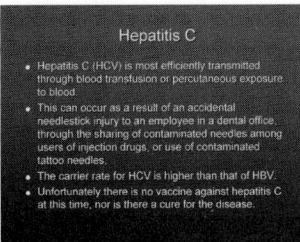

- Why is the use of standard precautions of the utmost importance when dealing with all patients, especially those with a history of HCV? (*HCV is caused by an enveloped RNA virus. The viral RNA can remain intact for at least seven days at room temperature.*)
- What is the incubation period of HCV? (*It is 2 to 26 weeks.*)
- Possible oral manifestations of HCV include: lichen planus, oral malignancy, and salivary gland disease.

Slide 48

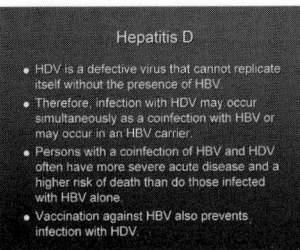

- HDV is the smallest animal virus known.
- What is the incubation period of HDV? (*It is 2 to 12 weeks.*)

Slide 49

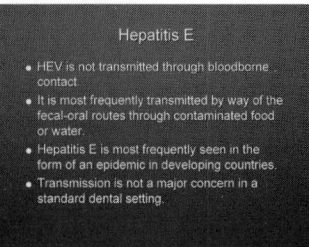

- HEV outbreaks are common in Africa, Asia, and Latin America.
- HEV does not pose a major risk of cross-contamination in dentistry.

Slide 50

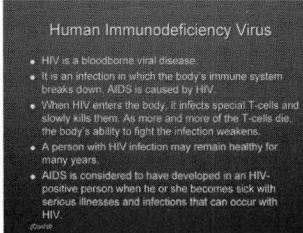

- T-cells are responsible for supporting immunity.
- HIV is spread via sexual contact with an infected person and by needle sharing among drug users.
- Before blood donor screening, HIV was transmitted during transfusions via infected blood products.
- HIV is destroyed easily by heat from an autoclave or hot-air oven.
- The virus can survive for 15 days at room temperature and at body temperature.
- Disinfectants, including 2% glutaraldehyde and hypochlorite, are effective in killing HIV on surfaces within a few minutes.

Slide 51

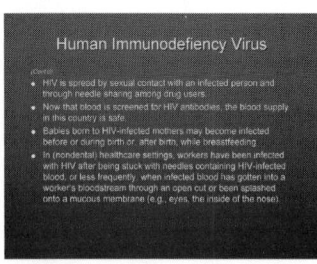

- The virus can enter the body through the lining of the vagina, vulva, penis, rectum, or mouth.
- The virus can also be transmitted through infected blood or other body fluids such as breast milk.
- Is saliva considered a body fluid which can transport HIV?
- What are the early orofacial manifestations of HIV infection?

Slide 52

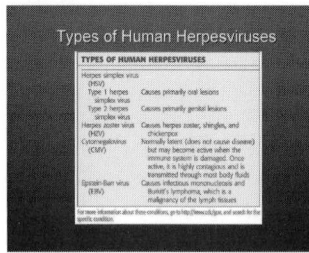

- The herpes virus is a double-stranded DNA virus that causes infections in humans.
- What are some common herpes infections?
- The virus may stay dormant for years and then become activated and cause disease.
- There are two types of herpes simplex virus. What are their names?
- Disease due to HSV are either primary infection due to first encounter with the virus, or a reactive or recurrent infection due to activation of the latent virus.
- Primary infections have an incubation period of 2 to 20 days.

ELSEVIER

Torres and Ehrlich Modern Dental Assisting, 9th ed.

Bird/Robinson

Slide 53

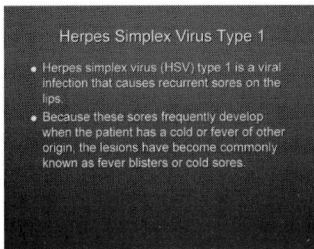

- Type I Herpes Simplex primarily causes oral lesions.

- Primary infectious lesions, called primary gingivostomatitis, are located on the lips and mouth.

Slide 54

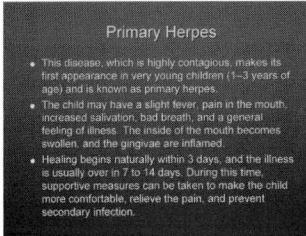

- What are some supportive measures to take when a patient is infected with primary herpes? (*Over-the-counter pain medication can be given to the child. Elimination of cross-contamination among family members should also be discussed: hand washing, no sharing of contaminated cups or utensils, etc.*)

Slide 55

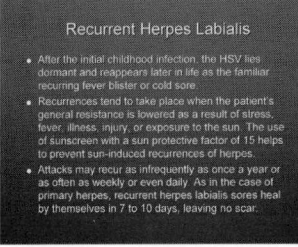

- About one-third of patients who have had primary infection develop herpes labialis in later life as a result of reactivation of the latent virus.

- Lesions develop at the mucocutaneous junction of the lip or on the skin adjacent to the nostrils.

Slide 56

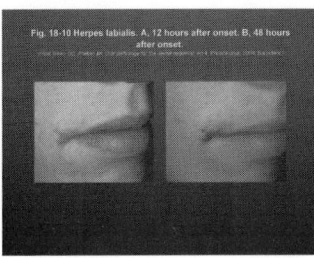

- Characteristically the lesions are preceded by some 24 hours by signs of itching, prickling, or a burning sensation.

- Blisters then develop, enlarge, coalesce, rupture, become encrusted and heal within 10 to 14 days.

- Intraoral recurrent herpetic infections are infrequent. If they occur, they usually involve the hard palate, alveolar ridges, and gingiva.

Bird/Robinson

Slide 57

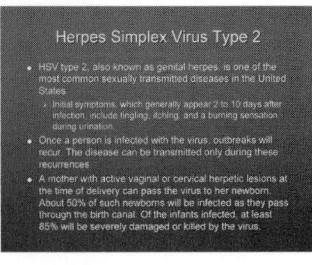

- The lesions are vesicular and painful.
- Additional herpes type viruses include:
    - Herpes zoster virus (HSV type 3): causes both varicella (chicken pox) and herpes zoster, also known as shingles.
    - Cytomegalovirus (CMV) (HSV type 5): rarely causes disease unless there are such factors present as a compromised immune system.
    - Epstein-Barr virus (HSV type 4): causes infectious mononucleosis, nasopharyngeal cancer, lymphoma, and oral hairy leukoplakia.

Slide 58

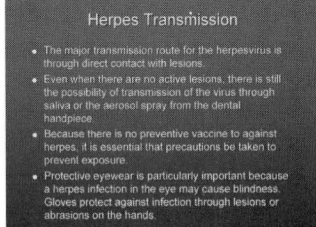

- The primary lesion is associated with fever and is more painful then the secondary lesions.
- Why would asymptomatic secondary lesions pose an increased danger? (*The spread of secondary lesions is more common because the person may be unaware that a breakout is occurring.*)

Slide 59

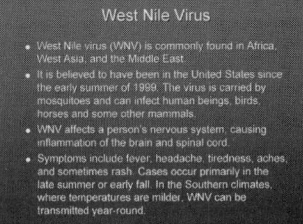

- Symptoms can last for as little as a few days, though even healthy people have been sick for several weeks.
- Approximately 80% of people (about 4 out of 5) who are infected with WNV will not show any symptoms at all.
- WNV is not spread through casual contact.
- People typically develop symptoms between 3 and 14 days after they are bitten by the infected mosquito.
- People over the age of 50 are more likely to develop serious symptoms of WNV if they do get sick, and should take special care to avoid mosquito bites.

Slide 60

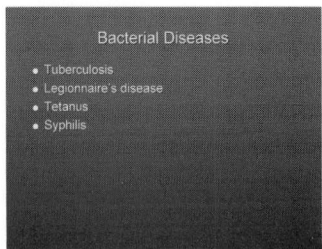

- Diseases caused by bacteria are also of concern for dental care workers.
- Bacterial diseases include: tuberculosis, Legionnaires' disease, tetanus, and syphilis.
- Bacterial diseases are also categorized as communicable diseases.

Slide 61

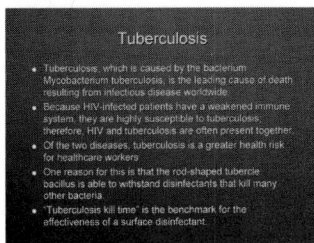

- What are the oral manifestations of tuberculosis? (*Oral lesions are usually secondary to primary infections commonly seen in the lungs. Oral lesions include: oral ulceration, tuberculous lymphadenitis, and periapical granuloma.*)

Slide 62

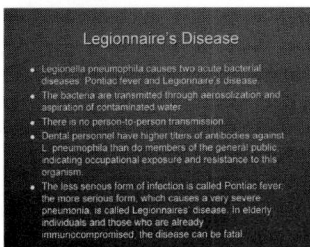

- Legionnaires' disease is also more commonly seen in heavy, middle-aged smokers.

Slide 63

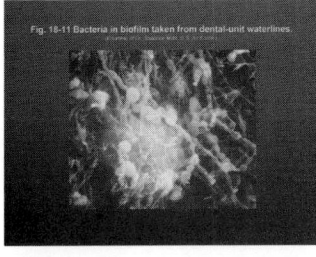

- The *L. pneumophilia* bacteria has been found to thrive in lakes, creeks, hot tubs, spas, air-conditioning systems, shower heads, water distillation systems, and the biofilm found in dental unit waterlines.
- Do you think that dental personnel are at greater risk of contracting a disease caused by the *L. pneumophilia* bacteria?

Slide 64

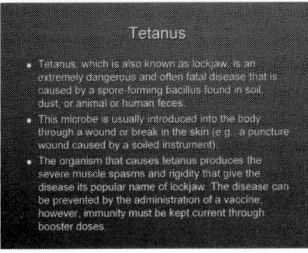

- What is the best way to protect yourself against contracting tetanus? (*Immunization with the vaccine tetanus toxoid, which is a component of the DTP vaccine, with follow-up boosters every 10 years.*)

Slide 65

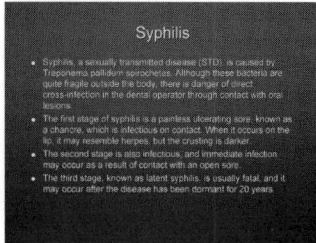

- An additional phase which falls between the second and third stage is called tertiary syphilis.

  - This phase occurs 3 to 10 years after the onset of primary syphilis.

  - Lesions appear as granulomatous nodules of the skin, mucosa, bone and internal organs.

  - This phase of the disease is very destructive.

Slide 66

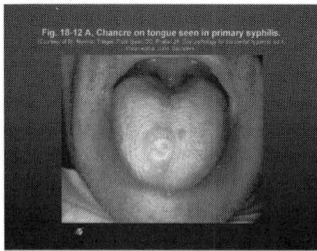

- The painless, ulcerated sore is also called a chancre.

- This lesion is very infectious on contact.

- Common oral sites include lips and tongue. Lesions forming on the gingiva and tonsillar area are not as common.

- The lesions usually heal 5 weeks after they first appear.

- Regional lymph nodes will also be enlarged.

Slide 67

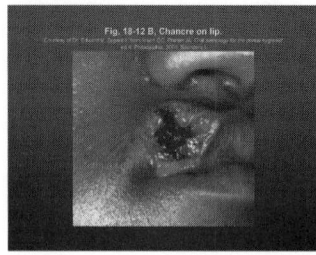

- This primary lesion resembles herpes when it is on the lip; however, the crusting is usually darker.

TEACHING FOCUS

This chapter gives students an opportunity to learn how to recognize the methods of disease transmission and to break the chain of infection that puts both the patients and dental team at risk. In addition, students will have the opportunity to learn how the immune system provides the body with resistance to infection and what to do in the event of exposure. CDC and OSHA standards and guidelines that minimize the risks of exposure and disease transmission will also be discussed.

MATERIALS AND RESOURCES

- ☐ adhesive bandage (Lesson 19.1)
- ☐ alcohol-based hand rub (Lesson 19.2)
- ☐ antiseptic cream or ointment (Lesson 19.1)
- ☐ chemical-resistant utility gloves (Lesson 19.3)
- ☐ disinfectant solution (Lesson 19.3)
- ☐ exposure incident report form (Lesson 19.1)
- ☐ computer and PowerPoint projector (all Lessons)

- ☐ gloves (Lesson 19.2)
- ☐ liquid soap in a dispenser (Lesson 19.2)
- ☐ nailbrush or orange stick (Lesson 19.2)
- ☐ paper towels (Lessons 19.1 and 19.2)
- ☐ protective clothing (Lessons 19.2 and 19.3)
- ☐ protective eyewear (Lessons 19.2 and 19.3)
- ☐ sink with running water (Lesson 19.2)
- ☐ soap and water (Lesson 19.1)
- ☐ surgical mask (Lessons 19.2 and 19.3)

LESSON CHECKLIST

Preparations for this lesson include:

- lecture
- evaluation of student knowledge and skills needed to perform all entry-level activities related to disease transmission and infection control, including:
  - ○ recognizing different infections and how they are spread
  - ○ natural and artificial immunities
  - ○ Universal and Standard Precautions
  - ○ CDC guidelines concerning infection control
  - ○ first-aid procedures in the event of exposure
  - ○ standard infection-control practices

ELSEVIER

Torres and Ehrlich Modern Dental Assisting, 9th ed.

Bird/Robinson

KEY TERMS

acquired immunity (p. 269)
acute infection (p. 267)
anaphylaxis (p. 291)
artificially acquired immunity (p. 270)
bloodborne disease (p. 270)
bloodborne pathogens (p. 267)
chain of infection (p. 266)
chronic infection (p. 267)
communicable disease (p. 269)
contaminated waste (p. 292)
direct contact (p. 270)
droplet infection (p. 270)
epidemiologic studies (p. 271)
hazardous waste (p. 292)
immunity (p. 269)
indirect contact (p. 270)

infectious disease (p. 267)
infectious waste (p. 292)
inherited immunity (p. 269)
latent infection (p. 267)
naturally acquired immunity (p. 269)
occupational exposure (p. 273)
OSHA Bloodborne Pathogens (BBP) Standard (p. 266)
pathogen (p. 267)
percutaneous (p. 273)
permucosal (p. 273)
personal protective equipment (PPE) (p. 279)
sharps (p. 274)
standard precautions (p. 272)
universal precautions (p. 272)
virulence (p. 266)

ADDITIONAL RESOURCES

PowerPoint slides (Evolve): 1-98
Multimedia Procedures DVD: Handwashing Techniques

Legend

CTQ
Critical
Thinking
Question

DVD
Multimedia
Procedures
Videos and
Animations

ESLR
EVOLVE
Student
Learning
Resources

IDO
Interactive
Dental
Office
CD-ROM

SW
Student
Workbook

TB
Test Bank
on the
TEACH
CD-ROM

PPT
PowerPoint
Slides

Class Activities are indicated in ***bold italic.***

ELSEVIER

Torres and Ehrlich Modern Dental Assisting, 9th ed.
Bird/Robinson

LESSON 19.1

PRETEST

1. The link in the chain of infection that refers to the strength of the organism is
   a. portal of entry.
   c. number of microorganisms.
   b. susceptible host.
   d. virulence.

2. A patient who had chickenpox as a child is now suffering from shingles (herpes zoster). This is an example of what type of infection?
   a. acute
   c. chronic
   b. latent
   d. opportunistic

3. Using moisturizers to maintain healthy skin helps to prevent which type of disease transmission?
   a. fecal-oral transmission
   c. splash or splatter
   b. airborne transmission
   d. chronic transmission

4. Aerosolized saliva, blood, or microorganisms created by use of the high-speed hand piece, air water syringe, and ultrasonic scaler can contribute to which mode of disease transmission?
   a. blood borne transmission
   c. airborne transmission
   b. indirect transmission
   d. fecal-oral transmission

5. Which type of immunity is present at birth?
   a. naturally acquired immunity
   c. passive immunity
   b. artificially acquired immunity
   d. inherited immunity

6. Leaving the dental office wearing contaminated attire and then hugging another person is an example of what type of disease transmission?
   a. dental team to patient
   c. patient to dental team
   b. dental office to community
   d. patient to patient

7. OSHA requires that every dental office and clinic protect its employees from potentially infectious material. The source for guidelines is
   a. OSHA's bloodborne pathogens (BBP) standard.
   b. the building's fire and emergency plan.
   c. material safety data sheets (MSDS).
   d. drug inserts for medications used in the office.

8. Areas of the hand that are frequently missed when washing with antimicrobial soap and water are the
   a. palm and wrist.
   c. tips of fingers and tip of thumb.
   b. knuckles and fingers.
   d. thumb and in between fingers.

9. Waterless antiseptic products that contain alcohol are most effective at what concentration?
   a. 10%-30%
   c. 60%-95%
   b. 30%-60%
   d. 95%-100%

10. In what order should personal protective equipment be put on?
    a. protective clothing, mask, protective eyewear, wash and dry hands, put on gloves
    b. wash and dry hands, put on gloves, protective clothing, protective eyewear, mask
    c. protective clothing, wash and dry hands, put on gloves, mask, protective eyewear
    d. protective eyewear, mask, wash and dry hands, put on gloves, protective clothing

Answers

| 1. d | 3. c | 5. d | 7. a | 9. c |
| 2. b | 4. c | 6. b | 8. d | 10. a |

ELSEVIER

Torres and Ehrlich Modern Dental Assisting, 9th ed.

Bird/Robinson

BACKGROUND ASSESSMENT

Question: What are overgloves, and when are they used in the dental office?

Answer: Overgloves, also known as "food handler gloves," are made of lightweight, clear plastic and are worn over contaminated treatment gloves to prevent clean objects that are handled during treatment from becoming contaminated.

Question: How can cross-contamination be eliminated when wearing treatment gloves?

Answer: To eliminate cross-contamination when wearing treatment gloves, set up the required instruments and materials ahead of time and use overgloves when it is necessary to touch a surface. Use overgloves in the operatory to open cabinets, pull out drawers, and obtain any unanticipated items. Use a paper towel or gauze to open containers with lids or caps. Always remove gloves and wash hands when leaving the treatment area/operatory. When you return to treatment area/operatory, wash and dry hands before regloving with fresh gloves. Change gloves if they become damaged, torn, ripped, or punctured. Never wash or use disinfectant on gloves because the latex barrier is broken down and no longer protects. Change gloves frequently. If a procedure is long, change gloves about once each hour.

CRITICAL THINKING QUESTION

A patient tells the dental assistant that she has not been to a dentist in over 10 years because she is afraid of contracting the AIDS virus. How should the dental assistant respond?

Guidelines: The best way to reduce anxiety and fear is to educate the patient about methods of infection control. Measures to prevent contraction from dental staff are the use of masks and gloves, hand washing, and immunizations. Control measures to prevent patient-to-patient contraction include surface barriers, hand washing, gloves, and use of sterile instruments. The dental assistant should ask the patient if she has any specific questions that can be addressed to help reduce her anxiety. Then, once her specific concerns have been discovered, her apprehension can be relieved by explaining the four links in the chain of infection: virulence, the number of microorganisms, a susceptible host, and a portal of entry. When any link in the chain of infection is broken, the infectious process is also broken. The dental assistant should also demonstrate an extensive knowledge of infection-control practices in order to earn the patient's trust and confidence.

OBJECTIVES	CONTENT	TEACHING RESOURCES
Prounounce, define, and spell the Key Terms.	■ Key terms (p. 265)	📘 SW Fill in the Blank questions 1-22 (p. 77) 💿 ESLR Electronic Flashcards ▶ Discuss each of the key terms in Chapter 19, focusing on the definition, pronunciation, and spelling of each term. *Class Activity Go around the room and have each student use one of the key terms in a clinically relevant sentence in order to define the term. Continue until all terms have been used; if students become stuck, have the rest of the class offer suggestions.*
Identify links in the chain of infection.	■ The chain of infection (p. 266) ☐ Virulence (p. 266) ☐ Number of microorganisms (p. 266) ☐ Susceptible host (p. 267) ☐ Portal of entry (p. 267)	🖥 PPT 5-11 🖥 TB questions 1-2 📘 SW Short-Answer Questions 1, 6 (p. 75) CDC: Overview of the CDC Infection-Control Recommendations for Dentistry (p. 266) Figure 19-1 At least one part must be removed to break the chain of infection (p. 267) ▶ Discuss the life cycle of pathogens. How can the body defend itself against infection?

Bird/Robinson

OBJECTIVES	CONTENT	TEACHING RESOURCES
		▶ Discuss Figure 19-1 (p. 267) and identify several ways to break the chain of infection. ▶ Discuss the role of government agencies in protecting dental assistants from occupational health hazards. ***Class Activity** Divide the class into groups. Have each group use the first letter of each link in the chain of infection to develop an acronym or other mnemonic device the help them remember the terms. Have each group share its device with the class.*
Describe the differences between a chronic infection and an acute infection.	■ Types of infections (p. 267) □ Acute infection (p. 267) □ Chronic infection (p. 267)	⊠ PPT 12 TB question 3 ▶ Discuss the differences between chronic and acute infections. ▶ Discuss what it means to be asymptomatic. ***Class Activity** Divide the class into groups. Have each group discuss the differences between chronic and acute infections and identify five chronic infections and five acute infections. Have groups share their findings with the class for discussion.*
Give an example of a latent infection.	□ Latent infection (p. 267) □ Opportunistic infection (p. 267)	⊠ PPT 12 SW Short-Answer Questions 3, 5 (p. 75) ▶ Discuss some examples of a latent infection. What conditions might cause a latent infection to surface? ▶ Discuss which groups of people might be particularly susceptible to opportunistic infections. ***Class Activity** Divide the class into groups, and have each group identify three examples of a latent infection. Have each group share its findings with the class, then have students brainstorm conditions that could cause the different infections to surface. Record student responses on the board for comparison.*
Describe the methods of disease transmission in a dental office.	■ Modes of disease transmission (p. 267) □ Direct transmission (p. 268) □ Indirect transmission (p. 268) □ Airborne transmission (p. 268) □ Aerosol, spray or spatter (p. 268)	⊠ PPT 13-16 TB questions 4-7 SW Short-Answer Questions 7 (p. 75) Primary Modes of Disease Transmission in Dentistry (p. 268) Figure 19-2 Pathogens can be transferred from staff to patient, patient to staff, and patient to patient from contaminated equipment (p. 267) ▶ Discuss how communicable diseases spread. What common bloodborne diseases are of particular concern in dentistry?

ELSEVIER

OBJECTIVES	CONTENT	TEACHING RESOURCES
	☐ Parenteral transmission (p. 268)	▶ Discuss the four primary ways infectious diseases are spread in dentistry.
	☐ Bloodborne transmission (p. 268)	*Class Activity Divide the class into groups, and assign each group one of the following modes of disease transmission: direct, indirect, splash or spatter, airborne, parenteral, bloodborne, food and water, fecal-oral. Have each group identify two ways that disease is spread via its assigned mode of transmission in a dental office and explain four ways that infection can be prevented. Have each group share its findings with the class for discussion.*
	☐ Food and water transmission (p. 269)	
	☐ Fecal-oral transmission (p. 269)	
Describe the types of immunity, and give examples of each.	■ The immune system (p. 269)	⊠ PPT 17-19
	☐ Naturally acquired immunity (p. 269)	TB questions 8-9
		SW Short-Answer Questions 4 (p. 75)
	☐ Artificially acquired Immunity (p. 270)	Figure 19-3 Acquired immunity (p. 269)
		Primary Modes of Disease Transmission in Dentistry: Immunizations Strongly Recommended for Healthcare Personnel (p. 268)
		▶ Discuss the differences between artificial and natural immunity. What are some examples of active and passive immunities?
		▶ Discuss which immunizations are strongly recommended for health care personnel.
		Class Activity Divide the class into groups. Have each group create a time line that outlines when the immunizations recommended for dental assistants should be administered and how often. Have groups share their timelines with the class for discussion.
Describe the methods of disease transmission in a dental office.	■ Disease transmission in the dental office (p. 270)	⊠ PPT 20-25
	☐ Patient to dental team (p. 270)	TB questions 10-11
		SW Short-Answer Questions 7; Multiple Choice questions 1-3 (pp. 75, 78)
	☐ Dental team to patient (p. 270)	Recall questions 1-3 (p. 271)
	☐ Patient to patient (p. 270)	▶ Discuss the methods of disease transmission in the dental office and compare and contrast each.
	☐ Dental office to community (p. 271)	*Class Activity Divide the class into groups, and assign each group one of the following methods of disease transmission in the dental office: patient to dental team, dental team to patient, patient to patient, dental office to community, community to dental office to patient. Have each group identify three ways in which disease could be spread via its assigned method of transmission and outline strategies for preventing disease transmission. Have each group present its findings to the class.*
	☐ Community to dental office to patient (p. 271)	

OBJECTIVES	CONTENT	TEACHING RESOURCES
Describe the roles of the CDC and OSHA in infection control.	■ Roles and responsibilities of the CDC and OSHA in infection control (p. 271) ■ Guidelines for infection control in dental health-care settings (p. 271)	▢▤ PPT 26-28 ▣ TB questions 12-14 📖 SW Short-Answer Questions 8; Multiple Choice question 7 (pp. 75, 78) CDC: Rankings of Evidence (p. 271) CDC: Overview of CDC Guidelines for Infection Control in Dental Health-Care Settings—2003 (p. 272) ♀ CTQ 1 (p. 297) ▸ Discuss the differences between OSHA's responsibilities and those of the CDC. ***Class Activity** Draw a Venn diagram on the board and label one side CDC Guidelines for Infection Control and the other OSHA Guidelines. Have students compare and contrast the two agencies' guidelines and ask student volunteers to fill in the diagram on the board.*

Describe the components of an OSHA Exposure Control plan.	■ OSHA bloodborne pathogens standard (p. 272)
	
	☐ Exposure-control plan (p. 272)
		▢▤ PPT 29
		
		▣ TB questions 15-16
		
		📖 SW Short-Answer Questions 8; Multiple Choice questions 4-5 (pp. 75, 78)
		
		Written Exposure-Control Plan Required by OSHA (p. 270)
		
		Recall questions 4-5 (p. 275)
		
		♀ CTQ 4 (p. 297)
		
		▸ Discuss the components of OSHA's Exposure-Control Plan. Why is this the most important infection-control law in dentistry?
		
		▸ Discuss the types of facilities required to implement OSHA's Exposure-Control plan.
		
		***Class Activity** Have students contact a local dental office to examine its exposure-control plan. Then have students outline how the plan addresses each of the following components and share their findings with the class:*
		
		   1. The use of universal precautions.
		
		   2. Required use of personal protective equipment.
		
		   3. Standardized housekeeping.
		
		   4. Laundering of contaminated protective clothing.
		
		   5. Standardized policy on cleaning and disinfection.
		
		   6. Policy on general waste disposal.

ELSEVIER

Torres and Ehrlich Modern Dental Assisting, 9th ed.

Bird/Robinson

OBJECTIVES	CONTENT	TEACHING RESOURCES
		7. Labeling procedure (secondary labeling).
		8. Policy on sterilization (including monitoring) and disinfection.
		9. Use of sharps containers and disposal system.
		10. Standardized hand washing protocol.
		11. HBV vaccination.
		12. Post-exposure evaluation and medical follow-up.
		(For students to prepare for this activity, see Homework/Assignments #1.)
Explain the difference between Universal Precautions and Standard Precautions.	☐ Standard and universal precautions (p. 272)	PPT 30 TB questions 17-18 SW Short-Answer Questions 2, 9; Multiple Choice question 6 (pp. 75, 78) ▸ Discuss why all human blood and body fluids should be treated as if they were contaminated. ▸ Discuss the differences between universal and standard precautions as they apply to dentistry. *Class Activity Divide the class into groups, and present students with the following questions to discuss:* *1. Which organization uses the term Universal Precautions?* *2. Which organization uses the term Standard Precautions?* *3. What are the differences between universal precautions and standard precautions?* *4. Which of the precautions applies to contact with blood?* *Have groups share their findings with the class and record student responses on the board for comparison.*
Explain the rationale for standard precautions.	☐ Standard and universal precautions (p. 272)	SW Short-Answer Questions 9; Multiple Choice question 6 (pp. 75, 78) CDC: Standard Precautions (p. 272) Recall question 6 (p. 275) ▸ Discuss the standard precautions that should be used in treatment of all patients. ▸ Discuss how standard precautions expanded upon the elements of universal precautions. What additional infectious materials are included in the standard precautions, and why is this important to dentistry?

Bird/Robinson

OBJECTIVES	CONTENT	TEACHING RESOURCES
		Class Activity Pose the following questions to the class and ask students to discuss their responses: *1. Are the standard precautions developed to protect patients or healthcare providers?* *2. What is the population in question 1 being protected against?* *3. What would happen if there were no standard precautions?*
Identify the OSHA categories of risk for occupational exposure.	☐ Categories of employees (p. 273)	PPT 31 TB question 19 SW Short-Answer Questions 10 (p. 75) Table 19-1 Occupational Exposure Determination (p. 273) ▸ Discuss Table 19-1 (p. 273). Why would an office manager or receptionist be considered part of Category II? *Class Activity Lead a class discussion about the OSHA categories of risk for occupational exposure. Ask students to identify the employees included in each category and to discuss the risks associated with each category. Are there any risks involved with Category III employees? Record student responses on the board for comparison.*
Describe the first aid necessary after an exposure incident.	☐ Postexposure management (p. 273) Procedure 19-1 First aid after an exposure incident (p. 274) (SW/ESLR Competency 19-1, p. 81) ☐ Employee training (p. 273)	PPT 32-33 TB question 20 SW Short-Answer Questions 11 (p. 75) SW/ESLR Competency 19-1 Applying First Aid After an Exposure Incident (p. 81) Management of an Exposure Incident (p. 273) OSHA Bloodborne Pathogens Standard Training Requirements (p. 273) Standard HBV Informed Refusal (p. 274) Recall question 7 (p. 275) ▸ Discuss what should be included in an employee's record concerning exposure-control training. ▸ Discuss what equipment should be on hand to ensure appropriate first aid after an exposure incident. *Class Activity Divide the class into groups. Have each group create a time line that outlines the first aid that should be performed after an exposure incident. Have each group present its timeline to the class.*

ELSEVIER

Torres and Ehrlich Modern Dental Assisting, 9th ed.

Bird/Robinson

OBJECTIVES	CONTENT	TEACHING RESOURCES
Discuss the rationale for hepatitis B vaccination for dental assistants.	☐ Hepatitis B immunization (p. 273) – Need for a booster (p. 274) ☐ Employee medical records (p. 274)	⊠▤ PPT 34-38 📖 TB questions 21-22 📑 SW Short-Answer Questions 12; Multiple Choice question 10 (pp. 75, 78) Follow-up Measures for Exposed Worker (p. 272) CDC: Postvaccine Testing (p. 274) Recall question 8 (p. 275) 💡 CTQ 4 (p. 297) ▸ Discuss OSHA's BBP standard training requirements. ▸ Discuss the BBP standard requiring employers to offer the hepatitis B vaccine. What happens if an employee declines the vaccine? ▸ Discuss the exceptions that would require an employee to receive an HBV booster. *Class Activity **Lead a class discussion about hepatitis B vaccinations for dental assistants and ask students to explain why HBV boosters are optional, not mandatory, for dental staff. Why might an employee decline the vaccination? What are the risks of not receiving the vaccination? How is hepatitis B transmitted? Record student responses on the board for comparison.***
Describe the proper handling and disposal methods for each type of waste generated in dentistry.	☐ Managing contaminated sharps (p. 274) – Preventing needlesticks (p. 275)	⊠▤ PPT 39-41 CDC: Guidelines for Needles (p. 275) Requirements for Employee Medical Records (p. 275) Figure 19-4 A puncture-resistant sharps-disposal container (p. 275) Figure 19-5 OneShot safety syringe (p. 275) Figure 19-6 ProTector disposable needle guard (p. 275) ▸ Discuss the proper way to dispose of contaminated sharps. ▸ Discuss safety devices available to prevent needlesticks. *Class Activity **Divide the class into groups. Have each group outline the precautions that should be taken when handling and disposing of sharps in a dental office. What should be done if a needlestick occurs? Have groups share and discuss their findings with the class.***

Torres and Ehrlich Modern Dental Assisting, 9th ed.

Bird/Robinson

19.1 Homework/Assignments:

1. Have students contact a local dental office to examine its exposure-control plan. Then have students outline how the plan addresses each of the following components and share their findings with the class: pick up list from p. 7.

19.1 Instructor's Notes/Student Feedback:

CRITICAL THINKING QUESTION

On the first day of work a dental assistant observes the following: (1) An assistant leaves the operatory with contaminated gloves, goes to the lab room, and then returns with contaminated gloves to restock sterile 2 x 2 gauze. (2) An assistant who has worked in the office for 20 years takes an impression on a patient and does not disinfect the impression before pouring up with plaster and sending it to the laboratory. (3) During a procedure, the dentist asks the new dental assistant to write in the patient's chart and the dental assistant notices that there are no overgloves. How should the dental assistant handle this situation?

Guidelines: The dental assistant should begin by exploring what OSHA education/training has been completed or offered to staff members; perhaps the staff needs to relearn infection-control procedures. It is important to make suggestions in small steps and to support concerns with facts. Using current OSHA information can be helpful when discussing breaks in the chain of infection control. It is also important to suspend judgment when approaching the dentist or staff members and to always follow proper infection-control procedures, which can provide an example for others to follow. The dental assistant could also provide suggestions for the specific breaks in the chain of infection, such as pointing out that gloves should always be removed upon leaving the operatory, and hands should be washed and a new pair of gloves put on upon returning to the operatory. Sterile gauze and other items should only be restocked using either uncontaminated gloves or overgloves. The dental assistant who made this mistake may not understand that she has cross-contaminated the sterile gauze by handling it with contaminated gloves. The new dental assistant should remind her that gloves are worn for the team's safety, as well as the patients' protection. The assistant who failed to disinfect the impression before pouring the plaster may have learned the procedure for taking impressions before the CDC established guidelines for dental laboratories. The new dental assistant should point out the guidelines set forth by the CDC and explain the steps involved in disinfecting impressions. Finally, overgloves are inexpensive and essential to have in every dental office because they prevent clean objects such as a pen or pencil from becoming contaminated by exam gloves. If overgloves are not available, another less effective option is to use a piece of paper toweling or tissue to hold the pen. The dentist should be approached gently and respectfully when informing him or her of concerns with the breaks in the chain of infection control.

OBJECTIVES	CONTENT	TEACHING RESOURCES
Explain the importance of hand care for dental assistants.	■ Infection-control practices (p. 275)	SW Short-Answer Questions 13 (p. 75) ▸ Discuss why it is necessary to use liquid soap in handwashing. ▸ Discuss how faucets and sinks can be modified to minimize cross-contamination. *Class Activity Divide the class into pairs, and have students inspect their partner's hands and respond to the following questions:* *1. Is the skin healthy and able to withstand the damaging effects of repeated washing and wearing of gloves, or is the skin dry?* *2. Is there any evidence of a latex allergy or contact dermatitis?* *3. Does the person use hand lotions or creams to minimize the occurrence of irritant dermatitis associated with hand antisepsis or hand washing?*

Torres and Ehrlich Modern Dental Assisting, 9th ed.

Bird/Robinson

OBJECTIVES	CONTENT	TEACHING RESOURCES
		4. Does the person wear artificial fingernails or extenders? *5. Is the natural tip less than one-fourth inch long?* *6. Does the person wear any rings?* *7. Are the cuticles rough or smooth?* *8. Are the fingernails free of nail polish?* ***Then have students share their findings with the class, discuss any areas of concern, and identify ways to improve their hand care and promote hand health.***
Explain proper hand hygiene for dental assistants.	☐ Hand hygiene (p. 275) – Handwashing guidelines (p. 275)	🖳 PPT 44-46 📽 Multimedia Procedures DVD: Handwashing Techniques 📖 TB questions 11, 23 📑 SW Short-Answer Questions 14 (p. 75) Figure 19-7 Areas of the hand not thoroughly washed because of poor hand-washing technique (p. 277) Figure 19-8 Sensing device automatically turns the water on and off with hands-free operation (p. 279) CDC: Hand Hygiene in Dental Health-Care Settings (p. 278) Recall questions 9-10 (p. 279) ▸ Discuss the procedure for thorough hand washing. ▸ Discuss general recommendations for hand hygiene in dentistry. Why are jewelry and long fingernails discouraged in dental offices? **Class Activity** *Divide the class into pairs, and have students use lotion or soap to practice proper hand-washing technique. How can students ensure that they will wash the commonly missed areas of the hands? Have students develop a hand-washing system to share with the class.*

Explain the advantages of alcohol-based hand rubs.	– Alcohol based hand rubs (p. 277)
	
	  – Hand care recommendations (p. 278)
	
	  Procedure 19-2 Handwashing before gloving (pp. 276-277) (SW/ESLR Competency 19-2, p. 83)
		🖳 PPT 47-49
		
		📖 TB question 24
		
		📑 SW Short-Answer Questions 15 (p. 76)
		
		📑 SW/ESLR Competency 19-2 Handwashing Before Gloving (p. 83)
		
		📑 SW/ESLR Competency 19-3 Applying an Alcohol-Based Hand Rub (p. 85)

OBJECTIVES	CONTENT	TEACHING RESOURCES
	Procedure 19-3 Applying alcohol-based hand rubs (pp. 280-281) (SW/ESLR Competency 19-3, p. 85)	Figure 19-9 Alcohol-based hand rub agents (p. 279) CDC: Special Considerations for Hand Hygiene (p. 281) CDC: Hand-Care Products (p. 281) ▶ Discuss how alcohol-based hand rubs compare to liquid hand soap. When would liquid hand soap be preferable to a waterless hand rub? ▶ Discuss the benefit of using alcohol-based hand rubs. *Class Activity Lead a class discussion about proper hand-washing technique. Ask students to compare and contrast the procedure for using liquid hand soap and alcohol-based hand rubs and explain the advantages and disadvantages of each. Record student responses on the board.*
Discuss the types of PPE needed for dental assistants.	☐ Personal protective equipment (p. 279) ☐ Protective clothing (p. 281) – Protective clothing requirements (p. 283) – Handling contaminated laundry (p. 283) ☐ Protective masks (p. 284)	PPT 50-55 TB question 26 SW Short-Answer Questions 16; Multiple Choice questions 12-13 (pp. 76, 78) SW Case Study questions 1-4 (p. 79) Recall questions 11-12 (p. 287) Figure 19-10 Water-based hand products will not break down latex (p. 279) Guidelines for the Use of Protective Clothing (p. 284) Figure 19-11 Appropriate clinical attire (p. 279) Figure 19-12 Depending on the task, the dental assistant's attire might be scrubs, lab coats, or surgical gowns (p. 285) Figure 19-13 Containers of contaminated laundry must be labeled with the universal biohazard symbol (p. 285) Figure 19-14 Fluid-impervious gown (p. 285) Figure 19-15 Dome-style face mask (p. 285) ▶ Discuss some examples of personal protective clothing. When must PPE be worn? Name some lower risk and higher risk situations when the PPE might vary. *Class Activity Divide the class into groups. Have each group list the different types of personal protective equipment and describe the indications for the use of each. Have groups share and discuss their findings with the class.*

OBJECTIVES	CONTENT	TEACHING RESOURCES

Demonstrate the proper sequence for donning and removing personal protective equipment.	Procedure 19-4 Putting on personal protective equipment (p. 282) (SW/ESLR Competency 19-4, p. 87)
	
	Procedure 19-5 Removing personal protective equipment (pp. 283-284) (SW/ESLR Competency 19-5, pp. 89-90)
		TB question 27
		
		SW Short-Answer Questions 17 (p. 76)
		
		SW/ESLR Competency 19-4 Putting on Personal Protective Equipment (p. 87)
		
		SW/ESLR Competency 19-5 Removing Personal Protective Equipment (pp. 89-90)
		
		▸ Discuss which order you should put on PPE and why. What item is probably changed more often than others?
		
		▸ Discuss the proper way to remove gloves.
		
		Class Activity Have personal protective equipment available for students, including protective clothing (scrubs, lab coats, and surgical gowns), surgical masks, face shields, protective eyewear, disposable patient-treatment gloves, and heavy-duty utility gloves. Present the following circumstances to the class and ask student volunteers to don the appropriate PPE for each in the proper order:
		
		  – ***Chair-side assisting a dentist in the removal of a deficient amalgam and the placement of a dental composite.***
		
		  – ***Assisting with high speed suction for the dental hygienist as he performs an air polishing procedure to remove tobacco stains.***
		
		  – ***Assisting the oral surgeon during a surgical extraction of an impacted wisdom tooth.***
		
		  – ***A "lunch-and-learn" in the staff lounge for which a dental supplier has brought in sandwiches to eat while he discusses new dental products.***

Discuss the types of PPE needed for dental assistants.	☐ Protective eyewear (p. 285)
	
	  – Face shields (p. 286)
	
	  – Patient eyewear (p. 286)
		PPT 56-60
		
		TB question 28
		
		SW Multiple Choice question 14 (p. 78)
		
		Guidelines for the Use of Protective Masks (p. 286)
		
		Figure 19-16 Safety goggles with protective side shields (p. 286)
		
		Figure 19-17 (A) Facemask and safety glasses; (B) Facemask and disposable face shield (p. 286)
		
		Recall question 13 (p. 287)
		
		Figure 19-18 A face mask is still required when assisting with aerosol-generating procedures (p. 286)
		
		Figure 19-19 Patients should be provided with protective eyewear (p. 287)

OBJECTIVES	CONTENT	TEACHING RESOURCES
		▸ Discuss why protective eyewear may be necessary for dental assistants. *Class Activity* **Divide the class into groups. Have each group identify the different types of protective eyewear for dental assistants and explain under what circumstances each is used. When should patients wear protective eyewear? Have groups share their findings with the class.**
Identify the various types of gloves used in a dental office.	□ Gloves (p. 287) – Examination gloves (p. 287) – Gloves damaged during treatment (p. 287) – Gloves damaged by dental materials (p. 288) – Overgloves (p. 288) – Sterile surgical gloves (p. 288) – Utility gloves (p. 289) – Non-latex containing gloves (p. 289) □ Maintaining infection control while gloved (p. 289) – Opening drawers and cabinets (p. 289) – Opening containers (p. 289)	PPT 61-73 TB questions 23, 29 SW Short-Answer Questions 18; Multiple Choice questions 15-18 (pp. 76, 78-79) Box 19-1 Types of Gloves in Dentistry (p. 287) CDC: Gloves (p. 287) Figure 19-20 Nonsterile exam gloves (p. 288) Guidelines for the Use of Gloves (p. 288) Guidelines for the Use of Overgloves (p. 288) CDC: Sterile Surgeon's Gloves (p. 289) Figure 19-21 Overglove worn over a latex exam glove (p. 288) Figure 19-22 Utility gloves are used when preparing instruments for sterilization (p. 289) Recall questions 14-17 (pp. 287, 290) CTQ 2 (p. 297) ▸ Discuss the different types of gloves available and when it is appropriate to use each. ▸ Discuss what to do if gloves are damaged during treatment. How else should you maintain infection control while gloved? *Class Activity* **Provide students with different kinds of gloves used in the dental office, including examination gloves, damaged exam gloves, overgloves, sterile surgical gloves, nonlatex gloves, and utility gloves. In groups, have students identify each type of glove and explain—without using their textbooks—when each is used. What should be done with damaged examination gloves, and how can punctures be avoided? Have groups share their findings with the class.**

19.2 Homework/Assignments:

19.2 Instructor's Notes/Student Feedback:

LESSON 19.3

CRITICAL THINKING QUESTION

A dental assistant is responsible for the office's waste management and has been assigned the task of developing a waste-management program. Where should the dental assistant begin, and how should the plan be implemented?

Guidelines: OSHA BBP standards require that all waste be disposed of according to applicable federal, state, and local regulations. The dental assistant should begin by contacting the city's waste-management department to determine specific guidelines for regulated medical waste. From those guidelines, the dental assistant should determine the classifications of office waste and designate and label waste receptacles for each of the following waste categories: general waste, hazardous waste, contaminated waste, infectious or regulated waste (biohazard), blood and blood-soaked materials, pathologic waste, and sharps. The dental assistant should then develop a medical-waste management program and schedule a training session for the entire dental team to discuss the classifications of waste and how contaminated waste products should be handled. The names of those who attend the training session should be documented, and employees should be retrained as needed. Annual changes from city, state, and federal levels should also be reviewed and regularly integrated into the waste-management program.

OBJECTIVES	CONTENT	TEACHING RESOURCES
Explain the types and symptoms of latex reactions.	■ Latex allergies (p. 290) □ Irritant dermatitis (p. 290) □ Type IV allergic reaction (p. 290) □ Type I allergic reaction (p. 291) □ Treatment (p. 291) □ Latex sensitive patients (p. 291)	PPT 76-83 TB question 30 SW Short-Answer Questions 19; Multiple Choice questions 8-9 (pp. 76, 78) Figure 19-23 Latex-free nitrile gloves (p. 289) CDC: CDC Guidelines for Contact Dermatitis and Latex Hypersensitivity (p. 290) Figure 19-24 Irritant dermatitis (p. 290) Care of Patients with Latex Allergies (p. 290) Recall questions 18-21 (p. 291) CTQ 3 (p. 297) ▸ Discuss the different types of allergic reactions to latex gloves. What are their symptoms, and how are they treated? ▸ Discuss the steps that should be taken if an employee is found to have a latex allergy. *Class Activity Lead a class discussion about latex reactions and ask students to differentiate between the signs and symptoms of irritant dermatitis and the different types of allergic reactions. How can these types of reactions be avoided, and how could a dental office achieve a latex-free environment? Record student responses on the board for comparison.*
Describe the proper handling and disposal methods for each	■ Waste management in the dental office (p. 291) □ Classification of	PPT 84-92 TB questions 31-34

OBJECTIVES	CONTENT	TEACHING RESOURCES
type of waste generated in dentistry.	waste (p. 291) – General waste (p. 291) – Contaminated waste (p. 292) – Hazardous waste (p. 292) – Infectious or regulated waste (biohazard) (p. 292) ☐ Handling of extracted teeth (p. 292) ☐ Handling contaminated waste (p. 292) ☐ Handling medical waste (p. 293) – Infectious waste (p. 293) – Disposal of medical waste (p. 293)	SW Short-Answer Questions 20; Multiple Choice questions 19-20 (pp. 76, 79) CDC: CDC Guidelines for Regulated Medical Waste (p. 291) Table 19-2 Classification of Waste (p. 292) CDC: CDC Guidelines for Handling Extracted Teeth (p. 292) Figure 19-25 Waste is separated into clearly marked containers. (p. 293) Recall questions 22-25 (p. 293) ▸ Discuss the CDC Guidelines for Regulated Medical waste and compare the different classifications of waste in Table 19-2 (p. 292). ▸ Discuss how handling contaminated waste is different from other medical waste. *Class Activity **Divide the class into groups, and assign each group one of the following categories of medical waste: general, hazardous, contaminated, or infectious. Have each group outline the types of materials that are included in its assigned waste category and explain how the waste should be handled and disposed. Have groups present their findings to the class for discussion.***
Describe the roles of the CDC and OSHA in infection control.	■ Additional infection-control practices (p. 293) ☐ OSHA Blood-Borne Pathogens Standard (p. 293)	PPT 93 Recall question 26 (p. 296) ▸ Discuss how dental offices are monitored for their compliance with OSHA standards and CDC recommendations for infection control. *Class Activity **Have students research OSHA BBP guidelines for dental offices and prepare a list of five to ten guidelines to share with the class. (For students to prepare for this activity, see Homework/Assignments #1.)***
Explain the CDC recommendations regarding the use of a saliva ejector.	☐ CDC guidelines-special considerations (p. 293) – Saliva ejectors (p. 293)	PPT 94 SW Short-Answer Questions 21 (p. 76) CDC: Saliva Ejector (p. 293) Recall question 27 (p. 296) ▸ Discuss the possible dangers of using saliva ejectors. How should patients be instructed in their use? *Class Activity **Pose the following situation to the class for discussion:***

Torres and Ehrlich Modern Dental Assisting, 9th ed.

Bird/Robinson

OBJECTIVES	CONTENT	TEACHING RESOURCES
		A patient of 10 years comes to the dental office for an exam and periodontal root debridement. As the dental assistant begins to explain the need for a preprocedural mouthrinse as well as the proper technique for removing fluid from the patient's mouth, the patient interrupts and says that she has been closing her lips around the suction for 10 years and that she has never caught a cold. Why should she stop now? *How could the dental assistant educate the patient about the CDC recommendations regarding the use of the saliva ejector?*
Explain the precautions necessary when treating an active tuberculosis patient.	☐ Dental laboratory (p. 293) ☐ Preprocedural mouthrinses (p. 294) Procedure 19-6 Disinfecting an alginate impression (p. 295) (SW/ESLR Competency 19-6, p. 91) ☐ *Mycobacterium tuberculosis* (p. 294)	PPT 95-96 TB question 35 SW Short-Answer Questions 24 (p. 76) SW/ESLR Competency 19-6 Disinfecting an Alginate Impression (p. 91) Figure 19-26 Pouch for lab cases with the biohazard label (p. 294) Figure 19-27 This denture has large amounts of calculus adhering to it (p. 294) Figure 19-28 Impression trays are heat-sterilized in individualized bags (p. 294) CDC: CDC Guidelines for Dental Laboratories (p. 295) CDC: CDC Guidelines for *M. tuberculosis* (p. 296) Recall questions 28-29 (p. 296) ▸ Discuss the scientific evidence surrounding the practice of preprocedural mouthrinses. What are the CDC's guidelines concerning rinsing before procedures? ▸ Discuss how to hand dental prostheses or impressions to minimize cross-contamination. ▸ Discuss how the *M. tuberculosis* bacterium can be spread during a dental treatment. **Class Activity** *Present the following situation to the class for discussion:* *A 42-year-old woman is a new patient and has just completed the medical history form. The form indicates that she was exposed to TB years ago, and that she reacts to tuberculin skin tests (TST). The patient confirms that she has a latent TB infection. After she is seated in the patient chair she begins to cough uncontrollably and she spits out some phlegm with blood in it. How should this situation be handled?*

OBJECTIVES	CONTENT	TEACHING RESOURCES
Describe the rationale of CDC recommendations regarding Creutzfeldt-Jakob disease and other prion-related diseases.	☐ Creutzfeldt-Jakob disease and other prion diseases (p. 295)	⊠▦ PPT 97 ▣ TB question 36 ▨ SW Short-Answer Questions 22 (p. 76) CDC: Creutzfeldt-Jakob Disease (p. 296) ***Class Activity** Have students research the pathophysiology, signs and symptoms, treatments, and CDC recommendations for Creutzfeldt-Jakob disease and other prion-related diseases and present their findings to the class. (For students to prepare for this activity, see Homework/Assignments #2.)*
Describe the rationale of CDC recommendations regarding laser plumes.	■ Laser/electrosurgery plumes or surgical smoke (p. 296)	⊠▦ PPT 98 ▨ SW Short-Answer Questions 23 (p. 76) CDC: Laser/Electrosurgery Plumes/Surgical Smoke (p. 296) Recall question 30 (p. 296) ▸ Discuss the potential risks to healthcare professionals associated with use of laser plumes. ▸ Discuss the CDC's recommendations regarding the use of electrosurgery. ***Class Activity** Present the following situation to the class for discussion:* *A friend of yours is considering enrolling in a dental assisting program, but is hesitant because he is afraid of contracting an infectious disease. He is particularly concerned about surgical smoke because of an article he read in a magazine. How could this friend be reassured and encouraged to pursue a career in dental assisting? What preventative measures can be taken to reduce the effects of exposure when assisting with a laser procedure? What recommendations has the CDC provided on the effects of exposure to laser plumes and dental healthcare professionals?*
Performance Evaluation		▣ TB ▨ SW questions (pp. 75-79) ▨ SW Case Study (p. 79) ▨ ℮ SW/ESLR Competency 19-1 Applying First Aid After an Exposure Incident (p. 81) ▨ ℮ SW/ESLR Competency 19-2 Handwashing Before Gloving (p. 83)

Bird/Robinson

OBJECTIVES	CONTENT	TEACHING RESOURCES
		SW/ESLR Competency 19-3 Applying an Alcohol-Based Hand Rub (p. 85)
		SW/ESLR Competency 19-4 Putting on Personal Protective Equipment (p. 87)
		SW/ESLR Competency 19-5 Removing Personal Protective Equipment (pp. 89-90)
		SW/ESLR Competency 19-6 Disinfecting an Alginate Impression (p. 91)
		ESLR Electronic Flashcards
		ESLR Practice Quiz
		ESLR Labeling Exercise 17: Areas of the Hand Missed During Hand Washing
		Recall questions (pp. 271-296)
		CTQ (p. 297)

19.3 Homework/Assignments:

1. Have students research OSHA BBP guidelines for dental offices and prepare a list of five to ten guidelines to share with the class.

2. Have students research the pathophysiology, signs and symptoms, treatments, and CDC recommendations of Creutzfeldt-Jakob disease and other prion diseases and present their findings to the class.

19.3 Instructor's Notes/Student Feedback:

Slide 1

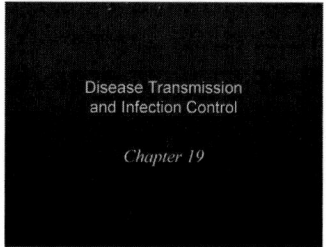

Disease Transmission
and Infection Control

Chapter 19

Slide 2

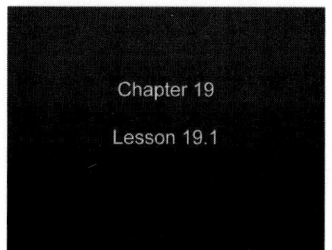

Chapter 19

Lesson 19.1

Slide 3

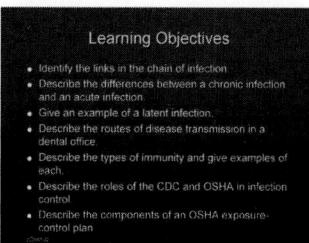

Learning Objectives

- Identify the links in the chain of infection.
- Describe the differences between a chronic infection and an acute infection.
- Give an example of a latent infection.
- Describe the routes of disease transmission in a dental office.
- Describe the types of immunity and give examples of each.
- Describe the roles of the CDC and OSHA in infection control.
- Describe the components of an OSHA exposure-control plan.

Slide 4

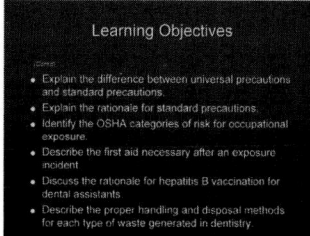

Learning Objectives

(Cont.)

- Explain the difference between universal precautions and standard precautions.
- Explain the rationale for standard precautions.
- Identify the OSHA categories of risk for occupational exposure.
- Describe the first aid necessary after an exposure incident.
- Discuss the rationale for hepatitis B vaccination for dental assistants.
- Describe the proper handling and disposal methods for each type of waste generated in dentistry.

Bird/Robinson

Slide 5

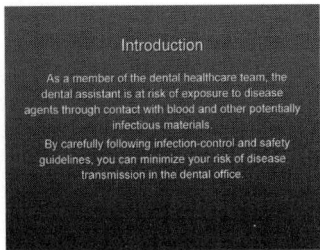

- Ask students how many of them have anxiety or concerns about their exposure to disease or infectious materials?

- Ask them who controls their safety, and how can they minimize their own risks in the dental office?

Slide 6

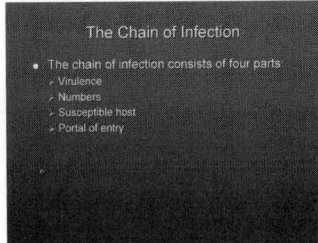

- Imagine a chain that has four links connected to one another. Break any link in the chain, and you stop the process of infection.

- Each link of the chain will be discussed at greater depth in a moment.

- Ask students whether they can guess what each of these four links represents.

Slide 7

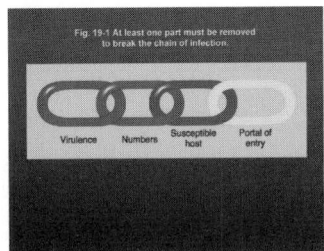

- Look at these four links in the chain of infection. Imagine them to be linked together until some strain is placed upon them, and then one of the links breaks or fails.

- What is a pathogen? *(A disease-causing organism.)*

Slide 8

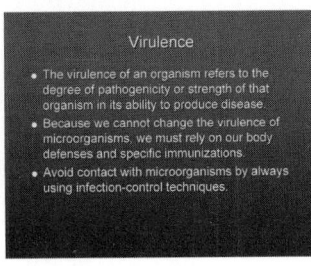

- Imagine an organism as a small round cell with an outer shell.

- The virulence of different organisms can be thought of as a difference in thickness of the outer shell. In order to reduce or eliminate an organism, you must break down its outer shell.

Torres and Ehrlich Modern Dental Assisting, 9th ed.

Bird/Robinson

Slide 9

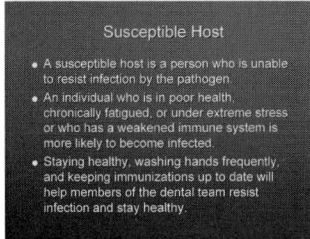

- Imagine I am telling you a war story, and there are 3 soldiers against 100. Who do you think won the battle, the group of 3 or the group of 100?

- By reducing the number of pathogens, the dental assistant can create a safer environment for the patient and the dental team.

Slide 10

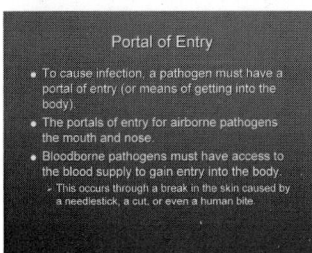

- An example of a susceptible host:

  - This person has been exposed to Herpes simplex, but has never had an outbreak. This person experiences stress from a major life change, such as going away to college. The stress is compounded by the fact that the person is staying up late cramming for exams and socializing and not getting enough sleep. In this stressful state, this person develops a herpetic lesion on the upper lip.

Slide 11

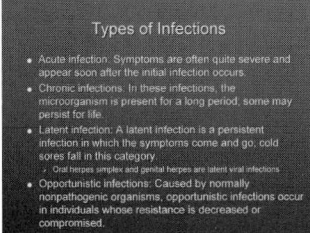

- In order to contract an infection, you must be exposed to pathogens, and those pathogens must have an entry point into your body.

- How can we protect the portals of entry to our bodies when working with patients?

Slide 12

- If a patient were to contract a common cold, which one of the four types of infection would he have?

- If a patient is undergoing chemotherapy for breast cancer, which one of the four types of infection would she be concerned about?

- Shingles is an example of which of the four types of infections?

- Hepatitis C virus is an example of what type of infection?

Bird/Robinson

Slide 13

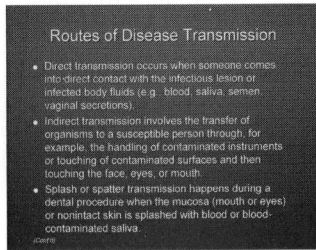

- Direct transmission is the most common method in the dental office environment. Why?
- Consider the following case: While assisting the dentist, using the high-speed evacuation system for a tooth extraction, you realize you have forgotten your protective eyewear on the counter. Just then the tooth cracks in half and blood splashes onto your face and eye area.
- How you would manage this situation and how you would avoid this scenario in the future?

Slide 14

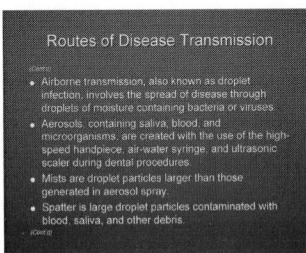

- Infections can be transmitted while assisting the dentist and inhaling aerosols produced by the air-water syringe, ultrasonic, or the handpiece. How can a dental assistant reduce the risk of infection?
- Every patient should be treated as though he or she is a carrier of disease, and PPE should always be worn.

Slide 15

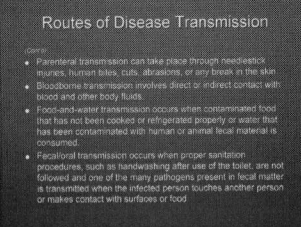

- Food and water transmission is an example of community-to-dental- office-to-patient transmission.
- Hepatitis is transmitted through fecal matter and can be easily controlled by simply washing hands thoroughly after use of the restroom.

Slide 16

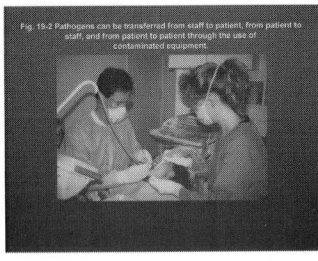

- Notice the plastic barriers on the cords of the suction and on the bracket tray. Barriers like these are used to protect surfaces that can be easily contaminated; they should be wiped down frequently with disinfectant wipes or spray.
- All surfaces touched with contaminated gloves or objects that cannot be sterilized with an autoclave should be protected with plastic barriers.

Slide 17

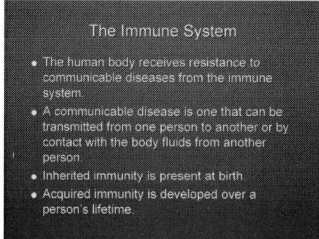

- The human body does a wonderful job of taking care of itself most of the time.

Slide 18

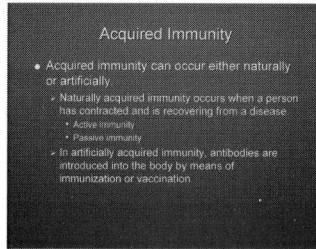

- The serum used to immunize a person can be created using the organisms from another person who has had the disease, or it can be developed artificially.

- The hepatitis B vaccine is an example of an artificially acquired immunization. The serum can be harvested from antigens from a person with hepatitis B, or they can be developed synthetically.

Slide 19

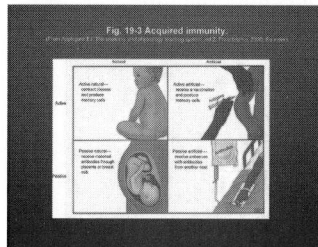

- Can students can think of any other examples of natural passive immunity? *(Through breast milk.)*

- Chicken pox was once an active natural disease; now there are immunizations to prevent it.

Slide 20

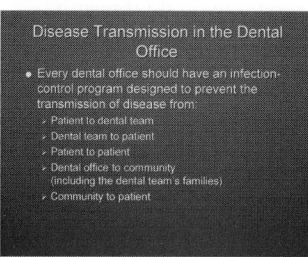

- It is critical to understand how disease transmission can occur in the dental office.

- The next five slides will discuss the various types of disease transmission, and ways to prevent them from occurring.

Bird/Robinson

Slide 21

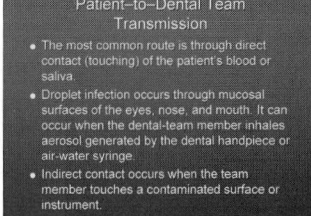

- A dental assistant will be in contact with many patients throughout the day.

- Some patients may be "carriers," or have a disease that the dental team members and the patient may not be aware of.

- It is important to use preventive measures on each patient.

Slide 22

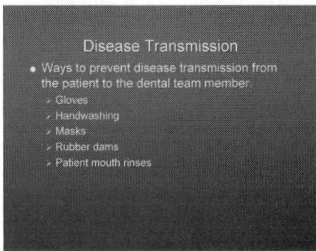

- Most patients believe that mouth rinse is used solely to reduce halitosis, or bad breath. Explain the benefits of mouth rinses to every patient.

- Rubber dams are used routinely for endodontic treatment (root canals) to isolate the individual tooth and prevent contamination of the canals. They can protect the dental team members by preventing a large number of pathogens from becoming airborne.

Slide 23

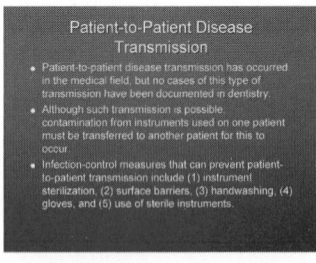

- Many patients are concerned that they may contract a disease from a prior patient. As a healthcare professional, it is important to communicate to patients that they are in a safe environment that practices standard infection control measures.

Slide 24

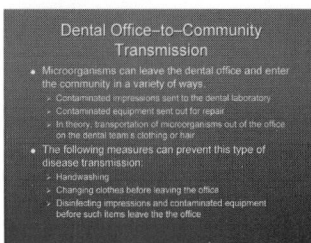

- The community includes members of the dental team's family.

- How would you feel about taking home bacteria that could transmit diseases to your family and friends?

Bird/Robinson

Slide 25

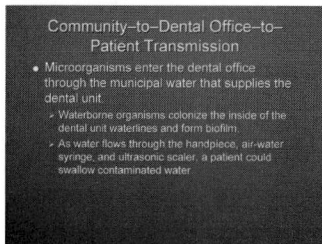

- One way to reduce the number of bacteria that colonize in water lines is to flush the handpiece, air-water syringe, and ultrasonic scaler for 60 seconds at the start of every day. This will reduce the number of bacteria present.

- There are also commercial products that use chemicals to help reduce bacteria and flush water lines.

Slide 26

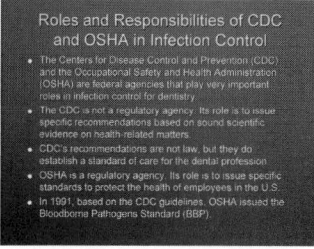

- For guidance on recommendations for infection control concerns, contact the Center for Disease Control (CDC).

- If you are ever concerned that a dental office is consistently noncompliant with regards to OSHA regulations, contact OSHA directly.

Slide 27

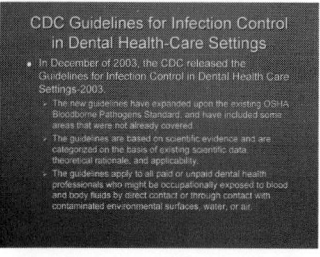

- The best way to stay abreast of the most recent updates and guidelines from the CDC and OSHA is to check their respective Web sites, www.cdc.gov and www.osha.gov.

- Which government agency is regulatory, and which only provides recommended guidelines?

Slide 28

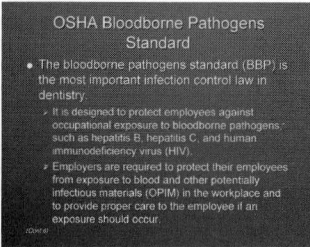

- OSHA requires that a copy of the BBP be present in every dental office and clinic.

- For a dental assistant's own protection and the health and safety of others, he or she should review the BBP regularly.

- Students can obtain a copy by visiting www.osha.gov.SLTC/bloodbornepathogens/.

ELSEVIER

Torres and Ehrlich Modern Dental Assisting, 9th ed.

Bird/Robinson

Slide 29

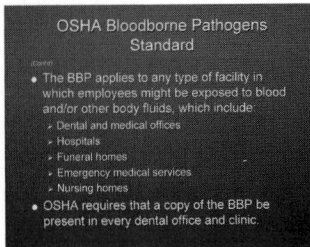

- Discuss office concerns and questions, then seek out answers within the BBP manual.

Slide 30

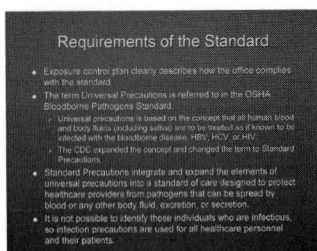

- Why do you think a dental office may not have a exposure plan?

- As a knowledgeable dental assistant, how can you encourage a dental office to develop a exposure plan that will comply with the requirements?

Slide 31

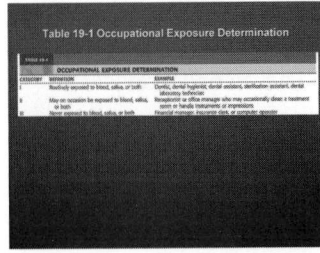

- Each category of the dental team should have specific training focusing on their particular occupational exposures.

- Why would a category III need training?

Slide 32

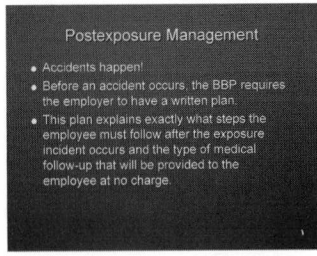

- How often should a dental office evaluate and update its exposure-control plan?

- What is another term for the BBP?

- Discuss the differences between Universal Precautions and Standard Precautions.

Slide 33

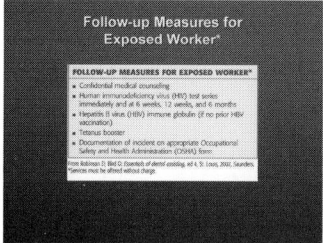

- It is an employee's right to have a medical follow-up after an occupational exposure. An employee's medical information is kept confidential from the employer.

Slide 34

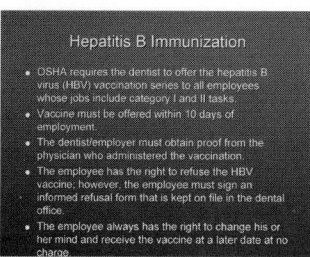

- Would you decline or accept the offer of the HBV vaccine? Why or why not?

Slide 35

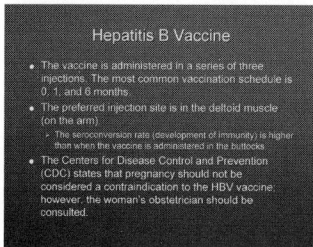

Slide 36

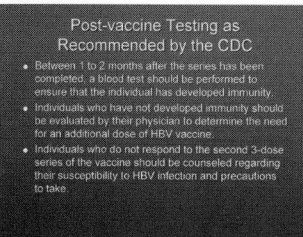

- What would the blood test show if your immunity to hepatitis B was properly developed?

Bird/Robinson

Slide 37

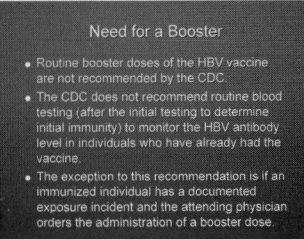

- Contact your physician if you have been exposed to a confirmed Hepatitis B patient, and you are concerned about your initial immunization.

Slide 38

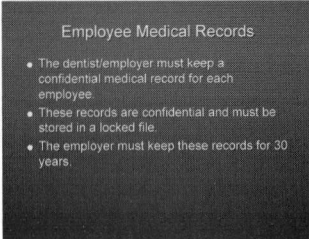

- The dental assistant should always keep the original and make copies as needed for changes in employment.

Slide 39

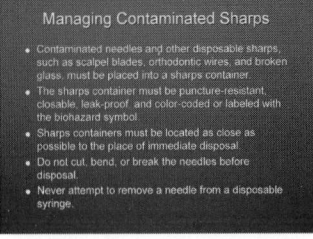

- Never overload a sharps container by forcing sharps into it.

Slide 40

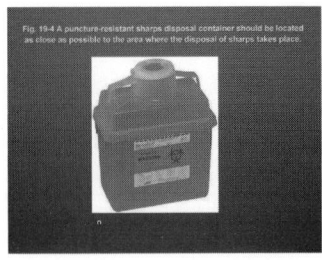

- Sharps containers come in a variety of sizes.
- Once container is full, close, seal, and dispose of the contents properly according to your state's laws.

Slide 41

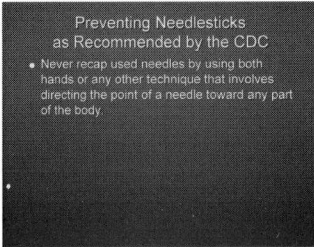

- What is the single-handed scoop technique?
- There are disposable, one-time-use needle guards available for dental professionals.

Slide 42

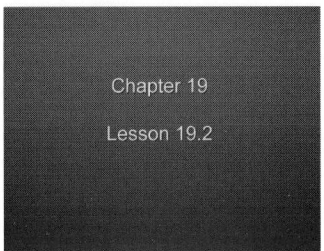

Slide 43

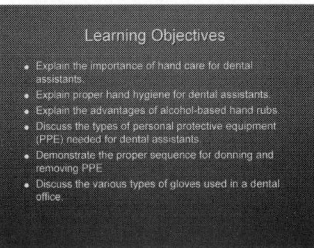

Slide 44

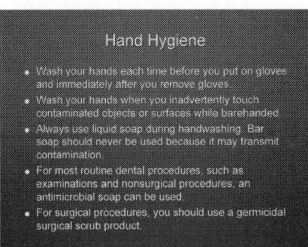

- When washing hands, strive to use hands-free faucets, which are activated either with foot pedals or electronically.

Torres and Ehrlich Modern Dental Assisting, 9th ed.

Bird/Robinson

Slide 45

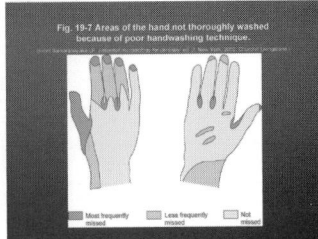

- Notice the areas most frequently missed.
- When washing hands, start with the frequently missed areas first to ensure thorough washing.

Slide 46

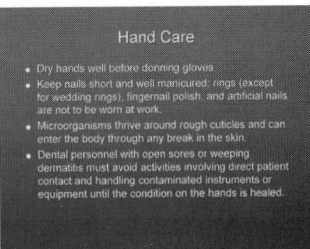

- Jewelry and long nails can puncture gloves, creating the potential for disease transmission.
- Powder in gloves can accumulate in jewelry clasps and crevices, causing damage.
- For health care providers using gloves, what is the maximum length for fingernail tips?

Slide 47

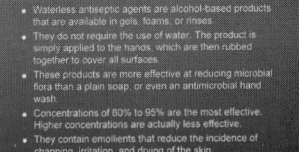

- Just as when using soap and water, remember to thoroughly apply the alcohol hand rub on areas that are frequently missed.
- What are the three advantages of using alcohol-based hand rubs over washing hands with soap and water?
- Ask students whether they can think of any other advantages.

Slide 48

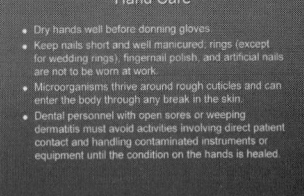

- The practice of general dentistry most likely uses a combination of routine hand washing with soap and water and alcohol-based, waterless hand rubs.
- Evidence suggests that alcohol-based antiseptic hand rubs are more effective at decontaminating the hands than washing with soap and water alone.
- Remember, if your hands are visibly soiled, you must wash with soap and water before applying an alcohol hand rub.

Slide 49

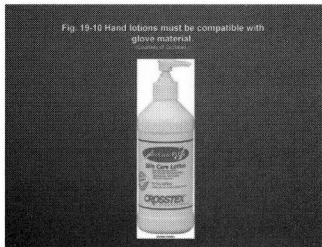

- Why is it important for a health care professional to use hand lotion?
- Having intact skin is the best defense against infection.
- What is meant by this caption: "Hand lotions must be compatible with glove material?"

Slide 50

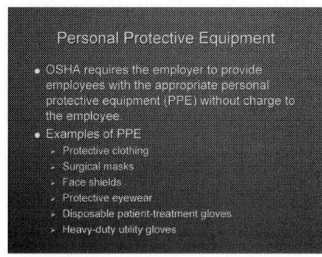

- PPE should be comfortable and functional. For example, if eyewear is too tight or too loose and fogs up, a dental assistant should try a different manufacturer or brand until one that fits properly is found.
- What is the purpose of PPE?

Slide 51

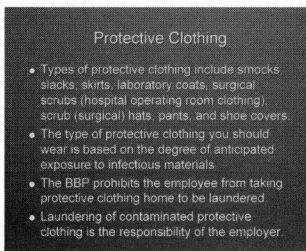

- Why should a health care professional not wear scrubs or lab coats or any other types of PPE to and from work?
- Contaminated PPE should be laundered at the dental office only if appropriate equipment is available and proper procedures are followed.

Slide 52

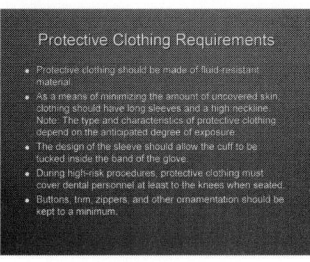

- If clothing becomes visibly soiled with blood or saliva, it must be changed immediately.
- The employer should have on hand an ample supply of scrubs and lab coats that are clean and fit properly.

Slide 53

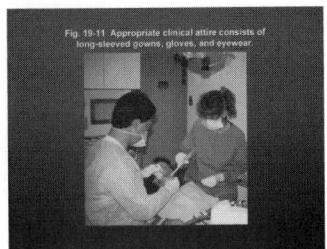

- There are many examples of proper infection control in this photo. *(Ask students to name them..)*

Slide 54

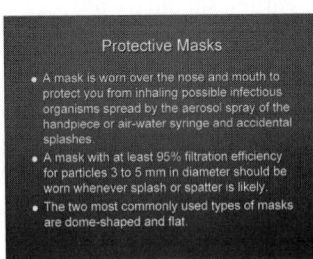

- Dental assistants should look at the mask manufacturer's box to ensure that the masks have at least 95% filtration efficiency; not all do.

- During what types of procedures should a protective mask be worn?

Slide 55

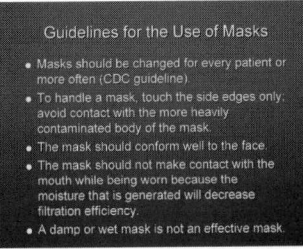

- Why wouldn't a face shield worn alone be adequate protection?

Slide 56

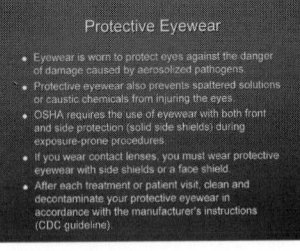

- If you wear prescription glasses, you must wear side and bottom shields or wear a full face shield over your glasses.

Slide 57

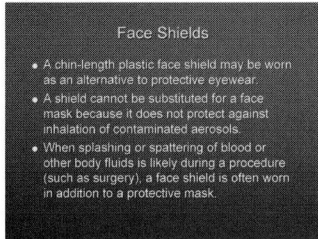

- Disposable combination shield and ear loop masks are available from dental supply companies.

Slide 58

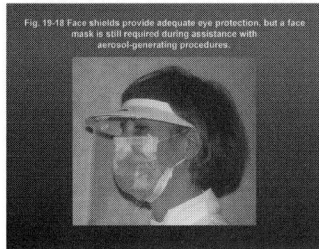

- This face shield is worn like a visor.

- Face shields must be able to withstand being properly washed with soap and water before and after every patient.

Slide 59

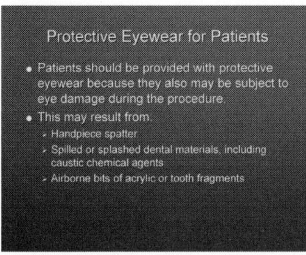

- Some patients may not feel comfortable wearing eyewear, as this may be a new protocol for them.

- Advise patients that the eyewear is for their protection.

- What is another procedure for which a patient must wear protective eyewear?

Slide 60

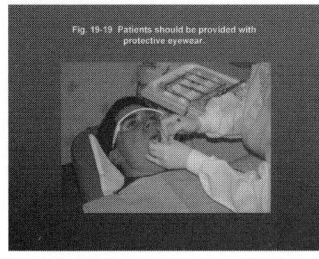

Torres and Ehrlich Modern Dental Assisting, 9th ed.

Bird/Robinson

Slide 61

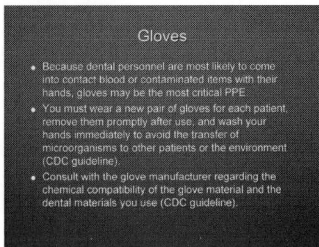

- Some putty impression materials may not be compatible with the powder found in gloves.
- Review manufacturer's guidelines for handling material while maintaining good infection control.

Slide 62

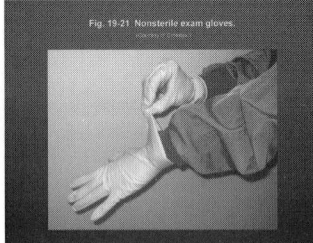

- Notice that the clinician is properly placing glove over sleeve to eliminate exposed skin, thereby reducing possible portal of entry sites.
- Nonsterile exam gloves are used most frequently for patient care.

Slide 63

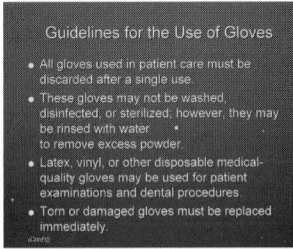

- Properly fitting gloves are essential for good patient care.
- Ambidextrous glove sizes range from XS to XL.
- Right- and left-handed gloves have a much better fit; however, they are more expensive.

Slide 64

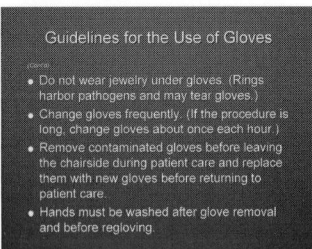

Slide 65

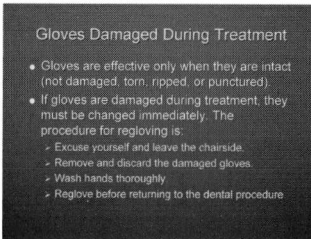

- Gloves can be torn or ripped during the manufacturing process. Always inspect both gloves before starting a procedure.

Slide 66

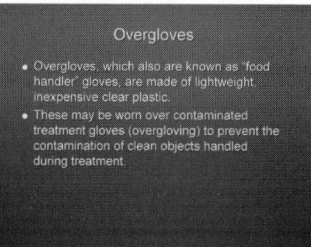

- Overgloves can greatly reduce cross-contamination and should be easily accessible in each treatment area.
- The following situations would necessitate the use of overgloves:
  - during a procedure, you must open a cabinet door to retrieve an instrument you forgot to lay out on the table;
  - you must open a drawer during a procedure;
  - you must take a phone call (and use the receiver) during a procedure.

Slide 67

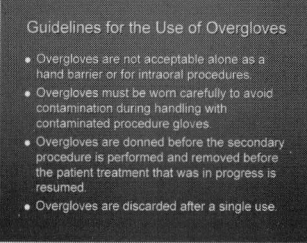

Slide 68

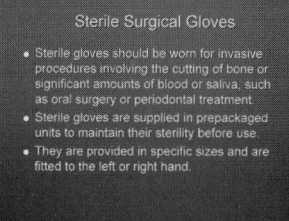

- Sterile surgical gloves are of a higher quality than treatment gloves and therefore more costly. CDC guidelines, and some state dental boards, require surgical gloves for surgical procedures.
- Some health care professionals choose to wear two pairs of sterile surgical gloves; this is not necessarily a CDC recommendation.

Slide 69

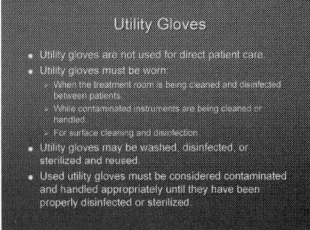

- Appropriately sized utility gloves should be used to ensure good control.

- After utility gloves are washed and disinfected, they should be hung on a hook until thoroughly dry before further use.

Slide 70

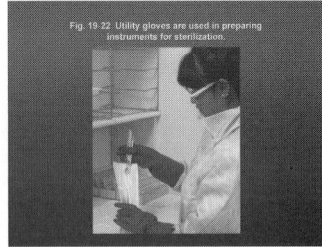

- Notice the assistant is properly wearing the utility gloves over the lab coat sleeve. Why is she doing this?

- Utility gloves should be thick enough to withstand possible instrument punctures.

Slide 71

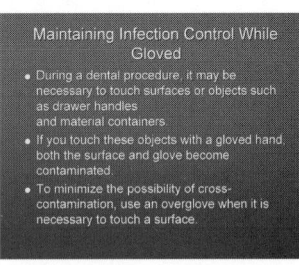

- A dental assistant should have all materials needed for each procedure out and ready for use to avoid cross-contamination.

Slide 72

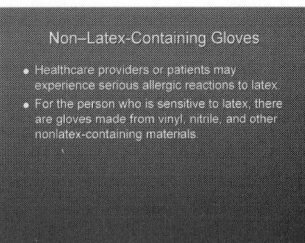

- Many dental clinics/offices are becoming latex-free to create a safer environment for those sensitive to latex.

Torres and Ehrlich Modern Dental Assisting, 9th ed.

Bird/Robinson

Slide 73

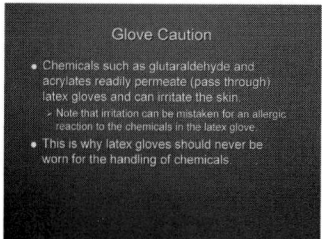

- If health care providers experience any skin irritation to latex gloves, they may want to try products from different manufacturers.

Slide 74

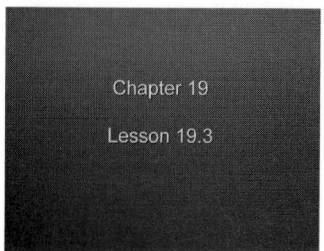

Slide 75

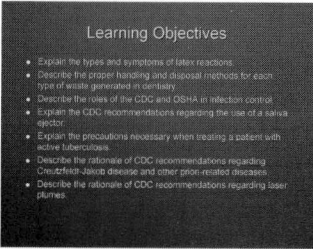

Slide 76

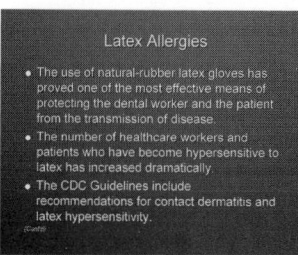

- Be certain to review patients' medical history to determine if they are allergic to latex before starting each procedure.

- Some patients may not be aware they are allergic to latex; watch for possible symptoms.

Slide 77

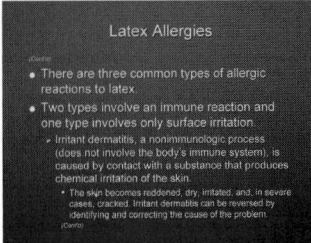

- Latex is present in many materials used in the dental office, such as the elastic ear loops of masks and prophy angle cups.

- What are symptoms of an immune reaction to latex?

- Is your office prepared if a patient has such an immune reaction?

Slide 78

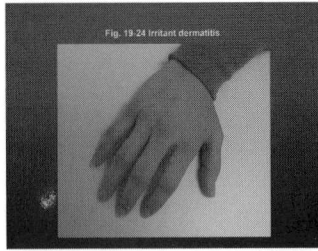

- This photo depicts the red, cracked, irritated skin caused from direct contact with latex or with irritants such as chemicals..

Slide 79

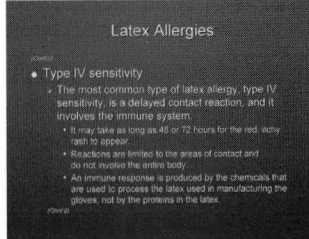

- Many healthcare workers confuse this type of reaction as a latex allergy.

- A patient should get an allergy test from a physician to rule out any confusion.

Slide 80

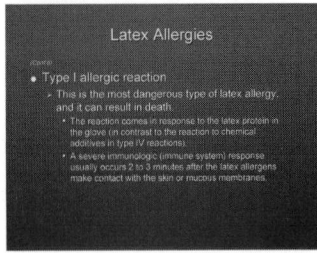

- Because this type of latex reaction is so severe, every dental office must have a first-aid kit and emergency protocol established.

- What causes death from this type of allergic reaction?

Slide 81

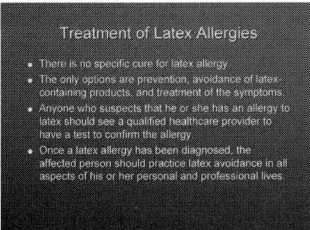

- Gloves made out of nonlatex materials such as vinyl and nitrile should be used on a latex-sensitive patient.

Slide 82

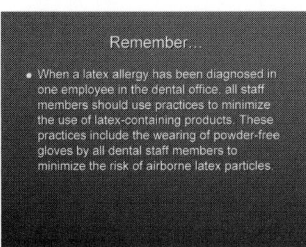

- When treatment gloves are removed or snapped off, they release airborne latex particles that can trigger an allergic reaction. Therefore, patients could experience a type I allergic reaction with or without direct latex contact.

Slide 83

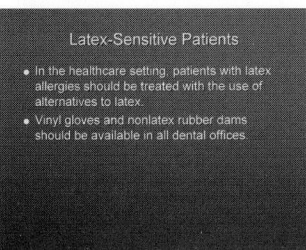

- Ask students the following question:
  - If you have a patient with a latex allergy, when should you schedule his or her appointment?

Slide 84

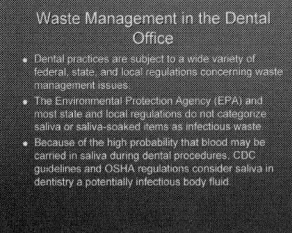

- It is the dental office's responsibility to stay current with specific federal, state, and local waste management regulations to avoid possible fines or penalties.
- Even though EPA does not categorize saliva or saliva-soaked items as infectious waste, dental offices should always treat them as such.

Slide 85

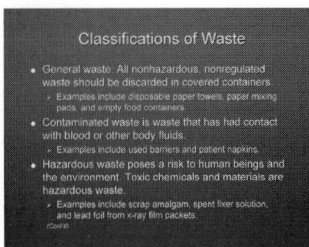

- A dental assistant must learn the different types of waste and how each is discarded when cleaning up, or processing, a dental treatment room.
- Waste containers must be labeled with the universal biohazard symbol when applicable.

Slide 86

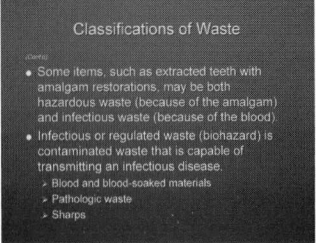

Slide 87

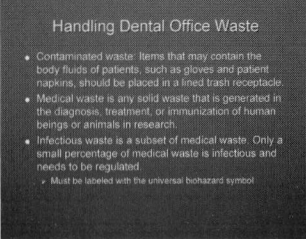

- What are the four areas of waste management with which a dental assistant needs to be concerned?
- Dental assistants need to wear appropriate PPE during waste management.

Slide 88

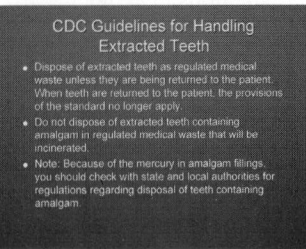

- If giving patients their extracted teeth, be certain to place the teeth in a sealed bag or sealed envelope.
- You may heat-sterilize the tooth if no amalgams are present.

Bird/Robinson

Slide 89

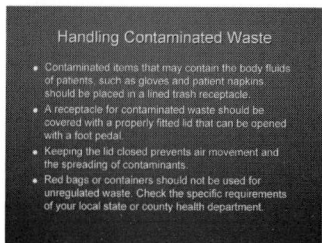

- When removing trash bags from receptacles, one must wear utility gloves.

Slide 90

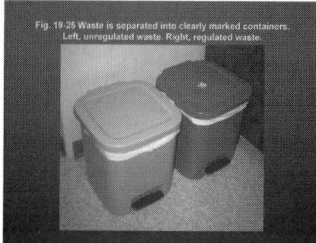

- Notice the foot pedals to avoid touching contaminated lids.
- Never compact waste with the foot.
- Biohazard stickers can be purchased through dental supply companies.

Slide 91

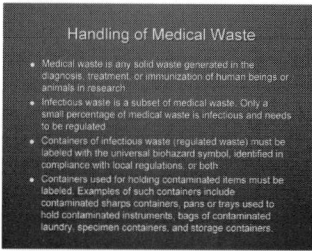

- The medical waste generated by most general dentistry practices is minimal and tends to consist mainly of sharps.

Slide 92

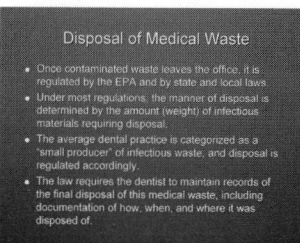

- A dental practice should direct any questions about waste management to the city where the dental practice is located.

ELSEVIER

Bird/Robinson

Slide 93

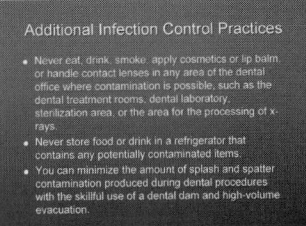

- When eating in the workplace, be sure to remove contaminated PPE.

Slide 94

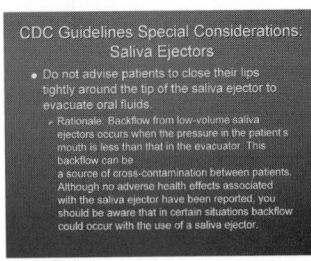

- Many patients have become accustomed to closing their lips around the suction.

Slide 95

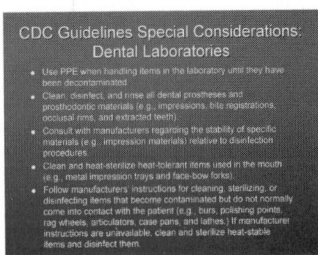

- It is easy to disinfect all lab materials that leave your office and clinic, and it takes very little time.

- Laboratory materials, such as impressions, can be damaged or distorted if not disinfected properly.

Slide 96

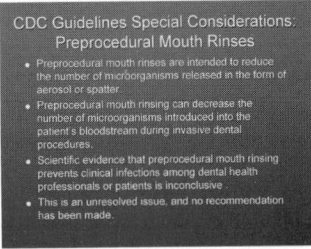

- The CDC has not made a recommendation about preprocedural mouth rinses in the dental office.

Slide 97

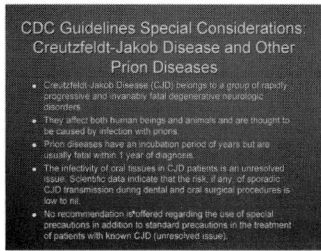

- Staying abreast of current research through professional journals and continuing education (CE) courses will create a safer environment for both you and your patients.

- Prion is a term for a protein particle that lacks nucleic acid and is the cause of neurologic disorders, such as CJD.

Slide 98

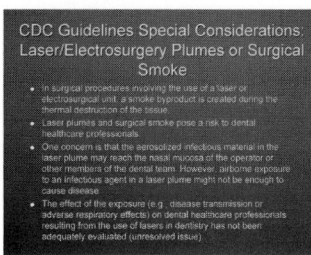

- Laser use is becoming more routine in general dentistry.

- Time, experience, and more research will help create more guidelines for this technology.

20 Lesson Plan
Principles and Techniques of Disinfection

TEACHING FOCUS

This chapter will introduce students to the principles and techniques of disinfecting a dental treatment area. Precleaning and disinfection of dental treatment room surfaces, housekeeping surfaces, and the use of surface barriers will be discussed. Students will also have the opportunity to learn the various types of disinfectants available and the EPA classifications for disinfectants, as well as CDC guidelines for their use.

MATERIALS AND RESOURCES

- ☐ computer and PowerPoint projector (all Lessons)
- ☐ liquid antimicrobial hand soap (Lesson 20.1)
- ☐ noncontaminated surfaces in dental treatment room (Lesson 20.1)
- ☐ paper towels (Lesson 20.2)

- ☐ personal protective equipment (including utility gloves, a mask, and goggles) (Lesson 20.2)
- ☐ plastic surface barriers (Lesson 20.1)
- ☐ utility gloves (Lesson 20.1)

LESSON CHECKLIST

Preparations for this lesson include:

- lecture
- evaluation of student knowledge and skills needed to perform all entry-level activities related to the principles and techniques of disinfection, including:
  - explaining why dental treatment-room surfaces need barriers or disinfection
  - determining what type of barrier or disinfectant is best for what surface
  - explaining the differences between disinfectant, sterilization, and antiseptics
  - identifying precautions needed when using chemical sterilants and disinfectants
  - describing CDC guidelines for disinfecting both housekeeping and clinical contact surfaces
  - demonstrating how to clean and disinfect treatment rooms and dental instruments

KEY TERMS

antiseptic (p. 305)
bioburden (p. 304)
broad-spectrum activity (p. 306)
chlorine dioxide (p. 309)
clinical contact surface (p. 300)
disinfectant (p. 305)
environmental surface (p. 299)
fungicidal (p. 305)
glutaraldehyde (p. 308)
high-level disinfectant (p. 309)
hospital disinfectant (p. 305)
housekeeping surface (p. 300)
immersion disinfectant (p. 308)
intermediate-level disinfectant (p. 300)
iodophor (p. 306)
low-level disinfectant (p. 310)

precleaning (p. 304)
residual activity (p. 305)
reuse life (p. 305)
shelf life (p. 305)
sodium hypochlorite (p. 307)
splash, spatter, and droplet surface (p. 300)
sporicidal (p. 305)
sterilant (p. 305)
sterilization (p. 305)
surface barrier (p. 300)
synthetic phenol compound (p. 306)
touch surface (p. 300)
transfer surface (p. 300)
tuberculocidal (p. 305)
virucidal (p. 305)

ADDITIONAL RESOURCES

PowerPoint Slides (Evolve): 1-43
Multimedia Procedures DVD:
    Placing and Removing Surface Barriers
    Treatment Room Cleaning and Disinfection

Legend

CTQ
Critical
Thinking
Question

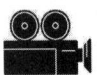

DVD
Multimedia
Procedures
Videos and
Animations

ESLR
EVOLVE
Student
Learning
Resources

IDO
Interactive
Dental
Office
CD-ROM

SW
Student
Workbook

TB
Test Bank
on the
TEACH
CD-ROM

PPT
PowerPoint
Slides

Class Activities are indicated in ***bold italic.***

Torres and Ehrlich Modern Dental Assisting, 9th ed.
Bird/Robinson

LESSON 20.1

PRETEST

1. Why is it important to use surface barriers and to disinfect treatment rooms?
   a. During patient treatment, equipment and surfaces may become contaminated with blood and saliva.
   b. Surfaces that are touched frequently, such as light and drawer handles, can act as reservoirs of microorganisms.
   c. Microorganisms can be transferred from surfaces to the dental team members and patients.
   d. All of the above.

2. Which of the following surfaces in the dental office are covered with barriers?
   a. x-ray control switches, light handles, drawer handles, bracket table
   b. the entire dental chair and the assisting chair
   c. carpet and flooring
   d. hard surfaces such as countertops and light handles

3. The two methods used to deal with surface contamination are
   a. autoclaving and glutaraldehyde.
   b. autoclaving and surface barriers.
   c. preclean and disinfect surfaces between patients, and surface barriers.
   d. preclean and disinfect at the beginning and end of each day, and surface barriers.

4. Using a chemical to reduce the number of microorganisms on living objects is called
   a. sterilization.   c. broad-spectrum activity.
   b. antisepsis.   d. disinfection.

5. An antiseptic is a(n)
   a. substance used to kill microorganisms found on the skin.
   b. chemical used to reduce the number of microorganisms on found on surfaces.
   c. product that is capable of killing fungi.
   d. EPA-registered, intermediate-level hospital disinfectant.

6. Which government agency is responsible for registering disinfectants?
   a. CDC   c. EPA
   b. OSHA   d. OSAP

7. Which of the following liquid disinfectants are considered to be intermediate-level?
   a. chlorine dioxide and glutaraldehyde
   b. iodophor and synthetic phenol compound
   c. sodium hypochlorite and phenol compound
   d. glutaraldehyde and sodium hypochlorite

8. When removing contaminated barriers and wiping down contaminated surfaces with an intermediate-level disinfectant after patient treatment is completed, which type of gloves should be worn?
   a. overgloves   c. treatment gloves
   b. utility gloves   d. treatment gloves and overgloves

9. Precleaning reduces the number of microbes and removes blood, saliva, and other body fluids called
   a. bioburdens.   c. pathogens.
   b. biohazards.   d. hazards.

10. When cleaning and disinfecting treatment rooms, it is important to spray the paper towel with product instead of spraying the surface directly because it
    a. reduces the amount of product used.
    b. saves time.
    c. reduces the amount of overspray and possible airborne transfer.
    d. all of the above.

Answers

1. d
2. a
3. c
4. d
5. a

6. c
7. b
8. b
9. a
10. c

BACKGROUND ASSESSMENT

Question: What are the different classifications of clinical contact surfaces, and how should they be maintained, according to OSAP's infection-control guidelines?

Answer: There are three clinical contact surfaces as classified by OSAP: touch surfaces, transfer surfaces, and splash, splatter, and droplet surfaces. Touch surfaces are areas that are directly touched and contaminated during patient care; they include drawer and light handles, dental unit controls, pens, telephones, x-ray buttons, and handles on the bracket tray. Transfer surfaces are areas that are not touched directly, but have contact with contaminated objects and instruments. These areas include: instrument trays, areas around the suction that are touched by saliva ejectors, and areas where the air and water syringes and handpieces rest. Touch and transfer surfaces should be cleaned and disinfected between patients, and barriers should be used wherever possible. Splash, splatter, and droplet surfaces are areas that do not come into contact with contaminated instruments, supplies, or dental team members. These surfaces include floors and countertops and should be cleaned at least once a day.

Question: How would you describe the classifications of chemical sterilants according to the EPA?

Answer: There are three classifications of disinfectants set forth by the EPA. High-level disinfectants provide a high level of disinfection when used with a short contact time, and serve as a sterilant when used with a prolonged contact time. High-level disinfectants are used on semicritical items that cannot be autoclaved. Intermediate-level disinfectants are hospital disinfectants that have tuberculocidal activity. These agents are used to clean noncritical items that have been contaminated with blood or saliva. Low-level disinfectants are nontuberculocidal and may be used to disinfect only surfaces that are not contaminated with blood.

CRITICAL THINKING QUESTION

In a dental office where patients are seen every hour, a dental assistant is asked to select a surface-disinfecting solution to clean the treatment room between patients. The dentist asks that the following criteria be considered: she does not want to use a product that can stain the fabric dental chair, and she wants the product to have a short contact time to ensure that the office stays on schedule. How should the dental assistant approach this decision?

Guidelines: The dental assistant should consider the following disinfectants when making a decision: Chlorines have the shortest contact duration (2 to 10 minutes); however, they may destroy fabrics. Complex phenols have a 10-minute contact time and are also safe for the fabric patient chair. Dual/synergized quaternary ammonium compounds have a 6- to 10-minute contact time, yet can damage some materials. Iodophors have a 10-minute contact time, but the iodine may stain the fabric chair. A phenol-alcohol combination has a 10-minute contact time, but can cause porous surfaces to crack. Halogens have a 5-minute contact time, but they are used to clean hard surfaces only. In order to satisfy the dentist's requirements, the dental assistant should eliminate chlorines, dual/synergized quaternary ammonium, and iodophors. Complex phenols would probably be the best choice. While they require a longer contact duration, they are the safest disinfectant for the fabric dental chair.

OBJECTIVES	CONTENT	TEACHING RESOURCES
Pronounce, define, and spell the Key Terms.	■ Key terms (p. 298)	SW Fill in the Blank questions 1-15 (p. 94) ESLR Electronic Flashcards ▸ Discuss each of the key terms in Chapter 13, focusing on the definition, pronunciation, and spelling of each term. ***Class Activity Have each student use one of the key terms in a clinically relevant sentence in order to define the term. Continue until all terms have been used; if students become stuck, have the rest of the class offer suggestions.***
Explain why dental treatment-room surfaces need barriers or disinfection.	■ Introduction (p. 299)	PPT 5 SW Short-Answer Questions 1; Multiple Choice question 1 (pp. 93, 95) CDC: Rankings of Evidence (p. 299) ▸ Discuss the lengths of time that various microorganisms can survive on environmental surfaces. ▸ Discuss the categories used by the CDC to rank scientific evidence supporting their recommendations. ***Class Activity Divide the class into groups, and ask students to respond to the following questions:*** *1. Why do barriers save time?* *2. What technique is used to save time and ensure that contaminated gloves do not touch the surface when removing barriers?* *3. What are some types of barriers that are available, and what are the advantages and disadvantages of each?* *4. What might have occurred before CDC recommendations regarding use of barriers in dental offices?* *5. What were dental assistants doing at that time to clean and disinfect challenging areas?* ***Have groups share their findings with the class for discussion.***
Describe the CDC guidelines for disinfecting clinical contact surfaces.	■ Environmental infection control (p. 300) ☐ Clinical contact surfaces (p. 300)	PPT 6-10 TB question 1 SW Short-Answer Questions 11; Topics for Discussion questions 1-2 (pp. 93, 96) CDC: CDC Recommendations for Environmental Infection Control (p. 300) Figure 20-1 (A) Touch surfaces; (B) transfer surfaces; (C) splash, spatter, and droplet surfaces (p. 300)

ELSEVIER

Torres and Ehrlich Modern Dental Assisting, 9th ed.

Bird/Robinson

OBJECTIVES	CONTENT	TEACHING RESOURCES
		▸ Discuss the differences between clinical contact surfaces and housekeeping surfaces. Which types of disinfectants are used for each?
		▸ Discuss the different categories of clinical contact surfaces.
		Class Activity Divide the class into groups, and assign each group one of the following clinical contact surfaces: touch; transfer; splash, spatter, and droplet. Have each group list 10 areas or surfaces in a treatment room for its assigned contact surface and present its findings to the class.
Describe the two methods to deal with surface contamination.	☐ Surface contamination (p. 300)	⊠▤ PPT 11 🖥 TB question 3 📖 SW Short-Answer Questions 3; Multiple Choice question 2 (pp. 93, 95) Figure 20-2 Smooth surfaces are easily sprayed and wiped (p. 301) ▸ Discuss which surfaces are easily cleaned and disinfected and which are not. *Class Activity Divide the class into four groups, and assign each group one of the following topics: advantages of surface barriers, disadvantages of surface barriers, advantages of precleaning/disinfecting, disadvantages of precleaning/disinfecting. Have each group list at least three examples to support its assigned topic and then present its findings to the class.*
List the types of surfaces in the dental office typically covered with barriers.	– Surface barriers (p. 301) **Procedure** 20-1 Placing and removing surface barriers (p. 303) (SW/ESLR Competency 20-1, p. 97)	⊠▤ PPT 12-18 🎥 Multimedia Procedures DVD: Placing and Removing Surface Barriers 🖥 TB questions 4-6 📖 SW Short-Answer Questions 2; Multiple Choice questions 3-4, 7; Topic for Discussion questions 3-4 (pp. 93, 95-96) 📖 *e* SW/ESLR Competency 20-1 Placing and Removing Surface Barriers (p. 97) Table 20-1 Comparison of Surface Barriers and Precleaning/Disinfection (p. 301) Figure 20-3 An example of water on a fluid-resistant material (p. 301) Surfaces Typically Protected with Barriers (p. 302) Recall questions 1-4 (p. 304)

Bird/Robinson

OBJECTIVES	CONTENT	TEACHING RESOURCES
		Figure 20-4 Surfaces touched during patient care should be covered with protective barriers (p. 302)
		Figure 20-5 Rolls of plastic tubing that can be cut to the desired length (p. 302)
		Figure 20-6 Tube socks provide barrier protection for diffucult-to-clean areas (p. 302)
		CTQ 1, 4 (p. 311)
		▸ Discuss which types of surfaces are better protected with surface barriers. Why should surfaces touched during patient care be covered with protective barriers?
		▸ Discuss the different types of materials used for barrier protection and where they might appropriately be used.
		Class Activity Lead a class discussion about surface barriers. Ask students to identify which surfaces in dental treatment areas are typically covered with barriers, and discuss which materials are best suited for each surface. Record student responses on the board for comparison.
Describe the two methods to deal with surface contamination.	– Precleaning and disinfection (p. 304) – Precleaning (p. 304) – Disinfection (p. 304)	PPT 19-22 TB questions 7-8, 12 SW Multiple Choice question 6; Topics for Discussion question 5 (pp. 95-96) CDC: Clinical Contact Surfaces (p. 304) CDC: Personal Protective Equipment (PPE) (p. 304) Recall questions 5-10 (pp. 304, 306) CTQ 2 (p. 311) ▸ Discuss the personal protective equipment that should be worn when precleaning or disinfecting. *Class Activity Divide the class into groups, and have each group discuss the differences between precleaning and disinfecting, and respond to the statement, "If a surface is not clean, it cannot be disinfected." Then have each group share its findings with the class.*
Explain the difference between disinfection and sterilization.	– Disinfection (p. 304)	PPT 22 SW Short-Answer Questions 5 (p. 93) ▸ Discuss the difference between sterilization and disinfection. ▸ Discuss the classifications of chemical disinfectants (Table 20-2, p. 305). *Class Activity Present the following list of dental items to the class, and have students identify whether each should be disinfected or sterilized:*

OBJECTIVES	CONTENT	TEACHING RESOURCES
		1. Contaminated dental instruments such as scalers used to remove plaque. (S)
		2. Contaminated countertops in patient treatment area. (D)
		3. Bite-wing film holders just used once on a patient. (S)
		4. Dental handpiece used to remove an old amalgam on a patient. (S)
		5. The suction handle that held a disposable saliva ejector. (D)
		6. The handle of the bracket table in contaminated treatment area. (D)
		7. The diamond burs used in the high-speed handpiece on a patient with diabetes. (S)
		8. The assistant chair. (D)
		9. The patients bib clips used to hold the patient napkin during an impression for whitening trays. (S)
		10. The utility gloves used to remove contaminated barriers. (D)
Explain the difference between a disinfectant and an antiseptic.	– Disinfection (p. 304)	PPT 23 SW Short-Answer Questions 6; Multiple Choice question 8 (pp. 93, 95) Recall question 8 (p. 304) ▶ Discuss the differences between antiseptics and disinfectants. Why should they not be used interchangeably? *Class Activity Divide the class into groups. Have each group explain the differences between disinfectants and antiseptics and list five examples of each. Then have each group present its findings to the class. Record student responses on the board for comparison.*

20.1 Homework/Assignments:

20.1 Instructor's Notes/Student Feedback:

CRITICAL THINKING QUESTION

A new patient who is a nurse at a local hospital asks the dental assistant to explain what is done between patients to prevent infection. The patient specifically asks how the disinfecting solution is selected, how long it stays on the surface, and what surfaces are covered with barriers. What is your response?

Guidelines: Because the patient is a nurse, the dental assistant can assume that he is knowledgeable about infection-control principles and procedures. The dental assistant should feel free to share which disinfecting solution is used and explain that it is left on the surface according to the manufacturer's suggestions and EPA guidelines. The dental assistant should also explain that when making the selection, the advantages and disadvantages of each product were weighed against the needs of the office, and that CDC recommendations were carefully considered to ensure proper environmental infection control. The patient should also be assured that the surface barriers used in the office are fluid resistant, and that all surfaces are carefully precleaned before barriers are put in place. Barriers are also carefully removed, but if a surface is inadvertently touched during barrier removal, the surface will be cleaned and disinfected. If the patient still feels unsure about the dental office's infection control, the dental assistant may allow the patient to observe the precleaning and disinfection process to ensure that proper infection-control measures are followed.

OBJECTIVES	CONTENT	TEACHING RESOURCES
Name the government agency that is responsible for registering disinfectants.	– Disinfectants (p. 305)	PPT 27-29 TB question 10 SW Multiple Choice questions 5, 9 (p. 95) Figure 20-7 Disposable premoistened wipes with tuberculocidal activity (p. 305) Table 20-2 Chemical Classification of Disinfectants (p. 305) Figure 20-8 Decreasing order of resistance of microorganisms to germicidal chemicals (p. 306) ▸ Discuss the EPA's classification of disinfectants (Table 20-2). ***Class Activity** Have students explore the EPA Web site to investigate how disinfectants are registered and listed and identify at least two examples of disinfectants that are not included on the Web site. Then have students share their findings with the class. (For students to prepare for this activity, see Homework/Assignments #1.)*
Demonstrate the process of precleaning contaminated dental instruments.	– Disinfectants (p. 305)	PPT 35-40 TB questions 11-12 SW Short-Answer Questions 9; Multiple Choice question 15 (pp. 93, 95) Recall questions 11, 15 (p. 310) ▸ Discuss Table 20-4 (p. 308). What are the advantages and disadvantages of the various instrument-immersion disinfectants for dentistry?

OBJECTIVES	CONTENT	TEACHING RESOURCES
		▸ Discuss the difference between sterilization and high-level disinfection. Why would you not use immersion disinfectants on surfaces? ***Class Activity** Divide the class into groups. Have each group discuss why contaminated instruments require precleaning; list several examples of instruments that can be disinfected using instrument immersion disinfectants; and discuss the personal concerns associated with immersion chemicals and how to manage them safely. Then have each group share its findings with the class.*
Explain the precautions when using chemical sterilants/ disinfectants.	– Disinfectants (p. 305)	PPT 35 TB questions 13-14 SW Short-Answer Questions 10 (p. 93) Disinfectant Precautions (p. 305) CTQ 3 (p. 311) ▸ Discuss what precautions you should take when preparing to sterilize heat-sensitive equipment. ▸ Discuss which chemical is highly toxic and must be followed with a thorough rinsing of water. Why is it used? ***Class Activity** Present the following situation to the class for students to discuss:* *A dental assistant is using on a patient a plastic bite-wing film holder that was recently treated with a high-level disinfectant.. The patient comments that the bite-wing holder that used to be white looks dirty because it is discolored with a yellow/brown tint. As the dental assistant places the film holder in the patient's oral cavity, the patient spits it out and states that it tastes bad.* ***What high-level disinfectant might have been used? Why is the patient experiencing such a bad taste, and how should the dental assistant proceed? Record student responses on the board for comparison.***
Identify chemical products used for intermediate-level and low-level surface disinfection, and explain the advantages and	– Ideal surface disinfectant (p. 305) – Iodophors (p. 306) – Synthetic phenol compounds (p. 306) – Sodium hypochlorite (p. 307)	PPT 30-34 TB questions 9, 11, 15 SW Short-Answer Questions 7; Multiple Choice questions 10-14 (pp. 93, 95) Table 20-3 EPA-Registered Surface Disinfectants for Dentistry (p. 307) Figure 20-9 Iodophor surface disinfectant (p. 306)

ELSEVIER

OBJECTIVES	CONTENT	TEACHING RESOURCES
disadvantages of each.	– Alcohol (p. 308) – Immersion disinfectants (p. 308) – Glutaraldehyde (p. 308) – Chlorine dioxide (p. 309) – Ortho-phthalaldehyde (p. 309)	Figure 20-10 Synthetic phenol disinfectant (p. 307) Figure 20-11 Sodium hypochlorite (household bleach) should not be used as a surface disinfectant (p. 308) Table 20-4 FDA-Cleared Instrument-Immersion Disinfectants for Dentistry (p. 308) Figure 20-12 Covered instrument tray for use with immersion disinfectants (p. 310) Recall questions 12-14 (p. 310) 💡 CTQ 5 (p. 311) ▸ Discuss the characteristics of an ideal surface disinfectant. What is meant by the term residual activity? *Class Activity Divide the class into groups, and assign each group one of the following disinfectants: chlorines, complex phenols, dual/synergized quaternary ammonium compounds, iodophors, phenol-alcohol combinations, other halogens. Have each group research its assigned disinfectant and identify three examples of the disinfectant and list its advantages, disadvantages, and instructions for use. Then have each group present its findings to the class for discussion.*
Demonstrate the process of cleaning and disinfecting a treatment room.	Procedure 20-2 Performing treatment room cleaning and disinfection (p. 309) (SW/ESLR Competency 20-2, p. 99) – Alcohol (p. 308) – Immersion disinfectants (p. 308) – Glutaraldehyde (p. 308) – Chlorine dioxide (p. 309) – Ortho-phthalaldehyde (p. 309)	📹 Multimedia Procedures DVD: Treatment Room Cleaning and Disinfection 📄 SW Short-Answer Questions 8 (p. 93) 📄 🅔 SW/ESLR Competency 20-2 Performing Treatment Room Cleaning and Disinfection (p. 99) ▸ Discuss how spreading bioburden can be avoided when cleaning large surfaces. *Class Activity Lead a class discussion about the process of cleaning and disinfecting a treatment room. Ask students to identify the equipment and supplies one should have on hand. Why is it important to check the manufacturer's instructions on all products? Record student responses on the board for comparison.*
Describe the CDC guidelines for disinfecting housekeeping surfaces.	☐ Housekeeping surfaces (p. 310) – Carpeting and cloth furnishings (p. 310)	🖥 PPT 41-43 💻 TB questions 16, 18 📄 SW Short-Answer Questions 11-12 (p. 93)

Torres and Ehrlich Modern Dental Assisting, 9th ed.

Bird/Robinson

OBJECTIVES	CONTENT	TEACHING RESOURCES
	– Spills of blood and body substances (p. 310)	CDC: Carpeting (p. 310) CDC: Managing Spills (p. 310) Recall questions 16-18 (p. 310) ▶ Discuss the type of disinfectant you would use for housekeeping surfaces. What must you do to avoid contaminating cleaning solutions? ▶ Discuss CDC recommendations for carpeting and cloth furnishings. *Class Activity Ask students to list different housekeeping surfaces and record responses on the board. Then have students explain how each surface should be disinfected and identify which products should be used.*
Performance Evaluation		🖥️ TB 📓 SW questions (pp. 93-96) 📓 🅔 SW/ESLR Competency 20-1 Placing and Removing Surface Barriers (p. 97) 📓 🅔 SW/ESLR Competency 20-2 Performing Treatment Room Cleaning and Disinfection (p. 99) 🅔 ESLR Electronic Flashcards 🅔 ESLR Practice Quiz 🅔 ESLR Labeling Exercise 18: Identify the Type of Surface Recall questions (pp. 304-310) 💡 CTQ (p. 311)

20.1 Homework/Assignments:

1. Have students explore the EPA Web site to investigate how disinfectants are registered and listed and identify at least two examples of disinfectants that are not included in the Web site. Have students share their findings with the class.

20.1 Instructor's Notes/Student Feedback:

20 **Principles and Techniques of Disinfection**

Slide 1

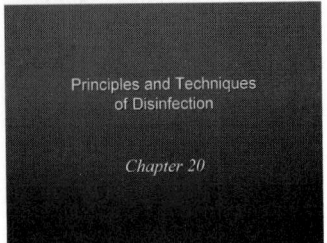

Principles and Techniques
of Disinfection

Chapter 20

Slide 2

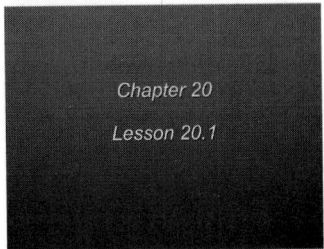

Chapter 20

Lesson 20.1

Slide 3

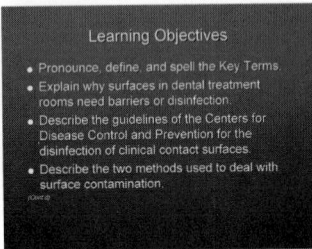

Learning Objectives

- Pronounce, define, and spell the Key Terms.
- Explain why surfaces in dental treatment rooms need barriers or disinfection.
- Describe the guidelines of the Centers for Disease Control and Prevention for the disinfection of clinical contact surfaces.
- Describe the two methods used to deal with surface contamination.

(Cont'd)

Slide 4

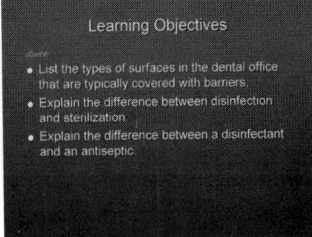

Learning Objectives

(Cont'd)

- List the types of surfaces in the dental office that are typically covered with barriers.
- Explain the difference between disinfection and sterilization.
- Explain the difference between a disinfectant and an antiseptic.

Slide 5

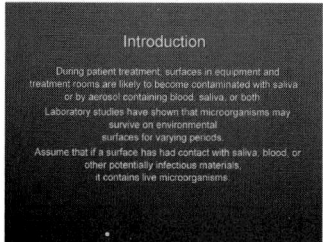

- What is one of the most difficult microorganisms to kill? *(Mycobacterium tuberculosis.)*

- How can exposure to microorganisms that survive on surfaces for long periods of time be reduced?

Slide 6

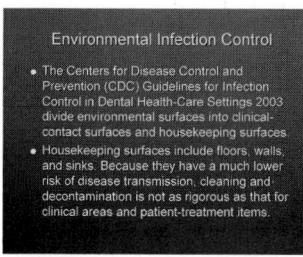

- Cleaning and decontaminating fabric used in carpet, draperies, and chairs is practically impossible without damaging the materials.

- What is a logical alternative to disinfecting these challenging housekeeping surfaces? *(Eliminate them from the clinical area.)*

Slide 7

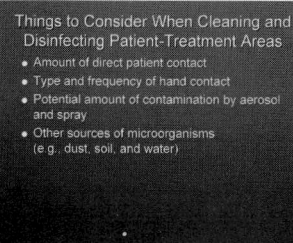

- Start cleaning and disinfecting the most contaminated areas first, and then move toward the least contaminated surfaces. Why is this the best sequence to use for disinfecting treatment areas?

Slide 8

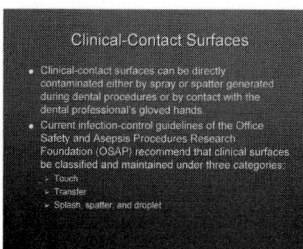

- What are the two divisions of environmental surfaces based on the CDC Guidelines (2003)? *(Clinical contact surfaces and housekeeping surfaces.)*

Bird/Robinson

Slide 9

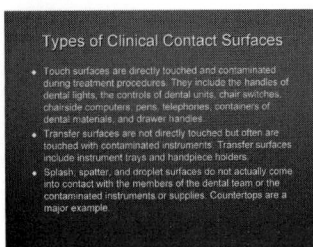

- Of these three categories, which area should be cleaned and disinfected first?
- *Touch surfaces* are directly touched and contaminated during treatment; they should be barrier-protected or disinfected between patients.
- *Transfer surfaces* are not directly touched but often are touched by contaminated instruments.
- *Splash, spatter, and droplet surfaces* do not come into direct contact with dental team members or contaminated instruments; they should be cleaned at least once daily.

Slide 10

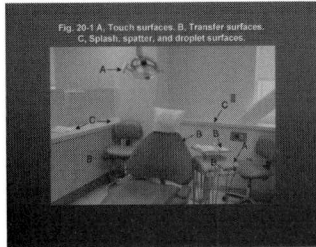

- This photo depicts the following categories of surfaces:
  - A areas: *touch surfaces* are directly touched and contaminated.
  - B areas: *transfer surfaces* are not directly touched but can be touched by contaminated instruments.
  - C areas: *splash, spatter and droplet surfaces* do not actually touch contaminated instruments or supplies.

Slide 11

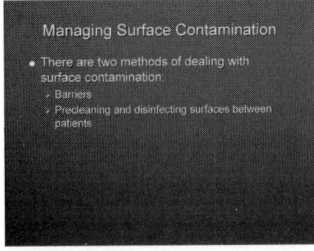

- Most dental offices and clinics will use a combination of precleaning and disinfecting surfaces along with use of barriers.

Slide 12

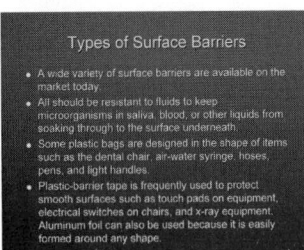

- When removing a contaminated barrier avoid touching a contaminated clean surface underneath the barrier.
- If a clean surface is inadvertently touched, the surface should be cleaned and disinfected.

Slide 13

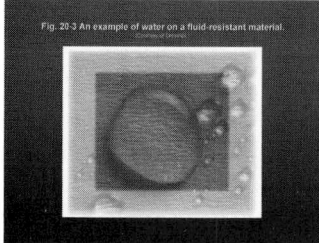

- Fluid, blood, and saliva should bead up on a fluid-resistant barrier.
- It should look like a freshly waxed car on a rainy day.

Slide 14

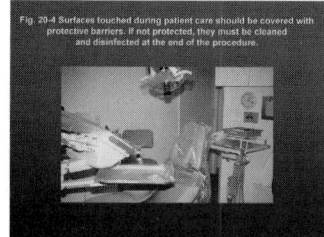

- As you can see in this photo, barriers can be purchased in many varieties of shapes and sizes.
- This variance helps ease application and removal, and it ensures a proper fit.
- Well-fitting barriers reduce contamination of surfaces underneath the barriers.

Slide 15

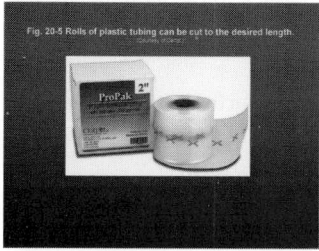

- Barriers can be dispensed in convenient boxes for easy access in treatment areas.

Slide 16

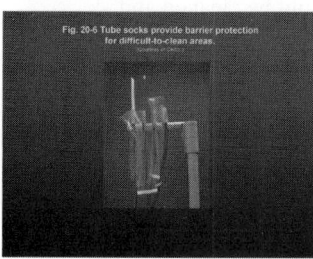

- Because cords can be a variety of lengths and thicknesses, tube socks are convenient to cut to a custom length.

Slide 17

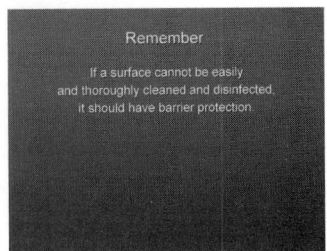

- Using barriers can actually save time and can create a safer environment compared to precleaning and disinfecting a surface.

Slide 18

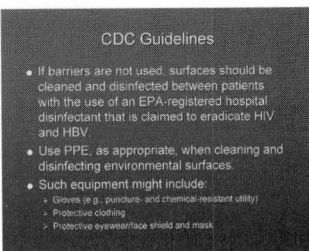

- Remember to spray disinfectant solution into a paper towel rather than directly on hard surfaces to avoid spreading chemical fumes.

Slide 19

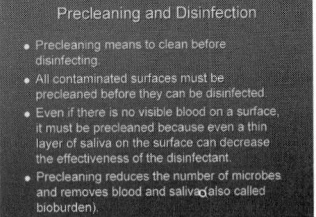

- Even though there are no cases of cross-infection linked to dental treatment room surfaces, the OSHA bloodborne pathogens standard requires that contaminated work surfaces be disinfected between patient visits.

- *Precleaning* is cleaning before disinfection: if a surface is not clean, it cannot be disinfected.

- Regular soap and water can be used for precleaning.

Slide 20

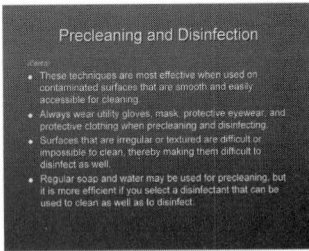

- If barriers are not used, or a combination of barriers and disinfecting is used to maintain surfaces, the surfaces should be cleaned and disinfected using an EPA-registered hospital disinfectant with HIV and HBV claim.

Torres and Ehrlich Modern Dental Assisting, 9th ed.

Bird/Robinson

Slide 21

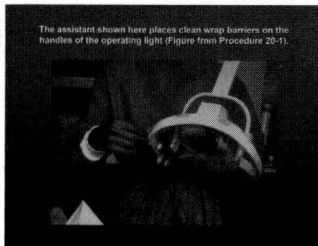

- Barriers can be placed with ungloved, washed hands.
- In this photo the assistant is using barrier tape on the light handles.

Slide 22

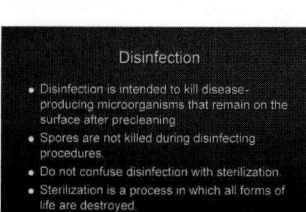

- Autoclave sterilization uses heat, pressure, and steam to kill all forms of life.

Slide 23

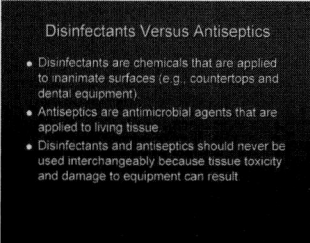

Slide 24

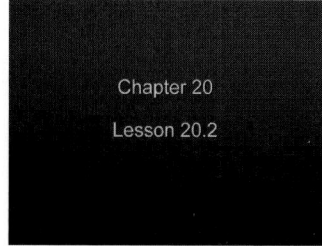

Bird/Robinson

Slide 25

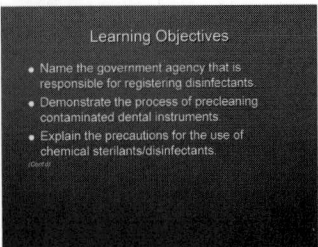

Slide 26

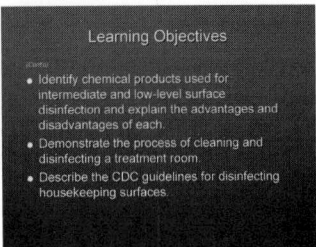

Slide 27

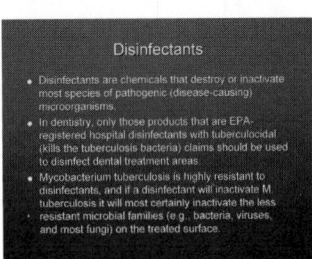

- Disinfectants are effective only when you follow the manufacturer's guidelines for contact time.

- Contact time is the amount of time the product should remain on the surface in order to destroy microorganisms.

- *Sporicidal*: a product that kills spores

- *Virucidal*: a product that kills some viruses

- *Fungicidal*: a product that kills fungi

Slide 28

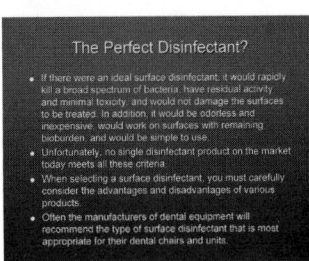

- Disinfectant choice will depend upon the type of equipment used in the office and on any other criteria the staff would like to apply, such as suggesting a product that does not require daily mixing.

Slide 29

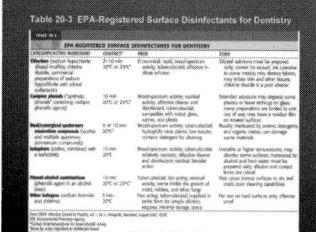

- This chart will be very helpful in determining which one of the EPA-registered surface disinfectants will work best for a specific set of office criteria.
- Note the contact time and the advantages and disadvantages of each product.

Slide 30

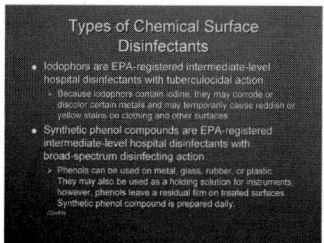

Slide 31

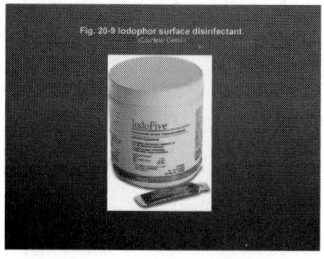

- This iodophor comes in prepackaged individual doses to assist in easy daily preparation.
- Typically the packet is placed in a spray container and water is added.

Slide 32

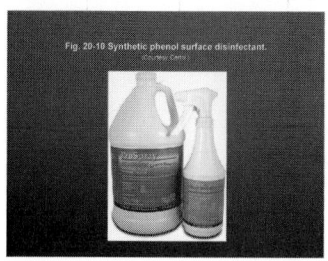

- The larger, gallon size allows one to measure the amount of disinfectant needed to pour into the spray bottle; water is then added.

Bird/Robinson

Slide 33

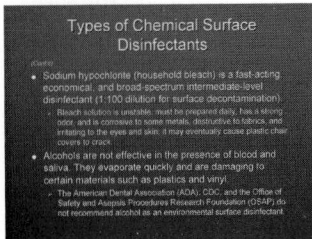

- In the past both of these chemicals were routinely used in the disinfection process.

- We now know they are not the best products to select. Why?

Slide 34

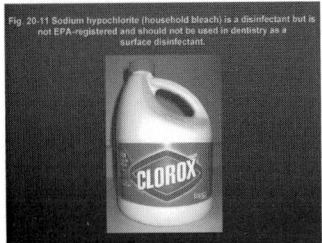

- Bleach can be damaging to plastic tubing if used to control biofilm. It is best to use less harsh alternatives.

Slide 35

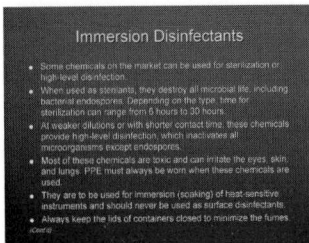

- If there are instruments that cannot withstand the heat from autoclaving and no disposable instruments are available, then immersion disinfectants may be used to sterilize the instruments.

Slide 36

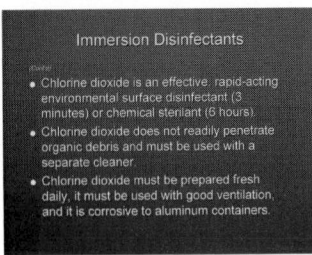

- It is important to maintain proper ventilation in a room in which immersion disinfectants are used.

ELSEVIER

Slide 37

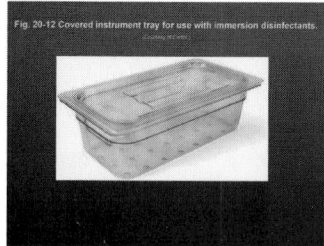

- Clear plastic instrument trays with lids are necessary to reduce fumes and evaporation.

Slide 38

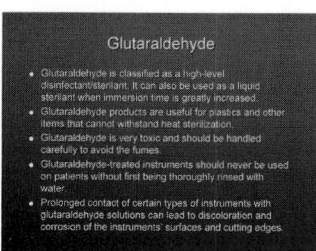

- Many states no longer allow glutaraldehyde to be used in the dental office or clinic unless proper ventilation is installed, and others suggest eliminating its use completely.

Slide 39

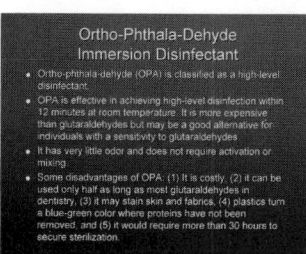

- All immersion disinfectants have disadvantages. Products that work best for the dental office should be selected, bearing in mind the amount of contact time needed and the type of ventilation available.

Slide 40

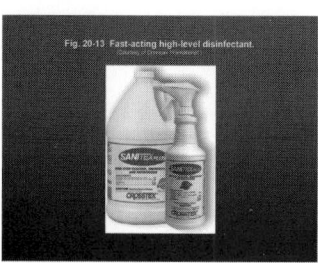

- This is a photo of a name-brand immersion disinfectant.

Slide 41

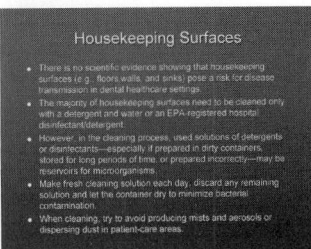

- To reduce aerosols, spray disinfectant directly into a paper towel.
- Clean the areas frequently to avoid dust buildup.

Slide 42

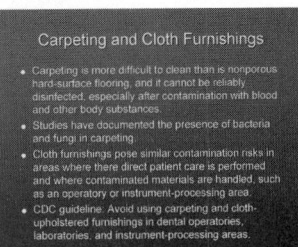

- Dental chairs made of fabric should be covered with a large plastic barrier.

Slide 43

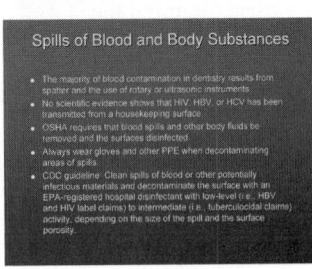

- What type of gloves should be worn when managing blood spills? *(Utility.)*
- Reduce spatter by using suction constantly during rotary or ultrasonic instrument use.

Lesson Plan

21 Principles and Techniques of Instrument Processing and Sterilization

TEACHING FOCUS

This chapter will give students the opportunity to learn about the principles and techniques of instrument processing and sterilization. The student will also have the opportunity to learn about classifying patient-care items, precleaning and packaging instruments, and methods of sterilization.

MATERIALS AND RESOURCES

- ☐ computer and PowerPoint projector (all Lessons)
- ☐ instruments and sterilization packing materials (Lesson 21.1)
- ☐ sterilization monitors (Lesson 21.2)

LESSON CHECKLIST

Preparations for this lesson include:

- lecture
- evaluation of student knowledge and skills needed to perform all entry-level activities related to the principles and techniques of instrument processing and sterilization, including:
  - ○ classification of patient-care items
  - ○ methods of sterilization
  - ○ precleaning and packaging instruments

ELSEVIER

Torres and Ehrlich Modern Dental Assisting, 9th ed.

KEY TERMS

autoclave (p. 323)
biologic indicators (p. 333)
biologic monitoring (p. 332)
chemical vapor sterilization (p. 327)
clean area (p. 316)
contaminated area (p. 316)
critical instrument (p. 314)
dry-heat sterilizer (p. 328)
endospore (p. 332)
event-related packaging (p. 336)

multiparameter indicator (p. 332)
noncritical instrument (p. 315)
process indicator (p. 332)
process integrator (p. 332)
semicritical instrument (p. 314)
single-parameter indicator (p. 332)
sterilant (p. 323)
sterilization (p. 315)
ultrasonic cleaner (p. 318)
use-life (p. 331)

ADDITIONAL RESOURCES

PowerPoint slides (IER, Evolve):1-87
Multimedia Procedures DVD:
    Autoclaving Instruments
    Operating the Ultrasonic Cleaner

Legend

CTQ	**DVD**	**ESLR**	**IDO**	**SW**	**TB**	**PPT**
Critical Thinking Question	Multimedia Procedures Videos and Animations	EVOLVE Student Learning Resources	Interactive Dental Office CD-ROM	Student Workbook	Test Bank on the TEACH CD-ROM	PowerPoint Slides

Class Activities are indicated in ***bold italic***.

Torres and Ehrlich Modern Dental Assisting, 9th ed.

Bird/Robinson

LESSON 21.1

PRETEST

1. An autoclave instrument sterilization process uses which sterilization agent?
   a. moist heat/steam
   b. hot formaldehyde vapors
   c. heated air
   d. ethylene oxide gas

2. What is classified as a critical instrument?
   a. mouth mirror
   b. amalgam condenser
   c. scalpel
   d. external x-ray head

3. The CDC recommends that sterilization devices used in the dental office be approved by what agency?
   a. ADA
   b. FDA
   c. OSHA
   d. EPA

4. What should not be located in the packaging area of the instrument processing area?
   a. set-up arrangement materials
   b. biologic monitoring materials
   c. stored, sterilized instrument packets
   d. instrument wrapping materials

5. When should holding solutions be used as part of the instrument processing procedure?
   a. after every dental procedure as part of routine instrument processing
   b. before every dental procedure as part of routine instrument processing
   c. only when instrument processing cannot be completed
   d. every morning as part of routine set-up of the instrument processing area

6. The purpose of the ultrasonic cleaner is to
   a. sterilize contaminated instruments.
   b. disinfect contaminated instruments.
   c. hold contaminated instruments until instrument processing can be completed.
   d. loosen and remove debris from contaminated instruments.

7. What is used to test the efficacy of the ultrasonic cleaner?
   a. lightweight aluminum foil
   b. physical indicator
   c. chemical indicator
   d. biologic indicator

8. What does a single-parameter chemical monitoring device indicate?
   a. exposure to pressure
   b. exposure to temperature/heat
   c. exposure to time
   d. exposure to pressure, heat, and time

9. What is a disadvantage of using an unsaturated chemical vapor sterilizer?
   a. cannot use closed containers
   b. long sterilization time
   c. corrodes instruments
   d. instruments take a long time to dry after the sterilization cycle

10. The typical steam sterilization temperature at 30 minutes is
    a. 50° F.
    b. 100° F.
    c. 150° F.
    d. 250° F.

Answers

1. a	3. b	5. c	7. a	9. a
2. c	4. c	6. d	8. b	10. d

Bird/Robinson

BACKGROUND ASSESSMENT

Question: What are the different levels of cleaning and preparing surfaces and instruments for use in the dental office? What are the different sterilization methods in a dental office setting?

Answer: High-level disinfection is the process that kills some but not all bacterial endospores and inactivates *Mycobacterium tuberculosis*. Intermediate-level disinfection inactivates *M. tuberculosis* and destroys less-resistant organisms such as hepatitis B virus and human immunodeficiency virus (HIV). Low-level disinfection is ineffective against *M. tuberculosis* and should be used in the dental office only for housekeeping purposes. Sterilization can be achieved by using a steam autoclave, chemical vapor sterilization, dry heat oven, or chemical disinfection/sterilization. Sterilization inactivates all microbial life, including bacterial spores, viruses, bacteria, and fungi.

Question: What are the seven steps for instrument processing? How can effectiveness of instrument processing be measured?

Answer: The seven steps for instrument processing are: (1) the contaminated instruments are transported to the processing area in a manner that minimizes the risk of exposure to persons and the environment; (2) the instruments are cleaned with a hands-free approach through the use of a mechanical cleaner such as an ultrasonic cleaner; (3) the instruments are packaged or wrapped in the clean section of the processing area; (4) the instruments are loaded into the sterilizer following manufacturer's guidelines where the sterilization process is carried through; (5) the sterilized instruments are stored in a clean, dry environment in a manner that maintains the integrity of the package; (6) the packages are delivered to the point of use in a manner that maintains sterility of the instruments until they are used; (7) an effective quality assurance program that documents proper training exercises, record-keeping, maintenance, and use of biological indicators. The effectiveness of the instrument processing steps can be measured by using three monitoring systems: (1) physical monitor, (2) chemical monitor, (3) biologic monitor. The first two steps must be used with the third monitoring system in order for true sterilization to be determined. Physical monitoring of the sterilization method involves looking at the gauges and readings on the sterilizer. Chemical monitoring (external and internal) involves the use of a heat-sensitive chemical that changes color when exposed to certain conditions. Biologic monitoring, or spore testing, involves testing a sample vial of bacteria and spores to see if they have been destroyed after being exposed to the sterilization process.

CRITICAL THINKING QUESTION

A dental assistant is given the task of designing an instrument-processing area in the dental office. She needs to purchase equipment and supplies and set up the area so that a step-by-step process can be completed consistently each time instruments must be prepared for sterilization. What sections should be included in the processing area? What tasks would be carried out in each section? What items and equipment would be found in each section?

Guidelines: The processing area would have three sections: (1) contaminated area, (2) packing area, (3) sterilization and storage area. Each section would be adequately labeled with a laminated sign to avoid confusion about which tasks should be completed in each. The tasks in the contaminated area would be to discard waste, place instruments in holding solutions, clean the instruments in the ultrasonic cleaning unit, rinse and dry the instruments, and place rust inhibitors on the instruments. The tasks in the packing area would be to arrange the tray setups, place the biologic monitors with each instrument setup, and wrap or package the instruments. The tasks in the third section include the sterilization and storage of instruments. In this section, record-keeping and the assembling of disposables on trays can also be completed. Each section of the processing area must also contain adequate supplies and equipment. The following items should be in the contaminated section: clean, protective eyewear, utility gloves, counter space, a sink, waste receptacles; holding solution; an ultrasonic cleaner; and an eye-wash station. The second section should include supplies for wrapping instruments before sterilization, such as biologic monitors, wrapping paper for cassettes, sterilization pouches, autoclave tape, and marking pens. The third section should be supplied with a sterilizer, sterilizing agents, storage areas and cabinets, record log, and supplies for assembling disposables on trays.

Bird/Robinson

OBJECTIVES	CONTENT	TEACHING RESOURCES
Pronounce, define, and spell the Key Terms.	■ Key terms (pp. 312-313) ■ Introduction (p. 313)	SW Fill in the Blank questions 1-17 (p. 102-103) ESLR Electronic Flashcards ▶ Discuss each of the key terms in Chapter 21, focusing on the definition, pronunciation, and spelling of each. *Class Activity Have students make flash cards of each key term, with the term on one side and the definition on the other. Then have the students quiz each other with the flash cards.*
Discuss the seven steps in processing dental instruments.	■ Introduction (p. 313)	PPT 5-8 SW Short-Answer Questions 1 (p. 101) Table 21-1 Seven Steps for Instrument Processing (p. 314) Terms Used in Instrument Processing (p. 315) CDC Rankings of Evidence (p. 315) ▶ Discuss the use of CDC rankings of evidence in dental assisting. ▶ Discuss what would happen if one of the seven steps for instrument processing were ignored. *Class Activity Divide the class into small groups, and assign each group one of the seven steps in processing dental instruments. Have each group outline the responsibilities and occurrence of its step and discuss its findings to the rest of the class.* *Class Activity Have students review the three levels of disinfection. Discuss which situations would call for a low-level, intermediate-level, or high-level disinfection.*
Describe the classification of instruments used to determine the type of processing.	■ Classification of patient-care items (p. 313) ☐ Critical instruments (p. 314) ☐ Semicritical instruments (p. 314) ☐ Noncritical instruments (p. 315) ☐ Personal protective equipment (p. 315)	PPT 9-15 TB questions 1, 3-4 SW Short-Answer Questions 11; Fill in the Blank questions 6-8; Multiple Choice questions 1-2 (pp. 101-103) Table 21-2 CDC Classification of Instruments and Procedures (p. 328) CDC Guidelines for Sterilization and Disinfection of Patient-Care Items (p. 315) Recall questions 1-2 (p. 315) Figure 21-1 PPE must be worn while preparing instruments for sterilization (p. 316) ▶ Discuss what would constitute personal protective equipment (PPE) and why it is necessary for a dental assistant.

OBJECTIVES	CONTENT	TEACHING RESOURCES
		Class Activity Have each student create a table with three columns: one for Critical Instruments; one for Semicritical Instruments; and one for Noncritical Instruments. Have students list the instruments used in the dental office that fall under each of the three categories and share their lists with the rest of the class.
Describe the Centers for Disease Control and Prevention (CDC) guidelines for sterilization and disinfection of patient-care items.	☐ Personal protective equipment (p. 315)	SW Short-Answer Questions 14 (p. 102) CDC Guidelines for Sterilization and Disinfection of Patient-care Items (p. 315) ▸ Discuss the merits of the CDC Guidelines for Sterilization and Disinfection of Patient-Care Items and why a dental assistant should know them. *Class Activity Have students research current CDC guidelines for sterilization and disinfection of dental instruments on the Internet. Have each student write a brief description of the guidelines and how these guidelines would fit into a dental office with which they are familiar. Students should share their findings with the rest of the class. (For students to prepare for this activity, see Homework/Assignments #1.)*
Describe the CDC guidelines for cleaning and decontamination of instruments.	■ Transporting and processing contaminated patient-care items (p. 315)	PPT 16 TB question 5 SW Short-Answer Questions 15 (p. 102) CDC Guidelines for Receiving, Cleaning, and Decontamination Procedures (p. 316) ▸ Discuss what hazards a dental assistant might face in transporting and processing contaminated patient-care items. ▸ Discuss why critical instruments should not be stored unwrapped. *Class Activity Have each student compare the cleaning and decontamination of instruments to the sterilization of instruments. Each student should list at least three differences. Have students share their findings with the rest of the class.*
Explain the purpose of a holding solution.	■ Instrument-processing area (p. 316) ☐ Workflow pattern (p. 316) ☐ Contaminated area (p. 316) ☐ Preparation and packaging area (p. 317)	PPT 17-30 TB questions 6-8 SW Short-Answer Questions 12; Fill in the Blank questions 9-10; Multiple Choice questions 3-4; Topics for discussion (pp. 101-103, 105) CDC Guidelines for Instrument-Processing Area (p. 316) Figure 21-2 Instrument processing areas (p. 317)

Torres and Ehrlich Modern Dental Assisting, 9th ed.

Bird/Robinson

OBJECTIVES	CONTENT	TEACHING RESOURCES
	■ Precleaning and packaging instruments (p. 318) ☐ Holding solution (p. 318)	Figure 21-3 Waste items are properly discarded (p. 317) Figure 21-4 A modern sterilization center (p. 317) Recall questions 3-4 (p. 321) ▸ Discuss how to set up an instrument processing area for the most efficient and safest use. ▸ Discuss the safest methods for preparing and packaging patient care instruments. ***Class Activity Divide the class into small groups. Each group should list the purpose of a holding solution and describe a situation in which one would be used.***
Understand the safety precautions necessary when operating an ultrasonic cleaner.	■ Precleaning and packaging instruments (p. 318) ☐ Holding solution (p. 318) ☐ Hand scrubbing (p. 318) ☐ Ultrasonic cleaning (p. 318) – Ultrasonic cleaning solutions (p. 320) Procedure 21-1 Operating the ultrasonic cleaner (p. 319) (SW/ESLR Competency 21-1, p. 107) – Care of the ultrasonic cleaner (p. 320) – Testing the ultrasonic cleaner (p. 321) ☐ Automated washers/disinfectors (p. 321) ☐ Drying, lubrication, and corrosion control (p. 321) ☐ Packaging instruments (p. 321) – Packaging materials (p. 322) ☐ Sterilization of unwrapped instruments (p. 322)	PPT 31-44 Multimedia Procedures DVD: Operating the Ultrasonic Cleaner TB questions 9-13 SW Short-Answer Questions 13; Fill in the Blank question 16; Multiple Choice questions 5-9 (pp. 101-103) SW/ESLR Competency 21-1 Operating the Ultrasonic Cleaner (p. 107) Figure 21-5 Commercial holding solutions for use in precleaning (p. 318) Figure 21-6 Ultrasonic cleaning system (p. 318) Figure 21-7 It is important to keep the ultrasonic cleaner covered (p. 320) Figure 21-8 A commercial all-purpose ultrasonic cleaner (p. 320) Figure 21-9 An enzyme ultrasonic cleaner in tablet form (p. 320) Figure 21-10 Special tartar and stain remover ultrasonic solution (p. 320) Figure 21-11 A Miele thermal disinfector (p. 321) CDC Guidelines for Preparation and Packaging (p. 321) CDC Guidelines for Sterilization of Unwrapped Instruments (p. 322) Recall questions 5-11 (pp. 321-322) ▸ Discuss the merits of ultrasonic cleaning and how a dental assistant can use the method to its best advantage. ▸ Discuss the effects of corrosion on patient-care instruments and how corrosion can be avoided. ***Class Activity Divide the class into pairs. Have one partner of each pair demonstrate the proper steps when using an ultrasonic cleaning unit and the other partner provide feedback. Have the pairs switch roles.***

Bird/Robinson

OBJECTIVES	CONTENT	TEACHING RESOURCES
Describe the precautions necessary when packaging materials for sterilization.	☐ Packaging instruments (p. 321) – Packaging materials (p. 322) ☐ Sterilization of unwrapped instruments (p. 322)	▣ PPT 45-50 ▣ TB questions 14-15 ▣ SW Short-Answer Questions 3; Multiple Choice question 11 (pp. 101, 104) Table 21-3 Packaging Materials and Types of Sterilization (p. 322) CDC Guidelines for Preparation and Packaging (p. 321) CDC Guidelines for Sterilization of Unwrapped Instruments (p. 322) Figure 21-12 Self-seal packages provide an excellent wrap for sterilized materials (p. 322) Recall questions 26-27 (p. 334) ▸ Discuss the different types of packaging materials available and their relative merits. ▸ Discuss when it would be appropriate to perform unwrapped sterilization. *Class Activity **Have each student prepare a summary of events that could cause injury during packaging instruments for sterilization; have them include preventive strategies. Have students share their thoughts with the rest of the class.***
Describe the CDC guidelines for preparation and packaging instruments for sterilization.	☐ Packaging instruments (p. 321) – Packaging materials (p. 322) ☐ Sterilization of unwrapped instruments (p. 322)	▣ SW Short-Answer Questions 16 (p. 102) CDC Guidelines for Preparation and Packaging (p. 321) CDC Guidelines for Sterilization of Unwrapped Instruments (p. 322) ▸ Discuss the importance of the CDC Guidelines for Preparation and Packaging to a dental assistant. ▸ Discuss why the CDC recommends that implanted devices should not be sterilized unwrapped. *Class Activity **Distribute instruments and sterilization packing materials to the class. Have each student demonstrate the proper steps in preparing and packaging instruments according to CDC guidelines.***

21.1 Homework/Assignments:

1. Have students research current CDC guidelines for sterilization and disinfection of dental instruments on the Internet. Have each student write a brief description of the guidelines and how these guidelines would fit into a dental office with which they are familiar. Students should share their findings with the rest of the class.

21.1 Instructor's Notes/Student Feedback:

LESSON 21.2

CRITICAL THINKING QUESTION

A dental assistant works in a dental office where numerous hinged instruments are used daily for surgery and other procedures. While preparing these instruments for sterilization, the assistant must determine which method is best for each one. The assistant must also be prepared to sterilize instruments quickly, either during a procedure or if needed for another patient, since this particular dental office does not have a large inventory of instruments. Which method will be used to sterilize each instrument, and what would be the best way to complete flash sterilization in this office?

Guidelines: Dental offices require the use of many specialized instruments to complete many different procedures and treatments. Hand instruments, surgical instruments, glass slabs, metal impression trays, and high-quality hinged pliers made of stainless steel can be sterilized using a steam autoclave or dry heat oven. When sterilizing hinged instruments, care must be taken to prevent corrosion and rust from building up in the hinged areas. Flash sterilization can be completed effectively using a dry heat sterilizer. A dry sterilizer is especially desirable in an office that uses a high volume of hinged instruments.

OBJECTIVES	CONTENT	TEACHING RESOURCES

Describe the three most common methods of heat sterilization and the advantages and disadvantages of each.	■ Methods of sterilization (p. 322)
	
	☐ Steam autoclave (p. 323)
	
	  – Packaging instruments (p. 323)
	
	Procedure 21-2 Autoclaving instruments (pp. 326-327) (SW/ESLR Competency 21-2, pp. 109-110)
	
	☐ Flash sterilization (p. 325)
	
	☐ Unsaturated chemical vapor sterilization (p. 327)
	
	  – Advantages (p. 327)
	
	  – Disadvantages (p. 327)
	
	  – Filtration and monitoring of chemical vapors (p. 327)
	
	  – Packaging (p. 328)
	
	  – Pressure, temperature, and time (p. 328)
	
	☐ Dry-heat sterilization (p. 328)
		⊠▀ PPT 53-68
		
		▄▄ Multimedia Procedures DVD: Autoclaving Instruments
		
		▀ TB questions 2, 21-22
		
		SW Short-Answer Questions 2; Fill in the Blank questions 1-3 (pp. 101-102)
		
		SW 𝒆 SW/ESLR Competency 21-2 Autoclaving Instruments (pp. 109-110)
		
		Table 21-4 Advantages and Disadvantages of Sterilization Methods (p. 323)
		
		Table 21-5 Sterilization and Disinfection Guide for Common Dental Items (pp. 324-325)
		
		Figure 21-13 Steam autoclave (p. 323)
		
		Table 21-6 Typical Steam Temperatures in Sterilizing Cycle (p. 325)
		
		Figure 21-14 Vacuum-type autoclave (p. 325)
		
		Figure 21-25 STAT/M sterilizer (p. 325)
		
		Recall question 12 (p. 330)
		
		▶ Discuss how an autoclave works and how it sterilizes instruments.
		
		▶ Discuss what measures a dental assistant should take to safely operate an autoclave.
		
		Class Activity Divide the class into small groups. Have each group write game questions relating to each of the heat sterilization processes. Each team will answer questions from opposing teams. Calculate which team earns the most points.

OBJECTIVES	CONTENT	TEACHING RESOURCES
	– Static air sterilizers (p. 328) – Forced air sterilizers (p. 329)	
Explain the primary disadvantage of flash sterilization.	☐ Flash sterilization (p. 325) ☐ Unsaturated chemical vapor sterilization (p. 327) – Advantages (p. 327) – Disadvantages (p. 327) ⎡Procedure⎤ 21-3 Sterilizing instruments with chemical vapor (p. 328) (SW/ESLR Competency 21-3, p. 111) – Filtration and monitoring of chemical vapors (p. 327) – Packaging (p. 328) – Pressure, temperature, and time (p. 328) ☐ Dry-heat sterilization (p. 328) – Static air sterilizers (p. 328) ⎡Procedure⎤ 21-4 Sterilizing instruments with dry heat (p. 329) (SW/ESLR Competency 21-4, p. 113) – Forced air sterilizers (p. 329)	🖥 PPT 58-59 💻 TB 19-20, 23-25 📄 SW Short-Answer Questions 7; Multiple Choice questions 18-19 (pp. 101, 104) 📄*e* SW/ESLR Competency 21-3 Sterilizing Instruments with Chemical Vapor (p. 111) 📄*e* SW/ESLR Competency 21-4 Sterilizing Instruments with Dry Heat (p. 113) Figure 21-16 Sterilant solution for a chemical vapor sterilizer (p. 327) Recall questions 13-15 (p. 330) ▶ Discuss and compare the advantages and disadvantages of flash sterilization, chemical vapor sterilization, and dry-heat sterilization. ▶ Discuss the advantages and disadvantages of a static air sterilizer and forced-air sterilizer. *Class Activity Have students make a table with three columns: one for Flash Sterilization, one for Chemical Vapor Sterilization, and one for Dry-heat Sterilization. Have students fill each column with the reasons each type of sterilization is used, and the pros and cons of each. Have students share their findings.*
Explain the limitation of chemical liquid sterilizers.	☐ Ethylene oxide sterilization (p. 329) ☐ Liquid chemical sterilants (p. 329) ⎡Procedure⎤ 21-5 Sterilizing instruments with chemical liquid (p. 331)	🖥 PPT 69-71 💻 TB question 27 📄 SW Short-Answer Questions 10; Fill in the Blank question 12; Multiple Choice question 22 (pp. 101-102, 104)

OBJECTIVES	CONTENT	TEACHING RESOURCES
	(SW/ESLR Competency 21-5, pp. 115-116)	SW/ESLR Competency 21-5 Sterilizing Instruments with Chemical Liquid (pp. 115-116) CDC Liquid Chemical Sterilants/High-Level Disinfectants (p. 330) Figure 21-17 Sporox II is a high-level disinfectant/sterilant (p. 330) Recall questions 16-17 (p. 330) ▶ Discuss when it would be appropriate to use chemical liquid sterilization. ▶ Discuss the importance of having MSDS sheets for chemical liquid sterilizers. *Class Activity Divide the class into small groups. Have the students write a few brief paragraphs in which they identify situations when chemical liquid sterilization should be used. Students should also include the limitations of chemical liquid sterilization and how to compensate for the limitations.*
Explain how sterilization failures can occur.	☐ Sterilization failures (p. 330)	PPT 72-73 TB question 26 SW Short-Answer Questions 9; Multiple Choice questions 16-17 (pp. 101, 104) Table 21-7 Results of Sterilization Errors (p. 331) Recall question 18 (p. 333) ▶ Discuss what could lead a dental assistant to improperly sterilize instruments. ▶ Discuss the consequences of sterilization failure to the dental office. *Class Activity Divide the class into five groups and assign each group one of the sterilization errors found in the textbook in Table 21-3. Each group should present, in the form of actual demonstrations or photos, examples of how the error can occur*
Describe the three forms of sterilization monitoring.	■ Sterilization monitoring (p. 330) ☐ Physical monitoring (p. 332) ☐ Chemical monitoring (p. 332) – Process indicators (p. 332)	PPT 74-82 TB question 17 SW Short-Answer Questions 8; Multiple Choice question 12 (pp. 101, 104) CDC Guidelines for Sterilization Monitoring (p. 330) Figure 21-18 (A) Unprocessed instruments; (B) Wrapped instruments after processing (p. 332)

Bird/Robinson

OBJECTIVES	CONTENT	TEACHING RESOURCES
	– Process integrators (p. 332) – Limitations (p. 332) ☐ Biologic monitoring (p. 332)	Recall question 19 (p. 333) 💡 CTQ 2 (p. 336) ▶ Discuss what constitutes physical monitoring of sterilization. ▶ Discuss why it is important to monitor the sterilization procedures in a dental office. ***Class Activity Bring the various forms of sterilization monitors into the classroom. As students view the monitors, have them discuss when and how each one is used.***
Explain the differences between process indicators and process integrators.	☐ Chemical monitoring (p. 332) – Process indicators (p. 332) – Process integrators (p. 332) – Limitations (p. 332) ☐ Biologic monitoring (p. 332)	🖥 PPT 76-79 📄 SW Short-Answer Questions 5; Fill in the Blank questions 14, 17; Multiple Choice question 13 (pp. 101, 103-104) CDC Guidelines for Sterilization Monitoring (p. 330) Figure 21-19 Integrator strips used inside packs to monitor time, temperature, and pressure (p. 332) Figure 21-20 The dental assistant inserts the integrator strip into the sterilization pouch with their instruments (p. 333) Recall questions 20-23 (p. 333) ▶ Discuss which types of process integrators might be the most convenient or reliable to use. ***Class Activity Divide the class into small groups. Have each group discuss the differences between process indicators and process integrators, and identify what each measures. What are the advantages and disadvantages of using them alone or in conjunction with other monitoring devices? Have groups present their conclusions to the class.***
Describe when and how biologic monitoring is done.	☐ Biologic monitoring (p. 332) Procedure 21-6 Performing biologic monitoring (p. 334) (SW/ESLR Competency 21-6, p. 117)	🖥 PPT 80-82 💻 TB question 18 📄 SW Short-Answer Questions 6; Fill in the Blank questions 4, 13, 15; Multiple Choice questions 14-15 (pp. 101-104) 📄💿 SW/ESLR Competency 21-6 Performing Biologic Monitoring (p. 117) CDC Guidelines for Sterilization Monitoring (p. 330) Figure 21-21 Use of a mail-in service is a convenient method of biologic monitoring (p. 333)

ELSEVIER

OBJECTIVES	CONTENT	TEACHING RESOURCES
		Figure 21-22 In-office biologic monitoring system (p. 333)
		Additional reasons for biologic monitoring (p. 333)
		▸ Discuss why it would be important to perform biologic monitoring in a dental office and how often it should be done.
		▸ Discuss the different types of biologic indicators and the most efficient use of each.
		*Class Activity **Have the students conduct Internet research on the various biological monitoring devices available for use in dental offices. Students should present their findings to the class, focusing on how and when the various devices are used.***

21.2 Homework/Assignments:

21.2 Instructor's Notes/Student Feedback:

ELSEVIER

Bird/Robinson

LESSON 21.3

CRITICAL THINKING QUESTION

The biologic monitor system used weekly in a dental office to monitor the success of sterilization processes has come back negative, indicating sterilization failure in the instrument-processing area. What are common errors found in the instrument-processing area and what might be their cause?
Guidelines: Five common errors could occur in the dental office instrument-processing area that would lead to a negative biologic reading: (1) inadequate instrument cleaning, (2) improper packaging, (3) improper loading of the sterilizer,(4) improper timing, or (5) improper temperature. Some examples of inadequate instrument cleaning are instruments that have dried blood or debris on them. In these cases, underlying organisms may be insulated from the sterilizing agents. If improper wrapping is a factor, the wrapping may be too thick, preventing the sterilizing agent from reaching the instruments. Another packaging error could occur if the packaging materials are not compatible with the sterilization method being used. For example, the packaging may melt, preventing the sterilizing agent from penetrating into the instruments. When the sterilizer is overloaded, the sterilizing agent cannot reach the instruments in the center of the load. Errors caused by improper timing mean that instruments were not exposed to the sterilization agent for a sufficient time, resulting in improper or incomplete instrument sterilization. And finally, insufficient heat will result in improper and incomplete sterilization. All of these errors will result in incomplete microorganism destruction and unsuccessful sterilization cycles.

OBJECTIVES	CONTENT	TEACHING RESOURCES
Describe the steps in cleaning and sterilization of the high-speed dental handpiece.	■ Handpiece sterilization (p. 334) ☐ Flushing techniques (p. 334) ☐ Sterilizing techniques (p. 334) *Procedure* 21-7 Sterilizing the dental handpiece (p. 335) (SW/ESLR Competency 21-7, p. 119)	PPT 85-87 TB questions 28-29 SW Short-Answer Questions 4; Multiple Choice questions 23-24 (pp. 101, 104) SW/ESLR Competency 21-7 Sterilizing the Dental Handpiece (p. 117) CDC Storage Area for Sterilized Items and Clean Dental Supplies (p. 336) Recall questions 24-25 (p. 334) Instruments and supplies stored in a closed cabinet (p. 336) Legal and Ethical Implications (p. 336) Eye to the Future (p. 336) ▸ Discuss the unique challenges facing the dental assistant in sterilizing the handpiece. ▸ Discuss how a handpiece can be damaged by improper sterilization techniques. *Class Activity Have students discuss the importance of proper handpiece sterilization. Review the materials that may get lodged in a handpiece and how the transfer of these materials might affect other patients.*

Bird/Robinson

OBJECTIVES	CONTENT	TEACHING RESOURCES
Performance Evaluation		TB
		SW questions (pp. 101-104)
		SW Topics for discussion (p. 105)
		SW/ESLR Competency 21-1 Operating the Ultrasonic Cleaner (p. 107)
		SW/ESLR Competency 21-2 Autoclaving Instruments (pp. 109-110)
		SW/ESLR Competency 21-3 Sterilizing Instruments with Chemical Vapor (p. 111)
		SW/ESLR Competency 21-4 Sterilizing Instruments with Dry Heat (p. 113)
		SW/ESLR Competency 21-5 Sterilizing Instruments with Chemical Liquid (pp. 115-116)
		SW/ESLR Competency 21-6 Performing Biologic Monitoring (p. 117)
		SW/ESLR Competency 21-7 Sterilizing the Dental Handpiece (p. 119)
		ESLR Electronic Flashcards
		ESLR Practice Quiz
		Recall questions (pp. 315-334)
		CTQ (p. 336)

21.3 Homework/Assignments:

21.3 Instructor's Notes/Student Feedback:

Torres and Ehrlich Modern Dental Assisting, 9th ed.

Bird/Robinson

Slide 1

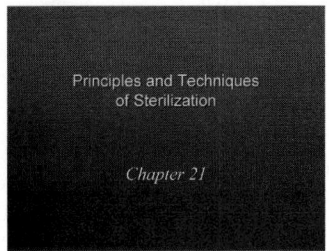

Principles and Techniques
of Sterilization

Chapter 21

Slide 2

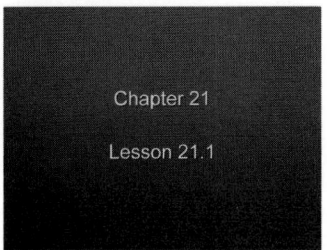

Chapter 21

Lesson 21.1

Slide 3

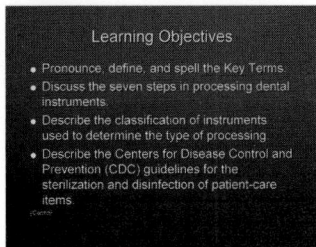

Learning Objectives

- Pronounce, define, and spell the Key Terms.
- Discuss the seven steps in processing dental instruments.
- Describe the classification of instruments used to determine the type of processing.
- Describe the Centers for Disease Control and Prevention (CDC) guidelines for the sterilization and disinfection of patient-care items.

(Cont'd)

Slide 4

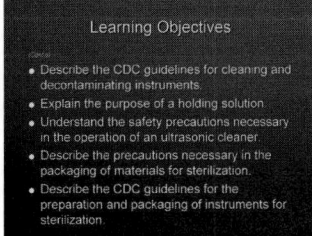

Learning Objectives

(Cont'd)

- Describe the CDC guidelines for cleaning and decontaminating instruments.
- Explain the purpose of a holding solution.
- Understand the safety precautions necessary in the operation of an ultrasonic cleaner.
- Describe the precautions necessary in the packaging of materials for sterilization.
- Describe the CDC guidelines for the preparation and packaging of instruments for sterilization.

Bird/Robinson

Slide 5

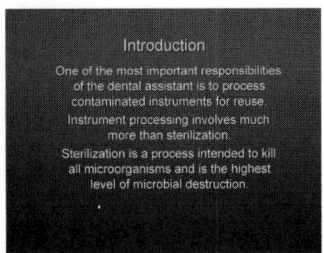

- Sterilization is one step in instrument processing.

- What are the other steps involved in instrument processing? (*Transport, cleaning, packaging, storage, delivery, and quality assurance.*)

- Many times the terms disinfection and sterilization are used interchangeably. Are these terms interchangeable? Why or why not?

Slide 6

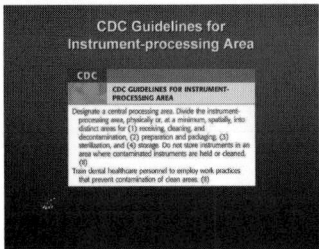

- The Centers for Disease Control and Prevention's mission is to promote health and quality of life by preventing and controlling disease, injury, and disability.

- Why does the CDC recommend a central processing area?

- Why is it recommended that instruments not be stored in an area where contaminated instruments are held or cleaned? (*This recommendation will reduce the chance of cross-contamination.*)

Slide 7

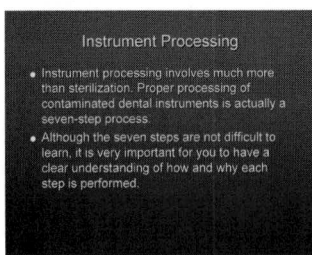

- Why is it important to have a clear understanding of how and why each of the seven steps is performed? (*Having a clear understanding will prevent error and the chance that a mistake could be made. A mistake could mean cross- contamination or injury to a dental care worker.*)

Slide 8

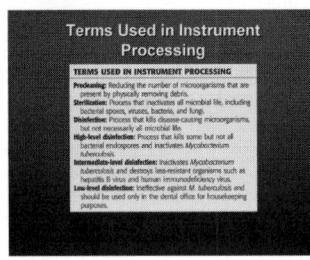

- Several key terms are used to describe tasks used during instrument processing. These terms are not used interchangeably.

- What are examples of items in the dental office setting that are disinfected after every procedure? (*Countertops, dental chair, dental light, etc.*)

- What are examples of items in the dental office setting that are sterilized after every procedure? (*Dental instruments, burs, handpiece, etc.*)

Slide 9

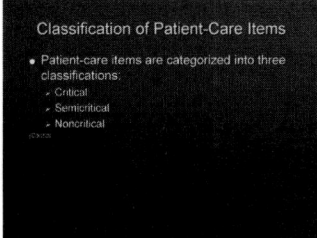

- These categories help determine which sterilization methods best ensure the safety of dental care workers and patients.

Slide 10

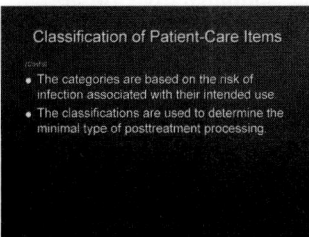

- What is the benefit of having these categories? (*To determine the proper method of disinfection and sterilization.*)

Slide 11

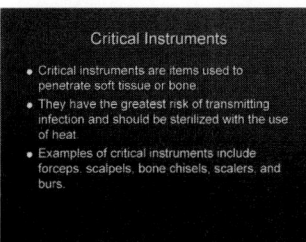

- Handling these instruments carefully during the seven-step instrument preparation process is essential to the safety and health of the dental care workers.

- If necessary, how should these instruments be disposed of? (*Place these items in a sharps container.*)

Slide 12

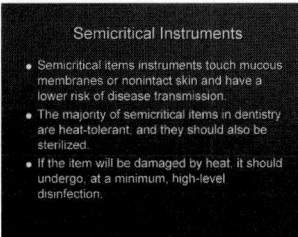

- What are examples of semicritical instruments? (*Plastic-handled brushes, high-volume evacuator (HVE) tips, rubber dam forceps, x-ray film holders, and amalgam carriers.*)

Bird/Robinson

Slide 13

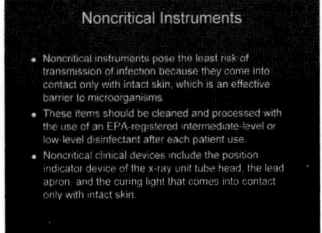

- Can you think of another way to maintain disinfection of these noncritical instruments? (*Use plastic barriers such as plastic bags or plastic tube sleeves.*)

- Do these items need to be disinfected when plastic barriers are used? (*Yes, a disinfection solution and disinfection techniques are still used if the surface below has become contaminated.*)

Slide 14

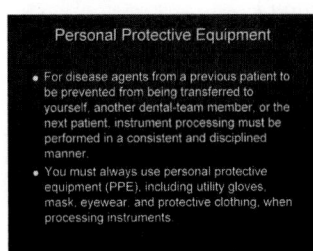

- PPE is intended to protect the dental worker from exposure that cannot be controlled through the use of engineering, administrative, or work practice controls.

- Household utility gloves such as the gloves worn for washing dishes are not specifically designed for protection when handling sharp objects.

Slide 15

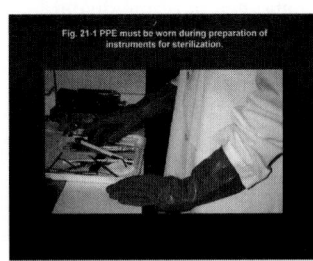

- Why is it recommended that PPE be worn during instrument preparation if care is taken during handling?

Slide 16

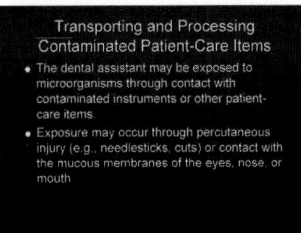

- Proper PPE must be worn during transport. A proper, rigid, leak-proof container must also be used to transport contaminated items.

- Care must be taken during cleaning, packaging, and sterilization to avoid injury or exposure.

ELSEVIER

Torres and Ehrlich Modern Dental Assisting, 9th ed.

Bird/Robinson

Slide 17

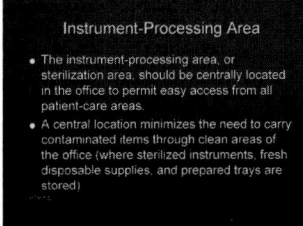

- Minimizing the need to carry contaminated items through other areas of the dental setting will minimize the opportunity for injury or exposure to occur.
- The CDC also recommends that the processing area have designated sections:
  - an area for receiving, cleaning, and decontamination
  - a preparation area for packaging the cleaned but contaminated instruments
  - a separate sterilization area for clean, packaged instruments only
  - a storage area should be away from the processing area to avoid cross-contamination of sterilized instruments with contaminated instruments

Slide 18

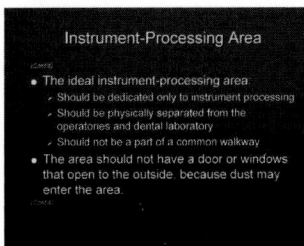

- Why should the processing area be dedicated to instrument processing only?
- Why should the processing area be separated from the treatment rooms?
- Why should the processing area be away from common walkways?
- Why should the window and/or door not open to the outside?

Slide 19

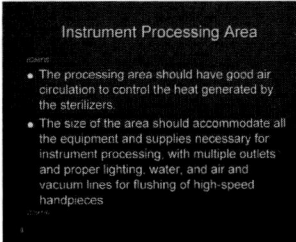

- Plenty of room should be available in the processing area to avoid bumping into coworkers or knocking over trays of contaminated instruments.
- What is the purpose of the air line and vacuum lines?

Slide 20

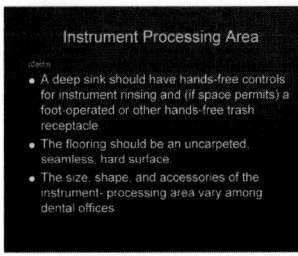

- Hands-free controls permit the operator to turn water on and off and open trash receptacles, thereby reducing the number of surfaces that can be contaminated by the dental worker's hands.
- If adequate space in unavailable in the processing area, what should you do to facilitate proper processing and instrument handling protocol?

ELSEVIER

Bird/Robinson

Slide 21

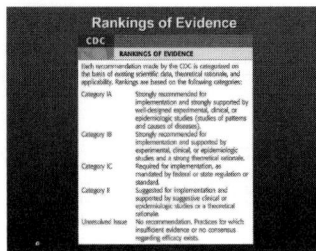

- Other factors influence the development of postoperative infection, especially in clean dental procedures for which the infection rate is generally low. Infections in these patients may be due solely to airborne exogenous microorganisms.

- In 1999, CDC's Health Care Infection Control Practices Advisory Committee published revised guidelines for the prevention of infections, as seen on this slide.

- These guidelines delve extensively into the literature concerning factors associated with postoperative infections.

Slide 22

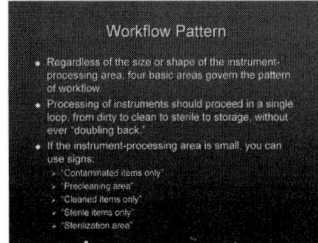

- How do signs enhance the workflow pattern in the processing area?

- The signs should be posted in a sequential and systematic manner.

- All signs should be laminated before posting to facilitate easy cleaning.

Slide 23

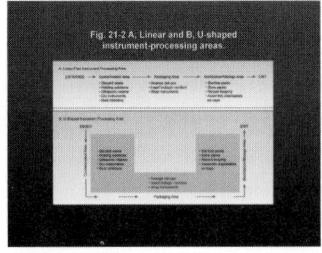

- Both of the pictured processing areas are designed following a systematic approach to instrument processing. Notice how both options have designated sections within the processing areas: (1) contaminated area; (2) packaging area; (3) sterilization/storage area.

- Notice how two doors are present: one entrance and one exit.

- Why are two doors recommended?

Slide 24

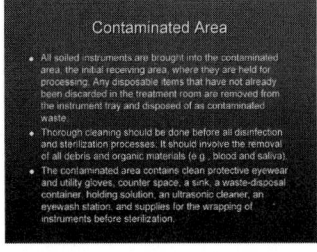

- Are blood-soaked items such as gauze or cotton rolls discarded with the rest of the trash?

- How do you remove debris from the soiled instruments?

- Why is the use of an ultrasonic cleaner recommended?

- Why is an eyewash station needed when protective eyewear is always worn?

Bird/Robinson

Slide 25

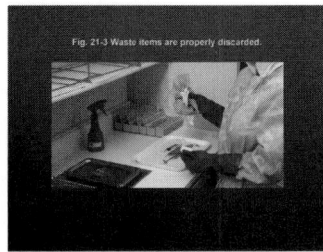

- What waste containers should be available in the processing area?
- Notice that the dental assistant is wearing heavy utility gloves that overlap the cuffed sleeves of the lab jacket. Why is this overlapping recommended?

Slide 26

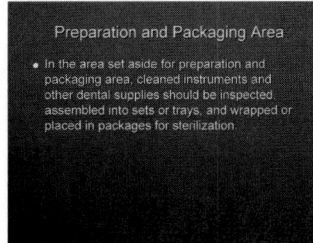

- The preparation and packaging area should have counter space and storage space for sterilized instruments, fresh disposable supplies, and prepared trays or instrument cassettes.
- What other items would you expect to see in this area?

Slide 27

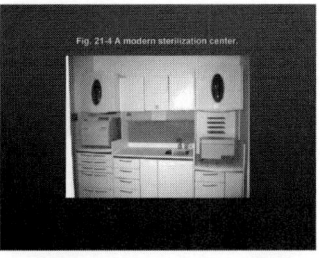

- What items do you expect to see in this area?

Slide 28

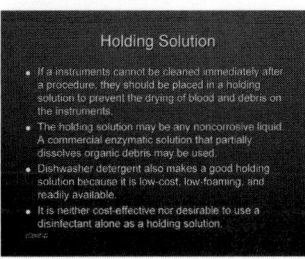

- Why is a nonfoaming detergent recommended?
- What could happen to the instruments if they are left in the holding solution too long?

Bird/Robinson

Slide 29

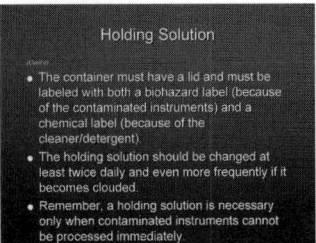

- How will you know if the holding tank solution has been changed or cleaned during the course of a busy day?
- When should the solution be changed?
- The holding tanks and solution should not be part of the normal routine of instrument processing. The holding tanks are used only when time does not permit the completion of instrument processing steps.

Slide 30

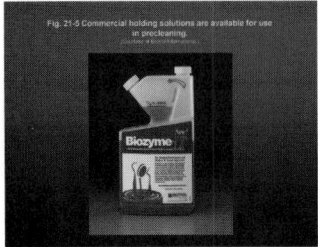

- Several commercial precleaning holding solutions are available but can be costly.
- Generally, these solutions are enzymatic detergent cleaners that dissolve blood and tissue within a few minutes in both room temperature and warm water.
- Most enzymatic cleaners are only effective in warm water. They can be used as a presoak and in the ultrasonic cleaning unit.

Slide 31

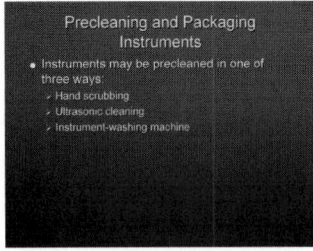

- Which of these three precleaning methods is most undesirable and why?
- Which method is least cost-effective?

Slide 32

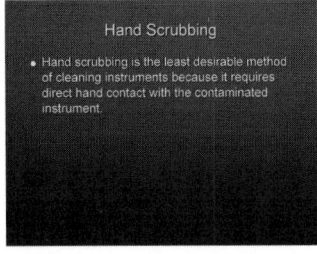

- As discussed earlier, injury can occur due to the handling and scrubbing of sharp instruments.
- If adequate ultrasonic or instrument washing equipment is unavailable, what would you do?

Bird/Robinson

Slide 33

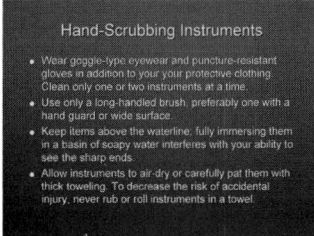

- If you absolutely must hand-scrub instruments, the precautions as listed on this slide must be taken.

- Remember to take care while scrubbing so injury is minimized.

- Scrub the instruments under running water to help eliminate aerosol production and to force debris down the drain.

Slide 34

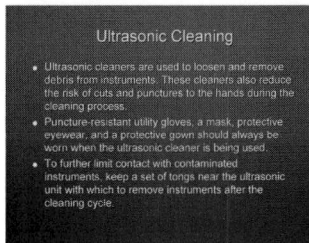

- Use of an ultrasonic cleaner is the most desirable method for removing debris and blood from dental procedure instruments.

- Remember to submerge the instruments completely so that all instruments are below the level of the ultrasonic solution.

Slide 35

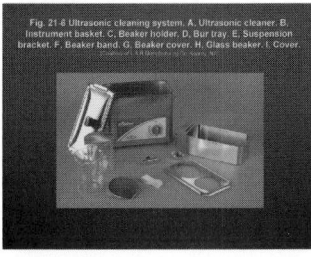

- Some ultrasonic units may sit on top of the counters in the processing area while others may be built into or recessed into the countertop.

Slide 36

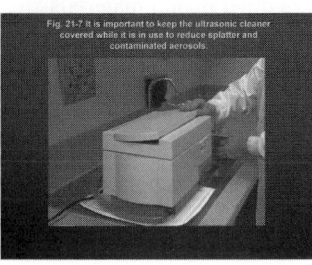

- Note how keeping the lid in place during use will minimize additional exposure of aerosols or splatter in the dental office environment.

- The ultrasonic solution may need to be changed several times during the day depending on the volume of instrument being cleaned. The solution should always be changed at the end of each day.

Slide 37

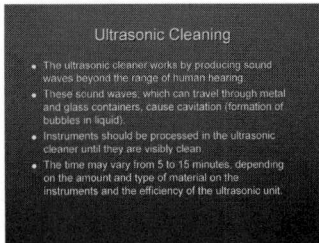

- Remember to use caution when loading the ultrasonic unit. Overloading the unit will inhibit the ability of the bubbles to collapse and create the turbulence necessary to effectively clean the surface of all of the instruments.

- What variables affect the time required to clean instruments in the ultrasonic unit?

Slide 38

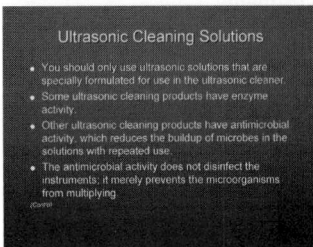

- What is the significance of solutions with enzymatic activity capabilities?

- Which type of solution might be changed fewer times during the day in high-volume dental offices and why?

Slide 39

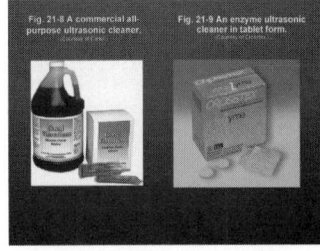

- Ultrasonic cleaning solutions come in a variety of sizes and types:
  - One-ounce packets
  - Tablets
  - Concentrate solutions
  - Ready-mixed gallon containers

- Which ultrasonic solution packaging would be most cost-effective in a busy, high-volume dental office?

Slide 40

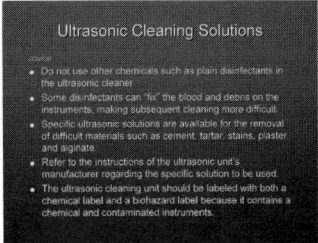

- Besides cleaning blood and tissue debris from dental instruments, the ultrasonic cleaner can also be used to remove other dental materials from instruments or trays.

- Do all dental instruments and equipment go into the ultrasonic cleaning unit?

Bird/Robinson

Slide 41

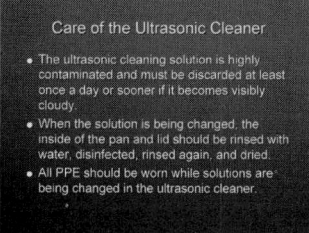

- What factors, along with solution appearance, should be considered to determine when the ultrasonic cleaning solution should be changed?
- Remember, the ultrasonic cleaner should be emptied and cleaned at the end of each day.

Slide 42

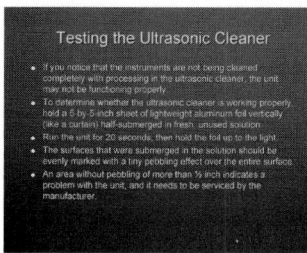

- Where should you document the maintenance check and schedule of the ultrasonic cleaner? (*In the record log that is kept in the instrument processing area.*)
- What causes the pebbling of the aluminum foil in a properly working ultrasonic cleaning unit? (*The turbulence caused by billions of tiny, collapsing bubbles.*)

Slide 43

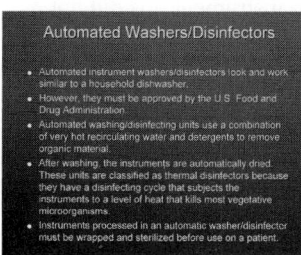

- After the washer/disinfector cycle is complete, PPE must be worn when removing the instruments. Why?
- In a low-volume dental office, do you think this method would be efficient and/or cost-effective?

Slide 44

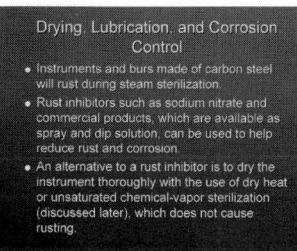

- Follow the manufacturer's guidelines when choosing a sterilization solution and sterilization method.
- Hinged instruments may need to be lubricated to maintain proper opening. Take care to remove all excess lubricant prior to heat sterilization.

Bird/Robinson

Slide 45

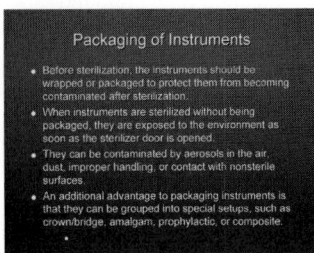

- Never store sterilized instruments open in a drawer or storage container. Once the sterilization container is opened, the sterilization of the instruments is compromised.

Slide 46

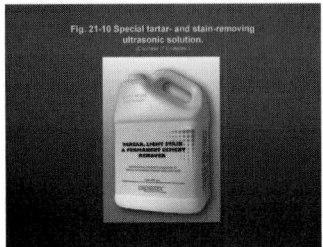

- When would you use tartar and stain remover ultrasonic solutions?

- How would you ensure asepsis when placing an appliance in an ultrasonic unit?

- Use caution when placing removable appliances in the ultrasonic unit. Always check the stability and condition of the denture or partial denture prior to placement in the ultrasonic unit.

Slide 47

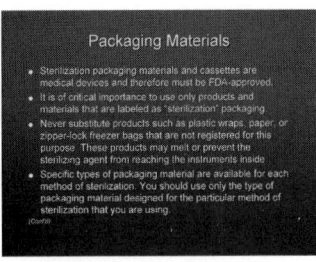

- Once the instruments are placed in sterilization pouches or bags, inspect the container to make sure that sharp instrument tips did not penetrate through.

- Always handle sterilization containers with care to avoid injury.

- Which sterilization container would minimize instrument tip breakage during the instrument processing cycle?

Slide 48

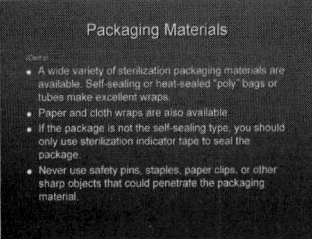

- Sterilization processing indicator tape looks much like masking tape prior to being exposed to the sterilization process. Once the tape has been exposed to sterilization, dark diagonal marking lines will appear on the tape.

- Do the dark marking lines indicate that sterilization has occurred and all microorganisms have been destroyed?

- Once cleaning and packaging are complete, the instruments are ready for sterilization.

Bird/Robinson

Slide 49

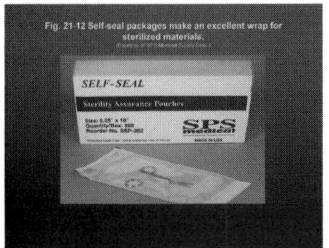

- Self-seal pouches allow you to view the contents of the package for easy storage and use.
- An internal indicator can be placed in the pouch facing out to indicate that the sterilization process has occurred. A change in the internal indicator means that the internal contents of the package have been exposed to heat and pressure.
- Why is one side of the packet paper?

Slide 50

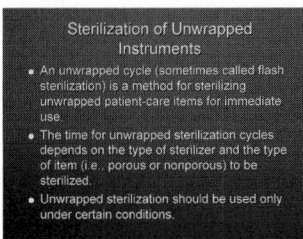

- Discuss with students the CDC recommendations for sterilization of unwrapped instruments.

Slide 51

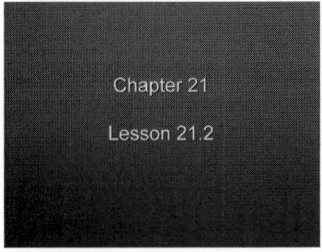

Slide 52

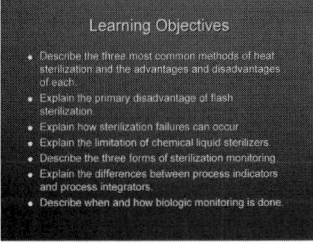

Torres and Ehrlich Modern Dental Assisting, 9th ed.
Bird/Robinson

Slide 53

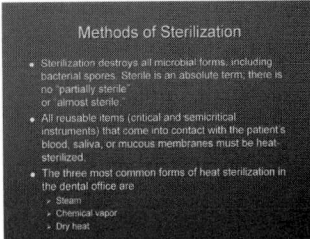

- Liquid sterilization may not be used to avoid damage to instruments that may be able to withstand heat sterilization.
- Critical and semicritical dental instruments must be sterilized using steam sterilization, chemical vapor sterilization, or dry heat sterilization.

Slide 54

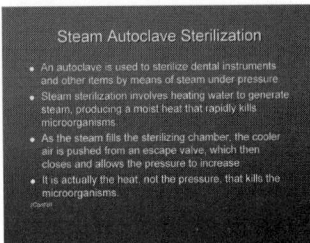

- The autoclave is the most common method of heat sterilization used in dental offices.
- What dental instruments can be sterilized in an autoclave?

Slide 55

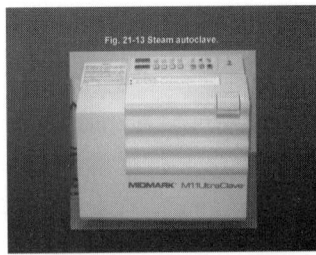

- It is important to read the manufacturer's guidelines before use.
- Different autoclaves will reach the proper temperature at different rates.
- The recommended time of exposure to the temperature required for sterilization does not include the time it takes for the autoclave to reach the proper temperature.
- Additional time is needed to allow depressurization of the chamber once the cycle has been completed.

Slide 56

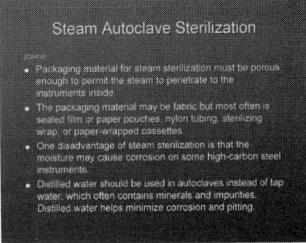

- Proper maintenance of the autoclave is important.
- Remember, allow the autoclave to complete the dry cycle and cool-down cycle. The dry cycle will help prevent rust and corrosion of instruments and the cool-down cycle will help prevent burn injury to the dental assistant.
- Which bacteria discussed in Chapter 18 is found in water distillation systems?

Slide 57

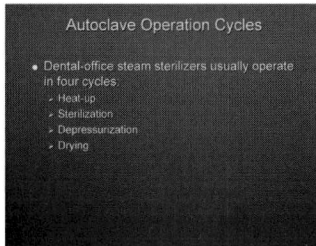

- The sterilization cycle is done using steam in a pressurized chamber, although it is the heat, not the pressure, that actually kills the microorganisms.

- The recommended time and temperature of a steam sterilizer is usually 121° C or 250° F, with pressures of 15 or 30 pounds per square inch (psi) for 20 minutes.

Slide 58

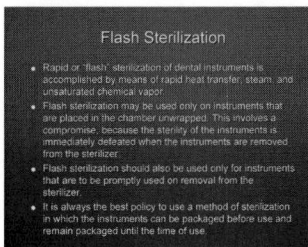

- When would flash sterilization be recommended?

- How long do the instruments stay sterilized once they are removed from the sterilizer after flash sterilization?

Slide 59

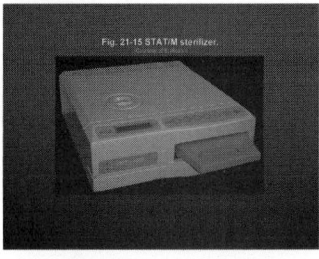

- The Statim sterilizer is recommended for flash sterilization techniques.

- It can also be used with unwrapped or wrapped instrument packets. The settings on the machine will compensate for instrument packets being used.

- Can you think of one disadvantage to using the Statim sterilizer?

Slide 60

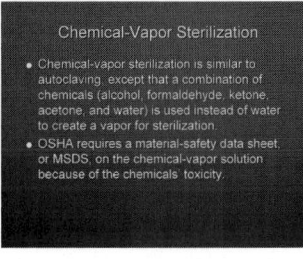

- It is recommended that chemical solutions prepared by the manufacturer be used in the chemical vapor sterilizer. Adequate chemical levels must also be maintained.

- Sealed containers or aluminum foils should not be used in the chemical vapor sterilizer.

ELSEVIER

Torres and Ehrlich Modern Dental Assisting, 9th ed.

Bird/Robinson

Slide 61

Advantages of Chemical-Vapor Sterilization
- The major advantage of the chemical-vapor sterilizer is that it does not rust, dull, or corrode dry metal instruments.
- The low water content of the vapor prevents destruction of items such as endodontic files, orthodontic pliers, wires, bands, and burs.
- A wide range of items can be sterilized routinely without damage.
- Other advantages include the short cycle time and the availability of a dry instrument after the cycle.

- Chemical vapor sterilizers are as easy to use as steam sterilizers.

Slide 62

Disadvantages of Chemical-Vapor Sterilization
- The primary disadvantage is that adequate ventilation is essential because residual chemical vapors containing formaldehyde and methyl alcohol may be released when the chamber door is opened at the end of the cycle.
- These vapors can temporarily leave an unpleasant odor in the area and may be irritating to the eyes.

- Chemical vapors leaking into the dental office can pose health risks to dental care workers and patients.
- Another disadvantage of the chemical vapor sterilizer is the cost of the chemicals.

Slide 63

Filtration and Monitoring of Chemical Vapors
- Newer sterilizers are equipped with a special filtration device that further reduces the amount of chemical vapor remaining in the chamber at the end of the cycle. Older models can usually be retrofitted.
- Formaldehyde-monitoring badges, similar to radiation monitoring devices, are available for employees. The badge measures personal exposure to formaldehyde for a period and is then mailed to the monitoring service, which sends a laboratory analysis to the employee.

- Filtration and monitoring information should be recorded in the record log that is kept in the instrument processing area.

Slide 64

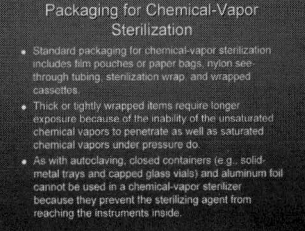

Packaging for Chemical-Vapor Sterilization
- Standard packaging for chemical-vapor sterilization includes film pouches or paper bags, nylon see-through tubing, sterilization wrap, and wrapped cassettes.
- Thick or tightly wrapped items require longer exposure because of the inability of the unsaturated chemical vapors to penetrate as well as saturated chemical vapors under pressure do.
- As with autoclaving, closed containers (e.g., solid-metal trays and capped glass vials) and aluminum foil cannot be used in a chemical-vapor sterilizer because they prevent the sterilizing agent from reaching the instruments inside.

- What items can be sterilized using chemical vapor sterilization techniques?

ELSEVIER

Bird/Robinson

Slide 65

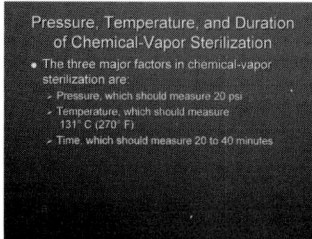

- What does "psi" stand for? (*Pounds per square inch.*)
- If the proper pressure, temperature, and time are achieved while using the chemical vapor sterilizer, is it safe to assume that all microorganisms have been destroyed?

Slide 66

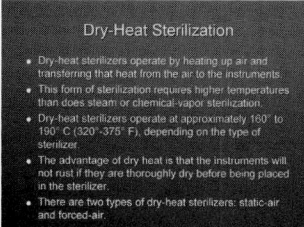

- It is important to use packaging materials that are designed for use in a dry heat sterilizer.
- Which packaging materials are acceptable to use in a dry heat sterilizer?
- Do not sterilize plastic items or adhesive tape in a dry heat sterilizer.

Slide 67

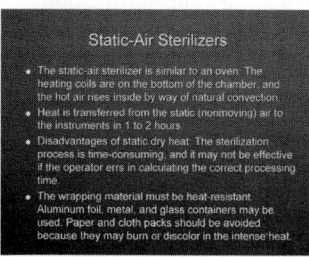

- The dental office will need to have a large instrument inventory if this method of sterilization is used. Why?

Slide 68

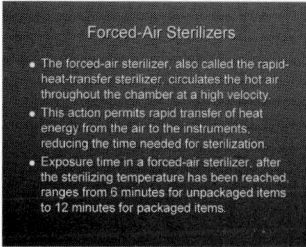

- What makes the forced-air dry heat sterilizer desirable for flash sterilization techniques? (*The low sterilization cycle time of 6 to 12 minutes offers quick sterilization when an instrument is needed quickly.*)

Bird/Robinson

Slide 69

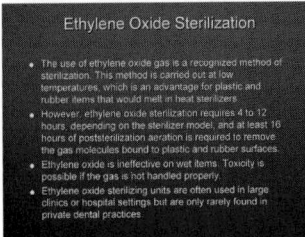

- This method of sterilization is not common in dental offices.
- Proper ventilation is required.
- The equipment needed is often large and costly.
- Toxicity is a problem along with the time required for completion of the sterilization process.

Slide 70

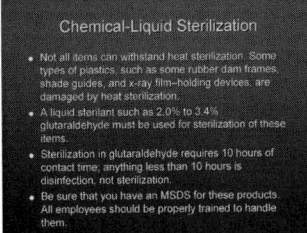

- Sterilization in glutaraldehyde is very time-consuming. The extended length of time will cause instruments to be unavailable for use for long periods of time.
- What is another disadvantage of using glutaraldehyde?

Slide 71

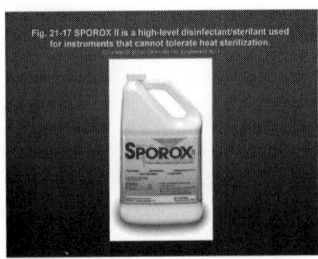

- What items can be sterilized using chemical disinfection/sterilization solutions?

Slide 72

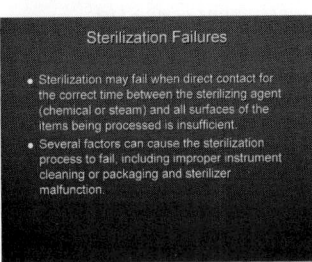

- What is the best way to determine if sterilization failure has occurred?
- Can physical monitoring or chemical monitoring systems be used to measure the success of the sterilization process?

Slide 73

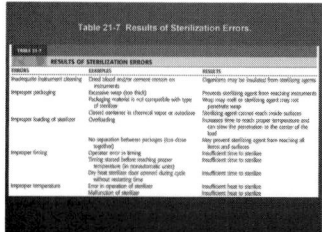

- Identifying errors is an important step in the sterilization process. What is even more important is that all dental workers are able to determine why the failure occurred and how to fix the problem.

Slide 74

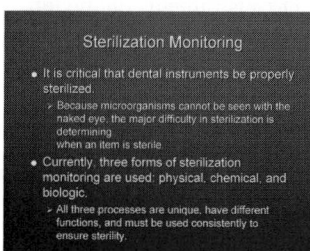

- Today more scientific monitoring systems are used, such as physical, chemical, and biologic systems.

- The monitoring of these systems should be documented and records should be maintained in the record log that is kept in the processing area.

Slide 75

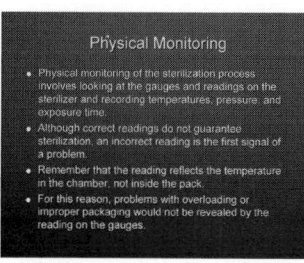

- After the sterilizer has started, the dental assistant should return periodically to the processing area to monitor the gauges outside the sterilizer for accurate time, pressure, and temperature readings.

- Why does overloading the sterilizer affect the temperature inside the instrument package?

Slide 76

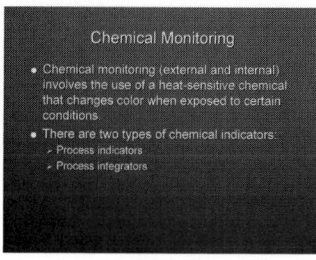

- Chemical indicators allow the dental team to determine that certain necessary measurements have been met.

- Chemical indicators should be used with every package of instruments in the sterilizer; one indicator per load is not adequate.

Bird/Robinson

Slide 77

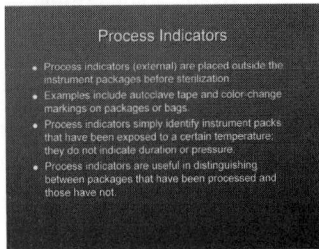

- What is another name for process indicators? (*Single-parameter indicators.*)

- Single-parameter indicators show that the packets have been exposed to one parameter of sterilization – temperature.

- Remember, when a change occurs in the process indicator, it does not ensure that sterilization has occurred and that all microorganisms have been destroyed.

Slide 78

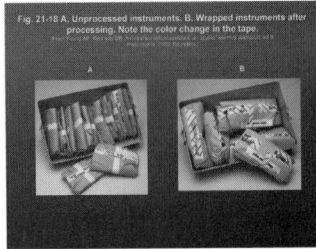

- At least we know that the instruments on the right have been through the process and have been exposed to heat. The instruments on the left have not gone through the process in the packaging that we see.

- What have the packets on the right been exposed to? (*Temperature only.*)

Slide 79

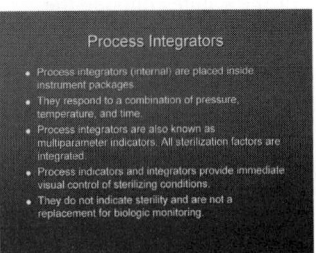

- What is another name for process integrators? (*Multiparameter indicators.*)

- Can you think of one advantage of using process integrators?

- If the process indicator on the outside of the instrument packet has changed colors along with the process integrator changes, would it be safe to assume that sterilization has occurred?

Slide 80

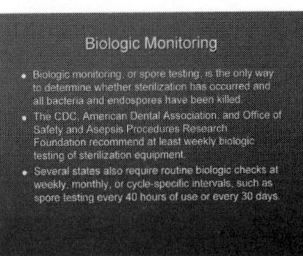

- What are some additional reasons to use biologic monitoring?

Slide 81

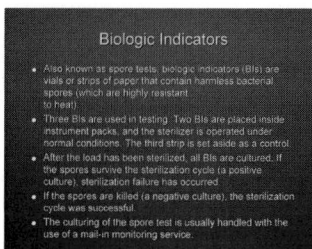

- The spores used to test steam sterilizers are different from those used to test chemical vapor sterilizers and are different from the bacteria used to test the dry heat and ethylene oxide sterilizers.
- What would be the best way to monitor the BI if you use different sterilization methods in your office and to avoid placing the wrong BI into the wrong sterilizer? (*Use dual-species BIs.*)

Slide 82

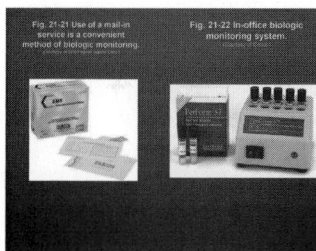

- All monitoring results and reports must be logged in the record log that is kept in the processing area.
- Can you think of an advantage of using the in-office culturing system?
- Can you think of a disadvantage of using the in-office culturing system?

Slide 83

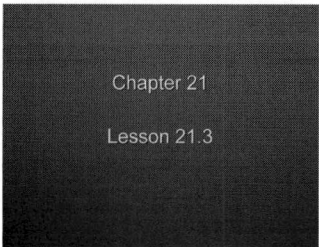

Slide 84

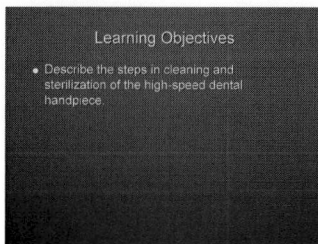

Slide 85

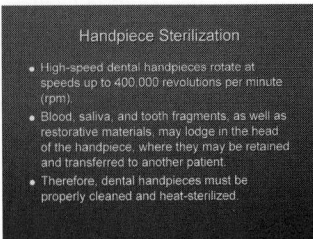

- Both high-speed handpieces and slow-speed handpieces have specific maintenance requirements.

- If a handpiece is not functioning properly, dental procedures will be hindered and patient safety may be affected.

- When a handpiece must be repaired or replaced because of inadequate maintenance, the cost-effectiveness of the dental office is decreased.

Slide 86

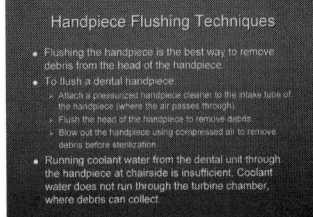

- The equipment and supplies needed to sterilize a handpiece include:
  - sterilizable handpiece
  - bur
  - ultrasonic cleaner (if recommended by the manufacturer)
  - lubricant (if recommended by the manufacturer)
  - cotton swab

Slide 87

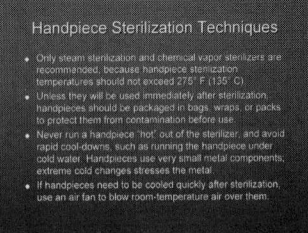

- What are the procedural steps for proper handpiece sterilization?

22 Regulatory and Advisory Agencies

TEACHING FOCUS

This chapter will give students the opportunity to learn about regulatory and advisory agencies for dentistry, including the roles of various professional associations and government agencies as they relate to dentistry. Students will also become acquainted with the differences between regulations and recommendations.

MATERIALS AND RESOURCES

☐ computer and PowerPoint projector (Lesson 22.1)

LESSON CHECKLIST

Preparations for this lesson include:

- lecture
- evaluation of student knowledge needed to understand the regulatory and advisory agencies related to dentistry, including:
  - ○ government agencies that apply to dentistry
  - ○ professional dentistry associations
  - ○ regulations and recommendations

ELSEVIER

Bird/Robinson

KEY TERMS

American Dental Association (ADA) (p. 339)

American Dental Assistants Association (p. 339)

American Dental Hygienists Association (p. 339)

Centers for Disease Control and Prevention (CDC) (p. 341)

Environmental Protection Agency (EPA) (p. 341)

Food and Drug Administration (FDA) (p. 341)

National Institute for Occupational Safety and Health (NIOSH) (p. 342)

National Institutes of Dental and Craniofacial Research (NIDCR) (p. 342)

National Institutes of Health (NIH) (p. 342)

Occupational Safety and Health Administration (OSHA) (p. 341)

Organization for Safety and Asepsis Procedures (OSAP) (p. 339)

ADDITIONAL RESOURCES

PowerPoint slides (Evolve): 1-16

Legend

CTQ
Critical
Thinking
Question

DVD
Multimedia
Procedures
Videos and
Animations

ESLR
EVOLVE
Student
Learning
Resources

IDO
Interactive
Dental
Office
CD-ROM

SW
Student
Workbook

TB
Test Bank
on the
TEACH
CD-ROM

PPT
PowerPoint
Slides

Class Activities are indicated in ***bold italic.***

ELSEVIER

Torres and Ehrlich Modern Dental Assisting, 9th ed.

Bird/Robinson

LESSON 22.1

PRETEST

1. Regulatory agencies issue
   a. recommendations with which dental offices should comply.
   b. rules and regulations with which dental offices should comply.
   c. rules and regulations with which dental offices must comply.
   d. recommendations with which dental offices must comply.

2. Nonregulatory agencies issue
   a. recommendations with which dental offices should comply.
   b. rules and regulations with which dental offices should comply.
   c. rules and regulations with which dental offices must comply.
   d. recommendations with which dental offices must comply.

3. The national professional organization for dentists is known as
   a. California Dental Association (CDA). c. International Dental Association (IDA).
   b. American Dental Association (ADA). d. Organization for Safety and Asepsis Procedures (OSAP).

4. The dentist's resource for infection control and safety is
   a. U.S. Occupational Safety and Health Administration (OSHA).
   b. American Dental Association (ADA).
   c. Centers for Disease Control and Prevention (CDC).
   d. Organization for Safety and Asepsis Procedures (OSAP).

5. The infection-control procedures practiced in dentistry are based on the
   a. Oral Health Services.
   b. Morbidity and Mortality Weekly Report.
   c. Guidelines for Infection Control in Dental Healthcare Settings.
   d. Centers for Disease Control and Prevention.

6. Which agency regulates the manufacturing and labeling of medical devices?
   a. U.S. Food and Drug Administration (FDA)
   b. U.S. Environmental Protection Agency (EPA)
   c. U.S. Occupational Safety and Health Administration (OSHA)
   d. U.S. Department of Health and Human Services (HHS)

7. What regulatory agency ensures the safety and health of America's workers?
   a. U.S. Environmental Protection Agency (EPA)
   b. U.S. Occupational Safety and Health Administration (OSHA)
   c. U.S. Department of Health and Human Services (HHS)
   d. National Institute for Occupational Safety and Health (NIOSH)

8. What nonregulatory agency focuses on the safety and health of America's workers?
   a. U.S. Environmental Protection Agency (EPA)
   b. U.S. Occupational Safety and Health Administration (OSHA)
   c. U.S. Department of Health and Human Services (HHS)
   d. National Institute for Occupational Safety and Health (NIOSH)

9. What agency serves as the dental research institute?
   a. National Institutes of Health (NIH)
   b. National Institute for Occupational Safety and Health (NIOSH)
   c. National Institute of Dental and Craniofacial Research (NIDCR)
   d. Centers for Disease Control and Prevention (CDC)

10. The agency that ensures the safety and effectiveness of disinfectants is the
    a. U.S. Occupational Safety and Health Administration (OSHA).
    b. U.S. Environmental Protection Agency (EPA).
    c. U.S. Department of Health and Human Services (HHS).
    d. U.S. Food and Drug Administration (FDA).

Answers

1. c	3. b	5. c	7. b	9. c
2. a	4. d	6. a	8. d	10. b

BACKGROUND ASSESSMENT

Question: What is the difference between OSHA and NIOSH?

Answer: The National Institute for Occupational Safety and Health (NIOSH) does not have regulatory authority. NIOSH is the only federal institute responsible for conducting research and making recommendations for the prevention of work-related disease and injury. The U.S. Occupational Safety and Health Administration (OSHA) is a regulatory agency that is part of the U.S. Department of Labor. OSHA sets and enforces standards that must be followed.

Question: When may OSHA inspect a dental office?

Answer: OSHA may inspect a dental office for any of the following three reasons. First, they may mount an inspection after receiving a complaint from an employee or patient. Second, OSHA is authorized to conduct random inspections for dental offices with more than 11 employees. Third, a dentist may request an inspection as part of an OSHA consultation.

CRITICAL THINKING QUESTION

A dental office is looking to develop an office policy for infection control. The dentists have assigned this task to a dental assistant. What resources would help the dental assistant to develop an office policy for infection control?

Guidelines: There are several resources available to develop an infection-control policy. One resource is the American Dental Association, which is the national professional organization for dentists. It offers infection-control recommendations that are updated regularly when new scientific information is available. Another organization that could be used as a resource is the Organization for Safety and Asepsis Procedures. This organization is a dentistry resource for infection-control procedures. Modern infection-control procedures practiced in dentistry are based on recommendations from the Centers for Disease Control and Prevention (CDC), a governmental resource. Using information from these three organizations will help the dental assistant develop an infection-control policy based on the highest quality scientific data.

OBJECTIVES	CONTENT	TEACHING RESOURCES
Pronounce, define, and spell the Key Terms.	■ Key terms (p. 338)	*ESLR* Electronic Flashcards ▸ Discuss how memorizing abbreviations can help an individual commit to memory the important professional organizations and government agencies related to dentistry. ***Class Activity** Have students develop a crossword puzzle using key terms. They can use a Web site such as www.puzzlemaker.com or create it on their own. Have students exchange their puzzles with classmates to solve them*

Torres and Ehrlich Modern Dental Assisting, 9th ed.

Bird/Robinson

OBJECTIVES	CONTENT	TEACHING RESOURCES
Explain the difference between regulations and recommendations.	■ Introduction (p. 339)	PPT 6-7 TB question 1 SW Short-Answer Questions 1 (p. 121) Government Agencies (p. 340) Professional Organizations (p. 340) Recall question 1 (p. 340) ▶ Discuss how a regulation differs from a recommendation and how the difference affects dentistry. ▶ Discuss the concept of an advisory agency and the application of such an agency to dentistry. *Class Activity Present the following information to the class. Ask the class to identify whether the information is a regulation or recommendation.* *1. OSHA Bloodborne Pathogens Standard* *2. American Dental Association infection control reports* *3. U.S. Food and Drug Administration rules on manufacturing and labeling of medical devices* *4. Centers for Disease Control and Prevention guidelines for infection control in dental healthcare settings*
Identify four professional sources for dental information.	■ Associations and organizations (p. 339) ☐ American Dental Association (p. 339) ☐ American Dental Assistants Association (p. 339) ☐ American Dental Hygienists Association (p. 339)	PPT 8-9 SW Short-Answer Questions 2; Fill in the Blank question 3 (pp. 121-122) Figure 22-1 Logo of the ADA (p. 339) Figure 22-2 Logo of the ADAA (p. 339) Figure 22-3 Logo of the ADHA (p. 340) CTQ 2 (p. 343) ▶ Discuss the roles of professional organizations and how they can benefit a dental assistant. ▶ Discuss what resources of the ADA would be beneficial to a dental assistant. *Class Activity Divide the class into four groups. Assign each group one of the four professional sources for dental information. Have each group discuss its assigned source. Then have each group share information with the rest of the class about its assigned source for dental information.*

Bird/Robinson

OBJECTIVES	CONTENT	TEACHING RESOURCES

Name the premiere infection-control educational organization in dentistry.	☐ Organization for Safety and Asepsis Procedures (p. 339)
	
	☐ State and local dental societies (p. 340)
		PPT 8-9
		
		TB question 2
		
		SW Short-Answer Questions 3; Fill in the Blank question 5 (pp. 121-122)
		
		Figure 22-4 Logo of OSAP (p. 340)
		
		Recall question 2 (p. 340)
		
		CTQ 1, 3 (p. 343)
		
		▸ Discuss how OSAP can be important to a dental assistant.
		
		▸ Discuss how OSAP can be beneficial in reducing infections in the dental office.
		
		Class Activity **Divide the class into small groups. Assign each group one of the following organizations and have it present information about the organization to the rest of the class. Next, ask the class to determine which organization is considered the premiere infection-control educational organization in dentistry and discuss why.**
		
		    1. Centers for Disease Control and Prevention
		
		    2. OSHA
		
		    3. FDA
		
		    4. American Dental Association

Describe the role of the Centers for Disease Control and Prevention.	■ Government agencies (p. 341)
	
	☐ Centers for Disease Control and Prevention (p. 341)
		PPT 10-11
		
		TB questions 3-4
		
		SW Short-Answer Questions 4; Fill in the Blank question 2; Multiple Choice question 1 (pp. 121-122)
		
		Figure 22-5 Logo of the CDC (p. 341)
		
		Recall question 3 (p. 343)
		
		CTQ 4 (p. 343)
		
		▸ Discuss other areas of healthcare besides dentistry that are affected by the CDC.
		
		▸ Discuss the role of the CDC in dentistry.
		
		Class Activity **Present the following information to the class. Ask the class to identify if the information presented is a role of the CDC.**
		
		    1. Develop regulations or laws for public health
		
		    2. Develop guidelines for public health
		
		    3. Information resource for dental professionals

Bird/Robinson

OBJECTIVES	CONTENT	TEACHING RESOURCES
		4. The lead federal agency for public health in the United States ***Next, encourage further discussion of the roles for the CDC.***
Describe the role of the Food and Drug Administration in relation to dentistry.	☐ Food and Drug Administration (p. 341)	PPT 12-13 TB question 5 SW Short-Answer Questions 7; Fill in the Blank question 1; Multiple Choice question 2 (pp. 121-122) Figure 22-6 Overview of a dental operatory showing items regulated by the FDA (p. 341) Figure 22-7 The FDA logo (p. 341) Recall question 4 (p. 343) CTQ 4 (p. 343) ▶ Discuss the areas of the dental office affected by the FDA. ▶ Discuss what other roles the FDA plays in healthcare. ***Class Activity Present the following information to the class. Ask the class to identify whether the information presented is a role of the Food and Drug Administration.*** ***1. Publishes morbidity and mortality reports*** ***2. Determines "good manufacturing practices"*** ***3. Regulates the manufacturing and labeling of medical devices*** ***4. Regulates antimicrobial handwashes and mouthrinses*** ***Next, encourage further discussion of the role of the Food and Drug Administration in relation to dentistry.***
Describe the role of the Environmental Protection Agency in relation to dentistry.	☐ Environmental Protection Agency (p. 341)	PPT 14 TB question 6 SW Short-Answer Questions 6; Fill in the Blank question 7; Multiple Choice question 3 (pp. 121-122) Figure 22-8 Logo of the EPA (p. 342) Recall question 5 (p. 343) CTQ 4 (p. 343) ▶ Discuss the primary role of the EPA in everyday life. ▶ Discuss how the EPA affects a dental office.

Bird/Robinson

OBJECTIVES	CONTENT	TEACHING RESOURCES
		Class Activity Divide the class into small groups. Ask each group to determine and discuss one role of the Environmental Protection Agency in relation to dentistry. Then, have each group share its information with the class.
Explain a primary difference between OSHA and NIOSH.	☐ Occupational Safety and Health Administration (p. 341)	PPT 15 ▧ TB questions 7-8, 10 📘 SW Short-Answer Questions 5; Fill in the Blank question 4; SW Multiple Choice question 4 (pp. 121-122) OSHA Inspections (p. 342) Figure 22-9 Logo of OSHA (p. 342) Recall question 6 (p. 343) 💡 CTQ 4 (p. 343) ▸ Discuss the impact of OSHA regulations on a dental office. ▸ Discuss what a dental assistant might do if he or she determines that the dental office is violating OSHA regulations. *Class Activity Present the following information to the class. Have the class determine if the information cited is considered the primary difference between OSHA and NIOSH.* *1. OSHA is a regulatory authority and NIOSH does not have regulatory authority.* *2. NIOSH makes recommendations for the prevention of injury and OSHA does not.* *3. OSHA provides educational outreach and training and NIOSH does not.* *4. NIOSH investigates hazardous work conditions and OSHA does not.* *Next, discuss why this distinction is considered primary.*
Describe the role of the National Institutes of Health.	☐ National Institutes of Health (p. 342)	📘 SW Short-Answer Questions 8 (p. 121) Figure 22-10 Logo of the NIH (p. 342) Recall question 7 (p. 343) 💡 CTQ 4 (p. 343) ▸ Discuss how the NIH affects a dental office. ▸ Discuss what other roles the NIH plays in the medical and scientific professions.

OBJECTIVES	CONTENT	TEACHING RESOURCES
		Class Activity Divide the class into small groups. Ask each group to determine and discuss one role of the National Institutes of Health. Then, have each group share its information with the class.
Describe the role of the National Institute of Dental and Craniofacial Research.	☐ National Institute of Dental and Craniofacial Research (p. 342)	SW Short-Answer Questions 9 (p. 121) Figure 22-11 Logo of the NIDCR (p. 342) Recall question 8 (p. 343) CTQ 4 (p. 343) ▶ Discuss how the NIDCR relates to the NIH. ▶ Discuss how the NIDCR affects the dental profession. *Class Activity Divide the class into small groups. Ask each group to determine and discuss one role of the National Institute of Dental and Craniofacial Research. Then have each group share its information with the class.*
Explain a primary difference between OSHA and NIOSH.	☐ National Institute for Occupational Safety and Health (p. 342)	PPT 16 TB question 9 SW Short-Answer Questions 5; Fill in the Blank question 6 (pp. 121-122) Figure 22-12 Logo of NIOSH (p. 343) Legal and Ethical Implications (p. 343) Eye to the Future (p. 343) CTQ 4 (p. 343) ▶ Discuss how NIOSH differs from OSHA. ▶ Discuss how NIOSH would affect a dental office. *Class Activity As a class, discuss the similarities and distinctions between OSHA and NIOSH. Based on the primary distinction, which body has more influence on the dental profession?*
Performance Evaluation		TB SW questions (pp. 121-122) ESLR Electronic Flashcards ESLR Practice Quiz Recall questions (pp. 340, 343) CTQ (p. 343)

Bird/Robinson

22.1 Homework/Assignments:

22.1 Instructor's Notes/Student Feedback:

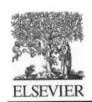

Torres and Ehrlich Modern Dental Assisting, 9th ed.

Bird/Robinson

Slide 1

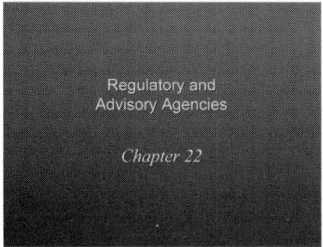

Regulatory and
Advisory Agencies

Chapter 22

Slide 2

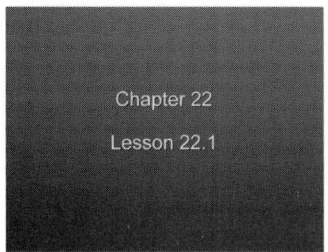

Chapter 22

Lesson 22.1

Slide 3

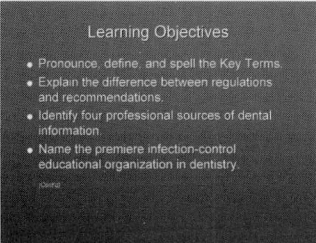

Learning Objectives

- Pronounce, define, and spell the Key Terms.
- Explain the difference between regulations and recommendations.
- Identify four professional sources of dental information.
- Name the premiere infection-control educational organization in dentistry.

Slide 4

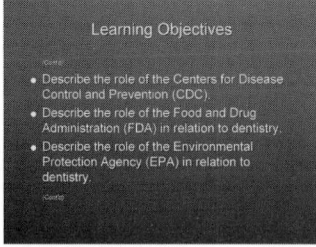

Learning Objectives

(Cont'd)

- Describe the role of the Centers for Disease Control and Prevention (CDC).
- Describe the role of the Food and Drug Administration (FDA) in relation to dentistry.
- Describe the role of the Environmental Protection Agency (EPA) in relation to dentistry.

(Cont'd)

Bird/Robinson

Slide 5

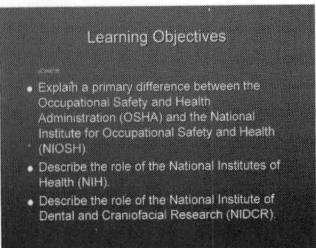

Slide 6

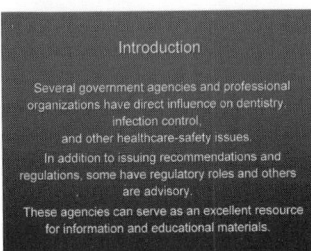

- Ask students to name the agencies and organizations they believe are involved with dentistry.

Slide 7

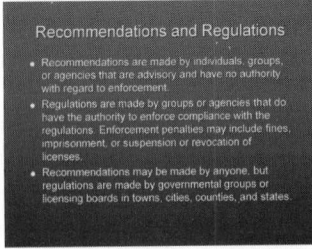

- Of the agencies and organizations named by the students, ask which provide regulations versus recommendations.

Slide 8

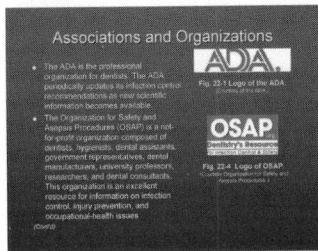

- Seven out of ten dentists are members of the ADA.

- Not only does the ADA provide information for dental professionals, but it also provides information for the public on oral health.

- OSAP is currently focusing on the issue of SARS – Severe Acute Respiratory Syndrome and the dental office.

  - Through December 2003, 161 confirmed or suspected cases were investigated in the United States and more than 8000 probable cases were reported worldwide, according to OSAP.

Slide 9

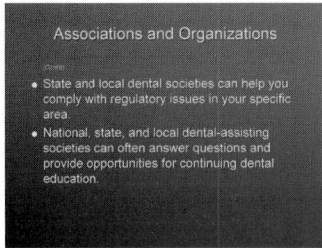

- In the state of Washington, the dental association is made up of 17 local component societies that play an important role in implementing projects and programs at the state and local level.

- Why is it important to be involved with the local dental society? *(It can answer questions and work with the dental professional or act as a liaison to the regulatory agencies.)*

Slide 10

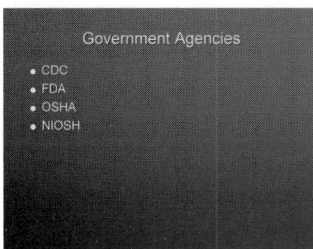

- Ask each student to name a dental product that is regulated by the FDA.

Slide 11

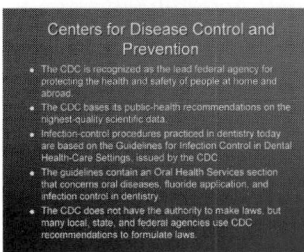

- Recently, the CDC published statistics on how many people in the United States visited the dentist in a year. What do you believe the statistics were? *(67.9% had; 32.1% had not.)*

Slide 12

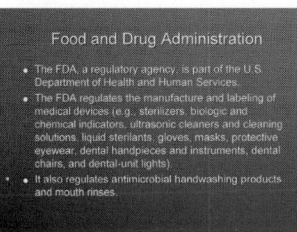

- Inform the students what should occur if the medical devices regulated by the FDA malfunction.

Torres and Ehrlich Modern Dental Assisting, 9th ed.

Bird/Robinson

Slide 13

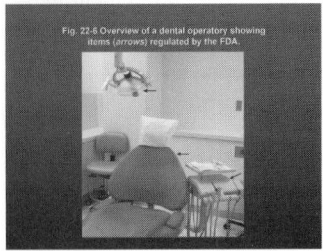

- Discuss other examples of medical products regulated by the FDA.

Slide 14

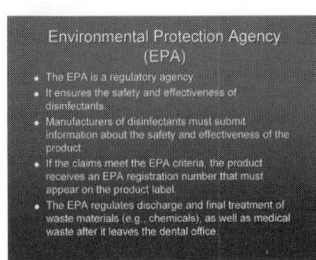

- Discuss different disinfectants and the information provided on the labeling.

Slide 15

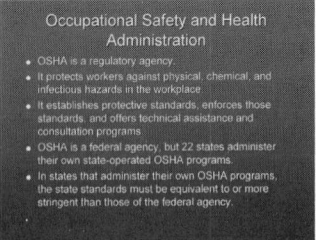

- What OSHA standards apply to dentistry? *(Bloodborne Pathogens, Hazard Communication, Occupational Exposure to Hazardous Chemicals in Laboratories, Medical Services and First Aid, Respiratory Protection, Personal Protective Equipment, Formaldehyde, Portable Fire Extinguishers, Nitrous Oxide, Ethylene Oxide.)*

Slide 16

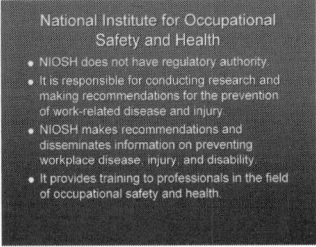

- The research branch is known as National Occupational Research Agency, or NORA.

- What projects or areas might NORA research that benefit dental professionals? *(Allergic and irritant dermatitis, infectious diseases, lower back disorders, emerging technologies, mixed exposures, control technology and personal protective equipment [PPE], exposure assessment methods, and risk- assessment methods.)*

ELSEVIER

Torres and Ehrlich Modern Dental Assisting, 9th ed.

Bird/Robinson

TEACHING FOCUS

This chapter introduces students to topics related to chemical and waste management in the dental office. The student has the opportunity to become acquainted with protection against hazardous chemicals, control of chemical spills, general precautions for storing chemicals, hazardous waste disposal, and dental office waste management. The elements of a hazard communication program, including chemical inventory, material safety data sheets, and employee training, are also discussed.

MATERIALS AND RESOURCES

- ☐ computer and PowerPoint projector (all Lessons)
- ☐ material safety data sheets (MSDS) for several chemicals (Lesson 23.2)

- ☐ protective equipment, including chemical-resistant nitrile gloves, chemical goggles, disposable respirator, rubber/neoprene apron (Lesson 23.1)
- ☐ secondary containers, MSDSs, and NFPA chemical labels (Lesson 23.2)

LESSON CHECKLIST

Preparations for this lesson include:

- lecture
- guest speakers: Occupational Safety and Health Administration (OSHA) representative
- evaluation of student knowledge and skills needed to perform all entry-level activities related to comprehension and application of chemical and waste management, including:
  - ○ short- and long-term effects of chemical exposure
  - ○ purpose of OSHA Hazard Communication Standard
  - ○ components of a hazard communication program
  - ○ purpose of material safety data sheets
  - ○ labels for a secondary container
  - ○ methods of personal protection
  - ○ storing chemicals
  - ○ types of toxic waste generated in a dental office
  - ○ packaging regulated waste for transport

ELSEVIER

Torres and Ehrlich Modern Dental Assisting, 9th ed.

Bird/Robinson

KEY TERMS

acute exposure (p. 346)
chemical inventory (p. 350)
chronic exposure (p. 346)
contaminated waste (p. 356)
Environmental Protection Agency (EPA)
   (p. 349)

Hazard Communication Standard (p. 349)
hazardous waste (p. 349)
infectious waste (p. 356)
material safety data sheet (MSDS) (p. 347)
regulated waste (p. 356)

ADDITIONAL RESOURCES

PowerPoint slides (Evolve): 1-35

Legend

  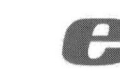

CTQ Critical Thinking Question	**DVD** Multimedia Procedures Videos and Animations	**ESLR** EVOLVE Student Learning Resources	**IDO** Interactive Dental Office CD-ROM	**SW** Student Workbook	**TB** Test Bank on the TEACH CD-ROM	**PPT** PowerPoint Slides

Class Activities are indicated in ***bold italic***.

Torres and Ehrlich Modern Dental Assisting, 9th ed.

Bird/Robinson

LESSON 23.1

PRETEST

1. The three primary methods of chemical exposure are
   a. gases, vapors, and dusts.
   b. absorption, gases, and direct.
   c. inhalation, ingestion, and skin contact.
   d. droplets, airborne, and gases.

2. Eating lunch in an area in which chemicals are used is a common way of chemical exposure through
   a. ingestion.
   b. inhalation.
   c. skin contact.
   d. vapors.

3. Dizziness, fainting, headache, and nausea are effects felt by an individual suffering from
   a. pregnancy.
   b. fear of the dentist's office.
   c. chronic toxicity.
   d. acute toxicity.

4. Liver disease can be an effect of
   a. acute toxicity.
   b. chronic toxicity.
   c. pregnancy.
   d. fear.

5. What type of gloves should be worn when using chemicals?
   a. cloth gloves
   b. utility gloves
   c. rubber kitchen gloves
   d. leather gloves

6. The proper face mask should
   a. repel fluids and provide respiratory protection.
   b. be snug fitting and flexible.
   c. be kept at work.
   d. fit all employees.

7. Mercury spill kits should be available
   a. by notifying the EPA.
   b. by notifying OSHA.
   c. in all dental offices.
   d. at the public works department.

8. Some manufacturers of eyewash units recommend a weekly flushing of how many minutes?
   a. 1 minute
   b. 3 minutes
   c. 5 minutes
   d. 10 minutes

9. The Occupational Safety and Health Administration Hazard Communication Standard is also known as
   a. the Hazard Communication Program.
   b. the written program.
   c. the Employee Right-to-Know Law.
   d. a material safety data sheet.

10. The four colors of the National Fire Protection Association (NFPA) hazardous chemicals labeling system are
    a. blue, orange, yellow, and white.
    b. yellow, red, orange, and green.
    c. blue, green, white, and red.
    d. blue, red, yellow, and white.

Answers

1. c	3. d	5. b	7. c	9. c
2. a	4. b	6. a	8. b	10. d

BACKGROUND ASSESSMENT

Question: Define a hazardous chemical. What characteristics make it hazardous?

Answer: A hazardous chemical is any chemical that can cause either a physical or health hazard. A chemical is considered hazardous if it (1) can ignite, (2) can react or explode when mixed with other substances, (3) is corrosive, or (4) is toxic.

Question: What are the classifications of dental waste?
Answer: Regulated waste contains sharps, blood, blood-soaked and blood-caked items, human tissue, and pathologic waste. Nonregulated waste includes contaminated waste materials as well as saliva-soaked gauze, used patient bibs, and surface barriers.

CRITICAL THINKING QUESTION

A dental office has taken shipment of a chemical. The dental assistant is reviewing the information on the material data safety sheet. Why is it important to review the material data safety sheet? Where should the sheets be organized?
Guidelines: Material data safety sheets (MSDS) provide comprehensive technical information and are a resource for employees working with chemicals. The sheets describe the physical and chemical properties of a chemical, health hazards, routes of exposure, precautions for safe handling and use, emergency and first-aid procedures, and spill-control measures. Material data safety sheets should be kept in binders in a central location so that all employees working with chemicals have ready access to them and can easily locate a particular MSDS.

OBJECTIVES	CONTENT	TEACHING RESOURCES
Pronounce, define, and spell the Key Terms.	■ Key terms (p. 344)	SW Fill in the Blank questions 1-11 (p. 124) ESLR Electronic Flashcards *Class Activity Have students develop a crossword puzzle using key terms. They can use an Internet Web site or create their own. Have students exchange puzzles with classmates to solve.*
Describe potential long-term and short-term effects of exposure to chemicals.	■ Hazardous chemicals (p. 345)	PPT 5-8 TB question 1 SW Short-Answer Questions 1; Fill in the Blank question 5; Multiple Choice questions 1, 8 (pp. 123-125) Recall questions 1-2 (p. 346) ▸ Discuss the properties used to classify a chemical as hazardous. ▸ Discuss the long-term and short-term effects on the body of exposure to chemicals. *Class Activity Divide the class into two groups. Ask each group to identify and discuss long-term and short-term effects of exposure to chemicals. Then have each group share its findings with the class for discussion.*
Describe three common methods of chemical exposure.	☐ Exposure to chemicals (p. 345)	PPT 9 TB question 2 SW Short-Answer Questions 3; Fill in the Blank questions 3-4; Multiple Choice question 2 (pp. 123-124) How Chemicals Enter the Body (p. 345) Figure 23-1 Chemical hazard warning labels (p. 346) Recall question 3 (p. 346)

ELSEVIER

Torres and Ehrlich Modern Dental Assisting, 9th ed.

Bird/Robinson

OBJECTIVES	CONTENT	TEACHING RESOURCES

		♀ CTQ 2 (p. 358)
		
		▸ Discuss exposure to chemicals from inhalation, skin contact, and ingestion and the physical damage that can occur from each method.
		
		Class Activity *Present the following characteristics to the class. Then, ask students to determine which method of chemical exposure the characteristic represents.*
		
		  – *Eating or drinking chemicals*
		
		  – *Direct skin contact with chemicals*
		
		  – *Inhaling chemical vapors*
		
		As a class, discuss the types of chemicals that are associated with each type of exposure. Are effects likely to be long term or short term?

Describe the difference between chronic and acute chemical exposure.	☐ Acute and chronic chemical toxicity (p. 346)	🖾 PPT 10 🖳 TB questions 3-4 📖 SW Short-Answer Questions 6; Multiple Choice question 3 (pp. 123-124) Recall question 4 (p. 346) ♀ CTQ 1 (p. 358) ▸ Discuss acute and chronic chemical toxicity, the potential for harm relative to the amount of dose and duration of exposure, and the effects on the body of each type of toxicity. **Class Activity** *Divide the class into two groups. Have one group discuss chronic chemical exposure and the other group discuss acute chemical exposure. What are the effects of exposure? What chemicals are likely to be involved in a dental office? Have each group present its findings to the class.*
Identify four methods of personal protection against chemical exposure.	☐ Hand protection (p. 346) ☐ Eye protection (p. 346) ☐ Protective clothing (p. 347) ☐ Inhalation protection (p. 347) ☐ Control of chemical spills (p. 347) ☐ Eyewash units (p. 347) ☐ Ventilation (p. 348)	🖾 PPT 11-21 🖳 TB questions 5-6 📖 SW Short-Answer Questions 7; Multiple Choice questions 4-5 (pp. 123-125) Figure 23-2 Clean room nitrile gloves (p. 346) Figure 23-3 Dental assistant wearing chemical goggles (p. 347) Figure 23-4 Disposable respirator (p. 347) Figure 23-5 Mercury spill kit (p. 347)

Bird/Robinson

OBJECTIVES	CONTENT	TEACHING RESOURCES
		Precautions When Working with Mercury (p. 348)
		Figure 23-6 Countertop eyewash and eye/face washes (p. 348)
		Recall questions 5-7 (p. 349)
		▸ Discuss hand, eye, and inhalation protection, control of chemical spills, and the importance of ventilation.
		▸ Discuss mercury spill kits and precautions to take when working with mercury and cleaning up a mercury spill.
		Class Activity *Present the following examples of personal protection against chemical exposure:*
		– Gloves
		– Goggles
		– Rubber apron
		– Mask
		Ask the class to identify the method of personal protection against exposure to specific types of hazardous substances.
Describe in general how chemicals should be stored.	☐ General precautions for storing chemicals (p. 348) – Follow instructions (p. 348) – Avoid exposure to light (p. 348) – Check expiration date (p. 349) – Rotate inventory (p. 349) ☐ Disposal of empty containers (p. 349) ☐ Hazardous waste disposal (p. 349)	PPT 22-24 SW Short-Answer Questions 8; Multiple Choice question 7 (pp. 123, 125) Guidelines for Minimizing Exposure to Chemical Hazards in the Dental Office (p. 349) Recall questions 8-9 (pp. 349-350) ▸ Discuss general precautions for storing and disposing of chemicals and disposing empty containers. Note that a basic policy is to store them in a cool, dry, dark place where they are not exposed to direct sunlight. ▸ Discuss the need to follow manufacturer instructions, check the expiration date, and rotate inventory. What are some signs that a chemical has deteriorated? **Class Activity** *Present the following situation to the class:* *A dental assistant is asked to review the practices of the office regarding storage of hazardous chemicals and disposal of empty containers. The assistant is asked to recommend improvements.* *What should the dental assistant look for? What elements should the "ideal" dental office incorporate?*

23.1 Homework/Assignments:

23.1 Instructor's Notes/Student Feedback:

CRITICAL THINKING QUESTION

A dental assistant is preparing to use a chemical that has a number 2 in a blue triangle on the chemical label. Before using the chemical, the assistant reads the chemical label and determines the special precautions needed when working with this chemical. What does the information on the chemical label indicate? What should the dental assistant do?

Guidelines: The chemical label indicates hazards to health, flammability, reactivity, and other special notice. A blue triangle on the chemical label represents health hazards. A number 2 in the health section of the chemical label indicates that the chemical is an inhalation hazard and that there is a need for a mask or special ventilation. The assistant should wear a mask and inform others working around the chemical of the inhalation hazard and ensure that proper protection is used. The dental assistant should also examine the ventilation to determine if it is adequate to prevent toxic exposure.

OBJECTIVES	CONTENT	TEACHING RESOURCES
Explain the purpose of the OSHA Hazard Communication Standard.	■ Hazard communication program (p. 349)	PPT 28 TB question 9 SW Fill in the Blank question 1; Multiple Choice question 9 (pp. 124-125) Recall question 10 (p. 350) ▸ Discuss the OSHA Hazard Communication Standard. ***Class Activity Lead the class in a discussion in which students explain the purpose of the OSHA Hazard Communication Standard. Why is it also known as the "Employee Right-to-Know Law"? Who benefits from the standard? What could be the consequences if it were not followed?***
Explain the record-keeping requirements of the Hazard Communication Standard.	■ Hazard communication program (p. 349)	SW Short-Answer Questions 2, 9 (p. 123) ▸ Discuss the OSHA Hazard Communication Standard while emphasizing the record-keeping requirements involved in each of the five parts of the hazard communication program. ***Class Activity Invite an OSHA representative to discuss the importance of record-keeping requirements and practical ways to develop and maintain good records in a dental office. Do local and state requirements vary? What are the responsibilities of the dental assistant? Ask students to prepare questions in advance.***
Describe the components of a hazard communication program.	■ Hazard communication program (p. 349) ☐ Written program (p. 350) ☐ Chemical inventory (p. 350)	PPT 29-31 TB question 10 SW Short-Answer Questions 4; Multiple Choice question 10 (pp. 123, 125) Responsibilities of Dental Assistant as Coordinator of Hazard Communication Program (p. 349)

ELSEVIER

OBJECTIVES	CONTENT	TEACHING RESOURCES

	☐ Material safety data sheets (p. 350)
	
	☐ Employee training (p. 350)
	
	☐ Labeling of chemical containers (p. 353)
		Recall question 11 (p. 350)
		
		▸ Discuss the five elements of the hazard communication program.
		
		▸ Discuss the responsibilities of the dental assistant as coordinator of the hazard communication program.
		
		***Class Activity** Divide the class into five groups. Assign each group one of the parts of the hazard communication program:*
		
		  – *Written program*
		
		  – *Inventory of hazardous chemicals*
		
		  – *MSDS for every chemical*
		
		  – *Proper labeling of containers*
		
		  – *Employee training*
		
		Ask each group to identify the components of its assigned part and to outline a plan for implementing the program in a dental office. Have groups present their plans. Evaluate as a class and incorporate appropriate elements from each part into a comprehensive class plan.

Explain the purpose of a material safety data sheet.	☐ Material safety data sheets (p. 350) ☐ Employee training (p. 350) ☐ Labeling of chemical containers (p. 353)	PPT 32-34 TB questions 11-12 SW Short-Answer Questions 5; Fill in the Blank questions 2, 6; Multiple Choice questions 11, 13-14 (pp. 123-125) SW Case Study question 5 (p. 126) Table 23-1 Sections of Material Safety Data Sheet (MSDS) (p. 350) Figure 23-7 Simulated material safety data sheet (MSDS) (pp. 351-352) Figure 23-8 Example of an MSDS binder (p. 353) Outline for Hazard Communication Training Program (p. 353) Table 23-2 Types of Dental Waste (p. 353) Recall questions 12, 14-15 (pp. 350, 354) ▸ Discuss the material safety data sheet, its purpose, the types of information included in its nine sections, and the importance of employee training for a successful hazard communication program. ▸ Discuss types of dental waste: medical waste, chemical waste, and general waste.

Torres and Ehrlich Modern Dental Assisting, 9th ed.

Bird/Robinson

OBJECTIVES	CONTENT	TEACHING RESOURCES
		Class Activity Divide the class into small groups, and give each group a different MSDS for a chemical commonly found in a dental office. Have each group discuss the information on the MSDS and what it means in practice for the dental assistant. What actions should the dental assistant take? How should the chemical be used? What record-keeping is necessary? Have each group share key points with the class for discussion and feedback.
Create a label for a secondary container.	☐ Labeling of chemical containers (p. 353) – National Fire Protection Association labels (p. 353) – Exemptions to labeling requirements (p. 354) Procedure 23-1 Creating an appropriate label for a secondary container (p. 354) (SW/ESLR Competency 23-1, p. 127)	PPT 35 TB question 13 SW Multiple Choice question 12 (p. 125) SW Case Study questions 1-4 (pp. 125-126) SW/ESLR Competency 23-1 Creating an Appropriate Label for a Secondary Container (p. 127) Figure 23-9 Chemical disinfectants *not* in their original containers must be clearly labeled (p. 354) Figure 23-10 Labeling and the National Fire Protection Association Rating System (p. 355) Recall question 13 (p. 354) CTQ 4 (p. 358) ▶ Discuss labeling of chemical containers, including secondary containers. ▶ Discuss National Fire Protection Association labels, including the system's use of four colored diamonds and numbering system. *Class Activity Divide the class into small groups, and provide each group equipment and supplies to label a secondary container. Identify several chemicals used in a dental office that may be stored in a secondary container, and assign each group a chemical. Then ask the groups to create an appropriate label. Students may refer to Procedure 23-1 (p. 373). Have groups present their labels, explain the steps they followed, and describe what they learned from performing the procedure.*
Identify types of regulated waste generated in a dental office.	■ Dental office waste management (p. 354) ☐ Classification of waste (p. 356) ☐ Extracted teeth (p. 356) ☐ Sharps (p. 356)	TB questions 14-16 SW Short-Answer Questions 10; Fill in the Blank questions 8-11; Multiple Choice question 15 (pp. 123-125) Dental Materials That May Be Regulated (p. 356) Figure 23-11 Classification of dental waste (p. 356) Figure 23-12 Biohazard bag and biohazard sharps container (p. 356)

OBJECTIVES	CONTENT	TEACHING RESOURCES
	☐ Scrap amalgam (p. 356) ☐ Photochemical waste (p. 357) – Radiographic fixer (p. 357) – Radiographic developer (p. 357) ☐ Lead contamination (p. 357) – Lead foil (p. 357) – Lead-lined boxes (p. 357) ☐ Disinfectants (p. 357) ☐ Nonhazardous waste management (p. 358)	Figure 23-13 Radiographic solutions in holding containers (p. 357) Figure 23-14 Lead-lined wooden box is a source of lead contamination (p. 357) Recall question 16 (p. 358) ▸ Discuss dental office waste management, including materials that may be regulated and why each is considered hazardous. What are proper procedures for disposing of extracted teeth, sharps, and scrap amalgam? ▸ Discuss the differences between regulated waste and contaminated waste. What is a main difference between OSHA regulations and EPA regulations? ***Class Activity** Ask the class to describe the classifications of dental office waste products. What is meant by regulated? Unregulated? Differentiate between medical waste and chemical waste. What are some examples of each type?*
Identify types of toxic waste generated in a dental office.	☐ Photochemical waste (p. 357) – Radiographic fixer (p. 357) – Radiographic developer (p. 357) ☐ Lead contamination (p. 357) – Lead foil (p. 357) – Lead-lined boxes (p. 357) ☐ Disinfectants (p. 357) ☐ Nonhazardous waste management (p. 358)	TB question 17 SW Short-Answer Questions 11; Multiple Choice question 6 (pp. 123, 125) Recall question 17 (p. 358) ▸ Discuss proper disposal methods for photochemical waste, lead contaminants, and disinfectants. ***Class Activity** Lead a discussion in which students identify the types of toxic waste generated in a dental office. What is the dental assistant's responsibility in using and disposing of these products?*
Describe how to package regulated waste for transport.	■ Waste disposal (p. 358)	TB questions 18-19 SW Short-Answer Questions 12; Fill in the Blank question 7 (pp. 123-124) Legal and Ethical Implications (p. 358) Eye to the Future (p. 358) CTQ 5 (p. 358) ▸ Discuss the characteristics of proper waste disposal containers, and describe state and local regulations for hazardous waste disposal.

OBJECTIVES	CONTENT	TEACHING RESOURCES
		▸ Discuss legal and ethical implications of improper waste management and why proper waste management is an important ethical consideration for the dental assistant. ***Class Activity** Divide the class into groups, and ask each group to identify options for disposing and transporting regulated waste from the dental office. What types of containers are required? What regulations must be followed? What resources are available? Ask groups to share their recommendations with the class.*
Performance Evaluation		TB SW questions (pp. 123-125) SW Case Study (pp. 125-126) SW/ESLR Competency 23-1 Creating an Appropriate Label for a Secondary Container (p. 127) ESLR Electronic Flashcards ESLR Practice Quiz ESLR Labeling Exercise 19: National Fire Protection Association Rating System Recall questions (pp. 346-358) CTQ (p. 358)

23.2 Homework/Assignments:

23.2 Instructor's Notes/Student Feedback:

ELSEVIER

Torres and Ehrlich Modern Dental Assisting, 9th ed.

Bird/Robinson

Slide 1

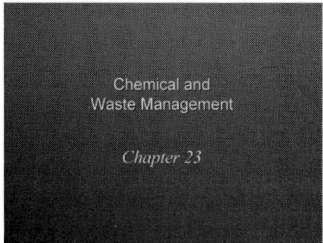

Slide 2

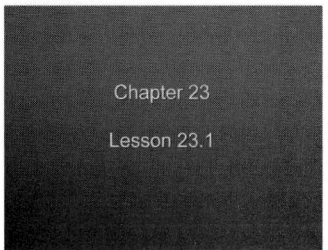

Slide 3

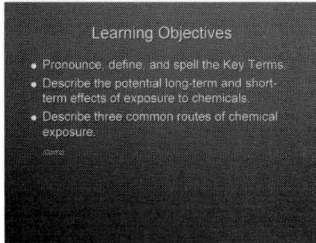

Slide 4

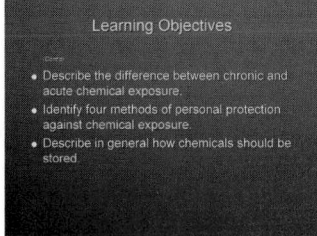

Torres and Ehrlich Modern Dental Assisting, 9th ed.

Bird/Robinson

Slide 5

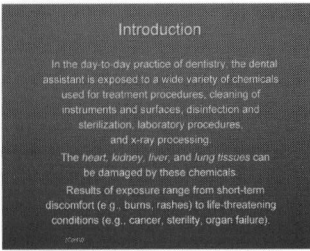

- What are some examples of items that require special disposal procedures? *(X-ray processing solutions, lead foil backing from film packets, scrap dental amalgam.)*

- Occupational Safety and Health Administration (OSHA) Hazard Communication Standard was designed to ensure chemical safety in the workplace.

Slide 6

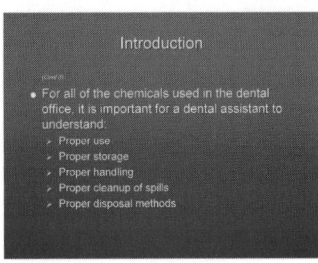

- In addition to understanding the proper use, storage, handling, cleanup, and disposal of chemicals, what knowledge should the dental assistant possess? *(First-aid procedures associated with chemicals.)*

- What is the nearest location where dental assistants can find OSHA-approved programs?

Slide 7

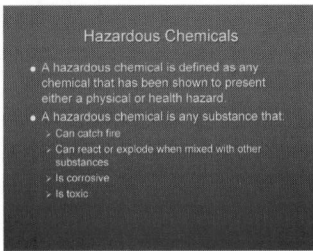

- What hazardous chemicals are used in dentistry? *(Mercury, powdered natural rubber latex, disinfectants, nitrous oxide, volatiles from resin-based materials, x-ray chemicals, cleansers, methyl metacrylate monomer, and elastomeric impression materials.)*

- Which chemical is of greatest concern? *(Mercury.)*

- What serious health consequences could result from exposure to hazardous chemicals?

Slide 8

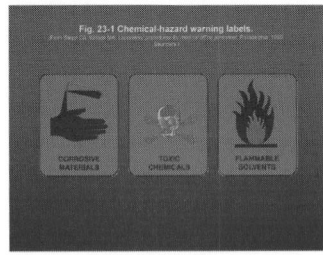

- What is the effect of corrosives? *(Corrosives can burn and destroy body tissues on contact.)*

- What materials are considered corrosive?

Bird/Robinson

Slide 9

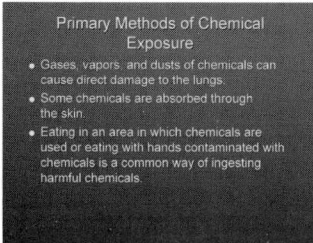

- What conditions can exposure cause or contribute to? *(Organ damage, respiratory disease, cancer, burns, sterility, dermatitis.)*
- Which hazardous chemicals are inhaled?
- Which are absorbed through the skin?
- Which are ingested?

Slide 10

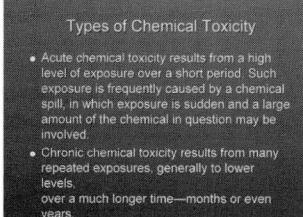

- The difference between acute and chronic toxicity: acute has a short duration and chronic lasts a long time.
- What are signs and symptoms of acute toxicity? *(Dizziness, fainting, headache, nausea, vomiting.)*
- What are the effects of chronic toxicity? *(Liver disease, brain disorders, cancer, infertility.)*

Slide 11

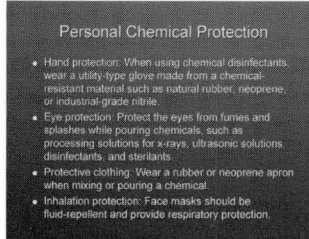

- Why are latex gloves worn during patient care insufficient when handling chemicals? *(Latex in the glove degrades and creates a sucking action that pulls contaminants and chemicals through the glove and onto the hands.)*
- What are the three types of eye/face protection? *(Safety glasses, face shields, and goggles.)*
  - Because of comfort, ease of use, and appearance, safety glasses are usually preferred over goggles.
- For what types of hazardous materials should the dental assistant wear protective clothing? Inhalation protection?

Slide 12

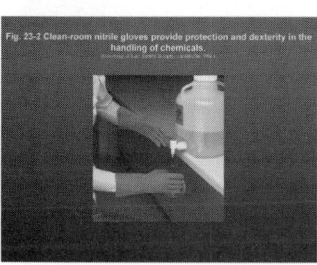

- Keep in mind that gloves were designed as protection against an occasional splash or spill, not for immersion in strong chemicals.
- What materials should be used to make gloves that are used by individuals who work with chemicals? Why?

Bird/Robinson

Slide 13

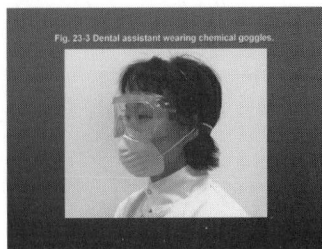

Fig. 23-3 Dental assistant wearing chemical goggles.

- According to a study published in the *Journal of Contemporary Dental Practice,* wearing eye protection was the least-practiced measure to control infection.

- What might be a common cause of damage to the eyes? *(Splatters and projectiles, including calculus and flying debris during cavity preparation.)*

Slide 14

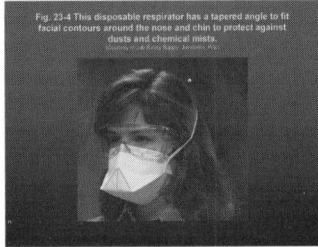

Fig. 23-4 This disposable respirator has a tapered angle to fit facial contours around the nose and chin to protect against dusts and chemical mists.

- Mist-respirator face masks must be approved by the National Institute of Occupational Safety and Health.

- The proper mask should repel fluids and provide respiratory protection.

- Under what circumstances should the dental assistant be sure to wear a mist-respirator face mask?

Slide 15

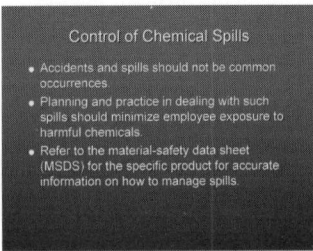

Control of Chemical Spills

- Accidents and spills should not be common occurrences.
- Planning and practice in dealing with such spills should minimize employee exposure to harmful chemicals.
- Refer to the material-safety data sheet (MSDS) for the specific product for accurate information on how to manage spills.

- What are the primary routes of exposure? *(Inhalation, skin contact, and ingestion.)*

- What information is provided on the material safety data sheet (MSDS)?

- For what types of chemicals are MSDSs required?

- How would a dental assistant use an MSDS?

Slide 16

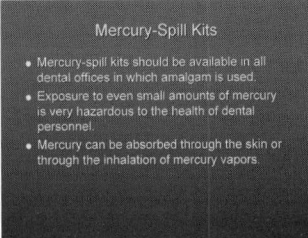

Mercury-Spill Kits

- Mercury-spill kits should be available in all dental offices in which amalgam is used.
- Exposure to even small amounts of mercury is very hazardous to the health of dental personnel.
- Mercury can be absorbed through the skin or through the inhalation of mercury vapors.

- What does a mercury spill kit contain? *(Mercury-absorbing powder, mercury- absorbing sponges, and a disposal bag.)*

- What are some precautions to take when working with mercury?

ELSEVIER

Torres and Ehrlich Modern Dental Assisting, 9th ed.

Bird/Robinson

Slide 17

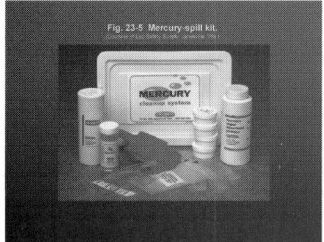

- A mask and utility gloves should be worn whenever cleaning up a mercury spill.

Slide 18

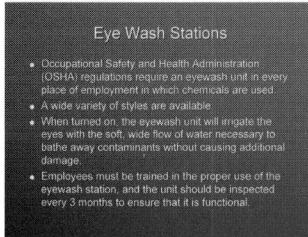

- Emergency eyewash stations provide on-the-spot decontamination and allow workers to flush away hazardous substances that can cause serious injury.

Slide 19

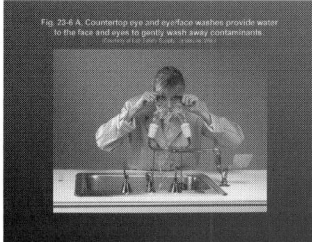

- Why do some manufacturers recommend a weekly, 3-minute flushing of the eyewash station? *(To reduce microbial content in the waterline.)*

Slide 20

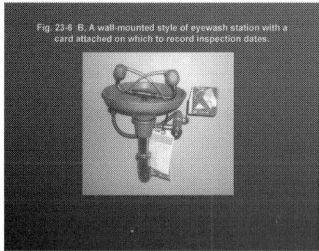

Slide 21

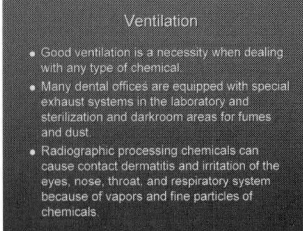

- Why is it important to have good ventilation in a dental office?
- Can good ventilation also help reduce incidence of airborne disease?
- How can a person tell if a dental office has good ventilation?

Slide 22

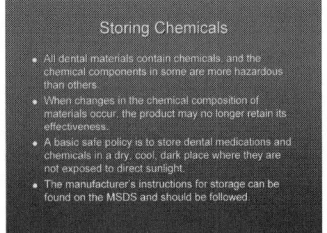

- What are four key points in storing chemicals? *(Follow manufacturer instructions, avoid exposure to light, check expiration date, and rotate inventory.)*
- What are some guidelines for minimizing exposure to chemical hazards in the dental office?

Slide 23

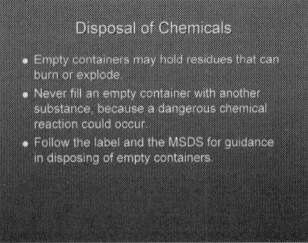

- What determines whether or not a substance is a hazardous waste? *(If it contains certain properties or chemicals that could pose dangers to human health and the environment after being discarded.)*
- What are the local and state regulations for disposal of hazardous waste?

Slide 24

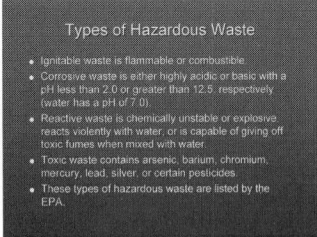

- Hazardous wastes can contaminate land, air, and water.
- What hazardous wastes are commonly generated by dental offices? *(Photo- processing wastes [x-ray fixer, developer, and cleaner; x-ray film; lead foils and shields] chemical disinfectants; line cleaner wastes; universal wastes [batteries, fluorescent lamps, mercury thermometers] amalgam wastes [scrap, capsules, extracted teeth, sludge].)*

Torres and Ehrlich Modern Dental Assisting, 9th ed.

Bird/Robinson

Slide 25

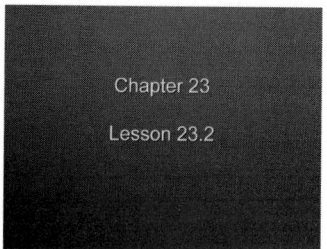

Slide 26

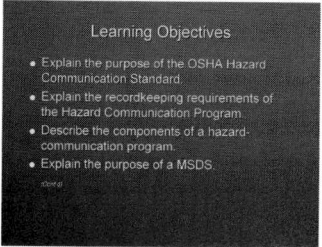

Slide 27

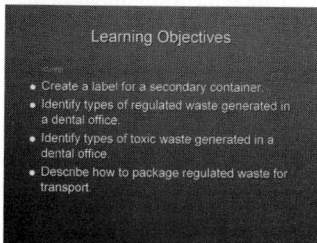

Slide 28

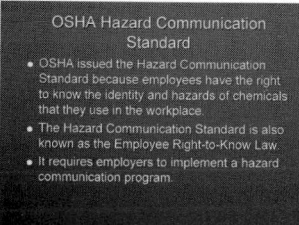

- It also ensures that employees know how to protect themselves from the chemicals.

- Why is the OSHA Hazard Communication Standard also known as the Employee Right-to-Know Law?

- What record-keeping elements are important? Why?

Slide 29

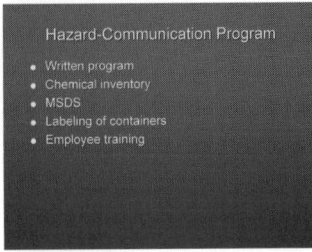

- In addition, the hazard communication program (HCP) should also address nonroutine tasks and exposure of other personnel, such as outside contractors.
- What are the dental assistant's responsibilities as coordinator of the office hazard communication program? *(Read and understand the OSHA Hazard Communication Standard and implement the written HCP. Compile a chemical inventory, obtain the MSDSs, and update the MSDS file as new products are added to the inventory. Inform other employees of the location of the MSDSs. Also label appropriate containers and provide training to other employees.)*

Slide 30

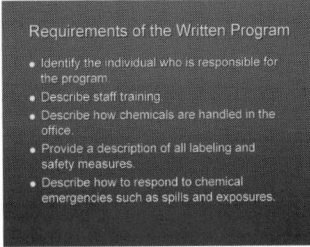

- The written program also requires that each individual who is exposed to hazardous chemicals be identified by name.

Slide 31

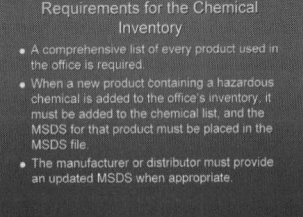

- Several companies offer software and bar code programs that keep track of the chemical inventory, where chemicals are stored, what is in stock, and MSDS information.
- What is included in the list of products that contain chemicals?

Slide 32

- The MSDS is meant to be an easy reference for information on hazardous substances.
- Why are MSDSs so important? *(Each employee has the right to know what types of substances he or she is working with and how to safely handle them.)*
- What are the nine sections of an MSDS?
- What information is included in each section?
- What is a good way to store MSDSs?
- Why are storage and accessibility of MSDSs important?

Slide 33

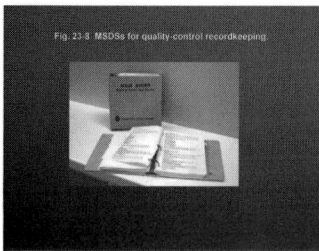

Slide 34

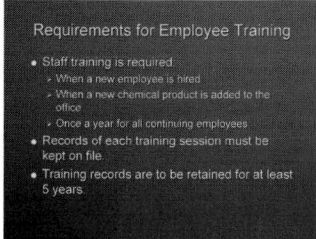

- What areas must be included in the chemical training program? *(The use of hazardous materials; all safety practices, including all warnings; required PPE; safe handling and disposal methods.)*

- Why is it important to train employees in the use and disposal of hazardous chemicals?

- What is included in a hazard communication training program?

Slide 35

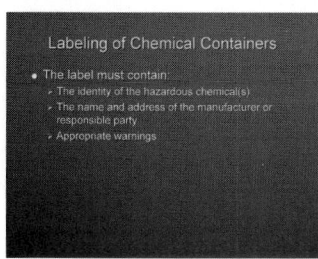

- The National Fire Protection Association has a labeling system that is frequently used to label containers of hazardous chemicals.

- What are the colors of the four diamonds and what does each represent? *(Blue – health hazard; red – flammable; yellow – reactivity; white – special hazard symbols.)*

- Is this an effective labeling system? Why or why not?

- What are the types of dental waste? How should each be labeled?

Bird/Robinson

24 Lesson Plan
Dental Unit Waterlines

TEACHING FOCUS

This chapter introduces the student to topics related to dental unit waterlines. The student will have an opportunity to learn about the microorganisms found in dental unit water; biofilm; methods for reducing bacterial contamination; and infection-control activities. The Centers for Disease Control and Prevention (CDC) recommendations for dental unit water quality and for the use of saliva ejectors will also be discussed.

MATERIALS AND RESOURCES

☐ computer and PowerPoint projector (all Lessons)

LESSON CHECKLIST

Preparations for this lesson include:

- lecture
- guest speaker: dental assistant
- evaluation of student knowledge and skills needed to perform all entry-level activities related to the principles underlying dental unit waterlines, including:
  - the role of biofilm in dental unit waterline contamination
  - the factors in bacterial contamination of dental unit water
  - methods to reduce bacterial contamination in dental unit waterlines
  - CDC recommendations for dental unit waterlines
  - the procedure for testing dental unit waterlines

Bird/Robinson

KEY TERMS

antiretraction device (p. 361)
biofilm (p. 361)
colony-forming units (CFUs) (p. 360)
dental unit waterline (DUWL) (p. 360)
heterotrophic bacteria (p. 364)

high-quality water (p. 363)
Legionella (p. 360)
microfiltration (p. 363)
planktonic (p. 361)
self-contained water reservoir (p. 363)

ADDITIONAL RESOURCES

PowerPoint slides (Evolve): 1-25

Legend

CTQ
Critical
Thinking
Question

DVD
Multimedia
Procedures
Videos and
Animations

ESLR
EVOLVE
Student
Learning
Resources

IDO
Interactive
Dental
Office
CD-ROM

SW
Student
Workbook

TB
Test Bank
on the
TEACH
CD-ROM

PPT
PowerPoint
Slides

Class Activities are indicated in ***bold italic.***

Torres and Ehrlich Modern Dental Assisting, 9th ed.

Bird/Robinson

LESSON 24.1

PRETEST

1. In community water, the number of waterborne bacteria is kept below
   a. 150 colony-forming units.
   b. 250 colony-forming units.
   c. 300 colony-forming units.
   d. 500 colony-forming units.

2. The number of CFUs found in water from air-water syringes and dental handpieces can frequently reach
   a. one-half the level found in community water.
   b. equal levels.
   c. 10 times that of community water.
   d. hundreds of thousands times that of community water.

3. Dental workers are at greater risk of exposure to what disease?
   a. legionella
   b. lymphoma
   c. fungus
   d. adult respiratory distress syndrome

4. The primary source of microorganisms in dental unit waterlines (DUWLs) is
   a. backflow.
   b. dirty hands.
   c. the public water supply.
   d. biofilm.

5. What are the two "communities" of bacteria in dental unit waterlines?
   a. algae and fungi
   b. planktonic bacteria and biofilm
   c. those inside dental tubing and dental plaque
   d. fungi and protozoa

6. Heating water in the dental line may enhance
   a. patient discomfort.
   b. patient pain.
   c. infection control.
   d. microorganism growth.

7. Compared to the water supplied to the office, the water that enters the dental unit is
   a. from a separate well.
   b. warmer.
   c. the same.
   d. colder.

8. How many times more resistant to germicides are bacteria in biofilm compared to planktonic bacteria?
   a. 250 times
   b. 500 times
   c. 750 times
   d. 1500 times

9. Biofilm cannot be removed by
   a. flushing alone.
   b. microfiltration cartridges.
   c. chemical treatment regimens.
   d. self-contained water reservoirs.

10. The rubber dam serves as
    a. the only waterline cleaning regimen.
    b. a protective barrier.
    c. a suction unit.
    d. a device to hold the mouth open.

Answers

1. d	3. a	5. b	7. c	9. a
2. d	4. c	6. d	8. d	10. b

BACKGROUND ASSESSMENT

Question: What is the only way to determine whether the waterline cleaning regimen is effective?
Answer: Testing the water coming out of the unit is the only way to know whether the waterline cleaning regimen is effective. Two options for testing dental unit water are a commercial testing service or an in-office test kit. Using a commercial testing service will result in a certificate if the sample is below 500 CFUs. The CDC recommends that dental offices follow the recommendations of the dental unit manufacturer or the treatment product to monitor the quality of the dental unit water.

Question: How do chemical agents control biofilm?
Answer: Biofilm is extremely resistant to chemical destruction; chemical treatments must be performed at least once a week. Two ways chemicals are used to control biofilm are periodic or shock treatment and continuous application. Periodic or shock treatment is the use of chemicals at levels that will kill microorganisms. Continuous application is the continuous use of chemicals at levels that will kill microorganisms but not harm humans. Always check with the dental equipment manufacturer to determine the recommended chemical product and maintenance protocol.

CRITICAL THINKING QUESTION

The staff at the dental office is developing a policy to reduce bacterial contamination of dental unit waterlines. What should be included in the policy?
Guidelines: Listed below are eight methods to reduce bacterial contamination of dental unit waterlines that should be included in the policy.

- Flush waterlines for several minutes at the beginning of the day and longer after weekends. In addition, flush for 20 to 30 seconds between patients.
- Use a self-contained water reservoir system.
- Use a self-contained water reservoir system combined with periodic or continuous application of chemical germicides as recommended by the equipment manufacturer.
- Use a separate (sterile water) system for surgical procedures.
- Purge the water from the dental lines and dry them with air at the end of each day.
- Use microfiltration cartridges in the waterlines.
- Stay current with new techniques and manufacturing technology for dental unit waterlines.
- Follow the recommendations for monitoring water quality provided by the dental unit manufacturer.

OBJECTIVES	CONTENT	TEACHING RESOURCES
Pronounce, define, and spell the Key Terms.	■ Key terms (p. 359)	▧ SW Fill in the Blank questions 1-8 (pp. 129-130) ✐ ESLR Electronic Flashcards ▸ Discuss each of the key terms in Chapter 24, focusing on the definition, pronunciation, and spelling of each term. *Class Activity Have students develop a crossword puzzle using key terms and then exchange their puzzles with classmates to solve them.*
Discuss why there is a renewed interest in DUWL contamination.	■ Background (p. 360)	▤▦ PPT 5-7 ▧ SW Short-Answer Questions 3; Fill in the Blank questions 1-2; Multiple Choice questions 1-4 (pp. 129-130) Figure 24-1 Close-up of dental tube opening (p. 360) Recall questions 1-3 (p. 361) ▸ Discuss outbreaks of waterborne disease. Note that a broad range of facilities is affected. ▸ Discuss categories of patients with lowered resistance to disease who might be at a higher risk of illness due to DUWL contamination. *Class Activity Invite a dental assistant to speak to the class. Ask the speaker to discuss why there is a renewed interest in dental unit waterline contamination. Encourage feedback from the class.*

OBJECTIVES	CONTENT	TEACHING RESOURCES
Explain why dental unit waterlines contain more bacteria than faucets.	■ Background (p. 360) ■ Microorganisms in dental unit water (p. 361)	▣🖥 PPT 7-8 🖥 TB question 1 📖 SW Short-Answer Questions 1; Fill in the Blank questions 5, 7-8 (pp. 129-130) Dental Patients with Lowered Resistance to Disease (p. 360) Table 24-1 Sample Amounts of Bacteria in Dental Unit Water at Various U.S. Sites (p. 361) Recall question 4 (p. 361) ▶ Discuss the exposure of dental workers to Legionella bacteria through inhalation of contaminated aerosol generated by the handpiece and air-water syringe. ▶ Discuss saliva as a source of microorganisms in dental unit water. Note that saliva may be retracted into waterlines during treatment (a process called "backflow"). ***Class Activity Divide the class into small groups. Ask each group to discuss and explain why dental unit waterlines contain more bacteria than faucets. Discuss the difference in the number of colony-forming units per milliliter in community water and that found in air-water syringes and dental handpieces. Have each group share its findings with the class.***
Identify the primary source of microorganisms in dental unit water.	■ Microorganisms in dental unit water (p. 361)	▣🖥 PPT 9 📖 SW Short-Answer Questions 5 (p. 129) 📖 SW Case Study question 1 (p. 131) ▶ Discuss the primary source of microorganisms in dental unit water: the public water supply. ***Class Activity Ask the class to identify the primary source of microorganisms in dental unit water. How does the concentration of microorganisms in dental unit water compare to the concentration in community water? Encourage further discussion with the class.***
Explain the role of biofilm in dental unit waterline (DUWL) contamination.	■ Biofilm (p. 361)	▣🖥 PPT 10-12 🖥 TB question 2 📖 SW Short-Answer Questions 2; Multiple Choice question 5 (pp. 129-130) Figure 24-2 (A) Biofilm formation on the walls of the tube; (B) Cross-section of biofilm formation in DUWL (p. 361)

Bird/Robinson

OBJECTIVES	CONTENT	TEACHING RESOURCES
		Recall question 5 (p. 362)
		▸ Discuss the microorganisms present in biofilm.
		▸ Discuss why the inside of dental tubing is an especially favorable environment for biofilm formation.
		***Class Activity** Divide the class into two groups. Ask each group to determine the role of biofilm in dental unit waterline contamination. Then have each group share its findings with the class.*

List the factors in bacterial contamination of dental unit water.	■ Biofilm in dental waterlines (p. 361)
	   □ Growth-promoting factors (p. 362)
	   □ Bacterial characteristics (p. 362)
		PPT 13-14
		
		TB question 3
		
		SW Short-Answer Questions 4; Fill in the Blank question 4; Multiple Choice questions 6-7 (pp. 129-130)
		
		Figure 24-3 Bacteria in biofilm taken from dental unit waterlines (p. 362)
		
		Figure 24-4 Bacteria in biofilm dropping into waterlines (p. 362)
		
		Recall question 6 (p. 362)
		
		CTQ 2 (p. 366)
		
		▸ Discuss the process of biofilm formation in DUWLs, noting that intermittent stagnation of water flow can lead to biofilm formation.
		
		▸ Discuss the use of water heaters in dental offices, noting that water heaters may contribute to the formation of biofilm.
		
		***Class Activity** Present the following information to the class. Ask the class to identify whether each of the items is a factor in bacterial contamination of dental unit water.*
		
		   – *Heating of the dental unit water*
		   – *Maze of waterlines*
		   – *Slow movement of water*
		   – *Increased use of antibacterial solution*

Describe the methods to reduce bacterial contamination in dental unit waterlines.	■ Methods for reducing bacterial contamination (p. 362)
	   □ Self-contained water reservoirs (p. 363)
	   □ Microfiltration cartridges (p. 363)
	   □ Chemical agents (p. 363)
		PPT 15-21
		
		TB questions 4-6
		
		SW Short-Answer Questions 6; Fill in the Blank questions 3, 6; Multiple Choice questions 8-9 (pp. 129-130)
		
		SW Case Study question 2 (p. 131)
		
		Methods to Reduce Bacterial Contamination of Dental Unit Waterlines (p. 362)
		
		Figure 24-5 Self-contained dental water unit (p. 363)

ELSEVIER

Torres and Ehrlich Modern Dental Assisting, 9th ed.

Bird/Robinson

OBJECTIVES	CONTENT	TEACHING RESOURCES
		Figure 24-6 Reservoir bottles and lines in self-contained water systems must be cleaned (p. 363)
		Figure 24-7 The DentaPure cartridge releases 2 to 6 parts per million of iodine (p. 363)
		Recall questions 7-10 (p. 364)
		CTQ 1 (p. 366)
		▸ Discuss self-contained reservoir systems. Describe how these systems work and note their advantages. Discuss microfiltration cartridges. Describe how cartridges work and emphasize that they must be changed daily.
		▸ Discuss chemical agents. Describe the two ways in which chemical agents are used to control biofilm formation.
		Class Activity *Divide the class into four groups. Assign each group one method for reducing bacterial contamination of the dental unit waterline. Have each group discuss its method and then present its conclusions to the class.*
Describe the Centers for Disease Control and Prevention (CDC) recommendations for dental unit water quality.	■ Methods for reducing bacterial contamination (p. 362) ☐ Self-contained water reservoirs (p. 363) ☐ Microfiltration cartridges (p. 363) ☐ Chemical agents (p. 363) ■ Infection control and dental unit water (p. 364) ☐ Using the proper water (p. 364) ☐ Flushing waterlines (p. 364) ☐ Minimizing aerosol (p. 364) ☐ Using protective barriers (p. 364) ☐ Monitoring water quality (p. 364) ☐ Use of saliva ejectors (p. 364)	SW Multiple Choice questions 10-11 (p. 130) SW Case Study question 4 (p. 131) SW/ESLR Competency 24-1 Testing Dental Unit Waterlines (p. 133) CDC Recommendations for Dental Unit Waterlines, Biofilm, and Water Quality (p. 364) CTQ 3 (p. 366) ▸ Discuss CDC recommendations for dental unit waterlines, biofilm, and water quality. **Class Activity** *Present the following information to the class. Ask the class to determine if each item is a CDC recommendation for dental unit water quality.* *– Use water that meets the EPA regulatory standards for drinking water.* *– Use surface-disinfect on handpieces and other intraoral instruments that can be removed from the air and waterlines of dental units.* *– After each patient, discharge water and air for a minimum of 20 to 30 seconds from any device connected to the dental water system that enters the patient's mouth.* *– Do not advise patients to close their lips tightly around the tip of the saliva ejector to evacuate oral fluids.*

ELSEVIER

Torres and Ehrlich Modern Dental Assisting, 9th ed.

OBJECTIVES	CONTENT	TEACHING RESOURCES
	Procedure 24-1 Testing dental unit waterlines (p. 365) (SW/ESLR Competency 24-1, p. 133)	
Explain the CDC recommendation for the use of saliva ejectors.	■ Infection control and dental unit water (p. 364) □ Using the proper water (p. 364) □ Flushing waterlines (p. 364) □ Minimizing aerosol (p. 364) □ Using protective barriers (p. 364) □ Monitoring water quality (p. 364) □ Use of saliva ejectors (p. 364)	▣ PPT 22-25 TB questions 7-9 SW Multiple Choice questions 12-15 (p. 130) SW Case Study question 3 (p. 131) Recall questions 11-15 (p. 365) Figure 24-8 Aquasafe water test kit (p. 366) CDC Recommendations for Dental Handpieces and Other Devices Attached to Air and Waterlines (p. 365) Legal and Ethical Implications (p. 366) Eye to the Future (p. 366) ▸ Discuss flushing waterlines, noting proper frequency and duration. Emphasize that flushing will not remove biofilm from the lines. ▸ Discuss protective barriers, including the rubber dam, masks, eye protection, and face shields. ▸ Discuss the purpose of testing dental unit water quality, and the two testing options available. ▸ Discuss the potential for backflow when using a saliva ejector. ***Class Activity** Divide the class into two groups. Ask each group to identify and discuss one CDC recommendation for the use of saliva ejectors. Then have each group share its recommendation with the class.*
Performance Evaluation		TB SW questions (pp. 129-131) SW/ESLR Competency 24-1 Testing Dental Unit Waterlines (p. 133) ESLR Electronic Flashcards ESLR Practice Quiz Recall questions (pp. 361-365) CTQ (p. 366)

24.1 Homework/Assignments:

24.1 Instructor's Notes/Student Feedback:

Slide 1

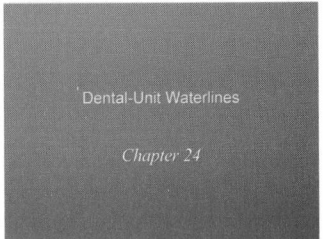

Dental-Unit Waterlines

Chapter 24

Slide 2

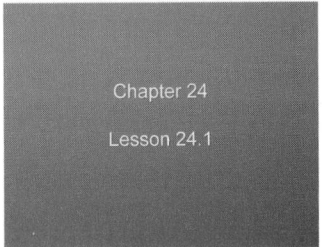

Chapter 24

Lesson 24.1

Slide 3

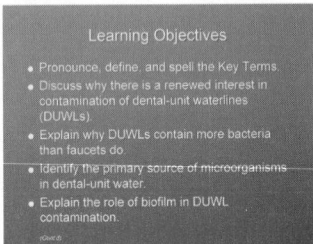

Learning Objectives

- Pronounce, define, and spell the Key Terms.
- Discuss why there is a renewed interest in contamination of dental-unit waterlines (DUWLs).
- Explain why DUWLs contain more bacteria than faucets do.
- Identify the primary source of microorganisms in dental-unit water.
- Explain the role of biofilm in DUWL contamination.

Slide 4

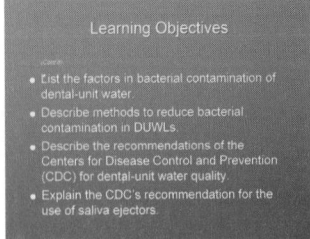

Learning Objectives

- List the factors in bacterial contamination of dental-unit water.
- Describe methods to reduce bacterial contamination in DUWLs.
- Describe the recommendations of the Centers for Disease Control and Prevention (CDC) for dental-unit water quality.
- Explain the CDC's recommendation for the use of saliva ejectors.

Torres and Ehrlich Modern Dental Assisting, 9th ed.

Bird/Robinson

Slide 5

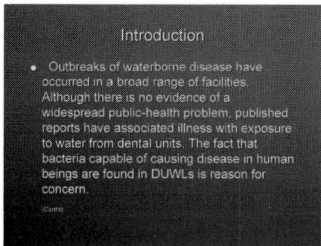

- The Centers for Disease Control recommend that dental water meet the same standards as drinking water.

Slide 6

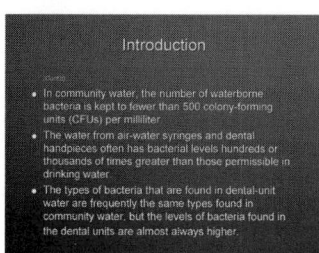

- Most organisms isolated from dental water systems originate from the public water supply and do not pose a high risk of disease for healthy persons.

Slide 7

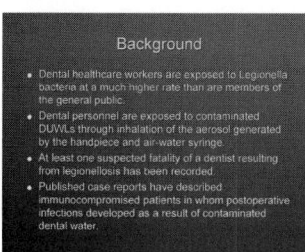

- What other pathogenic organisms are dental health care workers exposed to? *(Pseudomonas, CDC.)*

Slide 8

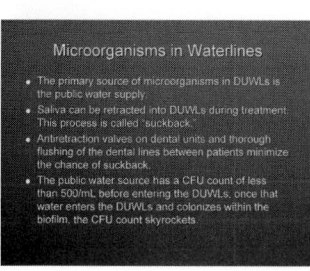

- How does biofilm function in the plastic tubing? *(It serves as a reservoir that dramatically increases the number of free-floating microorganisms in water.)*

- Monitoring of dental water quality can be performed with commercial, self-contained test kits.

Slide 9

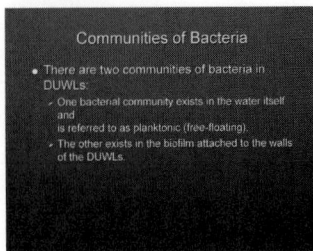

- How does biofilm form? *(Biofilm forms when bacteria attach to surfaces exposed to water and begin to excrete a slimy, glue-like substance.)*

Slide 10

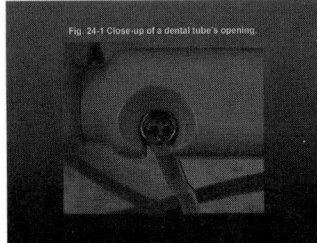

- The small bore tubing is ideal for biofilm formation.

- What is the most well-known biofilm? *(Dental plaque.)*

Slide 11

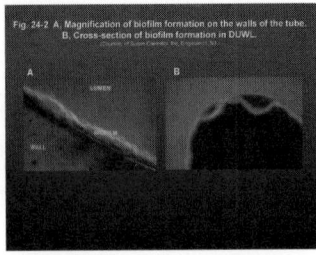

- Biofilm is responsible for diseases such as ear infection, bacterial endocarditis (infection of the inner surface of the heart and its valves), cystic fibrosis, and Legionnaires' disease.

- Biofilm may also be responsible for a variety of nosocomial (hospital-based) infections caused by infections at surfaces of catheters, medical implants, wound dressings, and other medical devices.

Slide 12

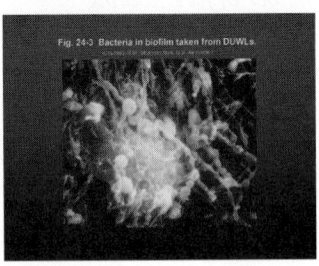

- Biofilm is highly resistant to antibiotics.

ELSEVIER

Torres and Ehrlich Modern Dental Assisting, 9th ed.

Bird/Robinson

Slide 13

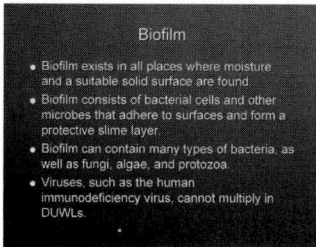

- Have students name five pathogens or organisms identified in dental water. *(Pseudomonas, Moraxella, Klebsiella, Legionella, Mycobacterium.)*

Slide 14

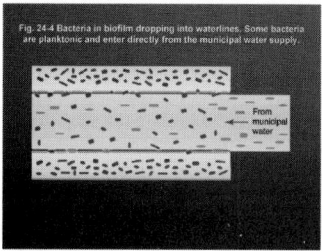

- Biofilm is notorious for causing pipe plugging, corrosion, and water contamination.

Slide 15

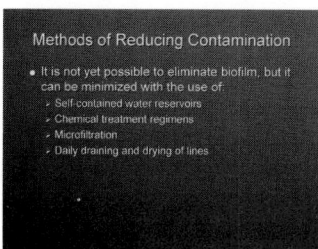

- The ADA and CDC recommend that waterlines be flushed for several minutes each morning.

- Handpieces should be flushed with air or water for 20 to 30 seconds between appointments.

- Some manufacturers may recommend installing antiretraction valves to prevent oral fluids from being drawn into the dental waterlines.

Slide 16

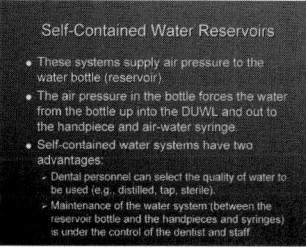

- This eliminates the need for inflow of municipal water and permits the introduction of chemical agents to remove or inactivate biofilm.

Bird/Robinson

Slide 17

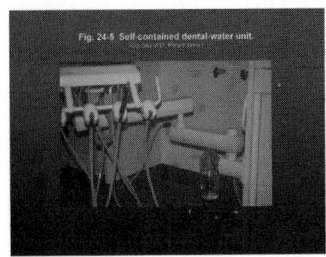

- Self-contained water systems require clearance by the Food and Drug Administration.

Slide 18

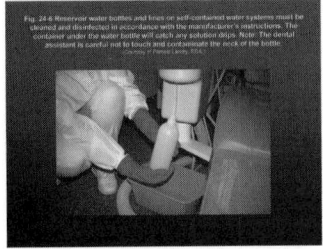

- Keep in mind that the water used on the patient is only as clean as the water entering the unit.

Slide 19

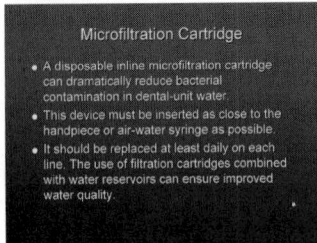

- The filter traps suspended organisms before they reach the surplus.
- Filtration cartridges require FDA clearance.
- Some filters also release germicides, which will require EPA registration.

Slide 20

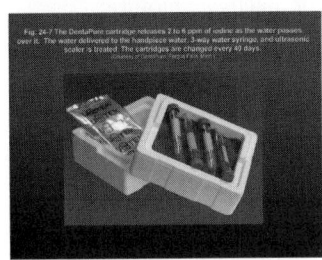

- Microfilters reduce the bacterial contamination of the water but do not affect the biofilm that colonizes the DUWLs.

Bird/Robinson

Slide 21

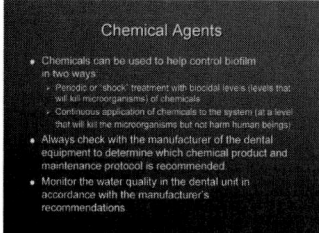

- Biofilm is extremely resistant to chemical destruction; therefore, chemical treatments must be performed regularly, usually once a week.

Slide 22

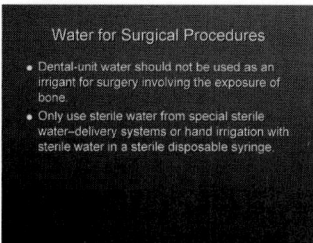

- Why is it important not to use dental unit water during surgery? *(Procedures like periodontal surgery, root canals, and tooth extractions are riskier because they expose the gum line. Introducing dental unit water could potentially introduce disease-causing bacteria.)*

Slide 23

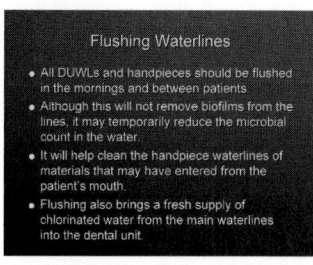

- Commercial devices and procedures designed to improve the quality of water used must be implemented to improve the quality of dental water.

- Flushing will not remove biofilm from the lines; biofilm can form while water is moving through the lines.

Slide 24

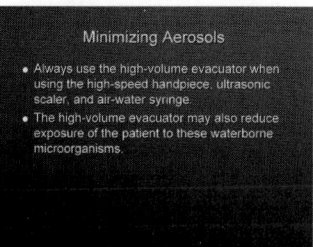

- Why should the high-volume evacuator be used? *(It will reduce contamination from the aerosol, spatter from the patient's saliva, and contamination from the water spray.)*

Slide 25

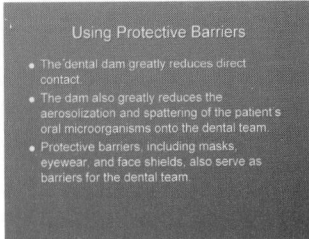

- What is the purpose of the rubber dam? *(It serves as a protective barrier for the patient from the dental unit water.)*

Torres and Ehrlich Modern Dental Assisting, 9th ed.

Bird/Robinson

25 Lesson Plan
Ergonomics

TEACHING FOCUS

This chapter will provide students with an opportunity to learn about the importance of ergonomics while performing tasks in the dental environment. The chapter illustrates preventive exercises to reduce muscle fatigue, eyestrain, neck strain, and musculoskeletal disorders. Students will also have the opportunity to examine carpal tunnel syndrome, a common injury caused by repetitive motion.

MATERIALS AND RESOURCES

☐ computer and PowerPoint projector (all Lessons)

LESSON CHECKLIST

Preparations for this lesson include:

- lecture
- evaluation of student knowledge and skills needed to perform all entry-level activities related to ergonomics, including:
  - demonstrating the proper (neutral) posture position
  - demonstrating accurate muscle-strengthening exercises for the hand, back, neck, and shoulders
  - identifying the proper reach techniques to reduce injury
  - identifying reach techniques that may be problematic
  - explaining the purpose and importance of ergonomics for the dental environment

Bird/Robinson

KEY TERMS

carpal tunnel syndrome (p. 370)
cumulative trauma disorders (p. 370)
ergonomics (p. 368)
maximum horizontal reach (p. 370)
maximum vertical reach (p. 370)
musculoskeletal disorders (MSDS) (p. 368)

neutral position (p. 369)
normal horizontal reach (p. 370)
sprains (p. 369)
strains (p. 369)
thenar eminence (p. 370)

ADDITIONAL RESOURCES

PowerPoint slides (Evolve): 1-38
Multimedia Procedures DVD:
    Body Strengthening Exercises

Legend

CTQ
Critical
Thinking
Question

DVD
Multimedia
Procedures
Videos and
Animations

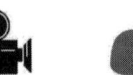

ESLR
EVOLVE
Student
Learning
Resources

IDO
Interactive
Dental
Office
CD-ROM

SW
Student
Workbook

TB
Test Bank
on the
TEACH
CD-ROM

PPT
PowerPoint
Slides

Class Activities are indicated in ***bold italic***.

ELSEVIER

Torres and Ehrlich Modern Dental Assisting, 9th ed.

Bird/Robinson

LESSON 25.1

PRETEST

1. Ergonomics deals with
   a. staying healthy.
   b. adaptation of the work environment to the human body.
   c. the finances of a dental practice.
   d. positioning of patients.

2. When the dental assistant first experiences pain, he or she should
   a. reduce inflammation and assist healing.   c. quit working.
   b. ignore it until it becomes more serious.   d. find a new occupation.

3. Posture affects the ability of the dental assistant to
   a. take periodic breaks.   c. reach, hold, and use equipment.
   b. perform less stressful procedures.   d. perform difficult procedures.

4. When turning is necessary, the dental assistant should
   a. reach behind his or her back and lift.   c. twist the top half of the body.
   b. rotate the chair.   d. lean forward.

5. The neutral position is established by
   a. sitting and leaning slightly forward.
   b. sitting upright and leaning to the side of preference.
   c. sitting and leaning slightly backward.
   d. sitting upright with weight evenly distributed.

6. Strains result from
   a. extreme stretching of muscles or ligaments.
   b. repetitive movements.
   c. sudden twists or wrenching of a joint with stretching or tearing of ligaments.
   d. reaching behind the body.

7. Sprains result from
   a. extreme stretching of muscles or ligaments.
   b. repetitive movements.
   c. sudden twists or wrenching of a joint with stretching or tearing of ligaments.
   d. reaching behind the body.

8. What is one of the most important factors in preventing CTS?
   a. stretching   c. deep breathing
   b. frequently resting the hands   d. maintaining a neutral position

9. To relieve eyestrain during a long procedure, for how many seconds should the dental assistant look up from a task?
   a. 5 seconds   c. 20 seconds
   b. 10 seconds   d. 45 seconds

10. Shoulder shrugging will help stretch
    a. shoulder muscles.   c. forearm muscles.
    b. neck muscles.   d. back muscles.

Answers

1. b	3. c	5. d	7. c	9. c
2. a	4. b	6. a	8. b	10. a

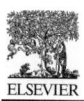

Torres and Ehrlich Modern Dental Assisting, 9ᵗʰ ed.

Bird/Robinson

BACKGROUND ASSESSMENT

Question: What is the neutral position?
Answer: The neutral position is the ideal way to work. This position is established by sitting upright with the weight evenly distributed and feet flat on the floor.

Question: What are the three categories of risk factors that contribute to musculoskeletal disorders?
Answer: Posture, repetition, and force. Posture affects the ability of the dental assistant to reach, hold, and use equipment. Repetitive motion, overflexion, and overextension of the wrist can significantly increase the risk of cumulative trauma disorders.

CRITICAL THINKING QUESTION

A dental assistant complains about lower back pain after sitting in a chair and bending over a patient while assisting the dentist. What steps could the assistant take to help prevent future complaints of lower back pain?
Guidelines: Poor position in the chair can contribute to the dental assistant's lower back pain. Proper positioning begins with making ceertain the chair is raised to a height that will allow for the dental assistant to sit straight while working on a patient. The dental assistant should also use the armrest to prevent further strain on the body and have the feet rest on the chair rail and not the floor. This will help to keep the back straight instead of bent over. Using the above recommendations will greatly reduce a recurrence of lower back pain due to poor positioning in the chair.

OBJECTIVES	CONTENT	TEACHING RESOURCES
Pronounce, define, and spell the Key Terms.	■ Key terms (p. 367)	*ESLR* Electronic Flashcards ▸ Discuss each of the key terms in Chapter 25, focusing on the definition, pronunciation, and spelling of each term. ***Class Activity** Have students develop a crossword puzzle using key terms. They can use a Web site such as www.puzzlemaker.com or do it on their own. Have them exchange their puzzles with classmates to solve them.*
Describe the goal of ergonomics.	■ Introduction (p. 368)	PPT 4-5 TB question 1 SW Short-Answer Questions 1; Fill in the Blank question 1; Multiple Choice questions 1-2 (pp. 135-136) Principle of Ergonomics (p. 368) Figure 25-1 Ergonomic factors in dentistry (p. 368) Recall questions 1-2 (p. 368) Legal and Ethical Implications (p. 373) CTQ 1 (p. 373) ▸ Discuss instances in which neglect of ergonomic factors has caused occupational injuries. ***Class Activity** Divide the class into six groups. Assign each group one of the ergonomic factors in dentistry. Have each group discuss and determine how their assigned factor plays a role in ergonomics. Then have each group share their factors with the class.*

Torres and Ehrlich Modern Dental Assisting, 9th ed.

Bird/Robinson

OBJECTIVES	CONTENT	TEACHING RESOURCES
Identify common symptoms of musculoskeletal disorders.	■ Ergonomics in the dental office (p. 368)	PPT 6 TB question 2 SW Short-Answer Questions 6; Fill in the Blank question 3; Multiple Choice question 3 (pp. 135-136) Figure 25-2 (A) Dental assistant in poor position; (B) in proper position (p. 368) Recall question 3 (p. 368) ▶ Discuss the types of musculoskeletal disorders that can occur when ergonomics are not practiced. ***Class Activity** Present the following symptoms to the class. Ask the class to identify whether it could be related to a musculoskeletal disorder and how.* – *Headache* – *Tingling in hands* – *Backache* – *Stiffness in joints*

25.1 Homework/Assignments:

25.1 Instructor's Notes/Student Feedback:

ELSEVIER

Torres and Ehrlich Modern Dental Assisting, 9th ed.

Bird/Robinson

LESSON 25.2

CRITICAL THINKING QUESTION

A dental assistant is complaining of wrist pain and the inability to grasp small dental instruments. The dental assistant has been employed with a busy dental practice for the past 10 years. The office manager has been notified. What do the signs suggest may be wrong with the dental assistant? What changes might the office manager make?

Guidelines: The signs that the dental assistant exhibits are consistent with carpal tunnel syndrome from repetitive motions. The office manager can make changes to the workplace, institute employee training, and allow adequate time for resting the hands to prevent or reduce the impact of carpal tunnel syndrome. In addition, the office manager can allow the dental assistant to have time for proper hand-stretching exercises. The dental assistant can also wear a brace that will immobilize the tendon, allowing it to rest and recover.

OBJECTIVES	CONTENT	TEACHING RESOURCES
Identify three categories of risk factors that contribute to increased risk for injury.	■ Ergonomics in the dental office (p. 368)	PPT 9-10 SW Short-Answer Questions 7; Multiple Choice question 4 (pp. 135-136) Recall question 4 (p. 368) Ergonomic Chairside Tips (p. 369) ▶ Discuss how repetition acts on the muscles to potentially cause injury. ***Class Activity** Divide the class into three groups. Assign each group one of the categories of risk factors that contribute to increased risk for injury. Have each group discuss and determine risk factors for its assigned category. Then have each group share its findings with the class.*
Demonstrate the neutral working position.	■ Posture (p. 369) ☐ Neutral position (p. 369) ☐ Deviations and problems (p. 369) ☐ Reaching movements (p. 370)	PPT 11-17, 19 TB questions 3-4 SW Short-Answer Questions 3; Fill in the Blank questions 4-8, 11; Multiple Choice questions 5-6 (pp. 135-136) Figure 25-3 Configuration of spine in seated dental assistant (p. 369) Figure 25-4 Small pieces of equipment should be in a location that does not require twisting or bending (p. 370) Optimal Dental Assistant Positioning (p. 369) Recall questions 5-6 (p. 370) CTQ 3-4 (p. 373) ▶ Discuss the proper posture for a dental assistant attending to patients over long periods..

OBJECTIVES	CONTENT	TEACHING RESOURCES
		Class Activity Divide the class into small groups. Have each group discuss and practice the neutral working position. Then have each group demonstrate the neutral working position to the class. Encourage further discussion on the importance of a neutral working position to prevent injuries.

Describe the symptoms of carpal tunnel syndrome.	■ Repetition and force (p. 370)
	
	□ Carpal tunnel syndrome (p. 370)
	
	□ Gloves (p. 370)
		⊠▪ PPT 18, 20-24
		
		TB questions 5-6, 9-11
		
		SW Short-Answer Questions 1; Fill in the Blank questions 9-10; Multiple Choice questions 7, 10 (pp. 135-136)
		
		Figure 25-5 Repetitive stress on the wrist from certain positions (p. 370)
		
		Optimal Operator Positioning (p. 369)
		
		Figure 25-6 (A) Cross-section of the wrist; (B) schematic view of the carpal tunnel (p. 371)
		
		Figure 25-7 Location of the thenar eminence (p. 371)
		
		Recall questions 7, 10 (pp. 370, 372)
		
		▸ Discuss the types of repetitive movements that are responsible for carpal tunnel syndrome. What positions or techniques tend to relieve pain associated with carpal tunnel?
		
		Class Activity Describe the following symptoms to the class. Ask the class to identify whether the symptom is related to carpal tunnel syndrome.
		
		   — *Abdominal pain*
		
		   — *Limited range of motion in the wrist*
		
		   — *Wrist pain*
		
		   — *Inability to grasp small objects*
		
		Next have the class identify and discuss other symptoms of carpal tunnel syndrome.

25.2 Homework/Assignments:

25.2 Instructor's Notes/Student Feedback:

LESSON 25.3

CRITICAL THINKING QUESTION

A dental assistant has been entering patient data into the computer for the past 6 hours. The dental assistant is complaining of eyestrain. What can the dental assistant do to help prevent eyestrain in the future?

Guidelines: The dental assistant most likely has eyestrain due to a prolonged intense focus at one depth of vision. An eye exercise that will help alleviate and prevent eyestrain is to have the dental assistant look up and at a distance for approximately 20 seconds. This allows the dental assistant to use the full range of vision. Practicing this exercise several times throughout the day will lessen eyestrain.

OBJECTIVES	CONTENT	TEACHING RESOURCES
Demonstrate the exercises that can reduce muscle fatigue and strengthen muscles.	■ Muscle-strengthening exercises (pp. 370-371)	PPT 27-32 Multimedia Procedures DVD: Body Strengthening Exercises TB questions 7-8, 12 SW Short-Answer Questions 2 (p. 135) Figure 25-8 Hand exercises (p. 372) Eye to the Future (p. 373) CTQ 2 (p. 373) ▸ Discuss various modifications of the hand exercises that also soothe, relax, and stretch muscles and joints. *Class Activity Divide the class into three groups. Have each group discuss and practice one exercise that can reduce muscle fatigue and strengthen muscles. Then have each group explain and demonstrate its exercise to the class.*
Demonstrate the exercises to reduce eyestrain.	■ Muscle-strengthening exercises (pp. 370-371)	PPT 33 Multimedia Procedures DVD: Body Strengthening Exercises SW Short-Answer Questions 4; Multiple Choice question 8 (pp. 135-136) Recall question 8 (p. 372) ▸ Discuss the role of lighting in the prevention of eyestrain. Does exposure to the bright light focused on the patient cause more or less eyestrain in the dental assistant over time? *Class Activity Divide the class into small groups. Have each group discuss and practice exercises to reduce eyestrain. Then have each group demonstrate exercises to reduce eyestrain to the class.*

ELSEVIER

Torres and Ehrlich Modern Dental Assisting, 9th ed.

Bird/Robinson

OBJECTIVES	CONTENT	TEACHING RESOURCES
Demonstrate the exercises to reduce neck strain.	■ Muscle-strengthening exercises (pp. 370-371)	⊠▤ PPT 34-38 📹 Multimedia Procedures DVD: Body Strengthening Exercises SW Short-Answer Questions 5; Multiple Choice question 9 (pp. 135-136) Figure 25-9 Full back release (p. 373) Figure 25-10 Shoulder shrugging (p. 373) Recall question 9 (p. 372) ▸ Discuss ways dental assistants can regularly practice these exercises to remain free of tension and minimize risk of injury. ***Class Activity** Divide class into three groups. Have each group discuss and practice exercises that can reduce neck strain. Then have each group demonstrate its exercise to the class.*
Performance Evaluation		🖥 TB SW questions (pp. 135-137) 🅔 ESLR Electronic Flashcards 🅔 ESLR Practice Quiz Recall questions (pp. 368-372) 💡 CTQ (p. 373)

25.3 Homework/Assignments:

25.3 Instructor's Notes/Student Feedback:

Bird/Robinson

Slide 1

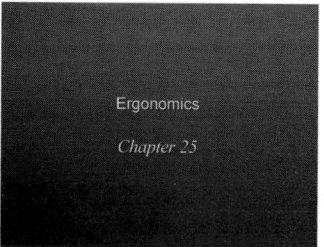

Slide 2

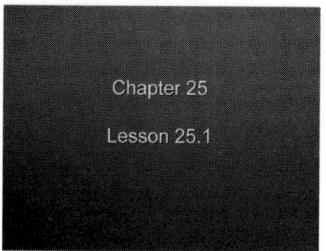

Slide 3

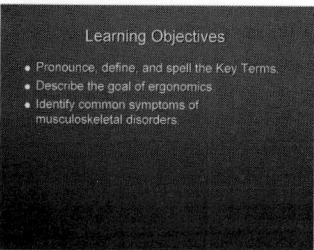

Slide 4

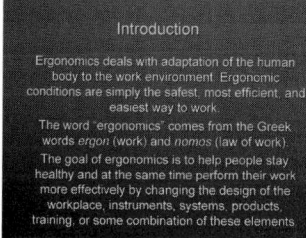

- OSHA has a comprehensive four-pronged approach: guidelines, enforcement, outreach and assistance, and a national advisory committee on ergonomics.

Slide 5

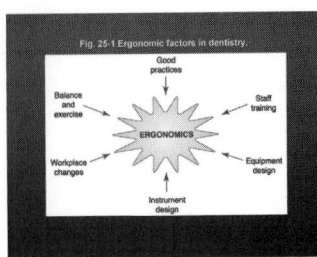

- Ask students to name eight ergonomic chairside tips.
- What is the importance of avoiding repetitive movements?

Slide 6

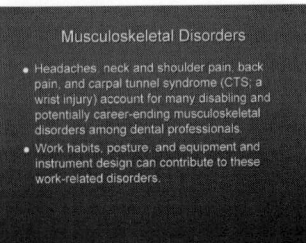

- What are some of the more common conditions identified as musculoskeletal disorders reported by employees? *(Tendinitis, tenosynovitis, epicondylitis, carpal tunnel syndrome, bursitis, deQuervain's disease, ganglion cyst, thoracic outlet syndrome, sprains, strains, tears, general pain.)*

Slide 7

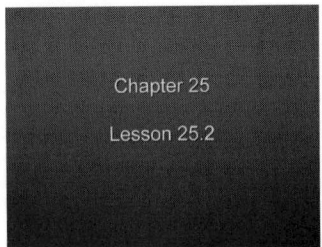

Slide 8

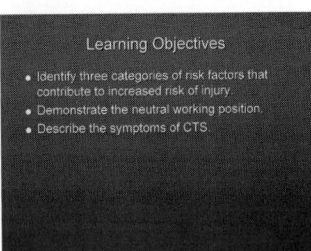

Slide 9

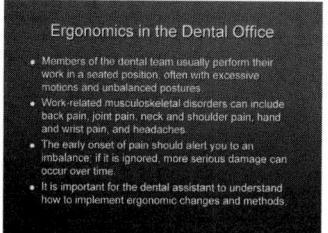

● What should the dental assistant do at the first experience of pain?

Slide 10

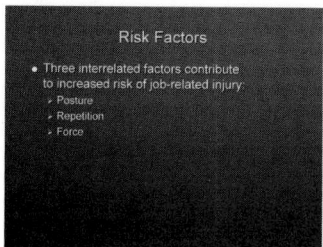

● In 1994 the Bureau of Labor Statistics recorded data on workplace-related injuries. How many cases do you think were the result of overexertion or repetitive motion? *(705,800 cases, which accounted for 32% of all cases)*

Slide 11

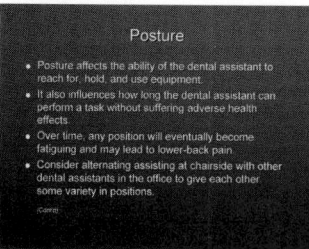

● Based on studies by the Department of Labor, strong evidence supports the relationship between posture and neck and neck/shoulder pain.

Slide 12

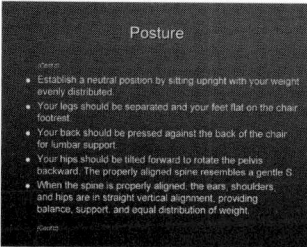

● Ask students to look around at the position of other students and practice sitting in the neutral position.

Torres and Ehrlich Modern Dental Assisting, 9th ed.

Bird/Robinson

Slide 13

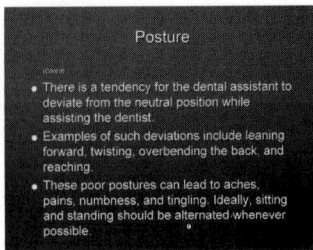

- Back pain is the most prevalent and expensive work-related musculoskeletal disorder among U.S. industries, according to NIOSH.

Slide 14

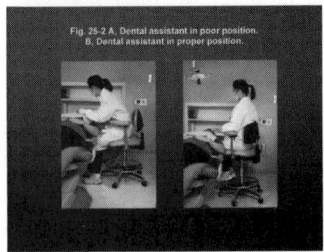

- Take a survey of the class asking them if they have chairs with lumbar support. in their workplaces.

Slide 15

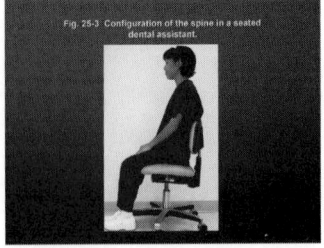

Slide 16

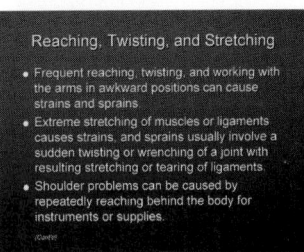

- Remind the students that reaching, twisting, and stretching for equipment or supplies can greatly increase their chances of sustaining an injury.

Torres and Ehrlich Modern Dental Assisting, 9th ed.

Bird/Robinson

Slide 17

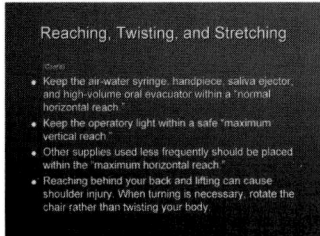

- Proper motion movement can prevent twisting and stretching injuries.

Slide 18

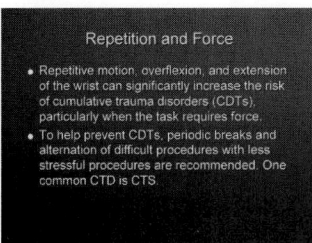

- Estimated costs of cumulative trauma disorders is $25 to $40 billion dollars a year.

Slide 19

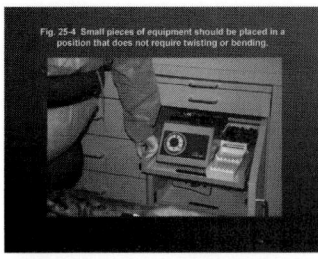

- Proper storage of small equipment can limit the potential for injuries from twisting or bending.

Slide 20

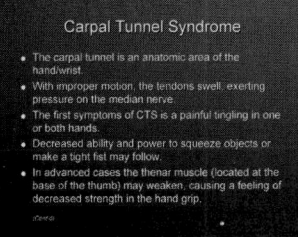

- Inform the students that braces can be worn that will splint the tendon, preventing movement. This will allow the tendon to rest and recover from the stress of repetitive motion.

Bird/Robinson

Slide 21

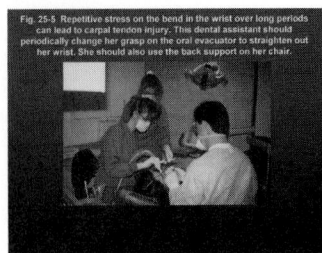

- Ask the class to suggest a better technique or use of equipment to prevent long term injury to the carpal tendon.

Slide 22

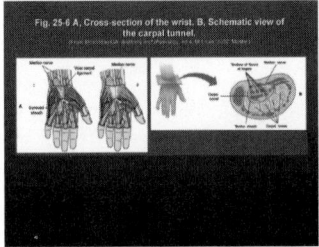

Slide 23

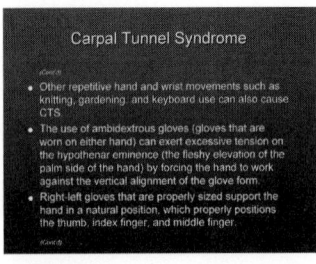

- Remind students of the dangers of repetitive hand and wrist movements.
- Encourage the proper use of equipment to minimize the stress on the tendon.

Slide 24

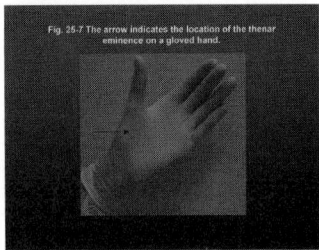

Slide 25

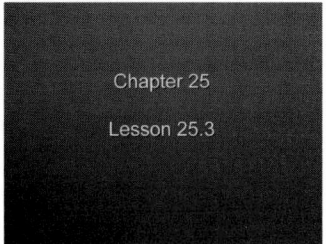

Slide 26

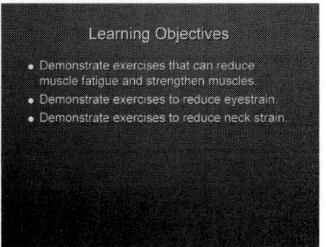

Slide 27

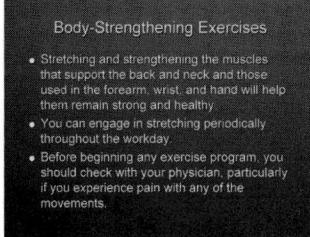

- Remind students of the importance of body-strengthening exercises to prevent injury.

Slide 28

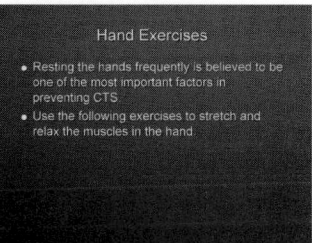

- Demonstrate the hand exercises to the class.

Slide 29

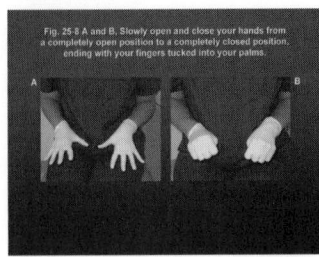

Fig. 25-8 A and B. Slowly open and close your hands from a completely open position to a completely closed position, ending with your fingers tucked into your palms.

- Discuss the benefits associated with this exercise.

Slide 30

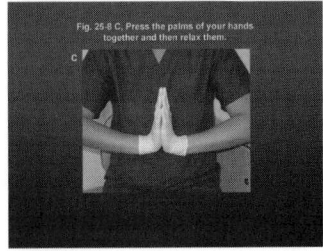

Fig. 25-8 C, Press the palms of your hands together and then relax them.

- What part of the body benefits from this exercise?

Slide 31

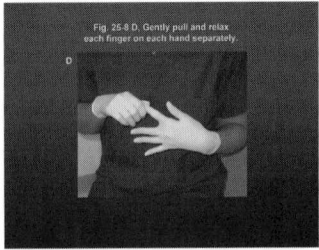

Fig. 25-8 D. Gently pull and relax each finger on each hand separately.

Slide 32

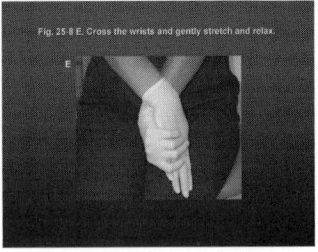

Fig. 25-8 E. Cross the wrists and gently stretch and relax.

- What repetitive motions in the dental office might cause pain in the wrists?

ELSEVIER

Torres and Ehrlich Modern Dental Assisting, 9th ed.

Bird/Robinson

Slide 33

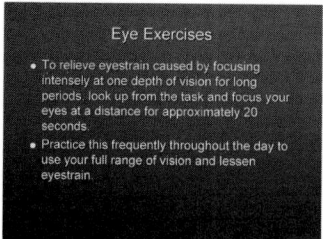

- Have the class practice this exercise in class.
- How frequently should this exercise be performed?

Slide 34

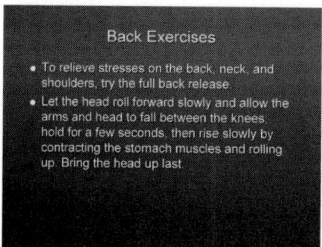

- Can these exercises be performed in the work setting?

Slide 35

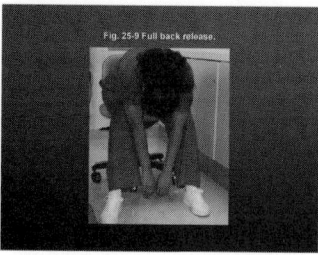

- Demonstrate full back release exercises to the class.

Slide 36

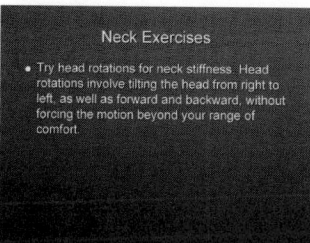

- Demonstrate neck exercises to the class.
- What might result if the motion is jerky or the head is tilted beyond a comfortable range?

Bird/Robinson

Slide 37

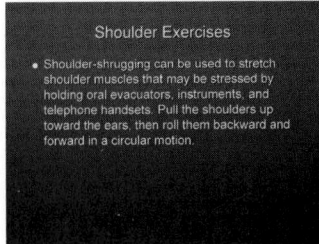

Slide 38

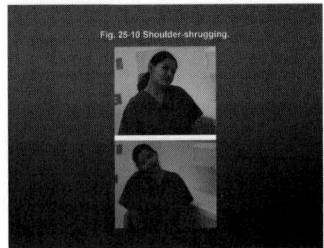

- Demonstrate shoulder-shrugging technique to the class.

TEACHING FOCUS

This chapter gives students the opportunity to learn about the maintenance and management of the patient record and its components. The multifaceted purpose of the patient record will be discussed along with exposure to important forms that must be included in the dental treatment record. Recording the dental treatment and chart correction are also discussed. Students will also have the opportunity to learn how to register a new patient and obtain a medical-dental health history.

MATERIALS AND RESOURCES

- ☐ computer and PowerPoint projector (all Lessons)
- ☐ copies of various forms included in a patient record (all Lessons)

LESSON CHECKLIST

Preparations for this lesson include:

- lecture
- guest speaker: dentist
- evaluation of student knowledge and skills needed to perform all entry-level activities related to patient records, including:
  - ○ explaining how a patient's record should be organized
  - ○ correctly identifying the appropriate forms that must be included in a patient's record
  - ○ demonstrating how to obtain a medical-dental health history
  - ○ demonstrating registering a new patient

Bird/Robinson

KEY TERMS

alert (p. 385)
assessment (p. 377)
chronic (p. 382)
chronologic (p. 380)
demographics (p. 380)

diagnosis (p. 377)
forensic (p. 377)
HIPAA (p. 377)
litigation (p. 380)
registration (p. 380)

ADDITIONAL RESOURCES

PowerPoint slides (Evolve): 1-28

Legend

CTQ
Critical
Thinking
Question

DVD
Multimedia
Procedures
Videos and
Animations

ESLR
EVOLVE
Student
Learning
Resources

IDO
Interactive
Dental
Office
CD-ROM

SW
Student
Workbook

TB
Test Bank
on the
TEACH
CD-ROM

PPT
PowerPoint
Slides

Class Activities are indicated in ***bold italic.***

ELSEVIER

Torres and Ehrlich Modern Dental Assisting, 9th ed.

Bird/Robinson

LESSON 26.1

PRETEST

1. What is the primary source of information that determines the overall quality of care the patient receives?
   a. insurance company
   b. patient record
   c. office equipment
   d. dental association

2. What is the minimum length of time that the signed acknowledgment must be kept in the patient's record?
   a. 2 years
   b. 6 years
   c. 10 years
   d. 20 years

3. Who owns the patient record in the dental office?
   a. dental board
   b. dentist
   c. patient
   d. insurance company

4. Which part of the patient record contains information relating to patient demographics and financial responsibility?
   a. HIPAA statement
   b. patient registration
   c. medical-dental history
   d. patient information and assessment form

5. Which part of the patient record allows cooperation between the professions so that the dental health care team can recommend treatment that takes into consideration the well-being of the total patient?
   a. HIPAA statement
   b. patient registration
   c. medical-dental history
   d. patient information and assessment form

6. Which of the following is an example of a medical alert to note in a patient dental record?
   a. likes mint-flavored fluoride
   b. uses an electric toothbrush
   c. female gender
   d. allergy to penicillin

7. Where is the medical alert to be posted on the patient dental record?
   a. outside cover
   b. inside cover
   c. outside spine
   d. file flag

8. Which of the following is used to record the course of treatment for the patient?
   a. patient registration
   b. treatment plan
   c. examination form
   d. progress notes

9. How does the dental assistant initially help the patient update the medical-dental history?
   a. form given to the patient for review
   b. patient asked to list changes on form
   c. patient is asked questions
   d. patient signs release forms

10. What is used to record statements in the progress notes of a patient dental record?
    a. black ink
    b. red ink
    c. red pencil
    d. black pencil

Answers

1. b	3. b	5. d	7. b	9. a
2. b	4. b	6. d	8. d	10. a

ELSEVIER

Torres and Ehrlich Modern Dental Assisting, 9th ed.

Bird/Robinson

BACKGROUND ASSESSMENT

Question: What type of information is the patient asked to provide in the dental history form?

Answer: The dental history form provides the dental health care team with information about the patient's previous dental treatment and concerns and also identifies fears. The patient is asked to provide information about the purpose of the visit, current dental problem, previous dentist, previous radiographs, brushing and flossing habits, previous orthodontic work, unpleasant dental experiences, and questions or concerns.

Question: How often should a patient's medical history be updated in the dental office? How is this done?

Answer: All patients returning for additional appointments are asked to update their medical histories. The patient's initial medical history form should be given to the patient for review. If there are any changes, a patient should record these on an additional form or a separate line in the treatment section of the patient record. The patient or parent/guardian must either indicate in writing "no change" or write a description of any changes in health status. The patient is then instructed to sign and date the form to indicate that the information is accurate and up to date.

CRITICAL THINKING QUESTION

A patient is moving back to the small town where he grew up. He wants to take his original patient record with him because he does not have time to wait for copies. In addition, he wants the dental assistant to cross out any references to his high blood pressure because his mother, who works at the new office, would be upset by his medical problem. What should the dental assistant do with the patient's record? What does the assistant need to ask the patient to do?

Guidelines: Because the dentist owns the patient record and it may not be removed from the dental practice, the dental assistant can only make copies of the record for the patient to take. The dental assistant cannot give the patient the original documents because original records and radiographs may not be given to anyone except through a court order. Furthermore, the dental assistant cannot change the patient record unless a mistake was recorded and the supervising dentist requested a change. The patient record is a legally binding document and cannot be altered in any way. The dental assistant will need to have the patient sign a written release to obtain the copy of the record before it can be given to him.

OBJECTIVES	CONTENT	TEACHING RESOURCES
Pronounce, define, and spell the Key Terms.	■ Key terms (p. 376)	🔵 ESLR Electronic Flashcards ▸ Discuss each of the key terms in Chapter 26, focusing on the definition, pronunciation, and spelling of each term. *Class Activity Have students make flash cards of the Key Terms with the terms on one side and the definitions on the other. Then have the students quiz each other with the flash cards; correct their pronunciation as needed.*
Identify the purpose of a patient record.	■ Introduction (p. 377) ■ Patient Compliance (p. 377) □ Permanent record (p. 377) □ Privacy (p. 377) □ Quality assurance (p. 380) □ Risk management (p. 380) □ Research (p. 380)	🖼 PPT 4-10 🖥 TB questions 1-6 📘 SW Short-Answer Questions 1; Fill in the Blank questions 1-2, 4-5, 7- 8; Multiple Choice questions 1-5 (pp. 139-140) Recall questions 1-5 (pp. 377, 380) Figure 26-1 Example of the patient record (p. 378) Figure 26-2 Notice of privacy practices form (p. 379) Figure 26-3 Business assistant reviewing a patient's health history form with a new patient (p. 380)

Bird/Robinson

OBJECTIVES	CONTENT	TEACHING RESOURCES
		Legal and Ethical Implications (p. 392) 💡 CTQ 1-2 (p. 393) ▶ Discuss the additional precautions that must be followed in a patient's record in light of recent HIPAA rules. ***Class Activity Divide the class into four groups. Assign each group one of the following:*** — ***Permanent record*** — ***Quality assurance*** — ***Risk management*** — ***Research*** ***Have each group discuss the purpose of the patient record in the context of its assigned subject. Then have each group share its findings with the class.***
Describe each form in the patient record.	■ Patient record forms (p. 380)	🖥 TB question 7 📖 SW Short-Answer Questions 2 (p. 139) ▶ Discuss ways that patients can be encouraged to completely fill out forms when resistance is offered. ***Class Activity In small groups, have students discuss the information that is included in each of the following forms that can make up the patient's record.*** — ***Patient registration*** — ***Medical-dental health history*** — ***Medical alert*** — ***Medical-dental health history update*** — ***Clinical examination*** — ***Treatment plan*** — ***Progress notes*** — ***Informed consent*** ***Have each group share its findings with the class.***
Supervise the completion of a new patient registration form.	☐ Patient registration (p. 380) ⬚Procedure⬚ 26-1 Registering a new patient (p. 382) (SW/ESLR Competency 26-1, p. 143)	⊠■ PPT 11-12 📖 SW Multiple Choice question 6 (p. 140) 📖 🅴 SW/ESLR Competency 26-1 Registering a New Patient (p. 143) Recall questions 6-7 (p. 382) Figure 26-4 Example of a patient registration form (p. 381)

OBJECTIVES	CONTENT	TEACHING RESOURCES
		▸ Discuss ways that accuracy can be achieved in the patient's record so that the practice is not exposed to any legal consequences. ***Class Activity** Obtain copies of a patient registration form from a local dentist's office. In pairs, have students take turns supervising the completion of the form with their partners. Check the forms for completion and accuracy.*

26.1 Homework/Assignments:

26.1 Instructor's Notes/Student Feedback:

Bird/Robinson

CRITICAL THINKING QUESTION

A new patient, who has a toothache, wants to see the dentist as soon as possible. He says he does not have time to fill out the medical-dental form. He says he takes prescribed medication and that is all the information the dentist needs. What can the dental assistant say to him to convince him that he needs to fill out this form?

Guidelines: The dental assistant will need to tell him that it is standard practice to provide the dentist with a patient's medical history before dental treatment in order to reduce an emergency risk. It is especially important in this case because the patient takes medication for an illness and might have a serious dental infection in addition. Careful review of the medical history will alert the dentist to possible interactions between dental treatment and medical treatment for this patient. His medical history will provide information that may require a consultation between his physician and the dentist. The dentist, and not the patient, would be liable for any complications that would occur if this standard of care is not met.

OBJECTIVES	CONTENT	TEACHING RESOURCES
Discuss the importance of the patient's medical-dental health history and its relevance to dental treatment.	☐ Medical-dental health history (p. 382) Procedure 26-2 Obtaining a medical-dental health history (p. 385) (SW/ESLR Competency 26-2, p. 145)	PPT 15-16 TB question 10 SW Short-Answer Questions 3; Multiple Choice question 7 (pp. 139-140) SW/ESLR Competency 26-2 Obtaining a Medical and Dental History (p. 145) ▶ Discuss at least three conditions that might affect the type of treatment a patient receives and why it is crucial to obtain information about these conditions at the first visit. ***Class Activity Invite a dentist from a local office to speak to the class about the patient's medical-dental history and how the information in the history typically affects dental care.***
Obtain a completed medical-dental health history form for a new patient.	– Medical history (p. 382) – Dental history (p. 382) ☐ Medical alert (p. 385) ☐ Medical-dental health history update (p. 385)	PPT 17-20 TB questions 8-9, 11-12 SW Short-Answer Questions 3; Fill in the Blank questions 3, 6; Multiple Choice questions 8-9; Case Study questions 1-3 (pp. 139-141) Figure 26-5 Example of a medical and dental health history form (pp. 383-384) Recall question 8-9 (pp. 382, 386) Figure 26-6 Examples of medical alert stickers (p. 385) Figure 26-7 Example of the medical-dental health history update form (p. 386) ▶ Discuss ways to verify that vague information recorded by the patient is accurately represented in the patient's medical-dental history.

Bird/Robinson

OBJECTIVES	CONTENT	TEACHING RESOURCES
		Class Activity *Obtain copies of a medical-dental history form from a local dental office. In pairs, have students take turns role-playing a dental assistant and patient completing the form. Students should provide plausible, but fictional, information.*

Prepare and organize a patient record.	☐ Clinical examination (p. 386)
	
	☐ Treatment plan (p. 386)
	
	☐ Progress notes (p. 386)
	
	☐ Informed consent (p. 386)
		⊠▪ PPT 21-28
		
		▦ TB questions 13-17
		
		▦ SW Multiple Choice question 10; Case Study questions 4-5 (pp. 140-141)
		
		Recall question 10 (p. 386)
		
		Figure 26-8 Example of a clinical examination form (p. 387)
		
		Figure 26-9 Example of a treatment plan form (p. 388)
		
		Figure 26-10 Example of a progress notes form (p. 389)
		
		Figure 26-11 Example of the informed consent form (p. 390)
		
		Standards and Criteria for Entering Data in a Clinical Record (p. 392)
		
		Eye to the Future (p. 392)
		
		♀ CTQ 3-5 (p. 393)
		
		▸ Discuss the most important standards that should be adhered to when it comes to keeping records.
		
		Class Activity *Obtain copies of each of the following forms from a local dental office. Divide the class into eight groups and assign each group one of the following forms:*
		
		  – Patient registration
		
		  – Medical-dental health history
		
		  – Medical alert
		
		  – Medical-dental health history update
		
		  – Clinical examination
		
		  – Treatment plan
		
		  – Progress notes
		
		  – Informed consent
		
		Next, have each group complete the form for the following patient: a 55-year-old patient receiving a filling who takes prescription medication for a heart condition and is extremely fearful of dental work. Provide additional information to groups where necessary. Next, collect each of the forms and organize the forms into a complete patient record to be reviewed and discussed by the class.

Bird/Robinson

OBJECTIVES	CONTENT	TEACHING RESOURCES
Chart the periodontal examination correctly.	☐ Entering data in a patient record (p. 391) Procedure 26-3 Recording the completed dental treatment (p. 391) (SW/ESLR Competency 26-3, p. 147)	SW/ESLR Competency 26-3 Recording the completed dental treatment (p. 147) Standards and Criteria for Entering Data in a Clinical Record (p. 392) ▸ Discuss the sequence that must be followed in recording examination information. *Class Activity Discuss a specific treatment procedure with the class. Then distribute blank patient dental records, and have each student record the treatment information in the record.*
Demonstrate how to make corrections on a patient's record.	Procedure 26-4 Correcting a chart entry (p. 391) (SW/ESLR Competency 26-4, p. 149)	SW/ESLR Competency 26-4 Correcting a chart entry (p. 149) ▸ Discuss the proper and improper ways to make corrections on a patient's record. What are the potential consequences of improper corrections? *Class Activity Give the students copies of a sample dental chart that includes an error. Have them practice correcting the chart error.*
Performance Evaluation		TB SW questions (pp. 139-141) SW Case Study (pp. 140-141) SW/ESLR Competency 26-1 Registering a New Patient (p. 143) SW/ESLR Competency 26-2 Obtaining a Medical and Dental History (p. 145) SW/ESLR Competency 26-3 Recording the completed dental treatment (p. 147) SW/ESLR Competency 26-4 Correcting a chart entry (p. 149) ESLR Electronic Flashcards ESLR Practice Quiz Recall questions (pp. 377-386) CTQ (p. 393)

26.2 Homework/Assignments:

26.2 Instructor's Notes/Student Feedback:

ELSEVIER

Torres and Ehrlich Modern Dental Assisting, 9th ed.

Bird/Robinson

Slide 1

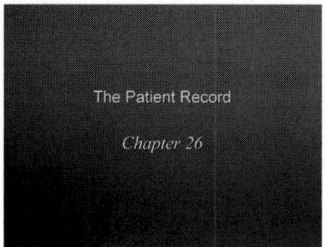

Slide 2

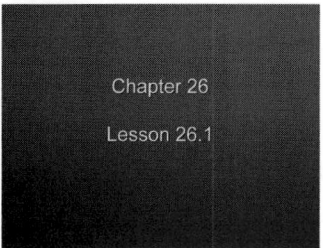

Slide 3

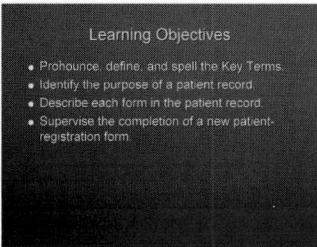

Slide 4

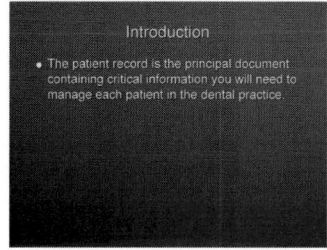

- The patient record is the first step in providing total care for your patient.

- What can the patient's record be used for?

- What would be considered "critical information"?

- What does the term "manage" mean in regard to patient care?

- Do offices have a different method for treating single-visit patients, such as for an emergency?

Bird/Robinson

Slide 5

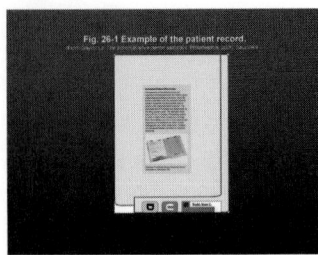

- What is the patient record?
- What does a patient record consist of?
- Have you ever seen your patient record at your dental office?
- What information must the dentist have from a patient before providing dental treatment?

Slide 6

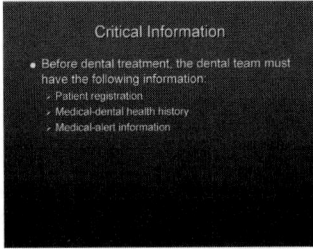

- Why must the dental team have this critical information before dental treatment?
- What is the first contact made with the patient concerning his or her patient record and how does interaction continue?
- How should information be recorded while talking to the patient?
- How should opinions about the patient be recorded?

Slide 7

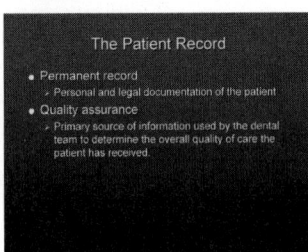

- Is the patient record a confidential document?
- How do you correct a patient record?
- Why would an office consider a patient record that is different for an adult than for a child?

Slide 8

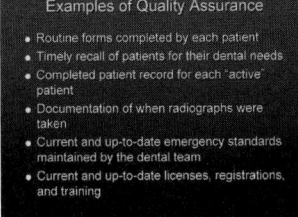

- What is quality assurance?
- Why does the chart need to be in the correct order?
- When you send a copy of the patient record, what should you note?
- How long should records be kept?

Slide 9

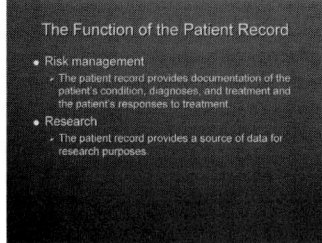

- Why is the dentist concerned about risk?
- If the clinic setting is large and busy, how does the dentist reduce his malpractice risk?
- Why is a patient record important in a research setting?
- Who owns the patient record?

Slide 10

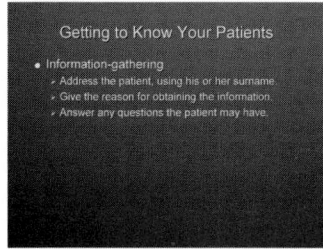

- What is a surname?
- When addressing patients, why do we use their surnames?
- What is the reason given to patients for obtaining information about them?
- All patients (new and existing) must sign an acknowledgment of receipt of notice of privacy practices. The signed acknowledgment must be kept in the patient's record for a minimum of 6 years.

Slide 11

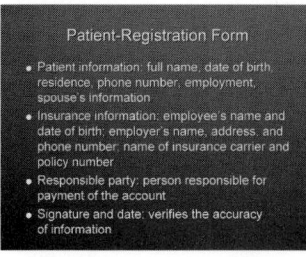

- What is registration? *(The act of completing forms with personal information.)*
- Where is the patient registration kept?
- Is the responsible party always a relative of the patient?

Slide 12

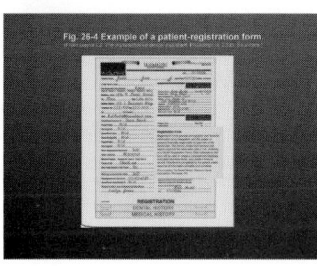

- Registration forms provide demographic and financial information about the patient and the person or persons financially responsible for payment of the dental fees.
- This form is divided into sections that help to organize the information. Data collected on this form will be used to create a computerized data base, to complete insurance forms, and to create a financial record.

Slide 13

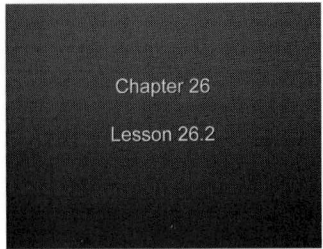

Slide 14

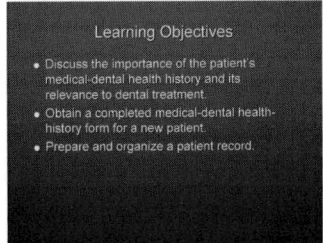

Slide 15

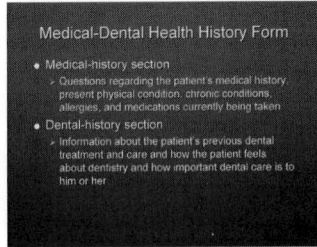

- Is the medical history all that is needed from a patient in order to deliver dental care?
- How is a medical history divided?
- Why would a dentist consult with the patient's physician?
- What is meant by chronic? *(Persisting over a long period.)*

Slide 16

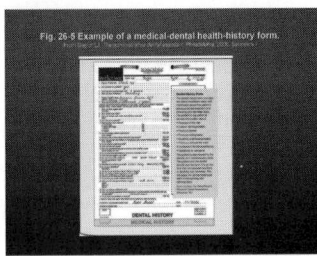

- Why do we need a patient's medical history?
- Why do we need a patient's dental history?
- What does a dental history include?

Bird/Robinson

Slide 17

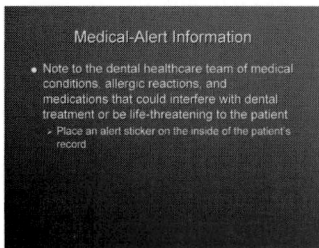

- What is meant by alert?

- Where should the medical alert be placed in the patient's records? *(To protect the confidentiality of the patient, alerts should not be placed on the outside of the folders where they may be read by other patients.)*

- Have you seen a medical alert sticker on a patient chart in a health care setting?

Slide 18

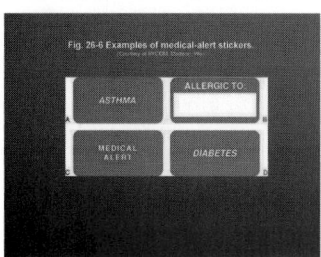

- Why is a medical alert sticker used in a dental office? *(The goal is to alert all members of the dental healthcare team and should be used in a manner that is consistent and easily visualized.)*

- What is an example of a medical alert in a dental office?

- How often should a patient update his or her medical-dental history?

Slide 19

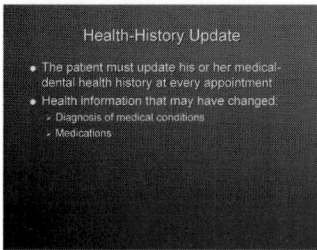

- Why do patients need to update their medical and dental history at every appointment?

- What is a diagnosis?

Slide 20

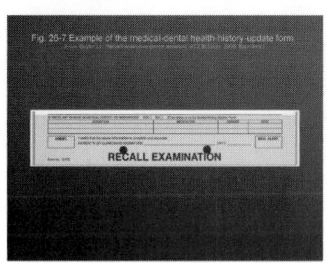

- The patient's initial medical-dental health history form should be given to the patient for review. If there are any changes, a patient should record these on an additional form or a separate line in the treatment section of the patient record.

- What form in the patient record would provide knowledge to the dental team of an existing restoration?

Torres and Ehrlich Modern Dental Assisting, 9th ed.

Bird/Robinson

Slide 21

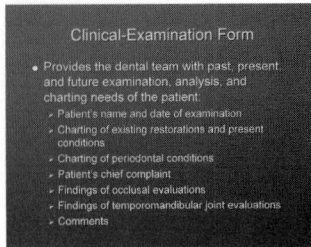

- What happens during the clinical examination of a patient? (*The dentist (1) assesses a patient's oral condition, (2) makes a diagnosis, (3) determines the type of treatment that would be best for the patient, (4) schedules appointments to provide treatment in a timely manner, and (5) follows through with the maintenance stages of the patient care process.*)

Slide 22

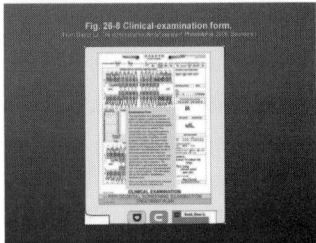

- Do you remember how teeth are charted? See the example of a clinical examination for this patient.

- What does a clinical examination form consist of?

Slide 23

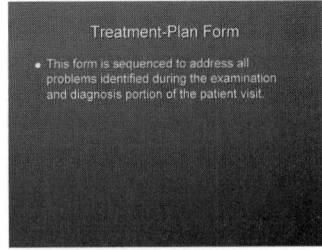

- How does the dentist form a treatment plan?

- Are there any differences between patients needing the same treatment?

Slide 24

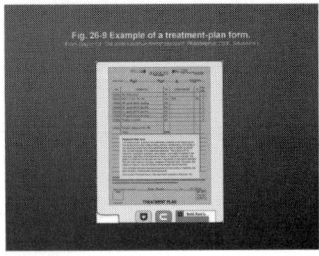

- How can a dental plan change?

- How is the treatment plan handled during the appointment?

Bird/Robinson

Slide 25

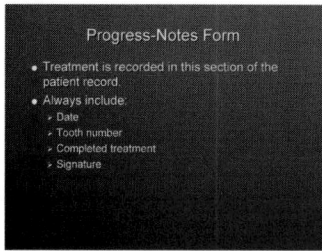

- Have students write down a progress note based on the following dictation from a dentist, using the Universal system of tooth numbering and correct caries classification:
  - "Today we worked on the upper right adult first molar by filling the top only."

Slide 26

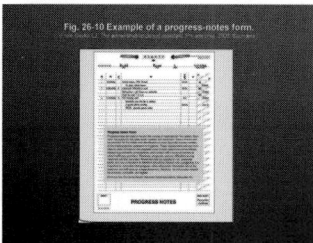

- What is a progress notes form?
- What specific areas should be noted on this form?
- What are progress notes used for and how are they recorded?

Slide 27

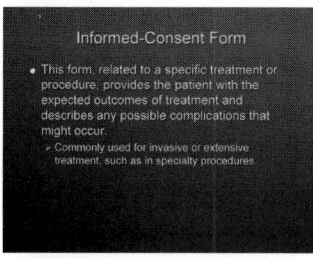

- When are these informed consent forms used? *(Examples of extensive treatment may include surgical procedures, orthodontics, endodontics, periodontics, and implants.)*

Slide 28

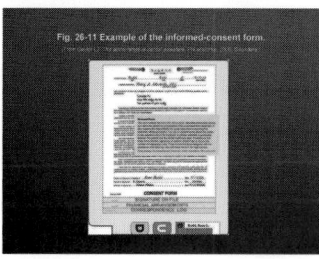

- What does an informed consent form consist of?
- What does the near future have in store for the patient record in a dental setting and how will it improve dental care for the patient?
- What is the term "paperless" office mean?

Bird/Robinson

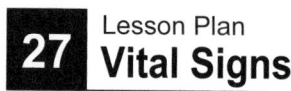
TEACHING FOCUS

This chapter will provide an opportunity for the student to understand the four vital signs commonly taken at the dental office. Temperature, pulse, respiration, and blood pressure will be discussed. Students will have an opportunity to learn how to take an oral temperature with a digital thermometer, take a patient's pulse, take a patient's respiration, and take a patient's blood pressure. Types of thermometers and electrocardiograms will be covered.

MATERIALS AND RESOURCES

- ☐ computer and PowerPoint projector (all Lessons)
- ☐ digital thermometer (Lesson 27.1)
- ☐ patient record for documenting temperature (Lesson 27.1)

- ☐ patient record to document findings (all Lessons)
- ☐ probe cover (Lesson 27.1)
- ☐ sphygmomanometer (Lesson 27.2)
- ☐ stethoscope (Lesson 27.2)
- ☐ watch with second hand (all Lessons)

LESSON CHECKLIST

Preparations for this lesson include:

- lecture
- evaluation of student knowledge and skills needed to perform all entry-level activities related to vital signs, including:
  - ○ factors affecting vital signs
  - ○ understanding body temperature, types of thermometers, and how to take an oral temperature reading with a digital thermometer
  - ○ understanding pulse and how to take a patient's pulse
  - ○ understanding respiration and how to take a patient's respiration
  - ○ understanding blood pressure and how to take a patient's blood pressure
  - ○ electrocardiogram procedures

Bird/Robinson

KEY TERMS

antecubital (p. 397)
arrhythmia (p. 398)
blood pressure (BP) (p. 400)
brachial (p. 397)
carotid (p. 397)
depth (p. 398)
diastolic (p. 400)
electrocardiogram (p. 403)
Korotkoff sounds (p. 400)
metabolism (p. 395)
palpate (p. 398)
pulse (p. 397)

radial (p. 397)
rate (p. 398)
respiration (p. 398)
rhythm (p. 398)
sphygmomanometer (p. 400)
stethoscope (p. 400)
systolic (p. 400)
temperature (p. 395)
thermometer (p. 396)
tympanic (p. 396)
volume (p. 398)

ADDITIONAL RESOURCES

PowerPoint slides (Evolve): 1-26
Multimedia Procedures DVD:
    Taking a Patient's Blood Pressure

Legend

CTQ
Critical
Thinking
Question

DVD
Multimedia
Procedures
Videos and
Animations

ESLR
EVOLVE
Student
Learning
Resources

IDO
Interactive
Dental
Office
CD-ROM

SW
Student
Workbook

TB
Test Bank
on the
TEACH
CD-ROM

PPT
PowerPoint
Slides

Class Activities are indicated in ***bold italic***.

ELSEVIER

Torres and Ehrlich Modern Dental Assisting, 9th ed.

Bird/Robinson

LESSON 27.1

PRETEST

1. Which of the following is one of the two major arteries on each side of the neck that carry blood to the head?
   a. aorta
   b. radial
   c. brachial
   d. carotid

2. Which of the following is the rhythmic contraction of the heart, especially noted in the ventricles?
   a. pulse rate
   b. diastolic measurement
   c. systolic measurement
   d. Korotkoff sounds

3. Which of the following is commonly used to measure blood pressure in the arteries?
   a. sphygmomanometer
   b. electrocardiogram
   c. tympanic device
   d. digital angel

4. Which of the following is a definition of the term arrhythmia?
   a. irregularity in the force or rhythm of the heartbeat
   b. rhythmic throbbing of the arteries produced by regular contractions
   c. act or process of inhaling and exhaling
   d. pressure exerted by the blood against the walls of the blood vessels

5. Where is a tympanic device gently placed?
   a. antecubital space
   b. eardrum
   c. wrist surface
   d. carotid artery

6. Which of the following pulse sites are used during CPR?
   a. aorta
   b. radial
   c. brachial
   d. carotid

7. Which of the following describes the pattern of the beats of the pulse, such as an occasional skipping, speeding up, or slowing down of the pulse?
   a. volume
   b. rate
   c. rhythm
   d. pattern

8. Which of the following experiences would result in blood pressure and respiration being much higher than a previous reading?
   a. drinking a hot beverage
   b. drinking a cold beverage
   c. a fearful episode
   d. a calm episode

9. What location on the body most often gives the lowest temperature reading?
   a. oral
   b. rectal
   c. tympanic
   d. axillary

10. What is the usual pulse reading per minute for a child?
    a. 20 to 50 beats
    b. 50 to 100 beats
    c. 70 to 120 beats
    d. 120 to 150 beats

Answers

1. d	3. a	5. b	7. c	9. d
2. c	4. a	6. d	8. c	10. c

Bird/Robinson

BACKGROUND ASSESSMENT

Question: When should the record of a patient's vital signs be updated in a dental setting and why? Which vital signs should be measured and updated in the patient's record?

Answer: If this is the patient's first visit, a 6-month recall, or an emergency situation, the clinical assistant should routinely take and record vital signs. Having this baseline provides the dental team with added assurance of the patient's well-being and health status. The vital signs that should be updated include the patient's respiration, blood pressure, temperature, and pulse reading

Question: If a patient experiences fear of an upcoming dental injection at the beginning of an appointment, what changes would you expect in the patient's vital signs? How do these changes relate to one of the responsibilities of the dental assistant?

Answer: The patient's temperature, pulse, respiration, and blood pressure would be elevated. When there is an increase in metabolism (such as when the patient experiences fear), vital signs will also typically increase. One of the responsibilities of a dental assistant is to recognize these situations and help the patient relax before measuring any vital signs. In addition, there may be a need to have these measurements taken more than once after the patient is reassured and becomes more calm. In addition, the dental assistant will need to inform the dentist as soon as possible about the patient's fear before the dental treatment has begun. There are many ways to reduce fear in the dental setting to avoid any unpleasant or emergency situations.

CRITICAL THINKING QUESTION

While updating the medical and dental history of a middle-aged male patient, the dental assistant learns that the patient has just begun a new exercise program that morning. He is still wearing his exercise clothes and is sweating profusely and breathing rapidly while the dental assistant takes his vital signs. Looking at the previous measurement of his vital signs in the patient record, the dental assistant notices that all the vital signs taken today are higher compared to his last appointment. What is the significance of this change and how should the dental assistant respond? What if the patient requests a cold beverage to cool down? Should the dental assistant remove the blood pressure cuff so that the patient feels more comfortable?

Guidelines: The dental assistant will have to take the vital signs of this patient again after the patient stops sweating, his breathing returns to normal, and he relaxes. When there is an increase in metabolism (such as with his new exercise regimen), vital signs will also typically increase and may not be typical for the patient. One of the responsibilities of a dental assistant is to recognize these situations and help the patient relax before taking vital signs, so that the measurements will be more accurate. After the patient consumes a cold beverage, it is necessary to postpone taking his temperature for a while so that the reading will be more accurate. The dental assistant should allow the deflated blood pressure cuff to remain on the patient for a minimum of 10 minutes before obtaining another reading or remove it completely. If the blood pressure is taken too soon, the reading may be incorrect. Communication with the supervising dentist regarding this situation is very important.

OBJECTIVES	CONTENT	TEACHING RESOURCES
Pronounce, define, and spell the Key Terms.	■ Key terms (p. 394)	🎓 ESLR Electronic Flashcards ▸ Discuss each of the key terms in Chapter 27, focusing on the definition, pronunciation, and spelling of each term. *Class Activity Call out a key term related to the vital signs, and ask students to respond with a short definition of that term.*
List the four vital signs commonly taken in the dental office.	■ Introduction (p. 395)	🖥 PPT 5 📺 TB question 1 🖊 SW Short-Answer Questions 1; Fill in the Blank question 3; Multiple Choice question 1 (pp. 151-152)

Torres and Ehrlich Modern Dental Assisting, 9th ed.

Bird/Robinson

OBJECTIVES	CONTENT	TEACHING RESOURCES
		SW Case Study questions 2, 4-5 (pp. 153-154)
		Legal and Ethical Implications (p. 405)
		Eye to the Future (p. 405)
		CTQ 2 (p. 405)
		▶ Discuss the four vital signs frequently taken in the dental office: temperature, pulse, respiration, and blood pressure. How are each of these vital signs measured?
		***Class Activity** Ask the students to work in groups to create a chart that could be used in the dental clinic displaying the normal values for the four vital signs. Have the class choose the best chart.*
Describe how metabolism affects a patient's vital signs.	■ Factors that affect vital signs (p. 395) ■ Temperature (p. 395) □ Temperature readings (p. 396)	PPT 6-7 TB question 2 SW Short-Answer Questions 2 (p. 151) Recall question 1 (p. 395) CTQ 1 (p. 405) ▶ Discuss the meaning of the term "metabolism." ▶ Discuss the ways that the body's metabolism can affect the vital signs. ***Class Activity** Have each student write a short scene in which a vital sign is affected by an incident such as drinking a hot beverage, exercising, experiencing fear, etc. Ask students to share their scenarios and discuss how the dental assistant should respond in each situation to obtain an accurate measurement of the vital signs.*
Discuss three types of thermometers.	□ Types of thermometers (p. 396) – Digital (p. 396) – Tympanic (p. 396) – Glass (p. 396)	PPT 8-9 TB questions 3-4 SW Short-Answer Questions 4; Fill in the Blank questions 11-12, 14; Multiple Choice questions 2-4 (pp. 151-152) Recall questions 2-4 (p. 397) Figure 27-1 Digital thermometer (p. 396) Figure 27-2 Tympanic thermometer (p. 396) Figure 27-3 Glass thermometer showing the mercury bulb (p. 397) ▶ Discuss the three types of thermometers: digital, tympanic, and oral. What are the advantages and disadvantages of each type?

ELSEVIER

Bird/Robinson

OBJECTIVES	CONTENT	TEACHING RESOURCES
		▸ Discuss how each type of thermometer is used. **Class Activity** *Divide the class into groups, and have them choose a type of thermometer and investigate its advantages and disadvantages. Have students research the range of costs of the thermometer from retailers and online vendors, as if they were buying it for their dental office. Then have each group report its findings to the class. (For students to prepare for this activity, see Homework/Assignments #1.)*
Take an oral temperature reading with a digital thermometer.	☐ Types of thermometers (p. 396) – Digital (p. 396) – Tympanic (p. 396) ⸤Procedure⸥ 27-1 Taking an oral temperature reading with a digital thermometer (p. 397) (SW/ESLR Competency 27-1, p. 155) – Glass (p. 396)	SW/ESLR Competency 27-1 Taking an Oral Temperature Reading with a Digital Thermometer (p. 155) Figure 27-1 Digital thermometer (p. 396) ▸ Discuss the steps needed to take an oral temperature reading with a digital thermometer. **Class Activity** *As a class, discuss the proper procedure for taking the oral temperature of the patient with a digital thermometer. Then have student pairs practice taking their own and each other's temperatures using the different types of thermometers.*
List the common pulse sites used for taking a pulse.	■ Pulse (p. 397) ☐ Radial artery (p. 397) ☐ Brachial artery (p. 397) ☐ Carotid artery (p. 397)	PPT 10-13 TB questions 5, 8 SW Short-Answer Questions 4; Fill in the Blank question 7; Multiple Choice question 7 (pp. 151-153) Figure 27-4 Location of the radial artery (p. 397) Figure 27-5 Location of the brachial artery (p. 398) Figure 27-6 Location of the carotid artery (p. 398) Recall questions 5-6 (p. 398) ▸ Discuss the three common pulse points and their locations. ▸ Discuss the process of taking the pulse from each pulse site. **Class Activity** *Ask for volunteers to demonstrate in front of the class the procedure for taking the pulse at each site. Then discuss general guidelines for obtaining an accurate measurement of the pulse.*

OBJECTIVES	CONTENT	TEACHING RESOURCES
Describe the characteristics of the pulse that you would look for in taking a patient's pulse.	☐ Pulse characteristics (p. 398) ☐ Pulse readings (p. 398)	⊠ PPT 14-15 TB questions 6-7 SW Short-Answer Questions 5; Fill in the Blank questions 4, 6, 15; Multiple Choice questions 5-6 (pp. 151-153) Recall question 7 (p. 398) CTQ 5 (p. 405) ▸ Discuss the three characteristics that must be noted in the patient record when documenting a pulse. ▸ Discuss the way to take a pulse reading, including how the patient should be situated. If the patient has been active just before arriving at the office, how will this affect the pulse? What is the proper procedure for taking the pulse in this situation? *Class Activity Have student pairs practice taking each other's pulses, making sure to measure the rate, volume, and rhythm of the pulse at each site. Ask volunteers to demonstrate the methods of taking the pulse and discuss the procedure for obtaining an accurate pulse measurement.*
Take a patient's pulse.	**Procedure** 27-2 Taking a patient's pulse (p. 399) (SW/ESLR Competency 27-2, p. 157)	TB question 8 SW Multiple Choice question 6 (p. 153) SW/ESLR Competency 27-2 Taking a Patient's Pulse (p. 157) CTQ 5 (p. 405) ▸ Discuss the procedure for taking a patient's pulse. What is the correct position of the dental assistant's fingers? *Class Activity Have small groups of students practice taking each other's pulses. Make sure all students have their pulses taken twice. Then have students compare their results, especially to see if each time a student's pulse was taken the measurement was the same.*

Torres and Ehrlich Modern Dental Assisting, 9th ed.

Bird/Robinson

27.1 Homework/Assignments:

1. Have students investigate the advantages and disadvantages of a specific type of thermometer. Students should research the range of costs of the thermometer from retailers and online vendors, as if they were buying it for their dental office.

27.1 Instructor's Notes/Student Feedback:

LESSON 27.2

CRITICAL THINKING QUESTION

The dental assistant is taking the vital signs of a 62-year-old woman who has a severe toothache. Her temperature using the digital thermometer is 101° F. Her blood pressure is 100 mm Hg systolic over 70 mm Hg diastolic. Her pulse reading is 75 beats per minute. Which vital signs taken by the dental assistant are not within the normal range? What is the likely cause of the abnormal reading? What characteristic of a digital thermometer should the assistant keep in mind when using it? How should the dental assistant respond to this information about the patient's vital signs?

Guidelines: The dental assistant should note on the patient's record that her temperature is not within the normal range. She has a slight fever since her temperature is above the average range of 97.6° F to 99° F for an adult. The elevated temperature may be an indication that her body is trying to fight the infection from the toothache. Her other vital signs are all in a normal range, since an adult resting pulse is 60 to 100 beats per minute and normal blood pressure is less than 120 mm Hg systolic over less than 80 diastolic mm Hg. It is important to remember that the digital thermometer has a timed feature because it may result in an inaccurate reading if the battery is low. This information should be conveyed to the dentist, in case there is a need to alter the patient's treatment for that day; and the dental assistant will record what is discussed in the progress notes of the patient's dental record.

OBJECTIVES	CONTENT	TEACHING RESOURCES
Describe the characteristics of respiration and how they affect a patient's breathing.	■ Respiration (p. 398) ☐ Respiration characteristics (p. 398)	PPT 18 TB questions 9-10 SW Short-Answer Questions 6; Fill in the Blank questions 8, 10, 13; Multiple Choice questions 8-10 (pp. 151-153) SW Case Study question 3 (p. 154) Recall questions 8-9 (p. 400) Figure 27-7 Respiration patterns (p. 400) ▸ Discuss the three characteristics of respiration that must be noted in the patient record when measuring a patient's total respiration. ▸ Discuss how each characteristic affects a patient's breathing. ***Class Activity** Have student pairs take turns role-playing a dental assistant recording a "patient's" respiration rate, rhythm, and depth while the patient is sitting normally. Then have the students record the respiration after the patient walks around the class for a few minutes to determine how the respiration is affected by the activity.*
Discuss the best way to obtain accurate readings of respiration.	☐ Respiration readings (p. 398)	SW Short-Answer Questions 7 (p. 151) Recall question 10 (p. 400) CTQ 4 (p. 405) ▸ Discuss the best way to obtain an accurate reading of respiration.

ELSEVIER

Torres and Ehrlich Modern Dental Assisting, 9th ed.

Bird/Robinson

OBJECTIVES	CONTENT	TEACHING RESOURCES
		▸ Discuss the normal respiration rate for a relaxed adult. What is the range of respiration rates resulting from various levels of activity?
		Class Activity Have each student write a paragraph on the best way to obtain an accurate respiration reading on each of the following patients: an older patient, a disabled patient, a child, and a pregnant woman.
Take a patient's respiration.	[Procedure] 27-3 Taking a patient's respiration (p. 399) (SW/ESLR Competency 27-3, p. 159)	TB questions 9-10
		SW Short-Answer Questions 7 (p. 151)
		SW/ESLR Competency 27-3 Taking a Patient's Respiration (p. 159)
		CTQ 4 (p. 405)
		▸ Discuss the procedure taking a patient's respiration.
		Class Activity Have student pairs take turns role-playing a dental assistant characterizing the respiration pattern, including rate, rhythm, and depth, of a patient. Then have students discuss what they learned from the activity.
Explain the importance of taking a patient's blood pressure.	■ Blood pressure (p. 400)	PPT 19-20
		Multimedia Procedures DVD: Taking a Patient's Blood Pressure
		TB questions 11-12
		SW Short-Answer Questions 8; Fill in the Blank question 5; Multiple Choice question 11 (pp. 151-153)
		Table 27-1 Blood Pressure Classifications for Adults (p. 400)
		Recall question 11 (p. 403)
		Patient Education (p. 405)
		CTQ 3 (p. 405)
		▸ Discuss the importance of obtaining a blood pressure reading. Discuss the definition of blood pressure, along with systolic and diastolic pressures.
		▸ Discuss the blood pressure readings for normal, prehypertension and hypertension stages.
		Class Activity Have students research high blood pressure and its significance for patients in the dental office. Students should research information obtained from the library or the Internet. Ask students how they would respond to a patient who is taking medication for hypertension. (For students to prepare for this activity, see Homework/Assignments #1.)

OBJECTIVES	CONTENT	TEACHING RESOURCES
Differentiate the Korotkoff sounds heard when taking a patient's blood pressure	■ Blood pressure (p. 400) □ Blood pressure equipment (p. 400) □ Blood pressure readings (p. 400) – Medical Considerations (p. 400)	PPT 21-24 TB questions 13-15 SW Short-Answer Questions 9; Fill in the Blank question 10; Multiple Choice questions 12-15 (pp. 151-153) Figure 27-8 Types of sphygmomanometers (p. 401) Figure 27-9 Stethoscope (p. 401) Figure 27-10 Automated electronic blood pressure device (p. 401) Table 27-2 Five Phases of Korotkoff Sounds in Blood Pressure Measurement (p. 401) Recall questions 11-15 (p. 403) ▸ Discuss the five phases of Korotkoff sounds in blood pressure measurement. Characterize the blood flow for each of the five phases. ▸ Discuss medical considerations that can affect blood pressure readings. ***Class Activity Lead a class discussion about the five phases of Korotkoff sounds. Ask students to identify the sound that is heard during each of the five phases. How is the blood flowing during each of the five phases?***
Take a patient's blood pressure.	*Procedure* 27-4 Taking a patient's blood pressure (pp. 402-403) (SW/ESLR Competency 27-4, pp. 161-162) ■ Advanced Monitoring Procedures (p. 403) □ Pulse Oximeters (p. 403) □ Electrocardiogram (p. 403)	PPT 25-26 TB question 13 SW Fill in the Blank question 9; Multiple Choice question 12 (pp. 152-153) SW/ESLR Competency 27-4 Taking a Patient's Blood Pressure (pp. 161-162) Pracitcal Suggestions for Monitoring the Pulse Oximeter (p. 404) Figure 27-11 The cardiac cycle in the electrocardiogram (p. 404) ▸ Discuss the procedure for taking a patient's blood pressure. What steps should be taken to ensure an accurate reading? ***Class Activity Ask students to correctly identify each of the steps involved in taking a patient's blood pressure. Have pairs of students take turns role-playing a dental assistant taking a patient's blood pressure. Then discuss factors that contribute to hypertension.***

ELSEVIER

Torres and Ehrlich Modern Dental Assisting, 9th ed.

Bird/Robinson

OBJECTIVES	CONTENT	TEACHING RESOURCES
Performance Evaluation		TB
		SW questions (pp. 151-13)
		SW Case Study (pp. 153-154)
		SW/ESLR Competency 27-1 Taking an Oral Temperature Reading with a Digital Thermometer (p. 155)
		SW/ESLR Competency 27-2 Taking a Patient's Pulse (p. 157)
		SW/ESLR Competency 27-3 Taking a Patient's Respiration (p. 159)
		SW/ESLR Competency 27-4 Taking a Patient's Blood Pressure (pp. 161-162)
		ESLR Electronic Flashcards
		ESLR Practice Quiz
		Recall questions (pp. 395- 403)
		CTQ (p. 405)

27.2 Homework/Assignments:

1. Have students research high blood pressure and its significance for patients in the dental office. Students should research information obtained from the library or the Internet. Ask students how they would respond to a patient who is taking medication for hypertension.

27.2 Instructor's Notes/Student Feedback:

Bird/Robinson

Slide 1

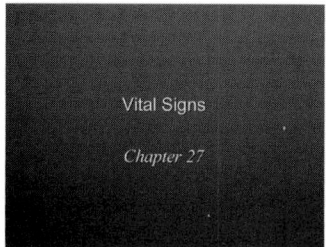

Slide 2

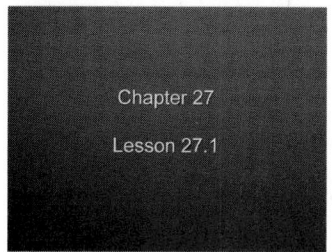

Slide 3

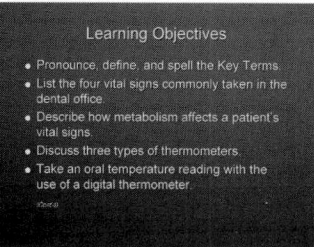

Slide 4

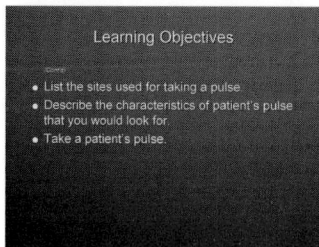

Torres and Ehrlich Modern Dental Assisting, 9th ed.

Bird/Robinson

Slide 5

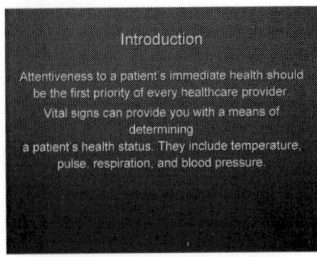

- What are vital signs? *(Certain tests, such as blood pressure, temperature, pulse, and respiration, that can help determine a person's condition.)*
- When should the clinical assistant take and document a patient's vital signs? *(After patient's first visit, the 6-month recall, or in an emergency situation.)*
- What is a baseline? *(A starting point or condition against which future changes are measured.)*

Slide 6

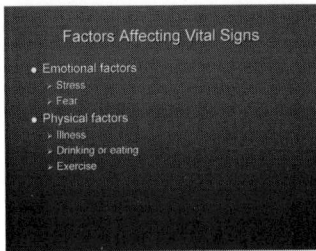

- How can patients' vital signs be affected by their present status? *(The human body is influenced by both emotional and physical factors.)*
- How can the dental assistant ensure that vital signs are not adversely affected by the patient's present status? *(Help the patient relax before taking vital signs. If the patient is normally calmer, provide reassurance, wait several minutes, and then retake the measurements.)*

Slide 7

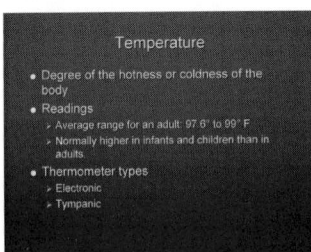

- How are temperature readings calibrated? *(In the Fahrenheit [F] scale, which is most frequently used in the United States, or the Celsius [C] scale, which is most frequently used in Canada and Europe.)*
- What is a fever? *(Fever, also known as pyrexia, is a medical symptom which describes an increase in temperature to levels that are above normal [37° C or 98.6° F].)*
- What are "goose bumps"? *(When there is a fever, blood vessels closest to the surface of the skin constrict and cause "goose bumps." The body shivers, beginning a chain reaction that causes the body to produce internal heat for warmth.)*

Slide 8

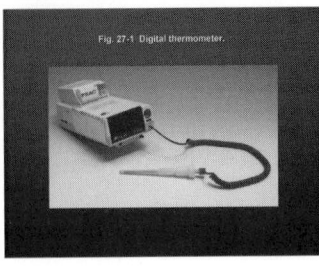

- How does a digital thermometer differ from a glass thermometer? *(It has a timing system that shows a digital reading after 30 seconds rather than a line of mercury that rises along a marked scale. Most digital thermometers "beep" to indicate completion. The reading then appears on the digital screen.)*
- What can cause an inaccurate reading on a digital thermometer? *(A low battery.)*
- How do you maintain infection control with a digital thermometer? *(With a disposable plastic sheath that slides over the probe before insertion.)*

Torres and Ehrlich Modern Dental Assisting, 9th ed.

Bird/Robinson

Slide 9

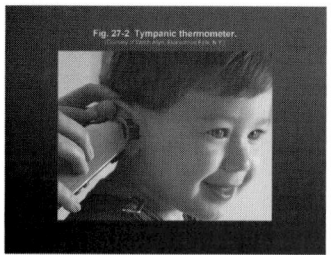

- How does a tympanic thermometer work? *(By means of a small probe that is gently inserted into the ear canal; an infrared signal is bounced off the eardrum, and a reading is provided within 2 seconds.)*

- What factors do NOT influence the tympanic temperature reading? *(Open mouth, hot or cold drinks, or nose congestion.)*

- This approach is very popular with children. The rapid measurement may be more accurate because of less patient movement.

Slide 10

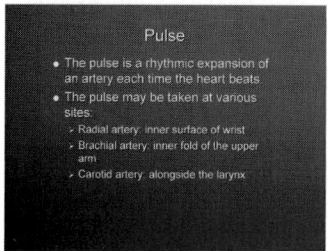

- What does the pulse represent? *(The pulse represents the beating of the heart, specifically the ejection of blood from the left ventricle into the general circulation of the body.)*

- Which site is the most common for taking a patient's pulse in the dental office? *(Radial artery.)*

Slide 11

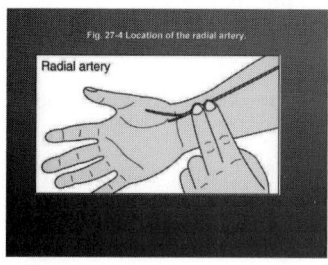

- How is the radial artery pulse taken? *(1) Place the tips of your index and middle fingers lightly on the patient's wrist between the radius [bone on the thumb side] and the tendon. This measures about one inch from the base of your thumb. (2) Feel for the patient's pulse before beginning to count, (3) Count the pulse for 30 seconds; then multiply by 2 to compute the rate for a 1-minute reading.)*

- Can you locate and feel the pulse of your radial artery?

Slide 12

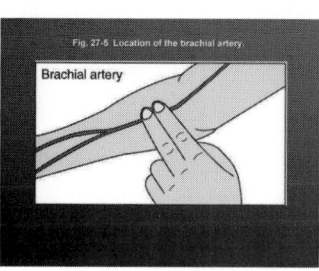

- Do not use your thumb to detect the patient's pulse. Your thumb has a fairly strong pulse of its own, and it may prevent an accurate reading.

- Where is the brachial artery located? *(On the inner fold of the arm, also referred to as the antecubital area of the elbow.)*

- This artery is also used to take a patient's blood pressure.

- Can you locate and feel the pulse of your brachial artery?

Slide 13

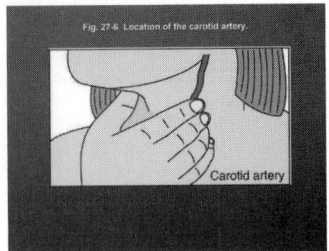

Fig. 27-6 Location of the carotid artery.

Carotid artery

- When is the carotid pulse commonly taken? *(When performing cardiopulmonary resuscitation.)*

- How is the carotid pulse taken? *(Place two fingers alongside the patient's larynx [Adam's apple] on the side of the neck nearest you. Move your fingers slowly down the groove to the soft area above the clavicle [collarbone] and then palpate this area gently to determine a pulse.)*

- Can you locate and feel the pulse of your carotid artery?

Slide 14

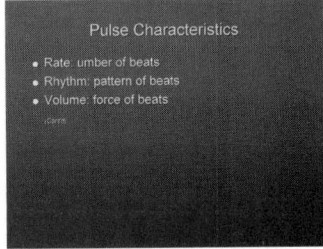

- The pulse represents the variation in blood pressure from diastole to systole. During diastole, blood pressure falls but increases after systole as the heart pumps more blood into the arteries.

- When taking a patient's pulse, look for any distinct changes in the pulse.

Slide 15

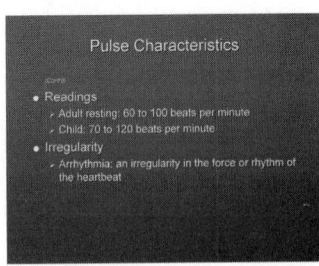

- Arrhythmia is not uncommon. Arrhythmia can occur in a healthy heart and be of minimal consequence. However, it may also indicate a serious problem and lead to heart disease, stroke, or sudden cardiac arrest.

- The term "tachycardia" refers to a heart rate of more than 100 beats per minute.

- The term "bradycardia" describes a heart rate of less than 60 beats per minute.

Slide 16

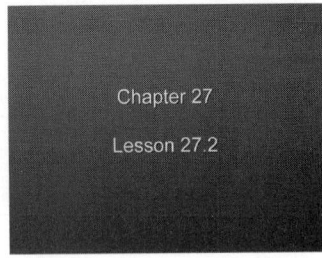

Chapter 27

Lesson 27.2

Torres and Ehrlich Modern Dental Assisting, 9th ed.

Bird/Robinson

Slide 17

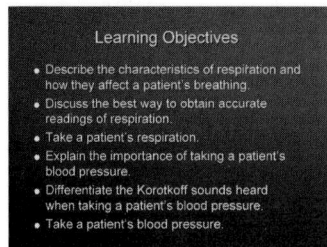

Slide 18

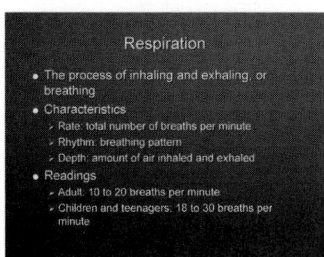

- How should a patient's respiration be assessed?

- What is the normal respiration rate for an adult?

- Is the respiration rate for a child or teenager lower or higher than an adult's?

Slide 19

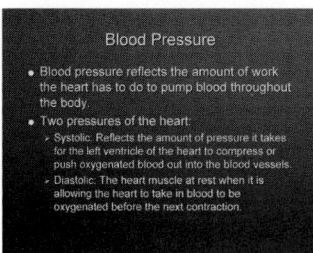

- How is blood pressure measured and recorded? *(Systolic and diastolic pressures are measured in millimeters of mercury [mm Hg]. The reading is recorded with the systolic value over the diastolic value.)*

- What is the range of a normal blood pressure reading for an adult?

- How important is accuracy when taking a blood pressure reading?

- What is a "white-coat reading"? *(A reading that is high because a healthcare professional is taking a blood pressure.)*

Slide 20

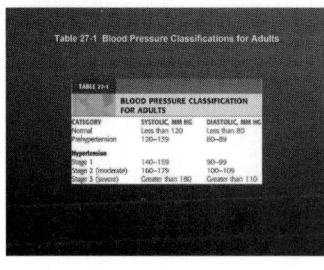

- If two or three blood pressure readings are needed to obtain an accurate or average reading, wait a minimum of 10 minutes before obtaining another reading. If taken too soon, the reading may be incorrect.

- What can elevate a patient's blood pressure? *(The stress and anxiety of a dental procedure.)*

- What should the dental assistant do if high blood pressure has been noted in a patient's medical history?

Slide 21

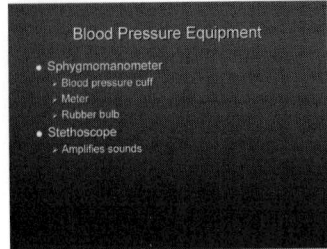

- What blood pressure device is similar to the sphygmomanometer without the stethoscope? *(Automated electronic blood pressure device.)*

- What might cause an inaccurate reading with the electronic blood pressure meter?

- What are Korotkoff sounds?

Slide 22

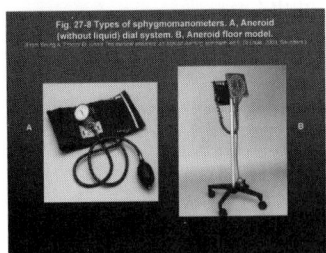

- The size of the inflation system can affect the accuracy of blood pressure readings. Choose the appropriate size cuff based on the circumference of the patient's bare upper arm. The bladder (inside the cuff) should encircle 80% of an adult's arm and 100% of the arm of a child under the age of 13. It is advisable to have a full range of cuff sizes available to accommodate dental office patients.

Slide 23

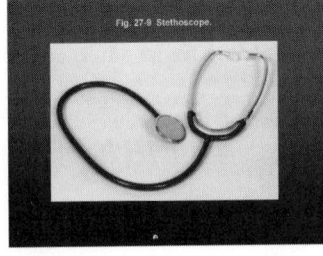

- Name the parts of the stethoscope.

Slide 24

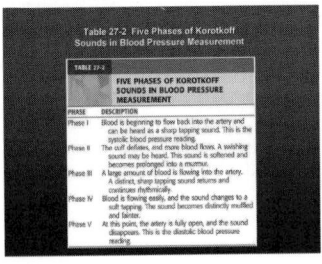

- How are Korotkoff sounds used for blood pressure readings? *(Systolic pressure is registered as the pressure at which the sounds are first heard [Phase I], and diastolic pressure is registered as the pressure at which the sounds disappear [Phase 5].)*

Slide 25

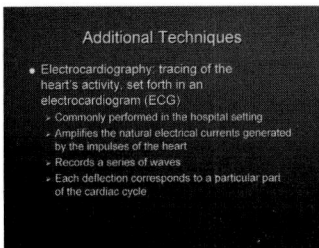

- What is an electrocardiogram (ECG or EKG) used for in dentistry?

- The ECG traces the pattern of the heartbeat on graph paper as it records a series of waves that move above or below a baseline.

- In most cases, a basic ECG takes about 5 to 10 minutes to complete and can be done in a doctor's office, in a laboratory, or in a hospital.

Slide 26

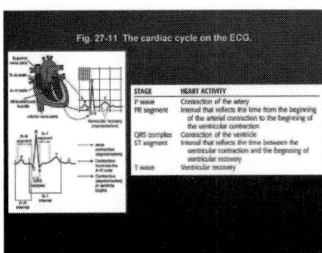

- What are the most common parts of the cardiac cycle that are observed?

- What is considered a normal electrocardiogram?

Torres and Ehrlich Modern Dental Assisting, 9th ed.

Bird/Robinson

28 Oral Diagnosis and Treatment Planning

TEACHING FOCUS

This chapater will give the student an opportunity to become acquainted with the examination and diagnostic techniques used for patient assessment, including visual evaluation, palpation, instrumentation, radiography, intraoral imaging, and photography. Recording the dental examination and charting will be discussed. The student will also have an opportunity to learn about the clinical examination of the patient. The types of treatment plans and treatment plan presentation will be covered.

MATERIALS AND RESOURCES

- ☐ air-water syringe (all Lessons)
- ☐ articulating paper (Lesson 28.1)
- ☐ articulating paper holder (Lesson 28.1)
- ☐ black ink pen (Lesson 28.2)
- ☐ clinical examination form (all Lessons)
- ☐ color pencils (red and blue/black) (Lesson 28.1)
- ☐ computer and PowerPoint projector (all Lessons)
- ☐ cotton pliers (Lesson 28.1)
- ☐ dental floss (all Lessons)
- ☐ eraser (Lesson 28.1)
- ☐ explorer (all Lessons)
- ☐ gauze sponges (2x2 and 4x4) (all Lessons)
- ☐ index cards (Lesson 28.1)
- ☐ mouth mirror (all Lessons)
- ☐ patient record to document findings (all Lessons)
- ☐ periodontal probe (Lesson 28.1)
- ☐ red pencil (Lesson 28.2)
- ☐ tongue depressor (optional) (Lesson 28.2)

LESSON CHECKLIST

Preparations for this lesson include:

- lecture
- guest speaker: general dentist
- evaluation of student knowledge and skills needed to perform all entry-level activities related to oral diagnosis and treatment planning, including:
  - ○ examination and diagnostic techniques
  - ○ recording the dental examination
  - ○ charting
  - ○ clinical examination of the patient
  - ○ the treatment plan
  - ○ recording the dental treatment

ELSEVIER

KEY TERMS

detection (p. 408)
extraoral (p. 407)
furcation (p. 422)
intraoral (p. 407)
mobility (p. 422)
morphologically, morphologic, morphology
    (p. 407)

palpation (p. 407)
probing (p. 408)
restoration (p. 407)
symmetric (p. 417)

ADDITIONAL RESOURCES

PowerPoint slides (Evolve): 1-31
The Interactive Dental Office CD-ROM: Todd Ledbetter

Legend

CTQ
Critical
Thinking
Question

DVD
Multimedia
Procedures
Videos and
Animations

ESLR
EVOLVE
Student
Learning
Resources

IDO
Interactive
Dental
Office
CD-ROM

SW
Student
Workbook

TB
Test Bank
on the
TEACH
CD-ROM

PPT
PowerPoint
Slides

Class Activities are indicated in ***bold italic.***

ELSEVIER

Torres and Ehrlich Modern Dental Assisting, 9ᵗʰ ed.

Bird/Robinson

LESSON 28.1

PRETEST

1. Which of the following is used by the dentist to detect imperfections in the enamel surface, which may be the beginning of decay?
   a. probe
   b. explorer
   c. spatula
   d. file

2. Which classification of decay is diagnosed as including the gingival third of facial or lingual surfaces of any tooth?
   a. Class II
   b. Class III
   c. Class V
   d. Class VI

3. Which numbering system begins with the maxillary right third molar and concludes at the mandibular right third molar, running from 1 to 32?
   a. Palmer Notation System
   b. International Standards Organization System
   c. Fédération Dentaire Internationale System
   d. Universal Numbering System

4. Which charting presentation uses a black or blue X drawn through the tooth to record it?
   a. root canal
   b. missing tooth
   c. drifting tooth
   d. fractured root

5. What method of assessment uses the examiner's fingers and hands to feel for texture, size, and consistency of hard and soft tissue?
   a. visualization
   b. instrumentation
   c. palpation
   d. probing

6. Which instrument does the dentist or dental hygienist need during a periodontal screening?
   a. probe
   b. spatula
   c. file
   d. UV light

7. Where does the dentist present the patient's treatment plan?
   a. reception area
   b. front desk
   c. sterilization center
   d. private office

8. Using the mobility scale, which of the following represents slight mobility in a tooth?
   a. 0
   b. 1
   c. 2
   d. 3

9. What happens directly after the treatment plan presentation?
   a. screening for periodontal and caries risk factors
   b. presentation of the fee estimate for each treatment option
   c. palpation of oral soft tissues
   d. examination of radiographs and typodonts

ELSEVIER

Torres and Ehrlich Modern Dental Assisting, 9th ed.

Bird/Robinson

10. During periodontal screening, how many surfaces of each tooth usually need to be recorded?
   a. 2
   b. 3
   c. 4
   d. 6

Answers
   1. b
   2. c
   3. d
   4. b
   5. c
   6. a
   7. d
   8. b
   9. b
   10. d

BACKGROUND ASSESSMENT

Question: What method of color-coded charting is used in the dental office? What types of pencils and pens does the dental assistant use for charting as the dentist makes notes on the patient's dentition?

Answer: In the color-coding method of charting, black or blue symbols represent dental work already completed. They can indicate dental work completed by another dentist or during previous appointments with the current dentist. Red symbols indicate treatment that needs to be completed at future dental appointments. Once this work is completed, the dental assistant erases or marks over the red with a blue or black notation to indicate that the work has been finished. The dental assistant should have colored pencils (possibly black or blue and red) to chart the dentition and a black ink pen to make notes available for use during the charting, as well as an eraser if that is the method used.

Question: What materials should be available during the presentation of the treatment plan? Where does the dentist present the treatment plan?

Answer: It is important to have the diagnostic tools used to present the case. The dentist should have readied the patient chart, radiographs, diagnostic casts, and treatment plans. Other visual aids might include before-and-after photographs, diagnostic casts of similar cases, and typodonts of proposed appliances, such as full or partial dentures, dental implants, or fixed crowns and bridges. The dentist should present the treatment plan to the patient in a private office or treatment area, but not at the front desk or in the reception area.

CRITICAL THINKING QUESTION

The dental assistant meets the first patient of the morning in the reception room. The patient, who is scheduled for a soft tissue examination, is wearing dark sunglasses and smells like alcohol. The dental assistant notices that the patient has difficulty getting up from a seated position and walking to the treatment room. When the dental assistant addresses the patient, the patient slurs his speech. What should the dental assistant do in this situation? How can the patient's behavior affect dental treatment?

Guidelines: The dental assistant must immediately notify the dentist what he or she has observed. The patient seems to be under the influence of alcohol. When escorting a patient to the treatment area for any examination, the dental assistant's role is to observe the patient's general appearance, speech, and behavior. If anything is unusual, it must be communicated immediately to the dentist, because the dentist does not have this early observation of the patient. This patient may be medically compromised by an addiction to alcohol or may have self-medicated because he is fearful about dental treatment. Alcohol abuse may indicate a risk for certain oral diseases and a possible change in future treatment planning.

OBJECTIVES	CONTENT	TEACHING RESOURCES
Pronounce, define, and spell the Key Terms.	■ Key terms (p. 406)	SW Fill in the Blank questions 1-12 (pp. 163-164) ESLR Electronic Flashcards ▸ Discuss each of the key terms in Chapter 28, focusing on the definition, pronunciation, and spelling of each term. *Class Activity Have the students make flash cards of the key terms by writing the terms on one side of an index card and the definitions on the other. Have the students quiz each other with the flash cards.*

Torres and Ehrlich Modern Dental Assisting, 9th ed.

Bird/Robinson

OBJECTIVES	CONTENT	TEACHING RESOURCES

List and describe the examination and diagnostic techniques used for patient assessment.	■ Examination and diagnostic techniques (p. 407)
	
	□ Visual examination (p. 407)
	
	□ Palpation (p. 407)
	
	□ Instrumentation (p. 408)
	
	   – Detection (p. 408)
	
	   – Probing (p. 408)
	
	□ Radiography (p. 408)
	
	□ Intraoral imaging (p. 408)
	
	□ Photography (p. 408)
		▦ PPT 5-14
		
		▥ TB questions 2-4, 18, 24
		
		▨ SW Short-Answer Questions 1; Fill in the Blank questions 1-2, 8; Multiple Choice questions 2-3, 5 (pp. 163-164)
		
		Figure 28-1 Detecting decay (p. 408)
		
		Figure 28-2 Using a periodontal probe to measure the sulcus (p. 408)
		
		Figure 28-3 Example of a bite-wing intraoral radiograph (p. 408)
		
		Figure 28-4 Example of a Panorex extraoral radiograph (p. 409)
		
		Figure 28-5 An intraoral imaging system is used to diagnose and educate the patient (p. 409)
		
		Figure 28-6 Photographs are taken to provide a visual evaluation of the patient (p. 409)
		
		Recall questions 1-4 (p. 409)
		
		Eye to the Future (p. 423)
		
		♈ CTQ 1 (p. 423)
		
		▸ Discuss the following examination and diagnostic techniques: visual examination, palpation, instrumentation, radiography, intraoral imaging, and photography.
		
		Class Activity Assign each student a diagnostic technique (such as digital radiography). Have the students conduct Internet research on the latest devices and techniques for the assigned technique and then write a short report to be presented in class. (For students to prepare for this activity, see Homework/Assignments #1.)

Discuss the role of the dental assistant in the clinical examination.	■ Recording the dental examination (p. 409)	▦ PPT 15 ▥ TB questions 14 ▨ SW Short-Answer Questions 2; Multiple Choice question 9 (pp. 163-164) Role of the Dental Assistant in Patient Examination and Treatment Planning (p. 407) Patient Education (p. 423) ▸ Discuss the activities the dental assistant performs with regard to patient examination and treatment planning.

Torres and Ehrlich Modern Dental Assisting, 9th ed.

OBJECTIVES	CONTENT	TEACHING RESOURCES
		Class Activity **Invite a general dentist to speak to the class about interesting clinical cases. Encourage students to ask questions. Then have students write a short report on the presentation.**
List the six categories of Black's classification of cavities.	■ Recording the dental examination (p. 409) □ Black's classification of cavities (p. 409)	☒▥ PPT 15-16 ▦ TB questions 5-6 ▣ SW Short-Answer Questions 3; Multiple Choice questions 6-7 (pp. 163-164) Figure 28-7 Black's classification of cavities (p. 411) ▸ Discuss the six categories of Black's classification of cavities, including the location and description of the cavities. *Class Activity* **Have students draw each class of cavity on prepared tooth outline figures, labeling each one correctly.**
Differentiate between an anatomic and a geometric diagram for charting.	□ Tooth diagrams (p. 410) □ Tooth-numbering systems (p. 410) – Universal numbering system (p. 410) – International Standards Organization System/Fédération Dentaire Internationale System (p. 410) – Palmer notation system (p. 410) □ Color coding (p. 410) □ Abbreviations (p. 410) ■ Charting (p. 410) □ Symbols (p. 410) ■ Clinical examination of the patient (p. 413) □ Soft tissue examination (p. 413) □ Examination and charting of teeth (p. 420)	☒▥ PPT 15, 17-24 ▦ TB questions 7-11, 13 ▣ SW Short-Answer Questions 4; Fill in the Blank questions 3-4, 9; Multiple Choice questions 4, 8, 10, 15; Charting questions 1-5 (pp. 163-165) Figure 28-8 Example of a geometric diagram for charting conditions of the mouth (p. 412) Figure 28-10 (A) Universal numbering system; (B) International Standards Organization System; (C) Palmer notation system (pp. 412-413) Recall questions 6-8 (p. 413) Legal and Ethical Implications (p. 423) ▯ CTQ 3-5 (p. 423-424) ▸ Discuss the anatomic diagram method of charting. ▸ Discuss the geometric diagram method of charting. *Class Activity* **Have students chart dentoforms with restorations in both the Universal and Palmer methods. Post similar charts in the International method so they can note the differences.**

Torres and Ehrlich Modern Dental Assisting, 9th ed.

Bird/Robinson

OBJECTIVES	CONTENT	TEACHING RESOURCES
Chart the correct restorative material for either an existing restoration or a required treatment.	*Procedure* 28-2 Charting of teeth (p. 421) (SW/ESLR Competency 28-2, p. 171)	PPT 15, 17-24 TB questions 6-8, 10-13 SW Multiple Choice questions 4, 8, 10, 15; Charting questions 1-5 (pp. 164-166) SW/ESLR Competency 28-2 Charting of Teeth (p. 171) Figure 28-8 Example of a geometric diagram for charting conditions of the mouth (p. 412) Figure 28-9 (A) Universal numbering system; (B) International Standards Organization System; (C) Palmer notation system (pp. 412-413) CTQ 3, 5 (pp. 423-424) ▸ Discuss the method of charting the correct restorative material for either an existing restoration or a required treatment. ***Class Activity** Divide the class into small groups, and have each group create a list of the supplies needed for charting of teeth. Then have the groups share their lists with the class.*
Chart the correct symbol for either an existing restoration or a required treatment.	*Procedure* 28-2 Charting of teeth (p. 421) (SW/ESLR Competency 28-2, p. 171)	PPT 17-24 TB questions 9 SW Short-Answer Questions 4; Charting questions 1-5 (pp. 163, 165-166) SW/ESLR Competency 28-2 Charting of Teeth (p. 171) Figure 28-8 Example of a geometric diagram for charting conditions of the mouth (p. 412) Figure 28-9 (A) Universal Numbering system; (B) International Standards Organization System; (C) Palmer notation system (pp. 412-413) CTQ 3, 5 (pp. 423-424) ▸ Discuss the method of charting the correct symbol for either an existing restoration or a required treatment. ***Class Activity** Have pairs of students take turns role-playing a dentist calling out specific notations during examination of a patient's teeth and a dental assistant recording those notations on the clinical examination form.*

OBJECTIVES	CONTENT	TEACHING RESOURCES
Explain the color coding of a chart diagram.	☐ Color coding (p. 410) ☐ Abbreviations (p. 410) ■ Charting (p. 410) ☐ Symbols (p. 410) ■ Clinical examination of the patient (p. 413) ☐ Soft tissue examination (p. 413) ☐ Examination and charting of teeth (p. 420)	⊠▤ PPT 15, 22-24 ▦ TB question 12 ▱ SW Short-Answer Questions 5 (p. 163) Figure 28-10 Example of color coding (p. 413) ▸ Discuss how color coding is used to represent and differentiate the treatment already completed and treatment that still needs to be completed. ▸ Discuss the benefits of color coding. *Class Activity **Have the students color code a chart of dentoforms with restorations. Then have the students exchange their charts and compare them.***

28.1 Homework/Assignments:

1. Assign each student a diagnostic technique (such as digital radiography). Have the students conduct Internet research on the latest devices and techniques for the assigned technique and then write a short report to be presented in class.

28.1 Instructor's Notes/Student Feedback:

Torres and Ehrlich Modern Dental Assisting, 9th ed.

Bird/Robinson

LESSON 28.2

CRITICAL THINKING QUESTION

A patient has had procedures in the dental office to improve his periodontal health. The patient had severe periodontal disease and has shown moderate improvement, although he states his "gums are still bleeding." The patient already has a series of radiographs, a periodontal chart, and intraoral photographs taken before the treatment began. What instruments and forms should the dental assistant have ready for the dentist for this patient's next examination? What must the dental assistant do during and after the examination?

Guidelines: The dental assistant must prepare for a periodontal screening, so that the dentist can examine the gingival tissues. The previous periodontal chart must be ready for the dentist, along with a black ink pen and red pencil. The chart will need to be dated again for the new readings. Any radiographs, especially any periapical ones, as well as the entire patient record, should be readily available for the dentist to consult. The dentist may also need referral forms for the periodontist. The dental assistant should prepare a tray with an explorer, probe, mirror, gauze sponges, dental floss, and possibly other items as requested (such as those used for an occlusal evaluation). The intraoral camera should be ready in case the dentist decides to take "after" intraoral photographs for the patient record. During the appointment, the assistant must use the air syringe to clear the mouth mirror and adjust the operating light as necessary, as well as record the probe readings, circling any reading where there is bleeding. Mobility, furcations, calculus, and sensitivity may also need to be recorded, and additional radiographs may need to be taken as requested by the dentist. At the completion of the procedure, the assistant should rinse and dry the patient's mouth and accurately document all information in the progress notes of the patient record.

OBJECTIVES	CONTENT	TEACHING RESOURCES
Describe the need for a soft tissue examination.	■ Clinical examination of the patient (p. 413) ☐ Soft tissue examination (p. 413) *Procedure* 28-1 The soft tissue examination (pp. 417-420) (SW/ESLR Competency 28-1, pp. 167-169) ☐ Examination and charting of teeth (p. 420)	PPT 27-30 TB questions 15-17 SW Short-Answer Questions 7; Fill in the Blank questions 6-7, 10, 12; Multiple Choice questions 11, 13-14 (pp. 163-165) SW/ESLR Competency 28-1 The Soft Tissue Examination (pp. 167-169) CTQ 2 (p. 423) ▸ Discuss what is involved in a soft tissue examination. ▸ Discuss the purpose of a soft tissue examination. ***Class Activity** Have pairs of students take turns examining each other's soft tissue and noting any abnormalities.*
Describe the pocket depth and bleeding index of the gingival tissues and how to record them.	■ Clinical examination of the patient (p. 413) ☐ Soft tissue examination (p. 413) ☐ Examination and charting of teeth (p. 420) ☐ Examination and charting of periodontium (p. 420)	PPT 27-28, 30 TB question 19 SW/ESLR Competency 28-3 Periodontal Screening: Examination of the Gingival Tissues (p. 173) SW Short-Answer Questions 6 (p. 163) Recall question 9 (p. 422)

OBJECTIVES	CONTENT	TEACHING RESOURCES
	<u>*Procedure*</u> 28-3 Periodontal screening: examination of the gingival tissues (p. 422) (SW/ESLR Competency 28-3, p. 173)	▸ Discuss how to record the pocket depth and bleeding index of gingival tissues. *Class Activity Have students periodontally chart three varying periodontally-involved cases using the dental clinic periodontal chart as you read out the probe readings, bleeding points, mobility, furcations, and notes on calculus and sensitivity.*

Discuss the importance of a treatment plan.	■ The treatment plan (p. 422)
	
	 ☐ Types of treatment plans (p. 422)
	
	   – Level I: Emergency care (p. 423)
	
	   – Level II: Standard care (p. 423)
	
	   – Level III: Optimum care (p. 423)
	
	 ☐ Treatment plan presentation (p. 423)
		⊠▤ PPT 31
		
		 ▤ TB questions 20-22
		
		 ▦ SW Short-Answer Questions 8 (p. 163)
		
		 ▸ Discuss the types of treatment plans and the reasons a treatment plan is important.
		
		 ▸ Discuss how to present a treatment plan to the patient.
		
		 Class Activity Have the students call out the items the dentist needs to present a treatment plan. List their responses on the blackboard.

Performance Evaluation		▤ TB ▦ SW questions (pp. 163-165) ▦ SW Charting (pp. 165-166) ▦ *e* SW/ESLR Competency 28-1 The Soft Tissue Examination (pp. 167-169) ▦ *e* SW/ESLR Competency 28-2 Charting of Teeth (p. 171) ▦ *e* SW/ESLR Competency 28-3 Periodontal Screening: Examination of the Gingival Tissues (p. 173) *e* ESLR Electronic Flashcards *e* ESLR Practice Quiz *e* ESLR Labeling Exercises 20-27 Recall questions (pp. 409-422) ⸙ CTQ (pp. 423-424)

Torres and Ehrlich Modern Dental Assisting, 9th ed.

Bird/Robinson

28.2 Homework/Assignments:

28.2 Instructor's Notes/Student Feedback:

Bird/Robinson

Slide 1

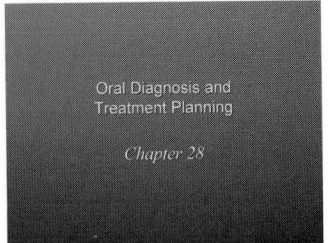

Oral Diagnosis and
Treatment Planning

Chapter 28

Slide 2

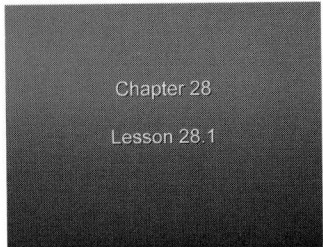

Chapter 28

Lesson 28.1

Slide 3

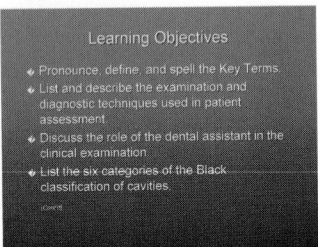

Learning Objectives

- Pronounce, define, and spell the Key Terms.
- List and describe the examination and diagnostic techniques used in patient assessment.
- Discuss the role of the dental assistant in the clinical examination.
- List the six categories of the Black classification of cavities.

(Cont'd)

Slide 4

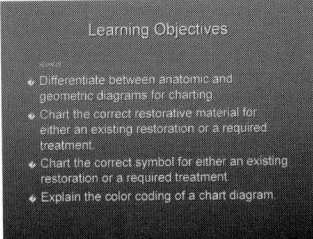

Learning Objectives

(Cont'd)

- Differentiate between anatomic and geometric diagrams for charting.
- Chart the correct restorative material for either an existing restoration or a required treatment.
- Chart the correct symbol for either an existing restoration or a required treatment.
- Explain the color coding of a chart diagram.

Torres and Ehrlich Modern Dental Assisting, 9th ed.

Bird/Robinson

Slide 5

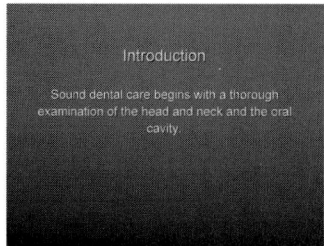

- What does a "thorough examination" mean?
- What is the clinical assistant's role during a dental examination procedure? *(To have the correct forms, instruments, and any additional supplies that may be needed by the dentist ready for use.)*

Slide 6

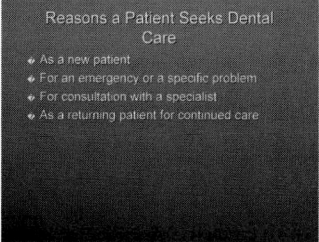

Slide 7

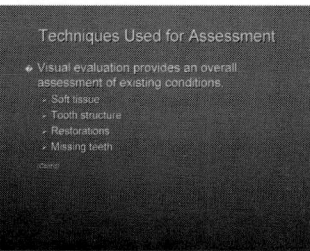

- What does assessment mean? *(Assessment is the process of making an official evaluation of someone or a situation.)*

Slide 8

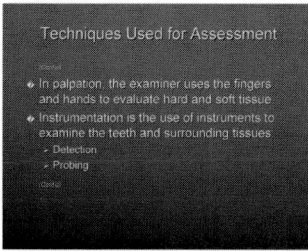

- How does the dentist use the explorer instrument? *(With the use of a sharp, pointed explorer, the dentist can detect imperfections in the enamel surface, which may be the beginning of decay. The dentist will also use an explorer to evaluate existing restorations for their stability and integrity.)*

Slide 9

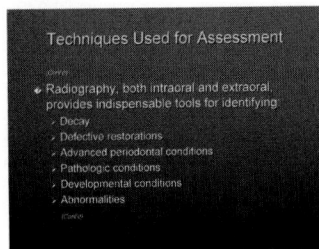

- What does *intraoral* mean?
- What does *extraoral* mean?

Slide 10

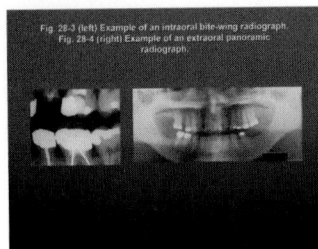

- What are radiographs used for in a dental practice, and how does the dentist decide which radiographs to prescribe?
- Radiographs have become indispensable tools for identifying decay, defective restorations, advanced periodontal conditions, pathology, developmental conditions, and other abnormalities.

Slide 11

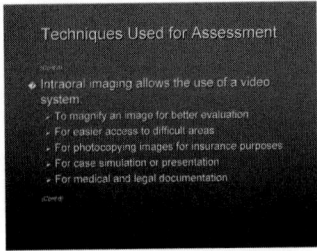

- What is intraoral imaging? *(Intraoral imaging is similar to the use of a miniature video camera.)*
- This technique allows the dentist to use a computer monitor as a complement to a video camera system, with a display of live video on a monitor screen.

Slide 12

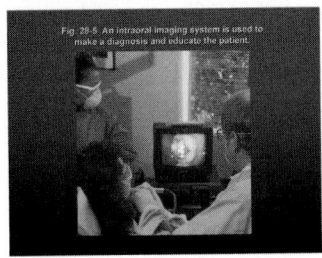

- Notice that the dental team members are practicing infection control while using the intraoral camera.

Bird/Robinson

Slide 13

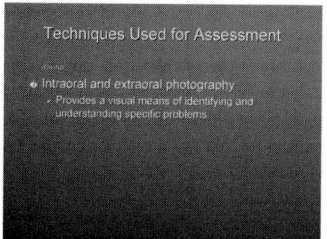

- For more comprehensive treatment, such as reconstructive or orthodontic procedures, a patient will have before-and-after photographs taken to see the changed results.

Slide 14

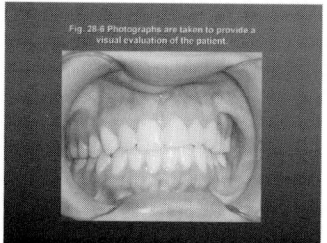

- What is being used to pull back the lips and cheeks to allow the teeth to show?

Slide 15

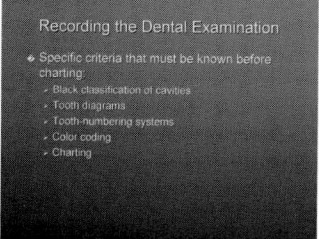

Slide 16

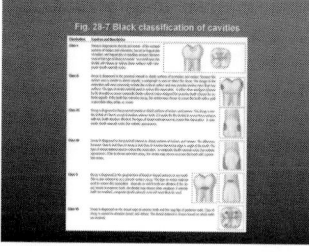

- Developed by G.V. Black in the early 1900s this standard classification system is universal to all dentists and is used to describe the location of decay and the best method for restoring the tooth. Black's original classification included Class I through Class V. Class VI was added later.

- What class in Black's classification system involves premolars and molars?

- What class in Black's classification system involves incisors?

Torres and Ehrlich Modern Dental Assisting, 9th ed.
Bird/Robinson

Slide 17

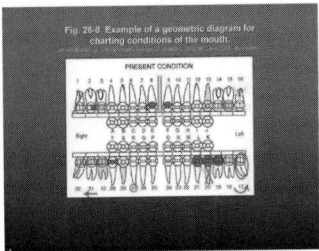

- The recording of the dental examination is often described as "shorthand" to note the dentist's findings.

- Symbols, abbreviations, and color coding are used in the recording to indicate various conditions and existing restorations.

- How is the dentition charted during a dental examination?

- What is a restoration? *(The use of a dental material to restore a tooth or teeth to a functional permanent unit.)*

Slide 18

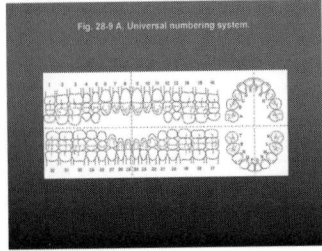

- When referring to the diagram, remember that the teeth are presented from the perspective of looking into the patient's mouth.

- What dental charting systems are available? *(A variety of diagram styles are available, but anatomic and geometric designs are most often used.)*

Slide 19

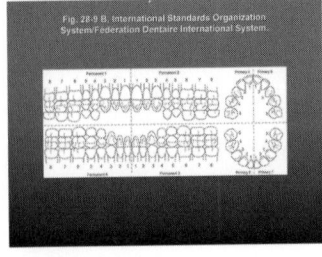

- How does this chart work? *(This numbering system [1-32] begins with the maxillary right third molar and concludes at the mandibular right third molar.)*

- Is this an example of an anatomic or geometric chart?

- Which charting system does your dentist use?

- Which charting system do you think would work best for you or the patient?

Slide 20

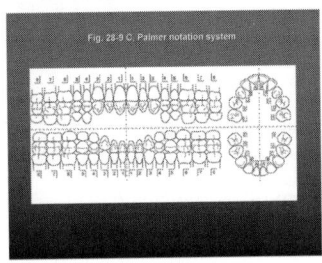

- How does this chart work? *(This numbering system assigns a two-digit number to each tooth: the first number is the quadrant; the second number is the tooth.)*

- Is this an example of an anatomic or geometric chart?

Bird/Robinson

Slide 21

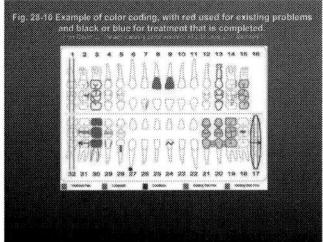

- How does this chart work? *(This numbering system uses a bracket to designate the four quadrants of the mouth.)*
- Is this an example of an anatomic or geometric chart?

Slide 22

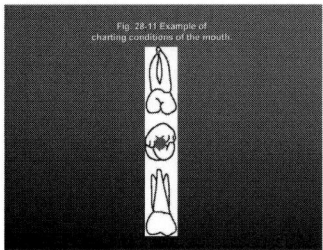

- Why does dentistry use color coding? *(To represent and differentiate the treatment already completed and treatment that still needs to be completed.)*
- This visual notation makes it easier to review the patient's dental status each time the patient is seen in the dental office.
- How does color coding work on a chart? *(Black or blue symbols indicate dental work already completed. Red symbols indicate treatment that needs to be completed at future dental appointments.)*
- Once this work is completed, the assistant will erase or mark over the red with blue or black to indicate the work has been finished.

Slide 23

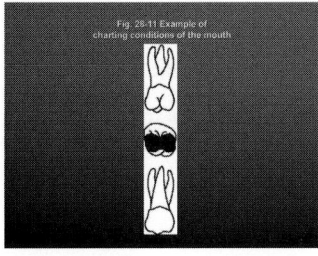

Slide 24

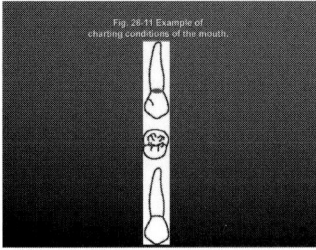

Slide 25

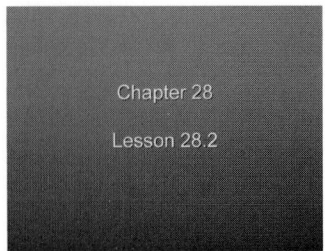

- Why are the cervical lymph nodes examined by the dentist?

- How is the temporomandibular joint evaluated? *(To evaluate in centric, lateral, protrusive, and retrusive movements, ask the patient to open and close the mouth normally and then to move the jaw from side to side. Palpate the tissues gently to detect lumps or similar abnormalities. To determine whether there is noise during movement, listen as the patient opens and closes the mouth. A stethoscope placed on the joint may be used.)*

Slide 26

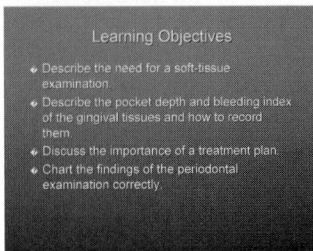

- What does the periodontium consist of?

- Who usually completes this part of the examination? What occurs during it? *(The dental hygienist completes this part of the examination, assessing the tissues that support the teeth, including the gingiva, cementum, periodontal ligament, and alveolar and supporting bone structures. The alveolar and supporting bone structures cannot be visually evaluated, so that updated periapical radiographs are required.)*

Slide 27

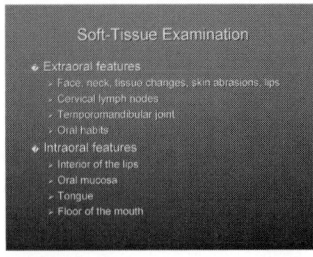

- What does the term *mobility* mean?

- When does mobility happen, and what should be recorded on the chart? *(If excessive bone loss is noticed on the radiograph, mobility may have resulted. Document any mobility on the examination form.)*

- During what portion of the oral diagnosis examination is tooth mobility evaluated?

Slide 28

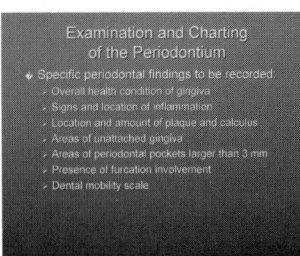

- How is the probe used? *(Using gentle pressure, the periodontal probe is inserted into the gingival sulcus until resistance is met. The probe is inserted into six specific sites for each tooth: mesiofacial, facial, distofacial, mesiolingual, lingual, and distolingual. The depth of insertion is read by noting the position of the markings on the probe while in the sulcus.)*

- How many probe readings of each tooth are usually recorded during a periodontal screening?

Torres and Ehrlich Modern Dental Assisting, 9th ed.

Bird/Robinson

Slide 29

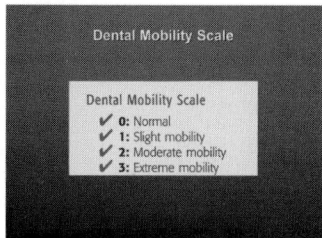

- When is the treatment plan presented to the patient, and how long does it last? *(On completion of a thorough clinical examination, an appointment will be scheduled to present the treatment plan to the patient. The type of treatment to be rendered will determine the length of the presentation. Typically, a 30-minute to a 1-hour appointment is scheduled for the patient.)*

Slide 30

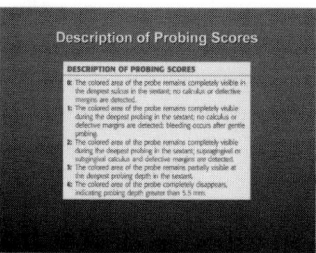

- How is the probe used? *(Using gentle pressure, the examiner inserts the periodontal probe into the gingival sulcus until resistance is met. The probe is inserted into six specific sites for each tooth: mesiofacial, facial, distofacial, mesiolingual, lingual, and distolingual. The depth of insertion is read by noting the position of the markings on the probe while it is in the sulcus.)*

- How many probe readings of each tooth are usually recorded during a periodontal screening?

Slide 31

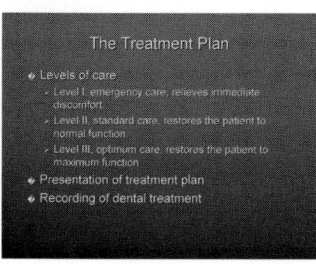

- When is the treatment plan presented to the patient, and how long does it last? *(On completion of a thorough clinical examination, an appointment will be scheduled to present the treatment plan to the patient. The type of treatment to be rendered will determine the duration of the presentation. Typically a 30-minute to 1-hour appointment is scheduled for the patient.)*

Torres and Ehrlich Modern Dental Assisting, 9th ed.
Bird/Robinson

29 | Lesson Plan
The Medically and Physically Compromised Patient

TEACHING FOCUS

This chapter will give the student an opportunity to understand the special needs of the medically and physically compromised patient. The classification of the aging population and the types of medical disorders that are associated with living longer will be discussed, as well as particular medical conditions that might affect oral health. Treatment modifications for specific medical disorders will also be described.

MATERIALS AND RESOURCES

- ☐ computer and PowerPoint projector (all Lessons)
- ☐ index cards (Lesson 29.1)
- ☐ list of older celebrities (Lesson 29.1)

- ☐ medical histories of physically compromised patients (all Lessons)
- ☐ photographs of incorrect wheelchair transfers (Lesson 29.2)
- ☐ wheelchair (Lesson 29.2)

LESSON CHECKLIST

Preparations for this lesson include:

- lecture
- guest speakers: representative from an organization that advocates for people with disabilities or the aging population
- evaluation of student knowledge and skills needed to treat aging and mentally or physically challenged patients, including:
  - identifying the classifications of the stages of aging
  - describing the orally related conditions that might affect the older population
  - detailing the importance of taking a medical history for the physically compromised patient
  - describing the major medical disorders that might affect a patient's oral health and identifying how to modify treatment for such patients
  - explaining how to transfer a wheelchair-bound patient to a dental chair

Bird/Robinson

KEY TERMS

Alzheimer's disease (p. 430)
anemia (p. 435)
angina (p. 432)
arthritis (p. 435)
asthma (p. 433)
atrophy (p. 435)
bacteremia (p. 433)
bronchitis (p. 435)
cannula (p. 435)
dementia (p. 430)
diabetes mellitus (p. 436)
emphysema (p. 435)

endocarditis (p. 433)
epilepsy (p. 430)
hemophilia (p. 435)
hyperplasia (p. 431)
hyperthyroidism (p. 436)
hypothyroidism (p. 436)
leukemia (p. 435)
myocardial infarction (p. 431)
seizure (p. 430)
stroke (p. 431)
xerostomia (p. 429)

ADDITIONAL RESOURCES

PowerPoint slides (Evolve): 1-32

Legend

CTQ
Critical
Thinking
Question

DVD
Multimedia
Procedures
Videos and
Animations

ESLR
EVOLVE
Student
Learning
Resources

IDO
Interactive
Dental
Office
CD-ROM

SW
Student
Workbook

TB
Test Bank
on the
TEACH
CD-ROM

PPT
PowerPoint
Slides

Class Activities are indicated in ***bold italic.***

LESSON 29.1

PRETEST

1. How long does a petit mal seizure last?
   a. no longer than 30 seconds
   b. 30 minutes
   c. longer than 1 hour
   d. a full day

2. Why are muscle relaxants such as diazepam prescribed for patients with multiple sclerosis?
   a. to inhibit salivary flow
   b. to control muscle spasms
   c. to sedate the patient
   d. to awaken the patient

3. What common oral side effect usually occurs from taking phenytoin?
   a. gingival recession
   b. increased saliva
   c. gingival hyperplasia
   d. tooth staining

4. What emergency situation is an angina patient at risk for?
   a. myocardial infarction
   b. cerebrovascular accident
   c. choking
   d. syncope

5. What is the most common form of hyperthyroidism?
   a. Heberden's nodules
   b. Raynaud's phenomenon
   c. Alzheimer's disease
   d. Graves' disease

6. Which of the following is caused by a sudden vascular lesion of the brain, such as hemorrhage, embolism, thrombosis, or ruptured aneurysm?
   a. Alzheimer's disease
   b. diabetes mellitus
   c. muscular dystrophy
   d. cerebrovascular accident

7. What is another name for hypertension?
   a. high blood sugar
   b. high cholesterol
   c. high blood pressure
   d. congestive heart failure

8. Which of the following medical histories usually leaves a patient with numbness, vertigo, visual disturbances, sweating, headache, and nausea?
   a. myocardial infarction
   b. Graves' disease
   c. bronchial asthma
   d. cerebrovascular accident

9. What is the cause of secondary dentin gradually reducing the size of the pulp chamber, making teeth more susceptible to fracture?
   a. increased hormone levels
   b. poor oral hygiene methods
   c. aging of the dentition
   d. increased blood sugar

10. Which category of physical assessment involves patients with medical conditions who require scheduling changes or shorter appointments?
    a. Category I
    b. Category II
    c. Category III
    d. Category IV

Answers

| 1. a | 3. c | 5. d | 7. c | 9. c |
| 2. b | 4. a | 6. d | 8. d | 10. b |

BACKGROUND ASSESSMENT

Question: What changes are noted in an aging oral cavity? What can be done to prevent these changes?

Answer: A patient with aging dentition will possibly have dry mouth, or xerostomia, which results from disorders or medications that cause a decreased flow of saliva. This condition can mean increased dental decay, especially root caries, because the aged dentition also has increased levels of gingival recession. A patient with aging dentition might also show signs of periodontal disease. If any teeth have been lost, there will be loss of the alveolar bone associated with the tooth. As a person ages, the teeth may also darken and become more brittle. This results from deposits of secondary dentin that have gradually reduced the size of the pulp chamber. Brittle teeth then become more susceptible to fracture. A patient can control age-related changes in the oral cavity by maintaining a sound diet, using fluoride products, sipping water, visiting the dental office, and practicing good oral hygiene. Finally, a patient may need to add strength to many teeth through new restorations.

Question: What is the category of patient assessment for most patients with heart disease? How must the dental staff modify treatment for patients with heart disease?

Answer: The patient with heart disease is usually a Category III patient. Such patients have medical conditions with lifelong implications and thus require modifications in dental treatment planning. First, the dentist may decide to consult a physician about the patient's heart disease before dental treatment. The dental staff must carefully schedule appointments so that heart disease patients avoid the stress of lengthy visits to the dental office. The dental staff must also obtain baseline vital signs before treatment begins, and then continue monitoring the patient throughout the procedure. The dentist may use premedication and nitrous oxide to help relieve stress, as well as supplemental oxygen throughout the procedure. Immediately before treatment, the dentist may consider using prophylactic sublingual nitroglycerin. The dentist can administer, within limits, epinephrine and other vasoconstrictors to patients who have mild to moderate cardiovascular disease. These patients may need to be seated in a semisupine rather than a supine position for greater comfort.

CRITICAL THINKING QUESTION

A dental assistant initially examines a teenager who has recently been diagnosed with diabetes, has had insulin prescribed, and wonders why his gums seem dry and sore. His physician recommends that the patient rest more to reduce future complications, but he feels that the patient's glucose levels are under control. In what physical classification is this patient? How will the dental assistant schedule him for his follow-up restorative appointments, modify his dental treatment, and discuss certain dental health recommendations with him and his guardians?

Guidelines: This patient has diabetes mellitus type 1, managed with insulin. His diabetes is under control, so the patient is in physical classification Category III, for patients who have medical conditions with lifelong implications. Therefore, the planned dental treatment might require modification. Before dental treatment begins the dentist may decide to consult with the patient's physician to address questions about the patient's control of the diabetes or complications that may be encountered. Because the patient displays some diabetes-related oral changes—such as dehydration of oral soft tissues resulting from xerostomia, and red, swollen, painful gingiva resulting from medication therapy—the dental assistant must explain these to the patient and his guardians. The dental assistant should plan morning appointments, keep them short to minimize patient stress, and consider using nitrous oxide sedation during the appointment. Finally, the dental assistant should instruct the patient and his guardians that normal dietary intake before dental appointments and a good oral hygiene routine are needed to reduce the risk of oral infections and hypoglycemia, the most common diabetes-related emergency arising from failing to eat.

ELSEVIER

Torres and Ehrlich Modern Dental Assisting, 9th ed.

Bird/Robinson

OBJECTIVES	CONTENT	TEACHING RESOURCES
Pronounce, define, and spell the Key Terms.	■ Key terms (pp. 425-426)	*E* ESLR Electronic Flashcards ▸ Discuss each of the key terms in this chapter, focusing on the definition, pronunciation, and spelling of each term. ***Class Activity** Divide the class into two groups, and have them create a Jeopardy-type game based on the medically and physically compromised conditions discussed in the textbook. Have the first group write down the answers on index cards. Then have its members take turns asking the other group to supply the questions.*
Describe the type of dental management a medically compromised patient would receive.	■ Introduction (p. 426) ■ Role of the dental assistant (p. 426)	PPT 5-6 TB question 1 ▸ Discuss when and why it is important for a dental team to be prepared to modify normal treatment practices. ▸ Discuss the purpose of the Americans with Disabilities Act. What is the American Dental Association's position on treating patients with physical or mental challenges? ***Class Activity** Divide the class into three groups, and assign each group one of the discussion points below, asking them to think about how a hearing-challenged patient would be treated in the dental office. After 15 minutes, have the groups share their findings with the class.* – *How does the Americans with Disabilities Act protect this patient?* – *What is the American Dental Association's position on treating this physically challenged patient?* – *Why should the dental office comply with the Americans with Disabilities Act and with the American Dental Association's position on treating medically compromised patients?*
Describe the stages of aging in the older population.	■ The aging population (p. 426) ☐ Stages of aging (p. 426)	PPT 7 TB questions 2-3 SW Short-Answer Questions 1; Fill in the Blank question 8; Multiple Choice questions 1-2 (pp. 175-176) Figure 29-1 Percentages of Americans age 65 and older in each state (p. 427) Recall questions 1-2 (p. 427) ▸ Discuss how the health expectations of "young-old" persons may be different from than that of "old" persons. ▸ Discuss how treatment of the older patient has changed and why.

Bird/Robinson

OBJECTIVES	CONTENT	TEACHING RESOURCES
		Class Activity Before the class meets, provide a list of older celebrities and ask the students to research the ages of those on the list, to place them in the stages of aging, and identify if the attitudes, characteristics, and needs of the celebrities match those of the typical person in their category. Have the class discuss their findings. (For students to prepare for this activity, see Homework/Assignments #1.)
Describe the orally related conditions affecting the older patient.	☐ Oral health of the aging (p. 427) ☐ Oral health conditions (p. 427) – Xerostomia (p. 429) – Periodontal disease (p. 429) – Tooth decay (p. 429) – Dark and brittle teeth (p. 429) – Bone resorption (p. 429)	PPT 8-12 TB questions 4-6 SW Short-Answer Questions 2; Fill in the Blank question 5; Multiple Choice questions 3-4 (pp. 175-177) Figure 29-2 Example of a medication profile for a patient (p. 428) Figure 29-3 Periodontal conditions of an older patient (p. 429) Figure 29-4 Root caries of a tooth in an older patient (p. 429) Figure 29-5 Darkened teeth associated with secondary dentin and aging (p. 429) Figure 29-6 Bone resorption with loss of teeth and alveolar ridge (p. 430) Recall questions 3-5 (p. 429) ▶ Discuss the oral health conditions specifically related to aging. Why is periodontal disease on the rise and how can it be prevented? ▶ Discuss why dental decay is more prevalent in older patients. *Class Activity Before the class meets ask students to conduct research on the Internet or in the library on one of the signs of aging in the oral cavity, and then write a short report on ways to prevent further oral damage. Have the class discuss the reports. (For students to prepare for this activity, see Homework/Assignments #2.)*
Describe the importance of the medical history for the medically compromised patient.	■ The medically compromised patient (p. 430)	PPT 13 TB question 7 SW Short-Answer Questions 3 (p. 175) ▶ Discuss the importance of taking a medical history. How is this different in older patients compared with the general population?

Bird/Robinson

OBJECTIVES	CONTENT	TEACHING RESOURCES
		▸ Discuss the importance of getting a patient's medication profile. How might some medications affect oral health directly? *Class Activity **Have the class prepare a brief summary for each category of medically compromised patients. Call on students to present to the class.***
Describe the major medical disorders that can affect a patient's oral health.	■ Specific illnesses of the medically compromised patient (p. 430) □ Neurologic disorders (p. 430) – Alzheimer's disease (p. 430) – Seizures (p. 430) – Multiple sclerosis (p. 431) – Stroke (p. 431) □ Cardiovascular disorders (p. 431) – Congestive heart failure (p. 431) – Hypertension (p. 431) – Angina (p. 432) – Endocarditis (p. 432)	⊠ PPT 14-21 TB questions 8-12, 16-17 SW Short-Answer Questions 4; Fill in the Blank questions 3, 6-7, 9 11, 15, 19; Multiple Choice questions 5-11 (pp. 175-176) SW Case Study questions 1-5 (p. 165) Treatment Plan Modifications for a Patient with Alzheimer's Disease (p. 430) Treatment Plan Modifications for a Patient with Epilepsy (p. 431) Treatment Plan Modifications for Patients with Multiple Sclerosis (p. 431) Recall questions 6-9 (p. 431) Treatment Plan Modifications for a Patient with Stroke (p. 446) Figure 29-7 Effects of a cerebrovascular accident (stroke) (p. 432) Figure 29-8 Incidence of heart disease (p. 433) Treatment Plan Modifications for a Patient with Heart Disease (p. 433) Figure 29-9 Effects of a blocked artery (p. 434) Recall questions 10-12 (p. 433) ⚲ CTQ 4 (p. 439) ▸ Discuss how illnesses may affect the mouth, both directly and indirectly. ▸ Discuss what a dentist should know about a patient with heart disease. What treatment modifications can help lessen stress and why is this important? *Class Activity **Divide the class into groups, and give each group a medical history of a patient with a type of neurological condition. Ask each group to list how it would accommodate the patient in a dental office setting. Then have the groups present their findings for class discussion and feedback.***

ELSEVIER

Torres and Ehrlich Modern Dental Assisting, 9th ed.

Bird/Robinson

OBJECTIVES	CONTENT	TEACHING RESOURCES
		Class Activity Divide the class into three groups, and have each group prepare: *– A short flyer discussing the interrelationships of cardiovascular disorders in oral health.* *– A chair-side reference that includes the antibiotic coverage for patients with a risk of endocarditis.*

29.1 Homework/Assignments:

1. Ask the students to research the ages of those on the list of older celebrities, place them in the stages of aging, and identify if the attitudes, characteristics, and needs of the celebrities match those of the typical person in their category.

2. Ask students to conduct research on the Internet or in the library on one of the signs of aging in the oral cavity, and then write a short report on ways to prevent further oral damage.

29.1 Instructor's Notes/Student Feedback:

LESSON 29.2

CRITICAL THINKING QUESTION

A dental assistant is speaking with an existing patient about her father, a new patient who does not hear well but is embarrassed about his problem. What must the dental assistant ask the daughter to assure the success of the father's initial examination? How must the dental assistant treat the patient when he arrives at the dental office, and how must the patient be scheduled?

Guidelines: The dental assistant must ask the daughter if her father wears hearing aids and if the hearing loss is related to any other condition. When the patient is in the office, the dental assistant should stand in front of him so that he can see face and lip movements clearly. Without shouting at him, the dental assistant and the rest of the dental staff must speak slowly and distinctly, keeping directions simple, and providing visual demonstrations. In addition to verbal instruction, the dental assistant will give him a written copy of all explanations. When scheduling him for his initial examination, the dental assistant must make the appointment longer to allow for his medical condition. The patient must be made to feel comfortable and not worried or embarrassed about his condition.

OBJECTIVES	CONTENT	TEACHING RESOURCES
Describe the major medical disorders that can affect a patient's oral health.	■ Specific illnesses of the medically compromised patient (p. 430) □ Pulmonary disorders (p. 433) – Allergies (p. 433) – Bronchial asthma (p. 433) – Chronic obstructive pulmonary disease (p. 435) □ Blood disorders (p. 435) □ Musculoskeletal disorders (p. 435) – Arthritis (p. 435) – Muscular dystrophy (p. 435) □ Endocrine disorders (p. 436) – Hyperthyroidism (p. 436) – Hypothyroidism (p. 436) – Diabetes mellitus (p. 436) □ Behavioral and psychiatric disorders (p. 437)	⊠ PPT 24-31 TB questions 13-15, 18 SW Short-Answer Questions 4; Fill in the Blank questions 1-2, 10, 12-14, 16-18, 20; Multiple Choice questions 12-15 (pp. 175-176) Treatment plan modifications for a patient with asthma (p. 433) Figure 29-10 Appearance of a patient with chronic obstructive pulmonary disease (COPD) (p. 435) Treatment plan modifications for a patient with COPD (p. 435) Treatment plan modifications for a patient with a blood disorder (p. 435) Treatment modifications for a patient with arthritis (p. 435) Figure 29-11 Effects of rheumatoid arthritis on the body (p. 436) Treatment modifications for a patient with muscular dystrophy (p. 436) Treatment modifications for a patient with hyperthyroidism (p. 436) Treatment plan modifications for a patient with diabetes (p. 437) Treatment plan modifications for a patient with a psychiatric disorder (p. 437) Recall questions 13-16 (pp. 435-436) CTQ 1-3 (p. 439)

ELSEVIER

Bird/Robinson

OBJECTIVES	CONTENT	TEACHING RESOURCES
		▸ Discuss what modifications you might make in the medications prescribed or used for a patient with asthma.
		▸ Discuss why patients with blood disorders may be particularly susceptible to infection. What precautions should be taken for a patient with a blood disorder and why?
		▸ Discuss what difficulties patients with arthritis and muscular dystrophy might encounter in the dental office.
		▸ Discuss what effects psychoactive drugs may have on the mouth.
		Class Activity Before the class meets ask students to research a blood disorder on the Internet and then write and bring to class a short report explaining why persons with the disorder may be particularly susceptible to infection. Have the class discuss the reports. (For students to prepare for this activity, see Homework/Assignments #1.)
		Class Activity Divide the class into three groups, and assign each group one of the discussion points below, asking them to refer to the Critical Thinking Question for Lesson 29.2. After 15 minutes, have the groups share their findings with the class.
		– *What is the physical classification system for this patient?*
		– *How will the patient be scheduled for his follow-up restorative appointments?*
		– *What modifications in the dental treatment of the patient must be made?*
		– *What dental health recommendations should be discussed with the patient and his guardians?*
		Class Activity Ask students to research newspaper articles about behavioral and psychiatric disorders that can affect oral health, and then write and bring to class a short report on their findings. Have the class discuss the reports. (For students to prepare for this activity, see Homework/Assignments #2.)
Describe the type of dental management a medically compromised patient would receive.	■ The physically compromised patient (p. 437) ☐ The wheelchair-bound patient (p. 437) ☐ The vision-impaired patient (p. 437)	▦ PPT 32 TB questions 19-20 SW Short-Answer Questions 5 (p. 175) SW Case Study questions 3-5 (p. 178) Figure 29-12 Escorting a vision-impaired patient (p. 437) Treatment modifications for hearing-impaired patients (p. 439)

ELSEVIER

Torres and Ehrlich Modern Dental Assisting, 9th ed.

Bird/Robinson

OBJECTIVES	CONTENT	TEACHING RESOURCES
	□ The hearing-impaired patient (p. 437)	CTQ 5 (p. 439) ▸ Discuss what modifications should be done for both vision-impaired and hearing-impaired patients. **Class Activity** ***Provide a medical history for a physically compromised patient whom students may encounter in the dental office. Have students prepare a chairside chart on daily oral hygiene for the patient.***
Demonstrate the correct transfer of a wheelchair-bound patient.	*Procedure* 29-1 Transferring a patient from a wheelchair (p. 438) (SW/ESLR Competency 29-1, p. 179)	TB question 20 SW Case Study questions 4-5 (p. 178) SW/ESLR Competency 29-1 Transferring a Patient from a Wheelchair (p. 179) ▸ Discuss what you should consider when making a dental office more accessible to a wheelchair-bound patient. ▸ Discuss what specific techniques you would use for transferring a patient in a wheelchair to the dental chair. **Class Activity** ***Display photographs of incorrect wheelchair transfers to the class and have the students call out what is wrong with each one.***
Describe the type of dental management a medically compromised patient would receive.	■ Assistance from organizations (p. 439)	Legal and Ethical Implications (p. 439) Eye to the Future (p. 439) ▸ Discuss the role of organizations in educating dental office staff about the special needs of compromised patients. **Class Activity** ***Have a representative from a local disability organization discuss access issues for patients with disabilities.***
Performance Evaluation		TB SW questions (pp. 175-177) SW Case Study (pp. 177-178) SW/ESLR Competency 29-1 Transferring a Patient from a Wheelchair (p. 179) ESLR Electronic Flashcards ESLR Practice Quiz Recall questions (pp. 427-439) CTQ (p. 439)

29.2 Homework/Assignments:

1. Ask students to research a blood disorder on the Internet, and then write and bring to class a short report explaining why persons with the disorder may be particularly susceptible to infection.

2. Ask students to research newspaper articles about behavioral and psychiatric disorders that can affect oral health, and then write and bring to class a short report on their findings.

29.2 Instructor's Notes/Student Feedback:

Slide 1

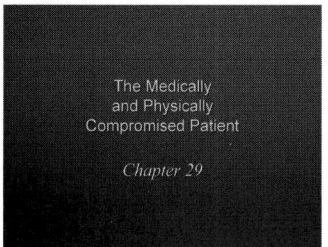

The Medically
and Physically
Compromised Patient

Chapter 29

Slide 2

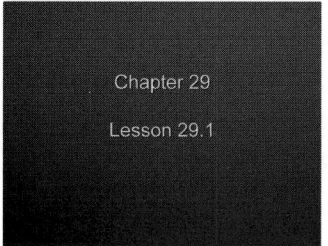

Chapter 29

Lesson 29.1

Slide 3

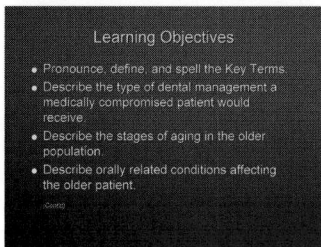

Learning Objectives

- Pronounce, define, and spell the Key Terms.
- Describe the type of dental management a medically compromised patient would receive.
- Describe the stages of aging in the older population.
- Describe orally related conditions affecting the older patient.

(Cont'd)

Slide 4

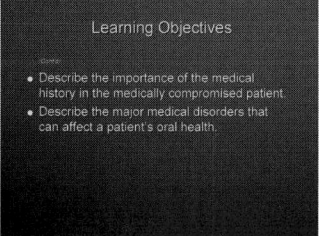

Learning Objectives

(Cont'd)

- Describe the importance of the medical history in the medically compromised patient.
- Describe the major medical disorders that can affect a patient's oral health.

Slide 5

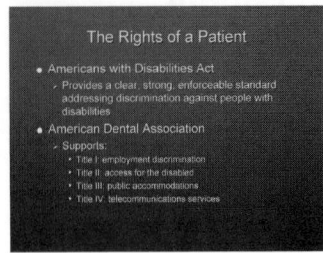

- Which law states that a dental practice, clinic, or school must provide appropriate access for disabled persons?
- Which law extends telecommunication services to hearing-impaired and speech-impaired persons?

Slide 6

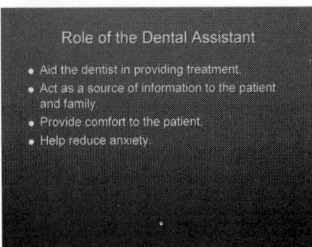

- What should a dental assistant expect with patients who have special needs? *(Patients who enter the dental practice may be very ill, in pain, or physically challenged. The dental assistant should use good judgment in helping these patients, which may mean bypassing some of the usual routines that take place during an appointment.)*

Slide 7

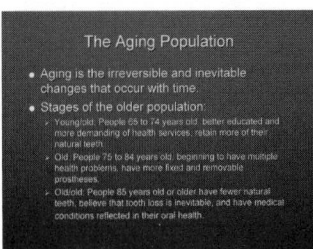

- What aging category would include a 76-year-old dental patient?
- What are the oral health conditions that affect the aging population?

Slide 8

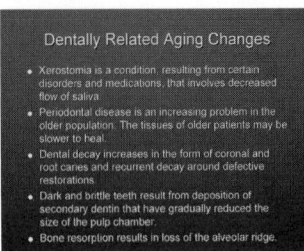

- What is xerostomia? How does it affect the oral cavity?
- What are root caries?
- Why does recurrent decay occur around defective restorations?

Torres and Ehrlich Modern Dental Assisting, 9th ed.

Bird/Robinson

Slide 9

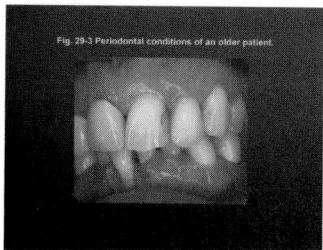

- What is the incidence of periodontal disease in older people?
- Can periodontal disease be prevented?
- In this photograph, what are the signs of periodontal disease?

Slide 10

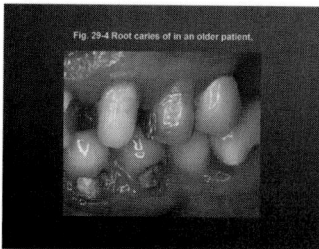

- What happens to a person's oral cavity with aging?
- Where are the root caries in this older person's mouth?
- Can root caries be restored? What type of restoration is first used in most cases of root caries?

Slide 11

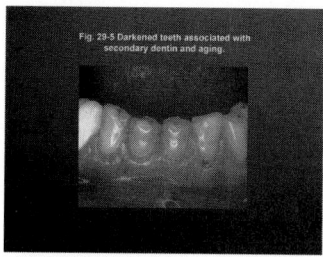

- What happens to the color of teeth as people age?
- In this picture, where are the dark teeth?
- Which teeth have been restored since they have fractured?

Slide 12

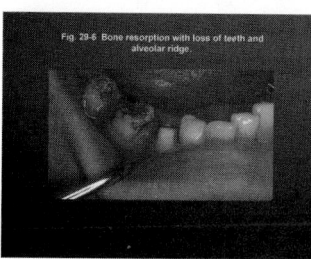

- How are tooth loss and changes in the jawbone related to age?
- Which teeth are missing in this photograph of an older person's mouth?
- What has happened to the alveolar bone that used to surround the missing teeth?

ELSEVIER

Torres and Ehrlich Modern Dental Assisting, 9th ed.

Bird/Robinson

Slide 13

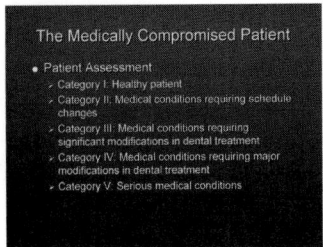

- What does it mean to be medically compromised?
- How does a medically compromised patient affect the dental office?
- Which categories of patient assessment may need a physician's consultation before dental treatment?
- What types of medical conditions may present an increased risk of emergencies in the dental office?

Slide 14

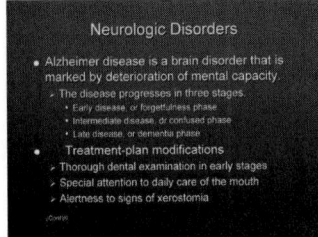

- What is dementia? Why would some patients who have dementia experience xerostomia?
- What challenges does a patient with dementia present for dental practitioners?
- In the later stages of the disease, who takes care of the patient's oral cavity?

Slide 15

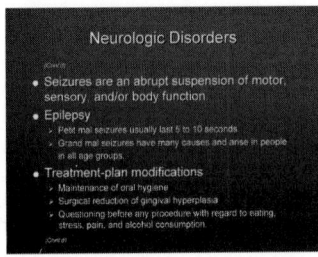

- What common side effect occurs from taking phenytoin?
- Why does a patient with a neurological disorder need to be questioned before treatment about eating, stress, pain, and alcohol consumption?

Slide 16

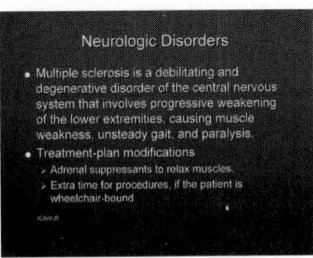

- Why would extra time be needed during a dental appointment if the patient with multiple sclerosis is in a wheelchair?
- Why is it important for dental office staff to encourage relaxed muscles in patients who have multiple sclerosis?

Slide 17

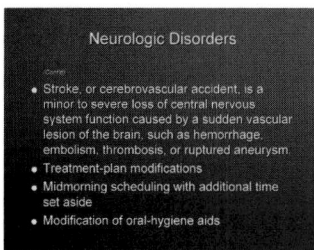

- What is another term for cerebrovascular accident?

- Why is a patient who has had a stroke scheduled for a dental visit in the morning?

- Why does this patient need modified oral hygiene aids?

Slide 18

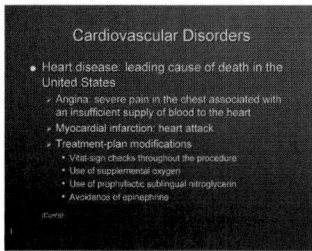

- What does it mean when the patient has a history of angina?

- How does treating a patient who has a history of angina affect dental office practices?

- What is another term for myocardial infarction?

Slide 19

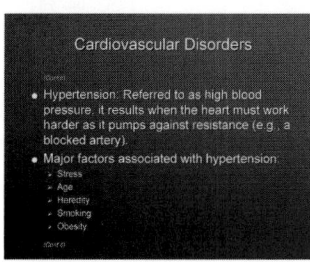

- What is another term for hypertension?

- How is high blood pressure treated?

- How can the dental office prepare for a patient who has hypertension?

Slide 20

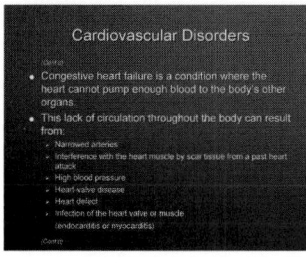

- How does high blood pressure affect the circulation of the body?

- What is endocarditis?

- What will be the appearance of a patient who has congestive heart failure?

- What precautions should the dental office take with a patient who has congestive heart failure?

Torres and Ehrlich Modern Dental Assisting, 9th ed.

Slide 21

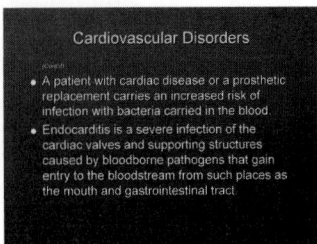

- How does the dental office reduce the risk of infection to a cardiac or joint prosthesis patient in the dental setting?
- How does the dental office prevent endocarditis in patients who are at high risk for this disorder?

Slide 22

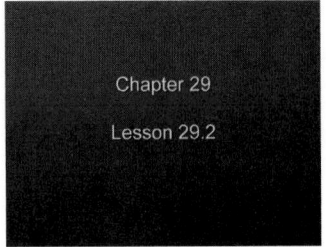

Slide 23

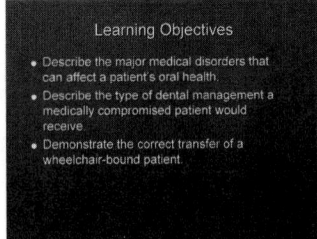

Slide 24

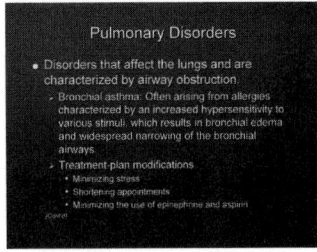

- Why should stress be minimized during the dental appointment of a patient with a pulmonary disorder?
- How is stress minimized in the dental office?
- Which organs are affected by pulmonary disorders?

Torres and Ehrlich Modern Dental Assisting, 9th ed.

Bird/Robinson

Slide 25

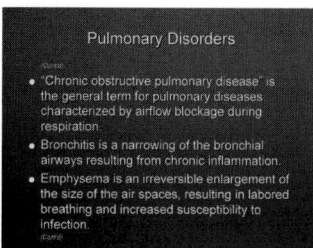

- What does the acronym COPD stand for?

- What is the appearance of a patient with COPD?

- What are the implications for dental treatment for patients who have pulmonary disorders?

Slide 26

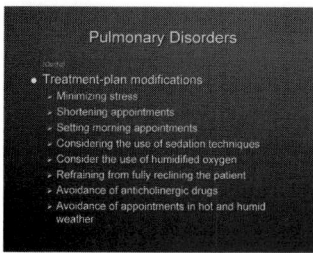

- Why should a patient with a pulmonary disorder NOT be fully reclined?

- How does hot, humid weather affect the patient who has a pulmonary disorder?

Slide 27

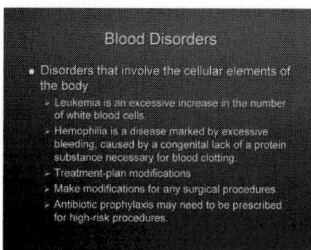

- How are bacterial infections prevented in patients who have blood disorders such as leukemia?

- Why would a bleeding disorder be a problem when a tooth is extracted and afterward during healing?

Slide 28

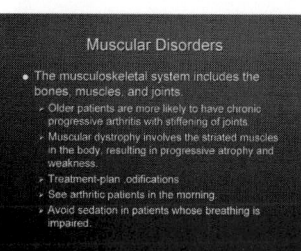

- What dental procedures may be difficult for a patient with arthritis?

- How does rheumatoid arthritis affect oral health and dental care?

- Should nitrous oxide, sedation, and general anesthesia be used on a patient with muscular dystrophy? Why or why not?

Bird/Robinson

Slide 29

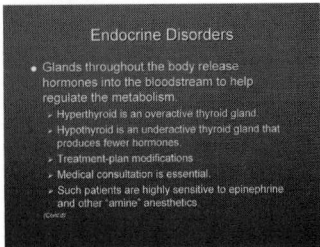

- How does hyperthyroidism affect the body?
- How does hyperthyroidism affect oral health and dental treatment?
- How does hypothyroidism affect dental treatment?

Slide 30

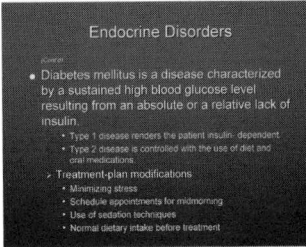

- How is a patient with type 2 diabetes classified in relation to the need for insulin?
- What are the oral manifestations of a patient with diabetes?
- What type of sedation techniques would be used on a diabetic patient to reduce stress during a dental appointment?

Slide 31

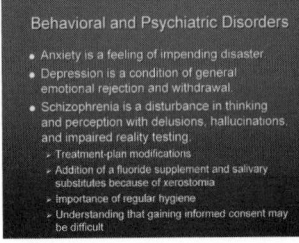

- Why do these patients have high risk of caries?
- Why is xerostomia a common occurrence in patients being treated for depression or schizophrenia?
- Why is informed consent difficult to obtain with patients who have behavioral and psychiatric disorders?

Slide 32

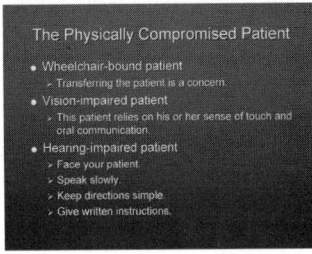

- How can the dental office accommodate wheelchair-bound patients?
- How can the dental office accommodate patients with vision impairment or hearing impairment?

Torres and Ehrlich Modern Dental Assisting, 9th ed.

Bird/Robinson

TEACHING FOCUS

This chapter will give the student an opportunity to learn the makeup of drugs, their uses, and the effects they produce. Drug names, how drugs are administered, and when a prescribed drug is used in the dental office setting are also discussed. Students will also have the opportunity to review the guidelines for dispensing prescription drugs and learn the role of the Drug Enforcement Agency in prescribing and dispensing drugs.

MATERIALS AND RESOURCES

- ☐ computer and PowerPoint projector (all Lessons)
- ☐ mock prescription pads (Lesson 30.1)
- ☐ drug reference handbook (all Lessons)

LESSON CHECKLIST

Preparations for this lesson include:

- lecture
- guest speaker: pharmacist
- evaluation of student knowledge and skills needed to perform all entry-level activities related to the principles of pharmacology, including:
  - ○ differentiating between a drug's chemical, generic, and trade name
  - ○ describing the stages a drug goes through once it enters the body
  - ○ listing the parts of a prescription and citing the factors in determining dosage
  - ○ describing various methods for administering a medication
  - ○ defining the Drug Enforcement Agency (DEA) and explaining the categories described in the Controlled Substances Act
  - ○ explaining the importance of drug reference materials
  - ○ describing the classifications of prescriptions and their effects, including possible adverse effects
  - ○ identifying when and why to use prophylaxis antibiotics

KEY TERMS

absorption (p. 443)
distribution (p. 443)
dosage (p. 443)
dose (p. 443)
drug (p. 441)
ethical drug (p. 441)
excretion (p. 443)
generic (p. 441)
inscription (p. 442)

metabolism (p. 443)
patent medicine (p. 441)
pharmacology (p. 441)
prescription (p. 441)
prophylaxis (p. 445)
signature (p. 442)
subscription (p. 442)
superscription (p. 442)
systemic (p. 443)

ADDITIONAL RESOURCES

PowerPoint slides (Evolve): 1-24

Legend

CTQ
Critical
Thinking
Question

DVD
Multimedia
Procedures
Videos and
Animations

ESLR
EVOLVE
Student
Learning
Resources

IDO
Interactive
Dental
Office
CD-ROM

SW
Student
Workbook

TB
Test Bank
on the
TEACH
CD-ROM

PPT
PowerPoint
Slides

Class Activities are indicated in ***bold italic***.

ELSEVIER

Torres and Ehrlich Modern Dental Assisting, 9th ed.

Bird/Robinson

LESSON 30.1

PRETEST

1. Which of the following is considered an over-the-counter drug?
   - a. prescription drug
   - b. ethical drug
   - c. patent drug
   - d. Schedule I drug

2. Which schedule of drugs does heroin belong to?
   - a. Schedule I
   - b. Schedule II
   - c. Schedule III
   - d. Schedule IV

3. On a written prescription, what does "p.c." stand for?
   - a. before meals
   - b. at bedtime
   - c. with water
   - d. after meals

4. Which of the following stands for taking a dose twice a day as noted on a written prescription?
   - a. qid
   - b. bid
   - c. pc
   - d. ac

5. Drugs on this schedule have clearly accepted medical usefulness and the lowest potential for abuse.
   - a. Schedule II
   - b. Schedule III
   - c. Schedule IV
   - d. Schedule V

6. Where is the prescription pad kept in the dental office when it is not in use?
   - a. by the telephone
   - b. on the operatory counter
   - c. on the dentist's desk
   - d. in a locked drawer

7. What type of drug slows blood clotting?
   - a. diuretics
   - b. anticoagulants
   - c. decongestants
   - d. bronchodilators

8. If a patient is allergic to penicillin, which drug is used for antibiotic prophylaxis?
   - a. amoxicillin
   - b. tetracycline
   - c. ampicillin
   - d. clindamycin

9. Which route of medication administration involves placing medications under the tongue?
   - a. sublingual
   - b. inhalation
   - c. transdermal
   - d. oral

10. Which drug can be ordered only with a written prescription?
   - a. bronchodilators
   - b. antibiotics
   - c. narcotics
   - d. antidepressants

Answers

1. c	3. d	5. d	7. b	9. a
2. a	4. b	6. d	8. d	10. c

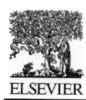
ELSEVIER

Torres and Ehrlich Modern Dental Assisting, 9th ed.

Bird/Robinson

BACKGROUND ASSESSMENT

Question: How is a drug identified? What are the two ways drugs are classified according to how they are dispensed?

Answer: Three names can be used to identify a drug. These names include (1) the drug's chemical name, which is the chemical formula of a drug; (2) the drug's generic name, which may be used by any company; and (3) the drug's brand name, or trade name, which is a registered trademark exclusively controlled by a company. Two categories are used for classifying drugs according to the way they are dispensed to patients: patent medicines and prescription drugs. Patent medicines are drugs that are obtainable without a prescription. These drugs are also referred to as over-the-counter (OTC) drugs. Prescription drugs, also called ethical drugs, can be supplied to patients only by a pharmacist who has been given a prescription from a physician or dentist.

Question: What is the main reason for dentists to prescribe antibiotic premedication before dental treatment? What type of patient medical history requires prescription of antibiotic prophylaxis before dental treatment? What are the three kinds of antibiotics usually prescribed for antibiotic prophylaxis?

Answer: The dentist uses antibiotic premedication mainly for the prevention of infective endocarditis, a rare heart infection for patients who may be at risk. Patient conditions that may warrant prophylactic antibiotics are the presence of a prosthetic heart valve, surgically constructed systemic-pulmonary shunts, organic heart murmur, and mitral valve prolapse with valvular regurgitation. The American Heart Association recommends the following three types of antibiotics for antibiotic prophylaxis: amoxicillin/penicillin, ampicillin, and clindamycin.

CRITICAL THINKING QUESTION

A patient calls the dental office asking that his usual premedication for dental anxiety be called into the pharmacy before his appointment for the following day. He is anxious to get the medicine as soon as possible and recounts how he almost got up out of the dental chair at his last visit, even with the medication. How should the dental assistant taking the phone call respond to this patient's request?

Guidelines: The dental assistant should let the patient know that he or she understands his concerns and should take the time to assure the patient that the dentist will be informed of the need for his anxiety medication. The dental assistant should continue to explain that only the dentist can contact the pharmacy with prescription information and that it is illegal for a dental assistant to "call in" a prescription. The dental assistant can call the pharmacy for the dentist and transfer the call to the dentist when the pharmacist comes to the phone, but the dental assistant should not try to relay information between them.

OBJECTIVES	CONTENT	TEACHING RESOURCES
Prounounce, define, and spell the Key Terms.	■ Key terms (p. 4440)	SW Fill in the Blank questions 1-15 (p. 182) ESLR Electronic Flashcards ▸ Discuss each of the key terms in Chapter 30, focusing on the definition, pronunciation, and spelling of each term. *Class Activity Divide the class into two teams. Provide key pharmacology terms, one term at a time. Have the students from either team call out the definition for the term. Keep score for correct definitions provided. At the end of the game, the group with the highest score is declared the winning team.*
Differentiate between a drug's chemical, generic, and brand or trade name.	■ Introduction (p. 441) ■ Overview of drugs (p. 441)	PPT 4-5 TB question 1 SW Short-Answer Questions 1; Fill in the Blank questions 6, 11, 15; Multiple Choice questions 1-2 (pp. 181-182)

ELSEVIER

OBJECTIVES	CONTENT	TEACHING RESOURCES
		Recall questions 1-2 (p. 441)
		Eye to the Future (p. 449)
		▸ Discuss the three names that identify a drug, giving an example of each.
		▸ Discuss the difference between an organic and inorganic drug.
		Class Activity Divide the class into small groups. Using a drug handbook, have the student groups locate 20 drugs and list their chemical, generic, and brand names and present their findings to the class.
Define the DEA and explain why drugs are categorized in five schedules of the Controlled Substances Act.	■ Dispensing of drugs (p. 441) □ Prescriptions (p. 441)	PPT 6-7 TB questions 3-4, 8 SW Short-Answer Questions 5; Fill in the Blank question 10; Multiple Choice question 5 (pp. 181-182) Recall questions 3-4 (p. 442) Legal and Ethical Implications (p. 449) ▸ Discuss the role of the Drug Enforcement Agency and who is authorized to write prescriptions. *Class Activity Invite a pharmacist to visit the classroom to discuss the ways that people try to pass off forged prescriptions and the methods used to spot them.*
List each part of a presciption.	– Prescription terminology (p. 441) – Recording prescriptions (p. 442) – Telephone guidelines (p. 442)	PPT 7-9 TB questions 5-7, 19 SW Short-Answer Questions 3; Fill in the Blank question 3; Multiple Choice question 6 (pp. 181-182) Table 30-1 Common Prescription Abbreviations (p. 442) Figure 30-1 Example of a prescription pad (p. 442) Recall questions 5-6 (p. 442) CTQ 2-3 (p. 449) ▸ Discuss the four parts of a prescription and explain the meaning behind the abbreviations (see Box 30-1 on p. 456). ▸ Discuss the guidelines a dental assistant needs to follow when interacting with a pharmacy on the telephone. Include discussion of what should be done if the pharmacist questions a patient's possible reaction to a drug. *Class Activity Divide the class into small groups. Using mock prescription pads, give the students verbal prescriptions and have them write out the prescriptions using the correct method of abbreviation. Ask the groups to exchange their written prescriptions with another group to check for completeness, accuracy, and clarity.*

OBJECTIVES	CONTENT	TEACHING RESOURCES
Describe the use of drug reference materials.	■ Drug reference materials (p. 443) ☐ Package inserts (p. 443)	PPT 10 TB question 9 SW Short-Answer Questions 7 (p. 181) Box 30-1 Information Included on a Package Insert (p. 443) CTQ 1 (p. 449) ▸ Discuss the drug reference material available to dentists and the importance of having more than just one reference on hand. Include discussion about how to ensure that the dental office has the most up-to-date information. ▸ Discuss what information may be found on a package insert. *Class Activity **Have each student investigate a commonly used drug in dentistry using a drug reference such as the PDR® or Internet resources. After the research is completed, ask for several volunteers to share findings with the class. (For students to prepare for this activity, see Homework/Assignments #1.)***

30.1 Homework/Assignments:

1. Have each student investigate a commonly used drug in dentistry using a drug reference such as the *PDR®,* Internet, online copy of the package insert, or the Web site of the company that sells the brand name of the drug.

30.1 Instructor's Notes/Student Feedback:

Bird/Robinson

LESSON 30.2

CRITICAL THINKING QUESTION

A new patient forgot to mention on the telephone that she has mitral valve prolapse with valvular regurgitation, even when she was asked by the dental office receptionist if she had any medical alerts to report. All she could remember to say at the time was that she had no allergies. The patient is now sitting in the operatory, ready for her initial appointment to have her severely bleeding gums looked at. How should the dental assistant handle this situation? Why does this patient warrant a change in dental treatment? What drug will need to be given to the patient?

Guidelines: The dental assistant should calmly explain to the patient that most of her initial appointment procedures will need to be rescheduled because of her risk for developing infective endocarditis due to her mitral valve prolapse with valvular regurgitation. The dental assistant should continue to explain that infective endocarditis is a rare heart infection that can occur when bacteria enter the bloodstream during an invasive dental procedure; this could possibly infect a patient's damaged heart. This makes antibiotic premedication necessary for the patient's safety. Before the patient leaves, she should also be given patient educational materials on personal oral hygiene methods to help reduce the bacteria that are entering her bloodstream from her periodontal disease. Finally, the patient will need a prescription from the dentist for amoxicillin (because she has no known drug allergies), which is to be taken one hour before her next dental appointment as an antibiotic prophylaxis. This will reduce her risk of infective endocarditis from dental treatment.

OBJECTIVES	CONTENT	TEACHING RESOURCES
Cite the factors in determining the dosage of a drug.	■ Drug dosage (p. 443)	PPT 13 TB question 10 SW Short-Answer Questions 9; Fill in the Blank question 4 (pp. 181-182) ▸ Discuss what factors must be considered when determining drug dosage. ▸ Discuss the different forms a drug can take, providing an example of each form. ***Class Activity** Have students choose any one of the factors that influence drug dosage. Have them research information on the factor and write one short paragraph about it. Have the students bring their paragraphs back to class for discussion. (For students to prepare for this activity, see Homework/Assignments #1.)*
Describe how medications are administered.	☐ Administration of medications (p. 443)	PPT 14-16 SW Short-Answer Questions 4; Fill in the Blank questions 1-2, 5, 7-9, 12, 14; Multiple Choice questions 7-8 (pp. 181-183) Eye to the Future (p. 449) ▸ Discuss the different routes in which a drug can be applied or administered, and identify the slowest route of absorption. ▸ Discuss the difference between a sublingual and subcutaneous drug and where they are administered.

OBJECTIVES	CONTENT	TEACHING RESOURCES
		Class Activity Divide the class into small groups. Have the students use a drug handbook to investigate drugs commonly prescribed in the dental office, focusing on how the drugs are administered. Challenge each group to find more than one drug for each route of administration discussed. Ask each group to share its findings with the class.
Describe the stages a drug goes through in the body.	☐ Administration of medications (p. 443)	☒▣ PPT 17 📖 SW Short-Answer Questions 2; Multiple Choice question 3 (pp. 181-182) Table 30-2 Stages of Drug Action in the Body (p. 442) Figure 30-2 Routes of drug administration (p. 444) Recall questions 7-9 (p. 443) ▸ Discuss Table 30-2 (p. 442) and what happens once the drug has entered the bloodstream. ▸ Discuss the various ways a drug leaves the body. *Class Activity Have the students use a drug handbook to investigate five commonly prescribed drugs in the dental office, focusing on the stages of drug action in the body. Direct the students to write brief reports describing the differing stages for each drug, as noted by the reference. Ask for volunteers to share their reports with the class for discussion.*
List the commonly prescribed drugs in dentistry.	■ Drugs commonly prescribed in dentistry (p. 443) ☐ Analgesics (p. 445) ☐ Antibiotics (p. 445) – Antibiotic prophylaxis (p. 445) ☐ Antifungal agents (p. 445) ☐ Antiviral agents (p. 445) ☐ Antianxiety agents (p. 446)	☒▣ PPT 19-22 ▣ TB questions 16-17 📖 SW Short-Answer Questions 9; Multiple Choice questions 11-12 (pp. 181, 183) 📖 SW Case Study questions 1-6 (p. 183) Table 30-3 American Heart Association Antibiotic Recommendations for a Dental Procedure (p. 446) Cardiac Conditions Associated with the Highest Risk of Adverse Outcomes from Endocarditis for which Prophylaxis with Dental Procedures is Recommended (p. 446 Recall questions 10-11 (p. 446) ▸ Discuss when it might be appropriate to use prophylaxis antibiotics. Name the three most common recommended by the American Heart Association. *Class Activity Divide the class into two teams. Have the students on one team write down "answers" related to the various types of prescription drugs, body system*

OBJECTIVES	CONTENT	TEACHING RESOURCES
		affected, drug actions, examples, and primary uses, and have the other team guess the "questions." After a reasonable time interval, have the teams switch roles and play another round.
List the commonly prescribed drugs in medicine.	■ Drugs commonly prescribed in medicine (p. 447) □ Cardiovascular drugs (p. 447) □ Respiratory drugs (p. 447) □ Gastrointestinal drugs (p. 447) □ Neurologic drugs (p. 447) □ Psychoactive drugs (p. 447) □ Endocrine/hormonal drugs (p. 448)	SW Fill in the Blank 13; Multiple Choice questions 13-14 (pp. 182-183) Recall questions 12-13 (p. 448)
Define the DEA and explain why drugs are categorized in five schedules of the Controlled Substances Act.	■ Controlled Substances Act (p. 448) □ Schedule I drugs (p. 448) □ Schedule II drugs (p. 448) □ Schedule III drugs (p. 448) □ Schedule IV drugs (p. 448) □ Schedule V drugs (p. 448)	PPT 18 TB questions 13-15 SW Short-Answer Questions 5, 8; Multiple Choice questions 4, 9 (pp. 169-170) Recall question 14 (p. 448) ▶ Discuss the five categories of schedule drug classification, including the factors that determine which category a drug would fit into. *Class Activity Have each student prepare a chart that states the schedule category, its explanation, and examples of each category, as stated in the textbook.*
Describe the effects of drug use.	■ Adverse drug effects (p. 448) □ Drug complications (p. 448)	PPT 23-24 TB question 18 SW Short-Answer Questions 6 (pp. 181) Common adverse effects of medications (p. 449) Recall question 15 (p. 448) Patient Education (p. 449) ▶ Discuss the different types of adverse effects a drug can have on the body and what precautions a dentist or dental assistant can take to avoid adverse reactions.

ELSEVIER

Torres and Ehrlich Modern Dental Assisting, 9th ed.

Bird/Robinson

OBJECTIVES	CONTENT	TEACHING RESOURCES
Performance Evaluation		TB TB SW questions (pp. 181-183) SW Case Study (p. 183) ESLR Electronic Flashcards ESLR Practice Quiz Recall questions (pp. 442-448) CTQ (p. 449)

30.2 Homework/Assignments:

1. Have students choose any one of the factors that influence drug dosage. Have each of them research information on the factor and write one short paragraph about their findings. Have the students bring their paragraphs back to class for discussion.

30.2 Instructor's Notes/Student Feedback:

Torres and Ehrlich Modern Dental Assisting, 9th ed.

Bird/Robinson

Slide 1

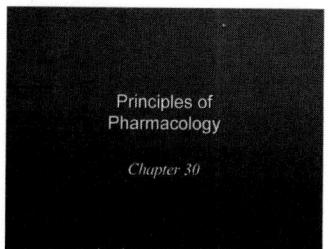

Principles of
Pharmacology

Chapter 30

Slide 2

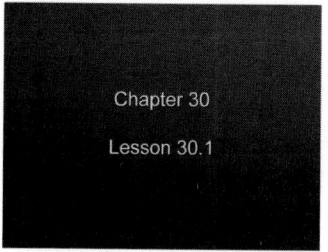

Chapter 30

Lesson 30.1

Slide 3

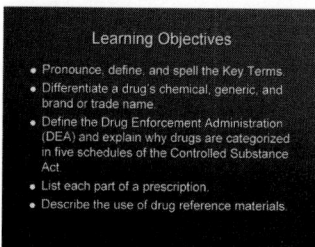

Learning Objectives

- Pronounce, define, and spell the Key Terms.
- Differentiate a drug's chemical, generic, and brand or trade name.
- Define the Drug Enforcement Administration (DEA) and explain why drugs are categorized in five schedules of the Controlled Substance Act
- List each part of a prescription.
- Describe the use of drug reference materials.

Slide 4

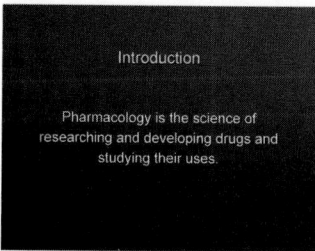

Introduction

Pharmacology is the science of researching and developing drugs and studying their uses.

Torres and Ehrlich Modern Dental Assisting, 9th ed.

Bird/Robinson

Slide 5

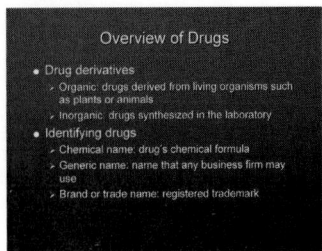

- Where do most drugs come from today?
- What is the chemical name for aspirin? *(Acetylsalicylic acid.)*
- What is the generic name for aspirin? *(Aspirin.)*
- What are some brand names for aspirin? *(Bayer, St. Joseph's.)*

Slide 6

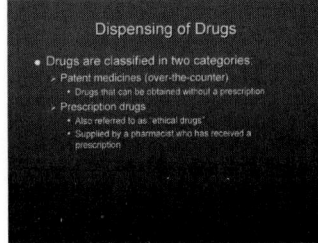

- Who is allowed to write prescriptions in the dental office?
- Give an example of an OTC and a prescription drug to treat the same illness (such as sore throat, allergy, pain).
- Why is the term "ethical" used for drugs that need a prescription?

Slide 7

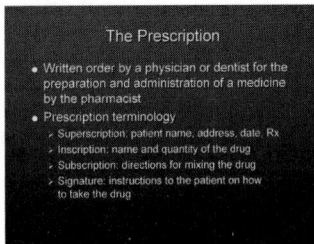

- What part of the prescription includes the name and quantity of the drug?
- What part of the prescription includes the instructions for the patient about how to take the drug?
- What part of the prescription includes the directions for mixing the drug?

Slide 8

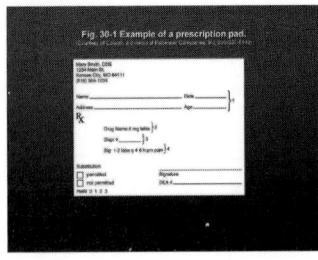

- Can a dental assistant prescribe medication to a patient?
- What is the role of the dental assistant regarding prescriptions?
- What does it mean to dispense "50"?
- What does "prn" mean for the patient as it relates to pain?

Bird/Robinson

Slide 9

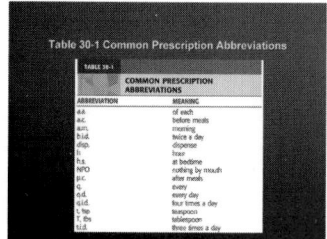

- What does the abbreviation bid stand for? How does that compare with tid or qid?
- How is documentation of a drug prescription done in the dental office?

Slide 10

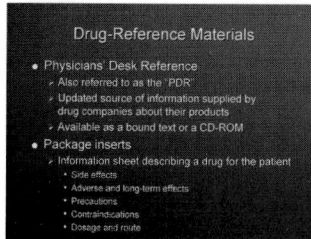

- Have you ever looked through the *PDR*?
- Do you look at the package insert before using a drug?

Slide 11

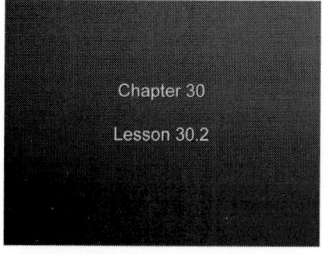

Slide 12

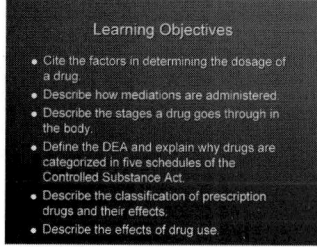

Slide 13

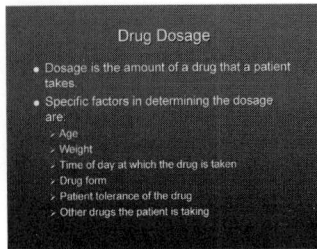

- What are the guidelines with respect to the telephone interaction of a dental assistant with a pharmacy?
- What should a dental assistant do when a pharmacist calls?

Slide 14

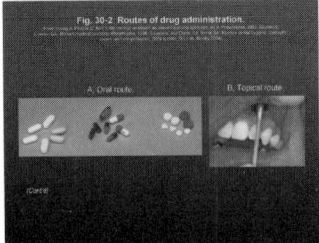

- What are three of the five ways that drugs are administered?
  - *Oral route in the form of pills, tablets, capsules, or liquids*
  - *Topical route by applying on the surface of the mucosa or skin*
  - *Transdermal route through a patch that continuously releases a controlled quantity of a medication through the skin*

Slide 15

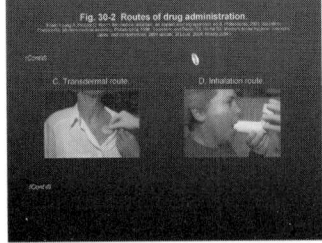

Slide 16

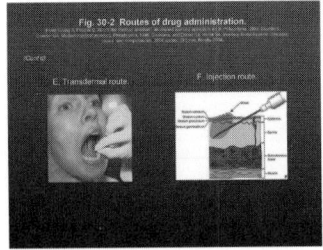

Slide 17

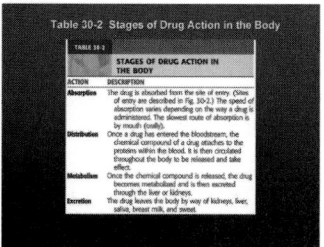

Slide 18

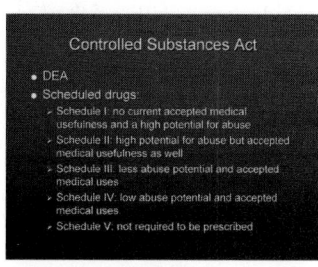

- What is a DEA identification number?
- Give examples of a Schedule I drug.
- Give examples of a Schedule II drug.
- Give examples of a Schedule IV drug.

Slide 19

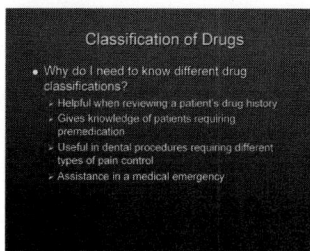

- What can the dental assistant do if patients do not know what drugs they are taking?
- What type of drug slows the clotting of blood?
- Why would a dentist prescribe an antibiotic?
- How would an antianxiety drug be used in a dental setting?

Slide 20

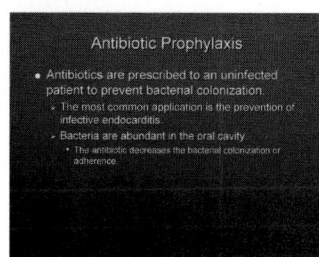

- What is infective endocarditis and who is at risk for it?
- What bacteria are mainly involved in infective endocarditis?
- How can the dental office prevent endocarditis in patients who are at risk?

Slide 21

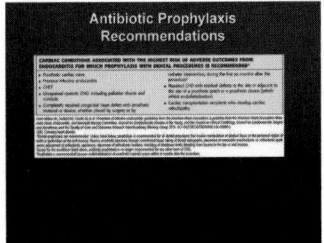

Slide 22

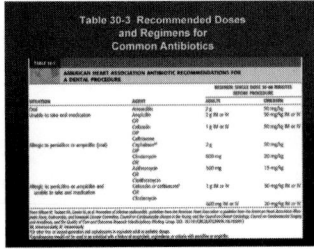

- What are the three drugs used for antibiotic prophylaxis?

- Why do patients need to take another drug besides amoxicillin if they are allergic to penicillin as an antibiotic premedication?

Slide 23

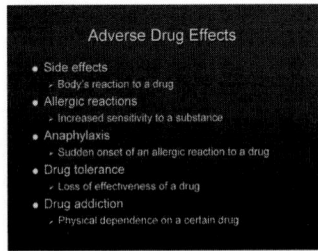

- What does it mean for a drug to have adverse effects?

- What is the drug that most commonly causes an anaphylaxic reaction? *(Penicillin.)*

Slide 24

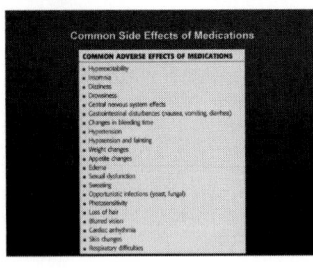

- How can these side effects alter dental treatment? Can they increase the risk of an emergency situation?

- Should a dental assistant evaluate a patient's reaction to a drug?

31 Assisting in a Medical Emergency

TEACHING FOCUS

This chapter will give students the opportunity to learn about assisting in medical emergencies that may occur in a dental office. Furthermore, students will have the opportunity to learn preventive measures to avoid medical emergencies, common signs and symptoms of medical emergencies, what equipment is needed to respond to medical emergencies, and how to respond to specific emergencies.

MATERIALS AND RESOURCES

- ☐ computer and PowerPoint projector (all Lessons)
- ☐ mannequins (Lesson 31.1)

LESSON CHECKLIST

Preparations for this lesson include:

- lecture
- guest speakers: general dentist, certified CPR trainer, oral surgeon, and emergency medical technician (EMT)
- evaluation of student knowledge and skills needed to understand how to assist in medical emergencies that may occur in a dentist office, including:
  - common signs and symptoms of medical emergencies
  - equipment needed to respond to a medical emergency
  - preventing a medical emergency
  - responses to specific emergencies

Bird/Robinson

KEY TERMS

acute (p. 463)
allergen (p. 465)
allergy (p. 465)
anaphylaxis (p. 465)
angina (p. 462)
antibodies (p. 465)
antigen (p. 465)
aspiration (p. 455)
asthma (p. 464)
cardiopulmonary resuscitation (CPR) (p. 454)
convulsion (p. 465)

epilepsy (p. 465)
erythema (p. 465)
gait (p. 453)
hyperglycemia (p. 468)
hypersensitivity (p. 465)
hyperventilation (p. 463)
hypoglycemia (p. 468)
hypotension (p. 462)
myocardial infarction (p. 463)
syncope (p. 462)
ventricular fibrillation (VF) (p. 455)

ADDITIONAL RESOURCES

PowerPoint slides (Evolve): 1-34
The Interactive Dental Office CD-ROM:
   Wendy Ledbetter
Multimedia Procedures DVD: 7 animations

Legend

CTQ
Critical
Thinking
Question

DVD
Multimedia
Procedures
Videos and
Animations

ESLR
EVOLVE
Student
Learning
Resources

IDO
Interactive
Dental
Office
CD-ROM

SW
Student
Workbook

TB
Test Bank
on the
TEACH
CD-ROM

PPT
PowerPoint
Slides

Class Activities are indicated in ***bold italic.***

ELSEVIER

Torres and Ehrlich Modern Dental Assisting, 9th ed.

Bird/Robinson

LESSON 31.1

PRETEST

1. What color coding is used for oxygen supplies in the dental office?
   a. red
   b. blue
   c. green
   d. yellow

2. What is the medical term used for fainting?
   a. postural hypotension
   b. hyperventilation
   c. syncope
   d. myocardial infarction

3. What is another term used for a cerebrovascular accident?
   a. stroke
   b. heart attack
   c. bruise
   d. coma

4. Which of the following statements is a sign of a patient's present condition during an emergency?
   a. "I feel dizzy."
   b. "I'm having trouble breathing."
   c. "My arm hurts."
   d. "My blood pressure is elevated."

5. What do most sudden cardiac arrest victims experience?
   a. severe coughing
   b. sudden syncope
   c. chronic coma
   d. ventricular fibrillation

6. Which of the following dental patient situations could lead to postural hypotension?
   a. pregnancy
   b. overweight
   c. allergies
   d. choking

7. Nitroglycerine is usually given in a dental setting for dealing with a(n)
   a. aura before an epileptic seizure.
   b. diabetic insulin overdose.
   c. angina attack.
   d. syncope condition.

8. Glucose is usually given to a patient in an emergency situation in a dental setting for dealing with a(n)
   a. aura before an epileptic seizure.
   b. diabetic insulin overdose.
   c. angina attack.
   d. syncope condition.

9. What does the tilt-lift method refer to in regards to CPR?
   a. tilting the chest forward and lifting the legs
   b. tilting the head back and lifting the chin
   c. tilting the chair back and lifting the armrests
   d. tilting the legs up and lifting the head to the chest

10. Which of the following emergency situations can be immediately life threatening in a dental setting?
    a. syncope
    b. hyperventilation
    c. anaphylaxis
    d. petit mal seizures

Answers

1. c	3. a	5. d	7. c	9. b
2. c	4. d	6. a	8. b	10. c

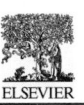

BACKGROUND ASSESSMENT

Question: What is syncope? How is an emergency situation such as syncope prevented in the case of a pregnant dental patient?

Answer: Syncope, commonly referred to as fainting, is one of the most frequent medical emergencies in the dental office. Syncope is caused by an imbalance in the blood distribution to the brain and the larger vessels within the body. This reduced blood flow to the brain causes the patient to lose consciousness. While in a supine position, the pregnant dental patient may feel dizzy or lightheaded and may faint (syncope). This reaction results from the pressure of the enlarged uterus on the abdominal veins. To prevent syncope, the pregnant patient should be turned onto her left side or moved into an upright sitting position. This change of position of the pregnant patient relieves the pressure on the involved blood vessels.

Question: What is diabetes mellitus and what are the signs and symptoms of this condition? What can possibly happen to a diabetic dental patient if he or she has eaten too many sugary foods? What serious complications can occur if this condition is not promptly treated?

Answer: Diabetes mellitus is a metabolic disorder resulting from disturbances in the body's normal insulin mechanism. An abnormal increase in the glucose (sugar) level in the blood can result in hyperglycemia, such as from eating too many sugary foods. The signs and symptoms of hyperglycemia include excessive urination, excessive thirst, dry mouth and skin, acetone breath (fruity smell), blurred vision and headache, rapid pulse, lower blood pressure, and possible loss of consciousness. If untreated, hyperglycemia may progress to diabetic ketoacidosis and a life-threatening diabetic coma.

CRITICAL THINKING QUESTION

During the placing of restoration on a young girl by the dentist, the patient jumps out of the dental chair and runs toward the reception area. The patient starts to grasp at her neck, making a high-pitched sound, with her face becoming bluish. What is happening to the patient and what needs to be done immediately? How can the dental office prevent this from happening again to this patient?

Guidelines: The child patient has made the universal sign for choking by grasping at her throat. She must have aspirated part of the restorative materials or devices when she got up out of the dental chair and now is choking on it. The office will need to begin its emergency protocol and perform the Heimlich maneuver on her until the aspirated object is expelled. At the same time, another staff member should place a call to emergency assistance. At the patient's future dental appointments, the dental office should reinforce the use of high-velocity suction, use of dental dam during routine treatment, and placement of a throat pack (gauze placed at base of throat) to prevent airway obstruction.

OBJECTIVES	CONTENT	TEACHING RESOURCES
Pronounce, define, and spell the Key Terms.	■ Key terms (pp. 450-451)	⊠ PPT 6 🅔 ESLR Electronic Flashcards ▸ Discuss each of the key terms, focusing on the definition, pronunciation, and spelling of each term. *Class Activity Have the students make flash cards of the key terms by writing the terms on one side of an index card and the definitions on the other. Have the students quiz each other with the flash cards.*
Describe the preventive measures taken for a medical emergency.	■ Introduction (p. 451) ■ Preventing a medical emergency (p. 451)	⊠ PPT 7 🖥 TB question 1 SW Short-Answer Questions 1; Fill in the Blank question 9; Multiple Choice questions 1-2 (pp. 185-186)

Bird/Robinson

OBJECTIVES	CONTENT	TEACHING RESOURCES
		Recall questions 1-2 (p. 452)
		Patient Education (p. 468)
		▸ Discuss the importance of maintaining updated patient records to prevent emergencies.
		▸ Discuss how a patient's stress can be reduced in the dental office.
		Class Activity In small groups, have students prepare a checklist to be used in a dental office setting to prepare for emergencies. The checklist should include the different roles that can be assigned to the various members of the dental team. Then have the groups share their lists with the class.
List the appropriate qualifications that a dental assistant must have for emergency preparedness.	■ Emergency preparedness (p. 452) ☐ Assigned roles (p. 452) ☐ Routine drills (p. 452) ☐ Emergency telephone numbers (p. 453)	PPT 8-10 TB questions 2-4 SW Short-Answer Questions 2; Multiple Choice questions 3-5 (pp. 185-186) Figure 31-1 It is important to have open communication with emergency personnel (p. 452) Figure 31-2 Preparing oxygen for an emergency (p. 452) Figure 31-3 The dental assistant has repositioned the patient (p. 452) Figure 31-4 Poster showing 911 (p. 453) Figure 31-5 EMS personnel on the scene (p. 453) Recall questions 3-5 (p. 453) Legal and Ethical Implications (p. 468) ▸ Discuss the concept of working as a team in dealing with a medical emergency in the dental office. ▸ Discuss how a medical emergency drill can be created and used to keep the dental staff prepared for an emergency. *Class Activity Invite an oral surgeon and a general dentist to speak to the class about emergencies that have occurred in their dental offices and the role that the dental assistant played during each emergency. Have the speakers discuss qualifications that dental assistants must have in emergency situations.*
Describe the common signs and symptoms of an emergency and how to recognize them.	■ Recognizing a medical emergency (p. 453) ☐ Signs and symptoms (p. 453) ■ Emergency care standards (p. 453)	PPT 11-13 TB questions 5-10 SW Short-Answer Questions 5; Fill in the Blank questions 3, 13; Multiple Choice questions 6-8, 20 (pp. 185-187)

OBJECTIVES	CONTENT	TEACHING RESOURCES
	☐ ABCDs of life support (p. 453) ☐ Cardiopulmonary resuscitation (p. 454) ☐ Choking (p. 455)	Recall questions 6-8 (p. 455) ▸ Discuss symptoms that would alert a dental assistant to a medical emergency. ▸ Discuss how a patient might choke in a medical office and what can be done to reduce the likelihood of choking. *Class Activity As a class, have students identify and discuss signs and symptoms that indicate a patient requires immediate emergency care. Write these symptoms on the board, and discuss the likely causes of and medical responses to each symptom.*
Accurately perform CPR on a simulated mannequin.	☐ Cardiopulmonary resuscitation (p. 454) Emergency Procedure 31-1 Performing cardiopulmonary resuscitation (pp. 454-455) (SW/ESLR Competency 31-1, pp. 189-190) ☐ Choking (p. 455)	PPT 13-16 SW/ESLR Competency 31-1 Performing Cardiopulmonary Resuscitation (pp. 189-190) ▸ Discuss the negative effects of CPR on the patient. *Class Activity In small groups, have students practice performing CPR on a mannequin. Correct the students' techniques as necessary. Next, have students perform CPR on a mannequin in front of a certified CPR trainer for possible certification.*
Accurately perform the Heimlich maneuver on a mannequin.	☐ Cardiopulmonary resuscitation (p. 454) ☐ Choking (p. 455) Emergency Procedure 31-2 Responding to a patient with an obstructed airway (p. 456) (SW/ESLR Competency 31-2, p. 191)	SW/ESLR Competency 31-2 Responding to a Patient with an Obstructed Airway (p. 191) ▸ Discuss how to properly perform the Heimlich maneuver to reduce patient injury during the procedure. *Class Activity In small groups, have students practice performing the Heimlich maneuver on a mannequin. Correct the students' techniques as necessary.*
Discuss the use of a defibrillator in an emergency.	☐ Automated external defibrillator (p. 455)	PPT 18-19 TB questions 12-13 SW Short-Answer Questions 4; Multiple Choice questions 10-11 (pp. 185, 187) Recall questions 9-10 (p. 457) ▸ Discuss other places automated external defibrillators might be used besides a medical office. ▸ Discuss how improperly using the automated external defibrillator might injure a patient or medical staff. *Class Activity Invite an emergency medical technician (EMT) to speak to the class abouthis or her experience swith emergency situations in which a defibrillator was .*

OBJECTIVES	CONTENT	TEACHING RESOURCES
Demonstrate use of the automated external defibrillator.	*Emergency Procedure* 31-3 Operating the automated external defibrillator (p. 458) (SW/ESLR Competency 31-3, p. 193)	PPT 18-19 SW/ESLR Competency 31-3 Operating an Automated External Defibrillator (p. 193) ▸ Discuss the importance of properly maintaining an automated external defibrillator. *Class Activity Ask the EMT from the previous Class Activity to demonstrate the proper use of an inactive defibrillator on a mannequin.*
List the basic items that must be included in an emergency kit.	■ Emergency equipment and supplies (p. 457) ☐ Oxygen (p. 457)	PPT 17, 18-19 TB question 11 SW Short-Answer Questions 3; Multiple Choice question 9 (pp. 185, 187) Figure 31-6 Standardized color-coded basic emergency kit (p. 457) Table 31-1 Drugs Used in Medical Emergencies (p. 457) Figure 31-7 Different sizes of oxygen cylinders (p. 462) Recall question 11 (p. 459) ▸ Discuss what drugs might be used most often in dealing with medical emergencies in a dental office. ▸ Discuss the importance of properly securing oxygen tanks in the dental office. *Class Activity Have students call out the basic items that must be included in an emergency kit in a dental office, and write them on the board. Next, have students identify other items that might be included in an emergency kit. Finally, discuss how each listed item is used.*
Demonstrate preparation and placement of oxygen.	*Emergency Procedure* 31-4 Preparing the oxygen system (pp. 460-461) (SW/ESLR Competency 31-4, p. 195)	SW/ESLR Competency 31-4 Preparing the Oxygen System (p. 195) ▸ Discuss the importance of properly preparing the oxygen system in a dental office. *Class Activity Using an empty oxygen canister, have small groups of students practice preparing the oxygen supply and placing the oxygen mask on other students in the group. Correct the students' techniques as necessary.*

ELSEVIER

31.1 Homework/Assignments:

31.1 Instructor's Notes/Student Feedback:

LESSON 31.2

CRITICAL THINKING QUESTION

The first patient on a Saturday afternoon is a mother of five children. Her medical history states that she is a diabetic patient on insulin therapy. She says that she has been driving her children to all their sports functions all morning and didn't eat lunch. But she has taken her insulin on time. Suddenly, she appears agitated. She is also sweating profusely. What is happening to the patient, and what needs to be done?

Guidelines: The patient is experiencing hypoglycemia. The signs and symptoms of hypoglycemia include mood changes, hunger, perspiration, increased anxiety, and possible unconsciousness. Hypoglycemia results from an abnormal decrease in the glucose (sugar) level in the blood. The most common causes of hypoglycemia are skipping a meal, taking too much insulin without adequate food intake, and exercising excessively without an appropriate adjustment of insulin and food intake. In this case, the patient has taken her insulin but has not eaten. The dental assistant does not have much time to act because this condition can manifest itself rapidly. The immediate response is to begin the dental office's emergency protocol, which includes a call for emergency assistance and informing the dentist. The patient should then be given a concentrated form of carbohydrate if she remains conscious, such as a sugar packet, cake icing, or concentrated orange juice so that the glucose (sugar) will be absorbed rapidly into her bloodstream. The dental assistant should prepare the emergency kit and oxygen for possible use by the dentist, help monitor and record the patient's vital signs, and be prepared to help provide basic life support (CPR) if the patient becomes unconscious.

OBJECTIVES	CONTENT	TEACHING RESOURCES
Describe how to respond to specific emergencies.	■ Emergency responses (p. 459) □ Syncope (p. 462) □ Postural hypotension (p. 462) □ The pregnant patient (p. 462) *Emergency Procedure* 31-5 Responding to the unconscious patient (p. 463) (SW/ESLR Competency 31-5, p. 197) □ Cardiac emergencies (p. 462) – Angina (p. 462) – Acute myocardial infarction (p. 463) □ Cerebrovascular accident (p. 463) *Emergency Procedure* 31-6 Responding to the patient with chest pain (p. 464) (SW/ESLR Competency 31-6, p. 199)	PPT 22-34 TB questions 14-21 Multimedia Procedures DVD: 7 animations SW Short-Answer Questions 6; Fill in the Blank questions 1-2, 4-7, 9-12, 14-18; Multiple Choice questions 12-19; Case Study (pp. 185-188) SW/ESLR Competency 31-5 Responding to an Unconscious Patient (p. 197) SW/ESLR Competency 31-6 Responding to a Patient with Chest Pain (p. 199) SW/ESLR Competency 31-7 Responding to a Patient Experiencing a Stroke (CVA) (p. 201) SW/ESLR Competency 31-8 Responding to a Patient with a Breathing Problem (p. 203) SW/ESLR Competency 31-9 Responding to the Patient Experiencing an Allergic Reaction (p. 205) SW/ESLR Competency 31-10 Responding to a Patient Experiencing a Convulsive Seizure (p. 207) SW/ESLR Competency 31-11 Responding to the Patient Experiencing a Diabetic Emergency (p. 209) Recall questions 12-19 (pp. 462, 464, 468)

OBJECTIVES	CONTENT	TEACHING RESOURCES
	Emergency Procedure 31-7 Responding to the patient experiencing a cerebrovascular accident (stroke) (p. 464) (SW/ESLR Competency 31-7, p. 201) ☐ Hyperventilation (p. 463) ☐ Asthma attack (p. 464) ☐ Allergic reaction (p. 465) ☐ Epileptic seizure (p. 465) *Emergency Procedure* 31-8 Responding to the patient with a breathing problem (p. 465) (SW/ESLR Competency 31-8, p. 203) *Emergency Procedure* 31-9 Responding to the patient experiencing an allergic reaction (p. 466) (SW/ESLR Competency 31-9, p. 205) ☐ Diabetes mellitus (p. 467) – Hyperglycemia (p. 468) – Hypoglycemia (p. 468) *Emergency Procedure* 31-10 Responding the patient experiencing a convulsive seizure (p. 466) (SW/ESLR Competency 31-10, p. 207) *Emergency Procedure* 31-11 Responding to the patient experiencing a diabetic emergency (p. 467) (SW/ESLR Competency 31-11, p. 209) ■ Documentation of an emergency (p. 468)	Eye to the future (p. 468) CTQ 1-5 (p. 468) ▸ Discuss the specific concerns a dental assistant should be aware of in dealing with a pregnant patient. ▸ Discuss what might cause a patient to lose consciousness while undergoing dental treatment. ▸ Discuss the differences between hyperglycemia and hypoglycemia and how to properly respond to each condition. ▸ Discuss what is involved in documenting an emergency and why it is important to maintain an accurate documentation of an emergency in a dental office. *Class Activity Present the following emergency situations to the class. In small groups, have the students identify what is happening to the patient and how a dental assistant should respond in each case. Have each group share its results with the rest of the class.* – *Syncope* – *Postural hypotension* – *Hyperventilation* – *Angina*

OBJECTIVES	CONTENT	TEACHING RESOURCES
Performance Evaluation		🖥 TB
		🎥 Multimedia Procedures DVD: 7 animations
		📘 SW questions (pp. 185-187)
		📘 SW Case Study (p. 188)
		📘 *e* SW/ESLR Competency 31-1 Performing Cardiopulmonary Resuscitation (pp. 189-190)
		📘 *e* SW/ESLR Competency 31-2 Responding to a Patient with an Obstructed Airway (p. 191)
		📘 *e* SW/ESLR Competency 31-3 Operating an Automated External Defibrillator (p. 193)
		📘 *e* SW/ESLR Competency 31-4 Preparing the Oxygen System (p. 195)
		📘 *e* SW/ESLR Competency 31-5 Responding to an Unconscious Patient (p. 197)
		📘 *e* SW/ESLR Competency 31-6 Responding to a Patient with Chest Pain (p. 199)
		📘 *e* SW/ESLR Competency 31-7 Responding to a Patient Experiencing a Stroke (CVA) (p. 201)
		📘 *e* SW/ESLR Competency 31-8 Responding to a Patient with a Breathing Problem (p. 203)
		📘 *e* SW/ESLR Competency 31-9 Responding to the Patient Experiencing an Allergic Reaction (p. 205)
		📘 *e* SW/ESLR Competency 31-10 Responding to a Patient Experiencing a Convulsive Seizure (p. 207)
		📘 *e* SW/ESLR Competency 31-11 Responding to a Patient Experiencing a Diabetic Emergency (p. 209)
		e ESLR Electronic Flashcards
		e ESLR Practice Quiz
		Recall questions (pp. 452-468)
		💡 CTQ (p. 468)

Torres and Ehrlich Modern Dental Assisting, 9th ed.

Bird/Robinson

31.2 Homework/Assignments:

31.2 Instructor's Notes/Student Feedback:

Slide 1

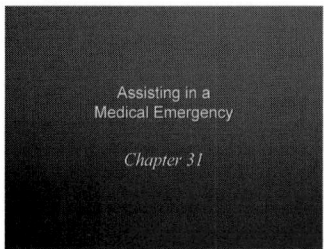

Slide 2

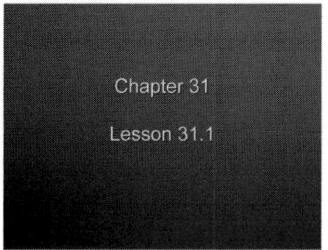

Slide 3

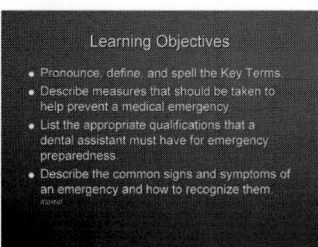

Slide 4

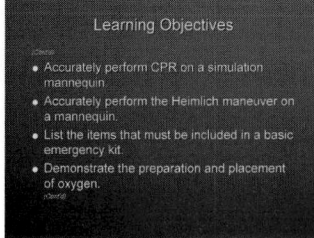

ELSEVIER

Torres and Ehrlich Modern Dental Assisting, 9th ed.

Bird/Robinson

Slide 5

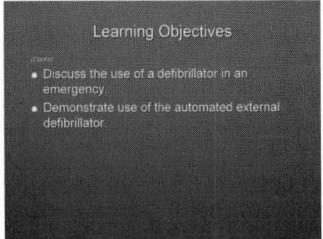

Slide 6

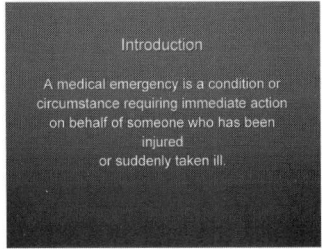

- What is an example of a medical emergency?
- Have you ever been involved in an emergency situation?
- What is the Good Samaritan Law?
- Why do medical emergencies occur in the dental office?

Slide 7

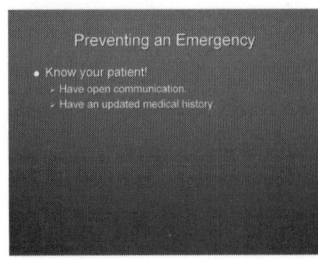

- What difference can open communication make in an emergency at a dental office?
- What difference can an updated medical history make in an emergency at a dental office?
- How does the dental assistant help in updating a medical history?
- What is a medical alert in the dental chart?

Slide 8

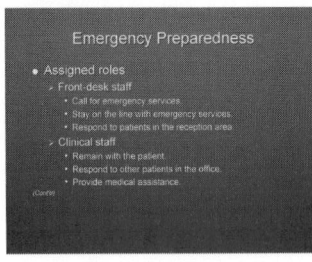

- Why should roles be assigned in the dental office with regard to emergencies, and who assigns these roles?
- Who in the dental office would most likely be in charge of calming down the patient?

Torres and Ehrlich Modern Dental Assisting, 9th ed.

Bird/Robinson

Slide 9

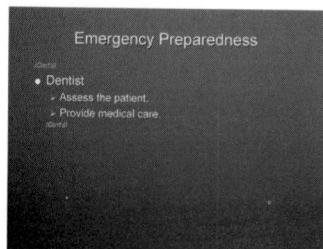

- How does the dental office prepare for future emergencies? *(Emergency first-aid protocols must be established and routinely practiced in the dental office.)*
- What are the physical changes most often seen during a dental office emergency?

Slide 10

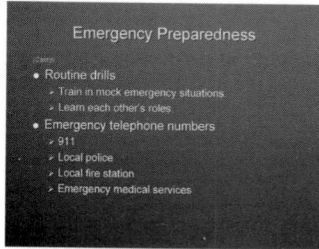

- Where should emergency phone numbers be kept?
- What is important to keep in mind with regard to the list of emergency telephone numbers?
- In addition to the standard emergency telephone numbers, what other numbers may be useful to a dental office in an emergency? Why?

Slide 11

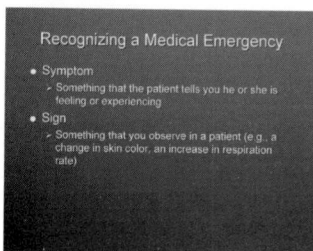

- What are examples of symptoms?
- What are examples of signs?
- Which is more objective, a sign or a symptom?
- What minimum credentials must a dental assistant have for emergency care standards?

Slide 12

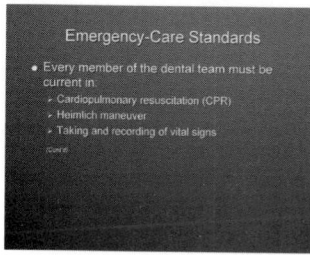

- What is choking?
- What does a person look like who is choking?
- How does the dental team prevent choking episodes?
- What is the Heimlich maneuver and what is it used for?
- What is another name for the Heimlich maneuver? *(Abdominal thrusts.)*

Slide 13

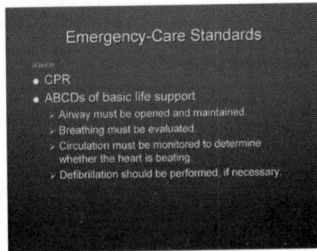

- What is CPR?
- CPR for small children and infants is similar to that for adults, but a few changes must be made to adapt to a child's anatomy and smaller body.

Slide 14

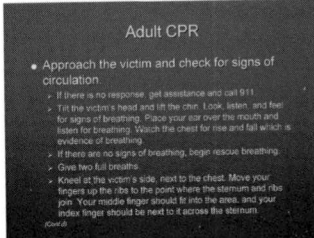

- How do you know a patient is breathing?
- How do you check for signs of circulation?
- Why do you tilt the victim's head and lift the chin at the beginning of CPR?
- Where is the sternum on the chest?

Slide 15

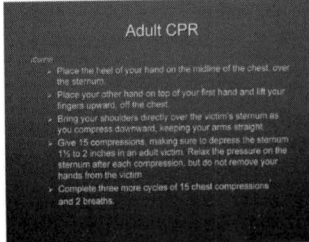

- How do you know a patient is breathing?
- How do you check for signs of circulation?
- Why do you tilt the victim's head and lift the chin at the beginning of CPR?
- Where is the sternum on the chest?

Slide 16

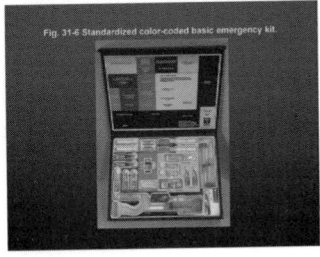

- What is a medical kit in a dental office, and who maintains it?
- If you do not have a standardized drug kit, the dentist will need to determine what emergency supplies and types of drugs should be maintained in the office.
- How is the medical kit maintained?

Bird/Robinson

Slide 17

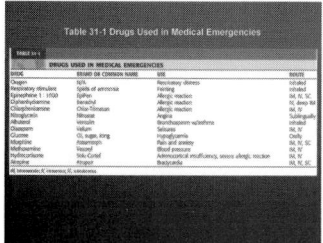

- What is the most frequently used "drug" in a medical emergency?
- What color is oxygen coded?
- Can the nitrous oxide unit be used to supply 100% oxygen in an emergency situation?
- What is important to remember when considering oxygen for emergencies?
- How can nitroglycerine be supplied? *(Tablets, spray, or topical cream.)*

Slide 18

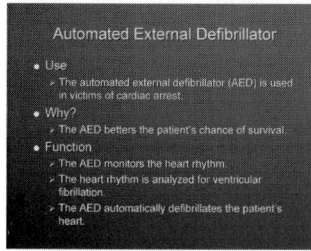

- What is ventricular fibrillation and how is it related to the AED?
- Most sudden cardiac arrest victims are experiencing what is called ventricular fibrillation (VF).
- VF is an abnormal, chaotic heart rhythm that prevents the heart from pumping blood.
- VF causes more cardiac arrests than any other rhythm.
- The sooner defibrillation begins, the better the victim's chances of survival.

Slide 19

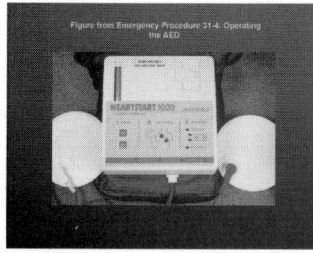

- How does an AED work?
- What powers an AED? *(A standard 110-volt current or battery powers this portable defibrillator.)*

Slide 20

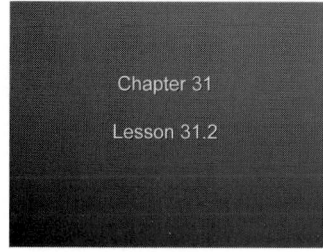

Slide 21

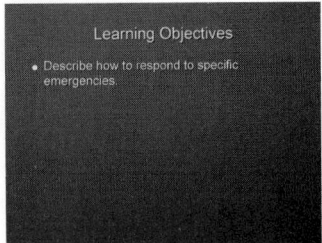

Slide 22

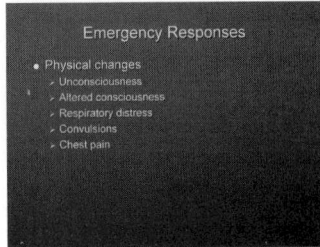

- How is a patient's responsiveness checked? *(Check for patient's responsiveness by tapping and shouting, pinching the muscles in the neck, or applying a sterna rub.)*

Slide 23

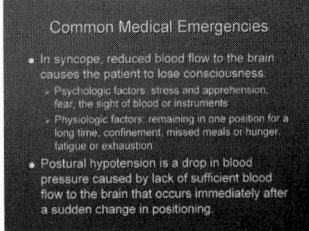

- What is the most common medical emergency in the dental office?
- What is another word for syncope? *(Fainting.)*
- What happens before a patient undergoes syncope, and is it serious?
- How is syncope treated in the dental office?
- How can syncope and postural hypotension be prevented in the dental office?

Slide 24

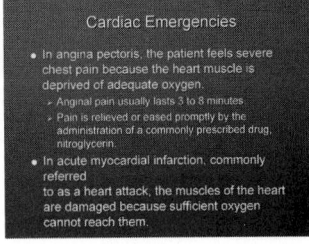

- What is the abbreviation for myocardial infarction?
- Do women have the same symptoms as men when they have a myocardial infarction?
- Why do the muscles of the heart need oxygen?
- Where does the dentist get the nitroglycerin for an emergency in the dental office?

Torres and Ehrlich Modern Dental Assisting, 9th ed.

Bird/Robinson

Slide 25

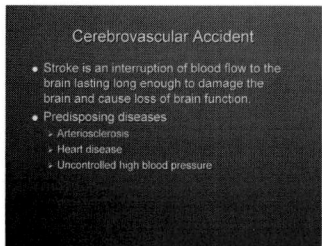

- What is the abbreviation for a cerebrovascular accident?

- Why does the brain become damaged without blood flow? How does this relate to the oxygen needs of the brain?

- What is arteriosclerosis?

Slide 26

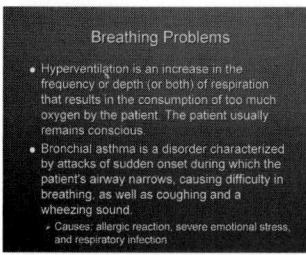

- What should be done by a person who is hyperventilating to help stop the faulty respirations?

- What does a person look like who is undergoing a bronchial asthma attack?

- What is used first by a person who is having a bronchial asthma attack?

Slide 27

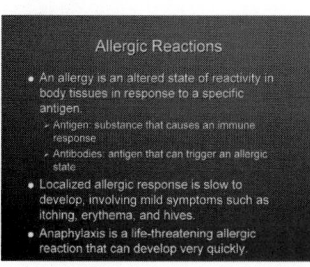

- Which allergic reaction is localized, and which one is systemic?

- What is now a common allergen found in the dental office? *(There is an increasing incidence of allergic reactions to the latex used in examination gloves and dental dams.)*

- What could happen to the patient who undergoes anaphylaxis? *(Without appropriate care, the patient could die within a few minutes.)*

Slide 28

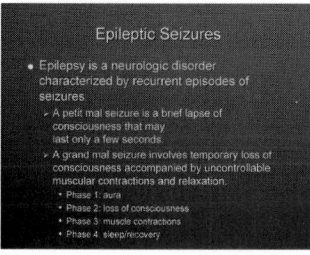

- What is an aura in relationship to epilepsy? *(The patient may experience a warning aura such as a peculiar smell, taste, vision, or sound before the seizure. This can last several seconds or several hours.)*

Slide 29

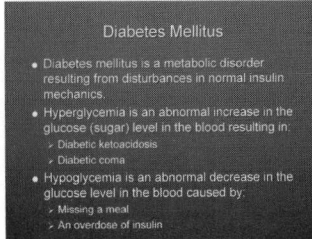

- What are the signs and symptoms of hyperglycemia and hypoglycemia?

- What would be important with regard to mealtimes when scheduling a diabetic patient?

- What would it be important to have in the emergency kit for emergencies because of hypoglycemia?

- Who retrieves the patient's insulin if it is needed, and who usually administers the insulin during a diabetic emergency?

Slide 30

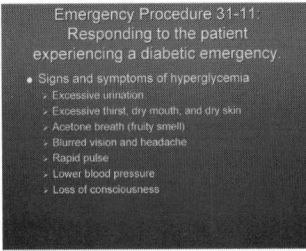

- Why does the diabetic need sugar in this emergency situation?

- What forms of sugar would be easiest to give to a diabetic in an emergency? *(Sugar packet, cake icing, or concentrated orange juice.)*

- What can you do in an emergency for an unconscious diabetic patient who needs sugar?

Slide 31

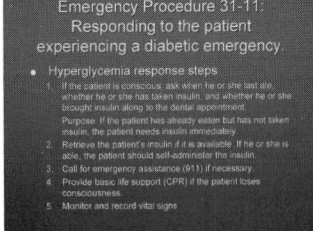

Slide 32

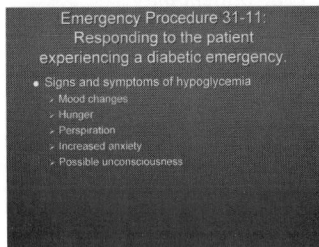

Bird/Robinson

Slide 33

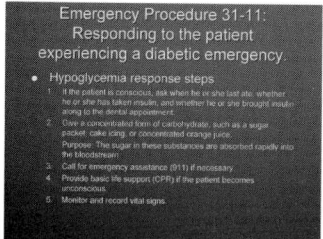

Slide 34

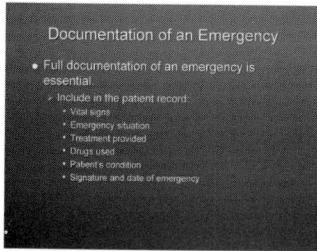

- Where in the patient record would you document an emergency that occurred in your dental office?

- What vital signs must be included in the report of an emergency in the dental office?

- If an emergency is not resolved in the dental office where it occurred, what will the dentist usually do?

TEACHING FOCUS

This chapter will give students an opportunity to learn about the different elements of the dental office, including the design of the dental treatment office, the clinical equipment most commonly found in a dental office, and the basic functions of the dental unit. The importance of the reception area and the areas of the dental environment in a professional office will also be explained.

MATERIALS AND RESOURCES

☐ computer and PowerPoint projector (all Lessons)

LESSON CHECKLIST

Preparations for this lesson include:

- lecture
- evaluation of student knowledge and skills needed to perform all entry-level activities related to the dental office, including:
  ○ areas of the dental environment
  ○ clinical equipment in dental treatment areas
  ○ dental reception and treatment areas
  ○ functions of the dental unit

Bird/Robinson

KEY TERMS

condensation (p. 479)
consultation room (p. 480)
dental operatory (p. 473)
rheostat (p. 476)

subsupine position (p. 475)
supine position (p. 474)
triturate (p. 478)
upright position (p. 474)

ADDITIONAL RESOURCES

PowerPoint slides (Evolve): 1-33

Legend

CTQ
Critical
Thinking
Question

DVD
Multimedia
Procedures
Videos and
Animations

ESLR
EVOLVE
Student
Learning
Resources

IDO
Interactive
Dental
Office
CD-ROM

SW
Student
Workbook

TB
Test Bank
on the
TEACH
CD-ROM

PPT
PowerPoint
Slides

Class Activities are indicated in ***bold italic.***

Torres and Ehrlich Modern Dental Assisting, 9th ed.

Bird/Robinson

LESSON 32.1

PRETEST

1. The ideal temperature for the clinical area of the dental office is
   a. 60° to 65° F.
   c. 75° to 80° F.
   b. 68° to 70° F.
   d. 80° to 85° F.

2. The recommended floor covering in the operatory or treatment room is
   a. vinyl.
   c. ceramic.
   b. carpeting.
   d. wood.

3. Which area of the dental office requires more security than the other areas?
   a. treatment areas
   c. administrative area
   b. reception area
   d. dentist's office

4. When the patient chair is positioned so that the patient's head is lower than the chest, this is called the
   a. upright position.
   c. anatomic position.
   b. subsupine position.
   d. supine position.

5. Which aspect of the dental assistant's stool could cause excessive leaning over the patient when the assistant is seated inappropriately?
   a. the foot platform
   c. the arm rest
   b. the cushion
   d. the abdominal arm

6. Which delivery system provides the easiest access to the dental handpiece without twisting of the body?
   a. front
   c. right side
   b. left side
   d. rear

7. The dental assistant should initially position the operating light
   a. on the patient's chest.
   c. over the patient's head.
   b. on the patient's mouth.
   d. toward the patient's feet.

8. Which oral evacuation system is used for less invasive procedures?
   a. high volume evacuation system with a standard tip
   b. cuspidor
   c. saliva ejector
   d. high volume evacuation system with a surgical tip

9. The instrument used to harden dental materials is the
   a. amalgamator.
   c. high-volume evacuator.
   b. central vacuum compressor.
   d. curing light.

10. Disposable traps should be changed
    a. daily.
    c. biweekly.
    b. weekly.
    d. monthly.

Answers

1. b	3. c	5. d	7. a	9. d
2. a	4. b	6. a	8. c	10. b

Bird/Robinson

BACKGROUND ASSESSMENT

Question: What aspects of the dental office environment should be considered to ensure a positive experience for the patient?

Answer: Several areas must be addressed to ensure that each patient has a positive experience in the dental office. These areas include temperature, lighting, wall and floor coverings, traffic control, sound control, and privacy. The temperature of the office should be comfortable, with the clinical area temperature slightly lower than that of the reception area. The lighting should be soft and easy on the eyes in the reception area and brighter in the administrative and clinical areas. Wall and floor coverings should be made of materials that are durable and easy to maintain and in colors that are calming and relaxing. The area where dental workers and patients walk must be free from clutter and should be easy to pass or walk through. Minimizing familiar "dental sounds" will keep the patients calm and minimize their apprehension. Privacy in both the clinical and administrative areas is also necessary to protect against disclosure of treatment and financial information.

Question: How does dental equipment design facilitate cleaning and infection-control procedures? What role does equipment maintenance play in office cleanliness and patient safety?

Answer: The dental office decor can either help or hinder infection-control steps and cleaning operations. The wall coverings should be durable and easily wiped down. Counter tops and cabinets should be smooth and easy to clean with minimal exposed hardware.. Floor coverings should be appropriate for each area of the dental office; the clinical areas should have vinyl-type flooring and the administrative and reception areas should have durable, stain resistant carpeting that doesn't show dirt. Dental equipment such as the patient chair and the dentist and dental assistant stools should have a seamless design and vinyl-type upholstery for easy cleaning and disinfection. Buttons on the patient chair should be flat and without crevices and ridges. Equipment maintenance is also important for office cleanliness and patient safety. The central vacuum compressor and central air compressor must be cleaned and maintained to eliminate the formation of condensation so that moisture, sediment, and algae do not build up. Waterlines and evacuator systems, including the disposable dental unit traps, must be cleaned to eliminate harmful bacteria and biofilm formation.

CRITICAL THINKING QUESTION

When telephoning patients who have not returned to the office for normal maintenance and recall appointments, several of the patients remark that the office has changed and that it isn't as nice as it used to be. The dentist instructs the dental assistant to create a list of improvements that would enhance the dental office setting. What aspects and areas of the dental office should be assessed, and what factors should be considered when making changes to the dental office environment?

Guidelines: The areas of the dental office that should be assessed for patient comfort and safety are the reception area, walkways, administration area, and treatment areas. The reception area should be well lit with adequate seating and a comfortable room temperature; it should have up-to-date reading materials; and it should be clean and well organized. There should also be an area for children that is well stocked with toys and books. Walkways throughout the dental office should be free of clutter. When walkways are cleared, the office will adopt a more professional, organized appearance and eliminate patient and worker safety issues. The administrative area should be well lit and private to allow financial and treatment discussions that take place between patients and dental staff and to enable patients to read and sign office forms without eye strain. Finally, the treatment rooms should always be clean and organized; patients who see dust, splatter, or clutter in a treatment area assume that measures to control infection are not being carried out. All areas of the office should be decorated in neutral or soft colors, and all the areas should be designed for minimal noise and sound. Temperature is also a factor. A comfortable temperature should be maintained throughout the dental office, with the temperature in the clinical areas slightly lower to accommodate for the close quarters of the operatory and the heat generated from the overhead dental lights.

Bird/Robinson

OBJECTIVES	CONTENT	TEACHING RESOURCES
Pronounce, define, and spell the Key Terms.	■ Key terms (p. 470)	SW Fill in the Blank questions 1-8 (p. 199) ESLR Electronic Flashcards *Class Activity **Go around the room and have each student use one of the key terms in a clinically relevant sentence in order to define the term. Continue until all terms have been used; if students become stuck, have the rest of the class offer suggestions.***
Describe the six areas of the dental environment in a professional office.	■ Office environment (p. 471) ☐ Temperature (p. 471) ☐ Lighting (p. 471) ☐ Wall and floor coverings (p. 471) ☐ Traffic control (p. 471) ☐ Sound control (p. 471) ☐ Privacy (p. 472)	PPT 4-8 TB questions 1-2 SW Short-Answer Questions 1; Multiple Choice questions 1-2; Case Study questions 1-4 (pp. 211-212) Figure 32-1 Design of the dental office using calming colors (p. 471) Specific areas of the dental office (p. 472) Recall questions 1-2 (p. 472) CTQ 1-2 (p. 481) ▸ Discuss how elements of the dental office environment can help calm a patient. ▸ Discuss the importance of traffic patterns between the specific areas of the dental office in optimizing efficiency. *Class Activity **Divide the class into groups and assign each group one of the following topics: temperature, lighting, wall and floor coverings, traffic control, sound control, or privacy. Have each group list and discuss the factors to be considered when assessing its assigned area and present its list to the class.***
Discuss the important qualities of the reception area.	■ Reception area (p. 472) ■ Administrative area (p. 472)	PPT 9-12 SW Short-Answer Questions 2; Multiple Choice questions 3-4 (pp. 211-212) Figure 32-2 Reception area of a dental office (p. 472) Figure 32-3 Part of a reception area designed for children (p. 472) Figure 32-4 Organization and design of the business area (p. 472) Recall question 3 (p. 475) ▸ Discuss how a part of the reception area can be made specifically for children. ▸ Discuss equipment needed for the administrative area of the dental office.

OBJECTIVES	CONTENT	TEACHING RESOURCES
		Class Activity Divide the class into groups, and have each group design a reception area for a mock dental office. Designs should include floor plans and a list of items and considerations to take into account when implementing the design. Have each group share and discuss its design with the class.
Describe the goals in designing the dental treatment area.	■ Treatment area (p. 473)	⊠▪ PPT 13-14 📺 TB questions 3-4 📖 SW Short-Answer Questions 3; Multiple Choice question 5 (pp. 211-212) Figure 32-5 Dental treatment area (p. 473) Recall questions 4-5 (p. 473) ▸ Discuss the primary goals in designing the treatment area. ▸ Discuss how the size of the dental treatment area can affect its setup and organization. *Class Activity Lead a class discussion about dental treatment areas. Ask students to explain how the dentist's Preferences influence the design of the room and how privacy and comfort can be promoted. What can be done when there are multiple dentists with different preferences? Record student responses on the board for comparison.*
List the clinical equipment most commonly found in dental treatment areas.	■ Clinical equipment (p. 473) ☐ Patient dental chair (p. 473) ☐ Operator's stool (p. 475) ☐ Dental assistant's stool (p. 475)	⊠▪ PPT 15-19 📺 TB questions 5-7 📖 SW Short-Answer Questions 4; Multiple Choice questions 6-7 (pp. 211-212) Figure 32-6 Patient dental chair (p. 473) Figure 32-7 Design of the headrest on a dental chair (p. 474) Figure 32-8 Control buttons on a dental chair (p. 474) Figure 32-9 Upright position of a patient in a dental chair (p. 474) Figure 32-10 Patient in a supine position in a dental chair (p. 474) Figure 32-11 Dental assistants' stool and operators' stool (p. 475) Recall questions 6-7 (p. 477) 💡 CTQ 3 (p. 481)

ELSEVIER

OBJECTIVES	CONTENT	TEACHING RESOURCES
		▸ Discuss the differences between the upright, supine, and subsupine patient positions in the patient dental chair and when each position might be used. ▸ Discuss how the operator's or dental assistant's stool can be adjusted to provide comfort for the operator or assistant and help prevent fatigue. ***Class Activity** Have students research clinical equipment commonly found in dental treatment areas, including their vendors, prices, and specifications. Have students share their findings with the class for discussion. (For students to prepare for this activity, see Homework/Assignments #1.)*

32.1 Homework/Assignments:

1. Have students research clinical equipment commonly found in dental treatment areas, including vendors, prices, and specifications. Have students share their findings with the class for discussion.

32.1 Instructor's Notes/Student Feedback:

Bird/Robinson

LESSON 32.2

CRITICAL THINKING QUESTION

The dental assistant has been assigned the responsibility of developing strategies to keep the office on task and to keep the equipment from breaking down. How can an efficient daily operation be established? What steps should be performed at the beginning and end of each day?

Guidelines: The best way to ensure a smooth day-to-day operation is to maintain equipment. The dental office has a significant amount of specialized equipment that must function properly so that the dental office can be effective and efficient in everything from patient scheduling to procedures. The dental assistant is responsible for coordinating the dental team, for keeping the dentist on track, and for maintaining a smooth-flowing schedule. In order to accomplish all of this, the dental assistant has responsibilities that must be carried out at the beginning and end of each day. The dental assistant should arrive at the dental office 30 minutes before the first scheduled patient of the day. The master switches for the central air compressor and vacuum units should be turned on; the treatment rooms should be inspected and prepared for patient care; and the appointment schedule should be rechecked. The dental assistant should also set up the treatment room for the first patient. At the end of the day the dental assistant is responsible for completing the operatory room exposure control clean-up and preparation protocols. All the equipment should be turned off; treatment rooms should be restocked and prepared for the next day; the next day's appointment schedule should be prepared and posted, and the sterilization room should be cleaned.

OBJECTIVES	CONTENT	TEACHING RESOURCES
Discuss the basic functions of the dental unit.	☐ Dental unit (p. 475) – Delivery systems (p. 475) – Rheostat (p. 476) – Waterlines (p. 476) – Air-water syringe (p. 476) – Operating light (p. 476)	PPT 22-25 TB question 8 SW Short-Answer Questions 5, Multiple Choice question 8 (pp. 211-212) Figure 32-12 Dental unit (p. 475) Figure 32-13 Diagram showing front delivery system (p. 476) Figure 32-14 Diagram showing side delivery system (p. 476) Figure 32-15 Diagram showing rear delivery system (p. 476) Figure 32-16 A rheostat controls the handpieces of the dental unit (p. 476) Figure 32-17 Air-water syringe (p. 477) Figure 32-18 Operating light (p. 477) Recall question 8 (p. 477) CTQ 4-5 (p. 481) ▸ Discuss the differences between front and side delivery systems, and explain when each system might be used. ▸ Discuss how the operating light is adjusted to provide maximum illumination without causing the patient discomfort.

OBJECTIVES	CONTENT	TEACHING RESOURCES
		Class Activity Divide the class into groups. Have each group identify the components of a dental unit, describe the functions of each, and explain the different delivery systems that can be used for different types of dental units. Have each group share its findings with the class.
List the clinical equipment most commonly found in the dental area.	☐ Oral evacuation system (p. 477) ☐ Curing light (p. 478) ☐ Amalgamator (p. 478) ☐ Dental radiograph unit (p. 478) – View box for radiographs (p. 478) ■ Care of dental equipment (p. 478) ☐ Central vacuum compressor (p. 479) ☐ Central air compressor (p. 479) ■ Central sterilization (p. 479) ■ Dental laboratory (p. 479) ■ Dentist's private office (p. 480) ■ Dental staff lounge (p. 480) ■ Morning and evening routines for dental assistants (p. 480)	⊠ PPT 25-27, 30-33 TB questions 9-12 SW Multiple Choice questions 9-10 (p. 212) Figure 32-19 Oral evacuation system (p. 477) Figure 32-20 Curing light is used to harden dental materials (p. 478) Figure 32-21 Amalgamator (p. 478) Recall questions 9-10 (p. 478) Figure 32-22 Radiograph unit (p. 479) Figure 32-23 View box (p. 479) Figure 32-24 Disposable traps (p. 479) ▶ Discuss the different operations that must take place daily to properly care for dental equipment. ▶ Discuss how staff can maintain the dentist's privacy while in his or her private office. ▶ Discuss items that might be put into a staff lounge. *Class Activity Divide the class into groups. Have each group first list the equipment commonly found in the dental area, and then outline the care and maintenance of the items. Have groups share their findings with the class for discussion.*
Prepare the dental treatment area for patient care in the morning before seeing patients.	Procedure 32-1 Performing the morning routine (opening the office) (p. 480) (SW/ESLR Competency 32-1, p. 215)	⊠ PPT 28 SW/ESLR Competency 32-1 Performing the Morning Routine (p. 215) ▶ Discuss the repercussions of failing to arrive at the dental office in time to properly prepare for the day's activities. *Class Activity Choose two student volunteers to role-play a dental assistant explaining how to perform the morning routine to a newly hired dental assistant. Have the rest of the class discuss the interaction and offer comments and suggestions.*

OBJECTIVES	CONTENT	TEACHING RESOURCES
Prepare the dental treatment area for patient care the next day.	Procedure 32-2 Performing the evening routine (closing the office) (p. 480) (SW/ESLR Competency 32-2, p. 217)	PPT 29 SW/ESLR Competency 32-2 Performing the Evening Routine (p. 217) ▶ Discuss ways the dental assistant can ensure that the evening routine for the dental office will properly prepare for the next day's activities. *Class Activity Lead a class discussion about the morning and evening routines that must be performed in a dental office. Have students identify the steps to be performed and compare and contrast the two routines. Record student responses on the board for comparison.*
Performance Evaluation		TB SW questions (pp. 211-212) SW Case Study (pp. 212-213) SW/ESLR Competency 32-1 Performing the Morning Routine (p. 215) SW/ESLR Competency 32-2 Performing the Evening Routine (p. 217) ESLR Electronic Flashcards ESLR Practice Quiz questions Recall questions (pp. 472-478) CTQ (p. 481)

32.2 Homework/Assignments:

32.2 Instructor's Notes/Student Feedback:

Slide 1

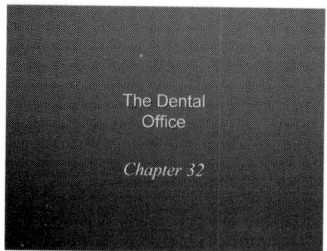

Slide 2

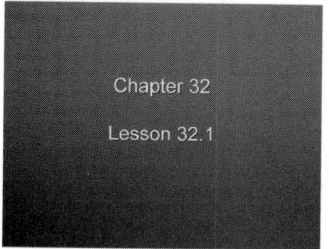

Slide 3

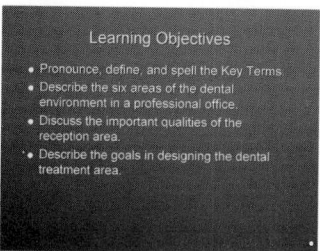

Slide 4

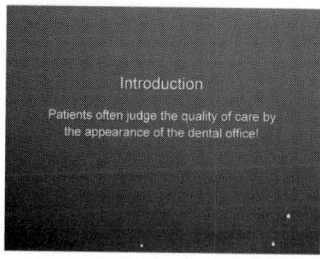

- The patient's first perception of a dental office will remain with that patient throughout future appointments.
- What are factors to consider when creating a positive experience for the patient? *(Details, organization, the manner in which you receive, treat, and dismiss the patient.)*
- All aspects of the dental office must be professional.

Slide 5

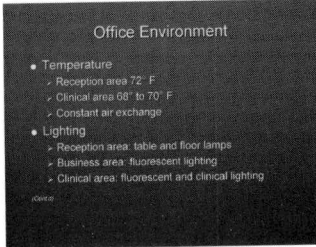

- Why do you think the temperature in the clinical area is higher? *(Usually, the clinical area is a smaller area and has an overhead dental light, which generates heat.)*
- What is a common statement from patients when air exchange is poor?

Slide 6

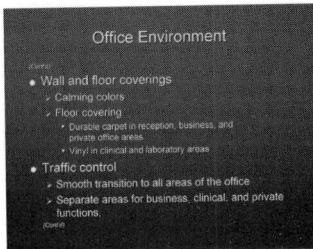

- The wall covering should not be too "busy." Wallpaper or paint are recommended.
- Why is a vinyl floor covering recommended for the clinical and laboratory areas instead of carpeting? *(Infection control. Vinyl flooring can be washed and disinfected.)*
- Why are separate areas recommended for the patients when they are checking out? *(Privacy; privacy is mandated under HIPAA regulations.)*

Slide 7

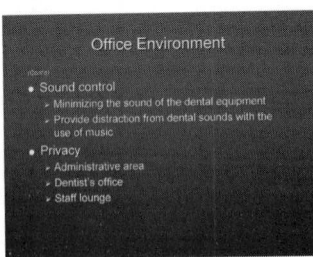

- Why is it important to keep specific sounds associated with the dental office from carrying throughout the dental office setting?
- Privacy: The Health Insurance Portability and Accountability Act of 1996 (HIPAA) took effect on April 14, 2003. The great challenge that HIPAA has created is the assurance that all patient account handling, billing, and medical records are HIPAA compliant.

Slide 8

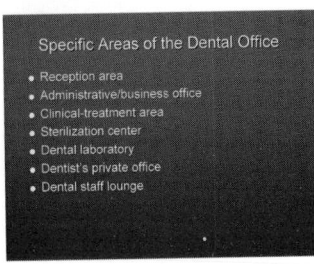

- The size of a dental practice varies. However, certain critical components are found in all dental offices.
- Dental offices must follow guidelines set forth by the American Dental Association (ADA) and the Americans with Disabilities Act when designing the office setting.

Torres and Ehrlich Modern Dental Assisting, 9th ed.

Bird/Robinson

Slide 9

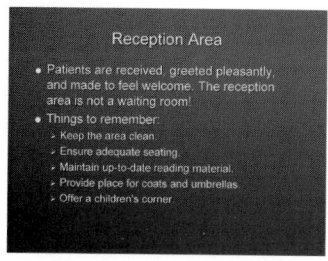

- What is one of the ways to assure that the reception area is not a "waiting room" ?

- If the reception room is dirty or outdated, what impression will patients have? *(That the dental office and treatment procedures are also dirty and out-of-date.)*

- Choose reading materials that will interest patients.

- Provide a place in the reception area where children can play with safe (plastic or soft) toys or read books. The toys should be kept away from traffic areas.

Slide 10

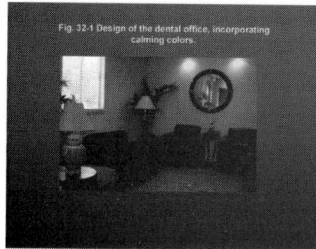

- What are the positive aspects of the reception room pictured?

- What are the negative aspects of the reception room? *(Light-colored carpet may be hard to maintain.)*

Slide 11

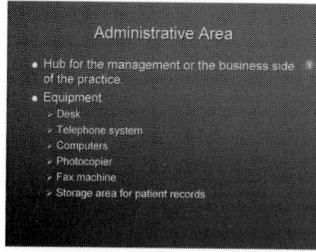

- The administrative area should be separate from the reception area and the clinical area to provide adequate patient privacy.

- No patient charts or information should be in plain sight or where other patients might have access to them.

Slide 12

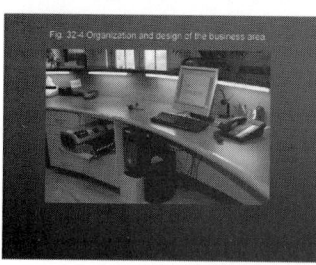

- What are the positive aspects of the administrative area pictured?

- What are the negative aspects of the administrative area pictured?

ELSEVIER

Torres and Ehrlich Modern Dental Assisting, 9th ed.

Bird/Robinson

Slide 13

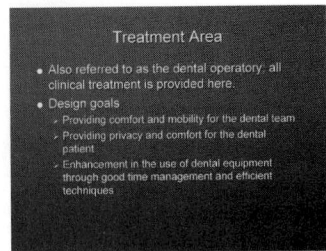

- The treatment area is the control center of the clinical area.

- Most dental offices have two or more dental treatment areas per dentist and one operatory for the dental hygienist.

- What is the purpose of having more then one operatory for each dentist? *(Increased efficiency.)*

- Arrangements of the operatories should be similar in design. Why? *(For easier access to items that may be kept in each room.)*

Slide 14

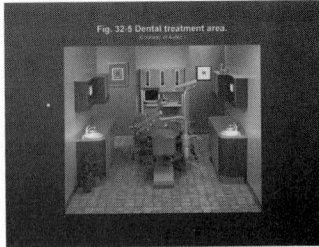

- What are the positive aspects of the treatment area pictured?

- What is a negative aspect of the treatment area pictured?

- Is this treatment room adequately equipped?

Slide 15

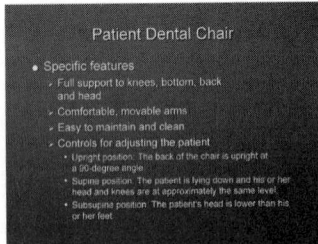

- Dental chairs are available in different sizes for adult and pediatric practices.

- The headrest can be adjusted for the patient's height and is used to support the patient's head securely.

- Chair arms can be moved aside when the patient is being seated or dismissed.

Slide 16

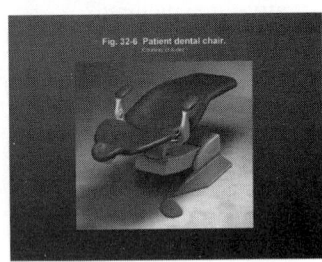

- Why should the dental chair have smooth, seamless surfaces and flat, smooth controls or buttons?

- Why are foot controls a positive design feature?

Bird/Robinson

Slide 17

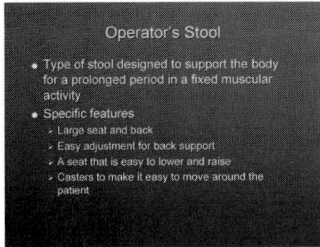

- What features of the operator's stool are important to reduce body and eye fatigue? *(The ability of the operator's stool to adjust both higher and lower and to move easily around the patient's chair.)*

- The minimum number of casters for adequate support and maneuverability on the operator's stool is five.

Slide 18

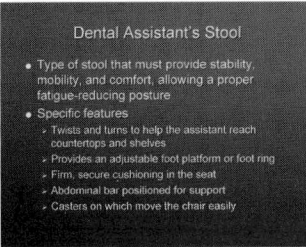

- Regardless of the assistant's height or stature, the stool should allow the assistant to twist and turn to easily reach countertops and shelves.

- What is the purpose of the abdominal bar? *(To help the assistant avoid lower back pain caused from leaning over during the dental procedure.)*

Slide 19

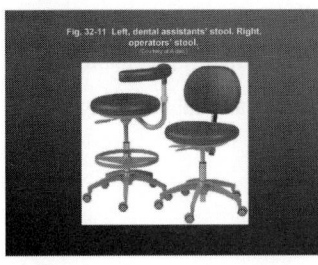

- Notice the multiple casters on both the operator's and the assistant's stools. They add stability and maneuverability.

- Notice the foot rest on the assistant's stool. It allows the assistant to raise the stool above the operator to increase visibility while supporting the assistant's weight. The feet are placed on the foot rest so that the assistant's thighs remain parallel to the floor for proper spine support.

Slide 20

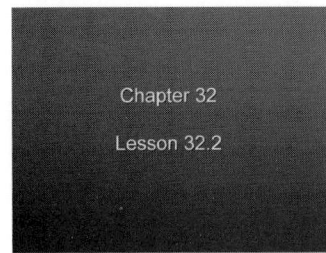

Bird/Robinson

Slide 21

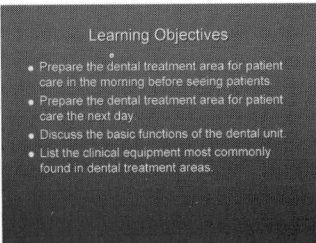

Slide 22

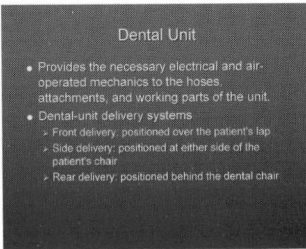

- What factors determine the type of dental unit placed in each operatory?

- Front delivery provides the operator with easy access to dental instruments and hand pieces without stretching or twisting.

- Side delivery allows the dental unit to be easily positioned for a left-handed clinician or a right-handed clinician.

- Rear delivery keeps dental instruments and hand pieces out of the patient's sight.

Slide 23

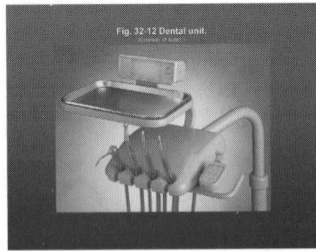

- The dental unit pictured, depending on where it is attached at the base of the chair, may swing to provide front, side, or rear delivery.

- Notice the smooth design with limited crevices to facilitate cleaning.

- Multiple attachments can be prepared and readily available during the dental procedures.

Slide 24

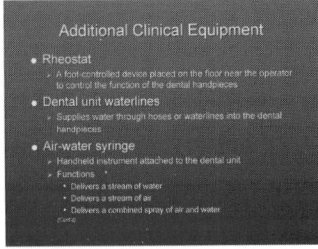

- The amount of pressure placed on the rheostat by the clinician's foot will determine the speed at which the hand piece revolves.

- The air-water syringe is necessary for every procedure. Often a dental unit will contain two air-water syringes, one close to the dentist and one close to the dental assistant.

ELSEVIER

Bird/Robinson

Slide 25

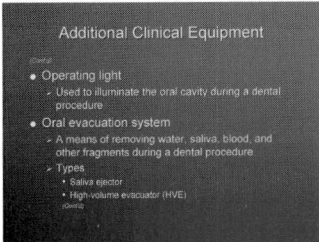

- Halogen bulbs are used in most operating lights. The light is attached to a flexible arm that is either track-mounted from the ceiling or attached to the wall or dental chair.

Slide 26

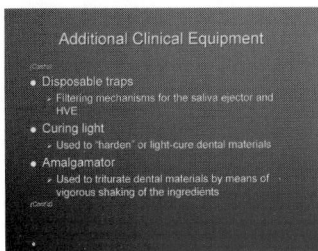

- Disposable traps collect large debris, tooth structure, or old restorative materials that may loosen during tooth preparation and keep them from becoming trapped in the plumbing pipes or expensive vacuum systems.
- The amalgamator and curing light can be mounted in a cabinet or under a countertop for easy access. However, the light cord must be able to reach chairside during dental procedures.

Slide 27

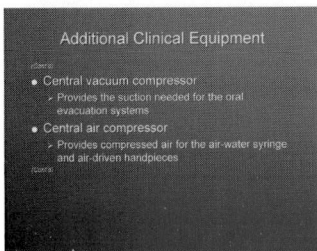

- The central vacuum compressor has two parts: (1) a compressor that creates air flow, (2) a vacuum tank that screens the flow of air to create suction.
- The central air compressor must be maintained routinely to avoid the buildup of condensation, which will result in the formation of algae and sediment in the air and water lines.

Slide 28

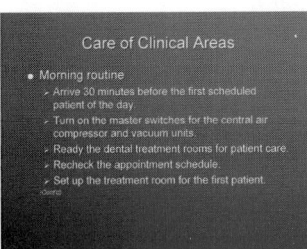

- Who is responsible for the care of the clinical areas before and after the scheduled patients? *(The dental assistant.)*
- Careful completion of the morning steps ensures the smooth flow of patient care throughout the day.

Bird/Robinson

Slide 29

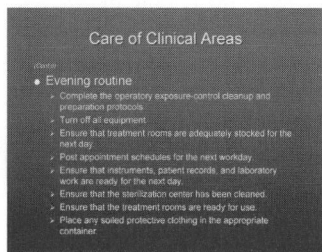

- Careful completion of the evening steps ensures that equipment will be maintained and the team will be prepared for the next day.
- Turning off dental equipment befpre closing the office each day will minimize overnight equipment problems or possible damage to the dental office by water leakage or fire.

Slide 30

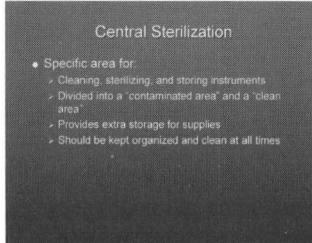

- The sterilization area is a crucial component of day-to-day operations.
- Step-by-step procedures and protocol must be followed to eliminate cross-contamination or problems of infection control that can injure a dental worker or patient.

Slide 31

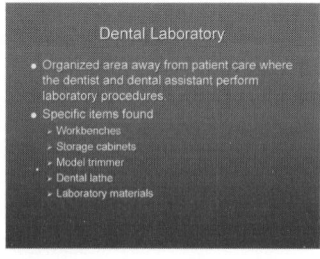

- What are some of the procedures performed in the dental laboratory? *(Pouring impressions, preparing diagnostic models, and creating custom impression trays.)*
- All contaminated materials (alginate impressions, removable appliances, etc.) should be disinfected before being handled in the lab.
- PPE should be worn during laboratory procedures.

Slide 32

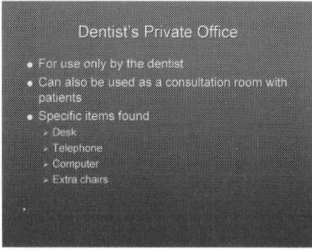

- What is a consultation room? *(A room where the dentist discusses diagnosis and treatment plans with the patient.)*

Bird/Robinson

Slide 33

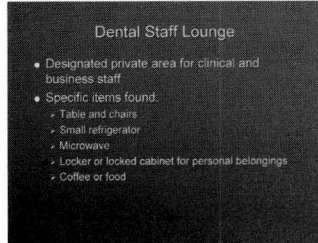

- This area can be used by the staff during personal time or for staff meetings.

- It is customary for the dentist to financially support a coffee service and food vendor.

- PPE should not be worn or taken into the staff lounge area.

TEACHING FOCUS

This chapter will introduce the student to topics related to delivering dental care. The student will become acquainted with the preparation for patient treatment, concepts of team dentistry, instrument exchange, and working as an operator in expanded functions. The student will have the opportunity to put the above information into context by participating in classroom activities and discussions.

MATERIALS AND RESOURCES

☐ computer and projector for Powerpoint (all Lessons)
☐ dental treatment area equipment (all Lessons)
☐ mouth mirror (Lesson 33.2)

LESSON CHECKLIST

Preparations for this lesson include:

- lecture
- evaluation of student knowledge and skills needed to perform all entry-level activities related to the principles underlying delivering dental care, including:
  - credentialing and responsibilities of the expanded-functions dental assistant
  - operating zones
  - preparation for care delivery, including reviewing the patient record, preparing the treatment area, and greeting and seating the patient
  - proper instrument transfer
  - team dentistry and principles of team positioning

KEY TERMS

delegate (p. 492)
direct supervision (p. 492)
expanded function (p. 492)
four-handed dentistry (p. 485)
fulcrum (p. 493)

grasp (p. 488)
indirect supervision (p. 492)
indirect vision (p. 492)
operating zones (p. 487)

ADDITIONAL RESOURCES

PowerPoint slides (Evolve): 1-30
Multimedia Procedures DVD: Transferring Instruments (Single-Handed)

Legend

CTQ
Critical
Thinking
Question

DVD
Multimedia
Procedures
Videos and
Animations

ESLR
EVOLVE
Student
Learning
Resources

IDO
Interactive
Dental
Office
CD-ROM

SW
Student
Workbook

TB
Test Bank
on the
TEACH
CD-ROM

PPT
PowerPoint
Slides

Class Activities are indicated in ***bold italic.***

ELSEVIER

Torres and Ehrlich Modern Dental Assisting, 9th ed.

Bird/Robinson

LESSON 33.1

PRETEST

1. What is the most common dental chair position for dental procedures?
   a. upright
   b. supine
   c. semi-reclined
   d. Trendelenburg

2. Where is the dental light directed when positioning the light and turning it on prior to treatment?
   a. over the patient's face
   b. over the patient's mouth
   c. over the patient's chest
   d. over the clinician's head

3. When the operator is positioned correctly, the thighs are _____ to the floor.
   a. parallel
   b. perpendicular
   c. at a 90°angle
   d. diagonal

4. What classification of motion is described as movement of fingers and wrist?
   a. Class I
   b. Class II
   c. Class
   d. Class IV

5. What is an example of Class III motion?
   a. picking up an instrument or single object.
   b. transferring an instrument using a pen grasp.
   c. using a slow-speed handpiece when performing coronal polishing.
   d. reaching for items in the mobile unit.

6. What is the transfer zone for a right-handed operator?
   a. The 1 to 4 o'clock position
   c. 36 position25 position 3 to 7 o'clock position

7. What is the static zone?
   a. the area where instruments and dental materials are exchanged
   b. the area where the person completing the procedure is seated
   c. the area directly behind the patient
   d. the area where the dental assistant is positioned

8. Who delegates expanded functions to the dental assistant?
   a. any member of the dental team
   b. another dental assistant
   c. the dental hygienist
   d. the dentist

9. What type of supervision is described as the presence of the dentist in the dental office area, but not necessarily present in the same treatment room?
   a. direct supervision
   b. indirect supervision
   c. general supervision
   d. universal supervision

10. What is the suggested positioning for the right-handed operator when treating the maxillary right buccal surfaces of the teeth?
    a. 2 to4 o'clock position
    b. 6 to 8 o'clock position
    c.10 to 12 o'clock position
    d.12 to 1 o'clock position

Answers

1. b	3. a	5. c	7. c	9. b
2. c	4. b	6. d	8. d	10. c

BACKGROUND ASSESSMENT

Question: What is the function of the mouth mirror? Why is it critical to the health of the clinician and dental assistant to properly use the mouth mirror?

Answer: The mouth mirror is a vital instrument when performing specific intraoral expanded functions. The mouth mirror is used to view indirect vision areas. It is critical to the health of the clinician and dental assistant to maintain posture, reduce eye strain, and complete specific functions.

Question: What is four-handed dentistry? How does four-handed dentistry fit into the team approach concept?

Answer: Four-handed dentistry is the process by which the operator and assistant work together to perform clinical procedures in an ergonomically structured environment. Four-handed dentistry originates from the concept that a qualified dental assistant is positioned across from the operator and they work together as a cohesive team. Throughout the procedure, the operator relies on the dental assistant to have all necessary supplies, instruments, and dental materials ready to be transferred into the operator's hands. The smooth, well-organized transfer of these items during the procedure is a team effort that requires coordination, communication, and practice between the operator and assistant.

CRITICAL THINKING QUESTION

You were just hired by Dr. Smith as a clinic assistant in his dental office. The operators you will assist are a dentist, Dr. Smith, and his wife, Mrs. Smith, a dental hygienist. You are nervous because you understand that it is your responsibility to prepare the treatment rooms and to assist the operators. You also understand that Dr. and Mrs. Smith are very particular about the efficiency of the office and expect the day to run smoothly and their patients to receive the best possible care. What can you do to ensure that all standards are met to avoid loss of production for the operators, inconvenience and discomfort for the patient, and unnecessary stress for everyone?

Guidelines: The clinic assistant should prepare in advance by obtaining the patient record, knowing the upcoming procedure, and having the supplies and equipment ready. Several tasks should be completed before greeting and seating the patient for dental care. First, obtain the patient record and identify whether any medical contraindications for dental procedures are noted. Review past dental experiences and procedures and current treatment plans. Determine if additional supplies will be needed for the up-and-coming procedure. You should always make sure the treatment room is clean, disinfected, and ready for the next patient. Prepare the patient's treatment record, radiographs, and laboratory case in the treatment room for easy viewing by the operator and assistant. Make sure the appropriate presterile instrument packets and other supplies are available. Place the dental chair in the appropriate position for receiving the patient. Once you are prepared, it is time to greet and escort the patient to the prepared treatment room. Greet the patient with polite conversation to help him or her feel at ease. When seating the patient, position the chair and surrounding objects so that the patient can safely enter the chair and be seated. Once the treatment procedure begins, you and the operator will position yourselves to allow access and visibility to all areas of the oral cavity. You can also employ motion economy principles by placing instruments and dental equipment within reach of both you and the operator to eliminate reaching, twisting and turning while seated in position.

OBJECTIVES	CONTENT	TEACHING RESOURCES
Define and spell the Key Terms.	■ Key terms (p. 482)	*e* ESLR Electronic Flashcards ▸ Discuss each of the key terms, focusing on the definition, pronunciation, and spelling of each term. ***Class Activity** Have the students write definitions of the terms in their own words and in laymen's terms. Then have them define the words using professional terms. Divide the class into pairs. Have each pair take turns role-playing a dental assistant talking with either a patient or a colleague. The dental assistant will explain the key terms to his or her partner in laymen's terms or*

Torres and Ehrlich Modern Dental Assisting, 9th ed.

Bird/Robinson

OBJECTIVES	CONTENT	TEACHING RESOURCES
		professional terms. The other student should ask questions to prompt further explanation by the dental assistant.
Discuss the importance of preparing a dental treatment room for a procedure.	■ Knowing your patients (p. 483) ■ Reviewing the patient record (p. 483) ■ Preparing the treatment area (p. 483)	☒ PPT 5-6 TB question 1 SW Short-Answer Questions 1; Multiple Choice question 1 (pp. 219-220) CTQ 1 (p. 496) ▸ Discuss issues that should be addressed by the dental team prior to the patient's arrival. ▸ Discuss the review of the patient's record and issues of particular importance to note prior to the patient's visit. **Class Activity** *Divide the class into groups of four for a role-play involving a dentist, a dental assistant, a receptionist, and a dental hygienist. Have students take turns in the roles and create scenarios for various patient preparation situations, including a variety of health history issues and proposed treatment strategies. The students should demonstrate how their team would prepare for the patient prior to the patient's arrival. Have each group of students perform one role-play in front of the class for discussion.*
Describe how to prepare the dental treatment area for a patient's arrival.	■ Preparing the treatment area (p. 483)	☒ PPT 7 TB question 2 SW Short-Answer Questions 2 (p. 219) ▸ Discuss what should be included in a treatment room preparation checklist. **Class Activity** *Select several students to demonstrate the preparation required prior to a patient's arrival in a dental office, including: obtaining the patient chart, reviewing the patient chart, preparing the treatment room, and setting up equipment and material. Then lead a class discussion on preparation of the treatment area.*
Demonstrate admitting and seating the patient.	■ Greeting and seating the patient (p. 483) *Procedure* 33-1 Admitting and seating the patient (pp. 484-485) (SW/ESLR Competency 33-1, p. 223)	☒ PPT 8-9 TB question 3 SW/ESLR Competency 33-1 Admitting and Seating a Patient (p. 223) ▸ Discuss the importance of putting a patient at ease by chatting about topics other than treatment. ▸ Discuss the importance of asking if the patient has any questions. Emphasize that patients may pose questions to the assistant that they may be reluctant to ask the dentist.

OBJECTIVES	CONTENT	TEACHING RESOURCES
		Class Activity **Have student pairs take turns role-playing an assistant greeting a patient. The assistant should greet the patient and escort the patient to the prepared treatment room. The assistant will then seat the patient in the dental chair, place the patient napkin on the patient, position the chair in a supine position, turn on the light and prepare for treatment to begin.**
Describe how the operator is positioned during treatment.	■ Team dentistry (p. 485) ■ Principles of team positioning (p. 485) ☐ Positioning the patient (p. 486) ☐ Positioning the operator (p. 486)	PPT 10-14 TB questions 4-5 SW Short-Answer Questions 3; Fill in the Blank question 6; Multiple Choice question 6 (pp. 219-220) Recall question 1 (p. 485) Figure 33-1 The concept of four-handed dentistry is shown in the positioning of the patient and dental team (p. 485) Figure 33-2 Distance of the operator's face to the patient's face when positioned correctly (p. 486) Figure 33-3 Position of the operator when seated correctly (p. 486) Recall question 3 (p. 486) CTQ 2-4 (p. 496) ▸ Discuss the concept of team dentistry, also known as four-handed dentistry. Note that the goal of this concept is to deliver high-quality, effective, and efficient care. ▸ Discuss principles of team positioning. Note that the goal of proper positioning is to ensure access to and visibility of all areas of the oral cavity while maintaining a position that offers optimal comfort and support. *Class Activity* **Divide the class into small groups, and have the groups discuss the philosophy of team dentistry. The discussion should include: how team dentistry works or does not work, what could enhance team dentistry, who benefits from the team dentistry approach, etc. Then have each group report its findings to the class for further discussion.**
Describe how the assistant is positioned during treatment.	☐ Positioning the dental assistant (p. 486) ■ Motion economy (p. 487) ☐ Classification of motions (p. 487)	PPT 15-20 TB questions 6-8 SW Short-Answer Questions 4; Fill in the Blank question 2; Multiple Choice questions 2-5; Labeling (pp. 219-220, 222) Figure 33-4 Position of the dental assistant when seated correctly (p. 486)

Bird/Robinson

OBJECTIVES	CONTENT	TEACHING RESOURCES
	■ Operating zones (p. 487)	Recall question 2 (p. 486)
	□ Operator's zone (p. 487)	Figure 33-5 Operating zones for a right-handed operator (p. 487)
	□ Transfer zone (p. 487)	Figure 33-6 Operating zones for a left-handed operator (p. 488)
	□ Assistant's zone (p. 487)	Recall questions 4-6 (p. 488)
	□ Static zone (p. 488)	▶ Discuss classification of motions, and note the need to eliminate or reduce Class IV and V motions.
		▶ Discuss operating zones. Note that operating zones are based on a clock concept and define the operator zone, transfer zone, assistant zone, and static zone for a right-handed and a left-handed operator.
		Class Activity Have students work in pairs. Have one student position himself or herself in the assistant stool to assist procedures in each area of a potential patient's mouth. The other student will observe and offer feedback about the positions of the student in the assistant stool. The feedback will focus on ergonomic principles and positioning within the assistant zone for instrument exchange for each area of a patient's mouth. Have the class discuss areas of strength and areas needing improvement.

33.1 Homework/Assignments:

33.1 Instructor's Notes/Student Feedback:

LESSON 33.2

CRITICAL THINKING QUESTION

After preparing the treatment room for the second patient of the day, you review the patient record and determine that the patient is scheduled for suture removal from an extraction that was completed six days ago. You also determine the patient is wheelchair-bound but is able to be transferred into the dental chair. What additional supplies and equipment will you prepare and what modifications will you make during the instrument exchange for efficient instrument transfer during the procedure? What patient preparation procedures would you modify?

Guidelines: The suture removal procedure requires additional equipment beyond the traditional examination instruments of a mirror, explorer, and cotton pliers. The dental assistant will also prepare a presterile packet containing scissors and a hemostat. The additional equipment will require a variation in instrument exchange. The scissors and hemostat are hinged instruments that are designed to have an open/closed use. These instruments will be held at their hinge. The hemostat is transferred by directing the handle into the dentist's palm. The scissors are transferred by positioning them over the dentist's fingers. Hinged instruments are often heavier than other instruments and a steady hand is necessary during the two-handed transfer. When greeting and escorting the patient to the treatment room, dental equipment and supplies must be placed out of the way to allow wheelchair access into the room. The dental chair is positioned so the wheelchair seat and the dental chair seat are aligned and parallel. The dental chair should be slightly lower than the wheelchair.

OBJECTIVES	CONTENT	TEACHING RESOURCES
Explain instrument transfer.	■ Instrument transfer (p. 488) □ Objectives of efficient instrument transfer (p. 488)	PPT 24 SW Multiple Choice question 12 (p. 221) ▸ Discuss the responsibilities of the dental assistant as they relate to instrument transfer. ▸ Discuss the benefits of a standardized operating sequence. ***Class Activity** Have the class brainstorm ideas regarding the dental assistant's role during instrument exchange. Have one student write the ideas on the board. Then have the class use the ideas to compile a list of responsibilities and roles of the dental assistant during instrument transfer.*
Demonstrate instrument transfer using a selection of instruments.	■ Instrument transfer (p. 488) □ Objectives of efficient instrument transfer (p. 488)	▸ Discuss objectives for efficient instrument transfer. ***Class Activity** Divide the class into student pairs. Have each student sit in the assistant's position and demonstrate instrument transfer to another student, who is seated in the operator's position, with each of the following instrument types: mirror and explorer, cotton pliers, handpiece, and hinged instruments.*
Specify three grasps used by the operator.	□ Grasping an instrument (p. 488)	PPT 25-26 TB question 9 SW Short-Answer Questions 6; Fill in the Blank question 7 (pp. 219-220) Figure 33-7. Basic instrument grasps (p. 489)

OBJECTIVES	CONTENT	TEACHING RESOURCES
		▸ Discuss the three basic instrument grasps.
		▸ Discuss circumstances and instruments for which each of the grasps would be used.
		Class Activity Have student volunteers sort through randomly chosen dental instruments and place them into groups according to how the instruments are used and the procedures performed with each instrument. Based on their groupings, have the class discuss which grasp would enhance the use of the instrument.
Demonstrate the correct grasp and use for hand instruments.	☐ Grasping an instrument (p. 488)	▸ Discuss grasps for mirror, explorer, cotton pliers, handpiece, and instruments with hinges.
		Class Activity Have each student demonstrate, using a typodont, the proper grasp and use of each of the following instruments: mirror and explorer, cotton pliers, handpiece, and hinged instruments.
Transfer instruments using the single-handed technique.	☐ Transfer technique (p. 489) ☐ Variations in instrument exchange (p. 489) – Mirror and explorer (p. 489) – Cotton pliers (p. 489) Procedure 33-2 Transferring instruments using the single-handed technique (p. 490) (SW/ESLR Competencies 33-2 and 33-3, pp. 225-227) – Handpiece (p. 491)	PPT 27-28 TB questions 10, 16 Multimedia Procedures DVD: Transferring Instruments (Single-Handed) SW Short-Answer Questions 5; Multiple Choice questions 7-8, 11, 13-15 (pp. 219-221) SW/ESLR Competencies 33-2 and 33-3 Transferring Instruments Using Single-Handed and Two-Handed Techniques (pp. 225-227) Figure 33-8. The dentist prepares to receive the mirror and explorer by positioning the hand on either side of the patient's head (p. 489) Figure 33-9. The assistant transfers the cotton pliers, ensuring the ends are together so as not to drop the item. (p. 489) Figure 33-10. Transferring the handpiece (p. 491) Recall questions 7-8 (p. 491) ▸ Discuss single-handed technique, and note when it is used. ▸ Discuss transfer of cotton pliers, noting that the working end of the pliers facilitates retrieval. ***Class Activity Divide the class into student pairs. Have each student sit in the assistant's position and demonstrate instrument transfer, using single-handed techniques, to another student, who is seated in the operator's position. The assistant should identify when single-handed techniques are used.***

Torres and Ehrlich Modern Dental Assisting, 9th ed.

Bird/Robinson

OBJECTIVES	CONTENT	TEACHING RESOURCES
Transfer instruments using the two-handed technique.	– Instruments with hinges (p. 491) ⌐Procedure⌐ 33-3 Transferring instruments using two-handed technique (p. 491) (SW/ESLR Competencies 33-2 and 33-3, pp. 225-227)	📺 TB question 11 📖 𝒆 SW/ESLR Competencies 33-2 and 33-3 Transferring Instruments Using Single-Handed and Two-Handed Techniques (pp. 225-227) Figure 33-11 Transferring scissors so that the dentist can grasp them correctly (p. 491) ▸ Discuss the transfer of instruments with hinges, noting that two-handed technique is often used due to the weight of these instruments. **Class Activity** *Divide the class into student pairs. Have each student sit in the assistant's position and demonstrate instrument transfer, using two-handed techniques, to another student who is seated in the operator's position. The assistant should identify when single-handed techniques are used. The operator should demonstrate the ready signal given to the assistant when simultaneous instrument exchange is desired.*
Identify five areas in which the assistant must have competency when practicing expanded functions.	■ The expanded-functions dental assistant (p. 492) □ Dental supervision (p. 492) ■ Working as the operator (p. 492) □ Operator positioning (p. 492)	🖾 PPT 29-30 📺 TB question 12 📖 SW Short-Answer Questions 7; Fill in the Blank questions 1, 4, 8-9 (pp. 219-220) 📖 SW Topics for Discussion questions 1-5 (p. 221) Table 33-1. Suggested Positioning of the Operator and Patient According to Areas of the Mouth (p. 493) 💡 CTQ 5 (p. 496) ▸ Discuss the benefits of delegating specific expanded functions. ▸ Discuss the dental anatomy topics that must be mastered by the expanded-function dental assistant. ▸ Discuss suggested positioning of the operator and patient according to areas of the mouth. **Class Activity** *Divide the class into small groups. Assign each group one or more of the areas in which the assistant must have competency when practicing expanded functions. Have each group describe the area, identify the reasons for additional knowledge in this area, and how this additional knowledge would enhance the EFDA abilities to perform intraoral procedures. Then have each group share its information with the class.*

OBJECTIVES	CONTENT	TEACHING RESOURCES
Demonstrate the proper use of a dental mirror.	☐ Developing mirror skills (p. 492) – Establish a working position (p. 492) – Establish preferred mirror-to-tooth position (p. 493) ☐ Using a fulcrum (p. 493) ☐ Understanding dental anatomy (p. 493) ☐ Understanding cavity preparations (p. 494) [Procedure] 33-4 Using the dental mirror intraorally (p. 494) (SW/ESLR Competency 33-4, p. 229)	☒ PPT 24 TB questions 13-14 SW Fill in the Blank questions 3, 5; Multiple Choice questions 9-10 (pp. 219-220) SW/ESLR Competency 33-4 Using the Dental Mirror Intraorally (p. 229) Figure 33-12. Positioning the mirror to reflect image of the teeth correctly (p. 492) Figure 33-13. Using a fulcrum to stabilize the hand and instrument (p. 493) Recall questions 9-10 (p. 495) ▸ Discuss the purpose of the dental mirror, and note the proper working position and preferred mirror-to-tooth position when using a dental mirror. ▸ Discuss the establishment of a fulcrum as a method of stabilizing the hand. Note the benefit of establishing a fulcrum as close to the working area as possible. *Class Activity Distribute to the class a maze printed on paper, and have the students make their way through with a pencil by looking into a dental mirror, to practice indirect vision skills.*
Demonstrate the use of a dental instrument intraorally.	☐ Adapting instrumentation (p. 494) ☐ Applying dental materials (p. 495) ☐ Evaluation of expanded functions (p. 495) [Procedure] 33-5 Using an instrument intraorally (p. 495) (SW/ESLR Competency 33-5, p. 231)	☒ PPT 24 TB question 15 SW/ESLR Competency 33-5 Using an Instrument Intraorally (p. 231) Patient Education (p. 495) Legal and Ethical Implications (p. 495) Eye to the Future (p. 496) ▸ Discuss the need to adapt the working end of the instrument to the tooth surface and then correctly move the instrument using one of two methods. ▸ Discuss different dental materials, their uses, and their proper applications. *Class Activity Have each student demonstrate the placement of a two-surface-amalgam restoration using a cotton forceps, mouth mirror, explorer, and amalgam instruments.*

Bird/Robinson

OBJECTIVES	CONTENT	TEACHING RESOURCES
Performance Evaluation		TB

SW questions (pp. 205-207)

SW/ESLR Competency 33-1 Admitting and Seating a Patient (p. 223)

SW/ESLR Competencies 33-2 and 33-3 Transferring Instruments Using Single-Handed and Two-Handed Techniques (pp. 225-227)

SW/ESLR Competency 33-4 Using the Dental Mirror Intraorally (p. 229)

SW/ESLR Competency 33-5 Using an Instrument Intraorally (p. 231)

ESLR Electronic Flashcards

ESLR Practice Quiz

ESLR Labeling Exercise 28: Identify the zones of the clock concept for a right-handed operator.

ESLR Labeling Exercise 29: Identify the zones of the clock concept for a left-handed operator.

Recall questions (pp. 485-495)

CTQ (p. 496) |

33.2 Homework/Assignments:

33.2 Instructor's Notes/Student Feedback:

Slide 1

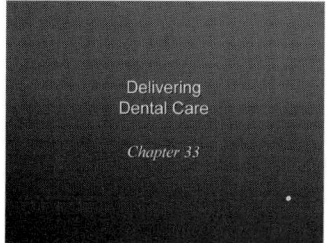

Delivering
Dental Care

Chapter 33

Slide 2

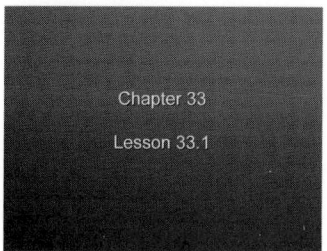

Chapter 33

Lesson 33.1

Slide 3

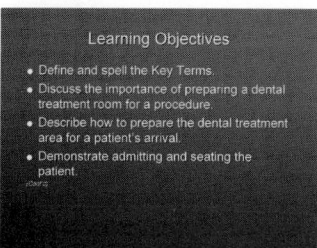

Learning Objectives

- Define and spell the Key Terms.
- Discuss the importance of preparing a dental treatment room for a procedure.
- Describe how to prepare the dental treatment area for a patient's arrival.
- Demonstrate admitting and seating the patient.

Slide 4

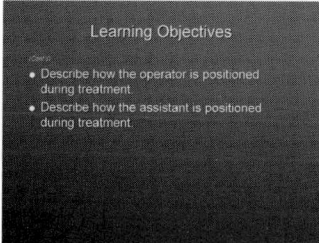

Learning Objectives
(Cont'd)

- Describe how the operator is positioned during treatment.
- Describe how the assistant is positioned during treatment.

Torres and Ehrlich Modern Dental Assisting, 9th ed.

Bird/Robinson

Slide 5

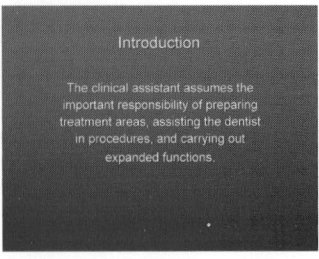

- What is four-handed dentistry? *(Process by which the operator and assistant work together to perform clinical procedures in an ergonomically structured environment.)*
- Can you list and discuss various advanced preparation procedures a dental assistant can complete to increase the smooth flow of patient care throughout the day? *(Obtain the patient record, know the upcoming procedure[s], and have the supplies and equipment ready.)*
- What could result from failure to meet the standards of these tasks? *(Loss of production for the dentist, inconvenience or discomfort for the patient, and unnecessary stress for everyone.)*

Slide 6

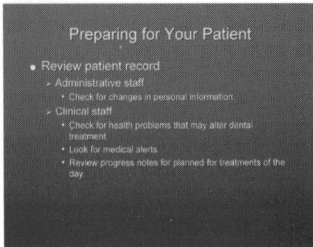

- What is the best way to know your patients and to be better prepared for their presence in the reception area? *(Have a brief meeting, or review the day's schedule before the patient arrives.)*
- Some of the issues that should be discussed among the dental team may include: Changes in the patient's dental history, additional supplies or equipment that may be needed, preparation for the apprehensive patient, and assignments of expanded functions.
- What are some of the tasks to complete when preparing for the apprehensive patient? *(Schedule longer appointments, use premedication, and use pain control measures, such as nitrous oxide administration.)*

Slide 7

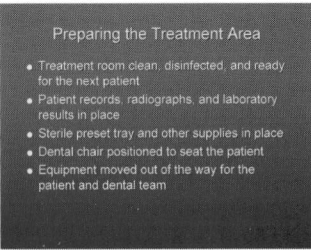

- Is it recommended that one wear PPE during treatment room cleaning and disinfection? *(Yes.)*
- Can you list the appropriate PPE? *(Safety eyewear; lab jacket with long, cuffed, sleeves; gloves, and face mask.)*
- Where should the radiographs be placed? *(Illuminated view box.)*
- When should the sterile preset tray be opened? *(After the patient is seated and before treatment.)*
- What is the proper dental chair position for receiving the patient? *(Upright and at the lowest height.)*

Slide 8

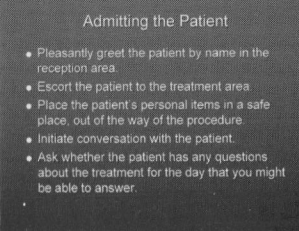

- The patients must be greeted in a courteous manner. Remember to call them by their last names and establish eye contact, smile, and introduce yourself.
- Where is the best place to put the patient's personal items?
- Why would you keep the items in the patient's sight?
- Why is initiating conversation with the patient important?
- Why should you ask the patients if they have any questions or need further information about the treatment?

Torres and Ehrlich Modern Dental Assisting, 9th ed.

Bird/Robinson

Slide 9

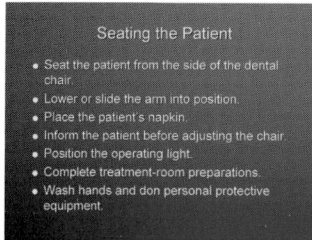

- Ask the patient to swing his or her legs onto the base of the chair after they are seated from the side of the dental chair, then place the patient napkin over the patient's chest and clasp the corners using a napkin chain.

- Why should you inform the patient before adjusting the chair?

- Move the chair slowly until the patient is in the right position.

- Turn on the light after positioning it so that it is aimed toward the patient's chest.

- Does the PPE for treatment setup differ from the PPE used during treatment procedures?

Slide 10

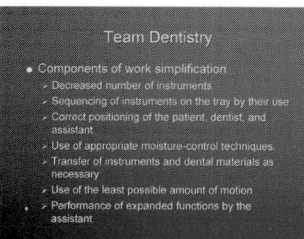

- What are the main goals of this concept? *(To deliver the best and most effective care to the patient and to increase productivity.)*

- How does ergonomics play a role in team dentistry?

- How do appropriate moisture control techniques simplify work? *(Vision of the work field in the mouth is increased.)*

- Expanded functions allow the dentist to use time more effectively and efficiently.

Slide 11

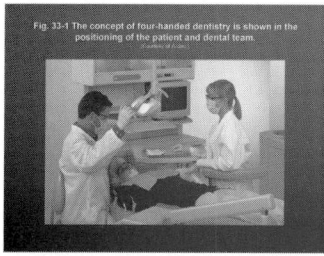

- How does four-handed dentistry affect ergonomics and the concept of team dentistry? *(Use of proper four-handed dentistry procedures enhances the treatment process by reducing stress and fatigue of both dentist and dental assistant. Four-handed dentistry practices also utilize the time of the dental team, which increases productivity.)*

Slide 12

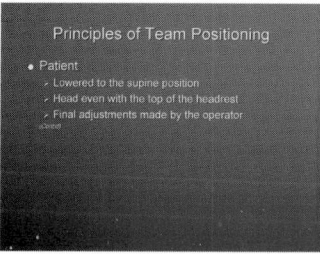

- Why is correct positioning of the dental team essential in the clinical area? *(Correct positioning habits allow access and visibility to all areas of the patient's mouth while providing maximum comfort and support to the dentist and dental assistant.)*

- What occurs when the dentist or dental assistant stretch to reach an instrument or gain access to the patient's mouth? *(Accumulated stress contributes to lower back pain, circulatory problems, and muscle aches and pain.)*

- What can you ask the patient to do to make access to specific areas of the mouth easier? *(Turn his or her head to the left or right.)*

Slide 13

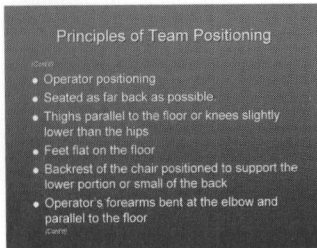

- What are the most essential qualities for the operator? *(Access and vision.)*

Slide 14

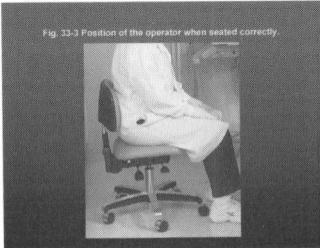

- Is this operator positioned correctly *(Yes.)*

- Note the neutral elbow position.

- Note how the weight of the operator is supported by the straight back and feet that are flat on the floor.

Slide 15

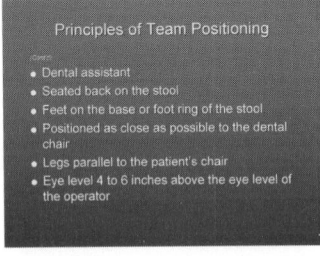

- The dental assistant must anticipate the needs of the dentist during treatment along with having access to the area of concentration.

Slide 16

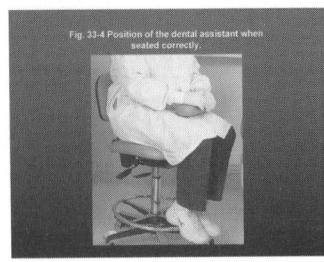

- Is the dental assistant positioned correctly? *(Yes.)*

- This position will allow the dental assistant to sit 4 to 6 inches above the clinician to allow the assistant to have access to the concentration area.

- Note the neutral elbow position.

- Note how the feet are supported by the ring at the base of the stool.

Bird/Robinson

Slide 17

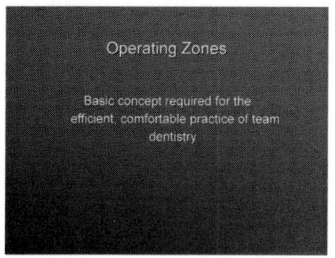

- Operating zones are based on a "clock concept." This concept offers the best way to identify the working position of the dental team, dental equipment, and supplies needed to perform a procedure.

- What affects the operator's position within the operating zone?

- The operator's zone is the zone in which the clinician is positioned.

- The transfer zone is the zone in which instruments and dental materials are exchanged between the clinician and the dental assistant.

- The assistant's zone is the area in which the assistant is positioned.

- The static zone is directly behind the patient. This is the area with rear delivery or a unit that holds the hand pieces, air-water syringe, and additional countertop space.

Slide 18

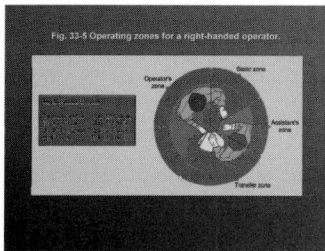

- What is the operator zone for a right-handed clinician? *(The 12 o'clock to 5 o'clock positions.)*

- What is the transfer zone for a right-handed clinician? *(The 4 o'clock to 7 o'clock positions.)*

- What is the assistant's zone for a right-handed clinician? *(The 2 o'clock 4 o'clock kpositions.)*

- What is the static zone for a right-handed clinician? *(The 12 o'clock to 2 o'cloc positionsk.)*

Slide 19

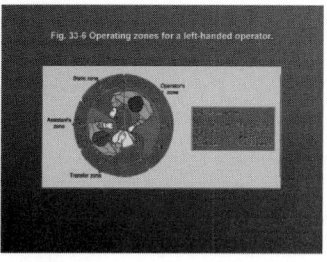

- What is the operator zone for a left-handed clinician? *(5 o'clock to 8 o'clock positions.)*

- What is the transfer zone for a left-handed clinician? *(5 o'clock to 8 o'clock positions.)*

- What is the assistant's zone for a left-handed clinician? *(8 o'clock to 10 o'clock positions.)*

- What is the static zone for a left-handed clinician? *(10 o'clock to 12 o'clock positions.)*

Slide 20

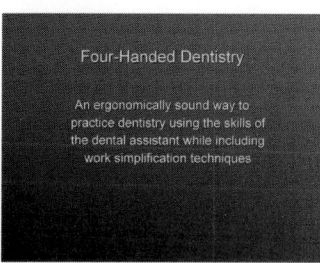

- What is the key term that describes the focus of four-handed dentistry?

- Instrument transfer or instrument exchange takes place in which zone?

- What is the role of the dental assistant during four-handed dentistry?

- Who benefits from a standardized operating sequence?

- How do the patient and the dental team benefit?

Bird/Robinson

Slide 21

Slide 22

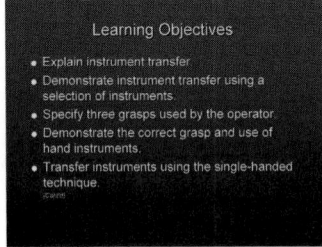

Slide 23

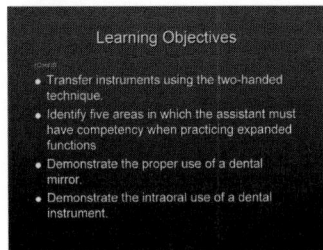

Slide 24

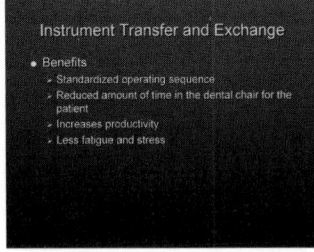

- Transferring instruments should be exchanged with a class I, class II and class III motion. These motions involve only the fingers, wrist and elbows.

- Describe a class I motion and give an example. *(Movement of fingers only.)*

- Describe a class II motion and give an example. *(Movement of wrist and fingers.)*

- Describe a class III motion and give an example. *(Movement of fingers, wrist, and elbow.)*

Torres and Ehrlich Modern Dental Assisting, 9th ed.

Slide 25

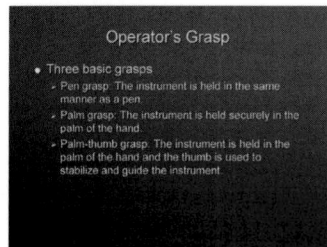

- Can you define the term *grasp*? *(Grasp is the correct way an instrument or handpiece is held.)*
- What affects the manner in which the operator grasps and holds an instrument? *(The instrument type, the way it is used, and the area of the mouth in which it is being used.)*

Slide 26

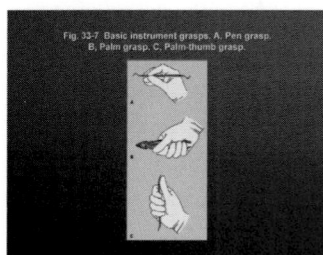

- Can you identify the grasps pictured on the slide? *(A: pen grasp; B: palm grasp; C: palm-thumb grasp.)*
- Can you identify when each grasp would be used? *(Pen grasp: explorer; palm grasp: surgical forceps; palm-thumb grasp: cotton pliers.)*

Slide 27

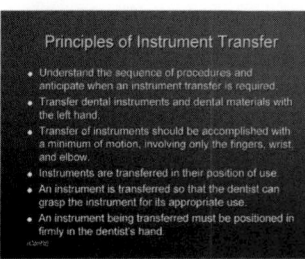

- If transferring of the dental instruments is done with the dental assistant's left hand, what is the function of the dental assistant's right hand? *(The right hand is kept free to suction and to ready the next materials and instruments.)*
- When transferring instruments, the working end or the position of use is pointed downward for mandible areas or pointed upward for maxillary areas.
- Why is it important to transfer instruments to the dentist in the position for use? *(So the dentist does not have to reposition the instrument in his or her hands before use.)*
- Assistant transfer technique is usually a single-handed technique.

Slide 28

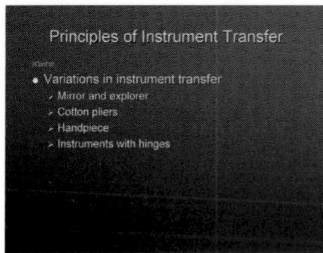

- Why are different instrument exchange procedures necessary? *(It is necessary because of variations in instrument design.)*
- The dental assistant delivers the mirror and explorer simultaneously, using a two-handed exchange.
- What signal is used by the dentist to indicate the need for the mirror and explorer? *(The dentist places one hand on each side of the patient's mouth in position ready to receive the instrument.)*
- The dental assistant delivers the pliers to the dentist while pinching the "beaks" to avoid dropping the item being held in the pliers.
- Take care to avoid tangling the hoses during handpiece transfer.
- Rubber dam forceps, surgical forceps, orthodontic pliers, and scissors should be transferred with care. Hold the instruments at the hinge and transfer by directing their handles into the dentist's palm *(Scissors are placed over the dentist's fingers.)*

Torres and Ehrlich Modern Dental Assisting, 9th ed.

Bird/Robinson

Slide 29

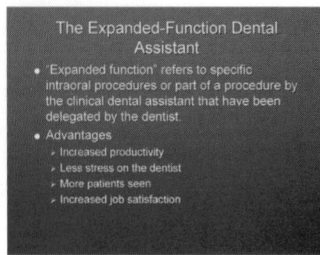

- Expanded-function dental assistants (EFDA) must be credentialed according to state guidelines. Most states require dental assistants to receive formal education before they can legally perform expanded function duties.
- What are approved educational training programs? *(Accredited dental assisting programs, programs approved by the state dental board but not accredited, specific course(s) approved by the state dental board.)*
- Who or what dictates if the expanded function must be under the direct or indirect supervision of the dentist? *(The dental practice act for that state.)*
- What is direct supervision? *(The dentist must be in the same treatment area as the EFDA for the assistant to perform the function.)*
- What is indirect supervision? *(The dentist must be in the dental office area, but not specifically in the same treatment room as the EFDA, and must be available to evaluate the assistant's expanded function.)*

Slide 30

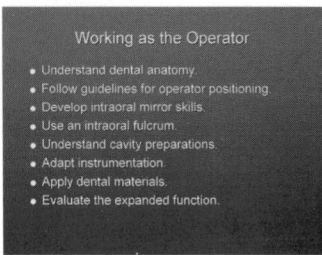

- A dental assistant carrying out an expanded function assumes the role of an operator.
- It is imperative that the EFDA become knowledgeable and competent in the areas listed on this slide.

34 Lesson Plan
Dental Hand Instruments

TEACHING FOCUS

This chapter will introduce the student to topics related to dental hand instruments. The student will be shown how to identify hand instruments and shown Black's instrument formula and instrument classification and sequencing. We will discuss examination instruments, hand-cutting instruments, restorative instruments, and accessory instruments and items,. The student will have the opportunity to put the above information into context by participating in classroom activities and discussions.

MATERIALS AND RESOURCES

- ☐ amalgam carrier (Lesson 34.2)
- ☐ amalgam knife (Lesson 34.2)
- ☐ articulating paper (Lesson 34.1)
- ☐ burnisher (Lesson 34.2)
- ☐ carver (Lesson 34.2)
- ☐ chisel (Lesson 34.1)
- ☐ composite placement instrument (Lesson 34.2)
- ☐ computer and PowerPoint projector (all Lessons)
- ☐ condensers (Lesson 34.2)
- ☐ cotton pliers (Lesson 34.1)
- ☐ dappen dish (Lesson 34.2)
- ☐ excavator (Lesson 34.1)

- ☐ explorer (Lesson 34.1)
- ☐ gingival margin trimmer (Lesson 34.1)
- ☐ hatchet (Lesson 34.1)
- ☐ hoe (Lesson 34.1)
- ☐ Hollenback carver (Lesson 34.2)
- ☐ Howe pliers (Lesson 34.2)
- ☐ mouth mirror (Lesson 34.1)
- ☐ nonlocking cotton pliers (Lesson 34.1)
- ☐ periodontal probe (Lesson 34.1)
- ☐ preset restorative tray (Lesson 34.2)
- ☐ scissors (Lesson 34.2)
- ☐ spatula (Lesson 34.2)
- ☐ spoon excavator (Lesson 34.1)
- ☐ storage tub (Lesson 34.2)

LESSON CHECKLIST

Preparations for this lesson include:

- lecture
- evaluation of student knowledge and skills needed to perform all entry-level activities related to dental hand instruments, including:
  - ○ Black's instrument formula
  - ○ design of instruments
  - ○ identification of instruments, including examination instruments, hand-cutting instruments, and restorative instruments
  - ○ instrument classification, including sequencing
  - ○ instrument setup

Torres and Ehrlich Modern Dental Assisting, 9th ed.

Copyright © 2009, 2006 by Saunders, an imprint of Elsevier Inc. All rights reserved.

Bird/Robinson

KEY TERMS

beveled (p. 503)
blade (p. 498)
handle (p. 498)
nib (p. 498)
plane (p. 503)

point (p. 498)
serrated (p. 498)
shank (p. 498)
tactile (p. 500)
working end (p. 498)

ADDITIONAL RESOURCES

PowerPoint slides (Evolve): 1-20

Legend

CTQ
Critical
Thinking
Question

DVD
Multimedia
Procedures
Videos and
Animations

ESLR
EVOLVE
Student
Learning
Resources

IDO
Interactive
Dental
Office
CD-ROM

SW
Student
Workbook

TB
Test Bank
on the
TEACH
CD-ROM

PPT
PowerPoint
Slides

Class Activities are indicated in ***bold italic.***

ELSEVIER

Torres and Ehrlich Modern Dental Assisting, 9th ed.

Bird/Robinson

LESSON 34.1

PRETEST

1. Hand instruments are designed with three specific parts. The three parts include the handle, shank, and
   a. working end.
   b. articulation.
   c. nib.
   d. angulation.

2. What does the third number of the G.V. Black's Instrument Formula describe?
   a. width of the blade
   b. angle of the blade
   c. length of the blade
   d. thickness of the blade

3. Which term describes the design of the tip of the explorer?
   a. thin, wire-like
   b. triangular in cross-section
   c. rigid
   d. nonflexible

4. The working end of the probe is calibrated in
   a. centimeters.
   b. millimeters.
   c. decimeters.
   d. inches.

5. Which instruments are set up for every procedure and are also called the examination setup?
   a. mirror, probe, explorer
   b. probe, scissors, explorer
   c. mirror, explorer, cotton forceps
   d. explorer, probe, cotton forceps

6. Which instruments are placed on the tray setup after the examination setup?
   a. hand-cutting instruments
   b. restorative instruments
   c. accessory instruments
   d. surgical instruments

7. Which instrument is considered a restorative instrument containing two wells on either end to transport freshly packed, mixed amalgam to a prepared tooth?
   a. amalgam burnisher
   b. amalgam carver
   c. amalgam condenser
   d. amalgam carrier

8. What restorative material is made from anodized aluminum and Teflon?
   a. amalgam
   b. composite
   c. gutta percha
   d. porcelain

9. This is a small glass bowl with different-sized wells on either side used to hold liquid dental materials.
   a. amalgam well
   b. spatula
   c. dappen dish
   d. storage tub

10. Which instrument is the instrument of choice to remove excess dental materials from interproximal spaces?
    a. Hollenback carver
    b. spoon excavator
    c. discoid-cleoid carver
    d. amalgam burnisher

Answers

1. a	3. a	5. c	7. d	9. c
2. b	4. b	6. a	8. b	10. a

Torres and Ehrlich Modern Dental Assisting, 9th ed.

Bird/Robinson

BACKGROUND ASSESSMENT

Question: What are dental instruments primarily made of and why? How are dental instruments identified?
Answer: Dental instruments are made primarily from stainless steel or carbon steel, plastic, or specialized metal because the instruments need to withstand constant use and sterilization procedures. Instruments are identified by name or with a three-number system known as G.V. Black's Instrument Formula. The first number identifies the width of the blade; the second number identifies the length of the blade; and the third number identifies the angle of the blade.

Question: What are the classifications of dental hand instruments? What is the recommended hand instrument sequence tray setup?
Answer: Dental hand instruments are classified into four categories: examination instruments, hand-cutting instruments, restorative instruments, and accessory instruments. These hand instruments are set up on the tray from left to right, starting with the examination instruments, followed by hand-cutting instruments, then restorative instruments. Accessory instruments should be situated on the counter top or within reach in an organized and sequenced manner. The rationale for this sequence is based on the way instruments are transferred and used throughout a dental procedure.

CRITICAL THINKING QUESTION

Dr. Smith has assigned one of the dental assistants the responsibility of setting up procedure trays to be sterilized and prepared for various procedures throughout the day. The dental assistant is responsible for putting together trays that are consistent and uniform, but which also meet the specific needs of all of the dentists in the office. Which instruments should the dental assistant place on the tray setup for an amalgam restoration, and in what sequence?

Guidelines: The examination instruments would be first, starting from the left side of the tray. The examination instruments would include the mouth mirror, double-ended explorer (right angle, pig tail and/or Shepard's hook explorer), cotton pliers, a periodontal probe, and articulating paper and paper holder. Next to the examination instruments would be the hand-cutting instruments, which are used to remove decayed tooth structures, smooth cavity walls and floors of preparations, and place retention grooves or bevels in dental materials. These include excavator (spoon and/or black spoon), hoes, chisels (straight, bin-angle, Wedelstaedt and/or angle-former), hatchets, and gingival margin trimmers. Next would be amalgam restorative instruments, which would include the amalgam carrier, condensers, burnishers (ball, football, T-ball, and/or the beaver tail), carvers (discoid-cleoid and/or the Hollenback), and the amalgam knife. The final instrument group on the tray (or within reach) would include accessory instruments such as spatulas (cement or single-ended), scissors (crown and bridge scissors with straight or curved blades), dappen dish/amalgam well, and/or Howe pliers/110 pliers.

OBJECTIVES	CONTENT	TEACHING RESOURCES
Define and spell the Key Terms.	■ Key terms (p. 497)	*e* ESLR Electronic Flashcards ▸ Discuss each of the key terms in Chapter 34, focusing on the definition, pronunciation, and spelling of each term. *Class Activity Have the students write definitions of the terms in their own words in lay terms. Then have them define the words using professional terms. Then divide the class into student pairs. Each pair of students will role-play, with one student acting as the dental assistant and the other as a patient, then a colleague. The dental assistant will explain the key terms to his or her partner in lay terms first and then in professional terms. Encourage the student playing the roles of the patient/colleague to ask questions to promote further explanation by the dental assistant.*

ELSEVIER

Bird/Robinson

OBJECTIVES	CONTENT	TEACHING RESOURCES
Describe the three parts of a dental hand instrument.	■ Identifying hand instruments (p. 498) ☐ Instrument number (p. 498) ☐ Instrument design (p. 498) – Handle (p. 498) – Shank (p. 498) – Working end (p. 498)	▣▤ PPT 5-8 ▥ TB questions 1-3, 13 ◆ SW Short-Answer Questions 1; Fill in the Blank questions 2-3, 5-7, 9-10; Multiple Choice questions 1-2 (pp. 233-234) Figure 34-1 Catalog or call number associated with Howe pliers (p. 498) Figure 34-2 Three parts of a dental hand instrument (p. 498) Recall questions 1-2 (p. 499) ▸ Discuss identifying hand instruments. Note that it is the dental assistant's responsibility to identify and set up hand instruments in a precise order of use. ▸ Discuss the three specific parts of hand instruments and the purpose of their design. *Class Activity **Have each student draw a dental hand instrument and label the three parts. Then have each student identify the parts and describe the parts in his or her own words.***
Describe the instrument formula designed by G.V. Black.	☐ Black's instrument formula (p. 498)	◆ SW Short-Answer Questions 2 (p. 233) Figure 34-3 Black's instrument formula (p. 499) Table 34-1 Numbers in G.V. Black's Instrument Formula (p. 499) Recall questions 1-2 (p. 499) ▸ Discuss Black's instrument formula that describes the angulations and dimensions of the working end of a hand instrument. Note that the three numbers in the formula identify the blade's width, length, and angle. ▸ Discuss the importance of learning instrument numbers. Note that dentists often refer to pliers and forceps by number rather than name. *Class Activity **Before class, assign each student a dental hand instrument using G.V. Black's Instrument Formula and have the students research the instruments on the Internet. In the classroom, the students will present their instruments and the design characteristics based on the three-number system. (For students to prepare for this activity, see Homework/Assignments #1.)***
Discuss the theory of placing an instrument in a	■ Instrument classification (p. 499) ☐ Instrument sequence (p. 499)	▣▤ PPT 9 ▥ TB questions 4-5

OBJECTIVES	CONTENT	TEACHING RESOURCES
specific sequence.		SW Short-Answer Questions 8; Multiple Choice question 3 (pp. 233-234) CTQ 1-2, 4 (p. 509) ▸ Discuss the four categories of instrument classification, and explain the general use of the instruments in each category. ▸ Discuss the dental assistant's use of the left hand when transferring instruments. *Class Activity Have each student list instruments according to how he or she would set them up on a tray. Have the students then share their tray sequence in class and discuss their rationale for the sequence.*
List the examination instruments and their uses.	☐ Examination instruments (p. 499) – Basic setup (p. 500)	PPT 10-11 TB question 6, 14 SW Short-Answer Questions 3; Fill in the Blank question 1; Multiple Choice questions 4-7 (pp. 233-234) SW Activity (p. 235) Figure 34-4 Tray setup showing appropriate sequence of instruments (p. 499) Figure 34-5 Examination instruments (p. 500) Figure 34-6 Uses for the mouth mirror (p. 501) Recall questions 3-7 (p. 501) Figure 34-7 Basic setup that includes mouth mirror, explorer, and cotton pliers (p. 501) Figure 34-8 . Transferring mirror and explorer simultaneously to operator (p. 502) CTQ 2 (p. 509) ▸ Discuss the basic setup, noting that the mouth mirror, double-ended explorer, and cotton pliers are set up for every procedure. ▸ Discuss the four major uses of the mouth mirror, including indirect vision, light reflection, retraction, and tissue protection. *Class Activity Divide the class into student pairs. Have each student create two index cards with the name of an examination instrument on one side and its use on the reverse. Have the students exchange their cards and critique each other's descriptions.*

OBJECTIVES	CONTENT	TEACHING RESOURCES
Identify examination instruments.	☐ Examination instruments (p. 499) – Basic setup (p. 500) Procedure 34-1 Identifying examination instruments (p. 502) (SW/ESLR Competencies 34-1 through 34-4, p. 237)	☐ *e* SW/ESLR Competencies 34-1 through 34-4 Identification of Dental Instruments for a Restorative Procedure (p. 237) ▸ Discuss the distinguishing features of the mouth mirror, explorer, cotton pliers, periodontal probe, articulating paper, and articulating paper holder. **Class Activity** *Divide the class into small groups. Have each group choose examination instruments randomly from a box of instruments supplied by the instructor. Have each group identify the name, number and function of the examination instrument.*
List the types of hand (manual) cutting instruments and their uses.	☐ Hand-cutting instruments (p. 501)	☒ PPT 12 TB question 7 (p. 408) SW Short-Answer Questions 4; Fill in the Blank questions 4, 8; Multiple Choice question 8 (pp. 233-234) Recall question 8 (p. 502) Figure 34-9. Hand (manual) cutting instruments (pp. 503-504) CTQ 3 (p. 509) ▸ Discuss hand (manual) cutting instruments. List these instruments and their uses. **Class Activity** *Before class, have each student research a cutting instrument on the Internet. In class, the students will present the instruments they identified and the uses, along with the instrument design features. (For students to prepare for this activity, see Homework/Assignments #2.)*
Identify hand (manual) cutting instruments.	☐ Hand-cutting instruments (p. 501) Procedure 34-2 Identifying hand (manual) cutting instruments (p. 502) (SW/ESLR Competencies 34-1 through 34-4, p. 237)	TB question 8 SW/ESLR Competencies 34-1 through 34-4 Identification of Dental Instruments for a Restorative Procedure (p. 237) ▸ Discuss the distinguishing features of the evacuator, hoe, chisel, hatchet, and gingival margin trimmer. **Class Activity** *Divide the class into groups of three or four. Have each group choose cutting instruments randomly from a box of instruments supplied by the instructor and identify the name, number, and function of each cutting instrument.*

34.1 Homework/Assignments:

1. Assign each student a dental hand-instrument using G.V. Black's Instrument Formula. Each student will research the instrument on the Internet.

2. Before class, have each student research a cutting instrument on the Internet.

34.1 Instructor's Notes/Student Feedback:

LESSON 34.2

CRITICAL THINKING QUESTION

You have just been hired in a dental practice where the restorative material of choice is amalgam. The hiring dentist has commented on how he and the other dentists struggle when placing amalgams because each of the dentists in the practice has his or her own sequence and instrument choice and the dental assistants can't keep each of their preferences straight. You have been assigned the task of preparing amalgam tray setups that will be placed in each of the operatories. These setups will be used by different dentists and dental assistants. It is important to have all of the trays set up in the same manner for convenience and efficiency. What specialized instruments are used to place an amalgam restoration? What variations of each of the instruments are available? What accessory items should be included to complete an amalgam restoration tray setup?

Guidelines: Restorative instruments are used to place, condense, and carve the restorative material back to the normal anatomy of that tooth. The amalgam trays will be set up from left to right, starting with examination instruments: dental mirror, explorer, and cotton forceps. Next, at least two hand-cutting instruments are placed on the tray (the spoon excavator and the Wedelstaedt chisel are two common hand- cutting instruments). Following the hand-cutting instruments will be the instruments used to place the amalgam: the amalgam carrier and the condenser. The amalgam carrier is a double-ended instrument with two wells to transport amalgam to the prepared tooth. The condenser is another double-ended instrument used to pack the amalgam into the prepared tooth. At least two different condensers will be available on the tray in varying sizes. Next on the tray, amalgam finishing instruments will be placed: the burnisher and the amalgam carver. The burnisher is used to smooth the freshly packed amalgam in the prepared tooth. At least two burnishers of varying shapes will be available: the ball- and football-shaped are the most commonly used. The amalgam carver is an instrument designed with a sharp edge to remove excess materials, contour surfaces, and carve anatomy into the amalgam. Most dentists prefer the discoid-cleoid carver and the Hollenback carver. The amalgam knife should be available on the tray for the removal of material along the margin between the filling and the tooth. Additional accessories should also be available on the tray during amalgam restoration placement, including the amalgam well, squeeze cloth, Howe pliers, matrix band and holder, and small crown and bridge scissors.

OBJECTIVES	CONTENT	TEACHING RESOURCES
List the types of restorative instruments and their uses.	☐ Restorative instruments (p. 502)	🗒 PPT 15 🖥 TB question 9 SW Short-Answer Questions 5; Multiple Choice questions 9-12, 15 (pp. 233-235) Figure 34-10 Restorative instruments (pp. 505-506) Recall questions 9-11 (p. 503) ▸ Discuss the sequencing of restorative instruments. ▸ Discuss the purpose and uses of double-ended instruments. *Class Activity Have each student create three different tables: one table for amalgam restorative instruments, a second table for composite instruments, and a third table for crown and bridge instruments. Have students complete their tables by filling in information pertaining to the type and function of each instrument. Have the students compare their tables with those of their classmates.*

OBJECTIVES	CONTENT	TEACHING RESOURCES
Identify restorative instruments.	☐ Restorative instruments (p. 502) ⎡Procedure⎤ 34-3 Identifying restorative instruments (p. 504) (SW/ESLR Competencies 34-1 through 34-4, p. 237)	💻 TB question 10 🖥️ 𝒆 SW/ESLR Competencies 34-1 through 34-4 Identification of Dental Instruments for a Restorative Procedure (p. 237) ▸ Discuss the distinguishing features of the amalgam carrier, condenser, burnisher, carver, amalgam knife, and composite placement instruments. *Class Activity Divide the class into small groups, and have each group choose restorative instruments randomly from a box of instruments supplied by the instructor. Then have each group identify the name, number, and function of each restorative instrument.*
Describe additional accessory instruments and items used in general dentistry.	☐ Accessory instruments and items (p. 503)	🖥️ PPT 16 🖥️ SW Short-Answer Questions 6; Multiple Choice questions 13-14 (pp. 233, 235) Figure 34-11 Accessory instruments and items (p. 507) Recall questions 12-14 (p. 503) 💡 CTQ 5 (p. 509) ▸ Discuss accessory items, noting that they are not necessarily on the tray setup but may be pulled from cabinets or tubs as needed. *Class Activity Have each student create a list of accessory instruments and describe the function and use of each instrument. Then have the students share their lists with the class.*
Identify accessory instruments and items.	☐ Accessory instruments and items (p. 503) ⎡Procedure⎤ 34-4 Identifying accessory instruments and items (p. 505) (SW/ESLR Competencies 34-1 through 34-4, p. 237)	💻 TB question 11 🖥️ 𝒆 SW/ESLR Competencies 34-1 through 34-4 Identification of Dental Instruments for a Restorative Procedure (p. 237) ▸ Discuss the distinguishing features of the cement spatula, impression spatula, scissors, dappen dish, amalgam well, and Howe pliers. *Class Activity Divide the class into small groups, and have each group choose accessory instruments randomly from a box of instruments supplied by the instructor. Have each group identify the name, number, and function of each accessory instrument.*
Describe the use of preset trays and tubs in dentistry.	☐ Preset cassettes (trays) (p. 508) ☐ Storage tubs (p. 508) ☐ Color-coding systems (p. 508)	🖥️ PPT 17-20 💻 TB question 12 🖥️ SW Short-Answer Questions 7 (p. 233) Figure 34-12 Preset restorative tray (p. 508)

Torres and Ehrlich Modern Dental Assisting, 9th ed.

Bird/Robinson

OBJECTIVES	CONTENT	TEACHING RESOURCES
		Figure 34-13 Storage tub holding additional items needed for a procedure (p. 508)
		Legal and Ethical Implications (p. 508)
		Eye to the Future (p. 508)
		⚲ CTQ 5 (p. 509)
		▸ Discuss the purpose of preset cassettes or trays, noting common procedures for which preset trays might be available.
		▸ Discuss the use of color-coding in organizing instruments and supplies for specific procedures.
		Class Activity Divide the students into pairs. Assign two treatment procedures to each pair. Each pair will create a list of the contents of preset trays or tubs for their assigned treatment procedures. Have the pairs share their lists with the class.
Performance Evaluation		🖥 TB
		📖 SW questions (pp. 233-235)
		📖 *e* SW/ESLR Competencies 34-1 through 34-4 Identification of Dental Instruments for a Restorative Procedure (p. 237)
		e ESLR Electronic Flashcards
		e ESLR Practice Quiz
		Recall questions (pp. 499-503)
		⚲ CTQ (p. 509)

34.2 Homework/Assignments:

34.2 Instructor's Notes/Student Feedback:

Slide 1

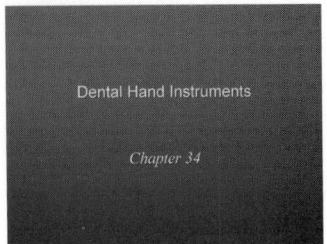

Dental Hand Instruments

Chapter 34

Slide 2

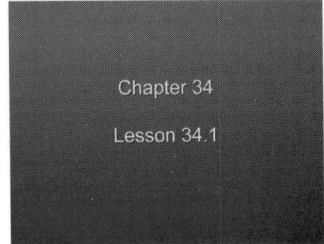

Chapter 34

Lesson 34.1

Slide 3

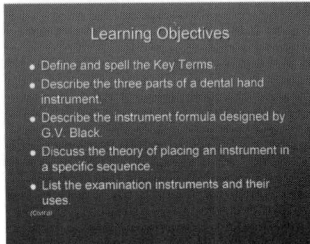

Learning Objectives

- Define and spell the Key Terms.
- Describe the three parts of a dental hand instrument.
- Describe the instrument formula designed by G.V. Black.
- Discuss the theory of placing an instrument in a specific sequence.
- List the examination instruments and their uses.

(Cont'd)

Slide 4

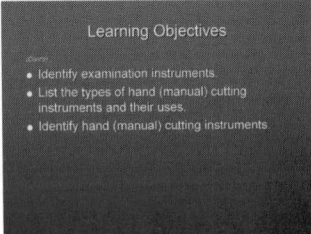

Learning Objectives

(Cont'd)

- Identify examination instruments.
- List the types of hand (manual) cutting instruments and their uses.
- Identify hand (manual) cutting instruments.

Slide 5

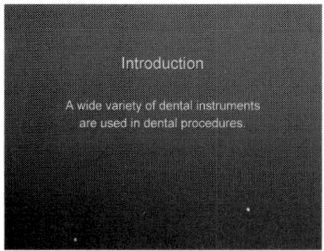

- Today's discussion will include the purpose of dental instruments that are most commonly used in dentistry for general restorative purposes.

Slide 6

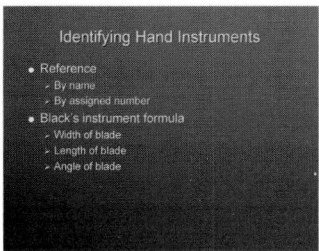

- Most hand instruments are made of stainless steel, carbon steel, plastic, or specialized metal.

- The dentist will refer to an instrument either by name or by number. This number is a universal representation of the instrument.

- G.V. Black designed a formula that describes the angulations and dimensions of the working ends of hand instruments.

- Why is it important that the dental assistant have knowledge regarding instrument design and usage?

Slide 7

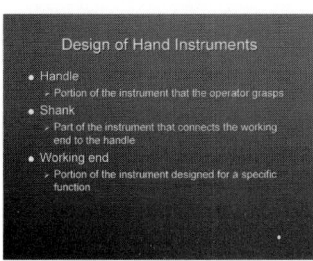

- What are the advantages to having a larger circumference handle? (*Larger handles are ergonomically designed to reduce fatigue and stress on hand muscles.*)

- Where would you use an instrument that had an angled shank? (*Posterior areas.*)

- The working end can have a point, blade, or nib. Instruments can also be single ended or double ended. Double-ended instruments are mirror images or have reverse angles.

- What are mirror imaged instruments called? (*Left and right instruments.*)

Slide 8

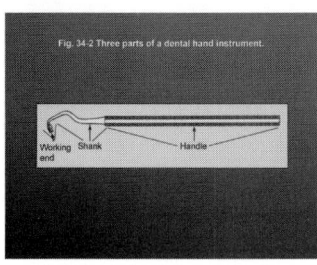

- Can you define each part of the instrument in your own words?

- What information is found on the handle of a dental instrument? (*Name of the instrument, manufacturer's name, and the universal identification number.*)

Slide 9

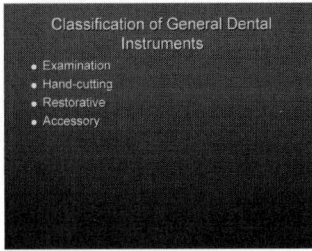

- In what procedures would an examination instrument be used? (*Caries examination, soft tissue oral inspection, periodontal assessment, etc.*)

- In what procedures are hand cutting instruments used? (*To cut bevels in the cavity prep, to remove decay lying close to the pulp, removal of soft dentin, etc.*)

- In what procedures are restorative instruments used? (*Amalgam placement, composite placement, etc.*)

- Can students name an accessory instrument?

Slide 10

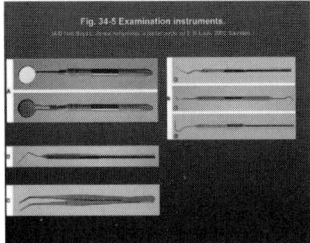

- Mouth mirror: Designed to have a straight handle, a slight angle to the shank, and a working end consisting of a round metal disk with a mirror on one side.

- Why is the tip so thin on explorer instruments? (*Tactile sensitivity is increased.*)

- Periodontal probe is used to measure sulcus and pocket depths of the periodontium of each tooth. The working end is calibrated in millimeters.

- Can you think of something else the periodontal probe can be used to measure? (*Oral lesions and the width of an anterior overjet.*)

Slide 11

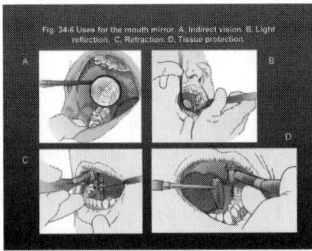

- What are the indirect areas of a patient's mouth for the right-handed operator?

- Light reflection/reflective illumination: Directs additional light into areas of the mouth.

- Retraction: Helps to maintain a clear field and protects the soft tissues from injury from the dental bur or hand instruments.

- What is another function of the dental mirror?

Slide 12

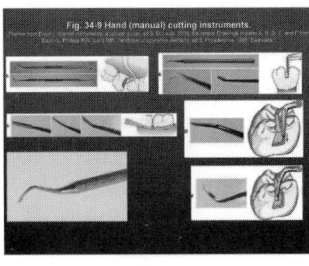

- Hand-cutting instruments are the group of instruments placed on the tray setup after the examination instruments.

- The spoon excavator is the most common excavator used.

- The hoe is similar in appearance to that of a garden tool. The blade is perpendicular to the handle.

- What function do you think the chisel has? Remember, it has a cutting edge. (*Cut enamel margins of the tooth preparation, form sharp lines and point angles, and place retention grooves.*)

Slide 13

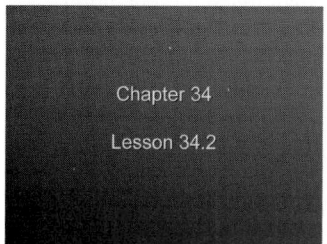

Slide 14

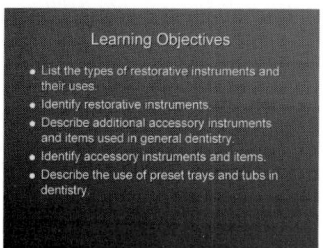

Slide 15

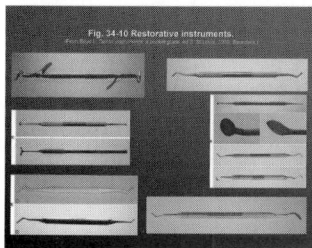

- Restorative instruments are used primarily to place, condense, and carve the restorative dental materials back to the normal anatomy of the tooth. They are primarily made of stainless steel:
  - Amalgam carrier
  - Condensers
  - Burnisher
  - Carvers
  - Amalgam knife
  - Composite placement instruments

Slide 16

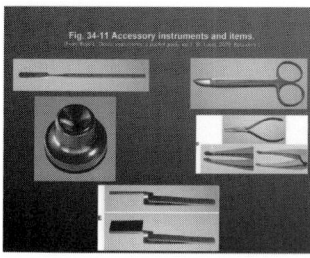

- Accessory instruments are not necessarily kept on the tray but should be readily available when needed:
  - Spatulas
  - Scissors
  - Dappen dish
  - Amalgam well
  - Howe pliers (also called 110 pliers)

Bird/Robinson

Slide 17

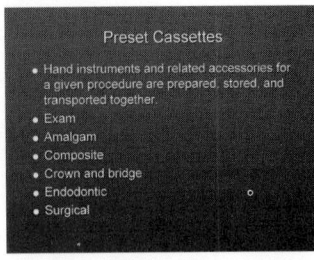

- A dental practice will have sufficient types of cassettes for most common procedures to allow adequate sterilization and preparation time before the tray is needed.

- Sterile trays or cassettes are taken into the treatment area as part of the advance preparation of the treatment room before seating the patient.

- How will you know which trays or cassettes to take into the treatment room prior to seating the patient? (*Look at the daily schedule and patient record to review the patient and the planned procedure.*)

Slide 18

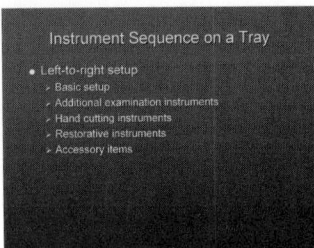

- How do you know what order to use when setting up the tray? (*The sequence is based on how instruments are transferred and used throughout a dental procedure.*)

Slide 19

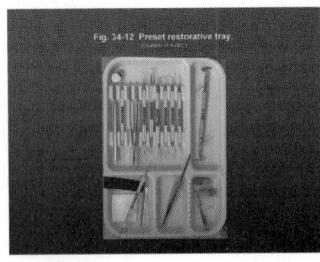

- Note how the examination instruments are placed on the tray, starting from the left. Following the examination instruments are the restorative instruments and then the accessory instruments.

- Based on the setup viewed on the slide, what procedure will be completed? (*Amalgam restoration placement.*)

Slide 20

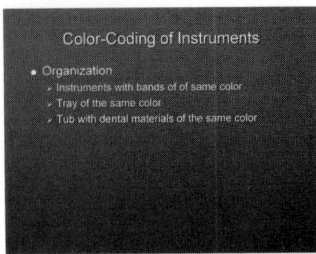

- Color coding the instruments with colored bands on the handles is a common way to organize instruments.

- What are two reasons for using a color-coding system? (*Convenience and efficiency.*)

Bird/Robinson

TEACHING FOCUS

This chapter will introduce the student to topics related to dental handpieces and accessories used in restorative and prosthodontic procedures. The student will become acquainted with dental handpieces, handpiece maintenance, rotary cutting instruments, and dental burs. Identifying and attaching dental handpieces, and identifying and attaching burs to rotary cutting instruments will be emphasized. The student will have the opportunity to put the above information into context by participating in classroom activities and discussions.

MATERIALS AND RESOURCES

- ☐ accessories and attachments for low-speed handpiece (Lesson 35.1)
- ☐ computer and PowerPoint projector (all Lessons)
- ☐ dental rotary instruments (Lesson 35.2)
- ☐ handpieces (all Lessons)
- ☐ index cards (Lesson 35.1)

LESSON CHECKLIST

Preparations for this lesson include:
- lecture
- evaluation of student knowledge and skills needed to perform all entry-level activities related to dental handpieces and accessories, including:
  - o identifying dental handpieces, including the low-speed handpiece, the high-speed handpiece, the ultrasonic handpiece, the laser handpiece, the air abrasion handpiece, and the laboratory handpiece
  - o attaching dental handpieces
  - o performing handpiece maintenance
  - o identifying rotary cutting instruments, including shank types, dental burs, diamond rotary instruments, finishing rotary instruments, abrasive rotary instruments, and laboratory rotary instruments
  - o attaching burs to rotary cutting instruments

ELSEVIER

Torres and Ehrlich Modern Dental Assisting, 9th ed.

KEY TERMS

bur (p. 517)
console (p. 513)
dental handpiece (p. 511)
flutes (p. 519)
laser (p. 513)

mandrel (p. 520)
rotary (p. 516)
shank (p. 516)
torque (p. 514)
ultrasonic (p. 513)

ADDITIONAL RESOURCES

PowerPoint slides (Evolve): 1-32
Multimedia Procedures DVD: Identifying and Attaching Handpieces

Legend

CTQ
Critical
Thinking
Question

DVD
Multimedia
Procedures
Videos and
Animations

ESLR
EVOLVE
Student
Learning
Resources

IDO
Interactive
Dental
Office
CD-ROM

SW
Student
Workbook

TB
Test Bank
on the
TEACH
CD-ROM

PPT
PowerPoint
Slides

Class Activities are indicated in ***bold italic.***

ELSEVIER

Torres and Ehrlich Modern Dental Assisting, 9th ed.

Bird/Robinson

LESSON 35.1

PRETEST

1. What is the definition of the term *mandrel*?
   a. part of an instrument in which the handle attaches to the working end
   b. metal shaft on which a sandpaper disk or abrasive material is mounted
   c. blades on a working end of a finishing rotary instrument
   d. mechanical radiant energy of water

2. When were rotary instruments introduced to dentistry?
   a. 1880s
   b. 1920s
   c. 1940s
   d. 1970s

3. Which handpiece is considered the most versatile handpiece used in dentistry?
   a. low-speed handpiece
   b. high-speed handpiece
   c. ultrasonic handpiece
   d. laser handpiece

4. The low-speed handpiece is available in speeds ranging from 10,000 rpm to
   a. 20,000 rpm.
   b. 30,000 rpm.
   c. 50,000 rpm.
   d. 75,000 rpm.

5. Which handpiece is used by the dentist in every restorative procedure?
   a. low-speed handpiece
   b. high-speed handpiece
   c. ultrasonic handpiece
   d. laser handpiece

6. How many rpm can the high-speed handpiece reach?
   a. 150,000 rpm
   b. 250,000 rpm
   c. 350,000 rpm
   d. 450,000 rpm

7. What mechanism is used to hold the bur in a high-speed handpiece?
   a. friction grip
   b. mandrel
   c. latch hook
   d. snap in

8. Which handpiece uses mechanical radiant energy of water and sound vibrations to create a pulsating effect on the tooth surface?
   a. low-speed handpiece
   b. high-speed handpiece
   c. ultrasonic handpiece
   d. laser handpiece

9. Which handpiece uses a beam of light to cauterize soft tissue or vaporize decayed tooth structure?
   a. low-speed handpiece
   b. high-speed handpiece
   c. ultrasonic handpiece
   d. laser handpiece

10. Because it comes into contact with blood, saliva, and tissue and must be sterilized before reuse, the dental handpiece is identified as a
    a. critical instrument.
    b. straight attachment.
    c. dental bur.
    d. latch-type shank.

Answers

1. b	3. a	5. b	7. a	9. d
2. c	4. b	6. d	8. c	10. a

Torres and Ehrlich Modern Dental Assisting, 9th ed.

Bird/Robinson

BACKGROUND ASSESSMENT

Question: When were handpieces and rotary instruments introduced to dentistry? How are they used in dentistry today? How have handpieces evolved since their introduction?

Answer: Handpieces and rotary instruments were introduced to dentistry in the 1940s. Handpieces are used to complement the use of hand instruments in the cutting, grinding, and polishing procedures performed daily in dentistry, Handpieces have come a long way since their introduction into dentistry. The first dental handpiece was belt driven. The long belt operated by running over a series of pulleys then back to a motor that continuously rotated the inserted rotary instrument. In the 1940s and 1950s, diamond cutting burs and tungsten carbide burs were invented, which greatly improved how the dentist cuts into hard tooth structures. Air-drive turbine handpieces were introduced in the 1950s.

Question: What types of handpieces are used in dentistry today?

Answer: Six different types of handpieces are used in dentistry today: the low-speed handpiece, high-speed handpiece, ultrasonic handpiece, laser handpiece, air abrasion handpiece, and laboratory handpiece. The low-speed handpiece, also known as the straight handpiece, is very versatile and can be used for laboratory or clinical procedures. The speed of this handpiece is relatively low, ranging from 10,000 to 30,000 rpm. The high-speed handpiece is used by the dentist in all restorative procedures. It operates with air pressure and reaches speeds up to 450,000 rpm. The ultrasonic handpiece uses mechanical radiant energy of water and sound vibrations to create a pulsating effect on the tooth surface to remove debris, stain, bonding materials, and cement. The laser handpiece uses a beam of laser light to cauterize soft tissue or vaporize decayed tooth structure. The air abrasion handpiece is a small version of the sandblaster. It has regained it popularity in dentistry because it is patient-friendly and requires no local anesthesia administration for dental procedures. The last handpiece, the laboratory handpiece, is designed for dental laboratories and operates at speeds up to 20,000 rpm.

CRITICAL THINKING QUESTION

The dental assistant is preparing a two-surface amalgam restoration on tooth #3. The patient's dental record indicates that the decay is surrounding a partially present existing restoration. The dentist has determined that the original filling is partially missing due to poor retention and undercuts in the original preparation. The patient's record also notes that the patient fears needles and administration of local anesthetic. What handpieces should the dental assistant prepare for the procedure, and why? Which rotary instruments should be used?

Guidelines: The high-speed handpiece should be the initial handpiece used in this procedure. In this situation, the high-speed is useful in removing decay and the existing faulty restoration. This handpiece can also be used to outline new retention grooves to mechanically lock the new filling into place. The second handpiece used to complete this procedure is the low-speed handpiece. It is used to remove any residual soft decay and to finish the cavity preparation, and also to polish the restoration after the new restoration is in place. When a patient fears needles and local anesthesia, the laser handpiece or the air abrasion handpiece generally can be used as alternatives. However, neither would be useful in this situation due to the existing restoration. These alternative handpieces are useful in removing decay without the use of local anesthesia but may not be successful in removing faulty restorative materials. The rotary instruments that should be used to remove old faulty restorations and decay include cutting burs with a round or inverted cone shape. Preparation of the internal walls can be established with a straight fissured bur. If retention angles need to be made, a tapered bur should be used. After the new restoration is in place, polishing or finishing may be needed.

OBJECTIVES	CONTENT	TEACHING RESOURCES
Pronounce, define, and spell the Key Terms.	■ Key terms (p. 510)	📖 SW Fill in the Blank questions 1-12 (pp. 239-240) 💿 ESLR Electronic Flashcards ▸ Discuss each of the key terms in Chapter 35, focusing on the definition, pronunciation, and spelling of each term.

ELSEVIER

Torres and Ehrlich Modern Dental Assisting, 9th ed.
Bird/Robinson

OBJECTIVES	CONTENT	TEACHING RESOURCES
		Class Activity Have students make flash cards for the key terms by writing the key terms on one side of an index card and the definitions on the other. Then have the students quiz each other with the flash cards.
Discuss the historical importance of the dental handpiece.	■ Evolution of rotary equipment (p. 511)	PPT 5-6 TB question 1 SW Short-Answer Questions 1; Multiple Choice question 1 (pp. 239-240) Figure 35-1 Belt-driven handpiece (p. 511) Recall question 1 (p. 512) ▸ Discuss the dental functions performed by rotary equipment. ▸ Discuss the advancements in rotary equipment that have been made since being introduced in the 1940s. *Class Activity Have the students conduct Internet research on the history of dental handpieces and how they have changed dental procedures. Have each student write a description of one dental procedure, explain how the procedure would have been performed before the introduction of the handpiece, and compare how it is carried out today. Have the students share their findings with the class. (For students to prepare for this Activity, see Homework/Assignments #1.)*
Describe the low-speed handpiece and its use in dentistry.	■ Dental handpieces (p. 511) □ Low-speed handpiece (p. 511) – Uses of the low-speed handpiece (p. 511)	PPT 7-10 TB questions 2-4 SW Short-Answer Questions 2; Multiple Choice questions 2-3 (pp. 239-240) Figure 35-2 Low-speed handpiece (p. 511) Recall questions 2-3 (p. 512) ▸ Discuss the different sizes and speeds of the low-speed handpiece. ▸ Discuss the clinical and laboratory uses of the low-speed handpiece. *Class Activity Have each student create a list of dental procedures and how each procedure is completed using the low-speed handpiece. Then have the students exchange their lists with classmates.*
Describe the attachments used on the low-speed handpiece.	– Straight attachment (p. 512) – Contra-angle attachment (p. 512) – Prophylaxis angle (p. 512)	PPT 11-13 TB question 5 SW Short-Answer Questions 3; Multiple Choice questions 4, 10; Topics for Discussion question 2 (pp. 239-241)

ELSEVIER

Torres and Ehrlich Modern Dental Assisting, 9th ed.
Bird/Robinson

OBJECTIVES	CONTENT	TEACHING RESOURCES
		Figure 35-3 Straight attachment slides onto the low-speed motor (p. 512)
		Figure 35-4 Contra-angle attachment (p. 512)
		Figure 35-3 Disposable prophy cup and brush (p. 512)
		Recall question 4 (p. 512)
		▶ Discuss the straight attachment. Describe the attachment and note its most common uses.
		▶ Discuss the purpose of the angle on the contra-angle attachment and the prophylaxis angle attachment. Note the circumstances under which each attachment is used.
		Class Activity Provide the class with a variety of attachments that can be used with a low-speed handpiece. Have the students identify the attachments and describe the uses of each.
Describe the high-speed handpiece and its uses.	☐ High-speed handpiece (p. 512) – Uses of the high-speed handpiece (p. 512) – Water coolant system (p. 513) – Bur adaptation (p. 513) – Fiberoptic lighting (p. 513)	⊠ PPT 14-16 ▣ TB questions 6-8 🗐 SW Short-Answer Questions 4; Fill in the Blank question 9; Multiple Choice questions 5-8; Topics for Discussion question 1 (pp. 239-241) Figure 35-6 High-speed handpiece (p. 513) Figure 35-7 Different styles of securing burs (p. 513) Figure 35-8 A fiber-optic light provides better illumination of an area for the operator (p. 513) Recall questions 5-8 (pp. 513, 516) ▶ Discuss uses of the high-speed handpiece. Note that it is used in every restorative procedure. Note that it does not have attachments. ▶ Discuss the difference in the locking system between the low-speed handpiece and the high-speed handpiece. *Class Activity Have each student create a list of dental procedures and how each procedure is completed with the high-speed handpiece. Then have the students exchange their lists with classmates.*
Review other handpieces used in dentistry.	☐ Ultrasonic handpiece (p. 513) ☐ Laser handpiece (p. 513) – Precautions in the care and handling of laser handpieces (p. 514)	⊠ PPT 17-25 ▣ TB questions 9-14 🗐 SW Short-Answer Questions 5; Fill in the Blank questions 2, 5, 10-11; Multiple Choice question 9; Topics for Discussion question 5 (pp. 239-241) Figure 35-9 Ultrasonic handpiece (p. 513)

OBJECTIVES	CONTENT	TEACHING RESOURCES
	□ Air abrasion handpiece (p. 514) □ Laboratory handpiece (p. 514) □ Handpiece maintenance (p. 516) – Handpiece sterilization (p. 516) – General considerations for handpiece sterilization (p. 516) – Sterilization procedure sheets (p. 516)	Figure 35-10 Laser unit (p. 514) Figure 35-11 Air abrasion handpiece (p. 514) Recall question 9 (p. 516) Figure 35-12 Lubrication system (p. 516) CTQ 1-2, 5 (pp. 522-523) ▸ Discuss the purpose and uses of the ultrasonic handpiece. ▸ Discuss the advantages and disadvantages of using the laser handpiece. ▸ Discuss precautions in the care and handling of laser handpieces. ▸ Discuss the advantages of air abrasion and note the circumstances under which the air abrasion handpiece is used. ▸ Discuss consideration in maintaining a handpiece. Note the problems with excessive or insufficient lubrication. ▸ Discuss considerations for handpiece sterilization. ***Class Activity** Have each student conduct Internet research on a different handpiece and its intended use. Then have the students share their findings with the class. (For students to prepare for this Activity, see Homework/Assignments #2.)*
Identify dental handpieces and correctly attach them to the dental unit.	Procedure 35-1 Identifying and attaching dental handpieces (p. 515) (SW/ESLR Competencies 35-1 and 35-2, p. 243)	Multimedia Procedures DVD: Identifying and Attaching Handpieces SW/ESLR Competencies 35-1 and 35-2 Identifying and Attaching Handpieces and Rotary Instruments (p. 243) ▸ Discuss the procedural steps involved in attaching dental handpieces. ***Class Activity** Provide the class with a variety of handpieces. Have the students identify the various handpieces. Then have student volunteers demonstrate proper attachment of the handpieces to a dental unit.*

Bird/Robinson

35.1 Homework/Assignments:

1. Have the students conduct Internet research on the history of dental handpieces and how they have changed dental procedures. Have each student write a description of one dental procedure, explain how the procedure would have been performed before the introduction of the handpiece, and compare how it is carried out today.

2. Have each student conduct Internet research on a different handpiece and its intended use.

35.1 Instructor's Notes/Student Feedback:

Torres and Ehrlich Modern Dental Assisting, 9ᵗʰ ed.

Bird/Robinson

LESSON 35.2

CRITICAL THINKING QUESTION

A dental assistant is working in a dental office equipped with an onsite dental laboratory. The administrative office has just informed the assistant that an additional patient has been added to the schedule. The patient is returning to the dental office because he is in pain. The patient received his new full upper denture two days ago. What process will be used to determine the cause of the patient's pain? What procedures will be completed to eliminate the cause of the patient's pain in the laboratory?

Guidelines: Review of the patient record is in order, including the most recent treatment. If the treatment was simply the delivery of the new full upper denture, the dental assistant can assume that the new prosthetic appliance is the cause of pain. It is not uncommon for adjustments to be made to full and partial dentures after delivery. When the patient arrives, the assistant should escort him to the treatment room and ask him to remove the denture. The assistant should receive the denture from the patient and place it to the side on the tray, remembering to follow infection control guidelines and to always wear PPE during the exchange. Next, the assistant should view the hard palate using the mouth mirror and dental light. If a sore spot is present, it will appear as a red, irritated area where the denture makes contact with the palate and alveolar ridge. An indicating stick should be used to mark the exact spot on the denture to be adjusted. Before bringing the denture into the laboratory for adjustment, the dental assistant should disinfect the appliance. In the laboratory, the assistant should still wear PPE. Numerous laboratory acrylic burs are available. Full upper denture adjustments can be made using the DMX 1 barrel, DMX 5 egg, DMX 15 pear, or DMX 17 round burs. The dental assistant should use the cone, pointed, or fissure-shaped burs with caution so as to not gouge the acrylic denture. Once the assistant adjusts the denture, polishing of the area is recommended using a rag wheel on the lathe. Finally, the assistant should recheck the denture for fit and comfort before dismissing the patient.

OBJECTIVES	CONTENT	TEACHING RESOURCES
Describe rotary instruments and how they are used.	■ Rotary cutting instruments (p. 516) ☐ Shank types (p. 516) – Neck (p. 517) – Head (p. 517)	⊠▤ PPT 28-29 ▣ TB questions 15-16 SW Short-Answer Questions 6; Fill in the Blank question 3 (p. 239) Figure 35-13 A-C Bur parts and types of shanks (p. 517) Recall question 10 (p. 517) ▸ Discuss the differences among the three basic shank styles. *Class Activity Divide the class into small groups. Have each group write questions and answers pertaining to each rotary instrument that is available for dental restorative procedures. Then have each group quiz the other groups. Keep track of which group answers the most questions correctly.*
List the parts of a bur.	■ Dental burs (p. 517) ☐ Bur shapes (p. 517)	⊠▤ PPT 30 ▣ TB questions 17-19 SW Short-Answer Questions 7; Fill in the Blank questions 1, 4, 6-8; Multiple Choice questions 11-12; Topics for Discussion questions 3-4 (pp. 239-241)

Bird/Robinson

OBJECTIVES	CONTENT	TEACHING RESOURCES
		Recall questions 11-12 (p. 517)
		Table 35-1 Burs for Restorative Dentistry (pp. 518-519)
		💡 CTQ 4 (p. 523)
		▸ Discuss the restorative procedures for which burs are used.
		▸ Discuss the various bur shapes, and note the procedures and purposes for which each is used.
		Class Activity Assign each student a different dental bur. Have each student create a drawing of the assigned dental bur and label its parts. Then have the students share their labeled drawings with the class.
Give the composition, shape, and use of the carbide and diamond burs.	■ Diamond rotary instruments (p. 517) ■ Finishing rotary instruments (p. 519) ■ Abrasive rotary instruments (p. 519) ☐ Accessories (p. 520 ■ Laboratory rotary instruments (p. 520)	🖥 PPT 31-32 📖 TB questions 20-24 📘 SW Short-Answer Questions 8; Fill in the Blank question 12; Multiple Choice questions 13-15 (pp. 239-241) Figure 35-14 Common designs and use of diamond burs (p. 537) Figure 35-15 Finishing burs (p. 520) Figure 35-16 A-E Abrasive materials for rotary instruments (p. 521) Figure 35-17 Types of mandrels (p. 522) Recall questions 13-15 (p. 522) Figure 35-18 Varying shapes of a laboratory acrylic bur (p. 522) Legal and Ethical Implications (p. 522) Eye to the Future (p. 522) 💡 CTQ 3 (p. 523) ▸ Discuss the benefits and disadvantages of diamond rotary instruments. ▸ Discuss the design and purpose of various finishing burs. ▸ Discuss the various abrasive materials and shapes of abrasive rotary instruments. *Class Activity Have each student conduct Internet research on a different carbide and diamond bur. Have each student report to the class the shape, design, and function of the bur researched. (For students to prepare for this activity, see Homework/Assignments #1.)*

Bird/Robinson

OBJECTIVES	CONTENT	TEACHING RESOURCES
Identify accessories and correctly attach them to the low-speed handpiece.	■ Diamond rotary instruments (p. 517) ■ Finishing rotary instruments (p. 519) ■ Abrasive rotary instruments (p. 519) ☐ Accessories (p. 520) ■ Laboratory rotary instruments (p. 520) Procedure 35-2 Identifying and attaching burs to rotary cutting instruments (p. 520) (SW/ESLR Competencies 35-1 and 35-2, p. 243)	Multimedia Procedures DVD: Identifying and Attaching Handpieces SW/ESLR Competencies 35-1 and 35-2 Identifying and Attaching Handpieces and Rotary Instruments (p. 243) ▸ Discuss types of mandrels. ▸ Discuss the procedural steps involved in attaching burs to rotary cutting instruments. *Class Activity Provide the class with a low-speed handpiece and a variety of accessories. Have the students identify and describe the various accessories that can be attached to a low-speed handpiece. Then have student volunteers demonstrate the attachment of the accessories to the low-speed handpiece.*
Identify rotary cutting instruments and correctly attach them to the appropriate dental handpiece or attachment.	■ Diamond rotary instruments (p. 517) ■ Finishing rotary instruments (p. 519) ■ Abrasive rotary instruments (p. 519) ☐ Accessories (p. 520 ■ Laboratory rotary instruments (p. 520)	Multimedia Procedures DVD Identifying and Attaching Handpieces ▸ Discuss the procedural steps involved in attaching rotary cutting instruments to the dental handpiece. *Class Activity Provide the class with a variety of rotary cutting instruments that can be attached to dental handpieces. Have the students identify and describe the various rotary cutting instruments. Then have student volunteers demonstrate the attachment of the rotary cutting instruments to the handpiece.*
Performance Evaluation		TB questions SW questions (pp. 239-241) SW/ESLR Competencies 35-1 and 35-2 Identifying and Attaching Handpieces and Rotary Instruments (p. 243) ESLR Electronic Flashcards ESLR Practice Quiz Recall questions (pp. 512-522) CTQ (pp. 522-523)

35.2 Homework/Assignments:

1. Have each student conduct Internet research on a different carbide and diamond bur. Have each student report to the class the shape, design, and function of the bur researched.

35.2 Instructor's Notes/Student Feedback:

Slide 1

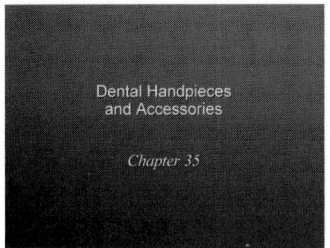

Slide 2

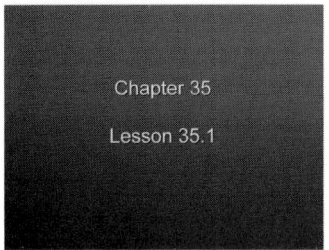

Slide 3

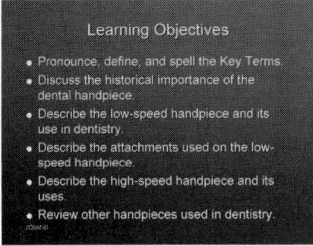

Slide 4

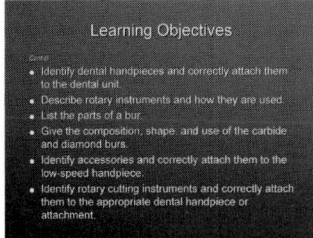

Slide 5

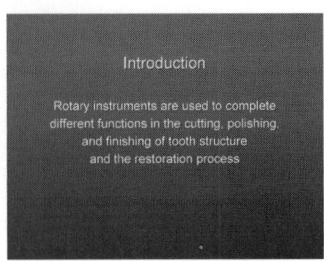

- What does the term rotary mean? (*Rotary is a part or device that rotates around an axis.*)
- In dentistry, rotary instruments are attached to a handpiece.
- Rotary instruments operate at different speeds: high speed and low speed.

Slide 6

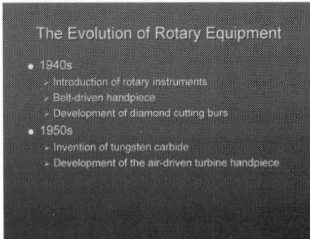

- Rotary instruments were first introduced to complement hand instruments in the cutting, grinding, and polishing procedures of operative dentistry.
- Electricity is the power source for rotary instruments.

Slide 7

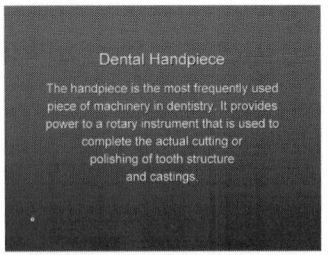

- Who primarily uses the high-speed handpiece? (*Dentist.*)
- Who primarily uses the low-speed handpiece? (*Dentist, dental hygienist, and expanded- function dental assistant.*)
- Always refer to your state practice act before using a handpiece for treatment or operative procedures.

Slide 8

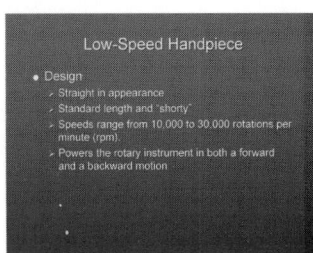

- Also referred to as the straight handpiece because of its design.
- The low-speed handpiece is one of the most versatile handpieces in dentistry.

Bird/Robinson

Slide 9

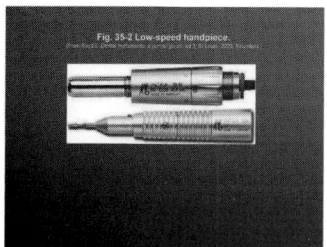

- The straight attachment slides onto the low-speed motor and locks into place.

- What is the straight attachment commonly used for? (*Laboratory procedures or for trimming removable prostheses, such as dentures, partial dentures, flippers, and orthodontic retainers.*)

Slide 10

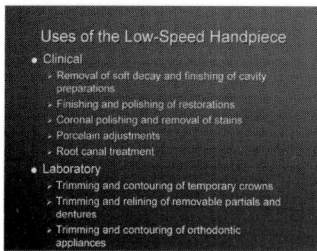

- Gloves, protective eyewear, mask, and appropriate garments must be worn when completing laboratory procedures.

Slide 11

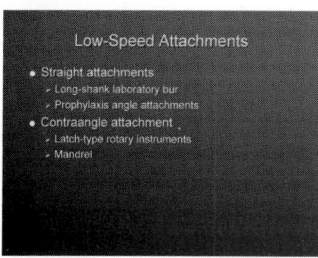

- What grasp is used with the straight attachment? (*Pen grasp or palm grasp.*)

- What grasp is used with the contra-angle attachment? (*Pen grasp or modified pen grasp.*)

- The angled shank of the contra-angle attachment provides ergonomic comfort. The operator can maintain proper neutral wrist position more readily during treatment procedures.

Slide 12

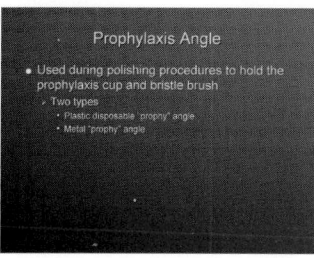

- Polishing procedures include prophylaxis, tooth prep before sealant placement, and amalgam polishing.

- What is an advantage of using disposable prophy angles in the dental office? (*Infection control. There is no need to clean and process the prophy angle for sterilization after use; simply dispose of the angle.*)

- What is a disadvantage of using disposable prophy angles in the dental office? (*Cost.*)

Slide 13

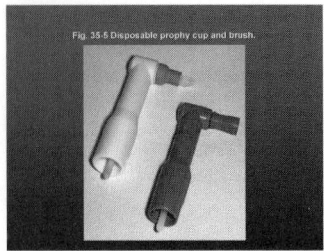

- This slide shows disposable prophy angles, one containing a brush and the other containing a rubber cup.

- The brush is used when polishing occlusal surfaces and lingual surfaces of anterior teeth.

- The rubber cup is used when polishing smooth tooth surfaces.

Slide 14

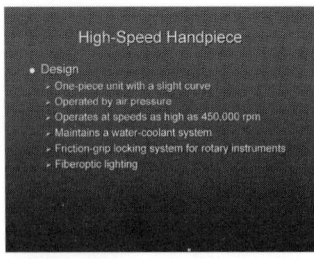

- The dentist uses the high-speed handpiece in every restorative procedure.

- What is the purpose of the water-coolant system? (*The high-speed handpiece generates a significant amount of heat and friction due to the high number of rpm. The water keeps the tooth cool to help avoid injury to the pulp during preparation.*)

- The fiber-optic light mounted in the head of the handpiece offers additional light to the operator and dental assistant during preparation of the tooth.

Slide 15

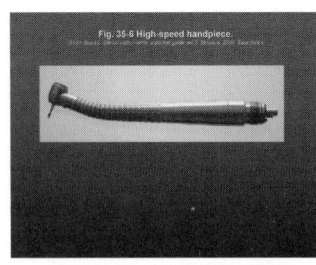

- Unlike the low-speed handpiece, the high-speed handpiece does not have attachments.

- The only additional items placed in the high-speed handpiece are rotary instruments.

- What are these rotary instruments called? (*Dental burs.*)

Slide 16

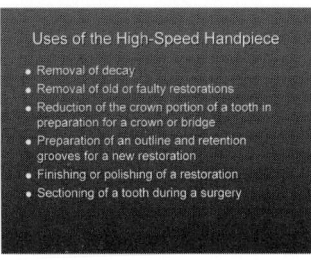

- The high-speed handpiece rapidly removes pathologic or decayed tooth structure.

- Often, the dentist will refine the tooth preparation with the low-speed handpiece after using the high-speed handpiece.

Bird/Robinson

Slide 17

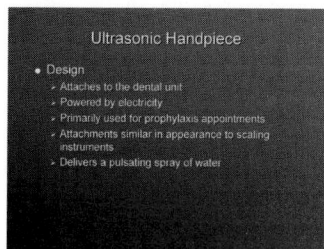

- The American Dental Association Council on Dental Materials, Instruments, and Equipment evaluates professional scaling devices. Ultrasonic tips are classified as acceptable or provisional acceptable.

- The ultrasonic handpiece uses mechanical radiant energy of water and sound vibrations to create a pulsating effect on a tooth surface.

Slide 18

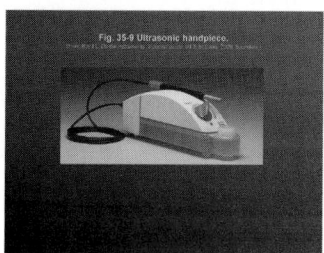

- There are three types of ultrasonic scalers: magnetostrictive, piezoelectric, and sonic.

- Magnetostrictive scaler: Vibrations range from 24,000 to 42,000 cycles per second.

- Piezoelectric scaler: Vibrations range from 29,00 to 50,000 cycles per second.

- Sonic scaler (pictured on this slide): Vibrations range from 2500 to 7000 cycles per second.

Slide 19

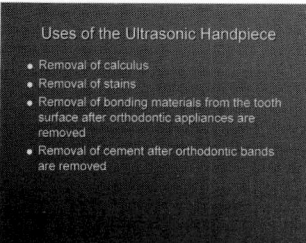

- The attachments for this handpiece are designed similarly to hand (manual) scaling instruments.

- A specific tip is selected depending on the surface and location of its use.

Slide 20

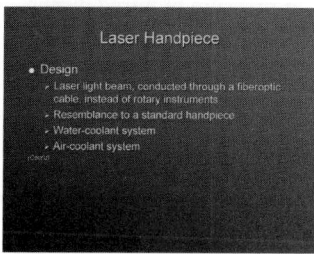

- Designed to perform special functions without changing or damaging the surrounding tissues or materials.

- Caution must be used when handling the laser handpiece: do not sharply bend the fiber-optic cord, do not touch the exposed fiber-optic cable, do not touch the end of the fiber-optic connector, and always keep the connecting parts clean.

Slide 21

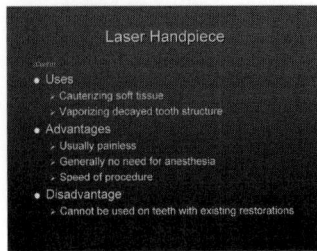

- Lasers are used in dentistry to remove decay from tooth structure, to cure bonding materials, in tooth whitening procedures, and in periodontal treatment.

- Very specific equipment and training are required to incorporate laser technology into the dental office.

Slide 22

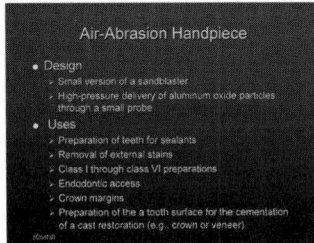

- The air abrasion system was introduced to dentistry in the 1940s. It was originally designed to remove stain and tooth decay.

- Considered a patient-friendly approach to restorative treatment

- Permits the dentist to remove enamel, dentin, and restorative materials without compromising healthy tooth structure.

Slide 23

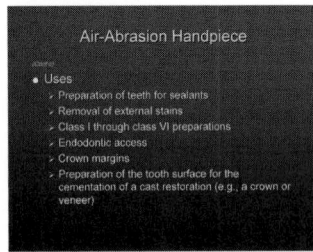

- An advantage to using air-abrasion handpieces is there is no need for local anesthesia.

- A disadvantage is the possibility of soft tissue (gingiva) damage if incorrect techniques are used.

Slide 24

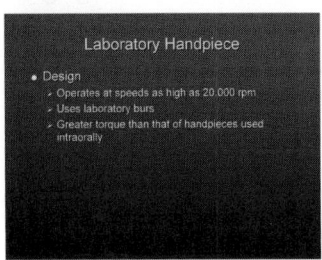

- What is torque? (*A twisting or turning force.*)

- Increased torque is better suited to the heavier pressure required during grinding and polishing procedures that take place outside the mouth.

Torres and Ehrlich Modern Dental Assisting, 9th ed.

Bird/Robinson

Slide 25

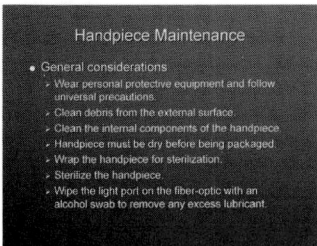

- What are the main reasons a handpiece fails or breaks? *(Improper cleaning and lubrication.)*

- Inadequate cleaning of the handpiece before sterilization can result in the collection of debris in the handpiece's internal parts. Debris creates wear on the handpiece motor and inner movable parts.

- Is it possible to lubricate a handpiece too much? (*Yes. Too much lubrication can be as damaging as not enough lubrication.*)

Slide 26

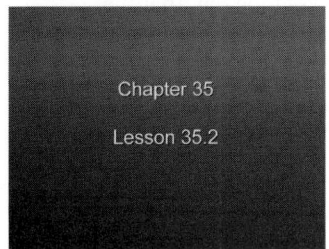

Slide 27

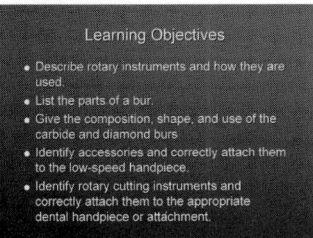

Slide 28

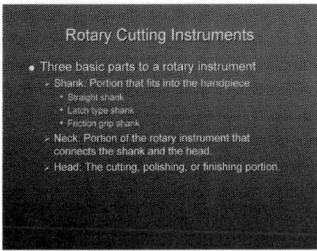

- Rotary cutting instruments are accessories intended for use with the dental handpiece.

- There are hundreds of different types of rotary instruments available in dentistry, and each is designed for a different task or use.

- It is important that the dental assistant know the dentist's preferences.

Slide 29

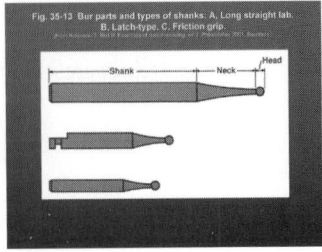

- Looking at the slide, what part makes up the largest section of the rotary instrument? (*Shank.*)
- The shank length will vary according to the specific function of the bur and the handpiece to which it is attached.

Slide 30

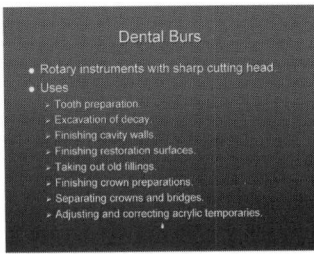

- A dental bur is classified as a "sharp." Care must be taken when placing the bur on the handpiece and removing the bur after the procedure. One should wear heavy utility gloves when removing a contaminated bur.
- Burs come in a variety of shapes. The shape is commonly referred to as the "contour" or "design."
- Burs are used to enter the tooth structure, remove decay, extend preparations, cut retention grooves, form internal walls of the prep, and provide angles to the wall prep.

Slide 31

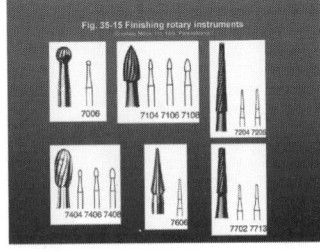

- Finishing rotary burs are similar in appearance to cutting burs except for one distinctive feature. What is that feature? (*The number of blades or flutes is increased on the finishing bur.*)
- The greater the number of cutting surfaces, the greater the polishing capability.
- The slide pictures the three most common finishing burs: round, tapered and flame-shaped.

Slide 32

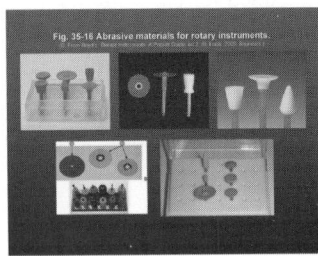

- Numerous abrasive materials are found on these instruments, from very coarse to fine.
- Abrasive discs and wheels are attached to a mandrel (a metal shaft), which is then attached to the dental handpiece.

ELSEVIER

Torres and Ehrlich Modern Dental Assisting, 9th ed.

Bird/Robinson

TEACHING FOCUS

This chapter will introduce the student to topics related to moisture control. The student will have the opportunity to learn about oral evacuation systems, rinsing the oral cavity, isolation of teeth, and the dental dam. Positioning the high-volume evacuator, performing a mouth rinse, placing and removing cotton rolls, and preparing, placing, and removing a dental dam will be emphasized.

MATERIALS AND RESOURCES

- ☐ air-water syringe (Lesson 36.1)
- ☐ basic setup (all Lessons)
- ☐ black spoon (Lesson 36.2)
- ☐ computer and PowerPoint projector (all Lessons)
- ☐ cotton rolls (all Lessons)
- ☐ crown and bridge scissors (Lesson 36.2)
- ☐ dental dam clamp or clamps with ligature attached (Lesson 36.2)
- ☐ dental dam clamp forceps (Lesson 36.2)
- ☐ dental dam napkin (Lesson 36.2)
- ☐ dental dam punch (Lesson 36.2)
- ☐ dental dam stamp and ink pad or template and pen (Lesson 36.2)
- ☐ dental tape or waxed floss (Lesson 36.2)
- ☐ lubricant for dam (Lesson 36.2)
- ☐ lubricant for patient's lips (Lesson 36.2)
- ☐ plastic barrier cover for high-volume evacuator (HVE) handle and hose (Lesson 36.1)
- ☐ precut 6-by-6-inch dental dam (Lesson 36.2)
- ☐ saliva ejector (Lesson 36.1)
- ☐ sterile HVE tip (Lesson 36.1)
- ☐ Young frame (Lesson 36.2)

LESSON CHECKLIST

Preparations for this lesson include:

- lecture
- evaluation of student knowledge and skills needed to perform all entry-level activities related to moisture control, including:
  - ○ understanding the purpose and use of oral evacuation systems
  - ○ positioning the high-volume evacuator
  - ○ performing a mouth rinse and using the air-water syringe
  - ○ placing and removing cotton rolls
  - ○ preparing, placing, and removing the dental dam
  - ○ understanding special applications of the dental dam

Bird/Robinson

KEY TERMS

aspirate (p. 532)   jaws (p. 535)
beveled (p. 526)   malaligned (p. 537)
bow (p. 535)   septum (p. 538)
exposed (p. 532)   stylus (p. 533)
invert (p. 541)   universal (p. 535)
isolated (p. 532)   winged clamp (p. 535)

ADDITIONAL RESOURCES

PowerPoint slides (Evolve): 1-43
Multimedia Procedures DVD:
    Positioning the High-Volume Evacuator
    Dental Dam Placement and Removal

Legend

CTQ
Critical
Thinking
Question

DVD
Multimedia
Procedures
Videos and
Animations

ESLR
EVOLVE
Student
Learning
Resources

IDO
Interactive
Dental
Office
CD-ROM

SW
Student
Workbook

TB
Test Bank
on the
TEACH
CD-ROM

PPT
PowerPoint
Slides

Class Activities are indicated in ***bold italic***.

ELSEVIER

Torres and Ehrlich Modern Dental Assisting, 9th ed.

Bird/Robinson

LESSON 36.1

PRETEST

1. What is the function of the saliva ejector?
   a. removes debris from the mouth
   b. removes excess fluid from the mouth
   c. removes excess dental materials from the mouth
   d. maintains a clear field at the surgical site

2. Where is the saliva ejector placed when it is stationary and shaped into a "candy cane"?
   a. under the tongue
   b. behind the retromolar pad
   c. at or near the maxillary tuberosity
   d. in the buccal vestibule

3. The high-volume evacuator should be held in the pen grasp or
   a. the thumb-to-nose grasp.
   b. in both hands.
   c. upside down.
   d. far from the tooth being treated.

4. Which oral rinsing technique is performed frequently as debris accumulates during the preparation and restoration of a tooth?
   a. full-mouth rinsing
   b. isolated tooth rinsing
   c. limited-area rinsing
   d. periodic-pause rinsing

5. Which isolation technique uses small, triangular absorbent pads?
   a. cotton roll/cotton holder isolation technique
   b. dental dam isolation technique
   c. two-by-two gauze isolation technique
   d. dry angle isolation technique

6. Dental dam material is available in a continuous roll or in two precut sizes of 6-by-6-inch squares or
   a. 5-by-5-inch squares.
   b. 4-by-4-inch squares.
   c. 3-by-3-inch squares.
   d. 2-by-2-inch squares.

7. What thickness of dental dam material is recommended during procedures for which tissue retraction and extra resistance are required?
   a. extra fine
   b. thin
   c. medium
   d. heavy

8. Which dental dam frame is recommended when radiographs may be required throughout the dental procedure?
   a. plastic U-shaped frame
   b. Young U-shaped frame
   c. Ostby frame
   d. black frame

9. What part of the dental dam punch is a rotary-type disk?
   a. stylus
   b. punch plate
   c. template
   d. clamp

10. What size hole should be punched to isolate a premolar tooth?
    a. 1
    b. 2
    c. 3
    d. 4

Answers

1. b	3. a	5. d	7. d	9. b
2. a	4. c	6. a	8. a	10. c

BACKGROUND ASSESSMENT

Question: Why is moisture control important? What is meant by the term *oral evacuation*? What evacuator systems are used in dentistry to manage moisture control?

Answer: One of the most important roles of the dental assistant is to maintain moisture control during a dental procedure. When the field in the patient's mouth where the dental procedure is being performed contains excess water, debris, saliva, and blood, visibility is decreased, which can hinder the successful completion of the procedure. Oral evacuation describes the process of removing excess fluid and debris from a patient's mouth before, during, and after a dental procedure. The dental evacuator systems used are the saliva ejector and the high-volume evacuator (HVE). The saliva ejector is a small, straw-type oral evacuator that is used during less invasive dental procedures to remove liquids from the mouth. The HVE is a more powerful evacuator system designed to remove saliva, blood, water, and debris during a dental procedure.

Question: When is the use of the dental dam indicated? How is the dental dam prepared?

Answer: The dental dam is an isolation technique that serves as an important infection-control barrier for the preparation of teeth. The dental dam is indicated when safeguards to protect the patient's mouth from contacting debris are needed. It is also indicated to control moisture, to protect the oral cavity from infection, to isolate an open tooth from microorganisms, and to maintain optimum visibility in the patient's mouth. The dental dam is prepared by stamping or marking the dam material using the template, inkpad, and stamp. Holes are then punched into the dam material using the dental dam punch.

CRITICAL THINKING QUESTION

A dental assistant is preparing the treatment room for extraction of a patient's #32 tooth. After preparing the necessary instruments and materials, the dental assistant sets up the unit with infection control barriers and evacuation system tips. Which evacuation system will be used during this procedure to maintain a clear field around the treatment area? Which evacuator tips will be used and why?

Guidelines: The high-volume evacuation (HVE) system will be used and held by the dental assistant to control moisture by removing water, debris, saliva, and blood. The HVE can also be used to retract the tongue if held on the lingual aspect of tooth #32 during this procedure. The surgical HVE tip should be attached to the high-volume hose. The surgical suction tip is a metal tip that is smaller in circumference. The metal tip is sterilized to control infection, and the smaller size is critical to placement within the surgical site.

OBJECTIVES	CONTENT	TEACHING RESOURCES
Define and spell the Key Terms.	■ Key terms (p. 524)	SW Fill in the Blank questions 1-10 (pp. 246-247) ESLR Electronic Flashcards ▶ Discuss each Key Term in Chapter 36, focusing on definition, pronunciation, and spelling. *Class Activity **Have students use each Key Term in a sentence.***
List isolation techniques used to decrease moisture during a dental procedure.	■ Oral evacuation systems (p. 525)	PPT 5 TB question 1 SW Short-Answer Questions 1 (p. 246) ▶ Discuss the importance of moisture control. Note that

OBJECTIVES	CONTENT	TEACHING RESOURCES
		moisture control is one of the most important roles of a dental assistant during a procedure. ***Class Activity Divide the class into small groups, and assign each group one isolation technique. Have each group create an outline describing the assigned technique, listing its pros and cons and the materials needed. Then, have the groups present their outlines to the class.***
Describe the two types of oral evacuation systems used in dentistry.	☐ Saliva ejector (p. 525) ☐ High-volume evacuator (p. 525) 　– Suction tips (p. 526) 　– Grasping the evacuator (p. 526) 　– Positioning the evacuator (p. 526) ☐ Daily maintenance of the evacuation system (p. 527)	🖵 PPT 6-10 📖 TB questions 2-5 📝 SW Short-Answer Questions 2; Fill in the Blank question 2; Multiple Choice questions 1-3 (pp. 246-247) Figure 36-1 Saliva ejector (p. 525) Figure 36-2 Saliva ejector placed under the tongue for a procedure (p. 526) Figure 36-3 High-volume evacuator suction tips (p. 526) Recall question 1 (p. 527) ▸ Discuss the saliva ejector. Note that it is not powerful enough to remove debris. ▸ Discuss the two ways the saliva ejector can be held or positioned. Note the use of a cotton roll to protect oral tissues. ▸ Discuss the use of the high-volume evacuator and note its three main purposes. ***Class Activity Have each student create a table comparing the two evacuation systems used in dentistry. The table should include at least three differences and three similarities. Then have the students share their tables with the class.***
Describe the grasp and positioning of the high-volume evacuator tip.	☐ High-volume evacuator (p. 525) 　– Suction tips (p. 526) 　– Grasping the evacuator (p. 526) 　– Positioning the evacuator (p. 526) ☐ Daily maintenance of the evacuation system (p. 527)	🖵 PPT 11-13 📖 TB questions 6-9 📝 SW Short-Answer Questions 3; Multiple Choice questions 13-14, 16, 20 (pp. 246, 247) Figure 36-4 Grasps used for operating the high-volume evacuator (p. 526) Recall questions 2-3 (p. 527) Figure 36-5 Operator and assistant positions in high-volume evacuation (p. 528) 💡 CTQ 2 (p. 543) ▸ Discuss the difference between the operative suction tip and the surgical suction tip, and note when each is used.

OBJECTIVES	CONTENT	TEACHING RESOURCES
		▸ Discuss the thumb-to-nose grasp and the pen grasp. Note that both methods provide adequate control. ▸ Discuss the alteration of evacuator positioning, and note that the assistant should grasp the evacuator with the right hand when assisting a right-handed dentist. *Class Activity Before class, ask students to find and print out a picture or photo of a grasp used in dentistry from the Internet. Then, have the students share their pictures and photos in class. (For students to prepare for this activity, see Homework/Assignments #1.)*
Perform the grasp and positioning of the high-volume evacuator during a procedure.	☐ High-volume evacuator (p. 525) – Suction tips (p. 526) – Grasping the evacuator (p. 526) – Positioning the evacuator (p. 526) ☐ Daily maintenance of the evacuation system (p. 527) Procedure 36-1 Positioning the high-volume evacuator during a procedure (p. 527) (SW/ESLR Competency 36-1, p. 249)	Multimedia Procedures DVD: Positioning the High-Volume Evacuator SW/ESLR Competency 36-1 Positioning the High-Volume Oral Evacuator During a Procedure (p. 249) ▸ Discuss specific guidelines for positioning the high-volume evacuator. ▸ Discuss differences in posterior and anterior placement. ▸ Discuss guidelines for maintenance of evacuation systems and the air-water syringe. *Class Activity Supply the class with high-volume evacuation tips. Have each student demonstrate the nose-to-thumb grasp and the pen grasp with a high-volume evacuation tip.*
Discuss the use of the air-water syringe.	■ Rinsing the oral cavity (p. 528) ☐ Limited-area rinsing (p. 528) ☐ Full-mouth rinsing (p. 528) ☐ Air-water syringe (p. 528)	PPT 14-15 TB questions 10-11 SW Short-Answer Questions 4; Multiple Choice question 4 (pp. 245-246) Recall question 4 (p. 529) CTQ 3 (p. 543) ▸ Discuss the purpose of frequent rinsing of the oral cavity. ▸ Discuss the difference between limited-area rinsing and full-mouth rinsing and when each technique is used. ▸ Discuss the purpose of the air-water syringe during rinsing of the oral cavity, and note guidelines for its use. *Class Activity Divide the class into small groups. Have each group discuss the uses of the air-water syringe during various dental procedures in a roundtable discussion format.*

OBJECTIVES	CONTENT	TEACHING RESOURCES
Perform limited-area and full-mouth rinses.	☐ Limited-area rinsing (p. 528) ☐ Full-mouth rinsing (p. 528) ☐ Air-water syringe (p. 528) Procedure 36-2 Performing a mouth rinse (p. 529) (SW/ESLR Competency 36-2, p. 251)	SW Multiple Choice question 19 (p. 247) SW/ESLR Competency 36-2 Performing a Mouthrinse (p. 251) ▸ Discuss the importance of the patient's head positioning during the full-mouth rinse. *Class Activity Divide the class into small groups and have students practice rinsing procedures using an air-water syringe and a typodont in class. Then, have students share feedback about the procedures they performed and observed.*
Place cotton rolls for isolation.	■ Isolation of teeth (p. 529) ☐ Cotton roll isolation (p. 529) – Using cotton rolls (p. 529) – Cotton roll holders (p. 531) Procedure 36-3 Placing and removing cotton rolls (p. 530) (SW/ESLR Competency 36-3, pp. 253-254) ☐ Dry-angle isolation (p. 531)	PPT 16-20 TB questions 12-15 SW Multiple Choice questions 5, 7; Case Study question 1 (pp. 246-247) SW/ESLR Competency 36-3 Placing and Removing Cotton Rolls (pp. 253-254) Figure 36-6 Cotton roll isolation in the mandibular quadrant (p. 531) Figure 36-7 Cotton roll holder (p. 532) Figure 36-8 Dry-angle placement in the buccal mucosa (p. 532) Recall questions 5-7 (p. 532) CTQ 1 (p. 543) ▸ Discuss the circumstances under which cotton roll isolation and dry-angle isolation are used. ▸ Discuss the advantages and disadvantages of using cotton rolls. ▸ Discuss the maxillary placement and mandibular placement of cotton rolls. *Class Activity Using a typodont, have each student demonstrate placement of cotton rolls with and without cotton roll holders. Have each student place cotton rolls to isolate different areas of the mouth. Have the students share feedback regarding the skills they performed and observed.*

36.1 Homework/Assignments:

1. Ask students to find and print out from the Internet.a picture or photo of a grasp used in dentistry

---

36.1 Instructor's Notes/Student Feedback:

Torres and Ehrlich Modern Dental Assisting, 9th ed.

Bird/Robinson

LESSON 36.2

CRITICAL THINKING QUESTION

An expanded-function dental assistant is scheduled to assist the dentist during a root canal procedure on tooth #25 and determines that placement of the dental dam would isolate the vulnerable tooth from the oral environment, which will eliminate further infection from developing in the tooth. The assistant prepares the dental dam for the anterior root. Which dental dam equipment will be used for placement of the dental dam? What are the necessary steps for placing the dental dam and for removing it after the root canal is complete?

Guidelines: Before placing the dental dam in the patient's mouth, the dentist administers local anesthesia. Next, a lubricating ointment is placed on the patient's lip, and the contacts of the teeth are flossed to remove any debris before dam placement. The dental dam material is slid between each contact. Finally, a ligature is placed at the opposite end of the anchor tooth to stabilize the rubber dam. When removing the dental dam, the assistant should release the stabilizing ligature first, slide his or her finger under the dam parallel to the arch, and pull outward to stretch the holes away from the isolated teeth. Using the crown and bridge scissors, cut from hole to hole and gently pull the dam material lingually to free the rubber from the interproximal spaces. Use the dental forceps to open the clamp to slide it off the tooth. Remove the dental dam and frame together. Inspect the dam to make sure that no material was left behind in the patient's mouth or between the teeth.

OBJECTIVES	CONTENT	TEACHING RESOURCES
Describe the dental dam and its role in moisture control.	■ The dental dam (p. 532)	PPT 24-25 TB questions 16-21 SW Short-Answer Questions 5; Fill in the Blank questions 3, 9-10; Multiple Choice questions 6, 8 (pp. 245-246) ▸ Discuss the purposes and benefits of a dental dam. List circumstances under which a dental dam would be used. *Class Activity Before class, have students research on the Internet the benefits of using the dental dam during dental procedures. Then, have the students share their findings with the class. (For students to prepare for this activity, see Homework/Assignments #1.)*
List the equipment and supplies for dental dam application.	□ Dental dam equipment (p. 532) – Dental dam material (p. 532) – Size (p. 532) – Color (p. 532) – Thickness (p. 532) – Dental dam frame (p. 533) – Dental dam napkin (p. 533) – Lubricants (p. 533)	PPT 26-41 SW Short-Answer Questions 6 (p. 245) ▸ Discuss the equipment and supplies for dental dam application. ▸ Discuss the material, size, color, and thickness of dental dams. Note considerations in choosing size (precut or roll), color, and thickness (thin, medium, heavy). ▸ Discuss the dental dam punch. Note the specific recommended uses for each hole size. *Class Activity Have each student create a list of the necessary equipment and supplies needed to prepare and place the dental dam in a patient's mouth. Then, have the students compare their lists with their classmates.*

Torres and Ehrlich Modern Dental Assisting, 9th ed.

Bird/Robinson

OBJECTIVES	CONTENT	TEACHING RESOURCES
	– Dental dam punch (p. 533) – Dental dam stamp and template (p. 534) – Dental dam forceps (p. 534) – Dental dam clamps (p. 535) – Dental dam stabilizing cord (p. 536)	
Identify the equipment and supplies used for dental dam application.	☐ Dental dam equipment (p. 532) – Dental dam material (p. 532) – Size (p. 532) – Color (p. 532) – Thickness (p. 532) – Dental dam frame (p. 533) – Dental dam napkin (p. 533) – Lubricants (p. 533) – Dental dam punch (p. 533) – Dental dam stamp and template (p. 534) – Dental dam forceps (p. 534) – Dental dam clamps (p. 535) – Dental dam stabilizing cord (p. 536)	☒▣ PPT 26-41 SW Fill in the Blank questions 1, 4, 8; Multiple Choice questions 9, 11-12, 17-18 (pp. 245-247) Figure 36-9 Dental dam material (p. 533) Figure 36-10 Dental dam frames (p. 533) Figure 36-11 Dental dam punch (p. 533) Figure 36-12 Size of holes for punching the dental dam and the coordinating teeth for the size of the punched holes (p. 534) Figure 36-13 Dental dam stamp (p. 534) Figure 36-14 Dental dam forceps (p. 535) Figure 36-15 Positioning the beaks of the dental dam forceps into the clamp properly (p. 535) Figure 36-16 Parts of the dental dam clamp (p. 535) Figure 36-17 Types of dental dam clamps (p. 535) Figure 36-18 Positioning the clamp on the tooth (p. 536) Figure 36-19 Ligature placed on the bow of the clamp for protective reasons (p. 536) Recall questions 8-10 (p. 536) ▸ Discuss the use of the dental dam stamp and template. Note the circumstances under which each is used. ▸ Discuss the purpose of the dental dam clamp. List the parts of the clamp and steps for proper fitting. Also explain the use of ligatures and the use of forceps to place and remove the clamp. ▸ Discuss the dental dam stabilizing cord. Note the circumstances under which the stabilizing cord might be used instead of the dental dam clamps. *Class Activity* ***Provide dental dam supplies and equipment to the class. Call on students to identify these supplies and equipment by name and function.***

OBJECTIVES	CONTENT	TEACHING RESOURCES
Describe the special preparation and placement of the dental dam.	■ Dental dam preparation (p. 536) ☐ Maxillary arch application (p. 536) ☐ Mandibular arch application (p. 536) ☐ Curve of the arch (p. 537) ☐ Malaligned teeth (p. 537) ☐ Teeth to be isolated (p. 537) ☐ Keypunch hole (p. 538) ☐ Hole sizing and spacing (p. 538)	PPT 42 SW Short-Answer Questions 7; Fill in the Blank questions 6-7; Multiple Choice questions 10, 15; Case Study questions 2-4 (pp. 245-247) Figure 36-20 Punching the dam for a maxillary application (p. 537) Figure 36-21 Punching the dam for a mandibular application (p. 537) Figure 36-22 Punching the dam for a malaligned tooth (p. 537) Recall question 11 (p. 542) CTQ 4 (p. 543) ▶ Discuss the six factors that must be included in the planning for the holes to be punched in the dental dam. ▶ Discuss the difference between the maxillary arch application and the mandibular arch application. ▶ Discuss how the curve of the arch may necessitate adjustments to the dental dam. *Class Activity Divide the class into pairs. Have each pair of students discuss the various steps in preparing and placing a dental dam.*
Have the dental dam prepared correctly for a procedure.	■ Dental dam preparation (p. 536) ☐ Maxillary arch application (p. 536) ☐ Mandibular arch application (p. 536) ☐ Curve of the arch (p. 537) ☐ Malaligned teeth (p. 537) ☐ Teeth to be isolated (p. 537) ☐ Keypunch hole (p. 538) ☐ Hole sizing and spacing (p. 538) – Troubleshooting hole size and spacing (p. 536)	SW/ESLR Competency 36-4 Preparing, Placement, and Removal of the Dental Dam (pp. 255-256) CTQ 5 (p. 543) ▶ Discuss steps for troubleshooting hole size and spacing. *Class Activity Provide the class with dental dam material, inkpads and stamps, templates, and dental dam punches. Assign each student specific teeth to isolate. Have each student prepare a dental dam by stamping it and punching the holes for the assigned teeth.*

OBJECTIVES	CONTENT	TEACHING RESOURCES
	Procedure 36-4 Preparation, placement, and removal of the dental dam (pp. 539-542) (SW/ESLR Competency 36-4, pp. 255-256)	
Place the dental dam as an expanded function.	■ Dental dam placement and removal (p. 538) Procedure 36-4 Preparation, placement, and removal of the dental dam (pp. 539-542) (SW/ESLR Competency 36-4, pp. 255-256)	Multimedia Procedures DVD: Dental Dam Placement and Removal SW/ESLR Competency 36-4 Preparing, Placement, and Removal of the Dental Dam (pp. 255-256) ▸ Discuss steps in placing the clamp and frame. ▸ Discuss steps in inverting the dental dam. *Class Activity Provide the class with the necessary materials, equipment, and typodonts for placement of a dental dam. Assign teeth for isolation to each student. Have each student practice placement of a dental dam on a typodont.*
Remove the dental dam as an expanded function.	■ Dental dam placement and removal (p. 538) Procedure 36-4 Preparation, placement, and removal of the dental dam (pp. 539-542) (SW/ESLR Competency 36-4, pp. 255-256) ■ Special applications for the dental dam (p. 538) ☐ Anterior teeth (p. 538) – Stabilizing the cervical clamp (p. 538) ☐ Fixed bridge (p. 542)	PPT 43 Multimedia Procedures DVD: Dental Dam Placement and Removal TB question 22 SW Case Study question 5 (p. 247) SW/ESLR Competency 36-4 Preparing, Placement, and Removal of the Dental Dam (pp. 255-256) Figure 36-23 Maxillary anterior dam application (p. 538) Figure 36-24 Compound wax used to stabilize anterior clamp (p. 542) Recall question 12 (p. 542) ▸ Discuss steps in removing the dental dam. Note the need to check for missing fragments of the dental dam. ▸ Discuss the change in isolation and application procedures when the dental dam is to be applied to anterior teeth. ▸ Discuss the specialized technique required for dental dam placement when a fixed bridge is in place. *Class Activity Provide the class with the necessary materials, equipment, and typodonts to work with a dental dam. Have each student practice dental dam removal and inspection of the dam materials after removal.*

Bird/Robinson

OBJECTIVES	CONTENT	TEACHING RESOURCES
Performance Evaluation		▦ TB questions
		📘 SW questions (pp. 245-247)
		📘 SW Case Study (p. 247)
		📘 *e* SW/ESLR Competency 36-1 Positioning the High-Volume Oral Evacuator During a Procedure (p. 249)
		📘 *e* SW/ESLR Competency 36-2 Performing a Mouthrinse (p. 251)
		📘 *e* SW/ESLR Competency 36-3 Placing and Removing Cotton Rolls (pp. 253-254)
		📘 *e* SW/ESLR Competency 36-4 Preparing, Placement, and Removal of the Dental Dam (pp. 255-256)
		e ESLR Electronic Flashcards
		e ESLR Practice Quiz
		Recall questions (pp. 527-542)
		💡 CTQ (p. 543)

36.2 Homework/Assignments:

1. Have students research on the Internet the benefits of using the dental dam during dental procedures.

36.2 Instructor's Notes/Student Feedback:

Torres and Ehrlich Modern Dental Assisting, 9th ed.

Bird/Robinson

Slide 1

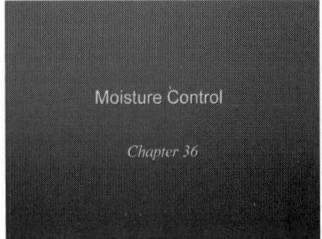

Moisture Control

Chapter 36

Slide 2

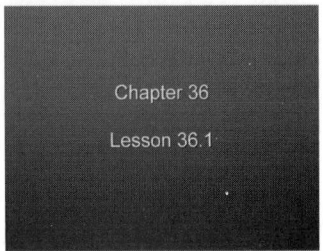

Chapter 36

Lesson 36.1

Slide 3

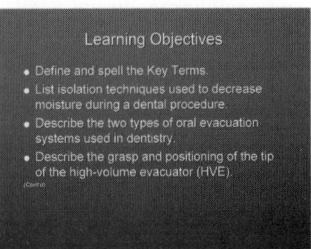

Learning Objectives

- Define and spell the Key Terms.
- List isolation techniques used to decrease moisture during a dental procedure.
- Describe the two types of oral evacuation systems used in dentistry.
- Describe the grasp and positioning of the tip of the high-volume evacuator (HVE).
(Cont'd)

Slide 4

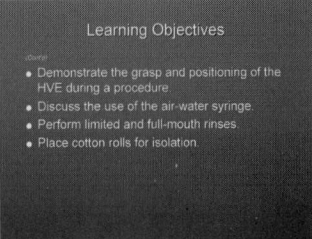

Learning Objectives
(Cont'd)
- Demonstrate the grasp and positioning of the HVE during a procedure.
- Discuss the use of the air-water syringe.
- Perform limited and full-mouth rinses.
- Place cotton rolls for isolation.

ELSEVIER

Torres and Ehrlich Modern Dental Assisting, 9th ed.

Bird/Robinson

Slide 5

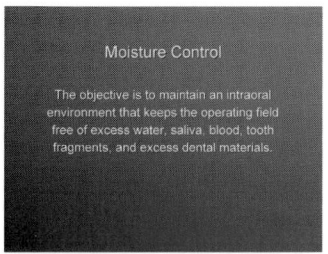

- One of the most important responsibilities of the dental assistant is to maintain moisture control during a procedure.
- Why is moisture control so important?
- The term oral evacuation describes the process of removing excess fluids from the mouth.
- When is an oral evacuator used? (*Before, during, and after dental procedures.*)
- The saliva ejector and the high-volume evacuator are the two types of evacuators used in dentistry.

Slide 6

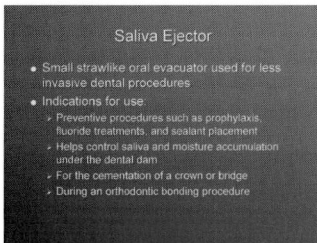

- What is the main function of the saliva ejector? (*Remove liquids from the mouth; it is not powerful enough to remove debris.*)
- The saliva ejector is made of a soft plastic tubing that can be shaped and easily placed in the oral cavity.

Slide 7

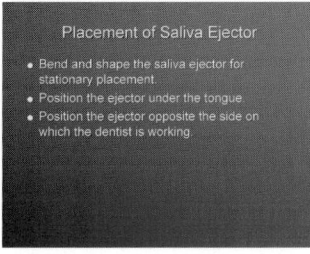

- Hold the saliva ejector throughout the procedure, repeatedly sweeping the mouth to remove fluids, or position the suction in the mouth during a procedure.
- When the saliva ejector is stationary, bend it into the shape of a candy cane. This shape allows for easy placement under the tongue.

Slide 8

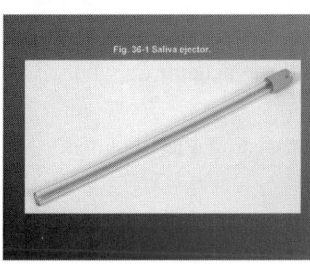

- Place the saliva ejector cautiously to avoid traumatizing soft tissue (floor of the mouth, frenums, mucosa, etc.).
- What common dental item can be used as a buffer to help avoid trauma? (*Cotton roll.*)
- Instruct the patient to avoid closing down on the saliva ejector and clamping off the vacuum suction.
- Tell the patient not to close the lips around the saliva ejector during suctioning.

Bird/Robinson

Slide 9

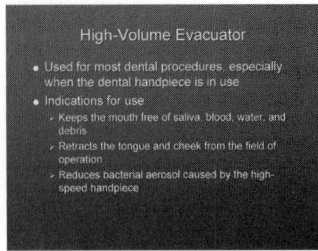

- The HVE, also known as the oral evacuator, works on a vacuum system.

- It is stronger than the saliva ejector and can remove debris because a high volume of air is moved into the vacuum hose.

- Two types of HVE tips are available. Each tip is specially designed for specific dental procedures.

Slide 10

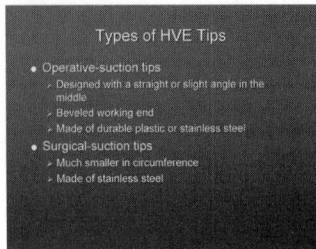

- What is an advantage and a disadvantage of a plastic operative tip? (*Advantage: disposable; Disadvantage: cost.*)

- Why does the surgical tip have a smaller circumference? (*So that it can operate within the limited space and visibility of surgical sites.*)

- What is the main function of the surgical tip? (*It removes blood, tissue, and debris instead of large amounts of water and fluids.*)

- The stainless steel tip is part of the surgical set-up tray.

Slide 11

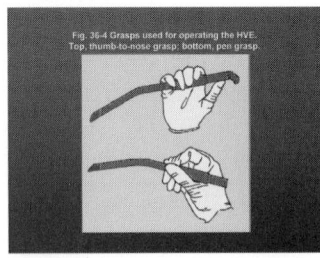

- Describe the two HVE grasps pictured in the slide. (*Top: thumb to nose grasp; Bottom: pen grasp.*)

- Both methods enable the dental assistant to control the tip.

- Why is it important to control the tip? *(For placement and to assure patient comfort and safety.)*

Slide 12

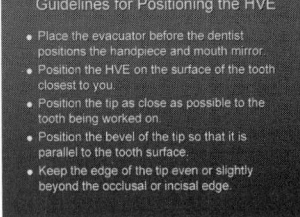

- Depending on how much the tissue resists retraction and depending on the area being treated, you may want to reduce dental assistant fatigue by changing the position of the evacuator.

- In which hand does the dental assistant hold the evacuator tip when assisting a right-handed dentist? (*Right hand.*)

- Hold the evacuator tip in the left hand when assisting a left-handed dentist.

ELSEVIER

Torres and Ehrlich Modern Dental Assisting, 9th ed.

Bird/Robinson

Slide 13

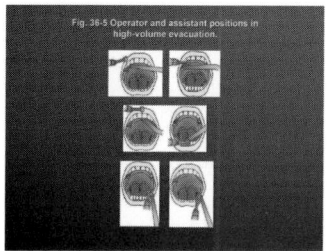

- The efficiency and effectiveness of the procedure depends on timing when suction is needed, when the HVE is positioned, and when to remove the suction tip.

- Notice how the suction tip is close to the working end of the handpiece.

- Why should the dental assistant position the HVE close to the handpiece? (*To catch water spray and debris before it collects in the patient's mouth.*)

Slide 14

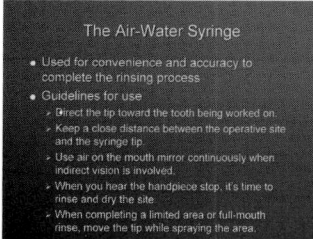

- Use the air-water syringe to increase visibility of the treatment area.

- The air-water syringe is attached to the dental unit; it directs air, water, or both through a small sterile metal tip or plastic disposable tip.

- Rinsing also removes debris from the patient's mouth before dismissal.

Slide 15

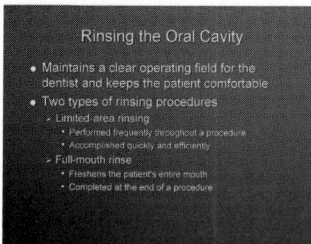

- Perform limited rinsing quickly and efficiently, without delaying the procedure, when the dentist exits the mouth and pauses for inspection.

- When the assistant is alone and rinsing the entire mouth, he or she can use the saliva ejector as an alternative to the HVE.

Slide 16

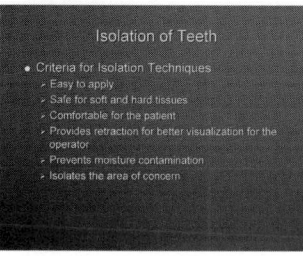

- For best results during a dental procedure, keep the area being treated dry and isolated from its normal environment.

- Why is isolation so important? (*The area or tooth being treated should be kept free from contaminants such as saliva, blood, and debris to avoid infection from a failed restoration.*)

- What are the three most common isolation techniques used in dentistry? (*Cotton roll isolation, dry-angle isolation, and dental dam placement.*)

ELSEVIER

Bird/Robinson

Slide 17

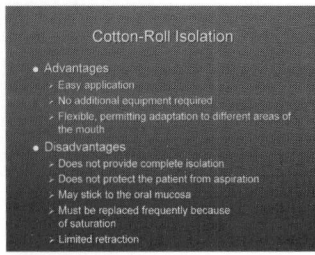

- Cotton rolls of tightly formed, absorbent cotton are preshaped to be positioned close to the salivary gland ducts.
- The cotton rolls are positioned to absorb the saliva flow and excess water.
- What is the best way to place or remove a cotton roll from the patient's mouth? (*Use cotton pliers or forceps.*)
- Use cotton roll holders, which are designed to hold multiple cotton rolls more securely, in the mandibular areas.
- Can you think of a time when cotton roll holders would be needed most? (*When the operator is working alone.*)

Slide 18

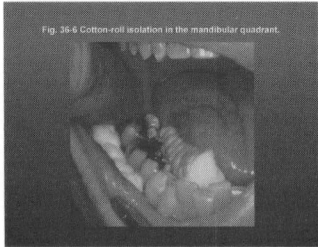

- Knowing salivary duct location is important to control proper moisture.
- Where are the salivary ducts on the maxillary arch and what are they called? (*The ducts are located in the buccal mucosa adjacent to the maxillary second molar buccal surfaces. These bilateral ducts are called the Stensen's duct.*)
- Where is the salivary duct on the mandibular arch located, and what is it called? (*The duct is located just under the tongue lingual to the mandibular anterior teeth. This duct is called the Wharton's duct.*)

Slide 19

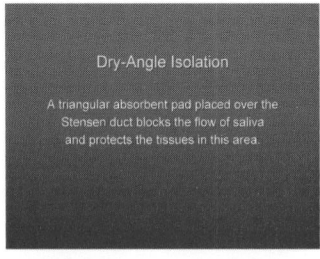

- Instead of placing a cotton roll along the buccal mucosa as an isolation technique, place a dry angle.
- This pad helps to isolate posterior teeth in both the maxillary and mandibular arches.
- Place the dry angle on the buccal mucosa over the Stensen's duct.
- What are the two functions of the dry angle? (*Block the flow of saliva, and protect the tissues in this area from injury from the dental bur or other dental instruments.*)

Slide 20

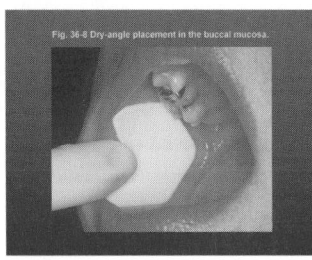

- Remember to follow manufacturer's instructions for placement.
- If the dry angle becomes soaked during the procedure, it may need to be replaced several times.
- Soaking the pad with water lets you easily remove and separate it from the tissues (buccal mucosa).
- Use the cotton pliers/forceps to replace the dry angle.

Slide 21

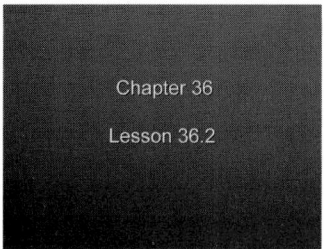

Slide 22

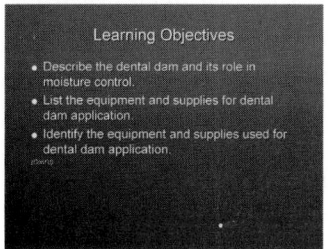

Slide 23

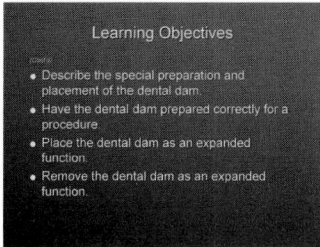

Slide 24

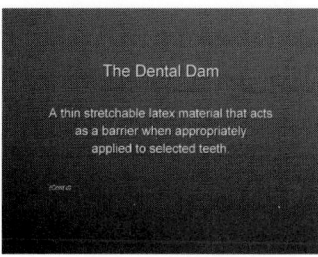

- When the dam is in place only selected teeth are visible through the dam.

- What are these isolated teeth called? (*Isolated or exposed teeth.*)

- The dam is placed after local anesthesia is administered and before the procedure begins.

- Use caution when using the dam on a patient allergic to latex, making sure the dental dam material is latex-free.

Bird/Robinson

Slide 25

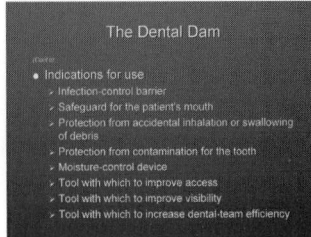

- The dental dam can be placed in about 2 minutes.
- The dental dam keeps debris from the preparation or treatment area away from the rest of the mouth.

Slide 26

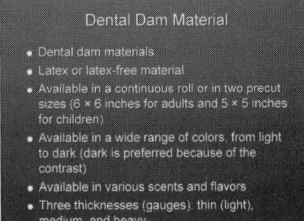

- Use thin dam materials most frequently for endodontic application, since only one tooth is isolated and minimal stretching of the material occurs.
- Often use medium thickness in operative procedures because it is easy to handle and can isolate selected teeth.
- Use heavy materials when tissue retraction and extra resistance to tearing is required. Also use heavier materials when you must isolate teeth with tight contacts.

Slide 27

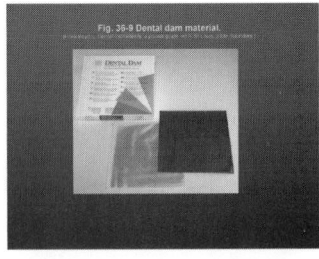

- Many different dental manufacturers or dental supply companies have dental dam materials available.
- Consider several factors when purchasing dental dam materials: cost, quality, availability, compatibility with dental dam napkins, lubricants, the dental dam punch, dental dam forceps and the dental dam frame.

Slide 28

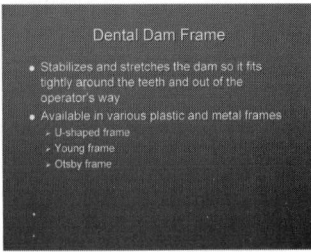

- The dental dam frame is a necessary component of dental dam placement.
- Both plastic and metal frames can be sterilized and reused.
- The plastic U-shaped frame is radiolucent, so it is not necessary to remove it before radiograph exposure. The frame is placed under the dam material.
- The Young frame is placed on the outside of the dam. Patients are more comfortable using this frame.

Torres and Ehrlich Modern Dental Assisting, 9th ed.

Bird/Robinson

Slide 29

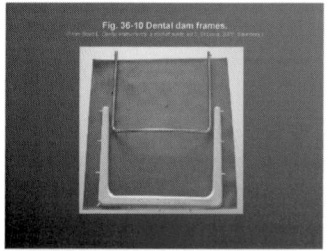

- Identify the two common dental dam frames in the slide. (*Both are U-shaped frames. The first is the metal Young U-shaped frame, and the second is a plastic U-shaped frame.*)
- The sharp projections hold the dental dam material in place.

Slide 30

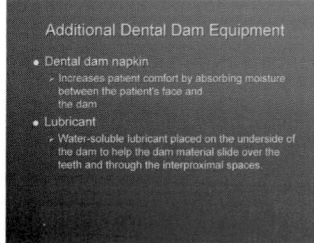

- Can you think of another advantage to using a dental dam napkin? (*It keeps the patient's face from contacting the dental dam material, which could cause skin irritation.*)
- Two dental dam lubricants can be used. One is used on the patient's lips to ensure patient comfort. The second is used to help the dam materials slide between the interproximal spaces without tearing or ripping.

Slide 31

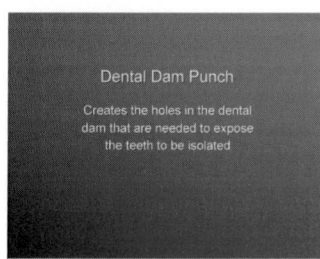

- The working end of the dental punch has an adjustable stylus.
- What is a stylus? (*Cutting tip.*)

Slide 32

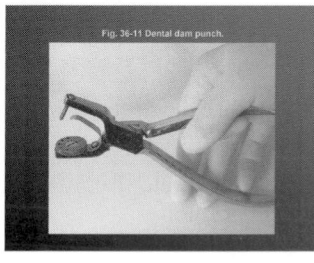

- Notice how the punch plate is a rotary plate form with five or six holes of different sizes cut into the face of the plate.
- These holes are approximately 1mm deep with sharp edges to accommodate the stylus.
- Use caution to make sure the holes are cut cleanly. Holes with a ragged edge may tear easily when forced between interproximal spaces of the teeth to be isolated. Ragged edges on the holes may also irritate the gingiva.

Slide 33

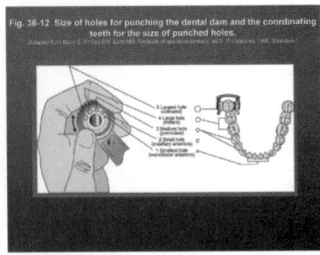

- The punch plate holes are numbered one (the smallest) through five (the largest), and fit around different size objects, as follows:
  - 1—mandibular anterior teeth
  - 2—maxillary anterior teeth
  - 3—mandibular and maxillary premolars
  - 4—larger teeth such as molars
  - 5—creates the hole that fits over the dental dam clamp
- How do you know where to punch the holes on the dental dam material? (*The dental dam stamp and template will guide the position of the holes to be punched.*)

Slide 34

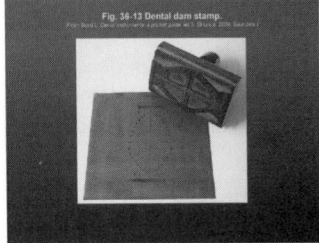

- The dental dam stamp and inkpad are used to mark the dental dam with predetermined markings for the average adult and pediatric arches.
- The template provides flexibility when one or more teeth in the arch are out of alignment.

Slide 35

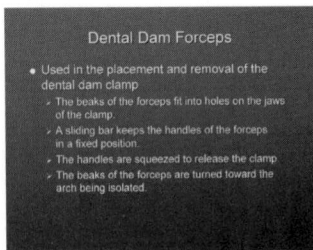

- The handles of the forceps work with a spring action.
- Why do you think the beaks of the forceps are turned toward the arch being isolated? (*This permits the operator to place or remove the clamp without having to rotate the forceps to put them into position.*)

Slide 36

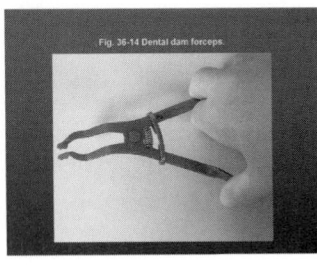

- Notice how the hand of the operator is stretched before squeezing the forceps.
- After squeezing the spring-action forceps, the operator holds the forceps in position with the sliding bar.
- The operator will squeeze the handles again to release the dental dam clamp.
- Notice the position of the beaks, which prevents the operator from having to rotate the forceps to place the clamp in position.

Bird/Robinson

Slide 37

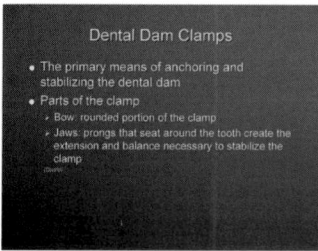

- The clamps are made of chrome or nickel-plated steel and can be sterilized and reused.
- The clamps are designed to hold the dental dam secure at both ends along with a dental dam stabilizing cord.
- Dental dam clamps are available in many sizes and designs to accommodate different needs.
- The jaws are designed to fit the cervical area or collar of the tooth.

Slide 38

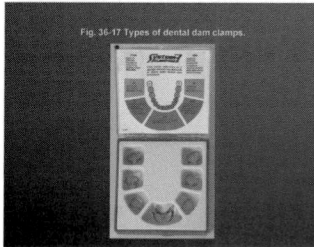

- Numerous clamps are available for various isolation needs:
  - Clamps 7 and W7 are universal mandibular molar clamps.
  - Clamps 8 and W8 are universal maxillary clamps.
  - Clamps 9 and W9 are designed for anterior teeth.
  - Clamps 00, W00, and 2 are designed for primary teeth.

Slide 39

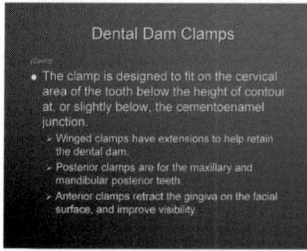

- Posterior and anterior clamps are available. The posterior clamp is universal and can be used on the same tooth in the opposite quadrant.
- Anterior clamps are designed to retract gingiva on the facial surfaces, improve visibility for class V restorations, and isolate an anterior tooth during endodontic treatment.

Slide 40

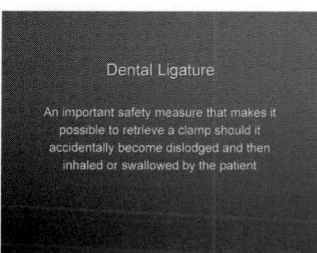

- A dental dam stabilizing cord can simply be a piece of dental floss or dental tape.

Slide 41

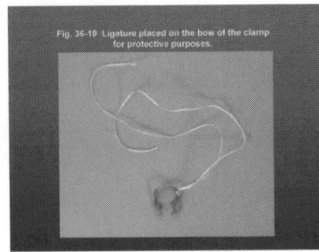

- The slide shows an example of ligating the dental dam clamp.
- Always cut a long enough piece so it can readily be grabbed if needed.
- Tie the other end of the ligature to the frame of the dental dam to ensure that you can easily find the end.

Slide 42

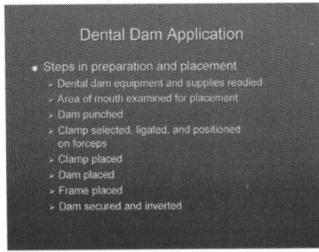

- Applications:
  - Maxillary arch application: Punch the holes one inch down from the upper edge of the dam.
  - Mandibular arch application: Punch the holes two inches from the edge.
- Curve of the arch: It may be necessary to make adjustments to accommodate an extremely narrow or wide arch.
- Use the one-step or the two-step method to place the dam. The main difference in the methods is the sequencing in the placement of the clamp and dental dam.

Slide 43

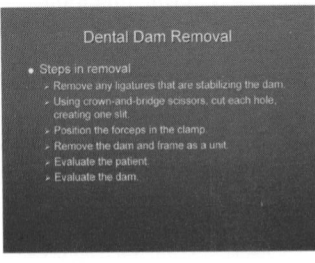

- Why is it important to evaluate the dental material after removal? (*Fragments of the dental dam left behind under the gingiva can cause gingival irritation.*)

Bird/Robinson

37 Anesthesia and Pain Control

TEACHING FOCUS

This chapter will give the student an opportunity to understand local anesthetic agents, including topical and local anesthesia. Injection techniques, local anesthesia setup, and complications and precautions will be discussed. The student will also have an opportunity to learn about electronic anesthesia, inhalation sedation, antianxiety agents, intravenous sedation, and general anesthesia. Documentation of anesthesia and pain control will be discussed.

MATERIALS AND RESOURCES

- ☐ computer and PowerPoint projector (all Lessons)
- ☐ equipment for measuring vital signs (Lesson 37.2)
- ☐ N₂O/O₂ system (Lesson 37.2)
- ☐ scavenger-type masks (adult and child sizes) (Lesson 37.2)
- ☐ sealed disposable needle or needles (Lesson 37.1)
- ☐ sterile assembled local anesthetic syringe (Lesson 37.1)

- ☐ sterile cotton-tipped applicators (Lesson 37.1)
- ☐ sterile gauze sponges (Lesson 37.1)
- ☐ sterile local anesthetic cartridges (Lesson 37.1)
- ☐ sterile syringe (Lesson 37.1)
- ☐ topical anesthetic ointment (Lesson 37.1)
- ☐ 2x2-inch cotton gauze sponges (Lesson 37.1)

LESSON CHECKLIST

Preparations for this lesson include:

- lecture
- guest speaker: dental assistant
- evaluation of student knowledge and skills needed to perform all entry-level activities related to anesthesia and pain control, including:
  - local anesthesia
  - topical anesthesia
  - vasoconstrictors in anesthesia
  - injection techniques
  - local anesthesia setup
  - complications and precautions
  - electronic anesthesia
  - inhalation sedation
  - antianxiety agents
  - intravenous sedation
  - local anesthetic agents
  - general anesthesia
  - documentation of anesthesia and pain control

ELSEVIER

Torres and Ehrlich Modern Dental Assisting, 9th ed.

Bird/Robinson

KEY TERMS

analgesia (p. 561)
anesthesia (p. 545)
anesthetic (p. 545)
aspirate (p. 552)
diffuse (p. 546)
duration (p. 548)
gauge (p. 552)
induction (p. 548)
innervation (p. 548)

lumen (p. 552)
oximetry (p. 561)
permeate (p. 546)
porous (p. 548)
systemic toxicity (p. 554)
tidal volume (p. 559)
titrate (p. 558)
titration (p. 558)
vasoconstrictor (p. 547)

ADDITIONAL RESOURCES

PowerPoint slides (Evolve): 1-46
Multimedia Procedures DVD:
    Applying a Topical Anesthetic
    Assisting with Local Anesthesia

Legend

CTQ
Critical
Thinking
Question

DVD
Multimedia
Procedures
Videos and
Animations

ESLR
EVOLVE
Student
Learning
Resources

IDO
Interactive
Dental
Office
CD-ROM

SW
Student
Workbook

TB
Test Bank
on the
TEACH
CD-ROM

PPT
PowerPoint
Slides

Class Activities are indicated in ***bold italic***.

ELSEVIER

Torres and Ehrlich Modern Dental Assisting, 9th ed.

Bird/Robinson

LESSON 37.1

PRETEST

1. How many hours before receiving general anesthesia must a patient refrain from eating or drinking?
   a. 2 to 4 hours
   b. 6 to 7 hours
   c. 8 to 12 hours
   d. 24 hours

2. In what circumstance may local anesthesia be less effective?
   a. painless administration
   b. if used at room temperature
   c. administration into an infected area
   d. administration of topical anesthesia first

3. A patient with a medical history with which of the following conditions may require the use of a local anesthetic without a vasoconstrictor (e.g. epinephrine)?
   a. a fractured foot
   b. an allergy to penicillin
   c. a history of skin cancer
   d. a recent heart attack

4. During intravenous conscious sedation, how often should physiologic measurements such as level of consciousness, respiratory function, oximetry, blood pressure, heart rate, and cardiac rhythm be taken and recorded?
   a. every 5 minutes
   b. every 15 minutes
   c. every 30 minutes
   d. every 60 minutes

5. What part of the syringe must be engaged for proper aspiration during a mandibular block?
   a. the finger bar
   b. the harpoon
   c. the thumb ring
   d. the finger grip

6. What does the addition of a vasoconstrictor to a local anesthetic help with?
   a. increases bleeding during a surgical procedure
   b. shortens the effect of the anesthetic agent
   c. improves the taste
   d. decreases bleeding during a surgical procedure

7. What should be applied with a cotton-tipped applicator to dry gingival tissue before administration of local anesthesia?
   a. petroleum jelly
   b. topical anesthesia
   c. lidocaine HCl
   d. rubbing alcohol

8. To prevent diffusion hypoxia following the use of nitrous oxide, how long should 100% oxygen be administered?
   a. 1 minute
   b. 5 minutes
   c. 10 minutes
   d. 30 minutes

9. What step helps reduce the exposure to nitrous oxide by dental professionals?
   a. use of a scavenging system
   b. venting gas inside the dental operatory
   c. using a poorly fitting mask on patients
   d. encouraging patients to talk while receiving nitrous oxide

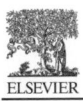

ELSEVIER

Torres and Ehrlich Modern Dental Assisting, 9th ed.

Bird/Robinson

10. Which of the following is an anxiolytic?
    a. Tylenol
    b. aspirin
    c. multivitamin
    d. Valium

Answers

1. c	3. d	5. b	7. b	9. a
2. c	4. b	6. d	8. b	10. d

BACKGROUND ASSESSMENT

Question: Lidocaine HCl with epinephrine is a commonly used local anesthetic in dentistry. What is epinephrine? Why is it added to local anesthetic? When should a local anesthetic with epinephrine be avoided, or used with caution?

Answer: Epinephrine is a vasoconstrictor that is added to a local anesthetic to help prolong the duration of action of the anesthetic. During surgical procedures, injection of a vasoconstrictor helps to decrease bleeding in the nearby tissues. Careful review of a patient's medical history is crucial. A history positive for cardiac conditions such as an irregular heart beat, congestive heart failure, a recent heart attack, or high blood pressure may indicate that a local anesthetic containing a vasoconstrictor should not be used.

Question: What is the most commonly used inhalational sedative used in dentistry? What are some of the advantages of inhalation sedation? What are some precautions?

Answer: Nitrous oxide and oxygen (N_2O/O_2) is the most common and safest type of the inhalational sedatives. N_2O/O_2 is inhaled through a nasal mask to provide a pleasant, relaxing environment for a patient receiving dental treatment. When administered properly, the patient remains awake and is able to communicate with the dental team throughout the entire procedure. N_2O/O_2 should be avoided during pregnancy and with individuals diagnosed with emphysema. A proper scavenging system should be in place at all times to collect and dispose of unused N_2O/O_2 to prevent unnecessary exposure of the dental team. At the end of the dental procedure, the N_2O should be discontinued, yet the patient should continue to have 100% O_2 delivered for 5 more minutes to prevent diffusion hypoxia.

CRITICAL THINKING QUESTION

You have just finished assisting the oral surgeon during multiple surgical extractions on a healthy 70-year-old man. This patient will now be visiting his general dentist a few floors down in the office building for insertion of an immediate partial denture. A copy of the clinical notes must accompany the patient. You have been asked to prepare the preliminary notes, which will ultimately be reviewed and signed by the oral surgeon. Both IV conscious sedation and local anesthesia were used. What information must be included in the patient notes?

Guidelines: First, it is important to state that the medical history has been reviewed. Any positive findings should be noted, including current medications, any known drug allergies, and any systemic concerns or past surgeries. The patient's vital signs (including the level of consciousness, blood oxygen concentration, and cardiac rhythm) should be clearly recorded on the sheet showing baseline vitals before surgery and during surgery (every 15 minutes) up to and including dismissal of the patient. This spreadsheet should highlight when IV anesthesia began, when it was stopped, when the IV was removed, the names, concentrations, and amounts of medications administered, as well as the amount of normal saline given over the course of IV conscious sedation. You should also mention into which arm the IV was placed. The sheet should also show the time local anesthesia was administered, the type, concentration, and amount of both local anesthesia and vasoconstrictor that was used and the method by which it was administered. You may also mention whether topical anesthesia was used first. In addition to a detailed description of the actual surgical procedure, it should also be noted whether there were any adverse events or complications, how the patient tolerated the procedure, any postoperative instructions given to the patient, any postsurgical follow-up planned, and whether anyone accompanied the patient.

OBJECTIVES	CONTENT	TEACHING RESOURCES
Pronounce, define, and spell the Key Terms.	■ Key terms (p. 544-545)	*e* ESLR Electronic Flashcards ▶ Discuss each of the key terms in Chapter 37, focusing on the definition, pronunciation, and spelling of each term. *Class Activity Divide the class into pairs, and have the students write a dialogue between an experienced dental assistant and a new assistant, about anesthesia and pain control using each of the key terms properly. Select several pairs to act out their prepared dialogue for the class. Encourage discussion and feedback, including teaching correct pronunciation and usage.*
Discuss the importance of pain control in dentistry.	■ Introduction (p. 545)	☒≣ PPT 5-6 ▣ TB question 1 ▓ SW Short-Answer Questions 1 (p. 257) ▶ Discuss the fact that a variety of procedures to control anxiety and pain has allowed the dental profession to extend oral health care to millions of individuals who would otherwise remain untreated. *Class Activity Have student pairs take turns role-playing a patient and a dental assistant in situations involving dental pain before, during, and after a procedure. Then have students discuss what they learned in the activity.*
Describe the composition and application of topical anesthetics.	■ Topical anesthesia (p. 545)	☒≣ PPT 7-8 ▣ TB questions 2-3 ▓ SW Short-Answer Questions 2; Fill in the Blank question 1; Multiple Choice questions 1, 19 (pp. 257-259) Recall question 1 (p. 546) Figure 37-1 Topical anesthetic (p. 546) ▶ Discuss how topical anesthetics work. ▶ Discuss how topical anesthetics are applied. *Class Activity Bring examples of various forms of topical anesthetics to class. Provide the students with photocopies of the manufacturer inserts for these various products. Ask students to find and highlight the composition of the products, as well as any special instructions. Then have students describe the information they found and compare all products.*
Demonstrate the placement of a topical anesthetic agent.	■ Topical anesthesia (p. 545) *Procedure* 37-1 Applying a topical anesthetic (p. 547) (SW/ESLR Competency 37-1, p. 261)	🎥 Multimedia Procedures DVD: Applying a Topical Anesthetic ▓ *e* SW/ESLR Competency 37-1 Applying a Topical Anesthetic (p. 261)

OBJECTIVES	CONTENT	TEACHING RESOURCES
		Figure 37-2 Topical gel patch (p. 546)
		♥ CTQ 2 (p. 562)
		***Class Activity** Provide each student with the appropriate material for topical anesthetic application (ointment type). Have student pairs take turns practicing drying the oral mucosa and applying small amounts of topical anesthesia on each other.*

Discuss the composition and application of local anesthetic agents.	■ Local anesthesia (p. 546)
	  □ Characteristics of local anesthetics (p. 563)
	  □ Method of action (p. 546)
	  □ Chemical composition of anesthetics (p. 546)
	  □ Vasoconstrictors in anesthetics (p. 547)
	    – Contraindications to vasoconstrictors (p. 547)
	  □ Time span of anesthetics (p. 548)
	■ Injection techniques (p. 548)
	  □ Maxillary anesthesia (p. 548)
	  □ Palatal anesthesia (p. 548)
	  □ Mandibular anesthesia (p. 548)
	  □ Periodontal ligament injection (p. 549)
	■ Local anesthesia setup (p. 549)
	  □ Anesthetic syringe (p. 549)
	  □ Anesthetic cartridges (p. 550)
	    – Color-coding of local anesthetic cartridges (p. 550)
	    – Guidelines for handling anesthetic cartridges (p. 551)
		⊠▤ PPT 9-18
		
		▣ TB questions 4-15
		
		▥ SW Short-Answer Questions 3; Fill in the Blank questions 3-4, 6-8, 10-13; Multiple Choice questions 2-7, 16-18, 20 (pp. 257-259)
		
		Box 37-1 Routinely Used Dental Anesthetics (p. 548)
		
		Recall questions 2-4 (p. 548)
		
		Figure 37-3 Maxillary injections (p. 549)
		
		Figure 37-4 Palatal injections (p. 549)
		
		Figure 37-5 Mandibular injections (p. 550)
		
		Figure 37-6 Periodontal ligament injection (p. 550)
		
		Figure 37-7 Anesthetic syringe (p. 551)
		
		Figure 37-8 Anesthetic cartridges (p. 551)
		
		Figure 37-9 Local anesthetic cartridges packaged in blister packs (p. 551)
		
		Figure 37-10 Anesthesia color codes (p. 551)
		
		Figure 37-11 Sterile needle (p. 552)
		
		Figure 37-12 Outer covering for the needle (p. 552)
		
		♥ CTQ 1, 3, 5 (p. 562)
		
		▸ Discuss the use of vasoconstrictors in anesthetics.
		
		▸ Discuss injection techniques for local anesthetics.
		
		***Class Activity** Bring examples of the various types of cartridges, syringes, and needles to class. Set up several stations around the classroom for the students to rotate through. At each station, have the students perform a different task:*
		
		– label various portions of the syringe with a number, and correctly pair numbers with a list of parts
		
		– pair up the appropriate color with the corresponding local anesthetic

OBJECTIVES	CONTENT	TEACHING RESOURCES
	☐ Disposable needle (p. 552)	*– practice safely decapping and recapping the needles in combination with safe transfers and proper disposal of sharps*
Demonstrate the preparation and management of the local anesthetic setup.	Procedure 37-2 Assembling the local anesthetic syringe (p. 553) (SW/ESLR Competencies 37-2 and 37-3, pp. 263-264)	TB question 16 SW/ESLR Competencies 37-2 and 37-3 Assisting in the Assembly and Administration of Local Anesthesia (pp. 263-264) ***Class Activity** Bring examples of various types of cartridges, syringes, and needles to class. Have the students practice safely assembling and disassembling the appropriate needle and cartridge into the aspirating syringe.*
Discuss the composition and application of local anesthetic agents.	■ Complications and precautions (p. 552) ☐ Injection into a blood vessel (p. 552) ☐ Infected areas (p. 552) ☐ Toxic reactions (p. 554) – Localized reactions (p. 554) – Systemic reactions (p. 554) ☐ Temporary numbness (p. 554) ☐ Paresthesia (p. 554)	PPT 19 TB questions 17-19 SW Multiple Choice question 8 (p. 257) Recall questions 5-8 (p. 552, 554) ▸ Discuss the characteristics of local anesthetics. ▸ Discuss the complications and precautions of local anesthetics. ***Class Activity** Divide the class into small groups, and have each group develop a set of educational materials on the possible toxic reactions to local anesthetic agents. Then have each group share its materials with the class.*
Assist during the administration of local anesthesia.	Procedure 37-3 Assisting in the administration of local anesthesia (p. 555) (SW/ESLR Competencies 37-2 and 37-3, pp. 263-264) ■ Electronic anesthesia (p. 556)	PPT 20 Multimedia Procedures DVD: Assisting with Local Anesthesia SW/ESLR Competencies 37-2 and 37-3 Assisting in the Assembly and Administration of Local Anesthesia (pp. 263-264) Figure 37-13 Electronic anesthesia (p. 556) ***Class Activity** Divide the class into small groups. Have each group discuss the procedural steps and rationales for each step of the administration of local anesthesia. Then have each group share its findings with the class.*

Torres and Ehrlich Modern Dental Assisting, 9th ed.
Torres and Ehrlich Modern Dental Assisting, 9th ed.

Bird/Robinson

37.1 Homework/Assignments:

37.1 Instructor's Notes/Student Feedback:

LESSON 37.2

CRITICAL THINKING QUESTION

At the end of your workday, you are reviewing tomorrow's schedule in order to have everything organized for the first patient. The first patient is a healthy, married, 30-year-old man with no allergies, nothing significant in his medical history, and who does not take any medications on a regular basis. He is scheduled for surgical extraction of nonrestorable, fractured tooth #2. Reading further, you note that the patient has reported extreme dental fear. He has been prescribed Valium to take the night before the morning of the procedure. Furthermore, the patient has requested nitrous oxide in addition to local anesthesia. List a few key points to keep in mind with respect to the oral anxiolytic, and describe how you would set up the room with respect to anesthesia and pain/anxiety control.

Guidelines: First, because this patient will have taken an oral sedative, he should be reminded that he should be accompanied to his appointment. Alternately, the patient may arrive one hour before the appointment and take the oral sedative at the office. Depending on office protocol, a telephone call the day before the appointment, not only for confirmation purposes, but to ask whether the patient has any other questions or concerns may be greatly appreciated by the patient. Have the written surgical consent form ready to be discussed and signed as well as a written postsurgical instruction sheet for the patient to take home. With respect to the local anesthesia, review the medical history with the dentist to assure that you have chosen the correct type. Because of the surgical nature of the procedure, a local anesthetic with a vasoconstrictor would be desirable. In this case, one or possibly two cartridges of local anesthesia will be required. Ensure that the syringe and a short needle (as anesthesia will involve various maxillary infiltrations) are available in addition to topical anesthesia, an applicator, and gauze. A blood pressure cuff will be needed, and a clock to record heart rate for presurgical vitals. All the surgical equipment should be chosen in advance to help expedite a smooth procedure, and thus help prevent undesirable patient concern. With respect to the N_2O/O_2, verify that that an adult-sized nose mask is in order, that the scavenging system is working, and that there is sufficient nitrous oxide and oxygen in the tanks. Assure that you are able to easily adjust the control on/off valves for proper titration; be sure the flow meters are accurate and that the reservoir bag is in good condition, with no leaks.

OBJECTIVES	CONTENT	TEACHING RESOURCES
Describe nitrous oxide/oxygen sedation and its use in dentistry.	■ Inhalation sedation (p. 556) □ Chemical makeup (p. 556) □ Contraindications to nitrous oxide use (p. 556) – Pregnancy (p. 556) – Nasal obstruction (p. 556) – Emphysema and multiple sclerosis (p. 556) – Emotional instability (p. 556) □ Equipment (p. 556)	⊠▤ PPT 24-29 TB. TB questions 20-22 SW Short-Answer Questions 4; Fill in the Blank question 14; Multiple Choice questions 9, 11-12, 15 (pp. 257-259) SW Case Study questions 1-5 (p. 260) Figure 37-14 Portable nitrous oxide system unit (p. 557) Figure 37-15 Nitrous oxide gas lines are color-coded blue, and oxygen gas lines are color-coded green (p. 557) Figure 37-16 Nasal mask used for inhalation (p. 557) 💡 CTQ 6 (p. 562) ▸ Discuss the chemical makeup of nitrous oxide. ▸ Discuss how nitrous oxide is administered. ***Class Activity Divide the class into small groups, and have them discuss clinical situations in which nitrous oxide may be helpful and others that may not warrant its use. Have the groups present their findings to the class.***

Bird/Robinson

OBJECTIVES	CONTENT	TEACHING RESOURCES
Discuss the importance of reducing the dental team's exposure to nitrous oxide.	– Scavenger system (p. 557) ☐ Reducing exposure to nitrous oxide (p. 557) ☐ Patient assessment and monitoring (p. 558) ☐ Patient education (p. 558) ☐ Administration (p. 558)	⊠ PPT 30-31 TB question 23-24 SW Short-Answer Questions 5; Fill in the Blank question 9; Multiple Choice question 10 (pp. 257-259) Recall questions 9-12 (p. 558) Figure 37-17 Scavenger system attached to mask and evacuation unit to redirect unused nitrous oxide gas (p. 558) ▸ Discuss the importance of reducing the dental team's exposure to nitrous oxide, along with ways to do so. *Class Activity Divide the class into small groups, and have each group develop an office checklist outlining safe usage of nitrous oxide. Have the students match guidelines with reasons why the guidelines are important. Have each group present its checklist to the class.*
Assist in the administration and monitoring of nitrous oxide/oxygen sedation.	Procedure 37-4 Assisting in the administration and monitoring of nitrous oxide/oxygen sedation (expanded function) (p. 559) (SW/ESLR Competency 37-4, pp. 265-266)	⊠ PPT 32-33 SW/ESLR Competency 37-4 Assisting in the Administration and Monitoring of Nitrous Oxide/Oxygen (pp. 265-266) *Class Activity Bring a portable nitrous oxide/oxygen unit into the classroom. Allow students to explore the various components and the proper names for each. Allow students to attempt placing a nasal mask on each other while adjusting for a proper and adequate fit of the scavenging component. Have students practice turning on and off the oxygen valve (but not while a mask is in use.)*
Discuss intravenous sedation and its use in dentistry.	■ Antianxiety agents (p. 558) ■ Intravenous sedation (p. 560)	⊠ PPT 34-38 TB questions 25-26 SW Short-Answer Questions 6; Fill in the Blank questions 2, 5 (pp. 257-258) Recall question 13 (p. 561) CTQ 4 (p. 562) ▸ Discuss how intravenous sedation works. ▸ Discuss the patient management and monitoring necessary during intravenous sedation. *Class Activity Invite a dental assistant who works in an oral surgery office to speak to the class. Have each student submit a paragraph at the end of the visit outlining the important points covered in the talk and listing any further questions they may have relating to IV conscious sedation.*

ELSEVIER

Bird/Robinson

OBJECTIVES	CONTENT	TEACHING RESOURCES
Discuss general anesthesia and its use in dentistry.	■ General anesthesia (p. 561) □ Four stages of anesthesia (p. 561) □ Patient preparation (p. 561) □ Patient education (p. 561) □ Patient recovery (p. 562) ■ Documentation of anesthesia and pain control (p. 562)	🖾 PPT 39-46 🖳 TB questions 27-29 📓 SW Short-Answer Questions 7; Multiple Choice questions 13-14 (pp. 257, 259) Recall questions 13-14 (pp. 561, 562) ▸ Discuss the four stages of anesthesia. ▸ Discuss the preparation, education, and recovery a patient needs when undergoing general anesthesia. ***Class Activity Divide the class into small groups, and have each group create a patient information sheet with preoperative and postoperative instructions. Have each group share its information sheet with the class for feedback and discussion.***
Performance Evaluation		🖳 TB 📓 SW questions (pp. 257-259) 📓 SW Case Study (pp. 259-260) 📓 *e* SW/ESLR Competency 37-1 Applying a Topical Anesthetic (p. 261) 📓 *e* SW/ESLR Competencies 37-2 and 37-3 Assisting in the Assembly and Administration of Local Anesthesia (pp. 263-264) 📓 *e* SW/ESLR Competency 37-4 Assisting in the Administration and Monitoring of Nitrous Oxide/Oxygen (pp. 265-266) *e* ESLR Electronic Flashcards *e* ESLR Practice Quiz questions Recall questions (pp. 546-562) ♀ CTQ (p. 562)

37.2 Homework/Assignments:

37.2 Instructor's Notes/Student Feedback:

Slide 1

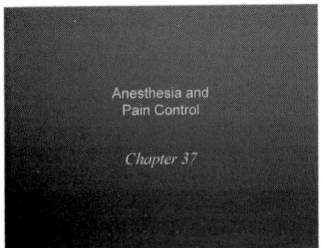

Slide 2

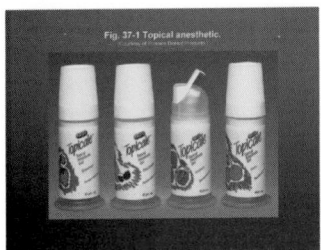

- Pain is one of the most feared aspects related to dentistry and one of the top reasons for avoiding dental treatment.

- Adequate and appropriate anesthesia and pain control for a patient during a dental procedure will make the delivery of dental treatment much easier and less stressful for the dental team, as well as for the patient.

Slide 3

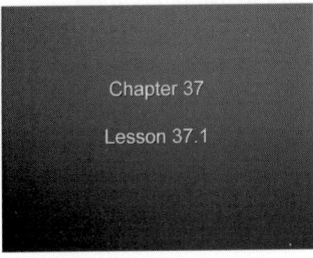

- Patients may not be able to adequately judge the caliber of dentistry delivered, but they are able to relay whether they experienced pain or discomfort.

Slide 4

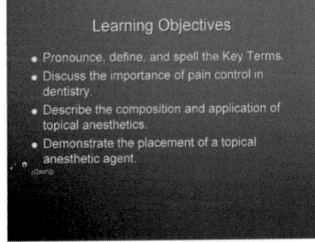

Slide 5

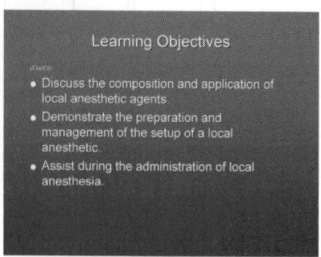

- What is an example of a psychological method to help prevent and treat pain and anxiety before, during, and after a dental procedure? *(Talking with the patient in a calm, gentle, and caring manner while addressing any questions about the anesthesia and procedure.)*

- What is an example of a physical approach? *(Gentle handling of the patient, avoiding fast, unexpected movements.)*

- Providing a patient with a painless dental experience will make future appointments more pleasant.

Slide 6

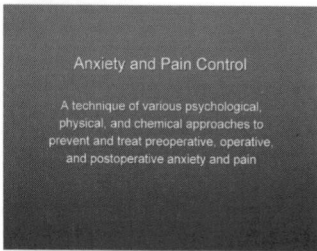

- Anesthetic agents include topical anesthetics *(jelly)* and local anesthetics *(injectables)*.

- Nitrous oxide and oxygen are the most common inhalational sedatives, but antianxiety medications may also be prescribed to be taken by mouth before the dental procedure.

- Medications may also be administered by IV alone or in combination with inhalational agents to provide deeper levels of analgesia and anesthesia.

Slide 7

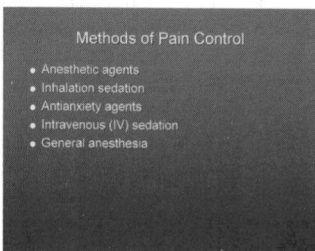

- Most commonly used is a jelly-like ointment, usually 20% benzocaine.

- Must be left on long enough to effectively permeate the oral mucosa before injecting a local anesthetic.

- What step helps promote effective penetration of the topical anesthetic? *(Drying the membranes with gauze to avoid dilution.)*

- Sprays are sometimes used for patients with extreme gag reflexes.

Slide 8

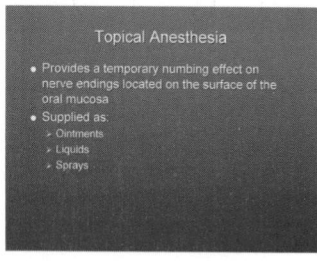

- Some topicals come in little jars. Dental assistants use cotton-tipped applicators to place the gel onto the oral mucosa.

- Following administration of both the topical and the local anesthetic, be sure to thoroughly rinse the patient's mouth, as even a small drip of local anesthetic holds a bitter taste and excess topical may temporarily cause an uncomfortable numbness of the throat.

Slide 9

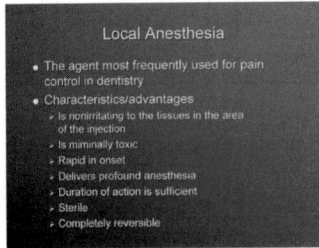

- Most patients experience minimal pain with the proper administration of topical anesthetic before injection of the local anesthetic.

- For children, is it important to know how much the child weighs, because the dentist must be careful not to exceed the maximum allowable dose, which is calculated by milligrams of the drug administered per kilogram, or pound, of body weight.

Slide 10

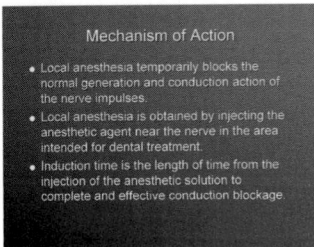

- The dentist will normally test for anesthesia before beginning the procedure by touching local and distant tissues that are normally nonresponsive with adequate anesthesia.

- It is also important to help the patient distinguish between pain and other unpleasant sensations such as vibrations, pressure, and noise. None of these problems can be resolved with additional local anesthesia.

Slide 11

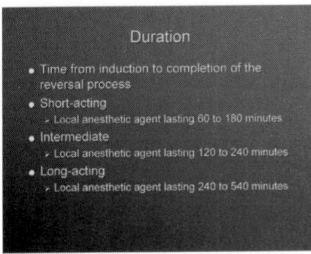

- What is a dental procedure that may require a short-acting local anesthetic? What may require longer anesthesia?

- Sometimes the procedure takes longer than anticipated; some people metabolize the anesthesia faster than anticipated, thus additional local anesthesia is administered.

- Remember that local anesthetic also has a different duration of action on the pulp of the tooth versus the soft tissue of the oral mucosa.

Slide 12

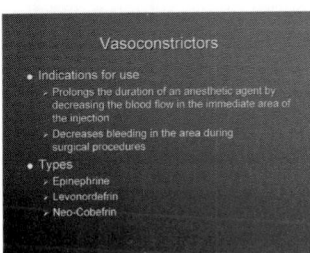

- During a surgical procedure, additional anesthetic may be injected directly into the surgical site, not because the patient is feeling pain but because additional hemostasis is required (to stop bleeding).

- Because a vasoconstrictor prolongs the duration of action, this allows for the use of less anesthetic.

- Epinephrine is one of the most common vasoconstrictors added to local anesthetics used in dentistry.

ELSEVIER

Slide 13

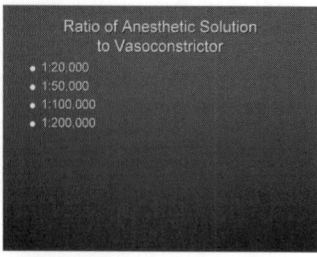

- What ratio represents a higher concentration of vasoconstrictor mixed with local anesthetic? *(1:20,000)*

- 1: 20,000 means that there is 1 g (or 1000 mg) of solute (drug) contained in 20,000 ml of solution (0.05mg/ml).

- Why use a higher concentration of vasoconstrictor? *(To prolong the effect of the local anesthesia and to decrease/control bleeding in the area.)*

Slide 14

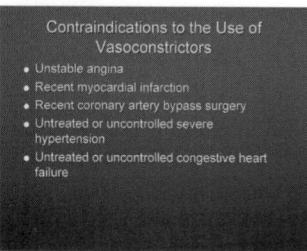

- In addition to the above contraindications for the use of a vasoconstrictor, numerous medications that a patient may be taking may also indicate limited or no usage of a vasoconstrictor.

- There are situations when an otherwise healthy person comes in for emergency treatment and, because of the vitals (elevated blood pressure due to extreme pain and/or lack of sleep), may need less vasoconstrictor than normal.

Slide 15

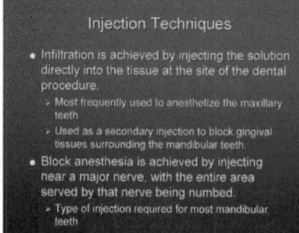

- When loading the syringe with a cartridge, what is important to consider with respect to the needle?

- With younger children, a short needle is usually used to administer all types of local anesthesia..

- Remember, when passing the loaded syringe to the dentist, keep it below the patient's chin, and away from the field of view. Keep the loaded syringe present throughout the procedure in the event that additional anesthesia is required.

Slide 16

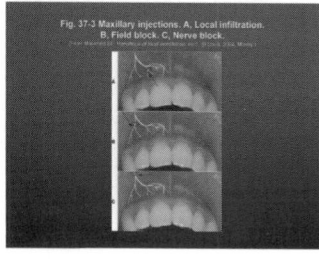

- The upper middle photo demonstrates the proper positioning of the needle during a posterior superior alveolar nerve block, which is used to anesthetize the maxillary first, second, and third molars.

- The bottom left photo highlights the approximate positioning of a lower right inferior alveolar nerve block of the mandible.

- The bottom right photo demonstrates interproximal insertion of the needle from the buccal toward the lingual to deposit additional anesthetic following the completion of an incisive nerve block.

Bird/Robinson

Slide 17

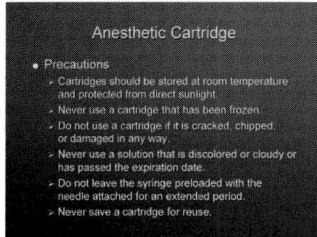

- Where should used or unused damaged anesthetic cartridges as well as needles be deposited? *(In a sharps container that is disposed of properly.)*
- Always check the expiration dates and, when restocking a treatment room, place the older cartridges at easy access for use before the newer ones.
- It is prudent to leave the used local anesthetic cartridges on the treatment tray until completion of the procedure so that an accurate account of the amount of anesthetic used is properly documented in the patient records.

Slide 18

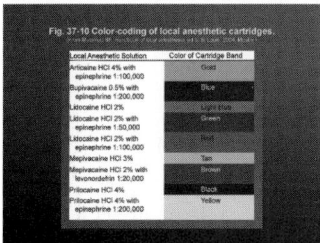

- This chart outlines the color-coded system developed by the ADA for the various types of local anesthesia with and without a vasoconstrictor. The chart corresponds to color bands on the cartridges.
- Although the bands offer a tool for quick recognition, dental assistants should always double-check by reading the label as well.

Slide 19

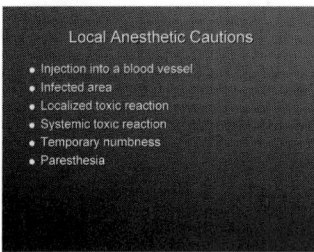

- How is injection of local anesthesia into a blood vessel prevented?
- Why is infiltration of local anesthesia into an infected area not advised? *(Inadequate anesthesia outcome due to different pH of infected tissues and risk of spreading infection.)*
- What is paresthesia? *(Loss of feeling—numbness that lasts beyond the expected duration of the local anesthetic.)*

Slide 20

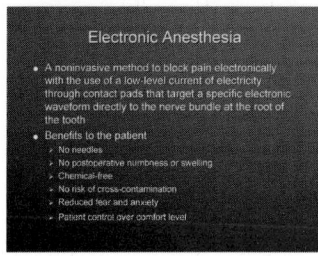

- What is a shortcoming of the above alternative to conventional local anesthesia?
- Local anesthesia is still the most widely used form of pain control in dentistry.
- In addition to what we have discussed as an alternative to the generic syringe, some dentists use a local anesthetic pump that delivers the anesthetic at a predetermined rate according to multiple variables.

Bird/Robinson

Slide 21

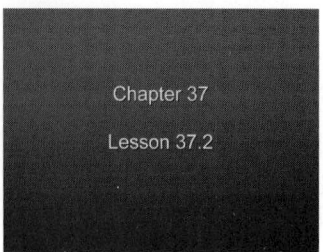

Slide 22

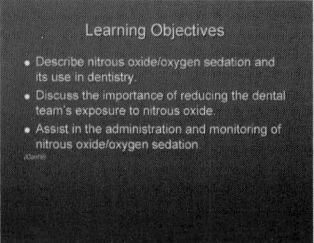

Slide 23

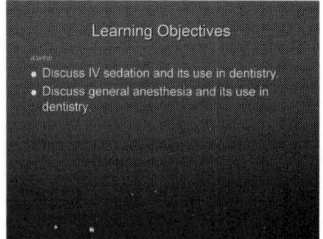

Slide 24

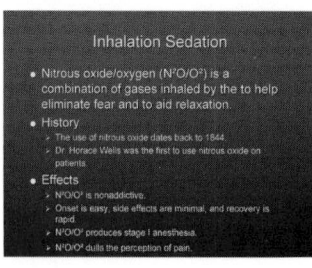

- Why should local anesthesia always be used in conjunction with nitrous oxide?

- Although nitrous oxide and oxygen are nonaddictive, dental professionals and the public may easily become addicted to the feeling experienced when inhaling this gas.

Torres and Ehrlich Modern Dental Assisting, 9th ed.

Bird/Robinson

Slide 25

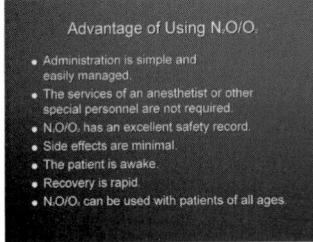

- It is important for the patient to remain awake throughout administration, allowing for proper titration of the gases according to the patient's signs and symptoms.

- When administering nitrous oxide to a child, be sure that children's nasal masks are available. Regardless of the patient's age, a qualified dental team member should stay with the patient at all times.

Slide 26

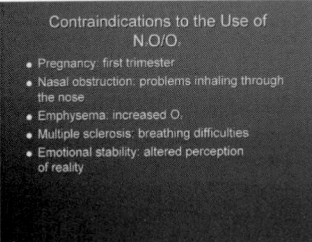

- What is an example of a common nasal obstruction? *(Deviated septum.)*

- There are some medical conditions in which nitrous oxide/oxygen is actually desirable because of the additional oxygen being delivered.

- The dental assistant should also be familiar with the unit because he or she may be required to deliver pure oxygen to a patient in an emergency.

Slide 27

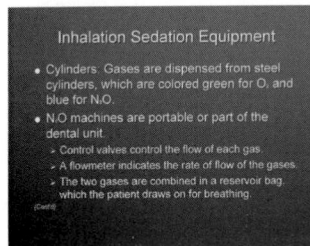

- If portable units are in place, the valves are not usually opened unless the unit is about to be used.

- Before using nitrous, both cylinders should be checked for adequate remaining gas levels.

- All parts of the delivery system should remain in acceptable working condition. The reservoir bag should be checked frequently for leaks.

Slide 28

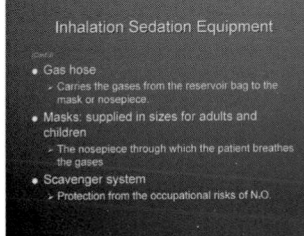

- Be aware that a large amount of facial hair (especially a moustache) may interfere with an adequate seal of the nosepiece, thus decreasing the amount of the sedative delivered to the patient, and perhaps increasing the amount of leakage to the surrounding environment, as well as exposure to the dental team.

- A scavenger system is essential for safely gathering and disposing of any unused or exhaled nitrous, outside of the building.

Bird/Robinson

Slide 29

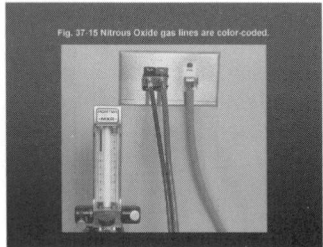

- What color represents nitrous oxide? *(Blue.)*
- What color represents oxygen? *(Green.)*
- The metal plate in the wall is an outlet for the nitrous oxide and the oxygen supplies, as well as an outlet for the scavenging system to prevent nitrous levels from accumulating.

Slide 30

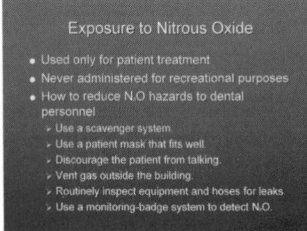

- Why is it important to discuss with patients before beginning a procedure the steps involved in the administration of nitrous oxide as well as what they may expect from the dental procedure itself?
- An office should have a schedule in place for routine inspection of nitrous equipment for safety and maintenance.

Slide 31

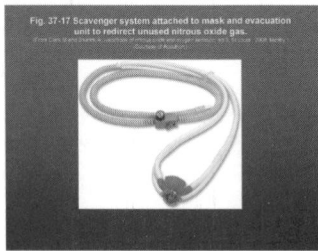

- This photo displays the nasal mask that is placed over the patient's nose to deliver nitrous in combination with the scavenging device that collects excess or exhaled nitrous.
- It is important that the mask be placed with the corresponding end over the bridge of the nose for a proper fit.
- The nosepiece is placed over the nose, and the tubing is secured behind the headset of the dental chair.

Slide 32

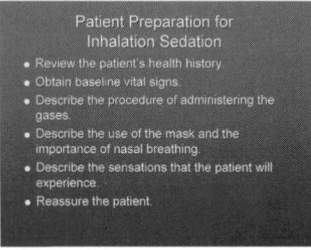

- Should the baseline vitals be recorded? If so, where?
- Discussing what patients may or should expect, as well as addressing their questions or concerns, will help alleviate and avoid any unwarranted anxiety during the procedure.

Bird/Robinson

Slide 33

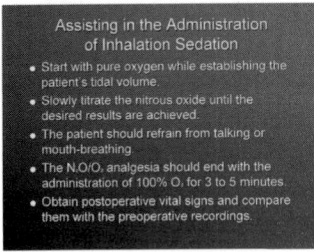

- The tidal volume is the amount of air inhaled and exhaled with every breath.

- Starting with pure oxygen will help patients get accustomed to having the nasal mask in place and practice breathing through their nose.

- What does inhaling 100% oxygen at the end of the procedure help to prevent? *(Diffusion hypoxia.)*

Slide 34

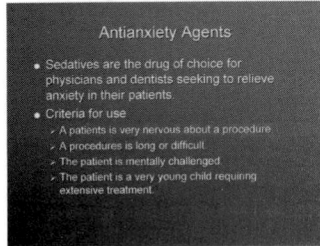

- Antianxiety medications are used as an adjunct to dental treatment.

- Patients with extreme dental fear may require this type of medication for the first few visits.

- Anxiolytics are also sometimes prescribed to mentally challenged patients who may be uncooperative.

Slide 35

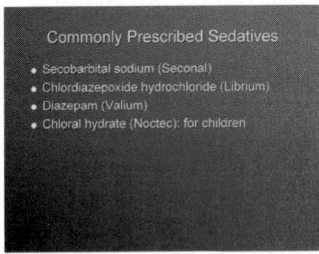

- Valium (diazepam) is a benzodiazepine that is available in 2, 5, and 10 mg tablets, and it may also be given IM/IV and via oral solution.

- Seconal is a sedative-hypnotic barbiturate; Librium is a benzodiazepine; and chloral hydrate is a sedative-hypnotic, used more often in pediatric dentistry.

Slide 36

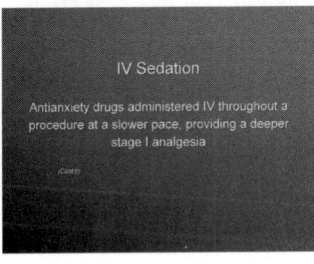

- Conscious IV sedation is frequently used by an oral surgeon during procedures such as the extraction of third molars, especially for difficult cases, such as when teeth are impacted and surgical removal of bone is necessary.

- Local anesthesia is administered once the patient is stable with IV conscious sedation. This also helps with postoperative pain until oral analgesics can be taken.

ELSEVIER

Bird/Robinson

Slide 37

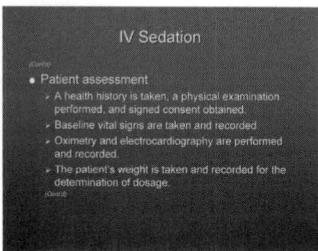

- All medications administered by way of an IV are calculated according to the patient's weight and are additionally titrated according to the vitals and feedback from the patient during the procedure.

- What is oximetry?

- A change in a patient's blood oxygen percentage throughout surgery may indicate that one of the medications (e.g., a narcotic analgesic) administered by IV is suppressing the respiratory drive.

Slide 38

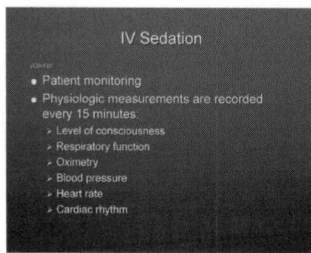

- In addition to the operating dentist and the assistant, a registered nurse is usually present to properly administer the medications through the IV and monitor the patient's vital signs throughout surgery.

- Although the vitals may be formally recorded only every 15 minutes, some dental offices choose to record them more frequently.

Slide 39

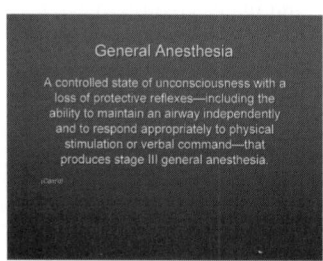

- General anesthesia is indicated for severely medically compromised or mentally disabled individuals who cannot be adequately treated in a regular dental setting.

- Due to the loss of protective reflexes, the patient is intubated, usually through the nose (to stay clear of the oral cavity) for delivery of the oxygen and anesthetic gases, while other medications are administered simultaneously by way of an IV line.

Slide 40

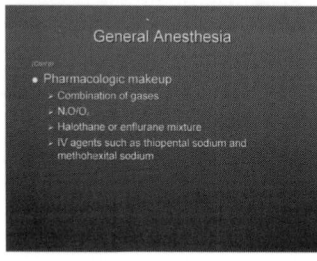

- A thorough preoperative examination including a physical examination, blood laboratory tests, and sometimes cardiac tests are performed and reviewed as part of the medical history before administration of general anesthesia.

- Both inhalational gases and intravenous agents are calculated and chosen according to the patient's health history, the anticipated length and type of surgery, and the anesthesiologist's preferences.

Bird/Robinson

Slide 41

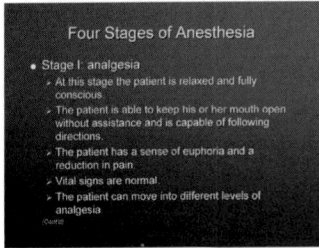

- What is an example of Stage I anesthesia? *(Nitrous oxide/oxygen.)*
- Monitoring the level of consciousness is important to assure that titration of the anesthetic is desirable.

Slide 42

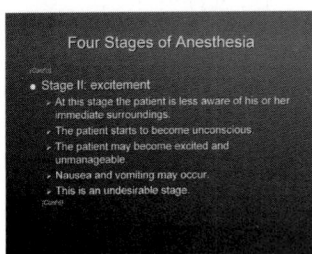

- Patients receiving intravenous conscious sedation should have their vital signs monitored carefully as they are placed in a deeper Stage I level of anesthesia.

Slide 43

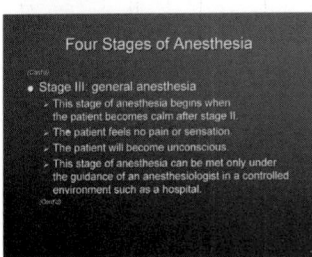

- Although a patient is thought to feel no pain, local anesthesia is usually administered to control bleeding throughout the procedure, and at or near the end to help with postoperative pain control.
- A throat pack is always placed so that the airway and esophagus are protected from instruments, irrigating solutions and blood, materials, free tissue debris, etc., as well as to protect the stomach from filling with liquid that may cause postoperative nausea and vomiting.

Slide 44

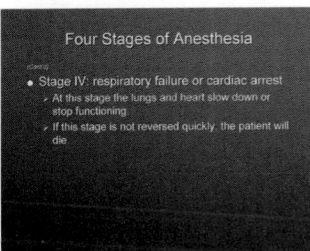

- Because of the risk, before choosing general anesthesia, it is very important that a patients is well-informed, has thoroughly discussed the dental office's consent form, and that all other anesthetic options have been exhausted or are found to be inappropriate.

Slide 45

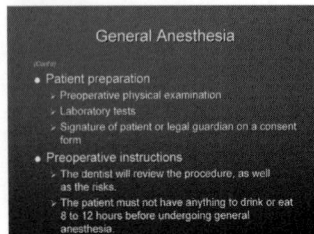

- NPO stands for a Latin abbreviation meaning nothing by mouth.

- Depending on the severity of the dental surgery and the outcome, most patients will be treated as day surgery patients; others will have to remain in the hospital, monitored in a controlled environment for a prescribed amount of time postsurgery.

Slide 46

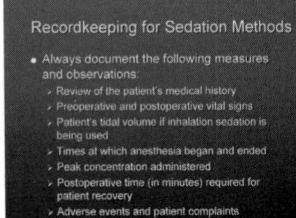

- Alongside a detailed account of the actual surgical procedure, the name, concentration, and amount of anesthesia used, time administered, and method of administration (e.g., local infiltration, IV, inhalation, etc.) should also be noted.

- For local anesthesia, remember to include whether or not it contained a vasoconstrictor, and if so, what type and in what concentration.

- In addition, any postoperative instructions should be documented.

Bird/Robinson

38 Foundations of Radiography, Radiographic Equipment, and Radiologic Safety

TEACHING FOCUS

This chapter will give the student an opportunity to understand the importance of dental radiographs as a diagnostic tool. The fundamentals of radiation physics (ionizing radiation). are discussed. The student will have the opportunity to learn about the hazards of exposure, including tissue damage, biologic effects, and the critical organs affected by radiation. Radiation safety for both patients and dental personnel will be covered..

MATERIALS AND RESOURCES

☐ computer and PowerPoint projector (all Lessons)
☐ examples of dental radiographs (Lesson 38.2)

LESSON CHECKLIST

Preparations for this lesson include:

- lecture
- guest speakers: dentist, dental assistant
- evaluation of student knowledge and skills needed to perform all entry-level activities related to radiography, radiographic equipment, and radiologic safety, including:
  - characteristics of the radiograph beam
  - dental x-ray machine
  - discovery of x-radiation
  - radiation effects
  - radiation measurement
  - radiation physics
  - radiation safety
  - types of radiation
  - x-ray production

KEY TERMS

ALARA concept (p. 581)
anode (p. 570)
atom (p. 567)
cathode (p. 570)
central ray (p. 571)
contrast (p. 574)
control panel (p. 569)
density (p. 575)
dental radiography (p. 565)
distortion (p. 575)
dose (of radiation) (p. 576)
electron (p. 568)
energy (p. 567)
extension arm (p. 569)
genetic effects (p. 576)
ion (p. 568)
ionization (p. 568)
ionizing radiation (p. 575)
kilovoltage peak (kVp) (p. 573)
latent period (p. 576)
lead apron (p. 579)

magnification (p. 575)
master switch, indicator light, selector buttons,
    exposure button (p. 571)
matter (p. 567)
milliampere (mA) (p. 575)
penumbra (p. 575)
photon (p. 568)
primary beam (p. 573)
primary radiation (p. 573)
radiation (p. 565)
radiograph (p. 566)
radiology (p. 566)
scatter radiation (p. 574)
secondary radiation (p. 574)
sharpness (p. 575)
somatic effects (p. 577)
thyroid collar (p. 579)
tubehead (p. 569)
tungsten target (p. 570)
x-radiation (p. 567)

ADDITIONAL RESOURCES

PowerPoint slides (Evolve): 1-94

Legend

CTQ
Critical
Thinking
Question

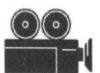

DVD
Multimedia
Procedures
Videos and
Animations

ESLR
EVOLVE
Student
Learning
Resources

IDO
Interactive
Dental
Office
CD-ROM

SW
Student
Workbook

TB
Test Bank
on the
TEACH
CD-ROM

PPT
PowerPoint
Slides

Class Activities are indicated in ***bold italic***.

Torres and Ehrlich Modern Dental Assisting, 9th ed.

Bird/Robinson

LESSON 38.1

PRETEST

1. What is the difference between E-speed film and the more recently developed F-speed film?
   a. E-speed film decreases a patient's exposure to x-radiation.
   b. F-speed film increases a patient's exposure to x-radiation.
   c. E-speed film has larger silver bromide crystals.
   d. F-speed film has larger silver bromide crystals.

2. What is the main advantage of using a rectangular collimator over a circular one?
   a. to make it easier to line up with the film
   b. to increase the size of the x-ray beam
   c. to reduce patient exposure
   d. for easier storage against the wall

3. What is the name given to the protective flexible lead shield that is placed over the neck region during x-ray exposure?
   a. blanket
   b. thyroid collar
   c. neck tie
   d. patient napkin

4. Which natural source of radiation provides the greatest amount of exposure per year?
   a. radon
   b. cosmic
   c. terrestrial
   d. internal

5. What is the purpose of aluminum filtration in the x-ray tubehead?
   a. to remove the low-energy, long-wavelength x-rays
   b. to remove the high-energy, long-wavelength x-rays
   c. to remove the low-energy, most penetrating x-rays
   d. to remove the low-energy, short-wavelength x-rays

6. What is the maximum permissible dose (MPD) of whole-body radiation for persons occupationally exposed to radiation?
   a. 500 mrem or 5 mSv per month
   b. 500 mrem or 5 mSv per year
   c. 5000 mrem or 5 rem per year
   d. 100 mrem per year

7. Which type of cells or tissue is the most sensitive to radiation?
   a. muscle
   b. nerve
   c. reproductive
   d. liver

8. What is the fuzzy or blurred area that surrounds an x-ray image?
   a. latent period
   b. halo
   c. umbrella
   d. penumbra

9. What is the positive electrode that acts as the target for the electrons in the x-ray tube called?
   a. cathode
   b. PID
   c. focusing cup
   d. anode

10. Which particles compose the nucleus of an atom?
    a. protons and photons
    b. electrons and photons
    c. protons and neutrons
    d. electrons and ions

Answers

1. d	3. b	5. a	7. c	9. d
2. c	4. a	6. c	8. d	10. c

BACKGROUND ASSESSMENT

Question: To what do the terms *radiolucent* and *radiopaque* refer?

Answer: Radiolucent refers to structures that appear dark on exposed and developed film because radiation was able to easily pass through them, in turn exposing the film in that area. Oral/dental structures that may appear radiolucent on a film include areas of tooth decay, the pulp, air spaces between and above teeth, abscesses, and soft tissues. Radiopaque refers to areas on the radiograph that are white or light gray where radiation was unable, or was not easily able, to pass through a structure and reach the film. Radiopaque images are usually formed with structures such as metal restorations, sound enamel, and dense areas of bone

Question: What is radiographic density, and what factors affect density?

Answer: Density is the overall blackness or darkness (degree of darkening) of a film exposed to x-rays that allows the dentist to evaluate and compare the black, white, and gray areas on the exposed film. The overall density depends on the number of photons absorbed by the film (emulsion). Increasing the milliamperage (mA), the kilovoltage (kVp), the exposure time, or reducing the source-film distance will increase the radiographic density. Subject thickness and subject density exposed to the film will also influence radiographic density, so a dentist should vary the exposure time according to the patient's size.

CRITICAL THINKING QUESTION

A 20-year-old man who smokes comes to your office for a new patient exam. The patient reports not having been to the dentist since he was about 10 years old. He claims to brush but not floss his teeth because his gums bleed when he flosses. He complains that a few of his teeth have recently become increasingly sensitive. After a brief initial extraoral and intraoral examination, the dentist orders a full mouth series of radiographs in order to proceed with the examination. While you are preparing the necessary films and holders, the patient asks you why you have to take so many radiographs. What are some of the reasons you can give him?

Guidelines: Because this patient has not been to the dentist in years, a baseline series of radiographs is important for various reasons. Radiographs are crucial for accurate diagnosis: without them a dentist cannot offer suitable treatment. Because caries, or decay, between the teeth or under existing restorations is generally not detectable by clinical examination. For this, radiographs are invaluable. This patient has even reported tooth sensitivity, which may be related to active decay. The series of radiographs will also help in the diagnosis of periodontal disease (the loss of supporting bone around the teeth), which may be very pertinent, especially with this particular patient, as his gums bleed, indicating gingivitis. Chronic uncontrolled gingivitis will usually lead to periodontitis. He is a smoker furthermore and smokers are at a greater risk of developing periodontitis. Dental radiographs are also useful for oral pathology screening in the jawbones and as a baseline for future comparisons. Asymptomatic lesions may be detected in very early stages when treatment and prognosis are more favorable. There are many systemic diseases that share an oral manifestation.

OBJECTIVES	CONTENT	TEACHING RESOURCES
Pronounce, define, and spell the Key Terms.	■ Key terms (pp. 564-565)	*ESLR* Electronic Flashcards ▸ Discuss each of the key terms in Chapter 38, focusing on the definition, pronunciation, and spelling of each term. *Class Activity Have each student create index cards for all key terms. These should have a key term on one side and the definition and a sentence using the key term correctly on the other. Pronounce a key term for the class and have students share their cards for that term with each other so they can compare their sentences. Repeat the drill until all key terms have been thoroughly reviewed.*

ELSEVIER

Torres and Ehrlich Modern Dental Assisting, 9th ed.

Bird/Robinson

OBJECTIVES	CONTENT	TEACHING RESOURCES
Describe the uses of dental radiographs.	■ Introduction (p. 565)	PPT 4-5 TB questions 1-2 SW Short-Answer Questions 1; Fill in the Blank questions 1, 6 (pp. 267-268) Uses of Dental Radiographs (p. 566) ▸ Discuss the six uses of dental radiographs. ***Class Activity** Divide the class into small groups, and have each group discuss why a radiograph would aid in the diagnosis in the following clinical situations:* – *a patient comes to the office with a tooth-related abscess or a severe trauma to the mouth* – *a new patient exam* – *a periodic oral examination* – *a procedure to confirm progress (e.g., root canal therapy, seating of a crown)* ***Have the groups share their findings with the class.***
Describe the discovery of x-radiation.	■ Discovery of x-radiation (p. 566)	PPT 6-8 TB question 3 SW Short-Answer Questions 2; Fill in the Blank questions 4-5; Multiple Choice question 1 (pp. 267-269) Figure 38-1 (A) Wilhelm Conrad Roentgen; (B) Crookes tube (p. 566) ***Class Activity** Before class, ask students to search the library or the Internet for more information about the discovery of x-radiation. Then, have students share one new piece of information each has discovered. Compile the list of newly researched information on the board. (For students to prepare for this activity, see Homework/ Assignments #1.)*
Name the highlights in the history of dental radiography.	☐ Pioneers in dental radiography (p. 567)	PPT 9 TB question 4 SW Fill in the Blank questions 2-3; Multiple Choice question 2 (pp. 268-269) Recall question 1 (p. 569) Figure 38-2 First radiograph of the human body (p. 566) Table 38-1 Highlights in the History of Dental Radiography (p. 569) ▸ Discuss how Otto Walkhoff made the first dental x-ray.

ELSEVIER
Torres and Ehrlich Modern Dental Assisting, 9th ed.

OBJECTIVES	CONTENT	TEACHING RESOURCES
		▸ Discuss the downside of C. Edmund Kell's contribution to dental radiographs. *Class Activity **Before class ask students to research the early development of dental radiography as well as recent changes in the field. Then, divide the class into groups and have them create educational materials for dental patients that describe their findings. Have each group share its materials with the class. (For students to prepare for this activity, see Homework/Assignments #2.)***

Explain what happens during ionization.	■ Radiation physics (p. 567)
	
	  □ Atomic structure (p. 568)
	
	    – Nucleus (p. 568)
	
	    – Electrons (p. 568)
	
	  □ Ionization (p. 568)
		🖼 PPT 10-20
		
		💻 TB questions 5-6
		
		📖 SW Short-Answer Questions 3; Fill in the Blank questions 2-3, 11, 14, 23-25; Multiple Choice questions 3, 14 (pp. 267-270)
		
		Recall question 3 (p. 569)
		
		Figure 38-3 Diagrammatic representation of an oxygen atom (p. 567)
		
		Figure 38-4 A molecule of water (H_2O) consists of 2 atoms of hydrogen connected to 1 atom of oxygen (p. 568)
		
		Figure 38-5 Ionization occurs when an electron is removed from the orbital shell of the electronically stable atom (p. 568)
		
		▸ Discuss atomic structure, including the nucleus and electrons.
		
		▸ Discuss the process of ionization.
		
		*Class Activity **Before class have students search the Internet for examples of ionization that occur in everyday living. In class discuss examples that may be useful to alleviating patient concerns. (For students to prepare for this activity, see Homework/Assignments #3.)***

38.1 Homework/Assignments:

1. Have students search the library or the Internet for more information about the discovery of x-radiation.

2. Ask students to research the early development of dental radiography as well as recent changes in the field.

3. Have the students search the Internet for examples of ionization that occur in everyday living.

38.1 Instructor's Notes/Student Feedback:

LESSON 38.2

CRITICAL THINKING QUESTION

Your office has just reopened after a week off for equipment repairs, the installation of some new dental chairs, and a thorough spring cleaning. You have been asked to retake a radiograph that you just took on a patient because the dentist reports that, although you captured the correct tooth, it is of nondiagnostic quality: the film is blurry and far too light. What are some of the variables that you can check in order to assure that the second exposure is of diagnostic quality?

Guidelines: Because the office has just undergone renovations and numerous workers who may not be familiar with the radiology equipment have been in the office, it may be prudent to check over the various components. First, check that the developing machine has been maintained properly. Old chemicals or the wrong temperature will change the quality of the developed image. Next, assure that the film you used is from a package with a valid expiration date and that the film has been stored at the proper temperature. Check that the settings on the control panel have not been altered. Many units hold a constant kilovoltage (kVp) and milliamperage (mA), yet allow the operator to adjust the exposure time. If your unit does allow for changes in the kVp or mA, check that these readings are desirable. Otherwise, focus your attention on ensuring that a proper exposure time is in place. Evaluate whether the exposure time may have to be increased from the previously selected setting, especially if your patient is a larger adult and/or is having a radiograph exposed in an area with more dense bone. You may also wish to check that the tubehead is not vibrating when lined up for exposure. Always remind the patient to remain as still as possible while exposing the radiograph. Just before leaving the room, check that the patient is not straining to hold the film holder in place, because this may also cause enough motion to distort the image. Extra cotton rolls or a more comfortable placement of the holder may be required for acceptable, motionless exposure.

OBJECTIVES	CONTENT	TEACHING RESOURCES
Describe the properties of x-radiation.	☐ Properties of radiographs (p. 568)	⊠ PPT 24-27
		TB question 7
		SW Short-Answer Questions 4; Fill in the Blank questions 1, 6, 11, 14-15, 23-25 (pp. 267-269)
		Box 38-1 Characteristics of X-Rays (p. 568)
		Figure 38-6 Electromagnetic spectrum, showing the various wavelengths of radiation typically used (p. 569)
		Recall questions 1-3 (p. 569)
		Figure 38-7 (A) Wavelength is the distance between the crest (peak) of one wave and the crest of the next; (B) The shorter the wavelength, the greater the energy and penetration (p. 569)
		▸ Discuss properties of radiographs.
		▸ Discuss the characteristics of x-rays.
		***Class Activity** Divide the class into small groups, and have each group discuss ways in which dental radiography has different characteristics from the other sources of electromagnetic radiation included in Figure 38-6, (p. 585) using the characteristics outlined in Box 38-1 (p. 585) as a guide. Then, have each group present its explanation to the class for feedback and discussion.*

OBJECTIVES	CONTENT	TEACHING RESOURCES
Label the parts of the dental x-ray tubehead and tube.	■ The dental x-ray machine (p. 569) ☐ Tubehead (p. 569) ☐ X-ray tube (p. 570) – Cathode (p. 570) – Anode (p. 570) ☐ Position indicator device (PID) (p. 571) ☐ Extension arm (p. 571) ☐ Control panel (p. 571) – Master switch and indicator lights (p. 571) – Exposure button (p. 573) – Milliamperage selector (p. 573) – Kilovoltage selector (p. 573)	⊠ PPT 28-41 TB. TB questions 8-9 SW Short-Answer Questions 6; Fill in the Blank questions 8-9, 15; Multiple Choice questions 4-7, 25 (pp. 267-270) Figure 38-8 Dental x-ray machine (p. 570) Figure 38-9 Diagram of the dental x-ray tubehead (p. 570) Figure 38-10 X-ray tube (p. 571) Figure 38-11 This x-ray tubehead has a rectangular PID (p. 571) Figure 38-12 Federal regulations require that the diameter of a collimated x-ray beam be restricted to 2.75 inches at the patient's skin (p. 571) Figure 38-13 Rectangular collimation (p. 572) Figure 38-14 The arrows point to the PID (p. 572) Figure 38-15 The operator stands at the central panel located outside the x-ray room (p. 572) Recall questions 4-7 (p. 573) ▸ Discuss the components of an x-ray machine. ▸ Discuss the parts of the dental x-ray tubehead and x-ray tube. ***Class Activity** Divide the class into small groups, and distribute to each group a copy of Figure 38-9 (p. 586) with the labels removed. Have the students work together to assign the correct names to the parts and discuss their functions. Then, have the groups share their findings with the class.*
Explain how radiographs are produced.	■ X-ray production (p. 573)	⊠ PPT 42-44 SW Short-Answer Questions 5; Fill in the Blank question 12 (pp. 267-268) Figure 38-16 The production of dental radiographs occurs in the x-ray tube (p. 573) Recall questions 8-9 (p. 574) ▸ Discuss the steps that occur during x-ray production. ***Class Activity** Create two sets of index cards. For each set, write the steps involved in x-ray production (p. 589), one step to a card. Divide the class in half, and provide each group with a set of cards. Have each group attempt to place the cards in order of occurrence. Have the groups present their results to the class for further discussion.*

Bird/Robinson

OBJECTIVES	CONTENT	TEACHING RESOURCES
Identify the range of kilovoltage and milliamperage required for dental radiography.	■ Types of radiation (p. 573) ■ Characteristics of radiograph beam (p. 574)	⊠▣ PPT 45-46 ▣ TB question 10 ▣ SW Short-Answer Questions 9; Multiple Choice question 9 (pp. 267, 270) ▸ Discuss the range of kilovoltage and milliamperage required for dental radiography. *Class Activity **Divide the class into small groups to discuss which combinations of kilovoltage and milliamperage settings are used in conjunction with which speed film. Ask them to discuss the standard ranges and why these ranges are chosen. Then have the groups share their findings with the class.***
Describe the effect of the kilovoltage on the quality of the x-ray beam.	■ Characteristics of radiograph beam (p. 574) ☐ Radiolucent and radiopaque characteristics (p. 574) ☐ Contrast (p. 574)	⊠▣ PPT 47-52 ▣ TB questions 11-13 ▣ SW Short-Answer Questions 7; Fill in the Blank question 10, 16; Multiple Choice questions 10-12 (pp. 267-270) Figure 38-17 Types of radiation interaction with the patient (p. 574) Figure 38-18 Bite-wing radiograph showing radiopaque (white) area of amalgam restoration and radiolucent (black) area of air and cheek tissue (p. 574) Figure 38-19 (A) Film produced with lower kilovoltage exhibits high contrast; (B) Film produced with higher kilovoltage exhibits low contrast (p. 575) ▸ Discuss how kilovoltage affects the x-ray beam. ▸ Discuss the contrast and gray scale of radiographs. *Class Activity **Divide the class into small groups. Distribute to each group several examples of dental radiographs that demonstrate a significant difference in contrast. Have the groups evaluate which radiograph shows a more desirable contrast, and, with all else being unchanged, which film was most likely exposed to a lower kilovoltage. Have the groups present their reasoning to the class.***
Describe how the milliamperage affects the quality of the x-ray beam.	☐ Density (p. 575) ☐ Geometric characteristics (p. 575)	⊠▣ PPT 53-56 ▣ TB questions 14-15 ▣ SW Short-Answer Questions 8; Fill in the Blank question 17; Multiple Choice question 13 (pp. 267, 269-270)

Torres and Ehrlich Modern Dental Assisting, 9th ed.

OBJECTIVES	CONTENT	TEACHING RESOURCES
		Table 38-2 X-Ray Beam Factors' Influence on Density and Contrast of Radiographs (p. 574)
		Recall questions 10-13 (p. 575)
		▸ Discuss how milliamperage affects the x-ray beam.
		▸ Discuss the density of radiographs.
		Class Activity Repeat the previous Class Activity using appropriate examples of paired films with significantly detectable differences in density that were achieved by changing only the milliamperes. Be sure to discuss what other variables may be altered to achieve a similar result.

38.2 Homework/Assignments:

38.2 Instructor's Notes/Student Feedback:

LESSON 38.3

CRITICAL THINKING QUESTION

You are assisting the dentist with an emergency patient, a 35-year-old woman who is five months pregnant. She has a large swelling associated with a lower right molar, is running a fever, and has not been able to eat or sleep for the past two days because of the pain associated with her tooth. After an initial clinical exam, the dentist orders a radiograph of the area. Once the dentist leaves the room, the patient becomes reluctant about having the radiograph taken because of her pregnancy. What information can you give her so that she better understands and appreciates the importance of acquiring the film, and the safety precautions in place to minimize exposure to her and her fetus?
Guidelines: First, reiterate that in her case, the benefits of an accurate diagnosis coupled with corresponding treatment far outweigh any risks of having a radiograph taken. Her dental infection has now spread to a systemic level (as indicated by the swelling and fever), which is very unfavorable for her and her fetus. Furthermore, a lack of sleep, the stress of pain, and deficiency in proper nutrition also pose a serious risk to the unborn child. If treatment is not sought at this point, the signs and symptoms, as well as the infection itself, may only worsen and may become an increasingly greater risk for both the patient and the fetus. Infections in the mandible run the risk of compromising the airway. Show the patient the lead apron that will cover her stomach completely and reach up over her neck, allowing no radiation to penetrate these protected areas. Inform her that even if she was not pregnant, the same precautions would be taken and the same advice would be offered. You may also wish to mention, if appropriate, that your office uses a fast-speed film, and a longer, rectangular positioning device, all of which help to decrease the already minimal exposure to the patient.

OBJECTIVES	CONTENT	TEACHING RESOURCES
Discuss the effects of radiation exposure on the human body.	■ Radiation effects (p. 575) □ Tissue damage (p. 576) – Ionization (p. 576) □ Biologic effects (p. 576) – Cumulative effects (p. 576) – Acute and chronic radiation exposure (p. 576) – Genetic and somatic effects (p. 576)	PPT 59-65 TB question 16 SW Short-Answer Questions 10; Fill in the Blank questions 7, 18-21, 26; Multiple Choice questions 15-16 (pp. 267-270) SW Topics for Discussion question 5 (p. 271) Figure 38-20 Sign indicating a radiation hazard area (p. 576) Figure 38-21 Comparison of somatic and genetic effects of radiation (p. 577) ▸ Discuss the tissue damage that can occur with radiation. ▸ Discuss the biologic effects that can occur with radiation. *Class Activity Before class, have students research daily environmental radiation exposure and its sources. In class, summarize their findings on the board and compare them to other sources of radiation, such as that from medical applications. (For students to prepare for this activity, see Homework/Assignments #1.)*
Identify the critical organs that are sensitive to radiation.	□ Critical organs (p. 577)	PPT 66 TB question 17

Torres and Ehrlich Modern Dental Assisting, 9th ed.

Bird/Robinson

OBJECTIVES	CONTENT	TEACHING RESOURCES
		SW Short-Answer Questions 12 (p. 267)
		Table 38-3 Disorders of Critical Organs Resulting from Cumulative Radiation Exposure (p. 576)
		Table 38-4 Relative Radiation Sensitivity of Cells and Tissues (p. 576)
		Recall questions 14-16 (p. 577)
		▸ Discuss the critical organs that are sensitive to radiation, covering the effect that radiation can have on each one.
		▸ Discuss the difference between genetic and somatic mutations.
		Class Activity Divide the class into small groups, and have the groups discuss the critical organs, how they are protected, and what types of environmental radiation may affect them. Then have the groups share their findings with the class for discussion.
Discuss the risks versus benefits of dental radiographs.	■ Radiation measurement (p. 577) ☐ Maximum permissible dose (p. 577) ■ Radiation safety (p. 578)	PPT 67-71 SW Short-Answer Questions 11; Multiple Choice questions 17-18 (pp. 267, 270) Table 38-5 Equivalent Traditional and SI Units of Radiation Measurement (p. 577) Recall questions 17-18 (p. 578) Table 38-6 Radiation Sources and Whole-Body Exposure (p. 578) Table 38-7 Absorbed Doses from Intraoral X-Rays (p. 578) CTQ 1-6 (p. 582) ▸ Discuss the ways to explain the risk versus benefits of x-rays to patients. ▸ Discuss the amount of radiation exposure to various sources that the average person receives each year. ***Class Activity Have student pairs take turns role-playing a dental assistant and a patient concerned about the dangers of x-rays. Have the dental assistant explain to the patient the risks and benefits of radiographs and respond to the patient's concerns. Then have the students discuss what they learned from the role-plays.***
Describe the methods of protecting the patient from excess radiation.	☐ Protective devices (p. 578) – Aluminum filtration (p. 579) – Collimator (p. 579)	PPT 72-83 TB questions 18-19 SW Short-Answer Questions 14; Multiple Choice questions 19-21 (pp. 268, 270)

Bird/Robinson

OBJECTIVES	CONTENT	TEACHING RESOURCES
	– Position indicator device (p. 579)	Dentist's Responsibilities for Dental Radiography (p. 578)
	☐ Patient protection (p. 579)	Figure 38-22 Compared with a short (8 inch) PID the longer (16 inch) PID is preferred because it produces less divergence of the x-ray beam (p. 579)
	– Lead apron and thyroid collar (p. 579)	Figure 38-23 The lead apron and thyroid collar must be large enough to cover the seated patient from the neck to above the knees (p. 596)
	– Fast-speed film (p. 580)	Figure 38-24 The patient's fingers are unnecessarily exposed to radiation when film holders are not used (p. 580)
	– Film-holding devices (p. 580)	Recall questions 19-22 (p. 580)
	– Exposure factor (p. 580)	▸ Discuss the ways the patient is protected from excessive radiation.
	– Proper technique (p. 580)	*Class Activity Divide the class into small groups, and have each group develop a safety checklist of the equipment used and actions taken to protect the patient from excess radiation. Then, have the groups present their checklists to the class, and incorporate all the ideas into one master checklist on the board.*
	☐ Pregnancy (p. 580)	
Describe the measures used to protect the operator from excess radiation.	☐ Operator protection and monitoring (p. 580)	PPT 84-91
	– Radiation monitoring (p. 580)	TB question 20
		SW Short-Answer Questions 15; Multiple Choice questions 22-23 (pp. 268, 270-271)
	☐ Equipment monitoring (p. 581)	Rules of Radiation Protection (p. 581)
		Figure 38-25 For safety, the dental assistant must stand out of the path of the primary beam (p. 580)
	☐ Pediatric patients (p. 581)	Figure 38-26 A film badge is used to monitor the amount of radiation that reaches the dental radiographer (p. 581)
		Figure 38-27 Child sitting on parent's lap for dental x-ray (p. 581)
		▸ Discuss the measures the dental assistant must take to avoid exposure to radiation.
		Class Activity Divide the class into small groups, and have each group discuss the ways in which dental personnel are protected from excessive radiation exposure. Have each group present its findings to the class for further discussion.
Discuss the ALARA concept.	☐ ALARA concept (p. 581)	PPT 92-94
		SW Short-Answer Questions 13; Fill in the Blank question 22; Multiple Choice question 24 (pp. 267, 269, 271)

Torres and Ehrlich Modern Dental Assisting, 9th ed.

Bird/Robinson

OBJECTIVES	CONTENT	TEACHING RESOURCES
		Recall questions 23-25 (p. 581)
		Patient Education (pp. 581-582)
		Legal and Ethical Implications (p. 5582)
		Eye to the Future (p. 582)
		▸ Discuss the concept of ALARA.
		***Class Activity** Have pairs of students take turns role-playing an operator performing all of the steps involved in taking dental radiographs on a patient. Have the operator (1) describe what he or she is doing and why, and (2) identify which actions are needed to keep radiation ALARA.*
Performance Evaluation		🖥️ TB
		📗 SW questions (pp. 267-271)
		📗 SW Topics for Discussion (p. 271)
		📗 SW Patient Case exercise (p. 271)
		💿 ESLR Electronic Flashcards
		💿 ESLR Practice Quiz
		💿 ESLR Labeling Exercise 30: Identify the components of an X-ray Tubehead
		💿 ESLR Labeling Exercise 31: Identify the components of an X-ray Machine
		Recall questions (pp. 569-581)
		💡 CTQ (p. 582)

38.3 Homework/Assignments:

1. Have students research daily environmental radiation exposure and its sources.

38.3 Instructor's Notes/Student Feedback:

ELSEVIER

Torres and Ehrlich Modern Dental Assisting, 9th ed.

Bird/Robinson

38 Foundations of Radiography, Radiographic Equipment, and Radiologic Safety

Slide 1

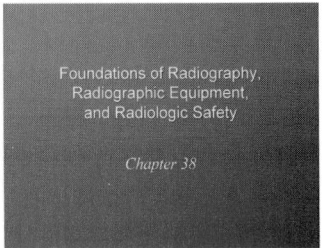

Foundations of Radiography,
Radiographic Equipment,
and Radiologic Safety

Chapter 38

Slide 2

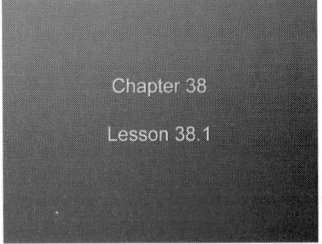

Chapter 38

Lesson 38.1

Slide 3

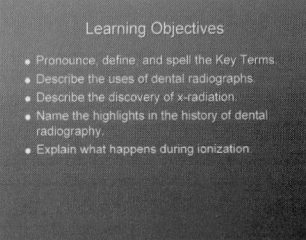

Learning Objectives

- Pronounce, define, and spell the Key Terms.
- Describe the uses of dental radiographs.
- Describe the discovery of x-radiation.
- Name the highlights in the history of dental radiography.
- Explain what happens during ionization.

Slide 4

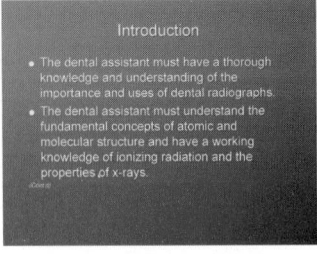

Introduction

- The dental assistant must have a thorough knowledge and understanding of the importance and uses of dental radiographs.
- The dental assistant must understand the fundamental concepts of atomic and molecular structure and have a working knowledge of ionizing radiation and the properties of x-rays.

- The dentist relies on the dental assistant to capture a radiographic image as accurately as possible in order for a proper diagnosis to be made.

- The dental assistant will also be responsible for documenting the number and type of radiographs taken in the patient's clinical record under a dated entry.

- It is important to learn the fundamentals of ionizing radiation to understand how the atomic structure of cells is changed by radiation.

Slide 5

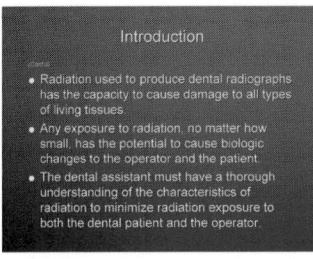

- While visiting the dentist, what steps have you noticed are taken to minimize radiation exposure to the patient and the operator? (This question should also be asked later on in the lesson where students can give additional, more sophisticated answers.)

- What everyday activities or objects are known to give off radiation that may also cause biologic changes in humans?

Slide 6

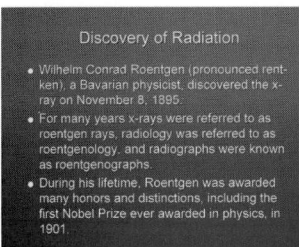

- Roentgen was experimenting in a darkened room with a vacuum tube and electrical screens that he found glowed a faint green color.

- After replacing the fluorescent screen with photographic plates, he was able to permanently capture images.

Slide 7

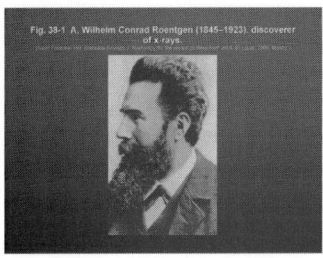

- Eventually, he placed his wife's hand on a photographic plate and exposed her to the rays for 15 minutes to show that he was able to permanently capture the image of the outline of her bones.

- This event was also recorded as the first radiograph of the human body.

Slide 8

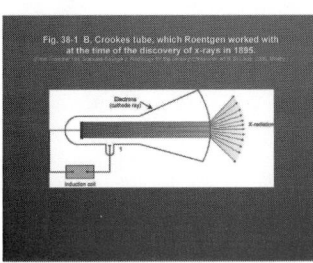

- This vacuum tube sent streams of electrons, using an electrical current, to expose special screens covered with a material that glowed when exposed.

Slide 9

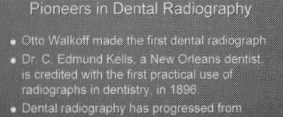

- Walkoff produced the first recorded dental radiograph by exposing a photographic plate in his own mouth for 25 minutes.

- Kells, after years of exposing his hands to x-rays every day, eventually developed cancerous tumors leading to the loss of his fingers, his hand, and later his arm.

- Many dental offices today use digital technology (beginning in 1987) instead of conventional radiography, offering new conveniences.

- Digital technology uses exposures 50% to 80% less than conventional film.

Slide 10

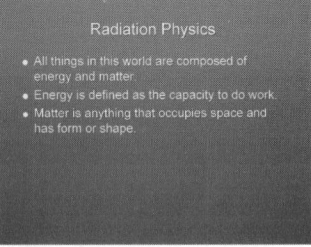

- What is an example of energy?

- What is an example of matter?

- What are the three forms of matter? *(Solid, liquid, and gas.)*

- What is an everyday example of matter in the three forms? *(Ice, water, and steam.)*

Slide 11

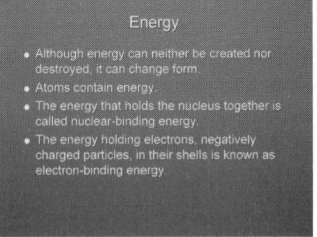

- What particles are found in the nucleus? *(Protons and neutrons.)*

- What charge do these particles have? *(Protons have a positive charge; neutrons have no charge.)*

- Where are electrons found? *(Outside the nucleus.)*

Slide 12

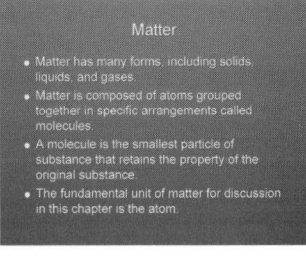

- It takes many molecules of matter, grouped together, to be able see them as a group with the naked eye.

Torres and Ehrlich Modern Dental Assisting, 9th ed.

Bird/Robinson

Slide 13

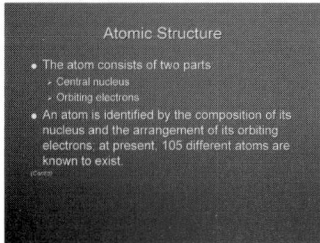

- What are found in the atom's nucleus? *(Protons and neutrons.)*
- Can anyone find the position of an oxygen atom on the periodic table of elements?

Slide 14

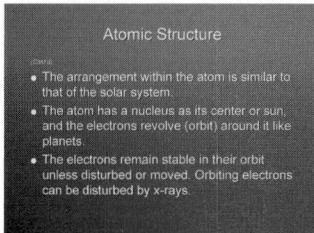

- What is holding the electrons in the shell? *(Electron-binding energy.)*
- What charge do the electrons have? *(A negative charge.)*

Slide 15

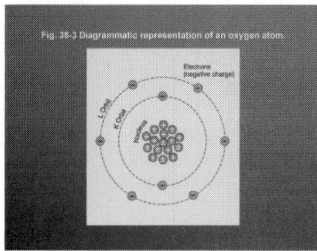

- Is the nucleus affected by x-rays? *(No, only the orbiting electrons.)*
- The various layers of shells are organized into orbits.

Slide 16

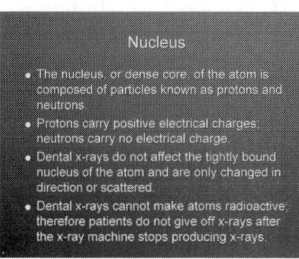

- Every atom has a nucleus.
- What is the force holding the nucleus together? *(Nuclear-binding energy.)*

Slide 17

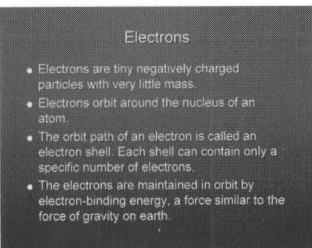

- It is the outer layer of electrons that may be disrupted during dental radiography.

- Every type of atom has a different number of electrons, giving each atom different overall characteristics.

Slide 18

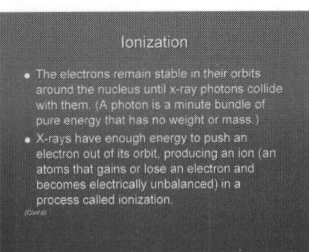

- Where does the photon come from for dental x-rays? *(From the tubehead of the dental x-ray machine. [Tubeheads will be reviewed later.])*

Slide 19

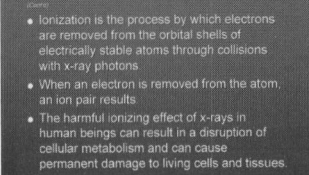

- A small change at the atomic or molecular level may lead to big changes at the cellular level.

- Other factors that affect the damage that may occur involve the amount of ionization that occurs over an amount of time (acute versus chronic).

- Ionization results from natural sources, not just from dental x-rays.

Slide 20

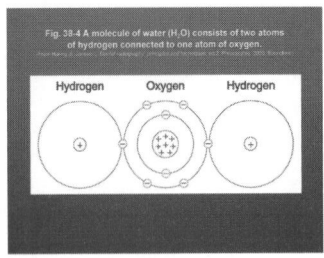

- The two hydrogen atoms are bonding to the oxygen atom by sharing electrons.

- The short form used for a water molecule is H_2O, which means that it is composed of two hydrogen atoms and one oxygen atom at the molecular level.

Torres and Ehrlich Modern Dental Assisting, 9th ed.

Bird/Robinson

Slide 21

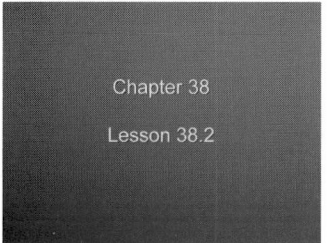

Slide 22

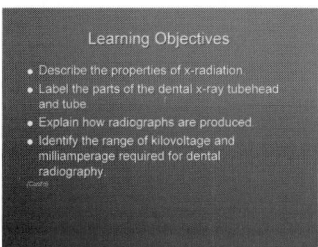

Slide 23

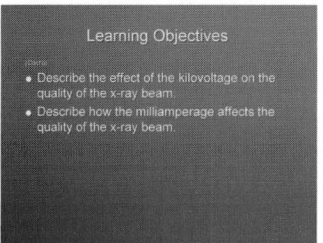

Slide 24

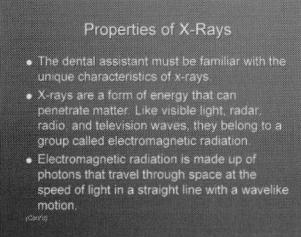

- A photon is a tiny bundle of pure energy that has no weight or mass and has the ability to collide with electrons found in the outer orbital shells of otherwise electrically stable atoms, resulting in ionization when an electron is lost.

- What are the characteristics of x-rays that make them unique? *(Refer to Box 38-1 on p. 568.)*

- Name a similarity between dental x-radiation and visible light.

Bird/Robinson

Slide 25

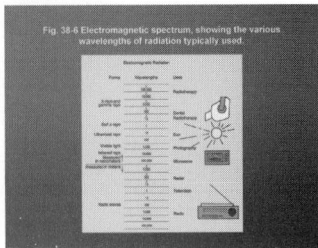

- The thick line through the middle marks a change in the unit of measure. Wavelengths are measured in nanometers (one billionth of a meter) above the line versus meters below the line.

- What type of electromagnetic radiation with a useful clinical application has an even shorter wavelength than the x-rays used for dental radiography? *(X-rays used for radiation therapy.)*

Slide 26

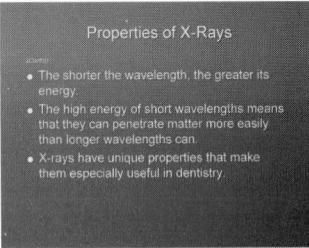

- The shorter the wavelength, the greater the penetration. Conversely, the longer the wavelength, the less penetrating its energy.

Slide 27

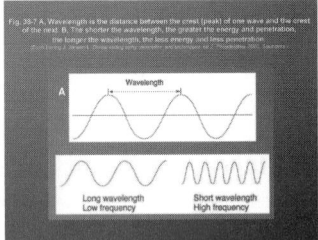

Slide 28

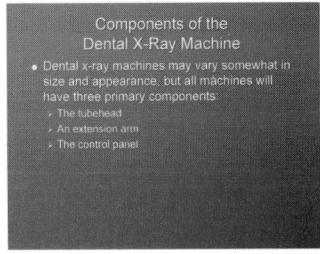

- What portion is the tubehead? *(The part that is lined up with the film holder and directed toward the patient's face.)*

- What portion is the extension arm? *(The portion connecting the tubehead to the control panel, allowing horizontal and vertical changes in the tubehead.)*

- What is the control panel? *(The portion, usually mounted on a wall, that allows the operator to turn the machine on or off and adjust the exposure time.)*

Bird/Robinson

Slide 29

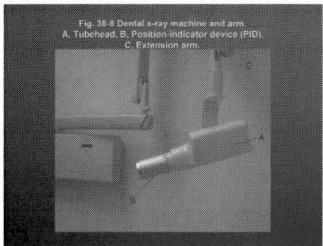

- For proper storage, the extension arm should be folded together and placed against the wall along with the tubehead.
- Why is proper storage important?
- What do the three letters (A, B, and C) point to? *(A: tubehead; B: PID [position indicator device]; and C: extension arm.)*

Slide 30

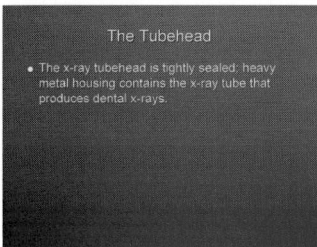

- The metal housing is filled with insulating oil to surround the x-ray tube.
- What is the tubehead attached to? *(The extension arm that allows the tubehead to be moved horizontally and vertically in order to properly position the opening of the collimator in the desired area to be x-rayed.)*

Slide 31

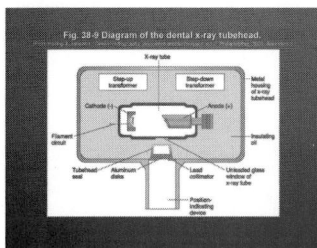

- What is the purpose of the cathode? *(Supplies the electrons necessary to generate x-rays.)*
- The hotter the filament becomes in the cathode, the more electrons are produced.
- Why does the insulating oil fill the metal housing and surround the x-ray tube? *(It prevents overheating by absorbing the heat generated by the production of x-rays.)*

Slide 32

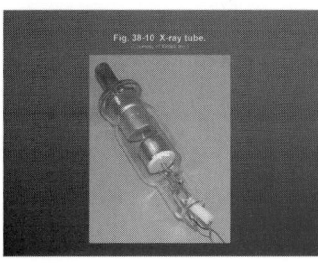

- This is a photograph of the x-ray tube, insulated by oil within the metal body of the tubehead. You will most likely never see one of these in real life.
- The anode is shown near the top left of the photograph whereas the cathode portion with the filament circuit is seen near the bottom right of the photograph.
- What encases the entire tube? *(Glass.)*

Bird/Robinson

Slide 33

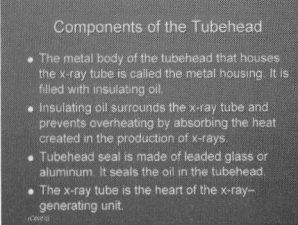

- The aluminum tubehead seal also acts as a filter to the x-ray beam.
- The x-ray tube contains the cathode with the filament circuit which generates electrons directed to the anode.

Slide 34

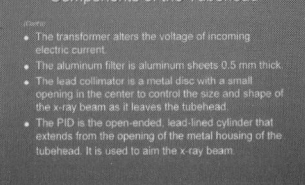

- A circular collimator limits the size of the x-ray beam to a two-inch circle.
- The dental patient is exposed to half the amount of radiation when a rectangular collimator slightly larger than the film is used.
- What are the various shapes and lengths of the PID? *(Round or rectangular; short or long.)*

Slide 35

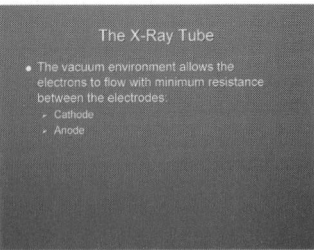

- Electrons travel from the cathode to the anode.

Slide 36

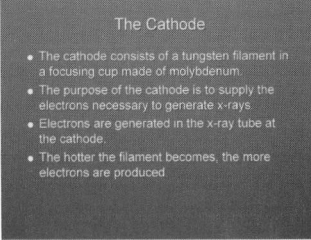

- What are electrons? *(The negatively charged particles that are found in the outer shell orbiting an atom.)*
- The focusing cup keeps the electrons ready near the cathode so that the instant the exposure button is activated, the circuit becomes complete and the electrons travel across the x-ray tube to the anode.

Torres and Ehrlich Modern Dental Assisting, 9th ed.

Bird/Robinson

Slide 37

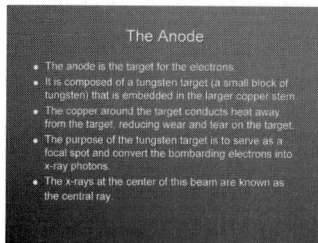

- Most of the x-rays (99%) are absorbed and given off as heat.
- The remaining one percent leaves the tubehead and is directed toward the patient.

Slide 38

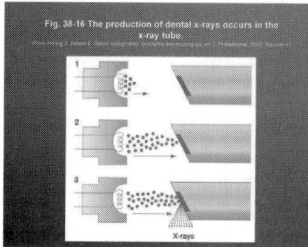

- Diagram 1 displays the electrons as red dots centered around a tungsten filament in the focusing cup of the cathode.
- Diagram 2 displays the electrons traveling toward the anode when the exposure button is activated, completing the circuit being formed.
- Diagram 3 shows that the electrons are transformed into photons, or x-rays, upon contact with the tungsten target of the anode.

Slide 39

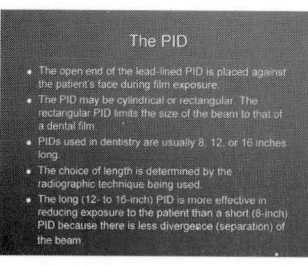

- The film holder has a metal connector piece with a ring on the end which serves as an extraoral target for the intraoral radiograph. There are notches on the ring which help the operator line up a round or a rectangular PID.
- More and more dental facilities are switching to a long rectangular PID to decrease the amount of x-ray exposure to the patient.

Slide 40

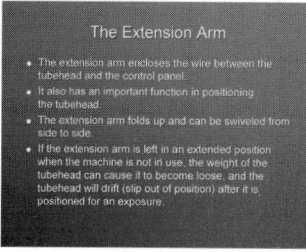

- The extension arm allows the operator to position the tubehead horizontally and vertically.
- Some dental treatment rooms share a common tubehead. The extension arm allows the operator to alternate the tubehead usage between two adjacent rooms.

Slide 41

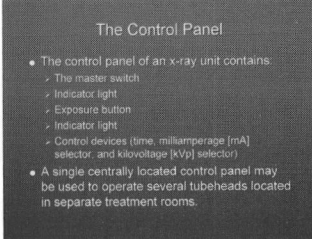

- When one control panel is used to operate multiple tubeheads, it is important for the operator to know which tubehead is being controlled at any given time, to avoid inadvertently exposing people to x-rays in an adjacent treatment room.

- Most dental x-ray units operate at a fixed milliamperage and kilovoltage. The exposure time is the variable most often adjusted according to patient age, size, and density.

Slide 42

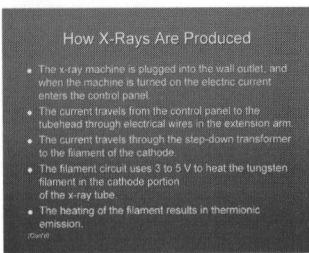

- All of this takes place without pressing the exposure button.

- What is the cathode? *(The negative electrode in the x-ray tube.)*

- Due to the energy used simply by keeping the machine on, the unit should be turned off every night and ideally during long periods of non-usage.

Slide 43

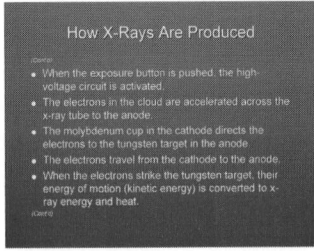

- How long does it take for this to happen? *(Much less than one second.)*

- The operator should remind the patient to stay as motionless as possible (at least until the beep or audible signal is heard) because even the smallest movement will distort the image and most likely result in a retake.

Slide 44

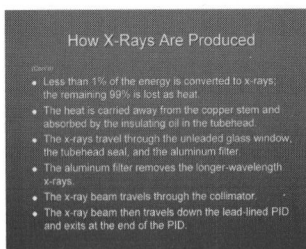

- At this point, the photons are directed through the patient's cheek, through the structures in question, and towards the film.

- Why are the longer wavelengths removed? *(They are less penetrating and thus not useful for dental radiography.)*

Torres and Ehrlich Modern Dental Assisting, 9th ed.

Bird/Robinson

Slide 45

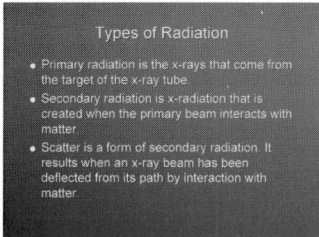

- The scatter portion of secondary radiation is dangerous and may expose any other patient tissues that are not protected by the lead apron.
- What is meant by "matter" here? *(Patient tissue.)*

Slide 46

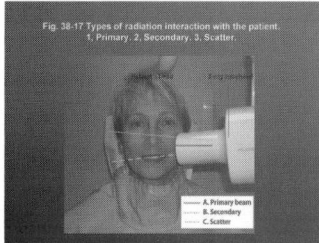

Slide 47

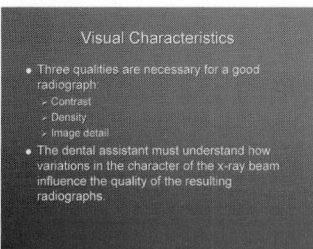

- It is important to know how to alter radiographic variables in order to change the contrast, density, and image detail.

Slide 48

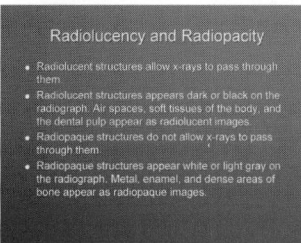

- These terms are relative. For example, although dentin is more radiopaque than dental pulp, it is more radiolucent than the overlying enamel.
- In order to ensure that these differences are noticeable, both contrast and density must be optimized.

Slide 49

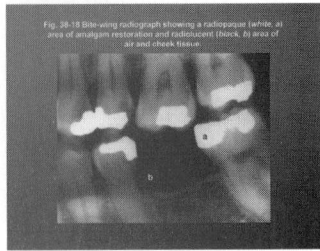

- Label "a" marks an amalgam restoration which appears radiopaque (white) on the film since no x-rays where able to pass through this material to reach the film.

- Label "b" marks a radiolucent (black) area on the film, an air space which allowed all x-rays to reach the film and expose it.

- Where are the areas of tooth decay evident on this film? *(Most noticeable are the large radiolucent areas on the distal-proximal of teeth #12 and #13.)*

Slide 50

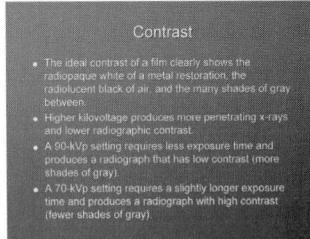

- A standard preset setting is commonly found to be 70 kVp coupled with 8 mA.

- When an x-ray machine has the above set readings, only exposure time may be altered.

Slide 51

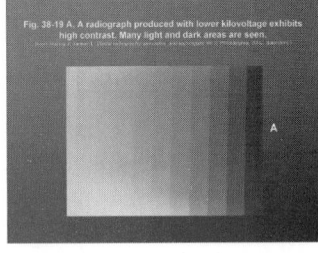

- Flip back and forth between this slide and the next one so that students may gain an appreciation for the difference between the two radiographs.

- Film A (lower kVp) shows a more drastic difference and thus more contrast from left to right compared to Film B (displayed on the next slide).

Slide 52

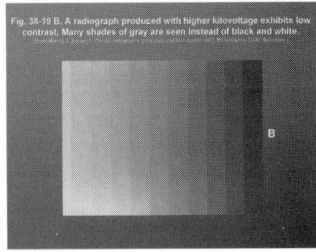

- Flip back and forth between this slide and the previous one so that students may gain an appreciation for the difference between the two radiographs.

- Film B (higher kVp) shows many shades of gray, getting darker from left to right. It shows less contrast compared to Film A on the previous slide.

ELSEVIER

Slide 53

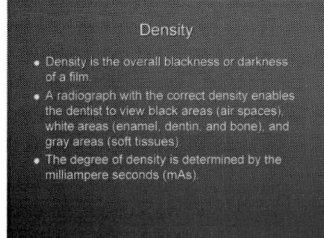

- Normal differences in bone densities are obvious between the maxilla and the mandible.

Slide 54

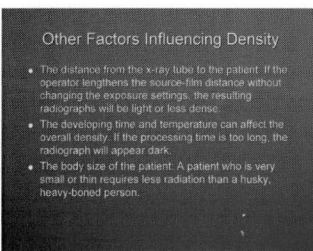

- If PIDs are changed on a tubehead, it is important to adjust the exposure time accordingly.

- A recommended maintenance schedule should be followed for the film developer, because old solutions will compromise the quality of the films.

Slide 55

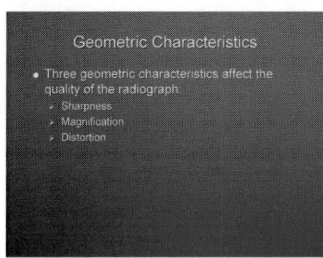

- A lack of sharpness can change a diagnosis dramatically. It may cause a problem to be undetected in an early stage when the prognosis would have been more favorable.

- Magnification is especially important when measuring the length of a tooth during root canal therapy.

- Distortion occurs when a radiograph is taken at a vertical angle that is greater than or less than necessary, resulting in a film image that appears either stretched out or shorter than it really is.

Slide 56

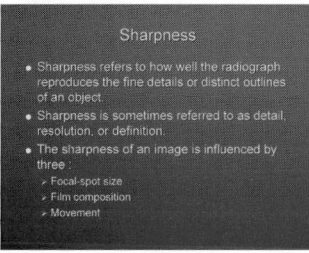

- Film speed may affect sharpness due to the different sizes in silver bromide crystals. A faster speed film has larger crystals.

- Name some sources of movement. *(The patient, the film not being held stably in the patient's mouth, or the x-ray unit.)*

- What is penumbra? *(The fuzzy or blurred area that surrounds an image.)*

Slide 57

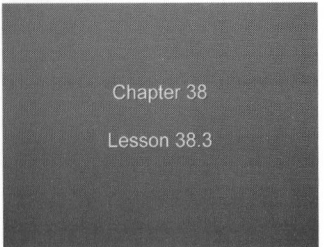

Slide 58

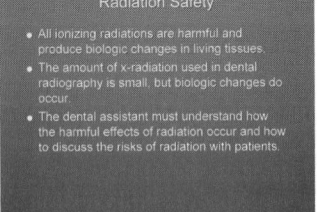

Slide 59

- Exercising radiation safety precautions will minimize radiation exposure to patients and operators alike.

- Radiograph retakes contribute to unnecessary exposure and are usually preventable when proper protocol is followed the first time.

- The benefits of dental radiography far surpass any risks.

Slide 60

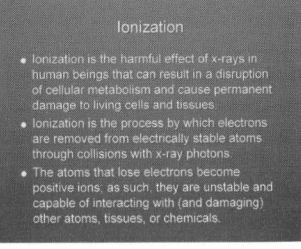

- We are exposed to background radiation every day, just from walking outside.

Torres and Ehrlich Modern Dental Assisting, 9th ed.

Bird/Robinson

Slide 61

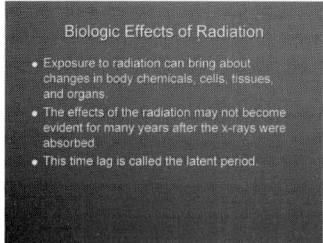

Biologic Effects of Radiation

- Exposure to radiation can bring about changes in body chemicals, cells, tissues, and organs.
- The effects of the radiation may not become evident for many years after the x-rays were absorbed.
- This time lag is called the latent period.

- Who was the dentist who exposed his hands to x-rays every day for years and eventually developed cancer as a consequence? *(C. Edmund Kells.)*

- What is one of the most common examples of chronic exposure to radiation? *(Radiation from the sun, which can cause skin cancer.)*

Slide 62

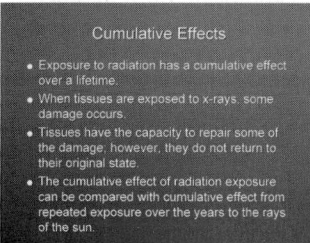

Cumulative Effects

- Exposure to radiation has a cumulative effect over a lifetime.
- When tissues are exposed to x-rays, some damage occurs.
- Tissues have the capacity to repair some of the damage; however, they do not return to their original state.
- The cumulative effect of radiation exposure can be compared with cumulative effect from repeated exposure over the years to the rays of the sun.

- With advancing technology, especially with the more widespread use of digital radiography, there is a decreasing amount of radiation exposure with dental radiographs.

Slide 63

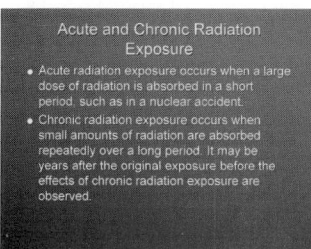

Acute and Chronic Radiation Exposure

- Acute radiation exposure occurs when a large dose of radiation is absorbed in a short period, such as in a nuclear accident.
- Chronic radiation exposure occurs when small amounts of radiation are absorbed repeatedly over a long period. It may be years after the original exposure before the effects of chronic radiation exposure are observed.

- What is a common example of chronic exposure? *(Sun exposure.)*

- What type of radiation exposure are dental patients and dental staff exposed to, regardless of how minimal and potentially insignificant? *(Chronic.)*

Slide 64

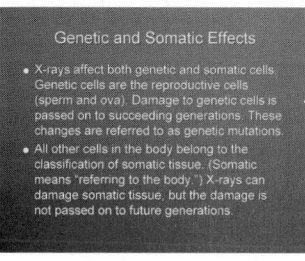

Genetic and Somatic Effects

- X-rays affect both genetic and somatic cells. Genetic cells are the reproductive cells (sperm and ova). Damage to genetic cells is passed on to succeeding generations. These changes are referred to as genetic mutations.
- All other cells in the body belong to the classification of somatic tissue. (Somatic means "referring to the body.") X-rays can damage somatic tissue, but the damage is not passed on to future generations.

- Genetic mutations are not apparent until the next generation, because the true function of these cells is to provide similar information from the contributing parent to the receiving child.

- Damage to somatic cells only has a chance of being expressed in that person's lifetime. Whether the damage will be expressed depends on an individual's genetic makeup and the degree of mutation.

Torres and Ehrlich Modern Dental Assisting, 9th ed.

Bird/Robinson

Slide 65

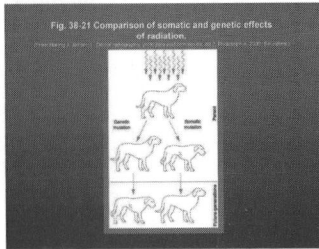

- This diagram uses squiggly red arrows to represent radiation to a dog.

- The left scenario shows the result of damage to a genetic cell that is passed on to the next generation—the parent dog exposed to the radiation is unaffected, while its progeny is small and sick.

- The scenario on the right shows the effect of a somatic mutation that is not inherited—radiation exposure affects the parent in an undesirable way, but the mutation is not passed on to its offspring.

Slide 66

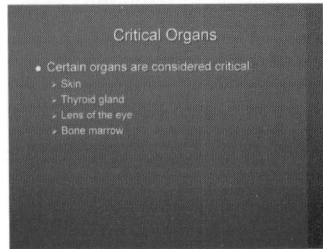

- Cell types that are most sensitive to radiation are those that generally (1) have a high mitotic rate [are dividing and duplicating fast in order to produce new cells just like them]; (2) will most likely undergo many future mitosis; and (3) are primitive in their differentiation [are younger, less differentiated cells that will most likely, with the proper genetic signals, turn into more mature cells with a distinct function].

- However, these generalizations do not apply to the following highly differentiated and non-dividing cells that are very radiosensitive: lymphocytes (immune system) and oocytes (female reproductive cells).

Slide 67

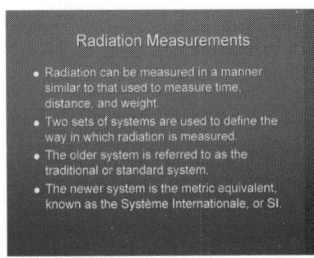

- These are not measurements that dental assistants will have to deal with very often.

- When radiation monitoring devices are checked, the radiation monitoring agency may use one of these systems to express measurement units in the resulting report.

Slide 68

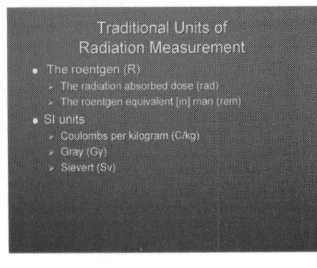

- Radiation exposure equivalents:
  - 1 roentgen (R) = 1 coulomb per kilogram (C/kg)
- Radiation absorbed dose equivalents:
  - 100 radiation absorbed doses (rad) = 1 gray (Gy)
- Radiation dose equivalence:
  - 100 roentgen equivalents in [hu]man (rem) = 1 sievert (Sv)

Torres and Ehrlich Modern Dental Assisting, 9th ed.

Bird/Robinson

Slide 69

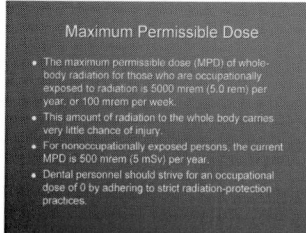

- Dental facilities should provide monitoring devices for their dental assistants and should make available the monthly reports received from the radiation monitoring agency.

Slide 70

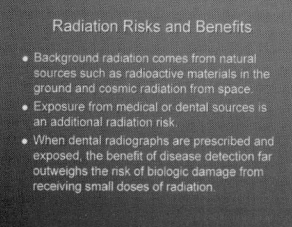

- Natural sources of radiation are unavoidable.

Slide 71

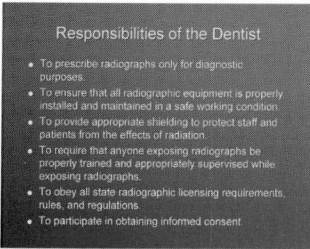

- It is important to stay current with the latest recommendations regarding dental workplace radiation exposure, protective methods, and new equipment developed to decrease exposure.

- Dental assistants need to be prepared to explain to a patient the importance of a diagnostic radiograph and should not hesitate to ask the dentist to reinforce the value of a radiograph for diagnostic purposes.

Slide 72

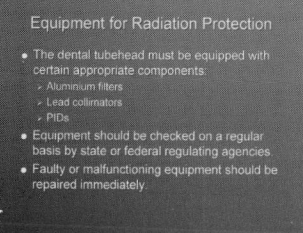

- If a patient expresses safety concerns, the dental assistant can mention how the design and maintenance of dental radiography equipment are created with radiation protection in mind.

- Radiographic equipment should be regularly monitored and, if need be, repaired as soon as possible to ensure optimal safety for the patient and the dental team.

Torres and Ehrlich Modern Dental Assisting, 9th ed.

Bird/Robinson

Slide 73

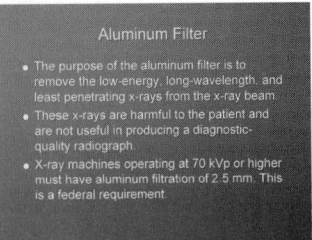

Aluminum Filter

- The purpose of the aluminum filter is to remove the low-energy, long-wavelength, and least penetrating x-rays from the x-ray beam.
- These x-rays are harmful to the patient and are not useful in producing a diagnostic-quality radiograph.
- X-ray machines operating at 70 kVp or higher must have aluminum filtration of 2.5 mm. This is a federal requirement.

Slide 74

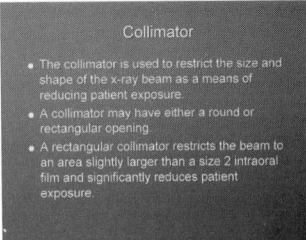

Collimator

- The collimator is used to restrict the size and shape of the x-ray beam as a means of reducing patient exposure.
- A collimator may have either a round or rectangular opening.
- A rectangular collimator restricts the beam to an area slightly larger than a size 2 intraoral film and significantly reduces patient exposure.

- Where is the collimator located? *(Between the x-ray tube and the position-indicating device.)*

Slide 75

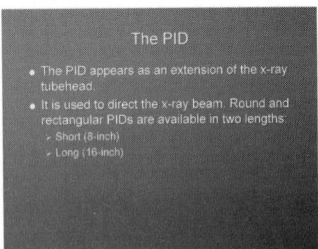

The PID

- The PID appears as an extension of the x-ray tubehead.
- It is used to direct the x-ray beam. Round and rectangular PIDs are available in two lengths:
  - Short (8-inch)
  - Long (16-inch)

- For infection control purposes, the PID, along with the tubehead, should be covered in plastic barriers and changed for each patient.

- The end of the PID should be positioned close to the extraoral portion of the film holder and lined up correctly in all three planes to ensure accurate exposure and image production on the film.

Slide 76

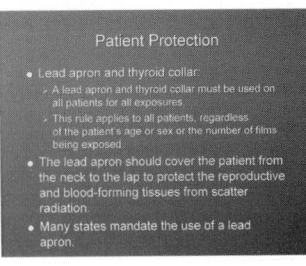

Patient Protection

- Lead apron and thyroid collar:
  - A lead apron and thyroid collar must be used on all patients for all exposures.
  - This rule applies to all patients, regardless of the patient's age or sex or the number of films being exposed.
- The lead apron should cover the patient from the neck to the lap to protect the reproductive and blood-forming tissues from scatter radiation.
- Many states mandate the use of a lead apron.

- Dental assistants should ensure that the lead apron and thyroid collar are stored properly and not folded, since creases may crack the lead.

- Newer, more lightweight and flexible versions of the apron are replacing the older and heavier versions.

- Care should be taken not to touch the apron with the same gloves that were used to place the film in the patient's mouth, as this will cause cross-contamination, compromising infection control.

ELSEVIER

Torres and Ehrlich Modern Dental Assisting, 9th ed.

Bird/Robinson

Slide 77

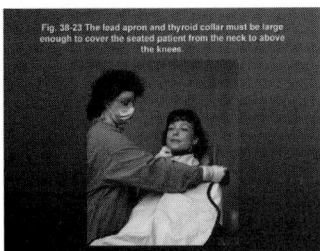

- The operator is placing the lead apron over the patient's upper body in addition to the lead thyroid collar around the neck.

- The operator should ensure that the patient removes any oral piercings, removable dental prostheses, or eye glasses that may distort or interfere with the desired image.

Slide 78

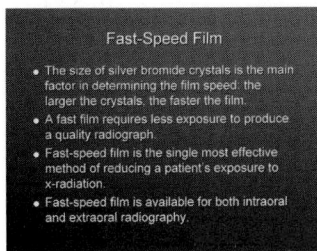

- With the onset of digital radiography, reusable sensors placed in the patient's mouth instead of film are attached to a computer software program which captures the image and displays it almost immediately on the computer screen. Digital radiography allows for an even more substantial decrease in patient exposure.

- Name a slight disadvantage to using F-speed film. *(Larger silver bromide crystals result in a slightly decreased contrast.)*

Slide 79

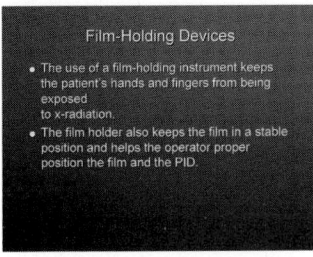

- Having edentulous or partially edentulous patients insert their denture or partial denture when taking periapical radiographs on the opposing arch will better stabilize the film holder.

- What may be placed in areas of missing teeth to help stabilize the film-holding instrument? *(Cotton rolls.)*

Slide 80

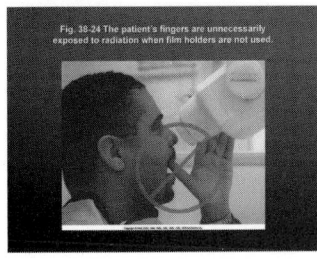

- When possible, a device should be used that aligns the intraoral film with the extraoral source, allowing precise capturing of the desired structure and avoiding "cone cuts." This also avoids distorting the image captured by the film when the PID is placed at the wrong angle to the film and anatomical structure.

- During times when it may be difficult to use this device (e.g., patient has on a rubber dam while receiving root canal therapy), the film may be held with surgical forceps, keeping the patient's hand at a reasonable distance from the x-ray source.

ELSEVIER

Torres and Ehrlich Modern Dental Assisting, 9th ed.

Bird/Robinson

Slide 81

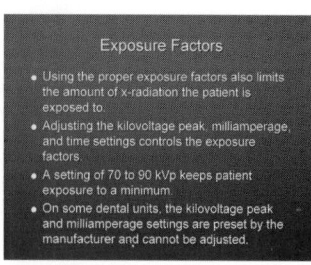

- What is the most likely factor that will require adjustment? *(Exposure time.)*

- What determines the exposure time? *(The speed of the film [very different for digital radiography], the size of the patient, and the denseness of the patient's anatomical structures.)*

- Structural denseness differs according to the region of the mouth; e.g., anterior central incisors require less exposure time than do mandibular molars.

Slide 82

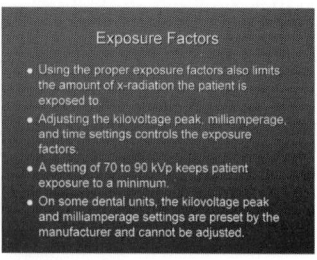

- Having to retake radiographs wastes time and is not relished by most patients.

- Although some retakes are unavoidable, most are preventable.

- If a retake is ordered, the dental assistant should know how to correct the error that resulted in the need for a retake.

Slide 83

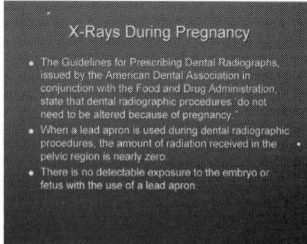

- When a radiograph is taken during pregnancy, the benefits of a proper dental diagnosis should outweigh the minimal risk of exposure from having a radiograph taken.

- An undiagnosed or improperly treated dental infection in a pregnant patient poses a far greater risk to the fetus than the minimal exposure from a dental radiograph.

Slide 84

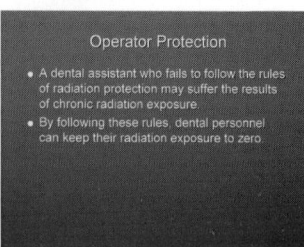

- Dental assistants must accept responsibility for their own radiation safety.

Bird/Robinson

Slide 85

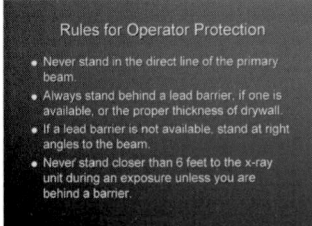

- Dental assistants working in an unfamiliar office or treatment room should familiarize themselves with the proper position to stand in while taking radiographs.
- Review where the exposure button is in addition to the control panel. These may be located in separate places.

Slide 86

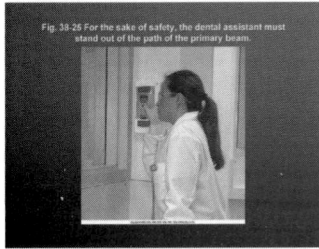

- Since dental facilities have different layouts for capturing dental radiographs, a different position may have to be taken to avoid exposure, depending on the facility.
  - There may be a lead wall to stand behind, or there may be a need to walk around the corner with a portable exposure button.
  - There may also be an exposure button positioned on a wall outside the room used for radiographs.
- When it is time to expose a film, the operator must ensure that visitors and other dental personnel are safely positioned.

Slide 87

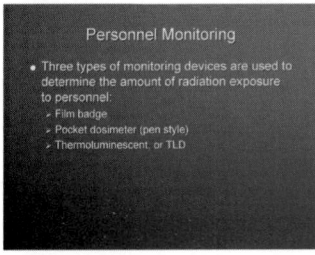

- These monitoring devices are small and light enough to be placed on the breast pocket of a lab jacket without interfering with normal duties.

Slide 88

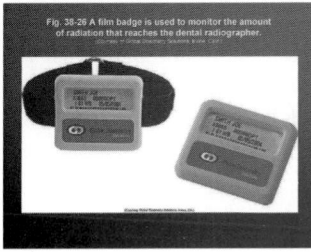

- Monitoring devices are usually sent to the agency monthly and a new one is returned to the operators along with a report to the dentist showing radiation exposure results for the individual.

Torres and Ehrlich Modern Dental Assisting, 9th ed.

Bird/Robinson

Slide 89

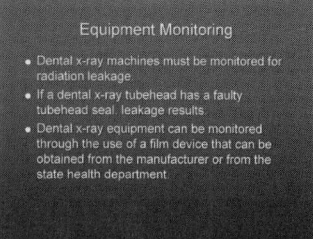

Equipment Monitoring

- Dental x-ray machines must be monitored for radiation leakage.
- If a dental x-ray tubehead has a faulty tubehead seal, leakage results.
- Dental x-ray equipment can be monitored through the use of a film device that can be obtained from the manufacturer or from the state health department.

- Suggest that students ask their dental office how the facility monitors the safety of its equipment and how often this safety check is performed.

- Has anyone ever seen what a monitoring device looks like or how it works?

Slide 90

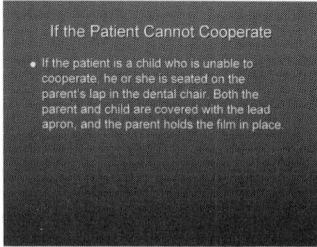

If the Patient Cannot Cooperate

- If the patient is a child who is unable to cooperate, he or she is seated on the parent's lap in the dental chair. Both the parent and child are covered with the lead apron, and the parent holds the film in place.

- Sometimes having children sit on the parent's lap helps with cooperation, and they may keep the film holder in their mouth without the parent's assistance.

- What simple analogies can be used to help gain the cooperation of young patients? *("Bite on the cookie" or "can you stay still and smile for the camera while we take a picture?")*

- What film size is appropriate for a pediatric patient? *(#0 or #1 size film is used with children with primary and mixed dentitions; #2 film is too large for bitewings on a small child and may hurt the child, promoting undesirable behavior.)*

Slide 91

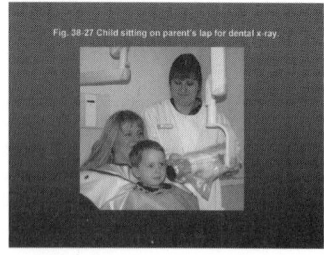

Fig. 38-27 Child sitting on parent's lap for dental x-ray.

- Both the child and his guardian are covered with a lead apron.

- What is missing around the child's neck? *(Thyroid collar.)*

- What type of collimator/PID is shown in this photo? *(Round/short, 8-inch.)*

- Why is there plastic over the tubehead? *(For proper infection control.)*

Slide 92

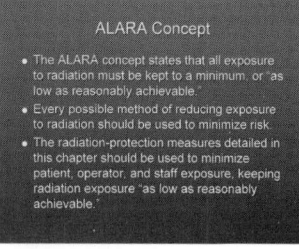

ALARA Concept

- The ALARA concept states that all exposure to radiation must be kept to a minimum, or "as low as reasonably achievable."
- Every possible method of reducing exposure to radiation should be used to minimize risk.
- The radiation-protection measures detailed in this chapter should be used to minimize patient, operator, and staff exposure, keeping radiation exposure "as low as reasonably achievable."

- What are some precautions taken to abide by the ALARA concept? *(Radiographs should be ordered only for diagnostic purposes; use the lowest possible kVp, mA, and exposure time; use F-speed film or digital radiography; use a longer PID with a rectangular shape; use a tubehead with an aluminum filter and a lead collimator; use a lead apron and thyroid collar; use film-holding devices; avoid retakes; and test equipment for efficiency and proper functioning.)*

Bird/Robinson

Slide 93

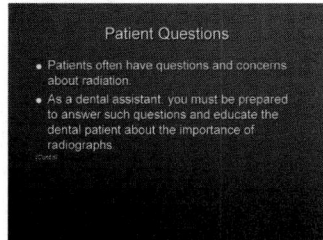

- Name some reasons why a dentist may need a radiograph.
  (As a baseline for a new patient's dental record; detection of dental decay, either new or recurrent, that may not be detectable clinically; diagnosis of periodontal disease by evaluating bone levels around the teeth; for forensic identification or for monitoring proper growth; for oral pathology screening; for diagnosis of problems that may involve the teeth, the soft or hard tissues, head or neck, or the entire body.)

Slide 94

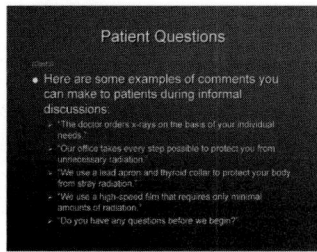

- It may prove useful to have educational brochures on hand that explain the importance of diagnostic dental radiographs and how their benefits far outweigh the minimal risks.

- Some dental facilities also have informative videos that can help educate patients about dental radiographs.

Bird/Robinson

39 Dental Film and Processing Radiographs

TEACHING FOCUS

This chapter will give students the opportunity to learn about dental film and processing radiographs and about types of film holders and devices. Students will also have the opportunity to describe the composition of dental x-ray film and the care and maintenance of processing solutions, equipment, and equipment accessories used in manual and automatic film processing. The component parts of an automatic film processor, common time and temperature errors, chemical contamination errors, film handling errors, and some common lighting errors during film processing will also be presented.

MATERIALS AND RESOURCES

- ☐ computer and PowerPoint projector (all Lessons)
- ☐ dental film (in and out of packaging) (Lesson 39.1)
- ☐ film holders (Lesson 39.1)

- ☐ hinged typodonts (Lesson 39.1)
- ☐ processing equipment (Lesson 39.2)
- ☐ unlabeled copies of Figure 39-22 (Lesson 39.2)

LESSON CHECKLIST

Preparations for this lesson include:

- lecture
- guest speaker: dental technician
- evaluation of student knowledge and skills needed to perform all entry-level activities related to dental film and processing radiographs, including:
  - ○ the role of the dental assistant in processing dental film
  - ○ how dental film works and its composition
  - ○ types of film and film processing (manual and automatic)

ELSEVIER

Torres and Ehrlich Modern Dental Assisting, 9th ed.

Bird/Robinson

KEY TERMS

automatic processor (p. 593)
beam alignment device (p. 584)
bite-wing (p. 588)
calcium tungstate (p. 589)
cassette (p. 588)
cephalometric film (p. 588)
duplicating film (p. 590)
emulsion (p. 585)
extraoral film (p. 588)
film holder (p. 584)
film speed (p. 586)

intensifying screen (p. 589)
intraoral film (p. 585)
label side (p. 587)
latent image (p. 585)
occlusal (p. 588)
panoramic film (p. 588)
periapical (p. 590)
processing (p. 591)
radiograph (p. 584)
tube side (p. 587)

ADDITIONAL RESOURCES

PowerPoint slides (Evolve): 1-85
The Interactive Dental Office CD-ROM:
    Miguel Ricardo
    Harriet Ross
    Lee Wong
Multimedia Procedures DVD:
    Automatic Processing of Dental Radiographs
    Duplicating Radiographs
    Manual Processing of Radiographs

Legend

CTQ
Critical
Thinking
Question

DVD
Multimedia
Procedures
Videos and
Animations

ESLR
EVOLVE
Student
Learning
Resources

IDO
Interactive
Dental
Office
CD-ROM

SW
Student
Workbook

TB
Test Bank
on the
TEACH
CD-ROM

PPT
PowerPoint
Slides

Class Activities are indicated in ***bold italic.***

Torres and Ehrlich Modern Dental Assisting, 9th ed.

Bird/Robinson

LESSON 39.1

PRETEST

1. A latent image is an image that
   a. exists on an exposed film before it is developed.
   b. appears on an exposed film after it is developed.
   c. appears on a developed film as a result of a developing error.
   d. appears when an unexposed film is exposed to light.

2. Extraoral film differs from intraoral film in that
   a. extraoral film is faster than intraoral film.
   b. intraoral film is less sensitive to radiation.
   c. extraoral film is sensitive to specific color light.
   d. extraoral film produces a sharper image.

3. Dental film speed increases as a result of a(n) _____ in the size of silver halide crystals, which results in a(n) _____ in the amount radiation used.
   a. decrease, increase
   b. increase, increase
   c. decrease, decrease
   d. increase, decrease

4. Which size film should be used for an occlusal x-ray?
   a. size #0
   b. size #1
   c. size #2
   d. size #4

5. Intensifying screens are used to
   a. increase the intensity of the x-ray beam for exposing intraoral films.
   b. increase the amount of radiation used in exposing extraoral films.
   c. decrease the amount of radiation used to expose extraoral films.
   d. decrease the amount of electricity used to produce an x-ray.

6. An exposed film left in the developer too long will
   a. appear similar to the way it would look if the solution were too hot.
   b. appear similar to the way it would look if the solution were too cold.
   c. have no effect on the final film.
   d. produce a more diagnostic film.

7. When removing film from a patient's mouth after exposure, the film should be
   a. placed on a bare countertop and sprayed heavily with disinfectant.
   b. wiped and placed in a clean container for transfer to the darkroom.
   c. immediately taken to the darkroom.
   d. sterilized before developing.

8. An advantage of digital x-rays is that they
   a. produce less radiation.
   b. are more sanitary.
   c. require less equipment.
   d. all of the above.

9. A radiograph used to show the crowns of both arches on a single film and commonly used to diagnose cavities is called
   a. periapical.
   b. occlusal.
   c. bite-wing.
   d. panoramic.

Torres and Ehrlich Modern Dental Assisting, 9th ed.

Bird/Robinson

10. The film layer that contains the latent image is the
    a. adhesive.   c. protective.
    b. base.   d. emulsion.

Answers

1. a	3. d	5. c	7. b	9. c
2. c	4. d	6. a	8. d	10. d

BACKGROUND ASSESSMENT

Question: What are the layers of a dental film? How do these layers vary in different types of film?

Answer: Dental film contains a transparent plastic base that is made from cellulose acetate, which is used to give the film its firm but flexible quality. On either side of the plastic base is an adhesive layer that is used to attach the emulsion layer, which is where the latent image is found after exposure. The outermost layer of dental film is a protective coating. These layers vary in different types of film. Intraoral and extraoral films have an additional emulsion layer on the front and back of the base to reduce the amount of radiation needed for exposure. Duplicating film has only one emulsion layer and is exposed via white light in a duplicating machine.

Question: How are dental films processed?

Answer: There are five steps in developing x-ray films: developing, rinsing, fixing, washing, and drying. Developing converts silver halide crystals that have been exposed to radiation to black metallic silver. Developing also softens the emulsion, which produces the black, radiolucent areas of the film. Rinsing is performed to remove the developer from the film in order to prevent overdevelopment, which produces a light film. Fixing removes the unexposed crystals from the film and hardens the emulsion, which produces the white or radiopaque areas. Fixer clears the film; by observing how easily light passes through the film, the dental assistant can determine if it has been adequately fixed. Washing removes the fixer solution from the film in order to prevent overfixing or underfixing. Drying is the final step in the process. After the dental film has been dried it can be filed in the patient's record.

CRITICAL THINKING QUESTION

A patient who is scheduled for an x-ray expresses concerns about being exposed to radiation because he witnessed the effects of radiation on his father, who died of cancer. How should the dental assistant respond to this patient's concerns?

Guidelines: Dental x-rays use much less radiation than do medical x-rays, and substantially less than is used in radiation therapy. Typically a person will receive more radiation from a day spent in the sun than is received during routine dental x-rays. Current film speeds decrease even further the amount of radiation used when taking x-rays, and use of XCPs ensures accurate films, which reduces the necessity for retakes. The PID also helps to direct the x-ray beam only where it is needed, and use of lead aprons further reduces the risks of exposure. If extraoral radiographs are necessary, the use of intensifying screens greatly reduces the radiation necessary for image generation. Digital x-rays use even less radiation than traditional intraoral films.

OBJECTIVES	CONTENT	TEACHING RESOURCES
Pronounce, define, and spell the Key Terms.	■ Key terms (p. 583)	⊠▤ PPT 5-6 ◳ SW Fill in the Blank questions 1-18 (p. 274) ◉ ESLR Electronic Flashcards *Class Activity Go around the room and have each student use one of the key terms in a clinically relevant sentence in order to define the term. Continue until all terms have been used; if students become stuck, have the rest of the class offer suggestions.*

OBJECTIVES	CONTENT	TEACHING RESOURCES
Identify the types of dental x-ray film holders and devices.	■ Dental film holders (p. 584)	PPT 7-11 TB question 1 SW Short-Answer Questions 1; Multiple Choice questions 1-2 (pp. 273, 275) Figure 39-1 Plastic-type and Styrofoam-type disposable bite-block film holders (p. 584) Figure 39-2 The EeZee-Grip film holder (formerly the Snap-A-Ray) (p. 585) Figure 39-3 The Endoray is designed to be used for radiographs of teeth with endodontic instruments in the canal (p. 585) Figure 39-4 Rinn XCP instruments are color-coded for easier assembly (p. 585) Recall questions 1-3 (p. 585) ▸ Discuss why film holders are used. ***Class Activity Divide the class into groups, and provide each group with a hinged typodont and different types of dental film holders. Have each group practice assembling (if necessary) and placing the holders in the typodont as it were a real patient. Have students discuss their actions and observations with the class.***

Describe the composition of a dental x-ray film.	■ Dental film (p. 585)
	  □ Film composition (p. 585)
	  □ Latent image (p. 585)
	  □ Film speed (p. 586)
		PPT 12-19
		
		TB questions 2-3
		
		SW Short-Answer Questions 2; Multiple Choice questions 3-4 (pp. 273, 275)
		
		Figure 39-5 Cross-sectional diagram of film base and emulsion (p. 585)
		
		Figure 39-6 Scanning electron micrograph of unprocessed emulsion of Kodak Ultra Speed dental film (p. 586)
		
		Figure 39-7 Insight is the new F-speed film available from Kodak (p. 586)
		
		▸ Discuss Figure 39-5 (p. 585), noting the relative thickness of dental x-ray film base and emulsion.
		
		Class Activity Divide the class into groups. Have each group diagram the layers that compose dental x-ray film and explain the functions of each. Then have each group present its diagram to the class.

OBJECTIVES	CONTENT	TEACHING RESOURCES
State the types of and indications for the three types of dental radiographs.	■ Types of film (p. 586)	⊠▤ PPT 20 📓 SW Short-Answer Questions 9 (p. 273) ▸ Discuss the contents of a dental film packet. *Class Activity **Divide the class into groups and assign each group one of the types of dental x-ray film: intraoral, extraoral, duplicating. Have each group discuss what its assigned type of x-ray is, when its use is indicated and how it is exposed and developed. Have each group present its findings to the class for discussion.***

Identify the five basic sizes of intraoral dental film.	☐ Intraoral film (p. 586)
	
	– Film packet (p. 586)
	
	– Packet information (p. 586)
	
	– Wrapper and lead sheet (p. 587)
	
	– Package positioning (p. 587)
	
	– Package disposal (p. 587)
	
	– Outer packet (p. 587)
	
	– Tube side (p. 587)
	
	– Label side (p. 587)
	
	– Film sizes (p. 587)
		⊠▤ PPT 21-27
		
		▣ TB question 4
		
		📓 SW Short-Answer Questions 10; Multiple Choice questions 5-7; Activity (pp. 273, 275)
		
		📓⦿ SW/IDO CD-ROM Patient Case Exercise questions 1-2 (pp. 276-277) (The Interactive Dental Office CD-ROM)
		
		Figure 39-8 Contents of a dental film packet: lead foil, radiograph film, and black paper (p. 586)
		
		Figure 39-9 The lead foil insert in this package has a raised diamond pattern across both ends (p. 587)
		
		Figure 39-10 A radiograph that was positioned backward in the mouth will have a herringbone pattern on it (p. 587)
		
		Figure 39-11 The white side of the film packet faces the tube (p. 587)
		
		Recall questions 4-8 (p. 588)
		
		💡 CTQ 1 (p. 599)
		
		▸ Discuss the information found in the film package.
		
		*Class Activity **Present the following situations to the class and have students identify which film size is most appropriate for each:***
		
		  1. A 23-year-old woman is having a full mouth radiographic survey.
		
		  2. A 2-year-old child is having occlusal radiographs.
		
		  3. A 43-year-old man is having a bite-wing examination.
		
		  4. A 37-year-old woman is having occlusal radiographs.
		
		  5. A 5-year-old child is having anterior radiographs.

OBJECTIVES	CONTENT	TEACHING RESOURCES
Explain the purpose of an intensifying screen.	☐ Extraoral film (p. 588) – Film packaging (p. 588) – Film cassette (p. 588) – Intensifying screen (p. 589) – Film types (p. 589)	PPT 28-37 TB questions 5-7 SW Short-Answer Questions 11; Multiple Choice questions 8-9 (pp. 273, 275) Figure 39-12 Panoramic x-ray film (p. 588) Figure 39-13 Cephalometric radiograph (p. 588) Figure 39-14 Boxes of extraoral x-ray film (p. 589) Figure 39-15 The dental assistant removes a film from a flexible film cassette (p. 589) Figure 39-16 Rigid-type film cassette with an intensifying screen (p. 589) Recall questions 9-11 (p. 590) ▸ Discuss the types and purposes of film cassettes. ***Class Activity Divide the class into groups, and assign each group one of the following types of intensifying screens: calcium tungstate, rare earth elements. Have each group diagram how its intensifying screen works and explain which types of film it is used in conjunction with and why. Then have each group present its findings to the class.***
Describe the process for duplicating radiographs.	☐ Duplicating film (p. 590) Procedure 39-1 Duplicating dental radiographs (p. 590) (SW/ESLR Competency 39-1, p. 279) ☐ Film storage (p. 590)	PPT 38-39 SW Short-Answer Questions 12; Multiple Choice questions 10-12 (pp. 273, 275) SW/ESLR Competency 39-1 Duplicating Dental Radiographs (p. 279) Figure 39-17 Example of a film duplicator (p. 590) Recall questions 12-14 (p. 591) ▸ Discuss the steps involved in duplicating dental radiographs. ▸ Discuss reasons why dental radiographs may need to be duplicated. ***Class Activity Lead a class discussion about duplicating film, and ask students to compare and contrast its layers and uses with the other types of film. Record student responses on the board for comparison.***

39.1 Homework/Assignments:

39.1 Instructor's Notes/Student Feedback:

Bird/Robinson

LESSON 39.2

CRITICAL THINKING QUESTION

A new assistant has just been hired and has been instructed to help the dental assistant prepare a full set of x-rays on two new patients. The dental assistant decides to take the x-rays herself and instructs the new assistant to develop the first set of x-rays while the dental assistant continues with the second patient. After developing the x-rays the new assistant presents the x-rays to the dental assistant. The x-rays are cloudy, chalky, and unreadable. How should this situation be handled? Should the x-rays be retaken?

Guidelines: Retaking x-rays is always a last resort. If x-rays are ever unclear, the first suspicion usually falls on the fixer solution. Because these films are cloudy and chalky, they were not left in the fixer long enough, the fixer solution was too cold, the films were inadequately washed, or the fixer solution was contaminated. The dental assistant should begin by checking the temperature and level of the fixer solution. If both are okay, the films should be placed in the fixer for an additional 2 minutes, washed, and allowed to dry. If placing them in the fixer for a longer period of time doesn't correct the problem, the dental assistant should next try fixing one film in a small cup of fresh solution. If this clears the film, the fixer solution should be changed completely and the remainder of the films should be fixed. If the film still appears cloudy and unreadable, the films may need to be retaken. Understanding potential processing errors is an enormous help to the dentist; it is one of the most important skills a good dental assistant can have.

OBJECTIVES	CONTENT	TEACHING RESOURCES
Describe the care and maintenance of the processing solutions, equipment, and equipment accessories used in manual and automatic film processing.	■ Film processing (p. 591) □ Five steps in processing (p. 591) □ Processing solutions (p. 591)	PPT 43-51 TB questions 8-9 SW Short-Answer Questions 3; Multiple Choice questions 13-15 (pp. 273, 275) Table 39-1 Developer Composition (p. 591) Table 39-2 Fixer Composition (p. 591) Recall questions 15-17 (p. 592) Figure 39-18 Concentrated solutions of film developer and fixer (p. 592) CTQ 2 (p. 599) ▸ Discuss the ingredients found in developer and fixer solutions. ***Class Activity Divide the class into groups. Have each group outline the steps involved in processing film, explain when and how processing solutions should be replenished, and discuss the dental assistant's roles and responsibilities. Then have each group share its findings with the class.***
Discuss the requirements necessary for the darkroom.	□ The darkroom (p. 592) – Lighting (p. 592) – Room lighting (p. 592) – Safe lighting (p. 592)	PPT 52-59 TB question 11 SW Short-Answer Questions 13; Multiple Choice questions 16-20 (pp. 273, 275-276) Requirements for a Film Processing Darkroom (p. 592)

ELSEVIER

OBJECTIVES	CONTENT	TEACHING RESOURCES
	– Processing tanks (p. 592)	Figure 39-19 A distance of a least 4 feet must separate the safelight from the working area (p. 593)
		Figure 39-20 Processing tanks showing developing and fixing tanks inserts in bath of running water (p. 593)
		Recall questions 18-20 (p. 593)
		Table 39-3 Processing Temperatures and Times (p. 594)
		▶ Discuss the equipment and materials necessary in a film-processing darkroom.
		Class Activity Divide the class into groups. Have each group design a darkroom for a dental office, outline all the factors and considerations that should be considered when constructing the darkroom, and develop a blueprint. Have each group present its design to the class for discussion.
List and identify the component parts of an automatic film processor.	□ Automatic processor (p. 593) – Components (p. 594) [Procedure] 39-2 Manual processing of dental radiographs (p. 595) (SW/ESLR Competency 39-2, pp. 281-282) – Processing solutions (p. 594) [Procedure] 39-3 Automatic processing of dental radiographs using daylight loader (p. 596) (SW/ESLR Competency 39-3, p. 283)	▣ PPT 60-64 ▣ Multimedia Procedures DVD: Automatic Processing of Dental Radiographs ▣ SW Short-Answer Questions 4 (p. 273) ▣ *e* SW/ESLR Competency 39-2 Processing Dental Radiographs Manually (pp. 281-282) ▣ *e* SW/ESLR Competency 39-3 Processing Dental Radiographs in an Automatic Film Processor (p. 283) Figure 39-21 (A) An automatic film processor (B) An automatic film processor equipped with a daylight film (p. 593) Figure 39-22 Component parts of the automatic processor (p. 594) Recall questions 21-23 (p. 594) ▶ Discuss the individual components of an automatic film processor, as shown in Figure 39-22 (p. 594). ***Class Activity Divide the class into groups, and provide them with unlabeled copies of Figure 39-22 (p. 594). Have students fill in the missing labels without using their textbooks, and then share their answers with the class for feedback.***
Describe common time and temperature errors during film processing.	■ Processing errors (p. 597)	▣ PPT 65, 67, 75-76, 79 ▣ TB question 10 ▣ SW Short-Answer Questions 5 (p. 273) Table 39-4 Time and Temperature Errors and Solutions (p. 596)

ELSEVIER

Bird/Robinson

OBJECTIVES	CONTENT	TEACHING RESOURCES
		Figure 39-23 Radiograph processing errors (p. 598) CTQ 3 (p. 599) ▶ Discuss the appearance of underdeveloped film, the cause, and the solution. *Class Activity **Divide the class into groups. Have each group identify three time or temperature errors that can occur when processing film and discuss ways the dental assistant could rectify the errors without retaking the radiographs. Have each group discuss its findings with the class.***
Describe chemical contamination errors during film processing.	■ Processing errors (p. 597)	PPT 65, 77, 79 SW Short-Answer Questions 6 (p. 273) Table 39-5 Chemical Contamination Errors and Solutions (p. 597) ▶ Discuss the appearance of fixer spots, the cause, and the solution. *Class Activity **Divide the class into groups, and have each group identify five ways in which chemical contamination errors can be avoided. Then have each group share its findings with the class.***
Describe film handling errors that can occur during film processing.	■ Processing errors (p. 597)	PPT 65, 69-74, 78-83 SW Short-Answer Questions 7 (p. 273) Table 39-6 Film Handling Errors and Solutions (p. 597) ▶ Discuss the appearance of a static electricity error, the cause, and the solution. *Class Activity **Lead a class discussion about processing errors, and have students compare and contrast the appearance of chemical contamination errors with errors in handling film.. How could film-handling errors be rectified without retaking x-rays? Record student responses on the board for comparison.***
Describe some common lighting errors during film processing.	■ Processing errors (p. 597)	PPT 65, 84-85 SW Short-Answer Questions 8 (p. 273) Table 39-7 Lighting Errors and Solutions (p. 599) ▶ Discuss the appearance of fogged film, the cause, and the solution. *Class Activity **Divide the class into groups. Have each group identify five ways in which lighting errors could be avoided and discuss the dental assistant's role in preventing these errors. Have groups present their findings to the class for discussion.***

ELSEVIER

Torres and Ehrlich Modern Dental Assisting, 9th ed.
Bird/Robinson

OBJECTIVES	CONTENT	TEACHING RESOURCES
Performance Evaluation		TB
		SW questions (pp. 273-276)
		SW/IDO Patient Case Exercises (pp. 276-277) (The Interactive Dental Office CD-ROM)
		SW/ESLR Competency 39-1 Duplicating Dental Radiographs (p. 279)
		SW/ESLR Competency 39-2 Processing Dental Radiographs Manually (pp. 281-282)
		SW/ESLR Competency 39-3 Processing Dental Radiographs in an Automatic Film Processor (p. 283)
		ESLR Electronic Flashcards
		ESLR Practice Quiz
		Recall questions (pp. 585-594)
		CTQ (p. 599)

39.2 Homework/Assignments:

39.2 Instructor's Notes/Student Feedback:

Slide 1

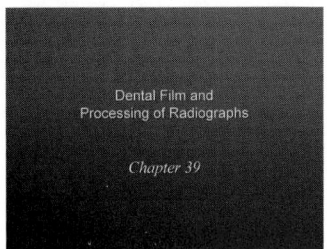

Slide 2

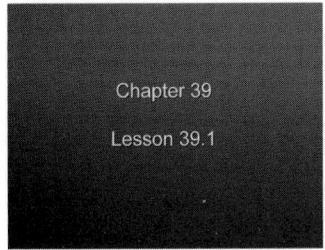

Slide 3

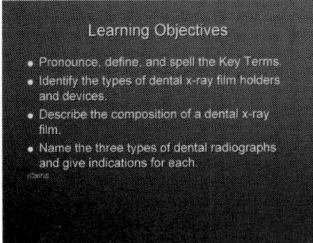

Slide 4

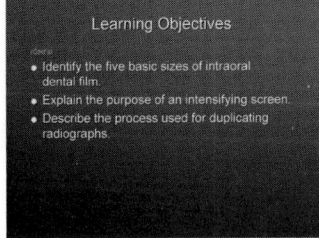

Slide 5

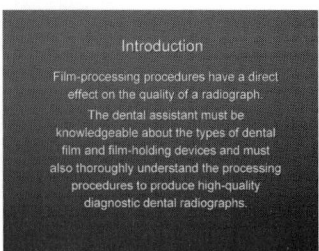

- Who is most often responsible for processing film? *(The dental assistant.)*

Slide 6

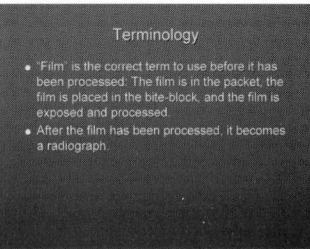

- Why is it important to use the correct terminology?
- What is the latent image?

Slide 7

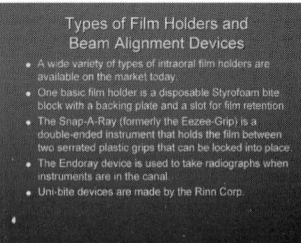

- What is a film holder?
- How do film holders reduce exposure? *(In two ways: by preventing cone cuts, thus reducing retakes; and by allowing the film to be held in place without the aid of the patient's finger in the field of radiation.)*
- Unibite is more commonly referred to as XCP (extension-cone paralleling).

Slide 8

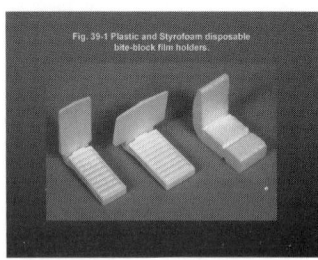

- What is the advantage of using the Styrofoam bite-block? *(It is disposable and does not need to be sterilized.)*

Slide 9

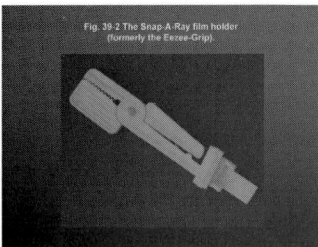

- It is used with the bisecting technique.
- It has the advantage of being able to be adjusted on the film for patients with jaws too shallow to accommodate the full depth of the film.

Slide 10

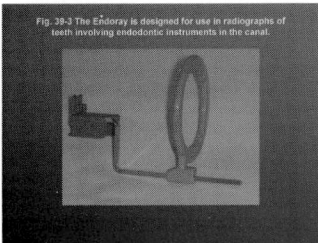

- How would an endodontic x-ray be taken if this device were not available? *(It is not uncommon to have patients use a finger or a hemostat to hold the film in place.)*

Slide 11

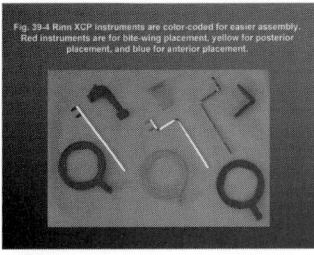

- The yellow (posterior) XCP requires flipping the ring when exposing opposite sides of the mouth (upper right/lower left vs. lower right/upper left).
- Therefore, the yellow ring lines up differently, depending on which way it is put on. The bite-block portion of the XCP should be in the center of the yellow ring after it has been assembled.

Slide 12

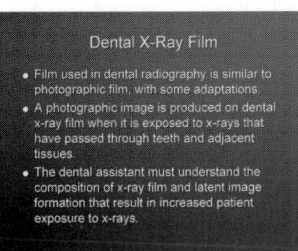

- How do skilled dental assistants reduce the patient's exposure to x-rays? *(By reducing the number of retakes.)*

Slide 13

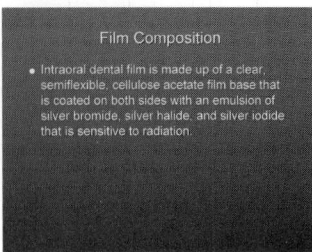

- Why is the film base a necessary component of the film composition? *(The chemical crystals are embedded in the film base.)*

Slide 14

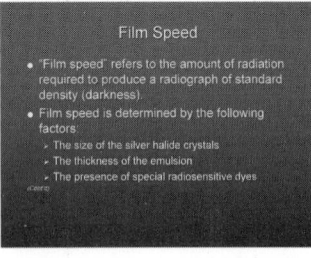

Slide 15

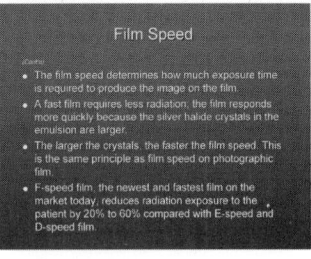

- What organization classifies film speed? *(The American National Standards Institute [ANSI].)*

Slide 16

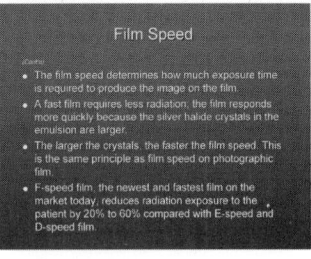

- How does the size of the crystals affect the resolution of the film? *(Larger crystals increase film speed, but slightly reduce image resolution.)*
- Where is the film speed indicated?

Slide 17

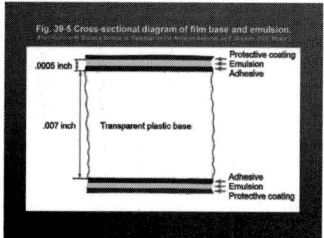

- Why are there two emulsion layers on intraoral films? *(This allows an image to be produced using less radiation.)*

Slide 18

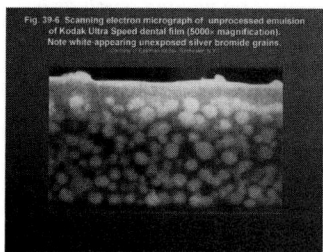

- Which portion of the developed radiograph will the exposed silver crystals become? *(They will become the black or dark portion of the radiograph. Areas that are dark on a radiograph are termed radiolucent, as this is the part of the field that radiation was allowed to pass through easily.)*

Slide 19

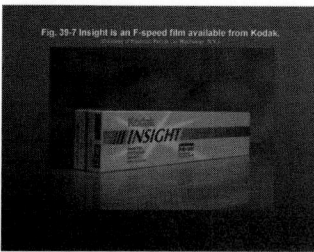

- F-speed film is the fastest film currently on the market.

- D- and E-speed film are still commonly used by cost-conscious dentists because the relative decrease in radiation exposure from F-speed is small when looking at only a few exposures.

Slide 20

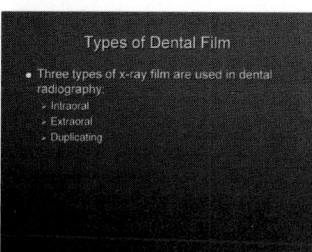

- Which of these three x-ray films is the most commonly used? *(Intraoral.)*

Torres and Ehrlich Modern Dental Assisting, 9th ed.

Bird/Robinson

Slide 21

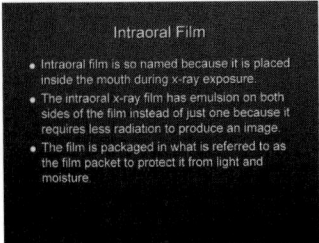

- Why does the film need to be protected from light? *(Light is a form of radiation and will expose and ruin the film.)*
- Light cannot pass through the packet, but x-rays can.
- The terms "film" and "film packet" are often used interchangeably.

Slide 22

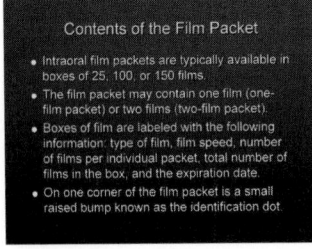

- Why do some packets contain two films? *(This allows for a copy to be made instantly when it is known that a copy will be needed, such as with certain insurance claims or specialty referrals.)*

Slide 23

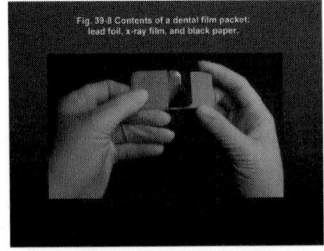

- What purpose does the lead foil serve? *(The lead foil protects the film from back-scattered radiation.)*
- What would happen if the lead foil was not there? *(The back-scattered radiation would fog the image.)*

Slide 24

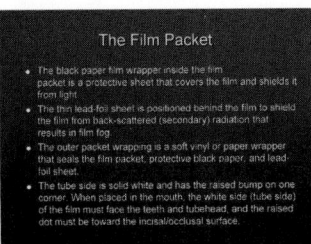

Torres and Ehrlich Modern Dental Assisting, 9th ed.
Bird/Robinson

Slide 25

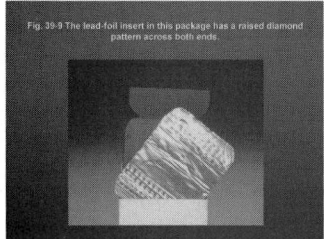

- What will the radiograph look like if it has been exposed backwards? *(It will have a herringbone pattern over the actual image.)*

Slide 26

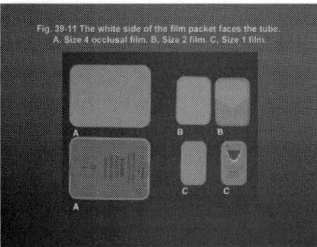

- Size #2 film is typically used for both anterior and posterior views because it will give a wider image that will overlap adjacent images. This allows for areas to be represented more than once in a set of x-rays, acting as a diagnostic backup. This reduces the need for retakes without increasing the amount of radiation exposure for the patient.

Slide 27

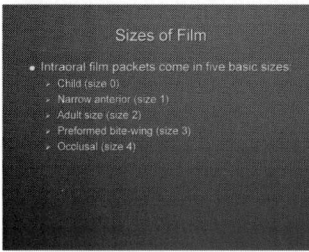

- Size #3 film is rarely, if ever, used.

- Bite-wings are usually taken with a size #2 film and a bite tab or red XCP.

Slide 28

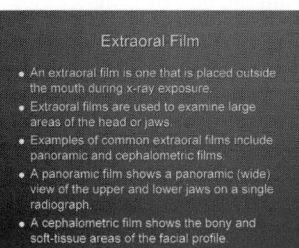

- What does "extraoral" mean?

Slide 29

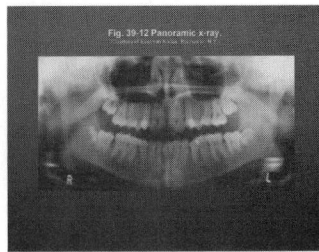

- Extraoral films are more common in specialty practices, such as orthodontic, pediatric, and oral surgery practices.

- Pediatric dentists use panoramic films to see the developing teeth because it is difficult for a child to sit through a full-mouth series of radiographs. It also exposes the child to less radiation than a full-mouth series.

Slide 30

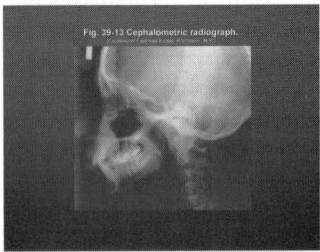

- Orthodontists commonly use cephalometric films to view the relationship of the jaw to the skull.

Slide 31

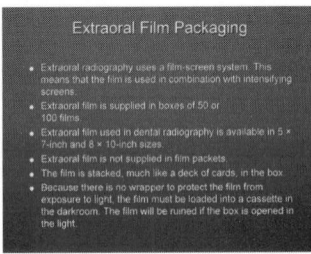

- Where should extraoral films be stored? *(Extraoral films should be stored in a darkroom. This will prevent them from being accidentally opened in a lighted room which can expose and ruin all the film in the box.)*

Slide 32

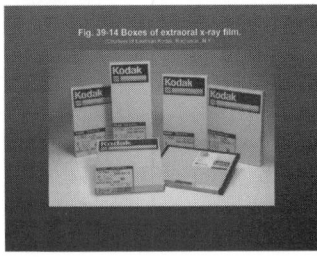

- It is advisable to seal an opened box with a rubber band to ensure that the cover doesn't accidentally fall off and ruin the box of film.

Slide 33

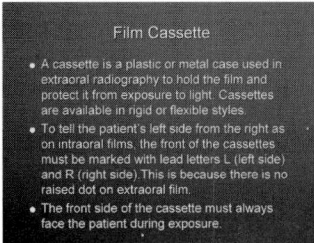

- The front side of the cassette is the side without the latch.

Slide 34

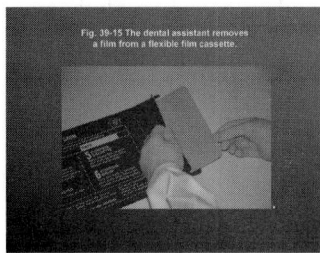

- What is the front side of the cassette typically made of?
- What is the back side of the cassette typically made of?

Slide 35

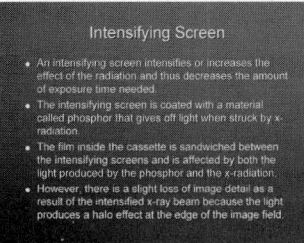

- This loss of detail makes panoramic x-rays unsuitable for caries diagnosis. For this reason, pediatric dentists take bite-wings in conjunction with the panoramic x-ray to make a pediatric full set.

Slide 36

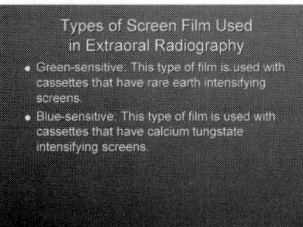

- These films are also sensitive to white light, as it contains every color of light in the visible spectrum.

Bird/Robinson

Slide 37

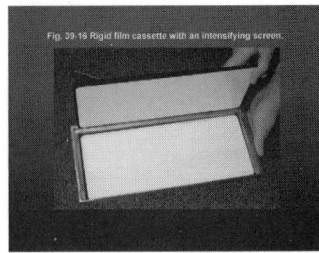

Fig. 39-16 Rigid film cassette with an intensifying screen.

- The front of this cassette is the side on the table; the back is the side with the latch.

Slide 38

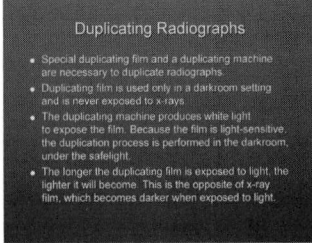

Duplicating Radiographs

- Special duplicating film and a duplicating machine are necessary to duplicate radiographs.
- Duplicating film is used only in a darkroom setting and is never exposed to x-rays
- The duplicating machine produces white light to expose the film. Because the film is light-sensitive, the duplication process is performed in the darkroom, under the safelight.
- The longer the duplicating film is exposed to light, the lighter it will become. This is the opposite of x-ray film, which becomes darker when exposed to light.

- What equipment is needed to duplicate dental radiographs?

Slide 39

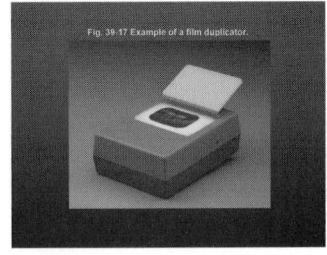

Fig. 39-17 Example of a film duplicator.

- How does duplicating film differ from standard intraoral film?
  (Unlike intraoral film, duplicating film has a single emulsion layer and is never exposed to x-rays—only to light.)

Slide 40

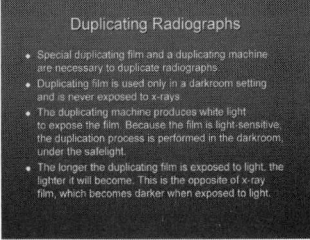

Duplicating Radiographs

- Special duplicating film and a duplicating machine are necessary to duplicate radiographs.
- Duplicating film is used only in a darkroom setting and is never exposed to x-rays
- The duplicating machine produces white light to expose the film. Because the film is light-sensitive, the duplication process is performed in the darkroom, under the safelight.
- The longer the duplicating film is exposed to light, the lighter it will become. This is the opposite of x-ray film, which becomes darker when exposed to light.

Slide 41

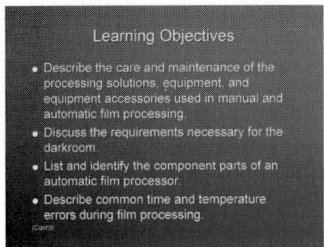

Slide 42

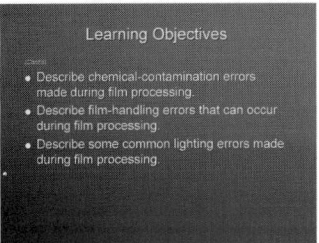

Slide 43

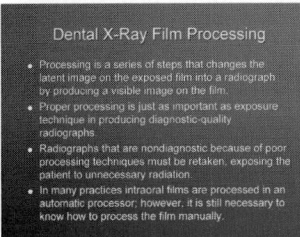

- Why is it necessary to know how to process the film manually in practices that have an automatic processor? *(There are two reasons: [1] to be able to identify and correct errors in processing; and [2] to have the ability to develop a film more quickly, as with endodontics. A film can be developed manually in about 2 minutes.)*

Slide 44

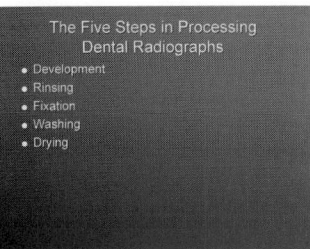

- Which step consumes the most time? *(Drying.)*

Torres and Ehrlich Modern Dental Assisting, 9th ed.

Bird/Robinson

Slide 45

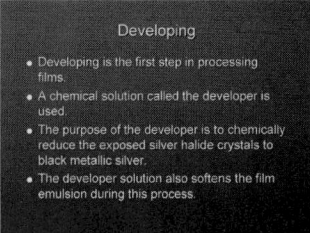

- When manually processing for endodontic procedures, the film is typically placed in the developer just long enough for an image to appear. This usually takes less than a minute. However, initial and final films should never be developed this way.

Slide 46

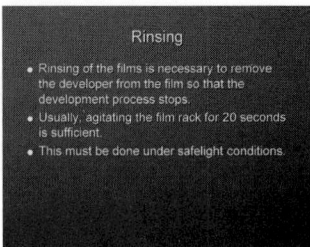

- When rinsing, unexposed crystals still remain on the film. Therefore, rinsing needs to be done under a safelight, since white light will expose those crystals and distort the image.

Slide 47

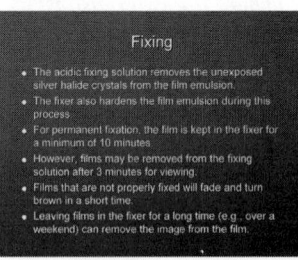

- A working film for endodontic procedures can be placed in the fixer for roughly one minute and will last long enough for the dentist to get the information he or she needs.

Slide 48

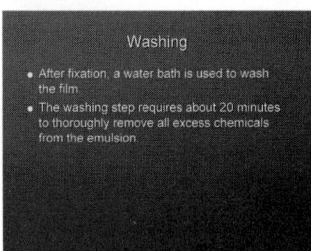

- This step no longer needs to be done in safelight. Why? *(Because the unexposed crystals have been removed, there is nothing to react with the white light.)*

Torres and Ehrlich Modern Dental Assisting, 9th ed.

Bird/Robinson

Slide 49

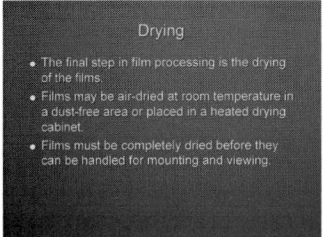

- Automatic processors use warm air to dry films more quickly.

Slide 50

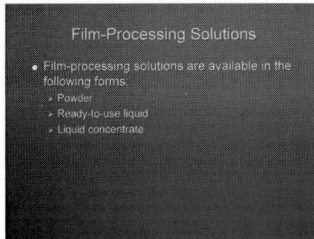

- Ready-to-use liquid is by far the most commonly used solution.

- Powder and concentrate require mixing, which most practices do not take the time to do.

Slide 51

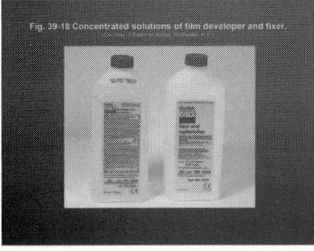

- Distilled water must be added to the concentrate before using.

- What would films look like if the developer solution was not diluted? *(The films would appear overdeveloped.)*

Slide 52

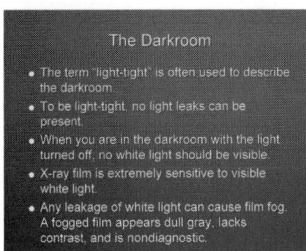

- What might cause a fogged film other than light leaks in the darkroom? *(The film may have been left in the x-ray room after the initial exposure and exposed to background radiation. Keep exposed films outside the radiography operatory.)*

Slide 53

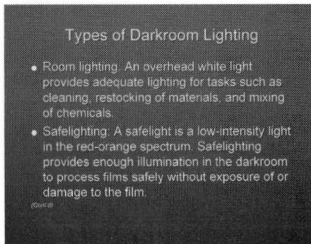

- At what distance from the working area should the safelight be placed? *(Four feet.)*

Slide 54

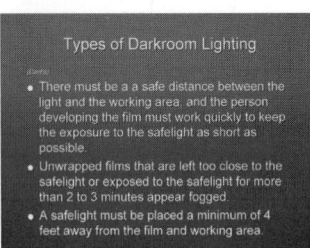

- Some safelights are made only for intraoral films, some for only extraoral films, and still others for both intraoral and extraoral films.

Slide 55

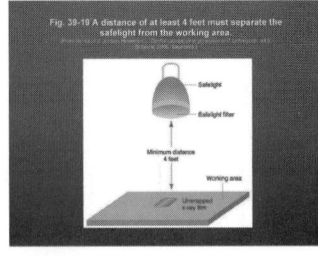

- Why does the safelight need to be placed at this distance? *(To decrease the intensity of the light reaching the undeveloped film. Safelight will still expose a film if left long enough or held close enough.)*

Slide 56

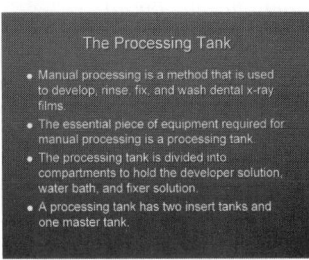

- What controls the temperatures of the developer and fixer solutions?
- What is the optimum temperature for the water bath in the insert tank?

Slide 57

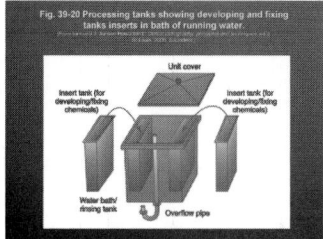

- What's the purpose of the cover? *(To keep solutions from evaporating when not in use.)*
- How often should solutions be changed? *(Every 3 to 4 weeks.)*

Slide 58

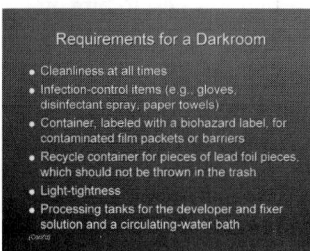

- What are the consequences of a room that is not light-tight? *(Film fog.)*

Slide 59

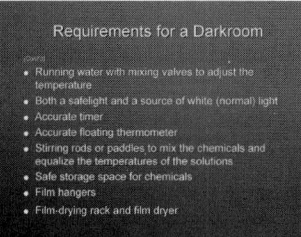

- What happens if the developer solution is too warm? *(Overdeveloped films.)*

Slide 60

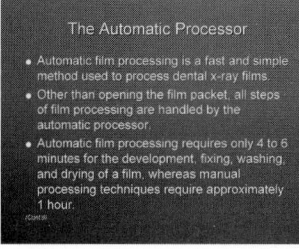

- Never open the automatic processor with the overhead light turned on if the film is still being processed.
- Should a film get stuck, open the automatic processor with the safelight on and try to locate the film. If necessary, reprocess the film or develop it manually.

Slide 61

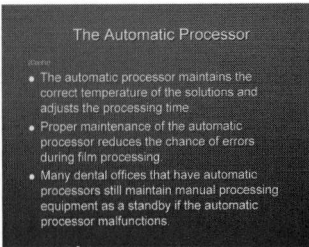

- Manual processing is commonly used to quickly develop working endodontic films.

Slide 62

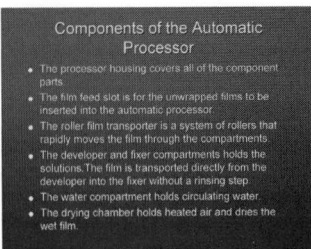

- When first turned on, most automatic processors require a period of time before they are ready to process. As a result, it is best to turn on the automatic processor first thing in the morning.

Slide 63

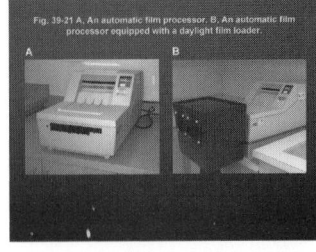

- The automatic processor pictured in Figure B displays a day loader, a device used to unwrap and process films without the need for a darkroom.

Slide 64

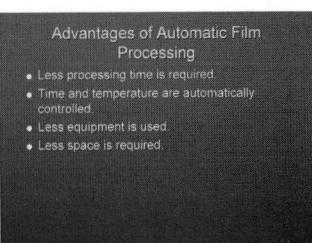

- There is also less chance of errors during film processing.

Slide 65

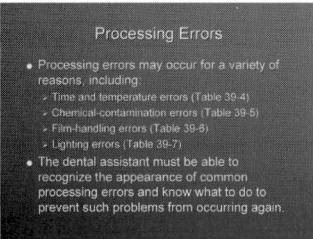

- In order for films to be of diagnostic use, they must be free of error.

Slide 66

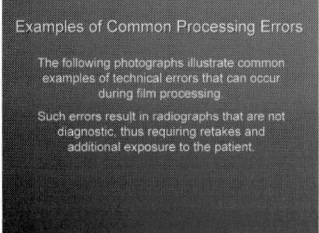

Slide 67

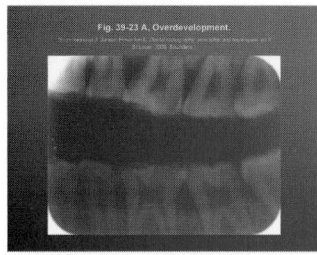

- What can cause overdeveloped film? *(Overdevelopment results from a developer solution that is too concentrated, or too warm, or film that is placed in the developer solution for too long.)*

Slide 68

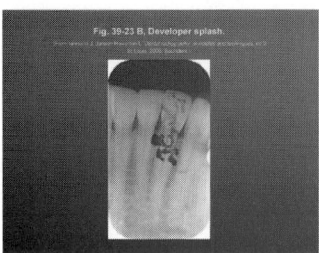

- A neat work area can prevent errors like developer splash.
- Give another example of an error caused by chemical contamination.

Slide 69

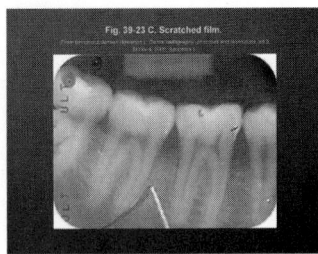

- Developer softens the emulsion, leaving it susceptible to scratches.
- Careful handling, especially before fixing, will prevent scratched film.

Slide 70

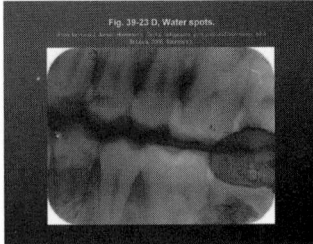

- How can this type of radiograph processing error be avoided?

Slide 71

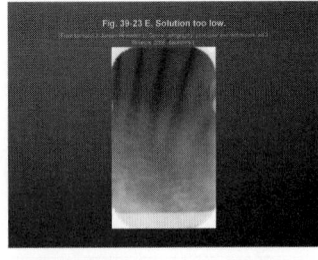

- How can this error be prevented?

Slide 72

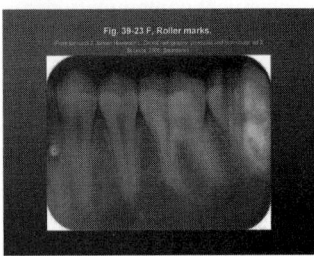

- What can the dental assistant do to prevent this type of error?

Slide 73

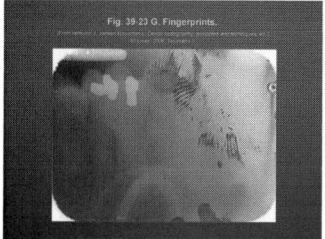

- Handle films by the edges until processing is complete.

Slide 74

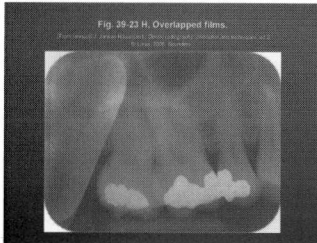

- This is a film-handling error caused by two films being in contact during processing.
- It can be prevented by separating films.

Slide 75

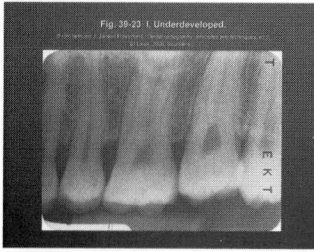

- Underdeveloped film is the exact opposite of overdeveloped film.
- What are some of the causes of underdevelopment?

Slide 76

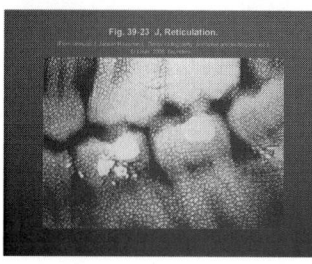

- This type of error is rare.
- Reticulation is caused by a sudden temperature change between solutions.

Bird/Robinson

Slide 77

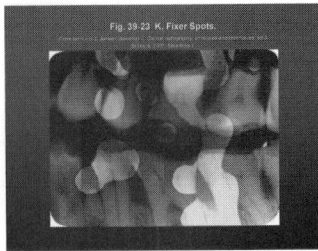

- A clean work area in the darkroom will help prevent fixer from contacting the film before processing.

Slide 78

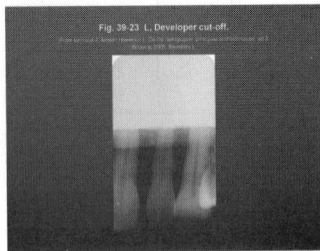

- The straight white border represents the undeveloped part of the film resulting from insufficient developer levels.

Slide 79

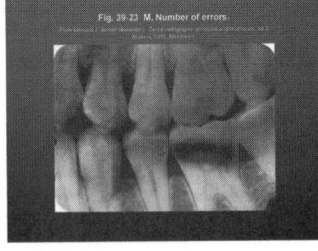

- Identify the errors represented here.

Slide 80

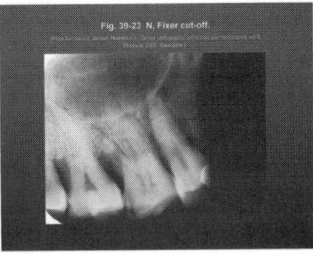

- The straight black border represents the unfixed part of the film resulting from insufficient fixer levels.

Slide 81

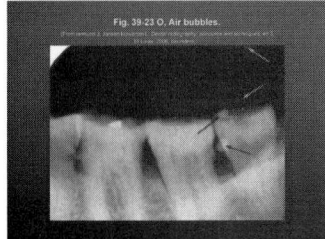

- What can prevent air bubbles from forming?

Slide 82

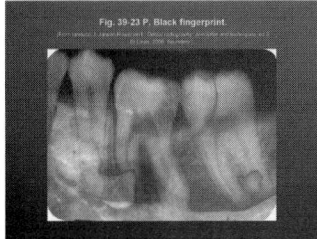

- This error in handling film is caused by touching the film with fingers contaminated with fluoride or developer.

- The solution is to wash and dry films thoroughly before processing. Also, only handle film by the edges until processing is complete.

Slide 83

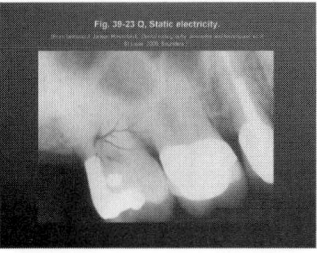

- Open film packets slowly to prevent static electricity damage to film.

Slide 84

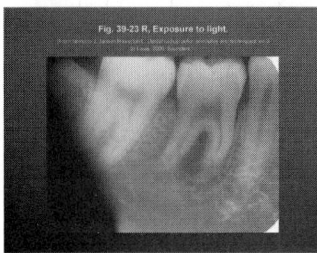

- What might the dental assistant check for to avoid this processing error?

Bird/Robinson

Slide 85

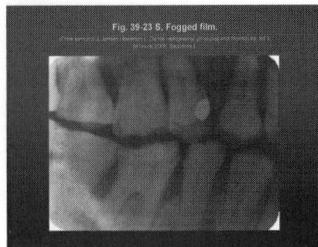

Fig. 39-23 8. Fogged film.

- Name one error that could cause fogged film? *(Storing film where it can be exposed to radiation.)*

- What might the dental assistant check for to avoid this processing error? *(See Table 39-7 Lighting Errors and Solutions on p. 599 in the textbook.)*

40 Legal Issues, Quality Assurance, and Infection Control

TEACHING FOCUS

This chapter will give students the opportunity to learn key terms relating to legal issues, quality assurance, and infection control. We will introduce students to informed consent regarding dental radiographs, the types of laws affecting dental radiography, and the Consumer-Patient Radiation Health and Safety Act. This chapter also discusses the eight annual tests recommended for x-ray equipment, the components of a quality assurance program, and the quality control tests for processing solutions. Students will have the opportunity to learn the use of a stepwedge radiograph, the purpose of a reference radiograph, and the infection-control requirements for preparing a radiography operatory. Finally, students will have the opportunity to implement the CDC guidelines for infection control in dental radiology.

MATERIALS AND RESOURCES

- ☐ computer and PowerPoint projector (all Lessons)
- ☐ copies of the Consumer-Patient Radiation Health and Safety Act (Lesson 40.1)
- ☐ developer solutions of various concentrations (Lesson 40.2)

- ☐ disclosing tablets (Lesson 40.3)
- ☐ scrubs (Lesson 40.3)
- ☐ stepwedge radiographs (undeveloped) (Lesson 40.2)

LESSON CHECKLIST

Preparations for this lesson include:

- lecture
- evaluation of student knowledge and skills needed to perform all entry-level activities related to legal issues, quality assurance, and infection control, including:
  - ○ knowledge of state and federal laws affecting dental radiography
  - ○ knowledge of certification needed to perform dental radiography
  - ○ explanation of the importance of quality assurance
  - ○ general knowledge of infection control and how it relates to dental radiography

Bird/Robinson

KEY TERMS

artifact (p. 612)
disclosure (p. 602)
informed consent (p. 602)
liable (p. 602)

quality assurance (p. 601)
quality control tests (p. 603)
stepwedge (p. 606)
viewbox (p. 604)

ADDITIONAL RESOURCES

PowerPoint slides (Evolve): 1-49

Legend

CTQ
Critical
Thinking
Question

DVD
Multimedia
Procedures
Videos and
Animations

ESLR
EVOLVE
Student
Learning
Resources

IDO
Interactive
Dental
Office
CD-ROM

SW
Student
Workbook

TB
Test Bank
on the
TEACH
CD-ROM

PPT
PowerPoint
Slides

Class Activities are indicated in ***bold italic***.

ELSEVIER

Torres and Ehrlich Modern Dental Assisting, 9th ed.

Bird/Robinson

LESSON 40.1

PRETEST

1. The Consumer-Patient Radiation Health and Safety Act requires that
   a. anyone taking x-rays obtain a state-issued license.
   b. anyone taking radiographs be trained and certified.
   c. anyone taking radiographs work no more than 35 hours per week.
   d. x-rays be taken under direct supervision of a dentist.

2. Key areas of risk management include
   a. consent.
   b. patient records.
   c. liability issues.
   d. all of the above.

3. Dental radiographs are
   a. owned by the patient and must be surrendered to the patient upon request.
   b. original, part of the patient's record, and never to be surrendered under any circumstances.
   c. not part of the accepted standard of care.
   d. taken without regard to patient radiation exposure.

4. Quality control tests alert the user regarding
   a. functional state of equipment.
   b. quality of supplies.
   c. a and b.
   d. cost of each x-ray.

5. A stepwedge radiograph is used to
   a. verify developer solution strength on a day-to-day basis.
   b. confirm film freshness.
   c. confirm x-ray beam strength.
   d. calibrate the x-ray beam focal distance.

6. The surfaces in the radiography operatory that are likely to become contaminated when exposing x-rays are the
   a. tubehead and PID.
   b. lead apron and chair controls.
   c. counter surfaces and exposure button.
   d. all of the above.

7. The major source of cross-contamination during radiographic procedures is the
   a. lead apron.
   b. PID.
   c. exposed film packet.
   d. film holder.

8. When transporting exposed films to the darkroom
   a. they should be placed in an aseptic container.
   b. gloves should be removed and hands washed.
   c. the area should be cleaned and the patient dismissed.
   d. all of the above.

9. Infection control guidelines are made by the
   a. CDC.
   b. FDA.
   c. EPA.
   d. NIH.

10. The person ultimately liable for what happens in the dental office is
    a. the patient.
    b. the office manager.
    c. the dental assistant.
    d. the dentist.

Answers

1. b	3. b	5. a	7. c	9. a
2. d	4. c	6. d	8. d	10. d

Torres and Ehrlich Modern Dental Assisting, 9th ed.

Bird/Robinson

BACKGROUND ASSESSMENT

Question: Why is quality assurance such an important function to be performed in the dental office? What are some common quality control tests performed in a dental office?

Answer: Quality assurance functions to ensure that everything possible is done to provide diagnostic quality radiographs while limiting the amount of radiation to which patients and auxiliaries are exposed. Maintenance schedules and logs are important aspects of quality assurance as they confirm that equipment and supplies are well-maintained. Quality control tests that are frequently performed include dental film tests to check freshness, x-ray machine calibration, checks of cassettes and screens for scratches, safelighting verified "light-tight," and change of automatic and manual processor solutions regularly.

Question: How is risk managed in a dental office?

Answer: Risk is managed at many different levels. At the state and federal levels it is managed by licensure and certification requirements to ensure that practitioners meet what is called the standard of care. On an interpersonal level it is managed by practicing informed consent, or ensuring that the patient has all the information needed to make an informed decision consenting to a given procedure. Patient education is equally important, especially when patients refuse necessary procedures based on a misinterpretation of the risk involved. X-rays are a common cause of exaggerated concern for some patients, and the assistant will likely have to explain this procedure to anxious patients. Patient records are a vital way of managing risk. An accurate record of patient interactions is often the best and only defense a dentist has in a malpractice suit.

CRITICAL THINKING QUESTION

A former patient comes into the dental office and states that she has recently been diagnosed with skin cancer. She demands her x-rays and treatment record, and claims that she was exposed to unnecessary radiation during her visits. How should the dental assistant respond? Can the dental assistant be held responsible?

Guidelines: In a situation like this it is important that the dental assistant remain calm even though the patient is upset. The dental assistant should begin by explaining to the patient that she must submit a request in writing regarding the x-rays and treatment record, as they are part of her patient record and the originals must remain at the office. The dental assistant should avoid getting into specifics about what happened with the agitated patient. Explain to the patient that while she is entitled to the information she requests, she must allow time for duplicates to be made. Because the dentist is ultimately responsible, the dental assistant need not worry. Although the likelihood of the patient's claim being true is minimal, when the patient is confrontational it is best to leave the matter to the dentist.

OBJECTIVES	CONTENT	TEACHING RESOURCES
Pronounce, define, and spell the Key Terms.	■ Key terms (p. 600)	SW Fill in the Blank questions 1-5 (p. 285) *e* ESLR Electronic Flashcards Recall question 2 (p. 603) Legal and Ethical Implications (p. 615) ▸ Discuss each of the key terms in Chapter 40, focusing on the definition, pronunciation, and spelling of each term. **Class Activity** *Have the students create crossword puzzles using the definitions of the key terms as clues. Have the students exchange puzzles and solve them.*
Describe the components of informed consent with regard to dental radiographs.	■ Legal considerations (p. 601) ☐ Federal and state regulations (p. 601) ☐ Licensure requirements (p. 601)	PPT 4-10 TB question 3 SW Short-Answer Questions 1; Fill in the Blank questions 1-2; Multiple Choice question 2 (pp. 285-286) Recall question 2 (p. 603)

ELSEVIER

Bird/Robinson

OBJECTIVES	CONTENT	TEACHING RESOURCES
	☐ Risk management (p. 601) ☐ Informed consent (p. 602)	▸ Discuss why disclosure and informed consent are crucial with regard to dental radiographs. ***Class Activity** Have two student volunteers role-play a dental assistant responding to a patient who is apprehensive about having x-rays. Discuss as a class what additional questions a patient might ask and whether the answers are necessary for informed consent.*
Describe the types of laws affecting the practice of dental radiography.	■ Legal considerations (p. 601) ☐ Federal and state regulations (p. 601) ☐ Licensure requirements (p. 601) ☐ Risk management (p. 601) ☐ Informed consent (p. 602) ☐ Liability (p. 602) ☐ Patient records (p. 602) – Ownership of dental radiographs (p. 602) ☐ Patient refusal (p. 602)	PPT 11-15 TB questions 1-2, 4 SW Short-Answer Questions 2-4; Fill in the Blank question 3; Multiple Choice questions 1, 3-4 (pp. 285-286) Recall questions 1, 3-4 (pp. 601, 603) Legal and Ethical Implications (p. 615) CTQ 3 (p. 615) ▸ Discuss the purpose of the legal consideration of risk management in the dentist's office. ***Class Activity** Divide the class into small groups. Have each group pretend that it is a government body responsible for setting x-ray safety regulations and discuss what laws are necessary to ensure patient and employee safety. Then have the groups share their findings with the class. Compare the findings to actual laws regarding x-rays.*
Describe the Consumer-Patient Radiation Health and Safety Act.	■ Legal considerations (p. 601) ☐ Federal and state regulations (p. 601) ☐ Licensure requirements (p. 601) ☐ Risk management (p. 601) ☐ Informed consent (p. 602) ☐ Liability (p. 602) ☐ Patient records (p. 602) – Ownership of dental radiographs (p. 602) ☐ Patient refusal (p. 60)	PPT 7 TB question 2 SW Short-Answer Questions 3; Multiple Choice question 1 (pp. 285-286) Recall question 1 (p. 601) ▸ Discuss how the federal government and state governments are involved in licensing persons who take dental radiographs. ***Class Activity** Distribute copies of the Consumer-Patient Radiation Health and Safety Act to the class. Have the students highlight important points in the act. Lead a class discussion by asking students to call out what they highlighted.*

Bird/Robinson

OBJECTIVES	CONTENT	TEACHING RESOURCES
Identify the individual that "owns" the dental radiographs.	☐ Liability (p. 602) ☐ Patient records (p. 602) – Ownership of dental radiographs (p. 602) ☐ Patient refusal (p. 602) ☐ Patient education (p. 603)	🖳 PPT 14-16 📺 TB question 4 📘 SW Short-Answer Questions 4; Multiple Choice question 4 (pp. 285-286) Recall question 4 (p. 603) Figure 40-1 The dental assistant explains the importance of radiographs and answers the patient's questions regarding the safety of dental x-rays. 💡 CTQ 3 (p. 615) ▸ Discuss what should be done with original radiographs when they are requested by a patient. ***Class Activity** As a class, discuss reasons why patients might believe they own their radiographs. Explain that when patients pay for their radiographs, they are paying for a diagnostic interpretation and not the actual radiographs.*

40.1 Homework/Assignments:

40.1 Instructor's Notes/Student Feedback:

LESSON 40.2

CRITICAL THINKING QUESTION

A dental assistant has just begun working at a new office. The staff tells the new assistant that in the past they have had problems with x-rays having to be retaken. The previous dental assistant in charge of quality assurance had trouble finding time to follow up on quality control tests and realized something was wrong only when the staff was busy attending to another patient. What sort of plan should the new dental assistant implement? How can the dental assistant ensure that the plan doesn't interfere with time allocated for patient treatment?

Guidelines: Ensuring that x-ray equipment works properly is vital to smooth operations in a practice. During the next staff meeting the dental assistant should determine what caused the past problems and try to ensure that those problems (e.g., tubehead drift) are fixed. A regular schedule should be implemented to ensure that films are fresh, x-ray equipment functions properly (tubehead steady, focal spot, timer, miliamperage, and kilovoltage are all accurate), and processing solutions are adequate. Whenever possible, these tasks should be performed in the morning before patient treatment. Delegating duties can help guarantee tasks are completed before treatment time. A good quality assurance plan will keep operations smooth and less stressful.

OBJECTIVES	CONTENT	TEACHING RESOURCES
Name the eight annual tests recommended for x-ray equipment.	■ Quality assurance in the dental office (p. 603) ☐ Quality control tests (p. 603) – Dental x-ray machines (p. 603) – Dental x-ray film (p. 604) – Screens and cassettes (p. 604) – Viewboxes (p. 604) – Darkroom lighting (p. 604) – Film processing (p. 605) ☐ Quality administration procedures (p. 606) – Description (p. 606) – Monitoring (p. 607) – Maintenance (p. 607) – Evaluation (p. 607) – Training (p. 607)	▨ PPT 19-23 ▥ TB question 7 X-Ray Machine Quality Control Steps (p. 604) ▸ Discuss annual tests that can be performed on dental x-ray machines by the dentist, the dental assistant, or the manufacturer's service representative. ***Class Activity** Divide the class into eight groups. Assign each group one of the annual tests recommended for x-ray equipment. Have each group explain how its test is performed and what the consequences would be if the test were never performed.*
Describe the components of a quality assurance program.	■ Quality assurance in the dental office (p. 603) ☐ Quality control tests (p. 603) – Dental x-ray machines (p. 603)	▨ PPT 19-23 ▥ TB questions 6-12 ▤ SW Short-Answer Questions 5-9; Fill in the Blank questions 4-5; Multiple Choice questions 5-15 (pp. 285-287) ▤ SW Topics for Discussion (p. 287)

Torres and Ehrlich Modern Dental Assisting, 9th ed.

Bird/Robinson

OBJECTIVES	CONTENT	TEACHING RESOURCES
	– Dental x-ray film (p. 604)	Types of Quality Control Tests (p. 603)
	– Screens and cassettes (p. 604)	X-Ray Machine Quality Control Steps (p. 604)
	– Viewboxes (p. 604)	Figure 40-2 Viewbox with clean Plexiglas and new bulb (p. 604)
	– Darkroom lighting (p. 604)	Recall questions 5-7, 13-15 (pp. 604, 606-607)
	– Film processing (p. 605)	Figure 40-3 (A) Unexposed film with coin on it; (B) Radiograph showing outline of coin (p. 605)
	☐ Quality administration procedures (p. 606)	Figure 40-4 Radiograph of a stepwedge (p. 606)
	– Description (p. 606)	Administrative Quality Control Steps (p. 606)
	– Monitoring (p. 607)	💡 CTQ 1-2 (p. 615)
	– Maintenance (p. 607)	▸ Discuss the Administrative Quality Control Steps.
	– Evaluation (p. 607)	***Class Activity** Divide the class into small groups. Have each group pretend it is an individual dental office and is conducting a staff meeting. Have each group devise a quality assurance plan, delegate duties, create schedules, and decide where logs should be kept.*
	– Training (p. 607)	
Describe quality control tests for processing solutions.	■ Quality assurance in the dental office (p. 603)	📺 PPT 19-23
	☐ Quality control tests (p. 603)	💻 TB questions 9-10
	– Dental x-ray machines (p. 603)	📖 SW Short-Answer Questions 7-9; Multiple Choice questions 12-13 (pp. 285-287)
	– Dental x-ray film (p. 604)	📖 SW Topics for Discussion (p. 287)
	– Screens and cassettes (p. 604)	Recall questions 11, 13 (p. 606)
	– Viewboxes (p. 604)	▸ Discuss when the dental assistant should check the processing solutions.
	– Darkroom lighting (p. 604)	***Class Activity** As a class discuss qualities of a processing solution that can change and affect radiograph development (e.g., temperature, concentration, contamination) and how to correct them.*
	– Film processing (p. 605)	
	☐ Quality administration procedures (p. 606)	
	– Description (p. 606)	
	– Monitoring (p. 607)	
	– Maintenance (p. 607)	
	– Evaluation (p. 607)	
	– Training (p. 607)	

ELSEVIER

Bird/Robinson

OBJECTIVES	CONTENT	TEACHING RESOURCES
Explain the use of a stepwedge.	■ Quality assurance in the dental office (p. 603) ☐ Quality control tests (p. 603) – Dental x-ray machines (p. 603) – Dental x-ray film (p. 604) – Screens and cassettes (p. 604) – Viewboxes (p. 604) – Darkroom lighting (p. 604) – Film processing (p. 605) ☐ Quality administration procedures (p. 606) – Description (p. 606) – Monitoring (p. 607) – Maintenance (p. 607) – Evaluation (p. 607) – Training (p. 607)	⊠▤ PPT 23 ▦ TB question 10 ✎ SW Short-Answer Questions 8; Multiple Choice question 12 (pp. 285-286) Recall questions 12-13 (p. 606) Figure 40-4 Radiograph of a stepwedge (p. 606) ♀ CTQ 1-2 (p. 615) ▸ Discuss the purpose of a stepwedge and how it is part of quality assurance. ***Class Activity** Expose a series of stepwedge radiographs. As a class demonstration prepare a series of developer solutions of varying concentrations. Label the concentrations and develop the stepwedge films to demonstrate how the developer solution affects the film density.*
Discuss the purpose of a reference radiograph.	■ Quality assurance in the dental office (p. 603) ☐ Quality control tests (p. 603) – Dental x-ray machines (p. 603) – Dental x-ray film (p. 604) – Screens and cassettes (p. 604) – Viewboxes (p. 604) – Darkroom lighting (p. 604) – Film processing (p. 605) ☐ Quality administration procedures (p. 606)	⊠▤ PPT 19-23 ▦ TB question 10 ✎ SW Short-Answer Questions 9; Multiple Choice question 12 (pp. 285-285) Recall questions 12-13 (p. 606) ♀ CTQ 1 (p. 615) ▸ Discuss the steps in making a reference radiograph, emphasizing the sequence of the process. ***Class Activity** Using the radiographs prepared for the previous activity, show the class that the first radiograph developed in the new undiluted solution is considered the reference radiograph.*

ELSEVIER

Torres and Ehrlich Modern Dental Assisting, 9th ed.

Bird/Robinson

OBJECTIVES	CONTENT	TEACHING RESOURCES
	– Description (p. 606)	
	– Monitoring (p. 607)	
	– Maintenance (p. 607)	
	– Evaluation (p. 607)	
	– Training (p. 607)	

40.2 Homework/Assignments:

40.2 Instructor's Notes/Student Feedback:

LESSON 40.3

CRITICAL THINKING QUESTION

A new patient waits outside the radiography operatory when the assistant is setting it up for use. The patient tells the assistant, "Isn't this overkill? I don't have anything wrong with me." How might the dental assistant educate this patient about infection control?

Guidelines: The dental assistant should offer the following explanation: The majority of patients do not appear to have anything wrong with them and do not appear to have any major communicable diseases. However, when a dental assistant takes radiographs, films and gloves come into contact with saliva. Even though it may not be visible, saliva can contain blood. Both blood and saliva contain bacteria and can also contain viruses, unknown to the patient. Normal bacteria in one patient can cause problems in another, as no two immune systems are exactly alike. Infection control standards require that all patients be treated as though they were sick because they do not always disclose information about their disease status. Therefore, to protect everyone involved, all patients are treated the same.

OBJECTIVES	CONTENT	TEACHING RESOURCES
Explain the infection-control requirements for preparing a radiography operatory.	■ Infection control (p. 607) □ Centers for Disease Control and Prevention guidelines (p. 607) □ The radiography operatory (p. 608) – X-ray machine (p. 608) – Lead apron (p. 608) – Dental chair (p. 609) – Work area (p. 609) □ Equipment and supplies (p. 609) – Film (p. 609) – Film packets (p. 609) – Film-holding devices (film holders) (p. 609) – Miscellaneous items (p. 609)	🖥 PPT 26-41 📗 SW Short-Answer Questions 10 (p. 285); Multiple Choice question 16 (p. 287) Recall questions 16-17 (p. 610) Checklist for Infection Control in Dental Radiography (p. 607) CDC Guidelines for Dental Radiology (p. 608) Surfaces Likely to Be Contaminated During X-Ray Procedures (p. 608) Figure 40-5 X-ray equipment with barriers in place (p. 608) Figure 40-6 Radiography operatory with barriers in place (p. 608) ▸ Discuss the importance of infection control in the radiography operatory. *Class Activity Have two students volunteer to role-play a patient and a dental assistant. Both participants should wear scrubs or clothes that can risk being stained. Set up a mock radiography room and have the assistant take four mock bite-wing x-rays. Before doing so, have the patient chew on a disclosing tablet. The student playing the dental assistant should mimic everything a dental assistant would normally do, including readjusting the tubehead and pressing the exposure button. Note to the class the "contamination" that occurs by what is stained by the disclosing tablet. Because saliva is clear, this activity should stress why infection control is so important.*

Bird/Robinson

OBJECTIVES	CONTENT	TEACHING RESOURCES

Implement the CDC guidelines for infection control in dental radiology.	■ Infection control (p. 607)
	
	□ Centers for Disease Control and Prevention guidelines (p. 607)
	
	□ The radiography operatory (p. 608)
	  – X-ray machine (p. 608)
	  – Lead apron (p. 608)
	  – Dental chair (p. 609)
	  – Work area (p. 609)
	
	□ Equipment and supplies (p. 609)
	  – Film (p. 609)
	  – Film packets (p. 609)
	  – Film-holding devices (film holders) (p. 609)
	  – Miscellaneous items (p. 609)
	
	□ Procedures during and after x-ray film exposure (p. 610)
	  – Operator preparation (p. 610)
	  – Drying of exposed file (p. 610)
	  – Collection of contaminated films (p. 610)
	  – Film-holding devices (p. 610)
	  – Disposal of contaminated items (p. 610)
	  – Handwashing (p. 610)
	  – Surface disinfection (p. 610)
	
	Procedure 40-1
	Practicing infection control during film
		PPT 42-49
		
		TB questions 13-14
		
		SW Short-Answer Questions 10; Multiple Choice questions 16-18 (pp. 285, 287)
		
		SW/ESLR Competency 40-1 Practicing Infection Control During Film Exposure (p. 289)
		
		SW/ESLR Competency 40-2 Practicing Infection Control in the Darkroom (p. 291)
		
		SW/ESLR Competency 40-3 Practicing Infection Control Using the Daylight Loader (p. 293)
		
		Checklist for Infection Control in Dental Radiography (p. 607)
		
		CDC Guidelines for Dental Radiology (p. 608)
		
		Surfaces Likely to Be Contaminated During X-Ray Procedures (p. 608)
		
		Figure 40-5 X-ray equipment with barriers in place (p. 608)
		
		Figure 40-6 Radiography operatory with barriers in place (p. 608)
		
		Figure 40-7 (A) Plastic surface barrier is placed over the work surface; (B) After each exposure, the dental assistant wipes the film dry (p. 609)
		
		Figure 40-8 Protective barrier on x-ray film (p. 609)
		
		Figure 40-9 The operator places the lead apron on the patient (p. 610)
		
		Recall questions 16-19, 21-22 (pp. 610, 613)
		
		Infection Control Steps in Dental Radiography (p. 613)
		
		▶ Discuss the necessity of CDC guidelines for infection control in dental radiology.
		
		Class Activity Divide the class into small groups. Have each group discuss what surfaces can be contaminated during x-ray procedures, and how those surfaces should be disinfected. Have each group share its findings with the class.

Bird/Robinson

OBJECTIVES	CONTENT	TEACHING RESOURCES
	exposure (p. 611) (SW/ESLR Competency 40-1, p. 289) □ Procedures during x-ray film processing (p. 613) – Transporting film (p. 613) Procedure 40-2 Practicing infection control in the darkroom (p. 612) (SW/ESLR Competency 40-2, p. 291) Procedure 40-3 Practicing infection control with use of daylight loader (pp. 613-614) (SW/ESLR Competency 40-3, p. 293)	
Performance Evaluation		TB SW questions (pp. 285-287) SW Topics for Discussion (p. 287) SW/ESLR Competency 40-1 Practicing Infection Control During Film Exposure (p. 289) SW/ESLR Competency 40-2 Practicing Infection Control in the Darkroom (p. 291) SW/ESLR Competency 40-3 Practicing Infection Control Using the Daylight Loader (p. 293) ESLR Electronic Flashcards ESLR Practice Quiz Recall questions (pp. 601-613) CTQ (p. 615)

Torres and Ehrlich Modern Dental Assisting, 9th ed.
Bird/Robinson

40.3 Homework/Assignments:

40.3 Instructor's Notes/Student Feedback:

Slide 1

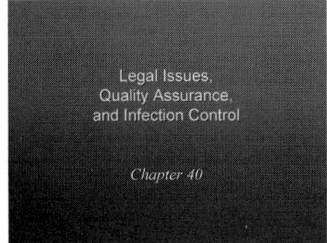

Slide 2

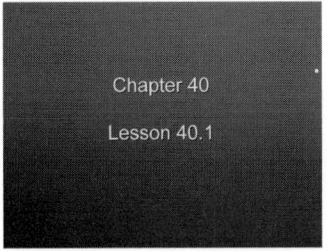

Slide 3

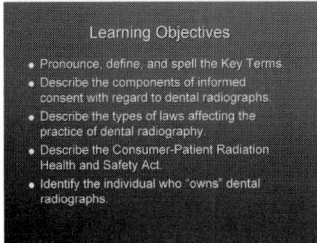

Slide 4

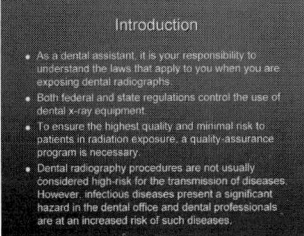

- Whom are infection control guidelines designed to protect? *(Both patients and employees.)*

Bird/Robinson

Slide 5

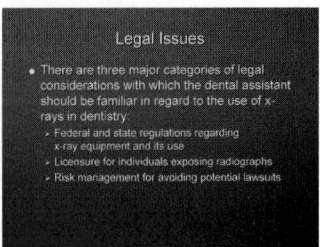

- Who determines the qualifications for licensure for individuals obtaining radiographs?
- What act requires those taking radiographs to be trained and certified?

Slide 6

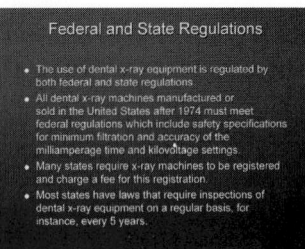

- What are some quality control tests that ensure x-ray equipment meets safety standards?

Slide 7

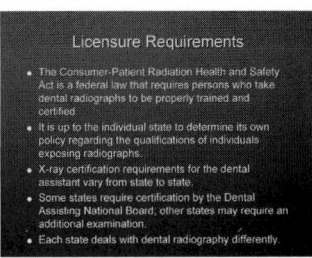

- What is the purpose of requiring licensure for persons who take radiographs?

Slide 8

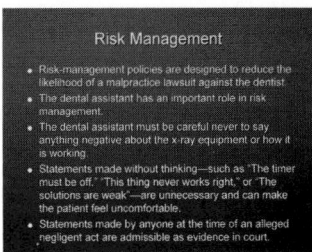

- Can a dental assistant be sued for malpractice or negligence? (*These liabilities are typically the dentist's responsibility, but there are some actions for which an assistant can be held accountable.*

- What is the dental assistant's role in risk management? (*He or she can help design quality assurance programs and, because assistants interact often with patients, it is important for them to project confidence and competence.*)

ELSEVIER

Torres and Ehrlich Modern Dental Assisting, 9th ed.

Bird/Robinson

Slide 9

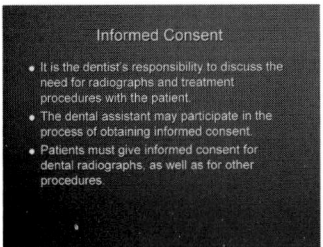

- What information is required for informed consent?

Slide 10

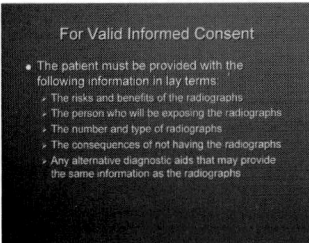

- The dental assistant must be very careful to use lay terms (e.g., for "amalgam" and "composite") in a way that clients understand.

- Dental assistants should not oversimplify an explanation.

- Calling radiation harmful might make a client uneasy. Explain to the client that many common things are harmful in excess. Radiation is something patients are exposed to every day from the sun.

Slide 11

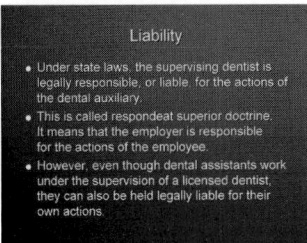

- When might an assistant be held liable? *(Anything done maliciously.)*

Slide 12

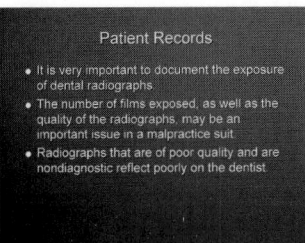

- Nondiagnostic radiographs are sometimes unavoidable, but a competent technician can keep these to a minimum.

Bird/Robinson

Slide 13

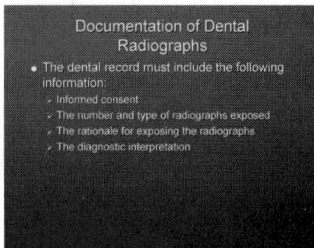

- The diagnostic interpretation must be made by the dentist.

Slide 14

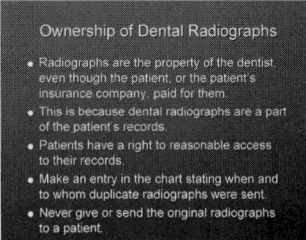

- Some patients may have trouble understanding that they do not own the radiographs. Explain to them that they are paying for the interpretation or diagnosis of those radiographs.

Slide 15

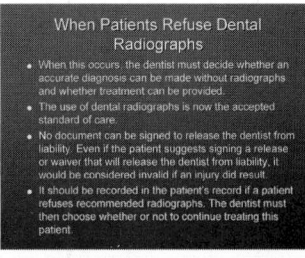

- A dentist should never work without a current radiograph of the problem area.

- Patients who refuse x-rays need to understand that the risk from radiation is minute compared to the risk of working without a radiograph.

Slide 16

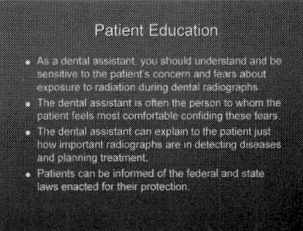

- Pamphlets can also be used as an educational aid.

Bird/Robinson

Slide 17

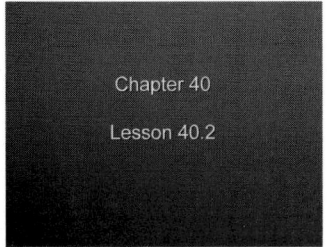

Slide 18

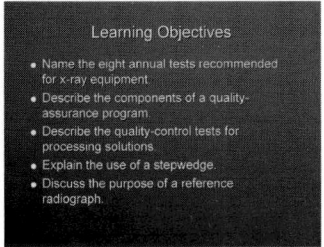

Slide 19

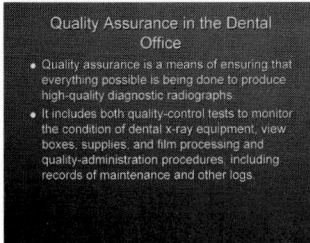

- Although the dentist is responsible for ensuring that these things are done, the tasks themselves are typically left for the assistants.

Slide 20

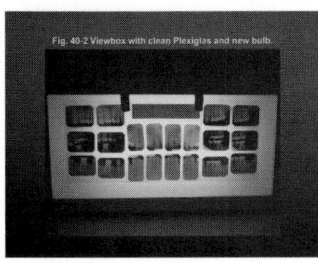

- Scratched Plexiglas or dim bulbs can make radiographs difficult to read.
- Maintenance of these items is part of quality assurance.

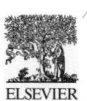

Slide 21

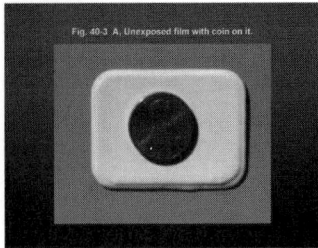

- This is used to test the safelight.

Slide 22

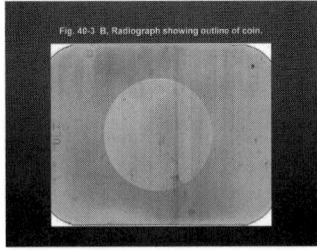

- The safelight is unsuitable for use.

Slide 23

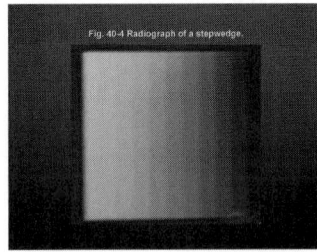

- This is used to ensure that the developer solution is of the proper strength.

Slide 24

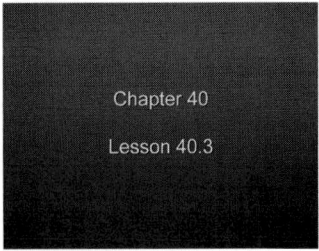

Slide 25

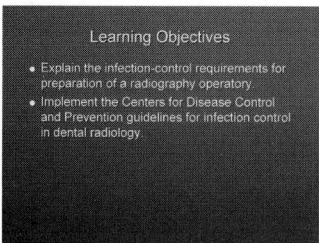

Slide 26

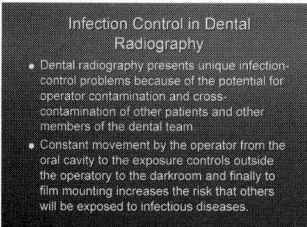

- When using film with an outer barrier, the barrier should be removed and the film placed in an aseptic container. This will keep the darkroom aseptic.

Slide 27

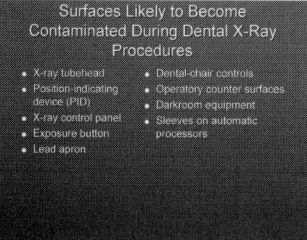

- All these surfaces should be covered.

Slide 28

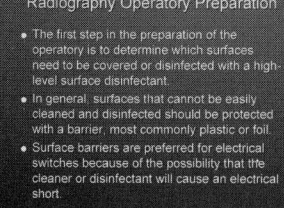

- The operatory should be completely prepared before the patient is brought in.

Slide 29

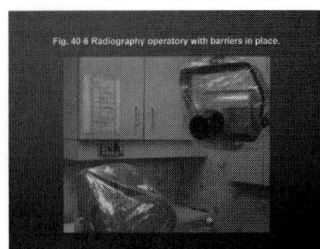

- The barriers should be changed after each patient.

Slide 30

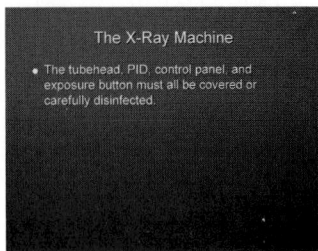

- Because disinfectant must sit on a surface for 10 minutes in order to work, it is best to use barriers in a busy operatory.

Slide 31

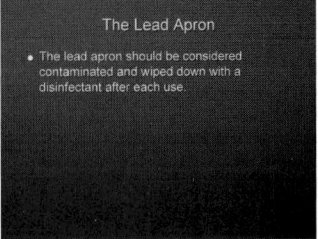

Slide 32

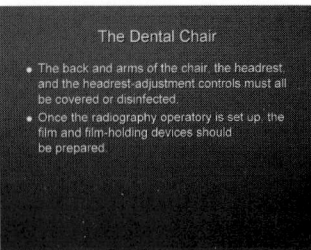

- Working neatly, especially when taking a full-mouth series, helps to speed up the series and ensures that the same area is not accidentally exposed twice.

Torres and Ehrlich Modern Dental Assisting, 9th ed.

Bird/Robinson

Slide 33

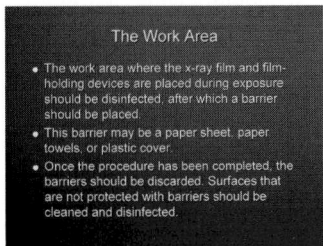

Slide 34

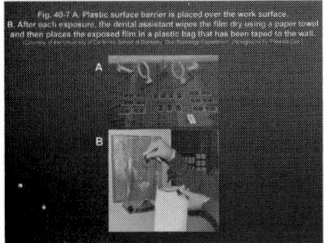

- An empty plastic cup works just as well.

Slide 35

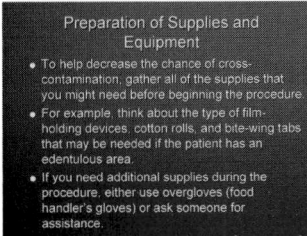

- Preparation is important for both infection control and time savings.

Slide 36

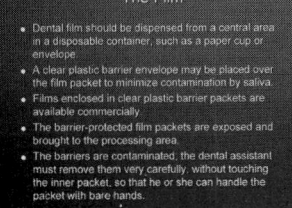

- It is best to dispose of the barrier before bringing the films to the processing area.

Slide 37

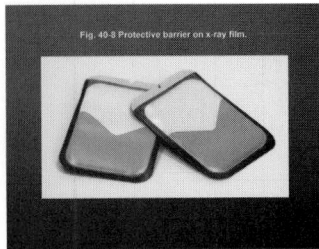

- Remove the barrier over an aseptic container, such as a plastic cup, and allow the exposed film to drop into the cup without touching it.

Slide 38

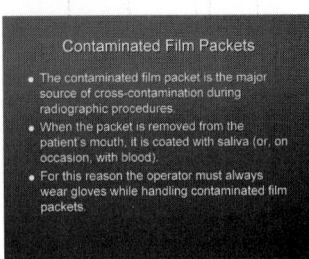

Contaminated Film Packets

- The contaminated film packet is the major source of cross-contamination during radiographic procedures.
- When the packet is removed from the patient's mouth, it is coated with saliva (or, on occasion, with blood).
- For this reason the operator must always wear gloves while handling contaminated film packets.

- Any film that goes into a patient's mouth— not just the films with blood on them—is considered contaminated,.

Slide 39

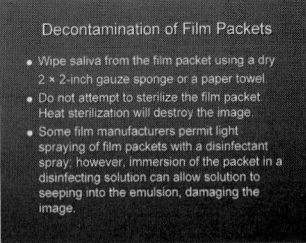

Decontamination of Film Packets

- Wipe saliva from the film packet using a dry 2 × 2-inch gauze sponge or a paper towel.
- Do not attempt to sterilize the film packet. Heat sterilization will destroy the image.
- Some film manufacturers permit light spraying of film packets with a disinfectant spray; however, immersion of the packet in a disinfecting solution can allow solution to seeping into the emulsion, damaging the image.

Slide 40

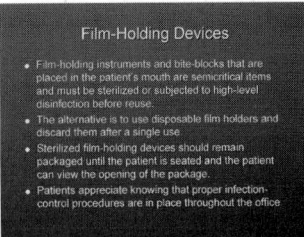

Film-Holding Devices

- Film-holding instruments and bite-blocks that are placed in the patient's mouth are semicritical items and must be sterilized or subjected to high-level disinfection before reuse.
- The alternative is to use disposable film holders and discard them after a single use.
- Sterilized film-holding devices should remain packaged until the patient is seated and the patient can view the opening of the package.
- Patients appreciate knowing that proper infection-control procedures are in place throughout the office.

- XCP devices should be placed in a sterilization pouch and steam sterilized.

Torres and Ehrlich Modern Dental Assisting, 9th ed.

Bird/Robinson

Slide 41

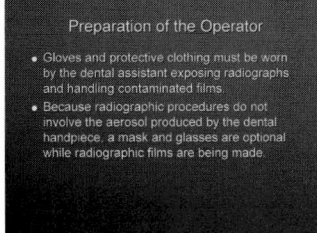

- Patients may wish to have tissues as well to wipe saliva from their faces. Saliva may get on a patient's face while removing films or from drooling while holding the bite-block in place.

Slide 42

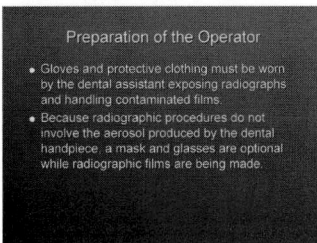

- If the patient has a cold or allergy, glasses and a mask should be worn.

Slide 43

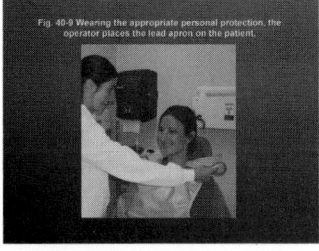

Slide 44

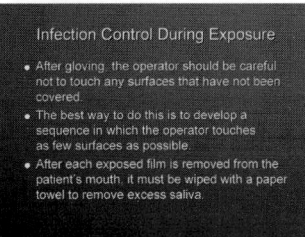

- Barrier films only need the barrier removed rather than wiped.

Slide 45

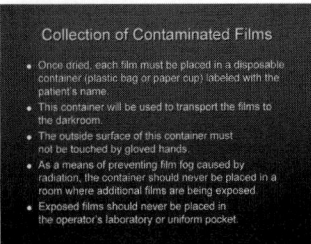

Slide 46

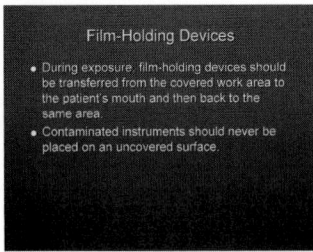

- What should the dental assistant do if he or she accidentally places a contaminated instrument on a covered surface? *(Use a high-level disinfectant on the surface for 10 minutes, then wipe clean.)*

Slide 47

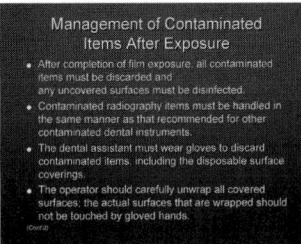

- For added infection control, lightly spray the uncovered surfaces before rewrapping.

Slide 48

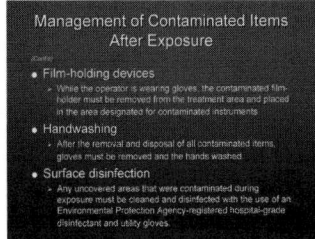

Slide 49

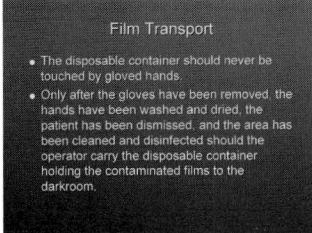

- Avoid leaving an operatory contaminated, even if there are plans to come back and clean it up later. The contaminated operatory can be entered by another person unaware of its contaminated status; that person might then contaminate other areas of the clinic.

Bird/Robinson

TEACHING FOCUS

This chapter introduces the student to topics related to intraoral radiography, including the paralleling, bisecting, bitewing, and occlusal techniques. The student will also become acquainted with the procedures for preparing the patient for dental x-rays, for assembling the XCP instruments, and for producing a full-mouth radiographic survey using both paralleling and bisecting techniques. The student will have the opportunity to learn how to accommodate patients with special medical or dental needs.

MATERIALS AND RESOURCES

- ☐ computer and PowerPoint projector (all Lessons)
- ☐ Rinn XCP instruments (Lesson 41.1)

- ☐ samples of film holders (all Lessons)
- ☐ samples of radiographs (all Lessons)
- ☐ typodont (all Lessons)

LESSON CHECKLIST

Preparations for this lesson include:

- lecture
- evaluation of student knowledge and skills needed to perform all entry-level activities related to intraoral radiography, including understanding how to:
  - accommodate patients with special medical or dental needs
  - assemble and use the XCP instruments
  - prepare the patient for dental x-rays
  - produce a four-film radiographic survey using the bite-wing technique
  - produce a full-mouth radiographic survey using both the paralleling and bisecting techniques
  - produce maxillary and mandibular radiographs using the occlusal technique

Torres and Ehrlich Modern Dental Assisting, 9th ed.

Bird/Robinson

KEY TERMS

angulation (p. 634)
bisecting technique (p. 618)
bite-wing (p. 638)
central ray (p. 618)
contact area (p. 620)
crestal bone (p. 638)
developmental disability (p. 652)
diagnostic quality (p. 655)
exposure sequence (p. 620)

interproximal (p. 618)
intersecting (p. 618)
long axis of the tooth (p. 618)
occlusal technique (p. 647)
parallel (p. 618)
paralleling technique (p. 618)
perpendicular (p. 618)
physical disability (p. 647)
right angle (p. 618)

ADDITIONAL RESOURCES

PowerPoint slides (Evolve): 1-96
The Interactive Dental Office CD-ROM:
 Christopher Brooks
 Antonio DeAngelis
Multimedia Procedures DVD:
 Bite-wing Technique
 Digital Radiography
 Mounting Dental Radiographs
 Occlusal Technique
 Paralleling Technique
 Positioning the Patient to Take Radiographs
 Preparing the Operatory/Equipment to Take Radiographs

Legend

CTQ
Critical
Thinking
Question

DVD
Multimedia
Procedures
Videos and
Animations

ESLR
EVOLVE
Student
Learning
Resources

IDO
Interactive
Dental
Office
CD-ROM

SW
Student
Workbook

TB
Test Bank
on the
TEACH
CD-ROM

PPT
PowerPoint
Slides

Class Activities are indicated in ***bold italic***.

ELSEVIER

Torres and Ehrlich Modern Dental Assisting, 9th ed.

Bird/Robinson

LESSON 41.1

PRETEST

1. What is the first step in obtaining quality radiographs?
   - a. exposure
   - b. mounting
   - c. placement
   - d. processing

2. What do the initials XCP represent?
   - a. x-ray cone paralleling
   - b. extension cone paralleling
   - c. x-ray crown positioning
   - d. extension cut positioning

3. When exposing films using the paralleling technique, which area should you begin with?
   - a. right posterior
   - b. left posterior
   - c. bite-wings
   - d. anterior

4. What is elongation on a radiograph the result of?
   - a. improper vertical angulation
   - b. improper horizontal angulation
   - c. improper film placement
   - d. improper film processing

5. Using the bisecting technique, what is the proper vertical angulation for maxillary premolar radiographs?
   - a. +50 - +55
   - b. +45 - +55
   - c. +40 - +50
   - d. +30 - +40

6. Using the bisecting techniques, what is the proper position of the patient during exposure?
   - a. supine
   - b. subsupine
   - c. midsagittal plane perpendicular to the floor
   - d. midsagittal plane parallel to the floor

7. What are bite-wing radiographs primarily used for?
   - a. to detect interproximal decay
   - b. to locate impacted teeth
   - c. to detect diseases of the pulp
   - d. to locate foreign objects in the mouth

8. What is the correct angulation used when obtaining bitewing radiographs?
   - a. -5°
   - b. 0°
   - c. +5°
   - d. +10°

9. What is the recommended film size for pediatric patients?
   - a. #0
   - b. #1
   - c. #2
   - d. #3

10. Which mounting technique is recommended by the ADA?
    - a. distal mounting
    - b. mesial mounting
    - c. labial mounting
    - d. lingual mounting

Answers

1. c	3. d	5. d	7. a	9. a
2. b	4. a	6. c	8. d	10. c

BACKGROUND ASSESSMENT

Question: Why is a full-mouth survey (FMX) so important in the dental examination?

Answer: A dental examination cannot be completed without dental radiographs, since we cannot see below the gum tissue. These radiographs are used for detecting interproximal decay, periodontal disease, recurrent decay underneath an existing restoration, pathological conditions of the oral cavity, tooth eruption, and tooth formation. An FMX generally contains 18 films: 14 periapical films and 4 bite-wing radiographs.

Question: Why is exposure sequencing so important when obtaining radiographs?

Answer: A full-mouth survey (FMX) requires 18 to 20 films. If these are not taken in a definite order, the radiographer is likely to omit an area. It is recommended that one start in the anterior portion of the mouth because it is easier for the patient to tolerate, and the patient is less likely to gag. After the anterior films have been obtained, the radiographer would then move to the posterior area, starting with the premolars. This area is also less likely to trigger the patient's gag reflex and is easier for the patient to tolerate. The molars would be the last radiographs in the sequence since they are most likely to trigger the patient's gag reflex.

CRITICAL THINKING QUESTION

A woman is scheduled for a full series of radiographs. The dental assistant is using the XCP instruments for the series and is prepared to start the procedure. Upon placement of the XCP and film in the patient's mouth, the patient appears to be very uncomfortable with the procedure and removes the XCP and film immediately, stating she is in pain. She says it hurts the roof of her mouth and she can't bite down to hold it in place. What adjustments will the dental assistant need to make with this radiographic technique?

Guidelines: The patient appears to have a very shallow palate, which is not a good indicator for use of the paralleling technique. The dental assistant should discontinue using the XCP instruments and opt for the use of an EeZee-Grip or Stabe bite-block film holder and continue taking the radiographs using the bisecting-angle technique. The bisecting-angle technique allows the film to be placed directly against the tooth rather than toward the middle of the oral cavity with the paralleling technique. This change should be more comfortable for the patient.

OBJECTIVES	CONTENT	TEACHING RESOURCES
Pronounce, define, and spell the Key Terms.	■ Key terms (pp. 616-617)	📇 ESLR Electronic Flashcards ▸ Discuss each of the key terms in Chapter 41, focusing on the definition, pronunciation, and spelling of each term. *Class Activity **Have students make flash cards with the key terms on one side and the definitions on the reverse. Then have the students quiz each other with the flash cards. Correct their pronunciation as needed.***
Explain the advantages and disadvantages of the paralleling and bisecting techniques.	■ Introduction (p. 617) ■ Full-mouth survey (p. 618)	🖥 PPT 5-14 💻 TB questions 1-4 📖 SW Short-Answer Questions 3; Fill in the Blank questions 4, 6-9 (pp. 295-296) Figure 41-1 Steps to quality radiographs (p. 618) Figure 41-2 Bitewing radiograph (p. 618) Figure 41-3 (A) Anterior periapical; (B) posterior periapical (p. 619) Figure 41-4 Mounted full-mouth series with eight anterior films using the parallel technique (p. 619)

ELSEVIER

Torres and Ehrlich Modern Dental Assisting, 9th ed.

Bird/Robinson

OBJECTIVES	CONTENT	TEACHING RESOURCES
		▸ Discuss the functions of a full-mouth survey.
		▸ Discuss the advantages and disadvantages of the paralleling and bisecting techniques. Which technique is recommended and why?
		*Class Activity **Divide the class into small groups and have each group discuss the advantages and disadvantages of the paralleling and bisecting techniques in the following scenarios: shallow palate, child, or large tori. Then have each group present its findings to the class.***
Name the two primary types of projections used in an intraoral technique and describe the differences.	■ Intraoral x-ray techniques (p. 618)	PPT 15 TB question 5 SW Short-Answer Questions 2; Fill in the Blank questions 1-2 (pp. 295-296) SW/IDO Patient Case Exercise: Brooks questions 1-2 (p. 299) (The Interactive Dental Office CD-ROM) Figure 41-5 Intraoral x-ray techniques (p. 619) ▸ Discuss the two primary types of projections used in an intraoral technique. How do they differ? *Class Activity **Divide the class into small groups, and have each group discuss how to appropriately identify which type of intraoral technique to use in the following circumstances: shallow palate; normal-sized mouth; small-sized mouth, large tori. Then have each group present its findings to the class.***
Explain the basic principle of the paralleling technique.	■ Paralleling technique (p. 618)	PPT 16 SW Short-Answer Questions 4; Fill in the Blank questions 10-15; Multiple Choice questions 1-5 (pp. 295-297) Recall questions 1-2 (p. 618) ▸ Discuss the importance of an exposure sequence for film placement. Why is it recommended that you start with anterior teeth? *Class Activity **Demonstrate the paralleling technique on a typodont. Then have the students use the typodont to practice the technique.***
State the five basic rules of the paralleling technique.	☐ Five basic rules (p. 618)	PPT 16-20 TB question 7 SW Short-Answer Questions 6 (p. 295) Figure 41-6 (A) Parallel lines; (B) Intersecting lines; (C) Perpendicular lines; (D) Right angle (p. 620)

OBJECTIVES	CONTENT	TEACHING RESOURCES
		Figure 41-7 (A) Long axis of maxillary incisor; (B) Long axis of mandibular premolar (p. 620)
		Figure 41-8 Position of the film, teeth, PID, and central ray of the x-ray beam in the paralleling technique (p. 620)
		Figure 41-9 X-rays pass through the contact areas of the premolars (p. 620)
		Figure 41-10 This radiograph demonstrates a cone cut (p. 621)
		▸ Discuss the five basic rules of the paralleling technique. What are some important guidelines for film placement?
		Class Activity **Divide the class into small groups, and have each group make a chart of the five basic rules of the paralleling technique that students can use during exposure on a typodont.**
Explain why a film holder is necessary with the paralleling technique.	☐ Five basic rules (p. 618)	PPT 16-20 TB question 15 SW Short-Answer Questions 5 (p. 295) Guidelines for Film Placement (p. 621) ▸ Discuss the importance of using a film holder with the paralleling technique. *Class Activity* **Demonstrate the use of a film holder with the paralleling technique, and have the students practice the technique on a typodont.**
Describe how to prepare a patient for dental x-rays.	☐ Patient preparation (p. 620) *Procedure* 41-1 Preparing the patient for dental x-rays (p. 621) (SW/ESLR Competency 41-1, p. 301)	PPT 21-22 Multimedia Procedures DVD: Preparing the Operatory/Equipment to Take Radiographs; Positioning the Patient to Take Radiographs SW Short-Answer Questions 1 (p. 295) SW/ESLR Competency 41-1 Preparing a Patient for Dental X-Rays (p. 301) ▸ Discuss the importance of properly preparing the patient for intraoral x-rays. What risks or problems can this avoid? *Class Activity* **Divide the class into small groups, and have the students practice on one another how to prepare patients for radiographs in the dental operatory.** – **Explain the procedure.** – **Ensure patient is seated upright in chair.** – **Adjust the headrest so that the midsagittal plane is perpendicular to the floor.**

OBJECTIVES	CONTENT	TEACHING RESOURCES
		– *Place the lead apron and thyroid collar on the patient.*
		– *Have patient remove objects that will interfere with the radiographs.*
		Have each group cycle through each preparatory stage until all students are familiar with all procedures.
Expose a full series of radiographs using the paralleling technique.	☐ Exposure sequence for film placement (p. 620) – Anterior exposure sequence (p. 620)	🖼 PPT 23-25 💻 TB questions 8-10 Figure 41-11 Anterior periapical film placement (p. 622) *Class Activity Divide the class into small groups, and have each group create educational materials to list and explain the anterior exposure sequence. Have each group share its materials with the class.*
Label and identify the parts of the Rinn XCP instruments.	*Procedure* 41-2 Assembling the XCP (extension-cone paralleling) instruments (pp. 623-624) (SW/ESLR Competency 41-2, p. 303)	📄 SW Short-Answer Questions 7 (p. 295) 📄 💿 SW/ESLR Competency 41-2 Assembling XCP (Extension-Cone Paralleling) Instruments (p. 303) ▸ Discuss the function and use of the XCP (extension-cone paralleling) instruments. *Class Activity Demonstrate the assembly of the Rinn XCP. Have students identify the parts of the Rinn XCP, then assemble it in the following sequence:* – *Anterior* – *Posterior* – *Right* – *Left*
Expose a full series of radiographs using the paralleling technique.	*Procedure* 41-3 Producing full-mouth radiographic survey using paralleling technique (pp. 625-633) (SW/ESLR Competency 41-3, pp. 305-308) – Posterior exposure sequence (p. 622) – Film placement (p. 634)	🖼 PPT 26-40 🎥 Multimedia Procedures DVD: Paralleling Technique 💻 TB question 11 📄 💿 SW/ESLR Competency 41-3 Producing a Full-Mouth Radiographic Survey Using the Paralleling Technique (pp. 305-308) Figure 41-12 Posterior periapical film placement (p. 634) Recall questions 3-5 (p. 634) *Class Activity Divide the class into four groups, and assign each group a quartile of the mouth. Have each group create a list of the procedural steps needed to produce a radiographic survey of a quartile using the paralleling technique.*

Bird/Robinson

41.1 Homework/Assignments:

41.1 Instructor's Notes/Student Feedback:

LESSON 41.2

CRITICAL THINKING QUESTION

After exposing and processing radiographs, the dental assistant notices that all four of the bite-wing radiographs have overlapped contact areas and cone-cuts. Why did these errors happen and what can the dental assistant do to correct them?

Guidelines: Bite-wing radiographs are used to detect interproximal decay, so it is very important that the central ray of the x-ray beam is directed through the contact areas of the teeth. To achieve the correct horizontal angulation, the operator can place his or her finger along the arch and align the open end of the position-indicating device (PID) to the finger. To correct the cone-cuts, the operator must position the PID so that the central ray is centered on the film to ensure that all areas of the film are exposed.

OBJECTIVES	CONTENT	TEACHING RESOURCES
Explain the procedural principles of the bisecting technique.	■ Bisecting technique (p. 634)	▣ PPT 44-45
		TB question 6
		SW Short-Answer Questions 11; Multiple Choice questions 6, 10 (pp. 295, 297)
		Figure 41-13 (A) A diagram of an anterior tooth; (B) A posterior tooth using the bisecting angle concept (p. 635)
		Recall questions 6-10 (p. 638)
		CTQ 1-2 (p. 659)
		▸ Discuss the bisecting technique and how it differs from the paralleling technique.
		▸ Discuss the most common indications for using the bisecting technique instead of the paralleling technique.
		Class Activity Demonstrate on a typodont the technique used in the bisecting technique. Then have the students practice the technique.
Identify the types of film holders that can be used with the bisecting technique.	☐ Film holders (p. 634)	▣ PPT 46
		Figure 41-14 EeZee-Grip (Rinn) film holder (posterior), Stabe anterior, Stabe posterior, and EeZee-Grip (Rinn) film holder (posterior) (p. 635)
		▸ Discuss the reason that a patient should not be asked to hold the film during radiography. What is the preferred alternative?
		Class Activity Have students manipulate the placement of these film holders on a typodont:
		– BAI
		– Stabe bite-block
		– EeZee Grip

Bird/Robinson

OBJECTIVES	CONTENT	TEACHING RESOURCES
Describe the appearance of opened and overlapped contact areas on a dental radiograph.	☐ Angulation of position indicator device (p. 634) – Horizontal angulation (p. 635)	PPT 48-53 TB question 13 SW Short-Answer Questions 10; Multiple Choice question 8 (pp. 295, 297) Figure 41-15 The arrows indicate movement in a horizontal direction (p. 635) Figure 41-16 Correct horizontal angulation (p. 635) Figure 41-17 Incorrect horizontal angulation (p. 636) Figure 41-18 Overlapped contact areas (p. 636) ▸ Discuss the concept of angulation and its importance to the bisecting technique. ▸ Discuss how to avoid a film with overlapped contact areas. *Class Activity **Divide the class into small groups, and have each group discuss how to correct overlapped contact areas on a dental radiograph in terms of horizontal angulation or vertical angulation. Have the groups present their findings to the class.***
Describe the correct vertical angulation.	– Vertical angulation (p. 636)	PPT 54-56 TB question 12 SW Short-Answer Questions 13 (p. 295) Figure 41-19 Vertical angulation of the position indicator device (p. 636) Table 41-1 Recommended Vertical Angulation Ranges for Bisecting Technique (p. 636) ▸ Discuss how vertical angulation differs in the bisecting technique from that in the paralleling technique. *Class Activity **Divide the class into small groups, and have each group create a chart indicating the correct vertical angulation to be used on intraoral radiographs. Have each group share its chart with the class for further discussion.***
Describe incorrect vertical angulation.	– Vertical angulation (p. 636)	PPT 57-58 TB question 14 SW Short-Answer Questions 14; Multiple Choice question 9 (pp. 295, 297) Figure 41-20 (A) If the vertical angulation is too steep, the image on the film is shorter than the actual tooth; (B) Foreshortened images (p. 637)

OBJECTIVES	CONTENT	TEACHING RESOURCES
		Figure 41-21 (A) If the vertical angulation is too flat, the image on the film is longer than the actual tooth; (B) Elongated images (p. 637) ▸ Discuss the problems that may occur when vertical angulation is incorrect. *Class Activity* **Divide the class into small groups, and have each group create a chart indicating the correct horizontal angulation to be used on intraoral radiographs. Have each group share its chart with the class for further discussion.**
Identify the film size used in the bisecting technique.	☐ Film size and placement (p. 637) ☐ Patient positioning (p. 637) ☐ Beam alignment (p. 638)	PPT 59-60 Multimedia Procedures DVD: Positioning the Patient to Take Radiographs SW Short-Answer Questions 12 (p. 295) ▸ Discuss film size and placement when using the bisecting technique. *Class Activity* **Show students the different-sized films that are available for intraoral radiography (#0, #1, #2, #3, #4). Then as a class, discuss the appropriate uses for each of the film sizes.**
Expose a full series of radiographs using the bisecting angle technique.	Procedure 41-4 Producing full-mouth radiographic survey using bisecting technique (pp. 638-646) (SW/ESLR Competency 41-4, pp. 309-314)	PPT 61-68 SW/ESLR Competency 41-4 Producing Full-Mouth Radiographic Survey Using the Bisecting Technique (pp. 309-314) *Class Activity* **Divide the class into four groups, and assign each group a quartile of the mouth. Have each group create a list of the procedural steps needed to produce a radiographic survey of a quartile using the bisecting-angle technique.**

Torres and Ehrlich Modern Dental Assisting, 9th ed.
Bird/Robinson

41.2 Homework/Assignments:

41.2 Instructor's Notes/Student Feedback:

LESSON 41.3

CRITICAL THINKING QUESTION

A patient comes to the office for a dental examination. He is hearing-impaired and is in a wheelchair. Dental x-rays must be taken today and the dental assistant is worried about a communication barrier and how the x-rays can be taken while the patient is in his wheelchair. The patient has come to the office without a caregiver, but can read lips. How should the dental assistant handle this situation?
Guidelines: The dental assistant will need to speak clearly and directly to the patient without a mask on so that he is able to lip-read. The dental assistant should explain the procedure as if the patient were not hearing-impaired, answering any questions that he may have regarding the radiographs. Since the patient came without a caregiver and cannot move out of his wheelchair on his own, the dental assistant will need to take the radiographs while the patient remains in his wheelchair. The dental assistant needs to place the patient as close to the x-ray machine as possible, using the extension arm to reach around the oral cavity to take the appropriate radiographs.

OBJECTIVES	CONTENT	TEACHING RESOURCES
Explain the basic rules for the bite-wing technique.	■ Bite-wing technique (p. 638)	PPT 72-78 Multimedia Procedures DVD: Bite-wing Technique; Digital Radiography TB questions 16-17 SW Short-Answer Questions 9; Fill in the Blank question 5; Multiple Choice questions 11-12 (pp. 295-297) ▸ Discuss the uses and principles of the bite-wing technique. ▸ Discuss the issues relating to the number and placement of bite-wing films. *Class Activity **Using a typodont, demonstrate the technique used for exposing bite-wing radiographs. Then have the students practice the technique.***
Explain the recommended vertical angulation for all bite-wing exposures.	☐ Film holder and bite-wing tab (p. 647) ☐ Angulation of position indicator device (p. 647) ☐ Exposure for film placement (p. 647)	PPT 72-78 SW Short-Answer Questions 8 (p. 296) Figure 41-22 Vertical angulation of +10 ° (p. 638) Figure 41-23 Bite-wing tab and film holder (p. 647) Recall questions 11-12 (p. 647) ▸ Discuss the importance of vertical angulation when using the bite-wing technique. *Class Activity **Divide the class into small groups, and have each group create a chart indicating the correct horizontal angulation to be used on bite-wing radiographs. Have each group share its chart with the class for further discussion.***

ELSEVIER

OBJECTIVES	CONTENT	TEACHING RESOURCES
Expose and mount a series of bite-wing radiographs.	Procedure 41-5 Producing four-film radiographic survey using bite-wing technique (pp. 648-649) (SW/ESLR Competency 41-5, p. 315)	SW/ESLR Competency 41-5 Producing a Four-Film Radiographic Survey Using the Bite-wing Technique (p. 315) *Class Activity* **Divide the class into two groups, and assign one group premolars and the other group molars. Have each group create a list of the procedural steps needed to produce a four-film radiographic survey of the premolars and molars, using the bite-wing technique.**
Explain the technique for exposing occlusal radiographs.	■ Occlusal technique (p. 647)	PPT 79-81 TB question 18 SW Short-Answer Questions 15; Multiple Choice questions 13-14 (pp. 296, 297-298) Recall questions 13-14 (p. 647) ▸ Discuss the uses and principles of the occlusal technique. *Class Activity* **Using a typodont, demonstrate the technique used for exposing occlusal radiographs on children and adults. Then have the students practice the technique.**
Expose a maxillary and mandibular occlusal radiograph.	Procedure 41-6 Producing maxillary and mandibular radiographs using occlusal technique (pp. 650-651) (SW/ESLR Competency 41-6, p. 317)	SW/IDO Patient Case Exercise: questions 1-3 (p. 299) (The Interactive Dental Office CD-ROM) SW/ESLR Competency 41-6 Producing Maxillary and Mandibular Radiographs Using the Occlusal Technique (p. 317) *Class Activity* **Divide the class into two groups, and assign one group the maxilla and the other group the mandible. Have each group create a list of the procedural steps needed to produce radiographs using the occlusal technique.**
Describe techniques for managing patients with physical and mental disabilities.	■ Patients with special medical needs (p. 647) 　□ Vision impairment (p. 651) 　□ Hearing impairment (p. 651) 　□ Mobility impairment (p. 651) 　□ Developmental disabilities (p. 652) ■ Patients with special dental needs (p. 652) 　□ Edentulous patient (p. 652)	PPT 82-91 TB questions 19-21 SW Short-Answer Questions 17; Multiple Choice questions 15-18, 20 (pp. 296, 298) Recall questions 15-16 (p. 652) Figure 41-24 Wheelchair-bound patient having x-rays taken (p. 652) Guidelines for Dental Treatment of Patients with Disabilities (p. 651) Figure 41-25 Mixed occlusal-periapical edentulous survey (p. 653) Figure 41-26 Extension-cone paralleling (XCP) instruments can also be used for the pediatric patient (p. 653)

Torres and Ehrlich Modern Dental Assisting, 9th ed.

Bird/Robinson

OBJECTIVES	CONTENT	TEACHING RESOURCES

	☐ Pediatric patient (p. 652)
	
	☐ Endodontic patient (p. 653)
		Figure 41-27 EndoRay II film holder is designed for use during endodontic procedures (p. 653)
		
		Guidelines for Dental Radiography of Pediatric Patients (p. 654)
		
		▶ Discuss ways to accommodate patients with special medical needs, such as vision or hearing impairment.
		
		▶ Discuss ways to accommodate patients with special dental needs, such as the pediatric or endodontic patient.
		
		Class Activity Divide the class into small groups, and have each group discuss how to handle patients with physical and mental disabilities and what adjustments must be made to obtain radiographs in the following scenarios:
		
		   – Vision impairment
		
		   – Hearing impairment
		
		   – Mobility impairment
		
		   – Developmental disabilities
		
		Have each group present its findings to the class.

Describe techniques for managing the patient with a hypersensitive gag reflex.	☐ Gagging patient (p. 654)
	
	  – Exposure sequencing (p. 654)
	
	  – Film placement (p. 654)
	
	☐ Extreme cases (p. 655)
		PPT 92
		
		TB questions 22, 25
		
		SW Short-Answer Questions 16; Multiple Choice question 19 (pp. 296, 298)
		
		Guidelines to Reduce Gag Reflex in Dental Patients (p. 654)
		
		Recall questions 17-21 (p. 655)
		
		▶ Discuss ways to accommodate patients with a hypersensitive gag reflexes. What are some useful guidelines in dealing with this situation?
		
		Class Activity Lead the class in a discussion on the precautions to take when using a topical anesthetic on a gagging patient, with particular attention to the possibility of inhalation, allergic reaction, or lasting effects.

Mount and label a full series of dental radiographs.	■ Radiographic technique errors (p. 655) ■ Mounting dental radiographs (p. 655) ☐ Recognizing anatomic landmarks (p. 655) ☐ Selecting the mount (p. 655) ☐ Methods of mounting (p. 655)	PPT 93-96 Multimedia Procedures DVD: Mounting Dental Radiographs TB questions 23-24 SW Fill in the Blank question 3; Multiple Choice questions 21-23 (pp. 296, 298) SW/ESLR Competency 41-7 Mounting Dental Radiographs (p. 319)

Torres and Ehrlich Modern Dental Assisting, 9th ed.

Bird/Robinson

OBJECTIVES	CONTENT	TEACHING RESOURCES
	Procedure 41-7 Mounting dental radiographs (p. 658) (SW/ESLR Competency 41-7, p. 319)	Guidelines for Mounting Radiographs (p. 655)
		Figure 41-28 Radiographic exposure errors (p. 656)
		Figure 41-29 Radiographic landmarks of normal anatomy (p. 657)
		Recall questions 22-25 (p. 659)
		Figure 41-30 With the labial mounting method, radiographs are viewed as though the dental radiographer were looking directly at the patient (p. 659)
		Legal and Ethical Implications (p. 659)
		Eye to the Future (p. 659)
		CTQ 3 (p. 659)
		▸ Discuss common radiographic technique errors and ways to avoid them.
		Class Activity ***Divide the class into small groups, and have each group practice mounting radiographs, using both methods.***
Performance Evaluation		TB
		SW questions (pp. 295-298)
		SW/IDO Patient Case Exercise (p. 299) (The Interactive Dental Office CD-ROM)
		SW/ESLR Competency 41-1 Preparing a Patient for Dental X-rays (p. 301)
		SW/ESLR Competency 41-2 Assembling XCP (Extension-Cone Paralleling) Instruments (p. 303)
		SW/ESLR Competency 41-3 Producing a Full-Mouth Radiographic Survey Using the Paralleling Technique (pp. 305-308)
		SW/ESLR Competency 41-4 Producing Full-Mouth Radiographic Survey Using the Bisecting Technique (pp. 309-314)
		SW/ESLR Competency 41-5 Producing a Four-Film Radiographic Survey Using the Bite-wing Technique (p. 315)
		SW/ESLR Competency 41-6 Producing Maxillary and Mandibular Radiographs Using the Occlusal Technique (p. 317)
		SW/ESLR Competency 41-7 Mounting Dental Radiographs (p. 319)

Torres and Ehrlich Modern Dental Assisting, 9th ed.

Bird/Robinson

OBJECTIVES	CONTENT	TEACHING RESOURCES
		ℯ ESLR Electronic Flashcards
		ℯ ESLR Practice Quiz
		ℯ ESLR Labeling Exercise 32 : Identify Correct Horizontal Angulation
		Recall questions (pp. 618-659)
		♨ CTQ (p. 659)

41.3 Homework/Assignments:

41.3 Instructor's Notes/Student Feedback:

Bird/Robinson

Slide 1

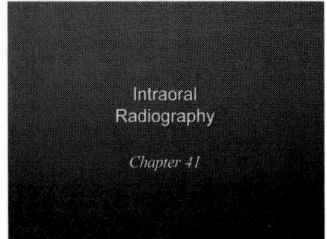

Intraoral
Radiography

Chapter 41

Slide 2

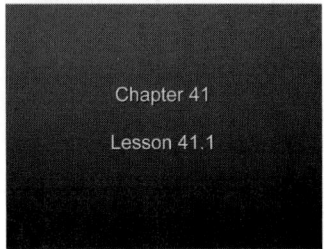

Chapter 41

Lesson 41.1

Slide 3

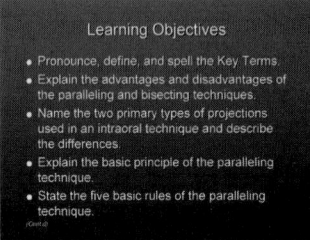

Learning Objectives

- Pronounce, define, and spell the Key Terms.
- Explain the advantages and disadvantages of the paralleling and bisecting techniques.
- Name the two primary types of projections used in an intraoral technique and describe the differences.
- Explain the basic principle of the paralleling technique.
- State the five basic rules of the paralleling technique.
(Cont'd)

Slide 4

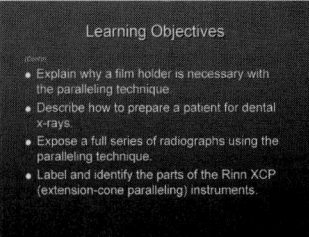

Learning Objectives

(Cont'd)
- Explain why a film holder is necessary with the paralleling technique.
- Describe how to prepare a patient for dental x-rays.
- Expose a full series of radiographs using the paralleling technique.
- Label and identify the parts of the Rinn XCP (extension-cone paralleling) instruments.

Slide 5

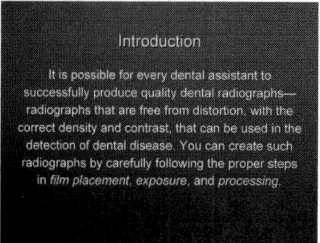

Introduction

It is possible for every dental assistant to successfully produce quality dental radiographs— radiographs that are free from distortion, with the correct density and contrast, that can be used in the detection of dental disease. You can create such radiographs by carefully following the proper steps in *film placement, exposure,* and *processing.*

Slide 6

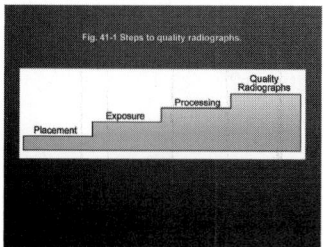

Fig. 41-1 Steps to quality radiographs.

- What are radiographs used to detect?

Slide 7

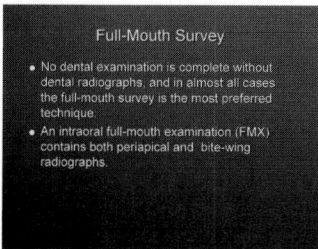

Full-Mouth Survey

- No dental examination is complete without dental radiographs, and in almost all cases the full-mouth survey is the most preferred technique.
- An intraoral full-mouth examination (FMX) contains both periapical and bite-wing radiographs.

- Dentist cannot see underneath the gum tissue.
- Used to detect disease, foreign objects, retained roots.
- What are periapical radiographs?
- What are bite-wing radiographs?

Slide 8

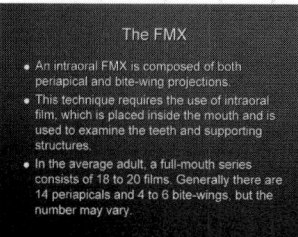

The FMX

- An intraoral FMX is composed of both periapical and bite-wing projections.
- This technique requires the use of intraoral film, which is placed inside the mouth and is used to examine the teeth and supporting structures.
- In the average adult, a full-mouth series consists of 18 to 20 films. Generally there are 14 periapicals and 4 to 6 bite-wings, but the number may vary.

- Film size selection is important.
- How many sizes are available for intraoral film?

ELSEVIER

Torres and Ehrlich Modern Dental Assisting, 9th ed.

Bird/Robinson

Slide 9

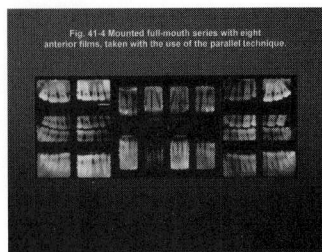

- How many periapicals are shown?
- How many bite-wings are shown?

Slide 10

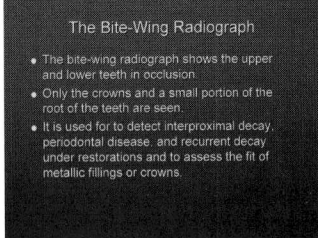

- Should show the crestal bone.
- Why would it be important to see the crestal bone in a bite-wing radiograph?
- Why are these unnecessary on edentulous patients?

Slide 11

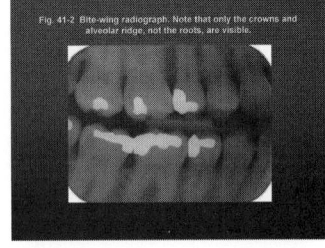

- Which teeth are the main focus of this radiograph?
- What are those "white spots"?
- Can you see the pulp chamber and pulpal canal?

Slide 12

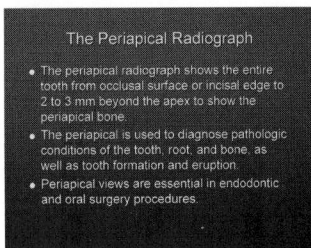

- What size film would be used for an adult?

Bird/Robinson

Slide 13

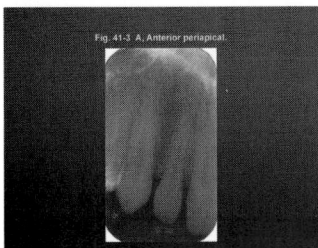

- Which teeth are the main focus of this radiograph?

Slide 14

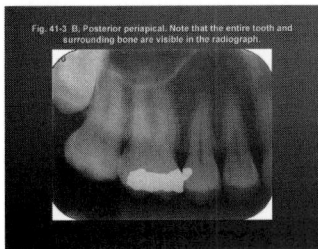

- Which teeth are the focus of this radiograph?
- Locate the sinus cavity.
- Identify the tooth impaction.

Slide 15

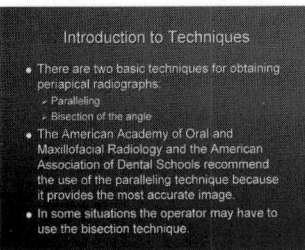

- The operator decides which technique to use according to the patient's needs.

Slide 16

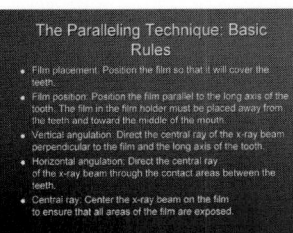

- Rules must be followed to obtain accurate radiographs.
- Why are accurate radiographs so important?

Slide 17

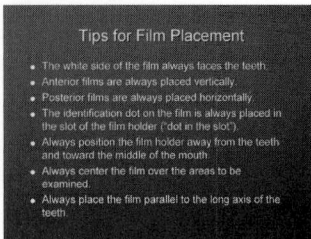

- Radiographs may not be of diagnostic quality if these tips are not followed.
- Why do you want to avoid retakes?

Slide 18

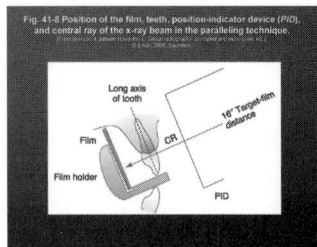

- What does the term *parallel* mean?
- What does the term *perpendicular* mean?

Slide 19

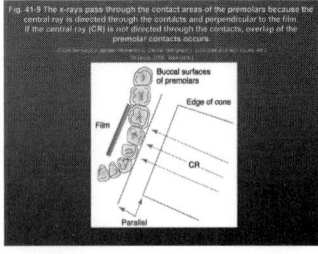

- The goal is to be able to see the contact areas without overlapping.

Slide 20

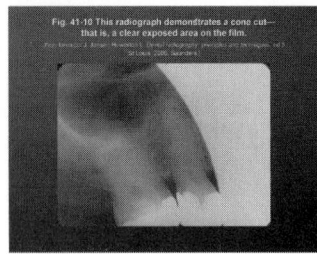

- Why did this cone cut occur?
- How can you correct this error?

Bird/Robinson

Slide 21

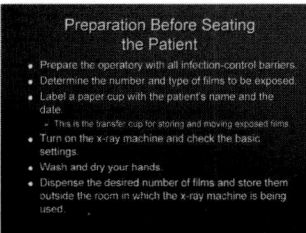

- Where would barriers be placed in the x-ray operatory?

Slide 22

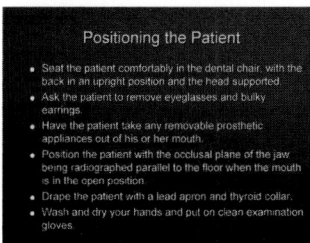

- The midsagittal plane should be perpendicular to the floor.
- Where is the midsagittal plane?
- Should tongue rings or studs be removed?

Slide 23

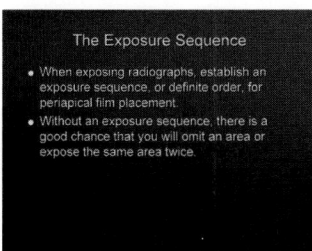

- How many periapicals are taken in a full-mouth series?
- How many bite-wings are taken in a full-mouth series?

Slide 24

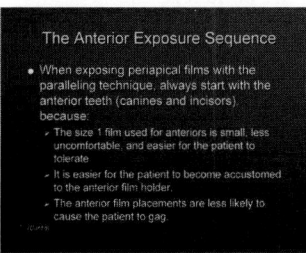

- If size #1 films are used seven or eight films are taken. What views are taken?
- If size #2 films are used six films are taken. What views are taken?
- Always ask the dentist what size film to use and how many anterior films to take.

Slide 25

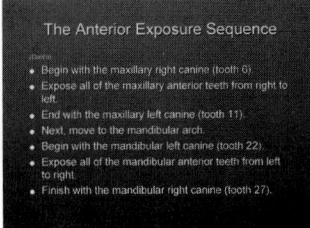

- Is it okay to start on the left and work to the right?
- Stick to a sequence: do not interchange from patient to patient.
- Make this sequence a habit for all radiographic exposures.

Slide 26

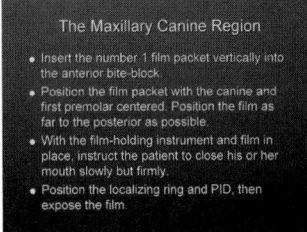

- Have the PID close to the patient so positioning of the ring will be quick.

Slide 27

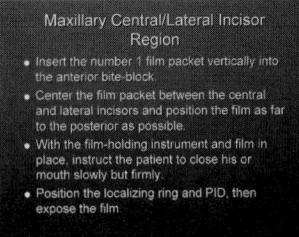

- Remind patient to hold still during exposure.
- Move swiftly; remove XCP from the oral cavity as soon as possible.

Slide 28

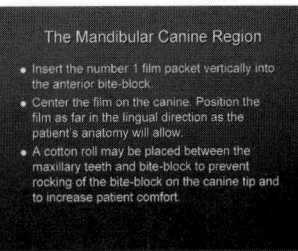

- Why is it important to have the PID close to the patient so that positioning on the ring will be quick?
- What other size film could be used?

Bird/Robinson

Slide 29

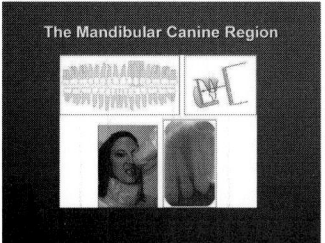

- Why is it important to remove the XCP from the oral cavity as soon as possible?.

Slide 30

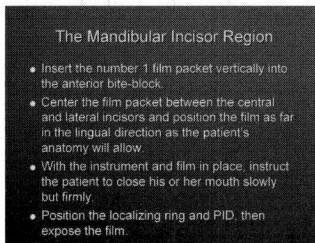

- What other size film can be used?

Slide 31

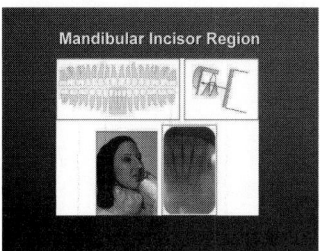

Slide 32

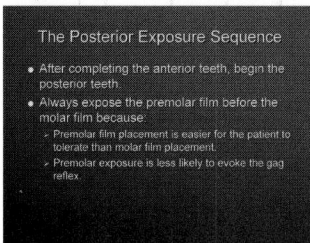

- What size film is used for posterior periapicals?
- How many premolar films will be taken in an FMX?

Slide 33

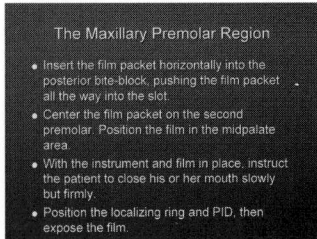

- Remind the patient not to open the mouth during exposure.

Slide 34

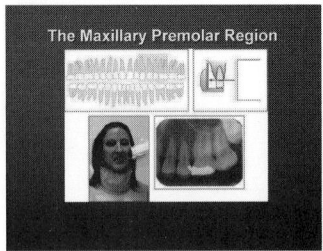

Slide 35

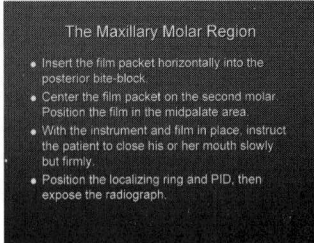

- As you move more posterior in the oral cavity, remind the patient to breathe through the nose (to avoid gagging).
- What size film is used for this area?

Slide 36

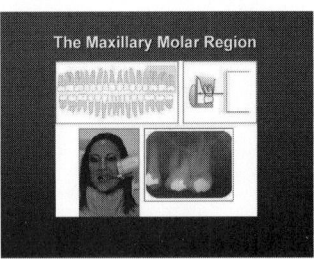

- Where is the ID dot placed?

Chapter 41 | Intraoral Radiography

Slide 37

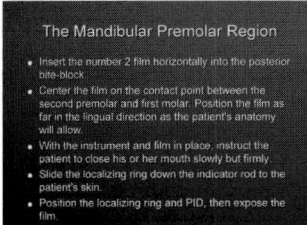

- Remind patient to not open during exposure and to breathe through the nose.

Slide 38

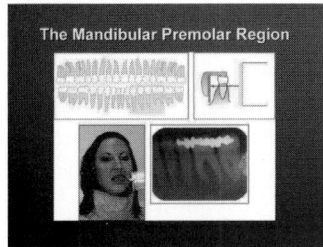

Slide 39

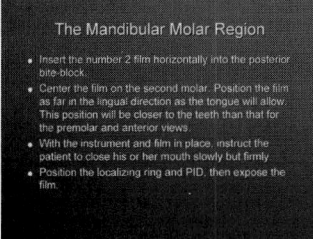

- What should the dental assistant do if the patient begins to gag ?

Slide 40

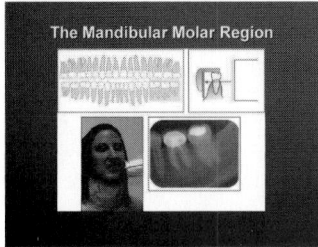

Slide 41

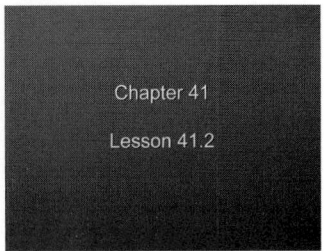

Slide 42

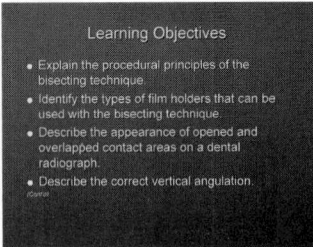

Slide 43

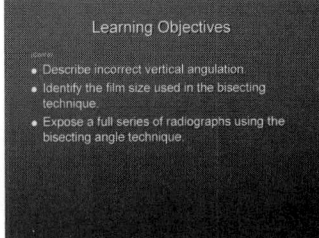

Slide 44

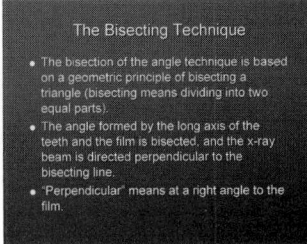

- Also known as the BAI technique or short-cone technique.

- What is the long axis of the tooth?

- Used as an alternative to the paralleling technique.

- Why would we use this method?

Slide 45

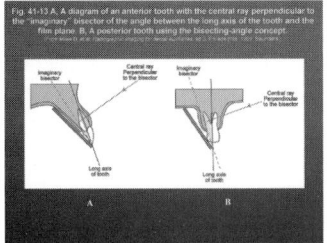

- Unlike paralleling, in which the film is placed away from the teeth, the bisecting angle places the film directly against the teeth.

- A disadvantage of this approach is that the images may be distorted.

Slide 46

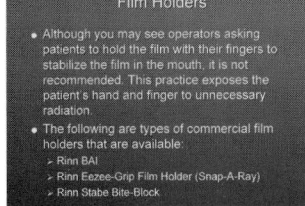

- BAI instruments include a metal indicator arm, plastic bite-blocks, and plastic aiming rings.

- The EeZee-Grip is the easiest to use with experience, and it is more comfortable for patient.

- The Stabe bite-block is disposable.

Slide 47

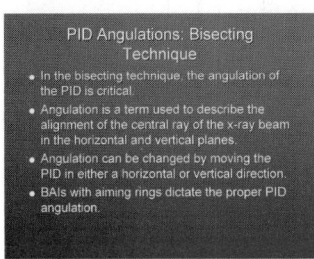

- What is the major disadvantage of using the bisecting technique?

- During the learning stages of this technique, the BAI instruments will be used.

Slide 48

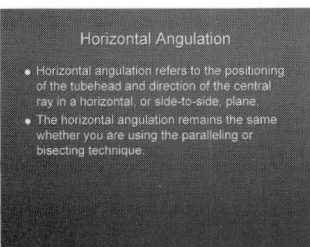

- What is the correct horizontal placement?

Bird/Robinson

Slide 49

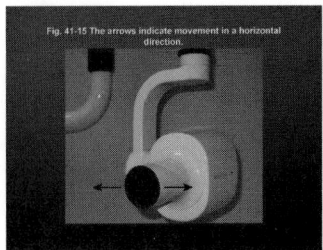

Slide 50

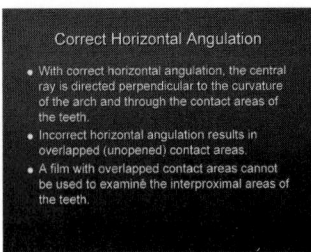

- Retakes would be necessary if there are overlapped contact areas.
- Why are retakes discouraged?

Slide 51

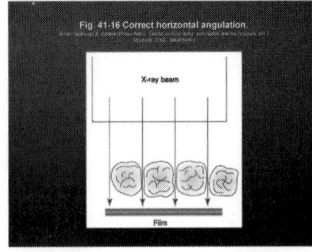

- X-ray beam is directed perpendicular to the film.
- Open end of the PID is aligned parallel to the film.

Slide 52

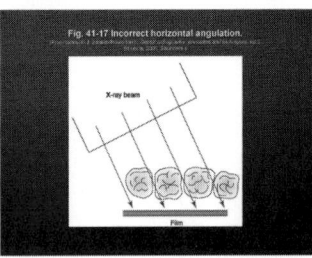

- What will the x-ray show if the horizontal angulation is incorrect?

Torres and Ehrlich Modern Dental Assisting, 9th ed.
Bird/Robinson

Slide 53

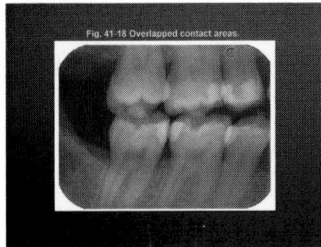

- What are contact areas?
- Why are they important in diagnosing treatment?

Slide 54

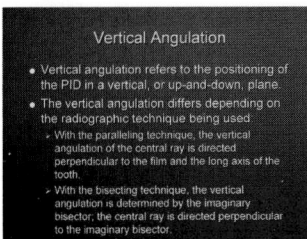

- Measurement of vertical angulation is marked on the outside of the tubehead.

Slide 55

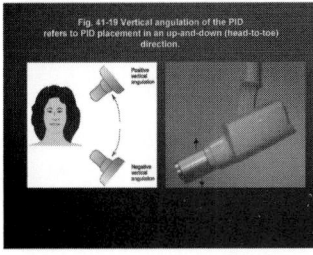

- When the open end of the PID is pointing downward, the PID has positive angulation.
- When the open end of the PID is pointing upward, the PID has negative angulation.

Slide 56

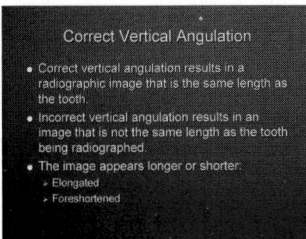

- What does the term *elongation* mean?
- What does the term *foreshortened* mean?

Bird/Robinson

Slide 57

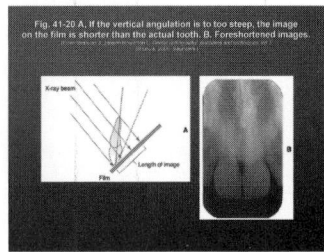

- Foreshortening occurs when there is excessive vertical angulation.

Slide 58

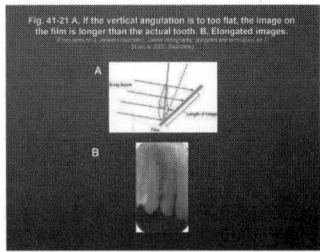

- Elongation occurs when there is insufficient vertical angulation.

Slide 59

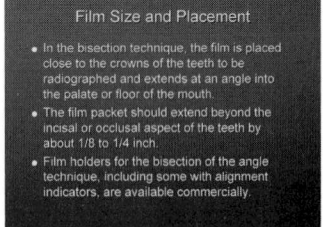

- What types of film holders are available for the bisecting-angle technique?
- What size film should be used on an adult?
- Where is the ID dot on the film placed?

Slide 60

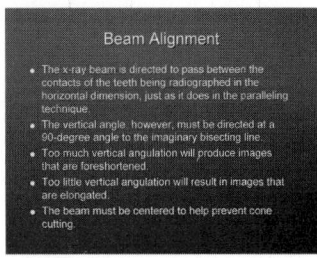

- Recommended vertical angulation:
  - Maxillary Canines: +45 to +55; Maxillary Incisors: +40 to +50
  - Maxillary Premolars: +30 to +40; Maxillary Molars: +20 to +30
  - Mandibular Canines: -20 to -30; Mandibular Incisors: -15 to -25
  - Mandibular Premolars: -10 to -15; Mandibular Molars: -5 to 0

ELSEVIER

Torres and Ehrlich Modern Dental Assisting, 9th ed.

Bird/Robinson

Slide 61

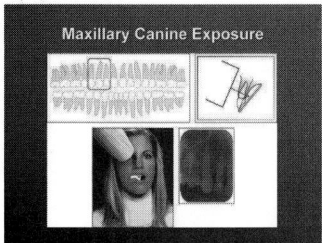

- What is the proper vertical angulation used for this film?
- Have the PID close to the patient so positioning on the ring will be quick.

Slide 62

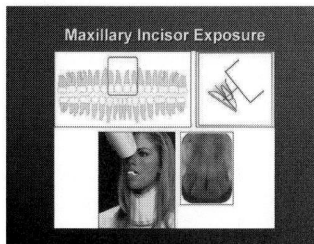

- What is the proper vertical angulation for this film?
- Remind patient to not open during exposure.

Slide 63

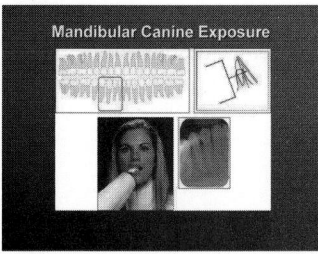

- What is the proper vertical angulation for this film?
- Remember that each patient is different. You will have to adjust for each one.

Slide 64

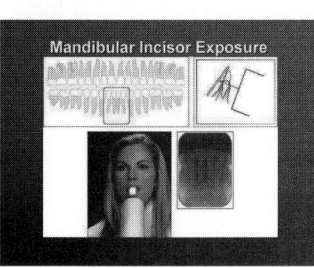

- What is the proper vertical angulation for this film?
- Remind patient to breathe through the nose.

Slide 65

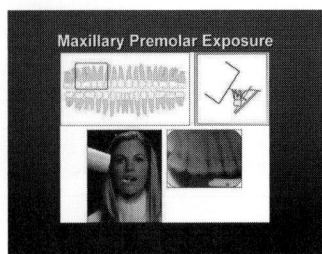

- What is the proper vertical angulation for this film?
- How will you know if you have the proper alignment?

Slide 66

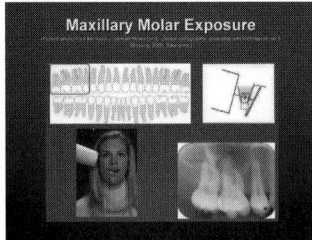

- What is the proper vertical angulation for this film?
- How do you keep the patient from moving during this procedure?

Slide 67

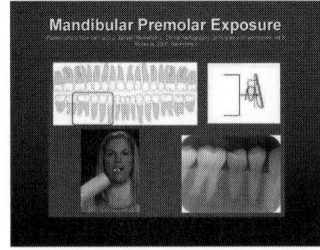

- What is the proper vertical angulation for this film?
- Remind patient not to move during exposure.
- How much time does it take to do a complete set of radiographs?

Slide 68

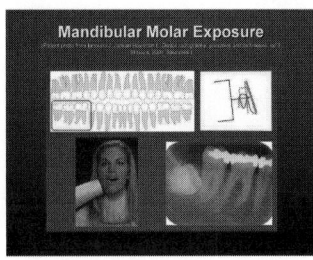

- What is the proper vertical angulation for this film?
- Why do you begin with the radiographs that are most comfortable for the patient?

Slide 69

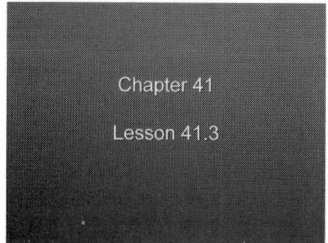

Slide 70

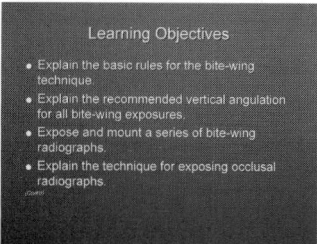

Slide 71

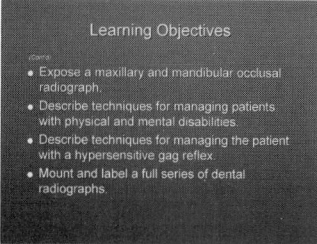

Slide 72

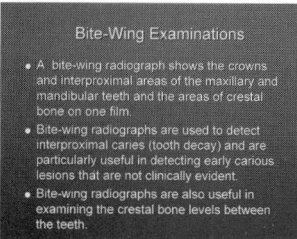

- How many bite-wings are taken on an adult?

- How many bite-wings are taken on a 5-year-old child?

- How many bite-wings are taken on an edentulous patient?

Slide 73

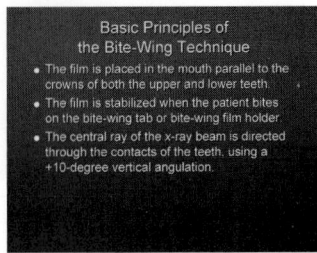

- What is the proper horizontal angulation for bite-wings?
- If the proper horizontal angulation is correct, what will be avoided?

Slide 74

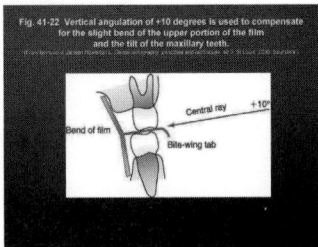

- The bite-wing tab stabilizes the film in the mouth when the patient bites together.

Slide 75

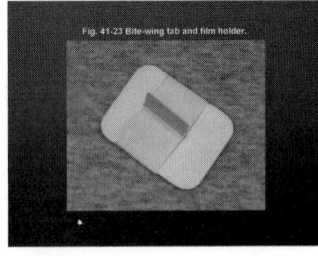

- This display is an example of a bite-wing loop.
- The bite-wing loop is also available in sticky tabs.
- It has the advantage that it can be reused for all four bite-wings in an adult.
- Bite-wing tabs are discarded after each patient.

Slide 76

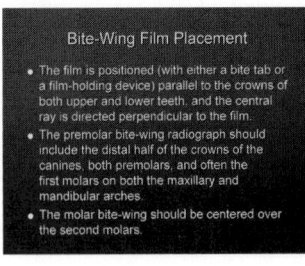

- Bite-wing tab or loop should be centered on the film before placement.
- Premolar films are taken first because they are less likely to trigger the gag reflex.

Slide 77

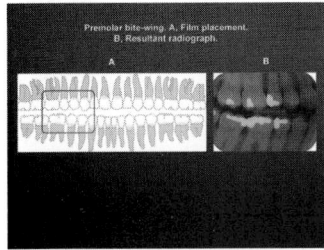

- Be sure the patient's occlusal plane is parallel to the floor; adjust as needed.
- Placement guideline: the most mesial portion of the film should align with the center of the mandibular canine.

Slide 78

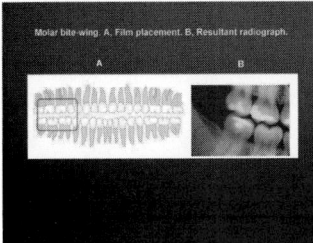

- Remind patient to remain still and to not move film with tongue.
- Placement guideline: ID dot toward the occlusal surface on all bite-wings.

Slide 79

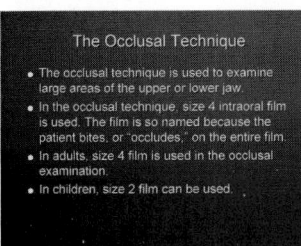

- Used to locate:
  - retained roots
  - supernumerary teeth
  - salivary stones
  - fractures
  - cleft palate

Slide 80

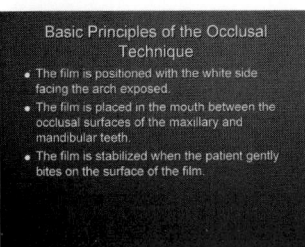

- Will the patient need to wear a lead apron for this type of film?
- Will the patient need to remove dentures, partials, or retainers?

Torres and Ehrlich Modern Dental Assisting, 9th ed.

Bird/Robinson

Slide 81

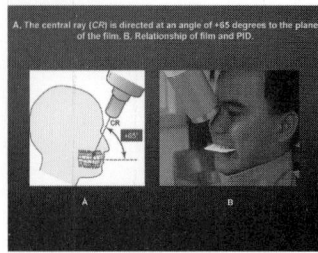

- Be sure the occlusal plane is parallel to the floor.
- The patient should be in an upright position.
- Patient should gently bite down; otherwise the patient can damage the film.

Slide 82

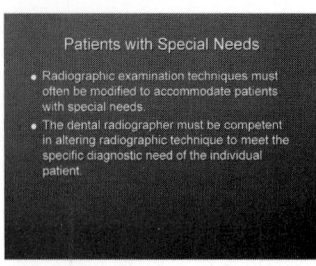

- Do not ask any unnecessary personal questions regarding patient's special needs.
- Be compassionate.

Slide 83

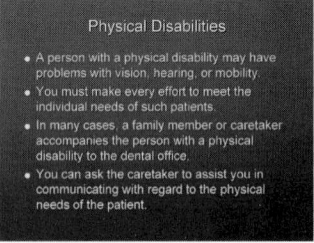

- Use terminology that can be understood by patient, but avoid "baby talk."
- Mobility: Ask if the patient needs your assistance.

Slide 84

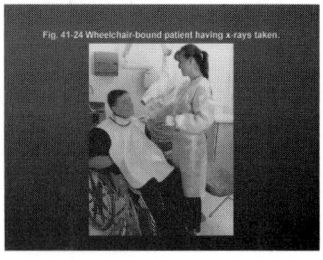

- Talk to the patient, not to the patient's caregiver.

Torres and Ehrlich Modern Dental Assisting, 9th ed.

Bird/Robinson

Slide 85

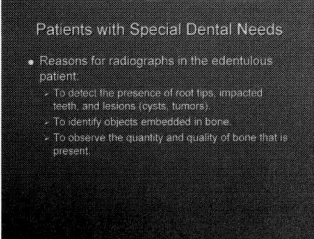

- What does the term *edentulous* mean?
- What are root tips?

Slide 86

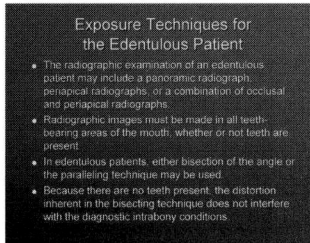

- For partially edentulous patients, cotton rolls may be used to stabilize the film holding devices.

Slide 87

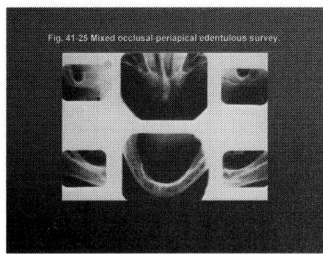

- What size film is used for periapicals?
- What size film is used for occlusals?

Slide 88

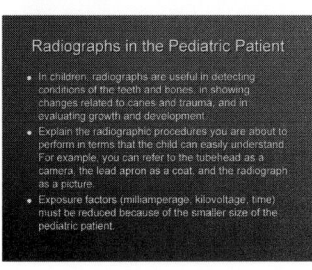

- Avoid "baby talk."
- Use positive reinforcement with children.
- Always commend them on a job well done.
- Must move quickly; have all settings ready; remind child to hold still.

Slide 89

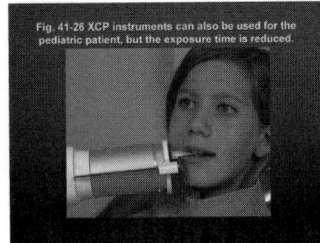

- What size films are used for children?
- Demonstrate actions for the child before you begin.
- May need to postpone films if child is uncooperative.

Slide 90

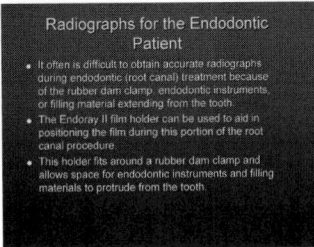

- Periapical film must be positioned to see 5 mm past the apex of the tooth.
- Tooth should be centered on the film.

Slide 91

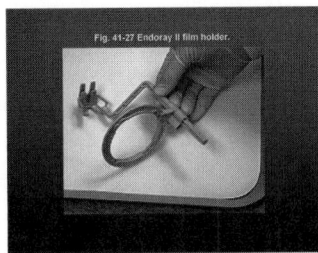

- What does this film holder resemble?
- Extension near film is to protect the materials used for endodontic procedure.

Slide 92

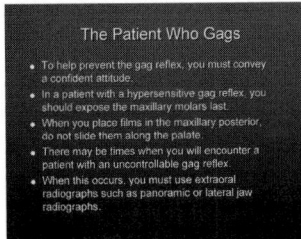

- Do not ask patient if he or she is a "gagger."
- Remind patients to breath through the nose.
- Commend patients on a job well done.
- Move quickly; remove films immediately from the mouth.
- What can be placed in the oral cavity to lessen a gag reflex?

Bird/Robinson

Slide 93

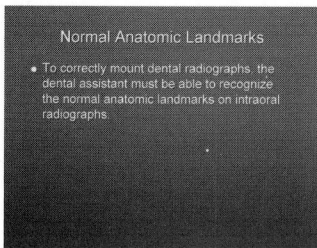

- Films are arranged on a mount for easy viewing.
- Films must be in order to avoid diagnostic errors.

Slide 94

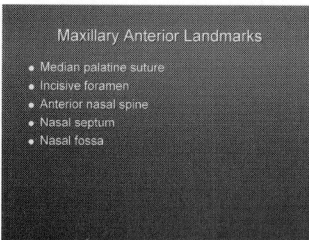

- Where are these landmarks located?
- What do they look like on a radiograph?

Slide 95

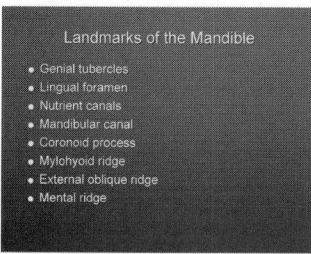

- Where are these landmarks located?
- What do they look like on a radiograph?

Slide 96

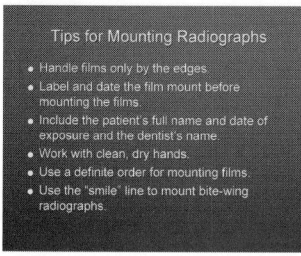

- What is labial mounting? What is lingual mounting?
- Which mounting is recommended by the ADA?
- What types of mounts are available? (*Plastic, cardboard.*)
- Double check mount for errors.

Bird/Robinson

42 Lesson Plan
Extraoral and Digital Radiography

TEACHING FOCUS

This chapter introduces the student to topics related to panoramic, extraoral, and digital radiography. This includes projections, films, intensifying screens, and equipment needed. Lateral jaw, skull, and temporomandibular joint (TMJ) radiography will be discussed. The student will also become acquainted with procedures for preparing equipment for panoramic radiography, for preparing the patient, and positioning the patient. Basic concepts, procedures, advantages, and disadvantages of digital radiography will be presented.

MATERIALS AND RESOURCES

☐ computer and PowerPoint projector (all Lessons)
☐ double-sided lead apron (or style recommended by the manufacturer) (Lesson 42.1)
☐ extraoral film (Lesson 42.1)

☐ index cards (all Lessons)
☐ infection control barriers (Lesson 42.1)
☐ panoramic cassette (Lesson 42.1)
☐ panoramic radiograph unit (Lesson 42.1)
☐ plastic container (Lesson 42.1)

LESSON CHECKLIST

Preparations for this lesson include:

- lecture
- evaluation of student knowledge and skills needed to perform all entry-level activities related to extraoral and digital radiography, including:
  - the uses and basic concepts of panoramic, extraoral, and digital radiography
  - how to prepare equipment for panoramic, extraoral, and digital radiography
  - how to prepare and position the patient for panoramic, extraoral, and digital radiography
  - the indications for various projections
  - the advantages and disadvantages of digital radiography

KEY TERMS

cephalostat (p. 670)
charge-coupled device (CCD) (p. 678)
digital radiography (p. 661)
digital images (p. 676)
digitize (p. 675)
exposure controls (p. 663)
extraoral radiographs (p. 661)

focal trough (p. 662)
Frankfort plane (p. 665)
midsagittal plane (p. 665)
sensor (p. 676)
temporomandibular joint (TMJ) (p. 675)
tomography (p. 662)

ADDITIONAL RESOURCES

PowerPoint slides (Evolve): 1-54
Multimedia Procedures DVD:
    Digital Radiography (four videos)
    Positioning Patient for Panoramic Radiography
    Preparing Panoramic Equipment
The Interactive Dental Office CD-ROM:
    Cindy Valladares
    Ingrid Pedersen
    Tiffany Cole

Legend

CTQ
Critical
Thinking
Question

DVD
Multimedia
Procedures
Videos and
Animations

ESLR
EVOLVE
Student
Learning
Resources

IDO
Interactive
Dental
Office
CD-ROM

SW
Student
Workbook

TB
Test Bank
on the
TEACH
CD-ROM

PPT
PowerPoint
Slides

Class Activities are indicated in ***bold italic.***

ELSEVIER

Torres and Ehrlich Modern Dental Assisting, 9th ed.

Bird/Robinson

LESSON 42.1

PRETEST

1. What does the term *extraoral* mean?
   a. inside of the mouth
   b. outside of the mouth
   c. spare
   d. exposure

2. What does a panoramic radiograph show?
   a. entire skull
   b. maxillary arch
   c. mandibular arch
   d. both maxillary and mandibular arches

3. What is a panoramic radiograph used for?
   a. to diagnose periodontal disease
   b. to diagnose dental decay
   c. to diagnose periapical lesions
   d. to observe tooth eruption patterns

4. An exaggerated smile line is when a patient's
   a. chin is tipped upward.
   b. chin is tipped downward.
   c. head is tilted to the left.
   d. head is tilted to the right.

5. Anterior teeth appear widened and blurred because a patient
   a. is not standing erect.
   b. does not have the tongue on the palate.
   c. is positioned too far back on the bite-block.
   d. is positioned too far forward on the bite-block.

6. What degree of angulation is used for lateral jaw radiography?
   a. -5 to -10
   b. -15 to -20
   c. +5 to +10
   d. +15 to +20

7. What is another term for the jaw joint?
   a. maxillary joint
   b. mandibular joint
   c. boney joint
   d. temporomandibular joint (TMJ)

8. A small detector that is placed intraorally to capture a radiographic image is a
   a. sensor.
   b. grid.
   c. panoramic film.
   d. periapical film.

9. What is a term for the imaginary plane that passes through the top of the ear canal and the bottom of the eye socket?
   a. midsagittal plane
   b. focal trough
   c. Frankfort plane
   d. TMJ

10. What is a cause of a ghost image?
   a. tongue
   b. movement by the patient during exposure
   c. metallic objects
   d. incorrect position of film

Answers

1. b	3. d	5. c	7. d	9. c
2. d	4. b	6. b	8. a	10. d

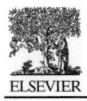

BACKGROUND ASSESSMENT

Question: Why are panoramic radiographs used in dentistry?

Answer: Panoramic radiographs are frequently used in dental offices to provide an overall view of the mandible and the maxilla, to observe tooth eruption patterns, and to locate impacted teeth. These patterns are not visible to the naked eye, and periapical radiographs show only a portion of the eruption patterns and impacted teeth; therefore, panoramic radiographs are used to evaluate these areas. Panoramic radiographs also are used to help detect lesions in the maxilla or mandible, and to help detect specific bone features. Panoramic radiographs are not used in diagnosing tooth decay, periodontal disease, or periapical lesions.

Question: How does digital radiography differ from traditional radiography?

Answer: Both digital radiography and traditional radiography are used to help diagnose dental disease. However, digital radiography does not require the use of film or film processing as with traditional radiography. Digital radiography uses an electronic sensor in place of film to record the images. Then the image data are sent to a computer that digitizes the impulses and produces a diagnostic image almost immediately. The sensor also allows the operator to use traditional radiographic techniques, such as paralleling and bisecting. Digital radiography can obtain panoramic and cephalometric images.

CRITICAL THINKING QUESTION

A 26-year-old woman came to the office for a panoramic radiograph. All procedural steps were followed for panoramic exposure, but upon processing, the film showed a large radiopaque area concealing a portion of the mandible. What is this type of error? What needs to be done in the future to avoid it?

Guidelines: This large radiopaque error was caused either by improper placement of the lead apron before obtaining the panoramic radiograph or by the use of a lead apron with a thyroid collar. To avoid this error in the future, a lead apron without a thyroid collar should be placed to protect the patient. This lead apron should be positioned low on the neck, so that it does not interfere with the x-ray beam.

OBJECTIVES	CONTENT	TEACHING RESOURCES
Pronounce, define, and spell the Key Terms.	■ Key terms (p. 660)	SW Fill in the Blank questions 1-8 (p. 322) ESLR Electronic Flashcards ▸ Discuss each of the key terms in Chapter 42. Focus on the definition, pronunciation, and spelling of each term. *Class Activity Go around the room and have each student use one of the key terms in a clinically relevant sentence in order to define the term. Continue until all terms have been used; if students become stuck, have the rest of the class offer suggestions.*
Describe the purpose and uses of panoramic radiography.	■ Introduction (p. 661) ■ Panoramic radiography (p. 661) □ Basic concepts (p. 662) □ Focal trough (p. 662)	PPT 4-8 TB questions 1, 3 SW Short-Answer Questions 1; Multiple Choice questions 1-2, 10 (pp. 321-323) SW Case Study question 2 (p. 323) Recall questions 1-3 (pp. 661, 668) Panoramic Radiographs in Dentistry (p. 661) Figure 42-1 (A) Panoramic radiograph; (B) Panoramic anatomy (p. 662)

OBJECTIVES	CONTENT	TEACHING RESOURCES
		Figure 42-2 The film and x-ray tubehead (p. 663)
		Figure 42-3 Example of an image layer (p. 663)
		▶ Discuss the appropriate uses of panoramic radiographs. When are intraoral radiographs preferred?
		▶ Discuss the concept of the focal trough. How does this relate to patient positioning?
		Class Activity Divide the class into groups. Assign each group one of the following tasks:
		– Locate impacted teeth
		– Observe tooth eruption patterns
		– Detect lesions in the jaw
		– Detect features in the bone
		– Provide an overall view of the mandible and maxilla
		Have each group discuss when panoramic radiography would be used in the dental office. Then, have each group report its conclusion to the class for discussion.
Describe the equipment used in panoramic radiography.	☐ Equipment (p. 663) – Tubehead (p. 663) – Head positioner (p. 663) – Exposure controls (p. 663) – Film and intensifying screens (p. 665) Procedure 42-1 Preparing equipment for panoramic radiography (p. 664) (SW/ESLR Competency 42-1, p. 325)	⊠▤ PPT 9-14 🎥 Multimedia Procedures DVD: Preparing Panoramic Equipment 💻 TB questions 2, 4 📖 SW Short-Answer Questions 2; Multiple Choice question 4 (pp. 321-322) 📖 *e* SW/ESLR Competency 42-1 Preparing Equipment for Panoramic Radiography (p. 325) Figure 42-4 Main components of a panoramic unit (p. 663) Figure 42-5 Head positioner (p. 665) Recall question 5 (p. 675) ▶ Discuss the similarities and differences between the panoramic x-ray tubehead and the intraoral tubehead. ▶ Discuss the components of the head positioner. Why is this needed for panoramic but not intraoral radiographs? ***Class Activity Before class ask students to bring in either photographs or copies of correctly identified equipment used in panoramic radiography. Have the class discuss the photos. (For students to prepare for this activity, see Homework/Assignments #1.)***

OBJECTIVES	CONTENT	TEACHING RESOURCES
Describe the steps for positioning patients in panoramic radiography.	*Procedure* 42-2 Preparing patient for panoramic radiography (p. 664) (SW/ESLR Competency 42-2, p. 327) *Procedure* 42-3 Positioning patient for panoramic radiography (p. 665) (SW/ESLR Competency 42-3, p. 329)	Multimedia Procedures DVD: Positioning the Patient for Panoramic Radiography SW Short-Answer Questions 3 (p. 321) SW/ESLR Competency 42-2 Preparing a Patient for Panoramic Radiography (p. 327) SW/ESLR Competency 42-3 Positioning Patient for Panoramic Radiography (p. 329) ▸ Discuss the procedure to prepare the patient for panoramic radiography. In what important ways does this differ from the preparations for intraoral radiography? ▸ Discuss the procedure to position the patient for panoramic radiography. What is the role of the bite-block, and how is it used in positioning the patient? *Class Activity Demonstrate proper patient positioning of panoramic radiography. Divide the class into pairs and have students practice on each other.*

Describe the errors caused during patient preparation and positioning during panoramic radiography.	☐ Common errors (p. 665)
	  – Patient preparation errors (p. 666)
	  – Patient positioning errors (p. 666)
		PPT 15-27
		
		TB questions 5-7
		
		SW Short-Answer Questions 5 (p. 321)
		
		SW/IDO Patient Case Exercise questions Valladares 1-2; Pedersen 1; Cole 1-2 (The Interactive Dental Office CD-ROM) (pp. 323-324)
		
		Figure 42-6 Large hoop earrings and "ghost" images (p. 666)
		
		Figure 42-7 On a panoramic radiograph, a lead apron artifact (p. 666)
		
		Figure 42-8 If the tongue is not placed on the roof of the mouth (p. 667)
		
		Figure 42-9 Patient's chin is tipped upward (p. 667)
		
		Figure 42-10 "Reverse smile line" (p. 668)
		
		Figure 42-11 Patient's chin is tipped downward (p. 668)
		
		Figure 42-12 "Exaggerated smile" (p. 669)
		
		Figure 42-13 Frankfort and midsagittal planes (p. 669)
		
		Figure 42-14 Patient is biting too far back on the bite-block (p. 669)
		
		Figure 42-15 The patient is positioned too far back on the bite-block (p. 669)
		
		Figure 42-16 The patient is positioned too far forward on the bite-block (p. 670)

Torres and Ehrlich Modern Dental Assisting, 9th ed.

Bird/Robinson

OBJECTIVES	CONTENT	TEACHING RESOURCES
		Figure 42-17 If the patient is not standing erect (p. 670)
		▸ Discuss the effects on the radiographs of errors in preparing the patient
		▸ Discuss the effects of patient positioning on the radiographs. What are the roles of the Frankfort and midsagittal planes in positioning?
		Class Activity Lead a class discussion about how to repair errors caused by positioning during panoramic radiography. Then divide the class into groups, and assign each group one of the following situations to discuss:
		– *Anterior teeth appear widened and blurred*
		– *Anterior teeth appear narrow and blurred*
		– *Superimposition of the cervical spine*
		– *Reverse smile line*
Discuss the advantages and disadvantages of panoramic radiography.	☐ Advantages and disadvantages (p. 667)	📺 TB question 8
		📖 SW Short-Answer Questions 4 (p. 321)
		Table 42-1 Advantages and Disadvantages of Panoramic Radiography (p. 668)
		▸ Discuss Table 42-1 Advantages and Disadvantages of Panoramic Radiography (p. 668).
		Class Activity Divide the class into groups, and have each group make index cards with the pros and cons of panoramics. Then, have groups exchange their cards with another group and quiz themselves using the set of cards they received.

42.1 Homework/Assignments:

1. Ask students to bring in either photographs or copies of correctly identified equipment used in panoramic radiography.

42.1 Instructor's Notes/Student Feedback:

ELSEVIER

Bird/Robinson

CRITICAL THINKING QUESTION

A 22-year-old man came to the office with jaw joint pain. He complained about a lot of discomfort in both ears, and about having trouble opening and closing his mouth. The patient also said that he heard popping and clicking sounds when he ate. What procedures could be performed to help diagnose the problem?

Guidelines: The patient is experiencing discomfort associated with his temporomandibular joints (TMJ). Identifying the problems he is having will require a series of radiographs. Radiography cannot be used to examine the articular disk and other soft tissues of this area; therefore, a transcranial TMJ radiograph can be performed in the office. This type of radiograph would show the bone and the relationship of the jaw joint. If the radiograph does not help to determine a diagnosis of the patient's condition, the patient should be referred to a specialist for magnetic resonance imaging (MRI) or computerized tomography (CT). A CT provides accurate imaging of the TMJ because it shows the extent of movement of the condyle as the mouth opens.

OBJECTIVES	CONTENT	TEACHING RESOURCES
Describe the purposes and uses of extraoral radiography.	■ Extraoral radiography (p. 668)	PPT 30 TB question 9 SW Short-Answer Questions 6, 8; Multiple Choice question 3 (pp. 321-322) Recall question 4 (p. 675) ▸ Discuss the most important uses of extraoral radiography. When might it be used instead of intraoral radiography? What is the disadvantage of this use? *Class Activity **Divide the class into groups. Have each group make flash cards of the key terms with the terms on one side and the definitions on the other. Then have the students quiz each other with the flash cards. Correct their pronunciation as needed.***
Describe the equipment used in extraoral radiography.	☐ Equipment (p. 670) ☐ Film and intensifying screens (p. 670) ☐ Grid (p. 670) ☐ Procedures (p. 671)	PPT 31-33 SW Multiple Choice question 5 (p. 322) Figure 42-18 A digital panoramic unit (p. 671) Figure 42-19 A grid decreases the amount of scatter radiation (p. 671) Recall question 6 (p. 675) ▸ Discuss the equipment used for intraoral radiography. What is the function of a grid? What is the risk of its use? *Class Activity **Provide the class with the following situations. Have them identify within 20 seconds when extraoral radiography would be used in the dental office. Discuss as necessary.***

OBJECTIVES	CONTENT	TEACHING RESOURCES
		– Identify trauma or fractures
		– Determine size and location of lesions
		– Identify TMJ disorders
		– Detect disease of jaw
		– Identify location of impacted teeth
		– Determine jaw growth and development
Identify the specific purpose of each of the extraoral film projections.	☐ Lateral jaw radiography (p. 671) – Body of mandible (p. 671) – Ramus of mandible (p. 671) ☐ Skull radiography (p. 673) – Lateral cephalometric projection (p. 673) – Posteroanterior projection (p. 673) – Waters projection (p. 673) – Submentovertex projection (p. 675) – Reverse Towne projection (p. 675) ☐ Temporomandibular joint radiography (p. 675)	⊠ PPT 34-45 TB question 10 SW Short-Answer Questions 7; Multiple Choice question 6 (pp. 321-322) Figure 42-20 (A) For the lateral jaw projection of the body of the mandible; (B) Lateral jaw radiograph of mandibular body (p. 672) Figure 42-21 (A) For the lateral jaw projection of the ramus of the mandible; (B) Lateral jaw radiograph of mandibular ramus (p. 672) Figure 42-22 (A) For the lateral cephalometric projection; (B) Lateral cephalometric radiograph (p. 673) Figure 42-23 (A) For the posteroanterior skull projection; (B) Posteroanterior skull radiograph (p. 674) Figure 42-24 (A) For the Waters projection; (B) This case of chronic maxillary sinusitis (p. 674) Figure 42-25 (A) For the submentovertex projection; (B) Submentovertex radiograph (p. 675) Figure 42-26 (A) For the reverse Towne projection; (B) Reverse Towne radiograph (p. 676) Figure 42-27 (A) As the tubehead and film move; (B and C) Corrected axial CT images (p. 677) Figure 42-28 Patient positioned for a transcranial radiograph of the temporomandibular joint (p. 677) Recall question 7 (p. 675) ▸ Discuss the purpose of lateral jaw radiography, including the two types of projections. ▸ Discuss the purpose of skull radiography, including the five types of projections. ▸ Discuss the purpose of temporomandibular joint radiography. When are other types of imaging preferred? **Class Activity** *Demonstrate the proper positioning of patient for lateral cephalometric projection.*

OBJECTIVES	CONTENT	TEACHING RESOURCES
Describe the purposes and uses of digital radiography.	■ Digital radiography (p. 675)	⊠▤ PPT 46 ▣ TB question 11 ▨ SW Short-Answer Questions 9 (p. 321) Figure 42-29 Digital radiographic system (p. 677) Recall question 8 (p. 680) ▸ Discuss the purposes and uses of digital radiography. What are the basic elements of a digital imaging system? *Class Activity **Bring a typodont to class, and have students practice placing sensors in the oral cavity.***
Discuss the fundamentals of digital radiography.	☐ Basic concepts (p. 676) ☐ Radiation exposure (p. 676)	⊠▤ PPT 47-54 ▣ TB question 12 ▨ SW Short-Answer Questions 10-11; Multiple Choice question 7 (pp. 321, 323) Figure 42-30 (A) Size of the electronic sensor; (B) Electronic sensor is protected with plastic barrier (p. 678) Figure 42-31 All types of radiographs may be produced in digital format (p. 678) ▸ Discuss the basic functions of a digital radiography system. How does it differ from film-based radiographic procedures? ▸ Discuss and compare radiation exposure in digital and film radiography. *Class Activity **Hand out blank sheets of paper, and have students draw a diagram of their understanding of a digital imaging system. Bring forward samples from the class and use them to point out the process of digital imaging systems.***
List and describe the equipment used in digital radiography.	☐ Equipment (p. 676) – X-ray machine (p. 676) – Intraoral sensor (p. 678) – Computer (p. 678) ☐ Types of digital imaging (p. 678) – Direct digital imaging (p. 678) – Indirect digital imaging (p. 678)	▦ Multimedia Procedures DVD: Digital Radiography (4 videos) ▨ SW Multiple Choice questions 8-9 (p. 322) Recall questions 9-10 (p. 680) Figure 42-32 Different digital imaging systems (p. 679) Figure 42-33 (A) The sensor is positioned in the bite-block with the alignment ring for use with the paralleling technique; (B) The digital Snap-A-Ray film holder has a notch in the bite-block for the sensor cable (p. 680) Figure 42-34 Sensor being placed in patient's mouth (p. 680)

OBJECTIVES	CONTENT	TEACHING RESOURCES
	– Storage phosphor imaging (p. 699) ☐ Procedures (p. 699) – Sensor preparation (p. 699) – Sensor placement (p. 699)	▸ Discuss the three types of digital imaging. ▸ Discuss some of the ways procedures differ in digital radiography versus standard radiography. ***Class Activity Divide the class into groups. Provide pictures of the equipment or the actual equipment without names. Then have the groups make labels to identify the equipment or pictures that you have displayed. Then have each group put its labels on the picture or equipment. The group with the most correct labels wins.***
List and discuss the advantages and disadvantages of digital radiography.	☐ Advantages and disadvantages (p. 679)	🖳 TB question 13 📖 SW Short-Answer Questions 12 (p. 321) Table 42-2 Advantages and Disadvantages of Digital Radiography (p. 680) Legal and Ethical Implications (p. 680) Eye to the Future (p. 681) 💡 CTQ 1-3 (p. 681) ▸ Discuss Table 42-2 (p. 680). If you were a dentist establishing a new practice, which type of radiography system would you choose and why? ▸ Discuss the legal and ethical implications of the use of digital radiography. ***Class Activity Before class have students conduct an Internet search on the digital radiographic systems available for dental offices. Then have them bring their results to class for discussion. (For students to prepare for this activity, see Homework/Assignments #1.)***
Performance Evaluation		🖳 TB 📖 SW questions (pp. 321-323) 📖 SW Case Study (pp. 304-323) 📖 SW/IDO Patient Case Exercises (pp. 323-324) (The Interactive Dental Office CD-ROM) 📖𝑒 SW/ESLR Competency 42-1 Preparing Equipment for Panoramic Radiography (p. 325) 📖𝑒 SW/ESLR Competency 42-2 Preparing a Patient for Panoramic Radiography (p. 327) 📖𝑒 SW/ESLR Competency 42-3 Positioning Patient for Panoramic Radiography (p. 329) 𝑒 ESLR Electronic Flashcards

OBJECTIVES	CONTENT	TEACHING RESOURCES
		ESLR Practice Quiz
		Recall questions (pp. 661-680)
		CTQ (p. 681)

42.2 Homework/Assignments:

1. Have students conduct an Internet search on the digital radiographic systems available for dental offices.

42.2 Instructor's Notes/Student Feedback:

Slide 1

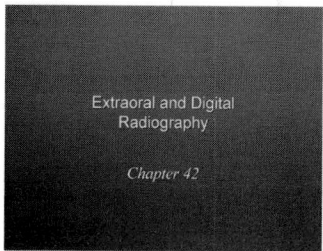

Slide 2

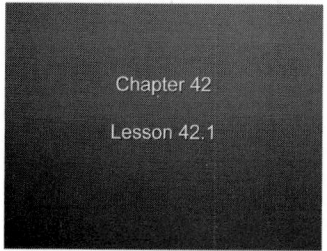

Slide 3

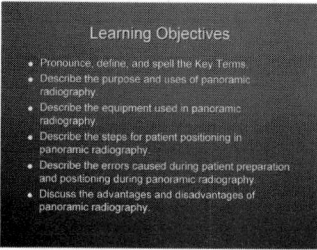

Slide 4

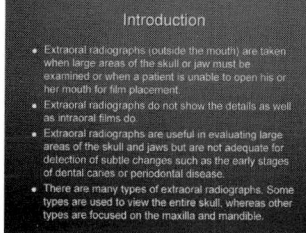

- Not used to detect decay, periodontal disease, or periapical lesions.
- Different types of extraoral radiographs are available.
- Depends on the area being radiographed.

Torres and Ehrlich Modern Dental Assisting, 9th ed.

Bird/Robinson

Slide 5

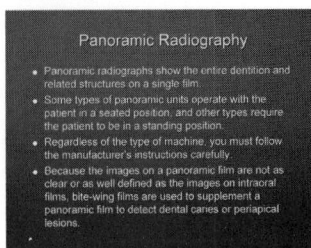

- Approximately 15 inches long
- Most panoramic units are operated while the patient is standing.
- Is adaptable for patients in wheelchairs.

Slide 6

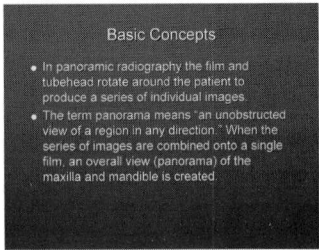

- Takes about 15 to 30 seconds to rotate around the patient's head.
- Requires the patient to hold still for the entire time.
- What are the indications for use of a panoramic radiograph? *(This type of radiograph can locate impacted teeth, show tooth eruption patterns, and detect lesions in the bone.)*
- What are the contraindications for use of a panoramic radiograph? *(This type of radiograph does not show caries, periodontal disease, or periapical lesions. The images are less sharp and more distorted than intraoral film.)*

Slide 7

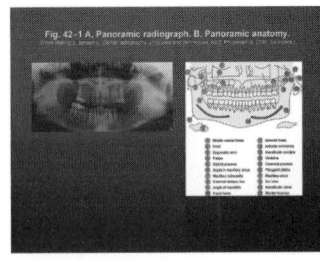

- Example of a panoramic radiograph.
- Shows maxillary and mandibular arch in one film.
- Make sure that students understand the importance of understanding the anatomical landmarks that are seen on a panoramic radiograph.

Slide 8

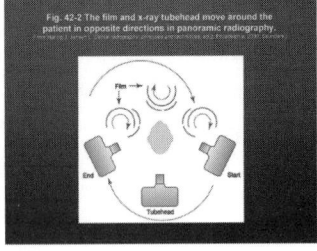

Torres and Ehrlich Modern Dental Assisting, 9th ed.
Bird/Robinson

Slide 9

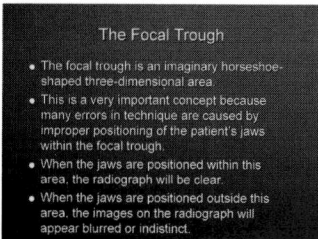

- Also known as an image layer.
- Check manufacturer's directions about positioning of patients.

Slide 10

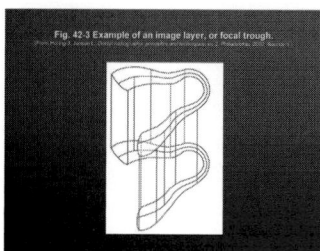

Slide 11

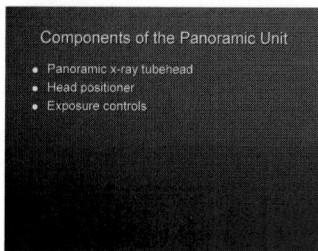

- Which of these is not used in traditional radiography? *(Head positioner.)*

Slide 12

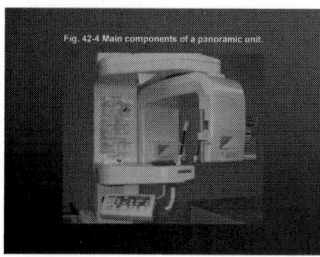

- Ask students to indicate the following:
  - Tubehead
  - Head positioner
  - Exposure control

Torres and Ehrlich Modern Dental Assisting, 9th ed.
Bird/Robinson

Slide 13

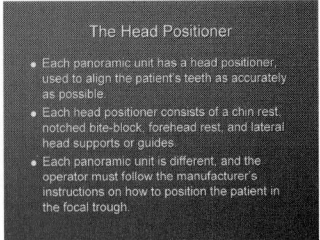

- Does this area need to be disinfected?

- Does this area need infection control barriers?

- Notched bite-block is heat-sterilizable.

Slide 14

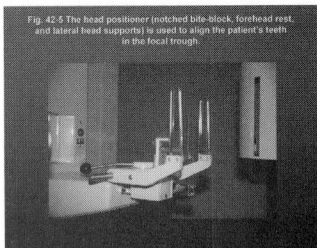

- The patient should stand as erect as possible while having a panoramic radiograph.

- Where should the patient's tongue be placed during exposure? *(Roof of the mouth.)*

Slide 15

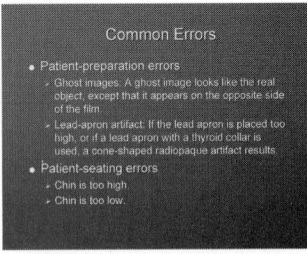

- Do patients need to remove items such as earrings, tongue rings, dentures, partials, and retainers before exposure? *(Yes.)*

Slide 16

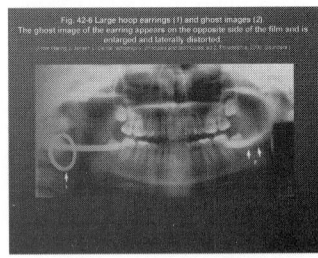

- What causes a ghost image? *(Patients who do not remove earrings, dentures, or other radiodense objects.)*

- Is this film of diagnostic quality? *(No.)*

Bird/Robinson

Slide 17

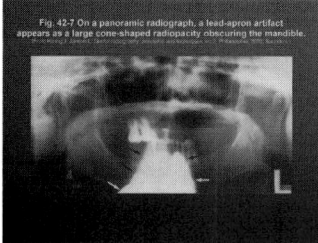

- What can be done to avoid this error in the future? *(Place the lead apron lower around the patient's neck.)*

Slide 18

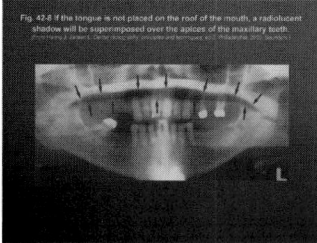

- Always remind the patient to swallow first, then place the tongue on the roof of the mouth.

Slide 19

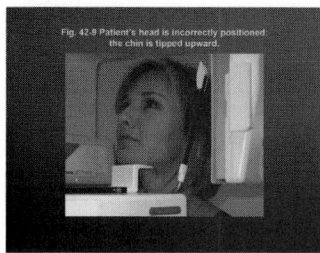

- What will be the end result of this error in positioning the patient? *(The radiograph will exhibit a "reverse smile line" and detail will be lost.)*

Slide 20

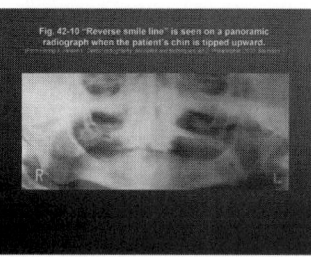

- Which plane is in the incorrect position before exposure? *(Frankfort plane.)*

Slide 21

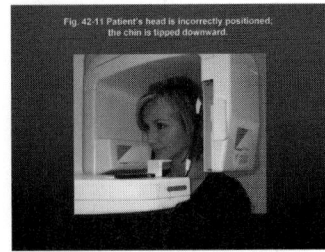

- What will the panoramic radiograph look like with patient positioned this way? *(The radiograph will exhibit an "exaggerated smile line," and the condyles will not be visible.)*

- What is the correct positioning? *(Midsaggital plane perpendicular to the floor, and Frankfort plane parallel to the floor.)*

Slide 22

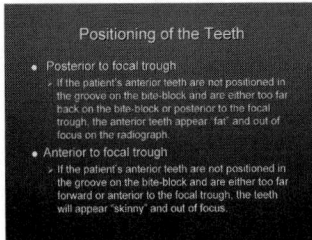

- What is the focal trough? *(An imaginary curved space, shaped like a horseshoe.)*

- What happens if the jaws are outside of this area? *(The radiograph will not be sharp.)*

- What happens if the jaws are inside this area? *(The radiograph images will be well defined.)*

Slide 23

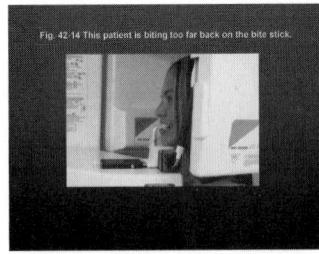

- Be sure the patient's anterior teeth are in the grooves of the bite stick.

- How do we obtain this film if a patient is missing all of his or her anterior teeth?

Slide 24

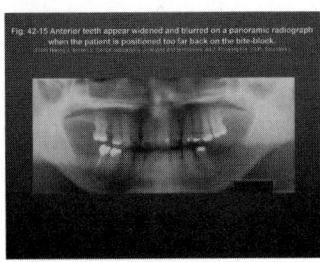

- What should be done to correct this error? *(Ask patient to bite more forward on the bite-block.)*

Slide 25

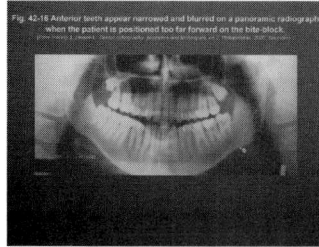

• What should be done to correct this error? *(Ask patient to bite farther back on the bite-block.)*

Slide 26

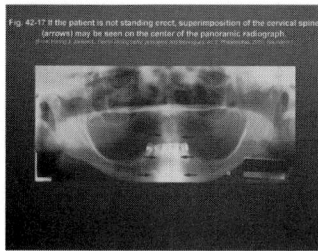

• Always remind patient to stand up straight and hold still during the exposure.

Slide 27

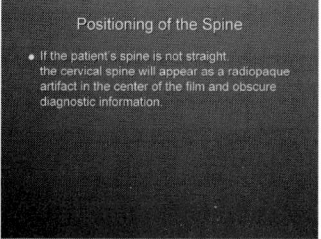

Slide 28

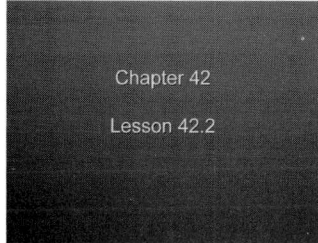

Torres and Ehrlich Modern Dental Assisting, 9th ed.

Bird/Robinson

Slide 29

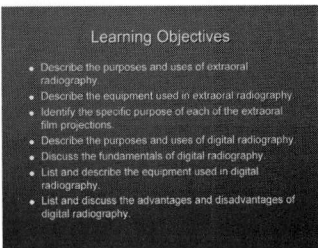

Slide 30

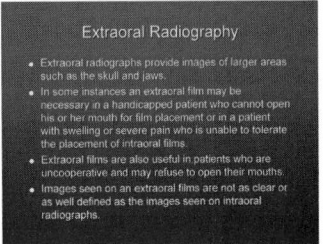

- Extraoral radiography is not used to detect decay, periodontal disease, or periapical diseases.

- What are extraoral radiographs used for? *(To detect fractures, lesions, diseases of the jaws, impacted teeth, and temporo-mandibular joint disorders.)*

Slide 31

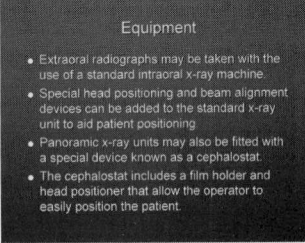

- Where is the cephalostat inserted when positioning the patient? *(Just inside the ears.)*

- Will the cephalostat need to be disinfected?

Slide 32

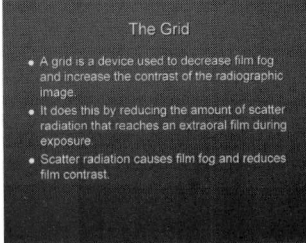

- What is scatter radiation? *(X-rays that bounce off bones and teeth.)*

- What does film fog look like on a radiograph?

- What is contrast? *(The gradations between dark and light areas on a radiograph.)*

Slide 33

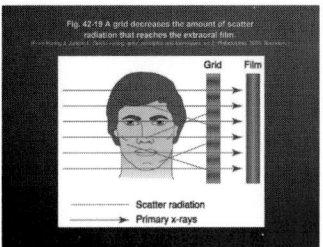

Slide 34

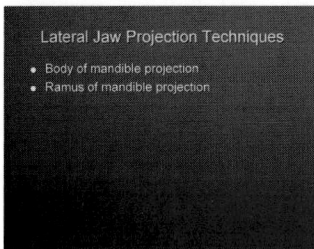

- Can be used on children.
- Not commonly used in dental offices.

Slide 35

- A standard intraoral radiograph machine can be used.
- What are these techniques designed to evaluate? *(Posterior region of the mandible, including impacted teeth, fractures, or lesions.)*

Slide 36

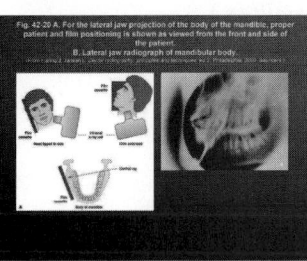

- Cassette is placed directly on patient's cheek.
- A disadvantage is that the patient must hold the cassette.

Torres and Ehrlich Modern Dental Assisting, 9th ed.

Bird/Robinson

Slide 37

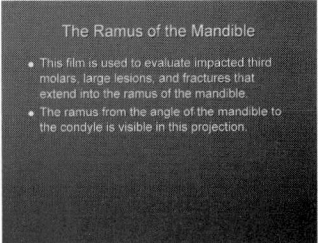

Slide 38

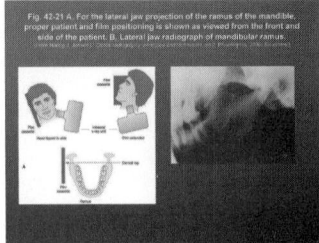

Slide 39

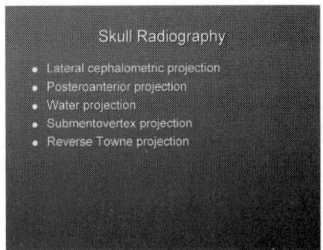

- Difficult to interpret these radiographs.
- A lateral cephalometric is the most common type of skull radiography.

Slide 40

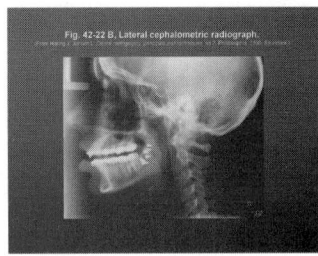

- What is this radiograph used to evaluate? *(Bones of the face and skull, including trauma, disease, or facial abnormalities.)*
- Used primarily for orthodontic purposes.

Slide 41

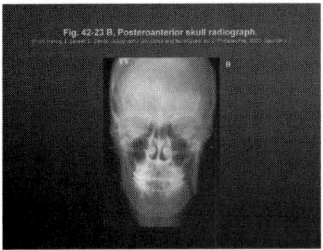

- What is this radiograph used to evaluate? *(Facial growth and trauma, disease, and facial development.)*

Slide 42

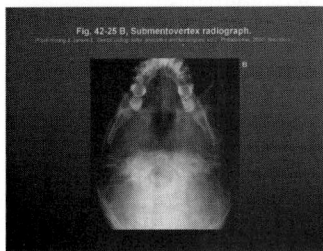

- Not commonly used in dental offices.
- What is this radiograph used to evaluate? *(Position of the condyles, base of the skull, and fractures of the zygomatic arch.)*

Slide 43

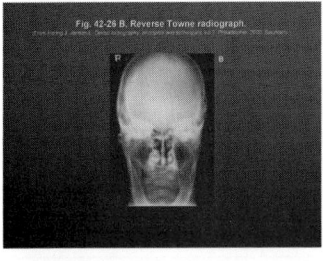

- Not commonly used in a dental office.
- What is this radiograph used to evaluate? *(Fractures of the condylar neck and ramus.)*

Slide 44

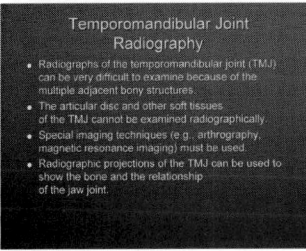

- Where is the TMJ located? *(It is the jaw joint.)*
- Patients usually sent to specialist who will obtain the special imaging techniques for diagnosis.

Slide 45

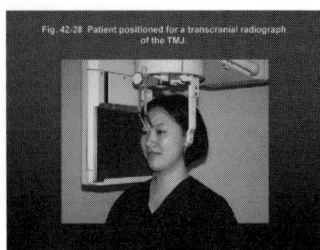

- Where is the cephalostat located? *(Around the patient's head.)*
- Should this patient have a lead apron on?

Slide 46

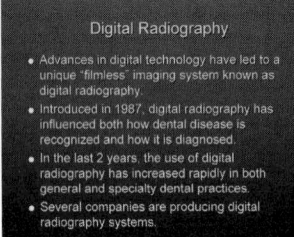

- This process is new technology.
- Does your particular dental office use digital radiography?
- This technology is currently an expensive investment for a dental office.

Slide 47

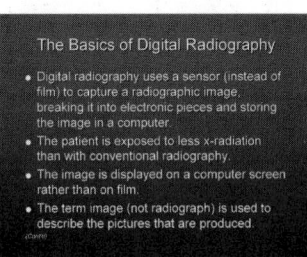

- What kind of film is used in digital radiography? *(No film is used.)*
- Are radiographic solutions used in digital radiography? *(No.)*
- How are the radiographs "processed"? *(An electronic sensor sends images to a computer.)*

Slide 48

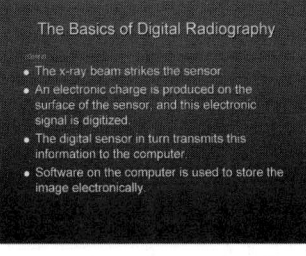

- What is a sensor? *(A small wired or wireless electronic square or rectangle.)*
- How long does it take for the sensor to transmit the information on the computer to display the image? *(Seconds.)*

Bird/Robinson

Slide 49

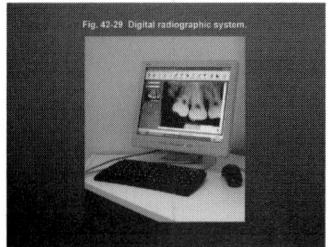

- What type of radiographic technique is used with digital radiography? *(The sensor picks up the x-rays and transmits an image to the computer, which digitizes the image and displays it in seconds.)*

Slide 50

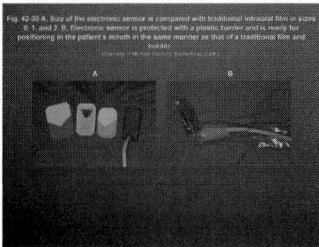

- Can you use an XCP with the sensor?

Slide 51

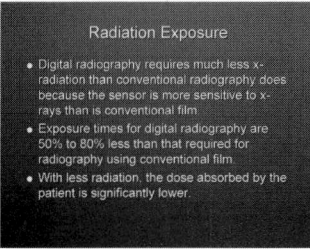

- Since there is less x-radiation used with digital radiography, does the patient still need to wear a lead apron? *(Yes.)*

Slide 52

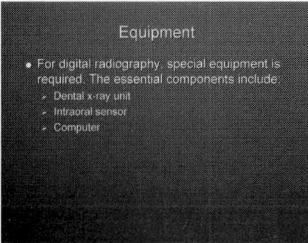

- Traditional dental radiograph machine can be used; timer must be calibrated.
- Sensor can be wireless.
- Computer must be up-to-date.

Slide 53

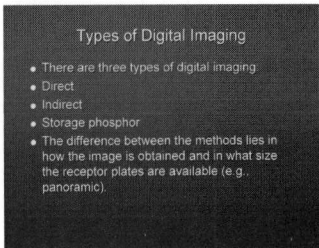

Slide 54

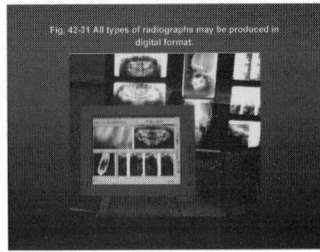

- Would each operatory need to be equipped with a computer monitor? *(Yes.)*

TEACHING FOCUS

This chapter introduces the student to topics related to restorative and esthetic dental materials. The student will become acquainted with properties of dental materials, including mechanical properties, thermal change, electrical properties, corrosive properties, solubility, and application properties. Direct restorations using amalgam and indirect restorations using gold-noble metal alloys and ceramic castings will be discussed.

MATERIALS AND RESOURCES

- ☐ alcohol gauze pads (Lesson 43.2)
- ☐ amalgam capsule (Lesson 43.1)
- ☐ amalgam carrier (Lesson 43.1)
- ☐ amalgam well or cloth (Lesson 43.1)
- ☐ amalgamator (Lesson 43.1)
- ☐ capsule activator (Lesson 43.1)
- ☐ composite instrument (Lesson 43.2)
- ☐ composite resin material (Lesson 43.2)
- ☐ computer and PowerPoint projector (all Lessons)

- ☐ curing light (Lesson 43.2)
- ☐ dappen dish (Lesson 43.2)
- ☐ dropper (Lesson 43.2)
- ☐ IRM liquid and dropper (Lesson 43.2)
- ☐ IRM powder and dispenser (Lesson 43.2)
- ☐ self-curing acrylic resin (Lesson 43.2)
- ☐ shade guide (Lesson 43.2)
- ☐ spatula (Lesson 43.2)
- ☐ treated paper pad or material dispenser (Lesson 43.2)

LESSON CHECKLIST

Preparations for this lesson include:

- lecture
- evaluation of student knowledge and skills needed for comprehension and application of principles underlying restorative and esthetic dental instruments, including:
  - general properties of dental materials and how these properties affect the application of each material
  - differences between direct and indirect restorative materials
  - properties of amalgam, composite resins, glass ionomers, temporary restorative materials, gold alloys, and porcelain
  - uses and application of amalgam, composite resins, glass ionomers, temporary restorative materials, gold alloys, and porcelain
  - use of tooth-whitening products

ELSEVIER

KEY TERMS

adhere (p. 687)
alloy (p. 689)
amalgam (p. 688)
auto-cured (p. 688)
ceramic (p. 703)
coupling agent (p. 695)
cured (p. 688)
curing (p. 688)
dual-cured (p. 688)
esthetic (p. 685)
filler (p. 695)
force (p. 686)
galvanic (p. 686)
gold (p. 702)
irregular (p. 689)

malleability (p. 702)
matrix (p. 695)
microleakage (p. 686)
palladium (p. 702)
pestle (p. 691)
platinum (p. 702)
porcelain (p. 703)
restorative (p. 685)
retention (p. 688)
spherical (p. 689)
strain (p. 686)
stress (p. 686)
trituration (p. 690)
viscosity (p. 687)
wetting (p. 687)

ADDITIONAL RESOURCES

PowerPoint slides (Evolve): 1-67
Multimedia Procedures DVD:
    Mixing and Transferring Amalgam

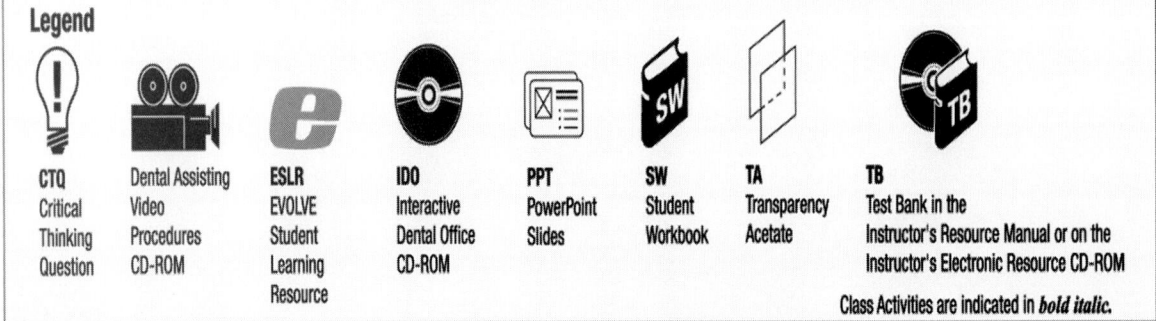

Legend

CTQ Critical Thinking Question

Dental Assisting Video Procedures CD-ROM

ESLR EVOLVE Student Learning Resource

IDO Interactive Dental Office CD-ROM

PPT PowerPoint Slides

SW Student Workbook

TA Transparency Acetate

TB Test Bank in the Instructor's Resource Manual or on the Instructor's Electronic Resource CD-ROM

Class Activities are indicated in ***bold italic.***

ELSEVIER

Torres and Ehrlich Modern Dental Assisting, 9th ed.

Bird/Robinson

LESSON 43.1

PRETEST

1. What is a favorable property of a dental material?
   a. high solubility
   b. galvanic action
   c. low solubility
   d. high contraction rate

2. Wetting, viscosity, surface characteristics, and film thickness are all characteristics that affect which of the following application properties?
   a. curing
   b. retention
   c. adhesion
   d. flow

3. Dental amalgam is composed of an alloy powder (made of silver, tin, copper, and zinc) that is triturated to be mixed in approximately equal parts with
   a. BIS-GMA.
   b. mercury.
   c. quartz.
   d. gold.

4. Which type of gold alloy is used for cast-removable partial dentures because of their hardness, malleability, and adaptability?
   a. type I
   b. type II
   c. type III
   d. type IV

5. IRM is the restorative material of choice for
   a. an anterior esthetic restoration.
   b. a final posterior restoration.
   c. a temporary sedative restoration.
   d. final cementing of a porcelain crown.

6. Which of the following dental restorative materials possesses the unique quality of fluoride release?
   a. glass ionomer
   b. amalgam
   c. composite resin
   d. porcelain

7. What makes composite resin a more favorable restoration than an amalgam?
   a. larger preparation needed for proper retention
   b. smaller cavity preparation needed due to bonding
   c. poor match with natural tooth
   d. the need to triturate material before use

8. Porcelain is chosen as an indirect restorative material for which of the following reasons?
   a. poor insulation
   b. galvanic action
   c. high coefficient of thermal expansion
   d. the esthetic colors for tooth matching

9. In addition to a shade guide, a curing light, and a composite instrument, what else may be useful during the preparation of a composite resin restoration?
   a. 2-x 2-inch alcohol gauze pads
   b. a spatula
   c. a liquid dropper
   d. a dappen dish

10. The organic matrix of composite resins is
    a. silica.
    b. quartz.
    c. glass.
    d. BIS-GMA.

Answers

1. c	3. b	5. c	7. b	9. a
2. c	4. d	6. a	8. d	10. d

BACKGROUND ASSESSMENT

Question: Tooth whitening is one of the most popular cosmetic procedures sought by the general public today. The dental assistant will be asked regularly about the various whitening methods that are available, including their differences. What are the three main options that are available? What are advantages and disadvantages of each method to help people decide which approach is best for them?

Answer: The three main tooth-whitening systems that are available are (1) over-the-counter, self-regulated tooth-whitening systems; (2) in-office treatment, dentist-supervised tooth whitening; (3) at-home treatment, dentist dispensed and supervised. The over-the-counter system has relatively low costs compared to a dentist-supervised treatment. It might not produce the same results as a dentist-supervised treatment due to poor adaptation of the universal shape delivery trays or systems to the teeth and it may also irritate the surrounding gingiva. The whitening solution changes only the color of natural tooth structure, not that of any tooth-colored directly or indirectly placed restorations. Despite a higher fee, dentist-supervised tooth whitening is recommended because the entire mouth should be evaluated before such a procedure. In-office tooth whitening is sometimes accomplished in a single visit, yet some individuals experience higher tooth sensitivity after the procedure as a result of the higher concentration of solution applied over a shorter amount of time. Alternatively, custom trays can be fabricated for use at home with a prescribed regimen. Although this treatment regimen usually takes a few weeks, the final results are very desirable and there is less tooth sensitivity.

Question: What are some of the most commonly used dental restorative materials? With respect to direct restorations, what are some of the indications and contraindications for both amalgam and composite restorations?

Answer: The most commonly used dental restorative materials include amalgam, composite resins, glass ionomers, temporary material, tooth-whitening products, gold alloys, and ceramic castings. All of these restorations have multiple indications and contraindications that depend on a multitude of variables such as the tooth or teeth to be restored (tooth condition, position in the mouth, the overall treatment plan); the dentist (personal preferences, styles, ability, educational background); the patient; current dental research; and recommendations from professional organizations such as the ADA. In general amalgam restorations remain indicated for both the primary and permanent dentition, especially in stress-bearing regions—most notably to restore small- to moderate-sized cavity preparations in posterior teeth. Amalgams are also chosen in some cases as a foundation for future indirect restorations in patients with poor oral hygiene, when cost is a consideration and when moisture control is a problem. Amalgams are contraindicated in most anterior teeth and when the patient has a true amalgam allergy. Composite resins are now widely used in both posterior and anterior regions, providing the most esthetic end result. However, composites should be placed only where adequate isolation from contaminants and moisture can be achieved and ideally in a patient with good oral hygiene.

CRITICAL THINKING QUESTION

The dental assistant looks over the day's schedule and notices that the first patient is scheduled for a class II posterior direct restoration on tooth #3. The dental assistant reads the notes in the chart and notices that the patient has not decided whether to have an amalgam or a composite filling. Although the patient has not arrived, the dental assistant wants to have the room set up to be ready for either situation. What should be included on the checklist?

Guidelines: The room should be prepared for placement of either an amalgam or a composite restoration. A clean environment with the appropriate barriers for the room, patient, and operators is the most important place to begin. If indicated, local anesthesia should be ready for use. Materials for isolation of the tooth to be restored, such as a rubber dam system or cotton rolls, should be available. Handpieces with both high and slow speed with the appropriate burs should be set up. A matrix, matrix holder, and wedges will be important for reestablishing proper tooth contours such as the proximal contact with the adjacent tooth. For amalgam placement, a varnish or dentin sealer with applicators and fresh capsules of amalgam should be ready. It is important to ensure that the amalgamator is functioning properly and that a dappen dish and carrier are available. Some hand instruments for condensing, burnishing, and carving amalgam are slightly different from those used for composite. A waste container for excess or unused amalgam scraps should be present. Articulating paper to check the bite and floss for checking the proximal contact will be used in both amalgam and composite procedures. For a composite, it will be necessary to have a shade guide with the corresponding appropriate composite resin shade and type, and also the acid etch, a bonding agent, and

Torres and Ehrlich Modern Dental Assisting, 9th ed.

Bird/Robinson

curing light. Various polishing tips will be useful as well. Finally, if the depth is greater than anticipated in a standard preparation after caries removal and/or removal of the previous defective restoration, additional materials such as liners or bases will be needed before placement of the amalgam or composite.

OBJECTIVES	CONTENT	TEACHING RESOURCES
Pronounce, define, and spell the Key Terms.	■ Key terms (pp. 684-685)	SW Fill in the Blank questions 1-20 (pp. 332-333) *E* ESLR Electronic Flashcards ▸ Discuss each of the key terms, focusing on the definition, pronunciation, and spelling of each term. ***Class Activity** Divide the class into small groups, and assign each group an equal number of terms. Have each group write a sentence using each term appropriately, and ask a group leader to read the sentences to the class.*
Discuss how a dental material is evaluated before being marketed to the profession.	■ Standardization of dental materials (p. 685) □ Criteria for a new dental material (p. 686)	PPT 5-6, 15 TB question 1 SW Short-Answer Questions 1; Fill in the Blank questions 6, 9; Multiple Choice question 1 (pp. 331-333) Recall question 1 (p. 686) ▸ Discuss common dental restorative materials. List the common materials used, and note that the dental assistant must perform the setup for each material and follow the manufacturer's recommendations for preparation. ***Class Activity** Provide the class with photocopies of manufacturer inserts found in the initial packaging of commonly used amalgam, composite resin, glass ionomer, temporary material, and tooth-whitening products. Divide the class into seven groups and assign each group one of the following dental materials: amalgam, composite resins, glass ionomers, temporary materials, tooth-whitening products, gold alloys, ceramic restorations. Include the corresponding manufacturer packaging insert or information provided by the manufacturing laboratory. Have each group make a report to the class.*
List the properties of dental materials and ways that they affect their application.	■ Properties of dental materials (p. 686) □ Mechanical properties (p. 686) – Types of stress and strain (p. 686) □ Thermal change (p. 686) – Contraction and expansion (p. 686)	PPT 7-14 TB question 2 SW Short-Answer Questions 2; Fill in the Blank questions 1, 3, 4, 11, 13-14, 18-19; Multiple Choice questions 2-5 (pp. 331-333) SW Case Study (p. 334) Figure 43-1 Types of stress and strain (p. 686) Figure 43-2 A galvanic action can occur when different types of metals touch each other (p. 687)

ELSEVIER

Torres and Ehrlich Modern Dental Assisting, 9th ed.

Bird/Robinson

OBJECTIVES	CONTENT	TEACHING RESOURCES
	☐ Electrical properties (p. 686) ☐ Corrosive properties (p. 687) ☐ Solubility (p. 687) ☐ Application properties (p. 687) – Flow (p. 687) – Adhesion (p. 687) – Retention (p. 688) – Curing (p. 688)	Figure 43-3 Corrosion can occur on certain metals (p. 687) Figure 43-4 Dental materials must withstand solubility of saliva in the oral cavity (p. 687) Figure 43-5 Light curing of a composite resin (p. 688) Recall questions 2-6 (p. 688) CTQ 3 (p. 704) ▸ Discuss the mechanical properties of dental materials. Note the need for restorative materials to withstand the biting and chewing forces of the mouth. ▸ Discuss the thermal properties of dental materials. Explain why thermal changes are of major concern, noting that each type of dental material expands and contracts at its own rate. ▸ Discuss the electrical properties of dental materials. List the conditions that allow electrical currents in the oral cavity. ▸ Discuss the corrosive properties of dental materials. List foods that may cause corrosion. ▸ Discuss the solubility of dental materials. Note that dental materials must have low solubility. *Class Activity Display textbook photos of various teeth and oral environments, e.g., anterior versus posterior, small cavity preparations versus grossly fractured or decayed, clean teeth versus teeth covered with heavy plaque, and a mouth with numerous restoration versus a mouth with no restorations. Have students identify a property that the dental material should possess in order to be applied in each situation.*
Describe the factors that affect how dental materials are manufactured for the oral cavity.	■ Properties of dental materials (p. 686) ☐ Mechanical properties (p. 686) – Types of stress and strain (p. 686) ☐ Thermal change (p. 686) – Contraction and expansion (p. 686) ☐ Electrical properties (p. 686) ☐ Corrosive properties (p. 687) ☐ Solubility (p. 687)	SW Short-Answer Questions 4 (p. 331) ▸ Discuss the application properties of dental materials. Describe issues related to flow, adhesion, retention, and curing. Discuss the difference between auto-cured and dual-cured material. ▸ Discuss the auto-cured, light-cured, and dual-cured processes. How does each process work? *Class Activity First ensuring the proper safety equipment, have students dispense in front of them a small sample of material set by each of the three curing methods. Have them record and compare how the material feels each minute after dispensing. Students should not manipulate the materials or change the lighting of the room between checks.*

Torres and Ehrlich Modern Dental Assisting, 9th ed.

Bird/Robinson

OBJECTIVES	CONTENT	TEACHING RESOURCES
	☐ Application properties (p. 687) – Flow (p. 687) – Adhesion (p. 687) – Retention (p. 688) – Curing (p. 688)	
Discuss the difference between direct and indirect restorative materials.	■ Direct restorative materials (p. 688)	PPT 16 TB question 3 SW Short-Answer Questions 3 (p. 331) ▸ Discuss direct restorations. Define a direct restoration and list materials that are used in direct restorations. *Class Activity Bring to class examples of commonly used materials for direct restorations as well as crowns or bridges that the students may handle and explore. Set up evaluation stations around the class that the students can systematically visit. Have a paper at each station that they may use to record observations for the other rotating students to see. After a full rotation discuss observations with the class as a whole.*
Describe the properties of amalgam and its application in restoring teeth.	☐ Amalgam (p. 688) – Indications for dental amalgam (p. 689) – Contraindications to dental amalgam (p. 689) – Composition of dental amalgam (p. 689) – High-copper alloys (p. 689) – Mercury-to-alloy ratios (p. 690) – Nonmercury alloys (p. 690) – Controversial issues in mercury (p. 690) – The application of dental amalgam (p. 690)	PPT 17-24 TB questions 4-5 SW Short-Answer Questions 5; Fill in the Blank questions 7, 12, 15-17; Multiple Choice questions 6-8 (pp. 331-333) Figure 43-6 Example of class II amalgam restorations (p. 688) Figure 43-7 The mercury and alloy powder are in their purest form before trituration (p. 689) Figure 43-8 Microscopic view of alloy powder particles (p. 689) Figure 43-9 Sources of mercury hazards in the dental operatory (p. 691) Table 43-1 Composition and Classification of Dental Amalgam Alloy Powders (p. 690) Box 43-1 Dental Mercury Hygiene Recommendations (p. 692) Recall questions 7-9 (p. 694) CTQ 2 (p. 704) ▸ Discuss how amalgam is made, its indications and

Torres and Ehrlich Modern Dental Assisting, 9th ed.

Bird/Robinson

OBJECTIVES	CONTENT	TEACHING RESOURCES
		contraindications, the composition of dental amalgam, and the main differences in the composition and classification of dental amalgam alloy powders. ▸ Discuss controversial issues related to the use of mercury. Note that patients are not harmed by the mercury within the amalgams placed in their teeth, but dental personnel need to be aware of the toxic effects of mercury vapors. ***Class Activity Divide the class in half. Have half the students individually list properties of amalgam on a piece of paper and hand them in to you. Make a list on the board of all the properties mentioned. Then have the other half of the class explain in writing why the listed properties would help in the application of the material.***
Mix and transfer amalgam.	– The application of dental amalgam (p. 690) Procedure 43-1 Mixing and transferring dental amalgam (p. 693) (SW/ESLR Competency 43-1 Mixing and Transferring Dental Amalgam, p. 335)	⊠ PPT 25-26 SW Fill in the Blank question 20; Multiple Choice questions 9-10 (p. 333) Multimedia Procedures DVD: Mixing and Transferring Amalgam SW/ESLR Competency 43-1 Mixing and Transferring Dental Amalgam (p. 335) Figure 43-10 Precapsulated amalgam (p. 691) Figure 43-11 Activator used to break the separating membrane in the capsule (p. 691) Table 43-2 Amalgamation Time (p. 691) Figure 43-12 Increments of amalgam placed (p. 694) Figure 43-13 Carving an amalgam restoration (p. 694) Recall questions 10-12 (p. 694) ▸ Discuss the application of dental amalgam. Explain the proper preparation, including trituration. ▸ Discuss condensation, carving, and finishing. ***Class Activity Divide the class into pairs. Have each pair take turns playing a dental assistant preparing amalgam and smoothly passing it to the operator, who then practices condensing the amalgam into a typodont. Have the operator pass the empty carrier back efficiently for more material until all the contents have been used.***

43.1 Homework/Assignments:

43.1 Instructor's Notes/Student Feedback:

LESSON 43.2

CRITICAL THINKING QUESTION

A 20-year-old woman in general good health comes to the office for a posterior composite restoration. After administering local anesthesia, the dentist has left the operatory to perform a checkup on another patient. At this time, the patient confides in the dental assistant that this is the first time she is having a tooth filled and that she is nervous about all of the materials and instruments arranged around her. She states that she would feel better if the dental assistant could briefly explain to her what she might expect when the dentist returns. How should the dental assistant respond?

Guidelines: Fortunately, the local anesthesia, which people seem to fear most, was administered in a comfortable manner for this patient. Assuming adequate anesthesia, the dental assistant should explain that when the dentist returns he will isolate the tooth to be worked on, perform the tooth preparation, and restore the tooth by placing a direct composite restoration. The best approach to take with most patients is to explain the steps in very general terms. The dental assistant might explain that first the tooth will be isolated (point out cotton rolls or a rubber dam); next, the cavity will be removed (show handpieces); next, the tooth with be cleaned or washed (acid etch); and then multiple layers of resin (prime and bond, composite) will be placed to replace any tooth structure that was removed and was carious. The resin will be set with a special light (curing light). Once the filling is placed, some adjustments might be made to ensure a comfortable bite and a smooth surface. Explanations may vary depending on the age and dental IQ of the patient. Anything the dental assistant does not feel comfortable discussing may be deferred to the dentist. Most dentists appreciate an assistant who plays an active, yet appropriate role in both educating patients and reducing dental fear.

OBJECTIVES	CONTENT	TEACHING RESOURCES
Describe the properties of composite resin materials and their application in restoring teeth.	☐ Composite resins (p. 694) – Composition of composite resins (p. 695) – The application of composites (p. 695)	PPT 31-37 TB questions 6-7 SW Short-Answer Questions 6; Multiple Choice questions 11-12 (pp. 331, 333) Figure 43-14 Class III composite restoration on tooth #10 (p. 694) Figure 43-15 Effect of particle size on surface finish of composite (p. 695) Figure 43-16 Summary of the historical evolution of dental composites, curing methods, and accompanying bonding systems (p. 696) Commercial examples of composite resins (p. 696) Recall questions 13-14 (p. 697) CTQ 5 (p. 704) ▸ Discuss composite resins. Note that they are typically placed in anterior teeth because of their esthetic qualities, and list their other qualities as well. ▸ Discuss composition of composite resins. Describe and state the purpose of the resin matrix, the filler, and the coupling agent. *Class Activity **Divide the class into four groups. Ask Group 1 to list the properties that make composite desirable. Ask Group 2 to list the desirable applications***

OBJECTIVES	CONTENT	TEACHING RESOURCES
		for composites. Ask Group 3 to list situations in which using composites would not be ideal. Ask Group 4 to list the required instruments and the sequence in which they are used for placing composite resin. Have each group report its findings to the class.
Prepare composite resin material.	– The application of composites (p. 695) – Polymerization (p. 697) – Steps in finishing a composite resin (p. 697) Procedure 43-2 Preparing composite resin materials (p. 698) (SW/ESLR Competency 43-2, p. 337)	PPT 38-40 TB question 8 SW Multiple Choice questions 13-15 (pp. 333-334) SW/ESLR Competency 43-2 Preparing Composite Resin Materials (p. 337) Figure 43-17 Use of a shade guide for color matching (p. 696) Figure 43-18 Composite resin kit (p. 697) Recall questions 15-17 (p. 697) ▸ Discuss the differences in the application techniques for amalgam restorations and composite restorations. Describe the process of polymerization and its role in the application of composites. ▸ Discuss the steps in finishing a composite resin. *Class Activity Have each student practice dispensing, manipulating, and light-curing a small sample of composite resin on a pad., Have students dispense material from the various carriers (tube, syringe, and from a pad), if available.* *Class Activity Have students use a shade guide to record the shade of their teeth in both natural and classroom light. Note differences. Have students compare shade differences between different teeth in their mouths (e.g., canines versus central incisors) and different parts of individual teeth (gingival versus incisal edge).*
Describe the properties of glass ionomers and their application in restoring teeth.	☐ Glass ionomers (p. 697) – Resin modified (p. 698) – Metal reinforcement (p. 698) – Fabrication and application (p. 698) – Cautions for placing glass ionomers (p. 698)	PPT 41-45 TB questions 9-10 (pp. 452-453) SW Short-Answer Questions 7 (p. 331) Figure 43-19 Setup for mixing glass ionomer liquid and powder (p. 699) Figure 43-20 Glass ionomers are supplied in tubes, cartridges, and tubs (p. 699) Recall questions 18-19 (p. 699) ▸ Discuss the advantages of glass ionomers, and note the applications for which glass ionomers are desirable. ▸ Discuss cautions for placing glass ionomers.

Torres and Ehrlich Modern Dental Assisting, 9th ed.

Bird/Robinson

OBJECTIVES	CONTENT	TEACHING RESOURCES
		***Class Activity** Have students work in small groups to prepare and submit charts to compare and contrast properties, indications, preparation, and application of glass ionomers, composite resins, IRM, and provisional coverage materials. Have each group summarize its findings and present them to the class.*
Describe the properties of temporary restorative materials and their application in restoring teeth.	☐ Temporary restorative materials (p. 699) – Intermediate restorative materials (p. 699) – Provisional restorative materials (p. 700)	PPT 46-49 TB questions 11-13 SW Short-Answer Questions 8; Multiple Choice questions 16-18 (pp. 331, 333-334) Figure 43-21 Placement of IRM into a molar (p. 699) Figure 43-22 Examples of provisional coverage materials (p. 700) Figure 43-23 Acrylic resin is supplied as liquid/powder, tubes, and automix cartridges (p. 701) Recall questions 20-23 (p. 701) CTQ 1 (p. 703) ▶ Discuss reasons why temporary restorative materials are used. ▶ Discuss the differences in composition and uses of intermediate restorative material and provisional restorative material. ***Class Activity** Using the information summarized in the previous Class Activity, have students make index cards with the name of the material on one side of the card. On the other side of the card, have them list four pieces of information about the material that would identify it.*
Mix intermediate restorative material.	– Intermediate restorative materials (p. 699) – Provisional restorative materials (p. 700) [Procedure] 43-3 Mixing intermediate restorative materials (p. 700) (SW/ESLR Competency 43-3, p. 339)	PPT 50-53 SW/ESLR Competency 43-3 Mixing Intermediate Restorative Materials (p. 339) ▶ Discuss the procedural steps required when mixing intermediate restorative material. ***Class Activity** Divide the class into three groups and, using the materials and instruments described in Procedure 43-3, have them gradually incorporate powder into the liquid. Group 1 should use less than the prescribed amount of powder; Group 2 should use more powder than prescribed; and Group 3 should use the exact amount of powder prescribed. Have one person in each group time the set after sufficient mixing according to the circumstances given. Have them note the setting times as well as the physical properties of each mixture at*

OBJECTIVES	CONTENT	TEACHING RESOURCES
		timed intervals. Then have each group present its findings to the class.
Prepare acrylic resin for provisional coverage.	– Provisional restorative materials (p. 700) Procedure 43-4 Mixing acrylic resin for provisional coverage (p. 701) (SW/ESLR Competency 43-4, p. 341)	SW/ESLR Competency 43-4 Mixing Acrylic Resin for Provisional Coverage (p. 341) ▸ Discuss the procedural steps required when preparing acrylic resin for provisional coverage. *Class Activity Group students according to supplies available and have each group practice assembling the acrylic resin automix cartridges onto the dispensing gun. Provide clear plastic stents of unprepared practice typodont teeth. Have students dispense acrylic resin as mentioned above into stents and place it over the corresponding prepared teeth until set.*
Discuss the use of tooth-whitening products.	☐ Tooth-whitening materials (p. 701) – Composition of whitening materials (p. 701)	PPT 54-58 TB questions 14-15 SW Short-Answer Questions 9 (p. 331) Commercial examples of bleaching products (p. 702) Figure 43-24 Before and after the use of a whitening product (p. 702) CTQ 4 (p. 704) ▸ Discuss the composition of whitening materials. List common substances that cause teeth to stain. ▸ Discuss different tooth-whitening treatment options and the advantages and disadvantages of each. *Class Activity Ask whether any students know people who have used any of the tooth-whitening products or who have had tooth-whitening procedures performed by the dentist. If so, have them describe to the class whether they are happy with the results and whether they have had any tooth or gingival sensitivity.*
Discuss the difference between direct and indirect restorative materials.	■ Indirect restorative materials (p. 702)	PPT 59 TB question 16 SW Multiple Choice question 20 (p. 334) Figure 43-25 Gold crown (p. 702) Recall question 25 (p. 703) ▸ Discuss indirect restorations. Define an indirect restoration and list the materials that are used in indirect restorations. *Class Activity Divide the class in half. Have Group 1 produce a list of direct restorative materials and prepare*

Torres and Ehrlich Modern Dental Assisting, 9th ed.

Bird/Robinson

OBJECTIVES	CONTENT	TEACHING RESOURCES
		a small class presentation about why and when these materials are selected. Assign Group 2 the task of listing various indirect restorative options. Have each group present its findings to the class.
Describe the properties of gold alloys and their application in restoring teeth.	☐ Gold-noble metal alloys (p. 702)	PPT 60-62 TB question 17 SW Short-Answer Questions 10; Fill in the Blank questions 5, 10; Multiple Choice question 19 (pp. 331-332, 334) Recall question 24 (p. 703) ▸ Discuss the three noble metals used for cast restorations. ▸ Discuss the description of gold alloys, and note the four types of gold alloys. *Class Activity Have students make a chart that lists the desirable and undesirable properties of gold as a restorative material. Then ask students to create a chart that lists the four types of alloys and their dental applications. Have students make their charts on index cards so they can use them for reference.*
Describe the properties of porcelain and its application in restoring teeth.	☐ Ceramic castings (p. 703) – Porcelain (p. 703)	PPT 63-67 TB question 18 SW Short-Answer Questions 11; Fill in the Blank questions 2, 8 (pp. 331-332) Figure 43-26 Porcelain crown (p. 703) Patient education (p. 703) Legal and ethical implications (p. 703) Eye to the future (p. 703) CTQ 5 (p. 704) ▸ Discuss ceramic castings, noting the four common combinations of ceramic-metal restorations. ▸ Discuss porcelain. Note its advantages compared to direct restorations. *Class Activity Display examples of porcelain crowns, inlays, onlays, and veneers to the class for the students to explore in addition to exploring porcelain fused to metal crowns and bridges.*
Performance Evaluation		TB SW questions (pp. 331-334)

OBJECTIVES	CONTENT	TEACHING RESOURCES
		SW Case Study (p. 334)
		Multimedia Procedures DVD: Mixing and Transferring Amalgam
		SW/ESLR Competency 43-1 Mixing and Transferring Dental Amalgam (p. 335)
		SW/ESLR Competency 43-2 Preparing Composite Resin Materials (p. 337)
		SW/ESLR Competency 43-3 Mixing Intermediate Restorative Materials (p. 339)
		SW/ESLR Competency 43-4 Mixing Acrylic Resin for Provisional Coverage (p. 341)
		ESLR Electronic Flashcards
		ESLR Practice Quiz
		Recall questions (pp. 686-703)
		CTQ 1-5 (pp. 703-704)

43.2 Homework/Assignments:

43.2 Instructor's Notes/Student Feedback:

Torres and Ehrlich Modern Dental Assisting, 9th ed.

Bird/Robinson

Slide 1

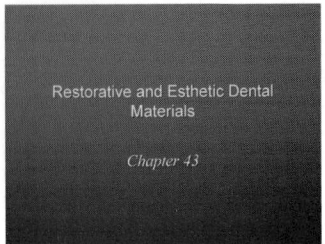

Slide 2

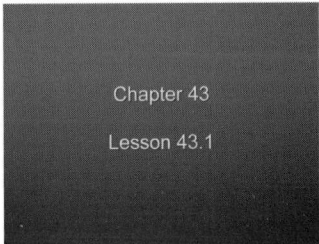

Slide 3

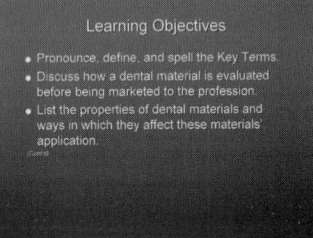

Slide 4

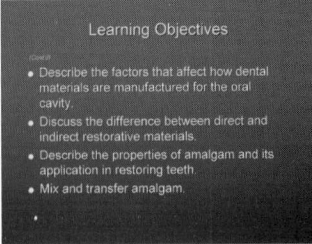

Slide 5

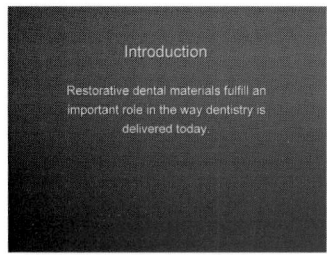

- As a clinical dental assistant, you will be spending much of your time working with various restorative and esthetic dental materials.
- It will be important to know which materials to have available, not only in the treatment rooms but also in the office supply room.
- It will be important to know how to dispense and mix these materials properly and perhaps apply some of them yourself.
- It will also be important to know how to properly clean the instruments used to prepare and place the materials and how to properly dispose of any leftover or expired materials.

Slide 6

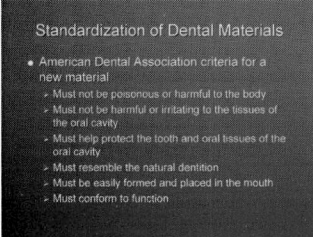

- The Council on Dental Materials, Instruments and Equipment, a subcommittee of the American Dental Association, works with federal agencies to ensure that strict specifications are followed by manufacturers in the development of new dental materials.
- What is an example of a dental material that has been the subject of a lot of public discussion about its safety?
- Many materials may be harmful to the oral cavity when in their unset or unmixed component form yet, if handled properly, provide a safe and desirable restoration once completed.

Slide 7

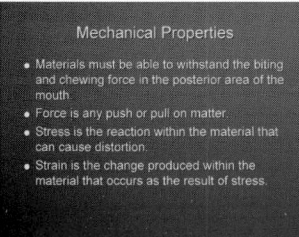

- Mechanical properties of a material placed in the anterior area should also withstand various forces caused by factors, including occlusion and a patient's habits.
- A restoration will eventually reach a breaking point, causing permanent deformation (change) after a certain amount of both stress and strain is applied over a certain amount of time.
- Stress is the amount of load per unit of a cross-sectional area. What is an example of stress?
- Remember that different materials have different properties under different types of force.

Slide 8

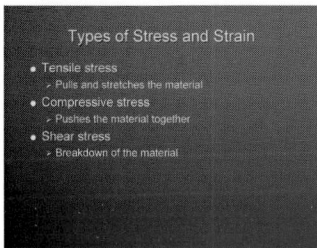

- What type of stress may a material undergo if subjected to the following scenarios?
  - A patient enjoys eating sticky candy. *(Tensile stress.)*
  - A patient reports clenching his teeth when he is concentrating hard at work. *(Compressive stress.)*
  - A patient has a habit of grinding her teeth at night, or nocturnal bruxism, *(Shear stress.)*

Bird/Robinson

Slide 9

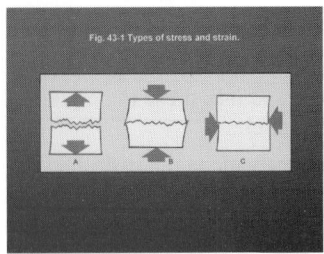

- What type of stress does diagram A represent? *(Tensile: eating sticky foods.)*

- What type of stress does diagram B represent? *(Compressive: clenching teeth.)*

- What type of stress does diagram C represent? *(Shear: nocturnal bruxism.)*

- These types of stresses may also be demonstrated to students using the palms of your hands.

Slide 10

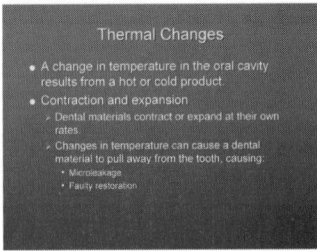

- Has anyone experienced sensitivity caused by a hot or cold food or drink in his or her mouth?

- When the restorative material and surrounding tooth structure have different rates of contraction and expansion, microleakage may occur. Space between the tooth and the restoration allows saliva or bacteria to enter, causing sensitivity and or breakdown of that interface and ultimately destroying the restoration and permitting decay in the tooth.

- he ideal restorative material is one that contracts and expands at a rate similar to that of the tooth within which it was placed.

Slide 11

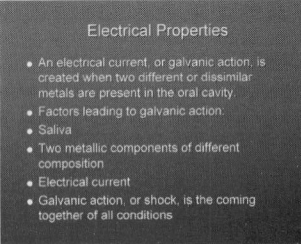

- What does galvanic shock feel like? *(An undesirable tingling sensation.)*

- One patient who may report such a feeling is someone who has teeth on opposing arches that contact each other in function. The teeth contain restorations composed of different metals (e.g., a full gold crown opposing a large amalgam).

- In the above scenario, the oral cavity acts like a battery, with saliva helping relay the electrical current.

Slide 12

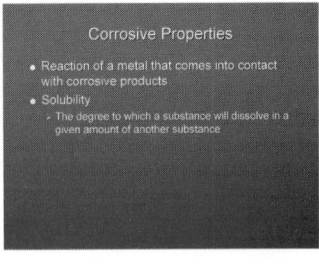

- What common drinks or foods have corrosive properties? *(Soft drinks, concentrated lemonade, and other products that create a highly acidic oral environment.)*

- Plaque that remains for an extended period on the margin between an amalgam and the tooth may also produce a more acidic environment locally.

- An acidic environment (lactic acid under dental plaque) drastically changes the solubility of tooth structure, such as enamel. Because enamel is the hardest substance in the body, the plaque must have been present for a considerable amount of time for a cavity to occur.

ELSEVIER

Slide 13

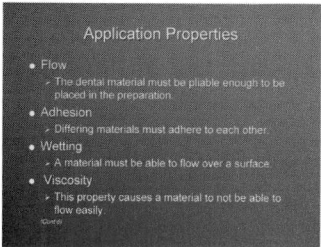

- When sealants that help prevent decay are placed on newly erupted permanent molars that are deeply fissured, the sealant material must flow well to plug up and protect areas that are not easily cleaned.

- Adhesion may be thought of as placing a piece of tape on a piece of paper.

- A consideration in wetting is whether two materials are hydrophilic (water-loving) or hydrophobic (water-hating). A hydrophilic surface would not be wet well by a hydrophobic liquid.

-

Slide 14

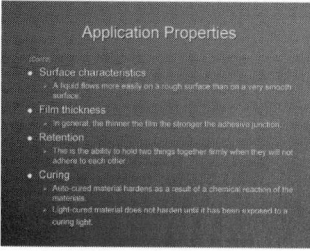

- For an example of ideal film thickness, think of piecing together a broken china ornament using Krazy Glue rather than the thicker glue used in gradeschool craft projects.

- Retention is very important in the preparation of teeth that are to receive amalgam fillings. One of the ways in which retention is achieved is preparing the opposing inside walls of the tooth to slant slightly inward so that when amalgam is placed and set it will not slide out.

- Bonded materials are set (hardened) by various means, including exposure to light of a particular wavelength, chemical reaction (auto), or a combination of the two.

Slide 15

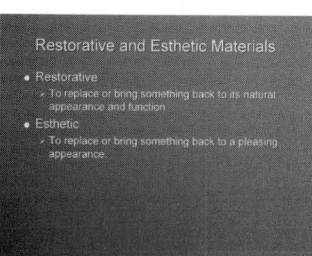

- Numerous materials fulfill most of the aforementioned criteria, yet there is an ongoing search for new materials and improvements to existing materials so that they may fulfill all criteria.

- Today much emphasis is placed on the esthetic aspect of restorative dentistry as patients seek to obtain, and dental professionals seek to create, a beautiful, natural-looking smile.

Slide 16

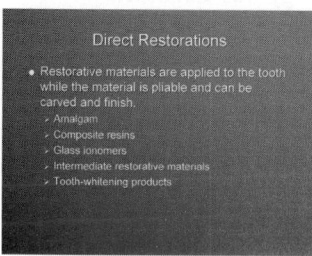

- The first four materials are placed in the mouth and adjusted to a desirable finish. They replace tooth structures that are missing as a result of cavity removal, fracture, or a deficiency at the time of the appointment.

- Tooth-whitening systems are examples of esthetic restorative dentistry.

- There are very distinct methods of dispensing, preparing, placing, and finishing these materials. All are very technique-sensitive and offer a wide range of treatment options.

Slide 17

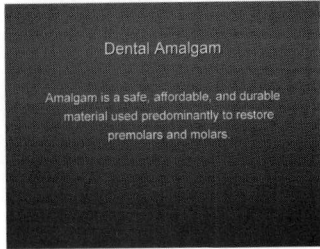

- Although amalgam has been used in restorative dentistry for many years, you may see fewer amalgam restorations placed as a result of esthetic concerns of patients and the ongoing controversy about the safety of amalgam use for both the patient and staff.

- Even if you see a minimal number of amalgam restorations being newly placed, you will surely see numerous existing amalgam restorations that remain in good condition for many years after placement.

Slide 18

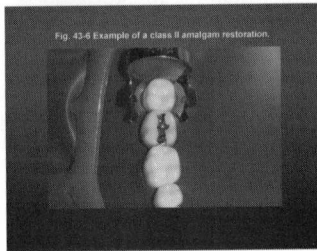

- This figure shows a lower right posterior arch isolated by means of a rubber dam (blue), a rubber dam clamp (metal ring), and rubber dam retainer (yellow plastic).

- A class II restoration is one that includes both the necessary portion of the occlusal surface and the proximal surface abutting the adjacent tooth, in this case the mesial.

- Ideally all teeth to be restored should be isolated with the use of a rubber dam in this manner. In reality, clinical circumstances do not always allow this.

Slide 19

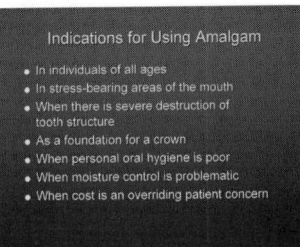

- The most convincing indication for amalgam placement continues to be when restoring an area where blood and saliva contamination is extremely difficult, beneath the gingiva, or both or in a poorly accessible, nonaesthetic region of the mouth where composites are contraindicated.

Slide 20

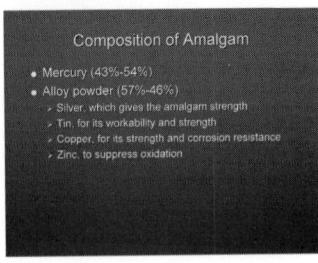

- A patient who present with an amalgam allergy should be questioned about the specific reaction and how the allergy was diagnosed.

- It is important to ask patients which type of restoration they prefer if choice is an option.

- If the patient opts for an unfavorable choice, the discussion should be documented.

- Once a restoration has been placed in the mouth, the materials used and methods followed must be documented in the patient's chart.

Slide 21

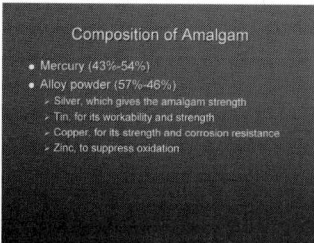

- The widely used Eames technique specifies a 1:1 ratio of mercury to alloy.

- If you have the opportunity to work with amalgam, you may eventually be able to distinguish between brands because of how they feel when properly triturated and how workable they are during condensation and carving.

Slide 22

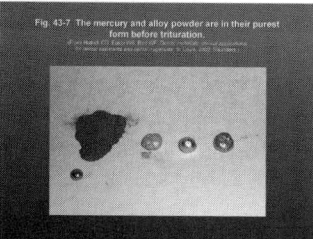

- This photo displays the mercury liquid and alloy powder, separated on the left, and at various stages of mixing to produce a final amalgam for placement.

- It is important to ensure that trituration is complete before amalgam is placed in a carrier for placement in the preparation. Different manufacturers call for different trituration times, depending on the components of their products.

- Other variables to keep in mind: Triturating machines sometimes malfunction, and stocked amalgam capsules may reach their expiration dates before being used.

Slide 23

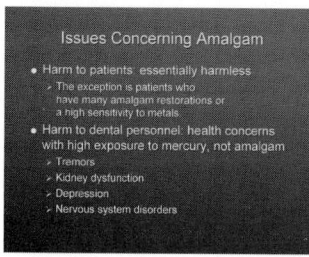

- It is important to stress to patients that once amalgam is set, the mercury content is inactive.

- Until the amalgam is set, though, components of the composite are toxic to tissues. The public is not aware of this because the irritating components are not commonly used words.

- It may be more detrimental to remove more tooth by replacing a sound amalgam restoration than to leave it alone. The oral environment may be reexposed with removal.

Slide 24

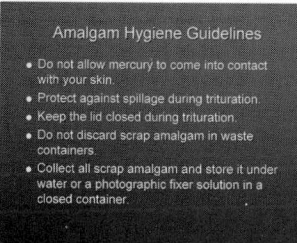

- It is very important to follow these guidelines for safe usage.

- Discard undermixed amalgam materials.

- The scrap-amalgam container should be disposed of properly, too.

Torres and Ehrlich Modern Dental Assisting, 9th ed.
Bird/Robinson

Slide 25

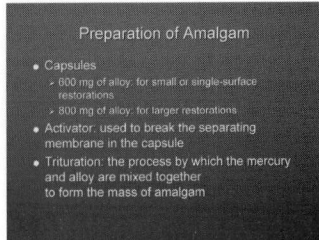

- Amalgam capsules come in different doses, so you should try to estimate what you need.

- Avoid triturating another dose of amalgam until the dentist is ready for it.

Slide 26

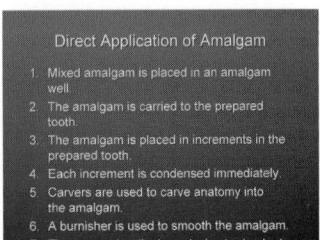

- If the restoration involves a proximal surface, a matrix band and wedge must be placed to reform the contour as necessary. The burnisher is used at this step to burnish the metal where contact will be reestablished with the adjacent tooth.

- Polishing of amalgams, if desired, is is done during a subsequent appointment with the use of a polishing cup and a slow-speed handpiece.

Slide 27

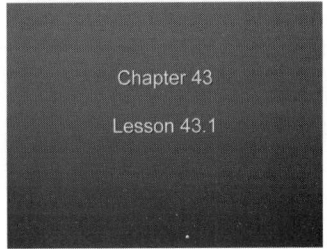

Slide 28

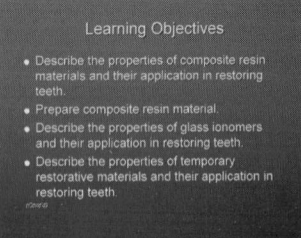

Torres and Ehrlich Modern Dental Assisting, 9th ed.

Bird/Robinson

Slide 29

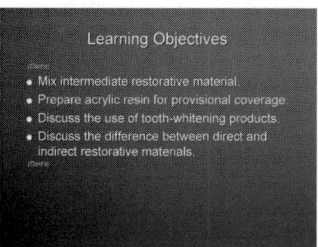

Slide 30

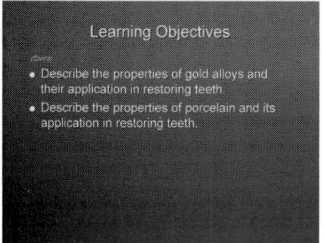

Slide 31

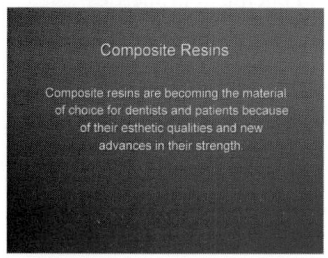

- Ask how many students have had composites placed in their mouths and if they are able to tell which teeth are composites by visual examination or touch.

Slide 32

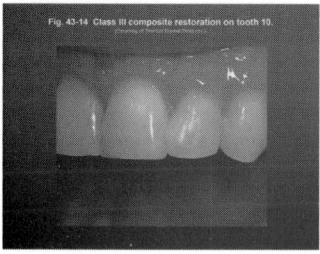

- The photograph depicts composite restorations on the mesial incisal facial of tooth 9 and the mesial facial of tooth 10.

- A skilled operator is able to disguise a composite restoration using color or color combination and by incorporating contours similar to the tooth's contralateral.

Torres and Ehrlich Modern Dental Assisting, 9th ed.

Bird/Robinson

Slide 33

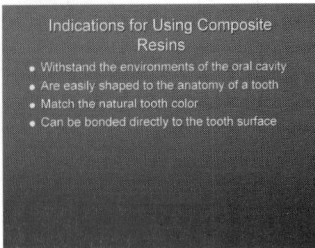

- What oral environments may be unfavorable for placement of a composite resin? *(Poor isolation, poor oral hygiene, tremendous bruxism, and lack of use of a night guard.)*
- Overall treatment-planning note: If the patient desires full-mouth whitening, it should be done before placement of any composites in an esthetic region, or the composites may no longer match after whitening.

Slide 34

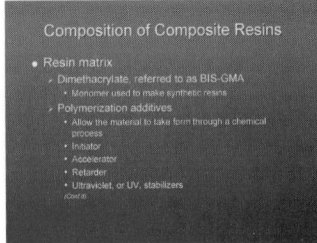

- Dimethacrylate is a tissue irritant in its monomer state.
- Polymerization is the process of bringing together multiple monomer units, using light as a catalyst.

Slide 35

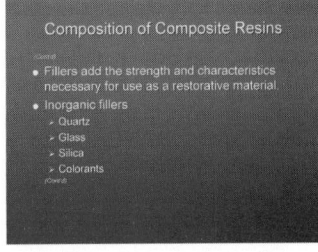

- Fillers come in many shapes and sizes and are used in different amounts to produce the desired physical and chemical properties.

Slide 36

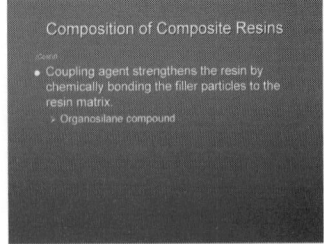

Torres and Ehrlich Modern Dental Assisting, 9th ed.
Bird/Robinson

Slide 37

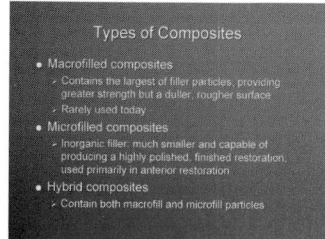

- Hybrid composites are widely used today for universal applications. They provide a happy medium of strength and polishing ability.

Slide 38

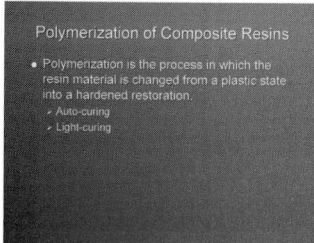

- Recall the definition of auto-curing.

- In light-curing, what determines the duration of curing? *(Manufacturer of* material *instructions, type of light being used, thickness and size of material being placed, shade of material being used.)*

Slide 39

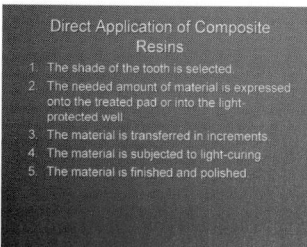

- The shade should be chosen before the tooth is prepared because dessication throughout the procedure changes the color.

- Some operators like to place the material directly into the tooth themselves with the use of the handheld applicator.

- Only 1- to 2-mm increments should be placed and light-cured at one time.

Slide 40

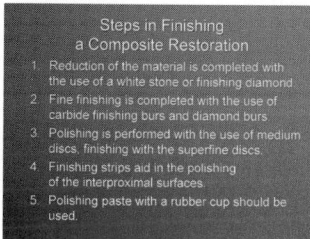

- Proper occlusion should be reestablished first.

- In addition to polishing discs, points and cups help shape the newly placed restoration.

Torres and Ehrlich Modern Dental Assisting, 9th ed.

Bird/Robinson

Slide 41

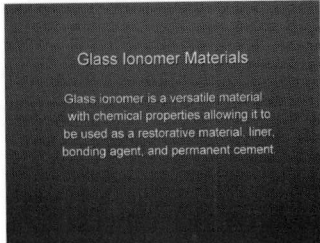

- Commercial examples of these are Vitrebond and Fuji LC.

Slide 42

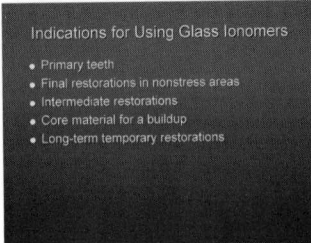

- In the restoration of a deep cavity preparation, CaOH (Dycal) may be placed in the deepest portion over the pulp as a liner, followed by glass ionomer (Vitrebond), which must be light-cured.

- The remaining preparation is then etched, bonded, and restored with the use of composite resin.

- Glass ionomer alone may also be placed on dentin in a slightly deep area of a preparation.

Slide 43

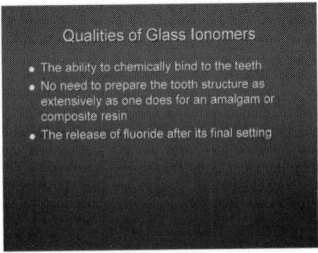

- Note that etching and other pretreatments are not necessary, so the smear layer remains.

- The components may be light-sensitive.

- The material is biocompatible.

Slide 44

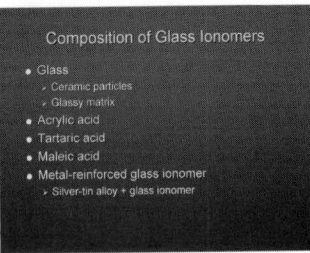

- Ionomers in the name "glass ionomers" refer to which ion-crosslinked polymers? *(acrylic, tartaric, and maleic acids)*

Slide 45

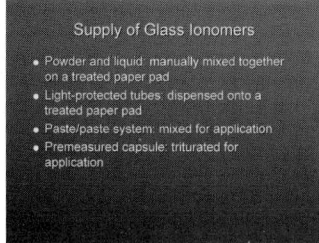

- Preparation tip: With powder and liquid components, such as Vitrebond, the powder is fluffed to loosen the components before being dispensed.

- Place with the use of a ball applicator (only on dentin).

- Half a millimeter or less should be placed first and cured, after which a second layer of as much as 2 mm may be placed.

- Components should be mixed in 10 to 15 seconds to allow ample working time (about 2 minutes). The mixture should then be light-cured for a minimum of 30 seconds.

- Remember, a higher room temperature will increase the setting time.

Slide 46

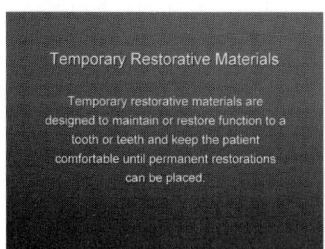

- These materials may also be used in emergency patients when insufficient time is allotted for definitive restoration.

- Eugenol, or oil of clove, provides a sedative effect.

Slide 47

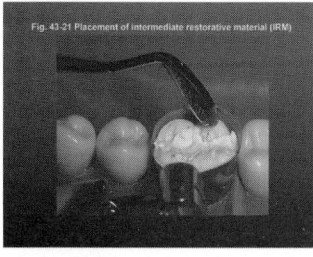

- This slide displays a molar isolated with the use of a rubber dam and surrounded by a matrix and matrix holder (bottom of photo), with and a wedge (blue) at the distal edge.

- The bright-white material, IRM, is being placed with the use of the instrument shown in the image.

- Newly mixed IRM has a puttylike consistency and must remain dry until it is completely set.

Slide 48

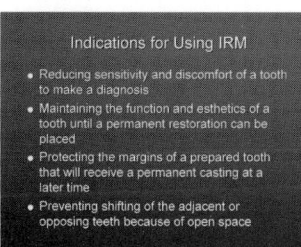

- *Describe clinical situations in which IRM may be placed:*

  - *A patient presents with a very sensitive posterior tooth. Caries removal extends deep toward the pulp and extensively throughout the tooth to the point that a crown is indicated.*

  - *IRM may be placed for 4 to 8 weeks to see whether symptoms decrease before final restoration (direct, indirect, or both). The necessity for a root canal can be evaluated before the final restoration.*

  - *IRM placement is also usefule in situations in which the diagnosis, the prognosis of the tooth, or both are unclear and under circumstances in which time is limited, such as in emergency treatment.)*

Torres and Ehrlich Modern Dental Assisting, 9th ed.

Slide 49

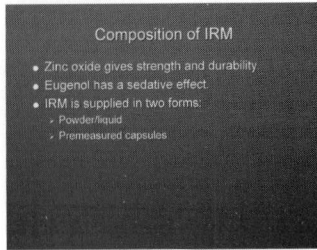

- Is IRM compatible with composite resin? *(No.)*
- If IRM is dispensed as a powder and a liquid, what is the ratio? *(One drop to one scoop, mixed with the use of a metal spatula.)*
- If IRM is dispensed in premeasured capsules, they are mixed by means of trituration, like amalgam capsules, in an amalgamator.
- Both of these methods may require the addition of more powder to improve manipulation.

Slide 50

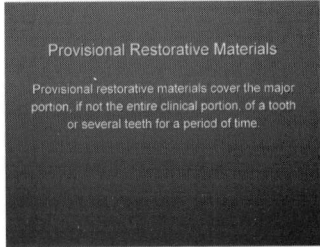

- You will need to be comfortable with dispensing and mixing this material if you assist in indirect restorative procedures.
- Knowledge of this material will also be important if you are asked to fabricate provisional restorations as an expanded-duty assistant.

Slide 51

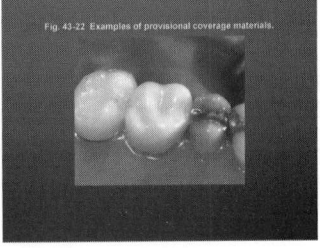

Slide 52

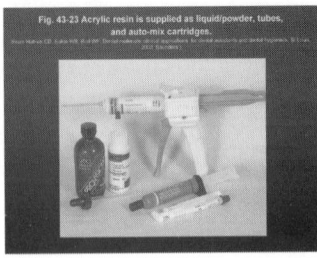

- At the bottom left are a liquid (dark bottle) and a powder (white bottle). The dropper is used to measure liquid into a dappen dish, to which the powder is gradually added to achieve the desired consistency.
- This photo displays a few of the dispensing methods for these materials, including an auto-mixing tip attached to a cartridge with two separate barrels, which is attached to a dispensing gun.

Slide 53

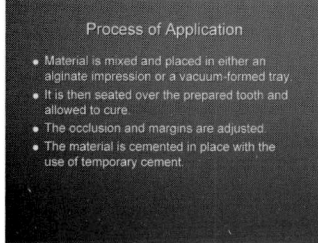

Process of Application

- Material is mixed and placed in either an alginate impression or a vacuum-formed tray.
- It is then seated over the prepared tooth and allowed to cure.
- The occlusion and margins are adjusted.
- The material is cemented in place with the use of temporary cement.

- Vacuum-formed tray: plastic stent formed over model of the tooth or teeth before preparation for an indirect restoration.

- Caution: Some materials set in an exothermic reaction (giving off heat) Therefore the necessary precautions, such as rinsing the tooth with cool water during setting, should be taken.

- Some provisional materials must be polished to a final luster.

Slide 54

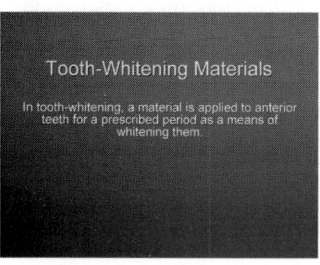

Tooth-Whitening Materials

In tooth-whitening, a material is applied to anterior teeth for a prescribed period as a means of whitening them.

- Ask the students how many of them have had their teeth whitened. If some have, ask them to share their experiences with the class.

- Tooth whitening is an important adjunct to overall treatment plans in cosmetic restorative dentistry.

- Besides the anterior teeth, all the facial/buccal surfaces of teeth that are visible when the patient is smiling can be whitened.

- Reminder: Only natural tooth structures will whiten. Indirect porcelain restorations and direct composite resins will not.

Slide 55

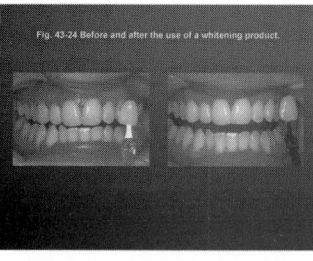

Fig. 43-24 Before and after the use of a whitening product.

- A shade guide is used to record the patient's baseline tooth shade before whitening.

- The baseline shade must be recorded in the patient's chart.

- Notes should also be made of other baseline characteristics, such as the shade of the canines which are usually darker than the rest of the dentition.

- Some practitioners also take clinical before-and-after photos.

Slide 56

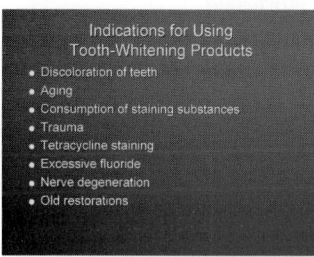

Indications for Using Tooth-Whitening Products

- Discoloration of teeth
- Aging
- Consumption of staining substances
- Trauma
- Tetracycline staining
- Excessive fluoride
- Nerve degeneration
- Old restorations

- Tooth whitening is contraindicated during pregnancy and lactation.

- For optimal results, teeth should be clean and free of plaque.

- Individuals with tetracycline staining (intrinsic) will have to wait longer than individuals whose teeth are discolored as a result of time, age, and extrinsic staining to wait longer to see results from whitening.

Bird/Robinson

Slide 57

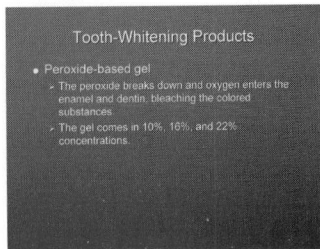

- In general, concentrations dispensed for at-home use are lower than those used for in-office tooth whitening.

Slide 58

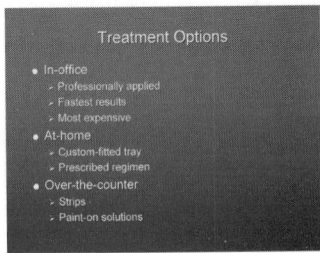

- Individuals who undergo in-office whitening, which involves the use of a higher concentration of solution over a short period, may experience a higher level of postprocedure sensitivity.

- Final whitening results appear a few weeks after the completion of treatment completion. At this time, nonmatching composite resins, veneers, and porcelain crowns are replaced with ones that match.

Slide 59

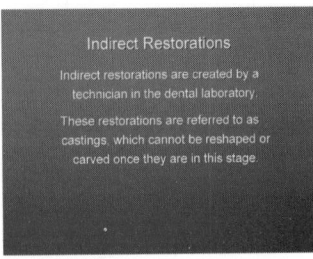

- What are some of the indications for the placement of an indirect restoration?

  - *A considerable amount of the natural tooth structure is missing as a result of trauma, decay, or fracture.*

  - *A tooth has been endodontically treated.*

  - *Cosmetics or function needs to be restored.*

  - *A surgically placed implant(s) must be restored.*

Slide 60

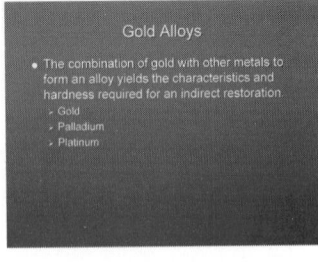

- Impressions of the prepared tooth structure are taken in the dental office and sent to a dental laboratory to be fabricated.

- Gold remains one of the best restorative materials and most biocompatible, despite esthetic concerns.

Bird/Robinson

Slide 61

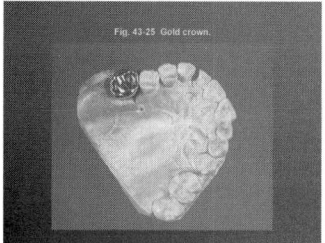

- This photo displays a stone model of a patient's maxilla with a full gold crown on tooth 3 before adjustment and final cementation in the patient's mouth.

Slide 62

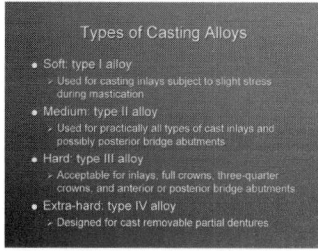

- Ask students whether they have any gold jewelry with the carat marking visible on the inside. Note that a 10K or 14K ring is more durable than a 24K ring, which has a higher gold content.

- One advantage of a type I alloy, used for inlays in areas bearing less stress, is that its margins can be burnished.

- A type IV alloy is much more durable when used as a framework to support the acrylic base and teeth.

Slide 63

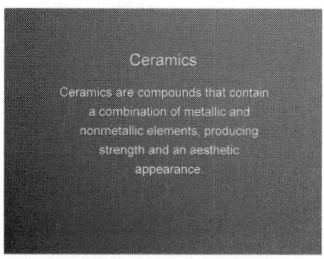

- Ceramics were incorporated into indirect restorative options for a more aesthetic result compared with the full metal crown previously shown.

- The preparation design differs slightly, according to where metal, porcelain, or both may be sought in the final preparation.

- Clinical cementing procedures and materials may differ, depending on whether the crown being cemented is made entirely of metal, of porcelain and metal, or of porcelain alone.

Slide 64

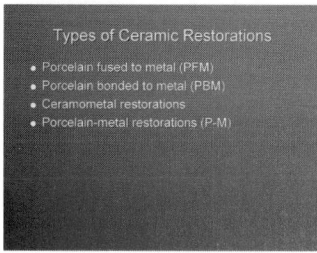

- The above are examples of restorations that are aesthetically conscious, for the most part. They use a tooth-colored material on the outside and are reinforced with metal on the inside.

- Porcelain-on-metal castings remain a popular choice for a full-coverage crown or a multiple-unit bridge, whereas all-porcelain crowns are being used more frequently now in the anterior region for aesthetic purposes.

- Remember to document the materials that were placed in the patient's mouth in the patient's chart.

Bird/Robinson

Slide 65

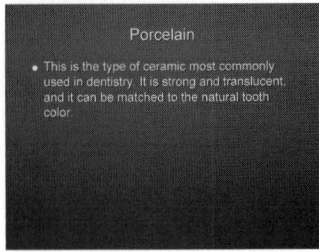

- More than one shade of porcelain may be used to create a more natural look, such as a darker shade near the gingival margin that gradually blends into a lighter and more translucent shade toward the incisal edge.
- As an assistant, you will most likely be asked to help write the laboratory scripts for the dental lab when sending an impression off for the fabrication of a porcelain crown. Some offices now send or e-mail intraoral photos to their dental labs to aid in crown fabrication.

Slide 66

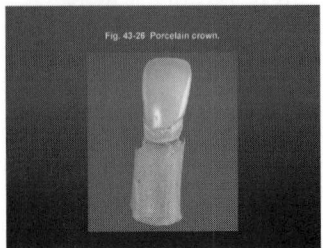

- The porcelain crown shown here is on a die of stone. The crown is fabricated as multiple layers of baked porcelain. The die is a replica of the prepared tooth that is being covered with a provisional restoration while the crown is being fabricated at the dental laboratory.
- Although most indirect restorations are fabricated by outside dental labs using intraoral impressions of the prepared teeth, you may work in an environment that has a machine used to mill ceramic restorations in the office from a computer-generated reproduction of a prepared tooth.

Slide 67

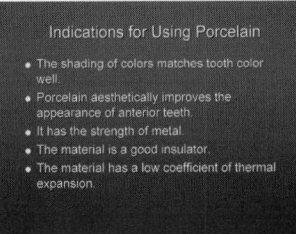

- Remember that shade selection for a porcelain crown should ideally take place in natural light, especially if the crown will be located in a region of aesthetic concern. If a nearby source of natural light is not accessible, the ideal is outside the office.
- Review: Porcelain has a low coefficient of thermal expansion. What would be a possible consequence if a material had a high coefficient of thermal expansion?

Bird/Robinson

Lesson Plan
44 Dental Liners, Bases, and Bonding Systems

TEACHING FOCUS

This chapter introduces the student to topics related to dental liners, bases, and bonding systems. The student will become acquainted with prepared tooth structures, dental liners, varnishes, dentin sealer, dental bases, and dental bonding. Procedures related to the application of dental liners, bases, and bonding systems will be discussed.

MATERIALS AND RESOURCES

- ☐ air-water syringe (Lessons 44.2 and 44.3)
- ☐ amalgam condenser (Lesson 44.2)
- ☐ applicator device or brush (Lesson 44.3)
- ☐ basic setup (Lessons 44.2 and 44.3)
- ☐ bonding agent (Lesson 44.3)
- ☐ calcium hydroxide applicator (Lesson 44.1)
- ☐ calcium hydroxide base and catalyst paste (Lesson 44.1)
- ☐ computer and PowerPoint projector (all Lessons)
- ☐ cotton pellets (Lesson 44.3)
- ☐ cotton rolls (Lesson 44.3)
- ☐ dental dam (Lesson 44.3)
- ☐ dental varnish (Lesson 44.1)
- ☐ dentin sealer materials (Lesson 44.2)
- ☐ etchant material (Lesson 44.3)
- ☐ eugenol liquid and dropper (Lesson 44.2)
- ☐ extracted teeth (Lessons 44.1 and 44.3)
- ☐ gauze pads (all Lessons)
- ☐ glass slab (Lesson 44.2)
- ☐ high-velocity evacuator (Lesson 44.3)
- ☐ micro brush applicators (Lessons 44.1 and 44.2)
- ☐ oral evacuation system (Lessons 44.2 and 44.3)
- ☐ plastic instrument (Lesson 44.2)
- ☐ polycarbonate liquid (Lesson 44.2)
- ☐ polycarbonate powder and dispenser (Lesson 44.2)
- ☐ prepared posterior teeth (Lesson 44.2)
- ☐ restorative textbook photos (Lesson 44.1)
- ☐ small ball instrument (Lesson 44.1)
- ☐ small paper mixing pad (Lesson 44.1)
- ☐ small spatula (Lessons 44.1 and 44.2)
- ☐ string (Lesson 44.3)
- ☐ syringe tip (Lesson 44.3)
- ☐ timer (Lesson 44.3)
- ☐ treated paper pad (Lesson 44.2)
- ☐ zinc oxide powder and dispenser (Lesson 44.2)
- ☐ zinc phosphate liquid and dropper (Lesson 44.2)
- ☐ zinc phosphate powder and dispenser (Lesson 44.2)

LESSON CHECKLIST

Preparations for this lesson include:

- lecture
- evaluation of student knowledge and skills needed for comprehension and application of principles underlying dental liners, bases, and bonding systems, including:
  - ○ how the sensitivity of a tooth determines the type of dental material selected
  - ○ the purpose and application of cavity liners
  - ○ the purpose and application of varnishes
  - ○ the purpose and application of dentin sealers
  - ○ the purpose and application of dental bases
  - ○ the etching process of a tooth
  - ○ the purpose and application of bonding systems

ELSEVIER

Torres and Ehrlich Modern Dental Assisting, 9th ed.
Bird/Robinson

KEY TERMS

dessicate (p. 717)
etchant (p. 715)
etching (p. 715)
eugenol (p. 711)
hybrid (p. 717)
insulating (p. 711)
micromechanical (p. 717)

obliterating (p. 717)
polymerize (p. 718)
retention (p. 715)
sedative (p. 711)
smear layer (p. 717)
thermal (p. 707)

ADDITIONAL RESOURCES

PowerPoint slides (Evolve): 1-28

Legend

CTQ
Critical
Thinking
Question

DVD
Multimedia
Procedures
Videos and
Animations

ESLR
EVOLVE
Student
Learning
Resources

IDO
Interactive
Dental
Office
CD-ROM

SW
Student
Workbook

TB
Test Bank
on the
TEACH
CD-ROM

PPT
PowerPoint
Slides

Class Activities are indicated in **bold italic.**

LESSON 44.1

PRETEST

1. Which type of dental base contains eugenol, which provides a sedative effect on irritated pulp?
   a. ZOE
   b. zinc phosphate
   c. polycarboxylate
   d. Vitrebond

2. Which dental material seals dentinal tubules, reduces leakage around restoration, and acts as a barrier against highly acidic cements?
   a. calcium hydroxide
   b. Dycal
   c. varnish
   d. zinc phosphate

3. Dentin sealer is also referred to as a
   a. varnish.
   b. desensitizer.
   c. phosphoric acid.
   d. dental liner.

4. Before restoring a tooth with composite resin, how long is the tooth etched?
   a. 5 to 10 seconds
   b. 15 to 30 seconds
   c. 45 to 60 seconds
   d. 1 to 2 minutes

5. Zinc phosphate cement is mixed
   a. on a gauze pad.
   b. on a cool glass slab.
   c. in the mouth.
   d. on a paper pad.

6. Stimulating the production of reparative or secondary dentin, protecting the pulp from chemical irritation, and compatibility with numerous types of restorative material are all characteristics of which dental liner?
   a. polycarboxylate
   b. calcium hydroxide
   c. fluoride varnish
   d. zinc phosphate

7. Thermal changes from hot and cold or electrical energy created by other metals coming into contact with the tooth are defined as which type of pulpal stimuli?
   a. biological
   b. chemical
   c. mechanical
   d. physical

8. Before dentin bonding, what function does acid etching have?
   a. closing the dentinal tubules
   b. burning the tooth
   c. addition of the smear layer
   d. removal of the smear layer

9. Which supplementary dental material may be placed to provide a protective, insulating, and sedative effect in a moderately deep cavity preparation before amalgam placement?
   a. fluoride varnish
   b. etchant
   c. Copalite
   d. dental base

ELSEVIER

10 .At which stage in cavity preparation and restoration should a dental varnish be applied?
- a. after the application of the liner
- b. after the placement of amalgam
- c. before the application of the liner
- d. before placement of composite resin

Answers

1. a	3. b	5. b	7. d	9. d
2. c	4. b	6. b	8. d	10. a

BACKGROUND ASSESSMENT

Question: List an example of a dental liner and a dental base. What are their main characteristics, and how are these materials applied?

Answer: Calcium hydroxide is a dental liner that is placed only on dentin over the deepest portion of the preparation in order to protect the pulp from chemical irritation and to stimulate the production of reparative or secondary dentin. It is compatible with most types of restorative materials. Zinc oxide-eugenol is a dental base with insulating and sedative properties that is not compatible with composite resins.

Question: One of the first steps of bonding composite resin to prepared dentin is acid etching. What is the usual composition of acid etch? What does the etch do to dentin? How is it applied and used? What is the next step following acid etching?

Answer: Acid etch is usually a 35% phosphoric acid gel that is dispensed into an isolated tooth preparation from a syringe tip. Depending on the situation, the etchant is left on the tooth for 15 to 30 seconds and later thoroughly washed off with the air-water syringe and high-speed suction. Care is taken not to completely desiccate the tooth, in order to avoid post-operative sensitivity. Etching helps provide a stronger mechanical bond between the prepared tooth structure and the bonded resins by way of enamel tags and removal of the smear layer to expose the dentinal tubules. Once etching is complete, a bonding agent is applied before the ultimate placement of the definitive composite resin.

CRITICAL THINKING QUESTION

A 35-year-old man in general good health arrives at the dental office complaining of upper right first molar tooth sensitivity for the past month; this is triggered when he drinks cold beverages or when he breathes cold air. This cold sensitivity does not last very long once the stimulus is removed. The tooth does not hurt when he bites. After a clinical examination and evaluation of a radiograph, the dentist informs the patient that there is a moderate-to-deep cavity in the tooth. The dentist decides to remove the cavity in order to better evaluate the patient's treatment and restorative options. How would the dental assistant set up the room with respect to restorative materials?

Guidelines: All of the appropriate materials should be available for a definitive amalgam or composite restoration (chosen by mutual agreement between the dentist and patient). However, in this situation, because of an anticipated caries removal depth beyond the standard (usually about 0.5 mm into dentin), a liner or a base should be available for placement as a protective feature before placing the chosen restoration. The assistant should anticipate that for a deep preparation a liner such as calcium hydroxide (commercially available example, Dycal) may be indicated, over which a base such as glass ionomer (commercially available example, Vitrebond) may be placed. In a moderately deep preparation, a base alone may be placed before the final restoration. Recall that calcium hydroxide will dry on its own, whereas a glass ionomer like Vitrebond will require light curing to achieve the final set. If placing an amalgam, a varnish or dentin sealer should be available as the next layer, whereas for composite resin, the acid etch and dentin bonding should be available.

OBJECTIVES	CONTENT	TEACHING RESOURCES
Pronounce, define, and spell the Key Terms.	■ Key terms (p. 705)	◪ SW Fill in the Blank questions 1-12 (pp. 343-344) ⓔ ESLR Electronic Flashcards ▸ Discuss each of the key terms, focusing on the definition, pronunciation, and spelling of each. *Class Activity **Have students work in pairs to write a mock dialogue between a dentist and the assistant using each***

OBJECTIVES	CONTENT	TEACHING RESOURCES
		of the key terms properly in a sentence. Have the student pairs recite their dialogues in front of the class. Correct their pronunciation if necessary.
Discuss how the sensitivity of a tooth determines what type of dental material is selected for a procedure.	■ Prepared tooth structures (p. 706) ■ Pulpal responses (p. 706) ☐ Types of pulpal stimuli (p. 707)	PPT 5 TB questions 1-2 SW Short-Answer Questions 1; Fill in the Blank question 2; Multiple Choice question 15 (pp. 343, 345) Table 44-1 Supplementary Dental Materials and Application in Order of Use (p. 706) ▶ Discuss the physical circumstances under which a tooth requires a shallow, moderately deep, or deep preparation and what dental materials can be used in each preparation. ▶ Discuss types of pulpal stimuli and how sensitivity drives the decision as to what type of dental material is selected. *Class Activity Organize stations around the classroom with displays of restorative textbook photos or a variety of extracted teeth, each of which demonstrates various preparations, shallow and deep, extensive and conservative. Have students rotate through the stations and record why they think a certain material or materials may be placed according to multiple variables, including depth and remaining tooth structure. Have various students share their thoughts on each example.*
Discuss how and why cavity liners are used in restoring tooth structure.	■ Dental liners (p. 707) ☐ Calcium hydroxide (p. 707)	PPT 6-10 TB question 3 SW Short-Answer Questions 2; Multiple Choice question 1 (pp. 343-344) ▶ Discuss the purpose of a dental liner. ▶ Discuss the characteristics of calcium hydroxide that make it a frequently selected type of cavity liner. *Class Activity Have each student draw a tooth in cross-section using different colors to represent different layers of the tooth, while leaving in the tooth a void representing the deep cavity preparation (similar to Fig. 44-1, p. 707). Have the students use a different color to show where in the prepared tooth the cavity liner should be placed (on dentin only, over deepest portion of pulpal floor). Students may also list the three distinctive characteristics of calcium hydroxide on their drawings. Have students keep the drawings for a future activity.*

Torres and Ehrlich Modern Dental Assisting, 9th ed.

Bird/Robinson

OBJECTIVES	CONTENT	TEACHING RESOURCES
Apply calcium hydroxide to a prepared tooth surface.	☐ Application (p. 707) **Procedure** 44-1 The application of calcium hydroxide (Expanded Function) (p. 708) (SW/ESLR Competency 44-1, p. 347)	⊠ PPT 9-10 SW Multiple Choice questions 2-3 (p. 344) SW/ESLR Competency 44-1 Applying Calcium Hydroxide (Expanded Function) (p. 347) Recall questions 1-3 (p. 707) Examples of commercial dental liners (p. 707) Figure 44-1 Placement of a liner (p. 707) ▸ Discuss the two types of liners available. Note that a liner is placed only on dentin and must be avoided on enamel or in retentive grooves. ▸ Discuss the application of calcium hydroxide. ***Class Activity Distribute paper on which you have marked several dots from the small size of a ballpoint pen mark to the size of a felt tip marker. (The dots represent the approximate range of diameters on the pulpal floor of dentin to which calcium hydroxide is usually applied). Have students practice dispensing small equal amounts of the base and catalyst of calcium hydroxide on a pad, mixing with a spatula and then using the appropriate small ball instrument to apply small amounts to the predrawn dots.***
Discuss how and why varnishes are used in restoring tooth structure.	■ Varnish (p. 707)	⊠ PPT 11-14 TB question 4 SW Short-Answer Questions 3; Multiple Choice questions 4-5 (pp. 343-344) Figure 44-2 Microscopic view of dentin structure with exposed dentinal tubules (p. 709) ▸ Discuss dental varnish and its purposes. ***Class Activity Ask the class to recite the three main reasons for varnish use, Write them on the board.***
Apply dental varnish to a prepared tooth surface.	☐ Application (p. 707) **Procedure** 44-2 The application of dental varnish (expanded function) (p. 710) (SW/ESLR Competency 44-2, p. 349) ☐ Fluoride varnish (p. 709)	⊠ PPT 13 SW/ESLR Competency 44-2 Applying Dental Varnish (Expanded Function) (p. 349) Figure 44-3 Location for placement of cavity varnish (p. 709) Examples of commercial varnishes (p. 709) Figure 44-4 Type of fluoride varnish currently used in the United States (p. 709) Recall questions 4-5 (p. 710)

OBJECTIVES	CONTENT	TEACHING RESOURCES
		▸ Discuss the application of dental varnish, noting that varnish is always placed after the liner is applied.
		▸ Discuss fluoride varnish and its advantages. Note the specific indications for the use of fluoride varnish.
		***Class Activity** Allow students to take turns applying two coats of dental varnish such as Copalite with microbrush applicators to all surfaces of a cavity preparation before amalgam placement. Have students time and record how long the varnish takes to evaporate.*

44.1 Homework/Assignments:

44.1 Instructor's Notes/Student Feedback:

Torres and Ehrlich Modern Dental Assisting, 9th ed.

Bird/Robinson

LESSON 44.2

CRITICAL THINKING QUESTION

A 50-year-old man comes to the office for an emergency visit complaining that an old, large silver filling fell out of his tooth this morning while he was eating breakfast. He can feel the void in his tooth and can see it when he opens his mouth and looks in the mirror, and the tooth is sensitive to cold. His concern is that he does not have time to stay for a long appointment today as he has a flight to catch in a few hours and will be away on business for the next week. The patient asks whether there is anything the dentist can do quickly to make him comfortable over the next week until he returns from his trip. What can be done?

Guidelines: With time for placement of a definitive restoration limited, IRM (zinc-oxide eugenol) is a good sedative restoration that will not only soothe a sensitive tooth (given that decay does not extend to the pulp, and that other potential problems such as fracture are ruled out) but will also temporarily help fill in voided areas that have exposed dentin and rough edges. IRM will keep bacteria from harboring in the preparation and causing further decay over time. It will also help hold the remaining tooth structure intact. Ideally, decay should be removed before placement. Recall that IRM is not bonded to the tooth but rather is held intact via mechanical retentive features. It must be allowed to set completely before final adjustments are made and the patient dismissed. Finally, IRM should not be kept in the tooth longer than from a few weeks to a couple of months because it will eventually dissolve in the oral environment, and the margins will deteriorate. IRM is not compatible with composite restorations.

OBJECTIVES	CONTENT	TEACHING RESOURCES
Discuss how and why desensitizers are used in restoring tooth structure.	■ Desensitizer (p. 710)	▣ PPT 17 ▦ SW Short-Answer Questions 4; Multiple Choice questions 6-7 (pp. 343-344) ▸ Discuss the purpose of a desensitizer. Note that it is also referred to as a "primer." ▸ Discuss the fact that no surface layer is formed when using a desensitizer, meaning that it can be used in all indirect restorations. ***Class Activity** Have students add to their drawings from Lesson 1. Ask them to list the main reason for placing a desensitizer.*
Apply desensitizer to a prepared tooth surface.	☐ Application (p. 710) Procedure 44-3 The application of a desensitizer (expanded function) (p. 711) (SW/ESLR Competency 44-3, p. 351)	▣ PPT 17 ▦ ℮ SW/ESLR Competency 44-3 Applying a Desensitizer (Expanded Function) (p. 351) Recall questions 6-7 (p. 711) ▸ Discuss the application of desensitizers. Note the steps involved in application. ▸ Discuss the components of desensitizer, emphasizing that it must be used sparingly and that no material is allowed to contact soft tissue. ***Class Activity** Have students apply desensitizer to a clean, prepared tooth surface with a microbrush applicator, waiting 30 seconds and being sure that the sealer is dry before the second application.*

Bird/Robinson

OBJECTIVES	CONTENT	TEACHING RESOURCES
Discuss how and why dental bases are used in restoring tooth structure.	■ Dental bases (p. 711)	⊠▤ PPT 18 TB question 5 SW Short-Answer Questions 5; Multiple Choice question 8 (pp. 343-344) Examples of commercial cement bases (p. 715) ▸ Discuss the circumstances under which dental bases are placed under a permanent restoration. ▸ Discuss the three ways in which a base is designed to provide pulpal protection. *Class Activity While performing the Class Activity below, have one student in each group give a narrative explaining the steps involved in placing a dental base and the reasoning behind each step. Have one of the members of each group hold the procedure notes and all members lend feedback. If a step is missed, performed incorrectly, or incorrectly stated, the operator should start over again.*
Mix and place three types of bases on a prepared tooth surface.	☐ Types of materials used (p. 711) ☐ Application (p. 711) Procedure 44-4 Mixing and placing zinc oxide-eugenol (ZOE) cement as a base (expanded function) (p. 712) (SW/ESLR Competencies 44-4 to 44-6, p. 353) Procedure 44-5 Mixing and placing zinc phosphate cement as a base (expanded function) (p. 713) (SW/ESLR Competencies 44-4 to 44-6, p. 353) Procedure 44-6 Mixing and placing polycarboxylate cement as a base (expanded function) (p. 714) (SW/ESLR Competencies 44-4 to 44-6, p. 353)	⊠▤ PPT 19-20 TB question 6 SW Fill in the Blank questions 4, 7, 11; Multiple Choice questions 9-11 (pp. 344-345) SW/ESLR Competencies 44-4 to 44-6 Mixing a Selected Type Of Cement for a Base in a Prepared Tooth (p. 353) Recall questions 8-11 (p. 715) Figure 44-5 Location for placement of a base (p. 715) ▸ Discuss types of materials used to form dental bases. Describe the circumstances under which each type of material is selected and note each material's advantages and disadvantages. ▸ Discuss the procedural steps involved in the application of zinc oxide-eugenol, zinc phosphate, and polycarbonate. *Class Activity Set up three work areas, each with a different base material to be evaluated. Divide the class into small groups. Have one student in a group manipulate the material while the other students provide feedback, as described above. Provide students with various prepared posterior teeth (molars and premolars, both maxillary and mandibular), and have them attempt dispensing, mixing, and placing the base found at their respective stations. Have students switch roles so that everyone has a chance to manipulate the materials. Have a class discussion at the end of the activity about whether manipulation or placement was more difficult.*
44.2 Homework/Assignments:		

ELSEVIER

Torres and Ehrlich Modern Dental Assisting, 9th ed.

Bird/Robinson

44.2 Instructor's Notes/Student Feedback:

LESSON 44.3

CRITICAL THINKING QUESTION

A 13-year-old boy with good oral hygiene and no previous cavities comes to the office for two small occlusal pit composite restorations on his upper left molars. The boy's mother is present in the treatment room and asks the dental assistant why the dentist recommended tooth-colored fillings instead of silver ones. How should the assistant respond?

Guidelines: Because the areas needing caries removal and restorations are very small and in non–stress-bearing areas, less tooth structure will have to be taken away in order to place the restoration. This more conservative preparation may be achieved because of the bonding abilities of the bonding agent and composite resin. The assistant should explain that if an amalgam were to be placed, more tooth structure would have to be removed in order to incorporate retentive features. In this case, with more natural tooth structure remaining, the tooth is stronger and generally at less risk for future complications such as fracture or sensitivity. Also, composite is tooth-colored and is thus more esthetic compared to amalgam. The assistant should also stress the importance of maintaining good oral hygiene.

OBJECTIVES	CONTENT	TEACHING RESOURCES
Describe the etching process of a tooth and its importance in the bonding of tooth and material.	■ Dental etchant (p. 715) ■ Dental bonding (p. 715)	PPT 23-27 TB questions 7-8 SW Short-Answer Questions 6; Fill in the Blank questions 5, 9, 12; Multiple Choice question 12 (pp. 343-345) Figure 44-6 Microscopic view of enamel tags after etching (p. 715) ▸ Discuss dental bonding and its improved retention properties. ▸ Discuss etchant and why it is critical for bonding. *Class Activity **Have students use their fingers to represent the surface area of dental bonding. Have them use pieces of string to measure and, later, compare the area if only the fingertips were exposed for bonding versus if the full outer surface of the individual fingers were exposed (etched enamel/dentin).***
Describe the bonding systems and how they provide a better adherence of dental materials to the tooth structure.	☐ Dentin bonding (p. 717) ☐ Enamel bonding (p. 717)	PPT 23-26 SW Short-Answer Questions 7; Fill in the Blank questions 1, 6, 8, 10; Multiple Choice questions 13-14 (pp. 343-345) Figure 44-7 Microscopic view in various stages of etching (p. 717) Recall questions 12-15 (p. 719) ▸ Discuss examples of enamel bonding and when each type is used. ▸ Discuss dentin bonding and the need to maintain a slight amount of moisture on the dentin. Discuss the need to remove the smear layer when bonding.

OBJECTIVES	CONTENT	TEACHING RESOURCES
		Class Activity Before class have students ask the dentists to whom they go which bonding system or systems they use and why. Students may also call their closest state dental school and inquire which bonding system it has chosen and why. Have student volunteers report back to the class. (For students to prepare for this activity, see Homework Assignments #1.)
Apply etchant material.	□ Application (p. 717) – Guidelines for clinical application of bonding products (p. 718) Procedure 44-7 Applying an etchant material (expanded function) (p. 716) (SW/ESLR Competency 44-7, p. 355)	PPT 27 SW Fill in the Blank question 3 (p. 343) SW/ESLR Competency 44-7 Applying an Etchant Material (Expanded Function) (p. 355) *Class Activity Using sterilized, extracted teeth with practice preparations in them, have students practice applying etchant to both dentin and enamel or to enamel only. Have them wait the prescribed amount of time, rinse thoroughly, and evaluate the surface.*
Apply a bonding system to the prepared tooth structure.	□ Application (p. 717) – Guidelines for clinical application of bonding products (p. 718) Procedure 44-8 Applying a bonding system (expanded function) (p. 718) (SW/ESLR Competency 44-8, p. 357)	PPT 27-28 SW Fill in the Blank question 3 (p. 343) SW/ESLR Competency 44-8 Applying a Bonding System (Expanded Function) (p. 357) Patient education (p. 719) Legal and ethical implications (p. 719) Eye to the future (p. 719) ▸ Discuss the procedural steps involved in the application of etchant. ▸ Discuss the different bonding systems and the general guidelines involved in the application of a bonding system. ▸ Discuss the questions the dental assistant might ask a patient who comes in with tooth sensitivity. *Class Activity Using the extracted teeth from the previous Class Activity, have students apply a bonding agent. Have them apply one coat to some teeth and multiple coats to other teeth. Ask them to note any surface differences between coats as well as before and after light curing, if indicated.*
Performance Evaluation		TB SW questions (pp. 343-345) SW Topics for Discussion (p. 345) SW/ESLR Competency 44-1 Applying Calcium Hydroxide (Expanded Function) (p. 347)

OBJECTIVES	CONTENT	TEACHING RESOURCES
		SW/ESLR Competency 44-2 Applying Dental Varnish (Expanded Function) (p. 349)
		SW/ESLR Competency 44-3 Applying a Desensitizer (Expanded Function) (p. 351)
		SW/ESLR Competencies 44-4 to 44-6 Mixing a Selected Type Of Cement for a Base in a Prepared Tooth (p. 353)
		SW/ESLR Competency 44-7 Applying an Etchant Material (Expanded Function) (p. 355)
		SW/ESLR Competency 44-8 Applying a Bonding System (Expanded Function) (p. 343)
		ESLR Electronic Flashcards
		ESLR Practice Quiz
		Recall questions (pp. 707-719)
		CTQ (p. 720)

44.3 Homework/Assignments:

1. Have students ask the dentists to whom they go which bonding system or systems they use and why. Students may also call their closest state dental school and inquire which bonding system it has chosen and why.

44.3 Instructor's Notes/Student Feedback:

Slide 1

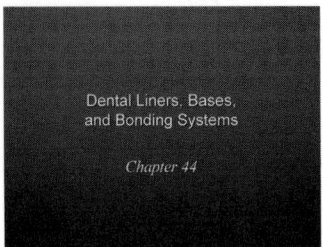

Dental Liners, Bases, and Bonding Systems

Chapter 44

Slide 2

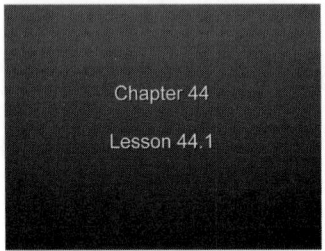

Chapter 44

Lesson 44.1

Slide 3

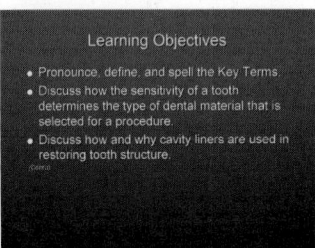

Learning Objectives

- Pronounce, define, and spell the Key Terms.
- Discuss how the sensitivity of a tooth determines the type of dental material that is selected for a procedure.
- Discuss how and why cavity liners are used in restoring tooth structure.

Slide 4

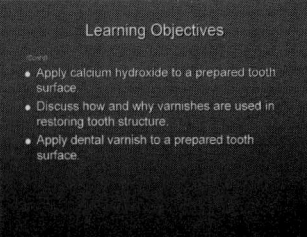

Learning Objectives

- Apply calcium hydroxide to a prepared tooth surface.
- Discuss how and why varnishes are used in restoring tooth structure.
- Apply dental varnish to a prepared tooth surface.

Slide 5

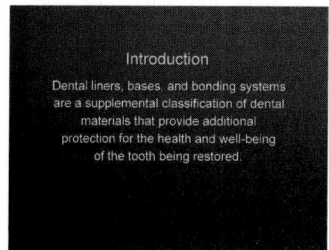

- Liners and bases can make a big difference in postoperative sensitivity and long-term pulpal prognosis when used appropriately.

- Liners and bases are even used in a cavity preparation that is small in circumference but deep.

Slide 6

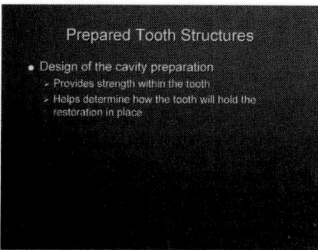

- This is different with amalgam, which relies primarily on retentive features such as removing enough tooth structure so that opposing walls are slanted slightly inward.

- Yet in general, the more natural tooth structure that remains, the stronger the tooth remains.

Slide 7

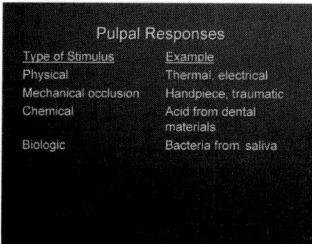

- The pulp is found inside the tooth and contains the nerve and blood supply that keep the tooth alive and supplied with nutrients.

- These are only a few of the stimuli that may trigger an unfavorable response from the pulp, either in a reversible or irreversible manner. Irreversible trauma to the pulp will require endodontic treatment (a root canal) to save the tooth.

Slide 8

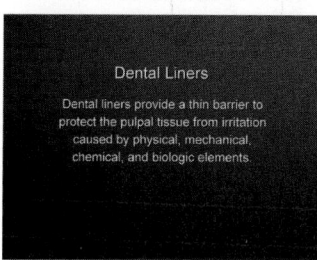

- Liners help protect the pulp from the irreversible irritations that may lead to endodontic therapy or an extraction.

Torres and Ehrlich Modern Dental Assisting, 9th ed.

Bird/Robinson

Slide 9

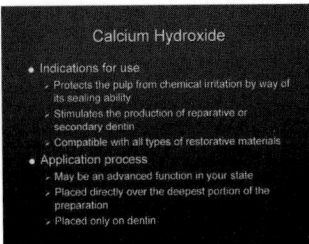

- The ability of calcium hydroxide to stimulate the production of reparative or secondary dentin is unusual among dental materials.

Slide 10

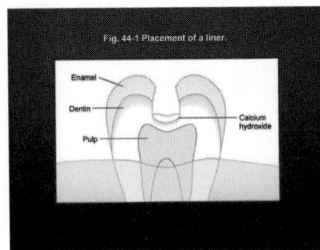

- This drawing represents a cross-section of a tooth with its various layers and the preparation in the middle.

- As shown, calcium hydroxide is placed over the deepest portion of the pulpal floor, and only on dentin.

Slide 11

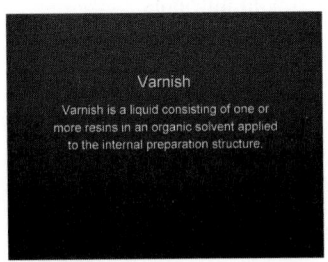

- If varnish is indicated, would it be placed before or after placement of calcium hydroxide? *(After.)*

Slide 12

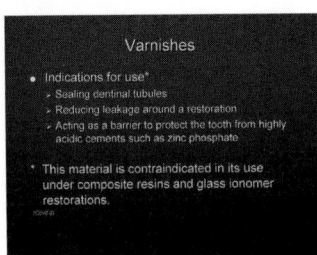

- A popular use is placing dental varnish such as Copalite throughout the preparation, just before amalgam placement.

- Note: Dental varnish has a distinct noxious smell that evaporates quickly. Care should be taken to replace the lid as soon as possible after dispensing it.

ELSEVIER

Torres and Ehrlich Modern Dental Assisting, 9th ed.
Bird/Robinson

Slide 13

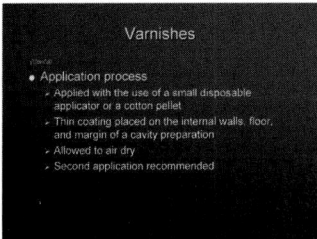

- For efficiency purposes, the dentist usually applies the varnish while the assistant carefully prepares the amalgam.

Slide 14

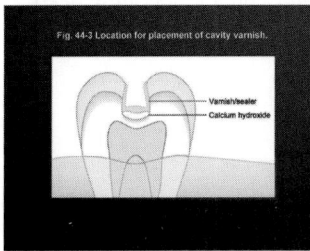

- This drawing reiterates that varnish or sealer is placed over the liner, which is applied first and is allowed to set.

- As you will see later in the lesson, a base is also sometimes placed after the liner, but before the sealer.

Slide 15

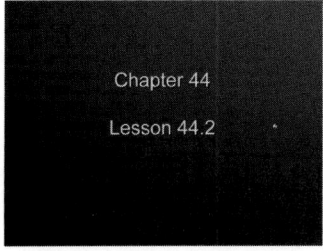

Slide 16

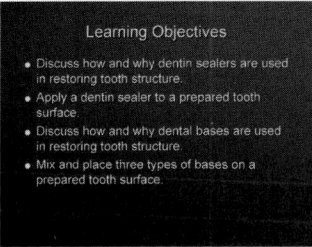

Slide 17

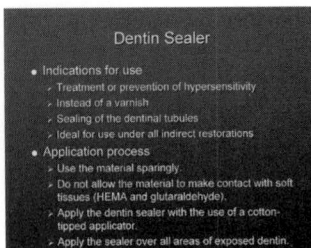

- Dentin sealer is used under restorations as per the listed indications.

- It may also be used as a temporary and conservative desensitizer in areas that may not be readily or immediately restored, for example, cervical abraction or in areas of toothbrush abrasion instead of doing a cervical/gingival composite.

Slide 18

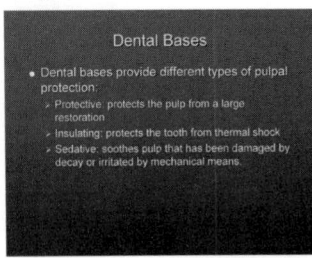

- Recall that for the reasons listed in this slide, a base would be applied over a liner (if a liner was indicated) or directly on a moderately deep dentinal floor. Following this, the varnish and/or sealer would be placed before final restoration.

Slide 19

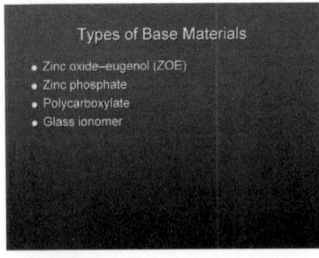

- Common commercial examples of dental bases include:

  - IRM (zinc-oxide-eugenol-ZOE)

  - Tenacin (zinc phosphate)

  - Durelon (polycarboxylate)

  - Vitrebond (glass ionomer). Glass ionomer is a popular option as it is compatible under composite resins and easy to manipulate and place.

Slide 20

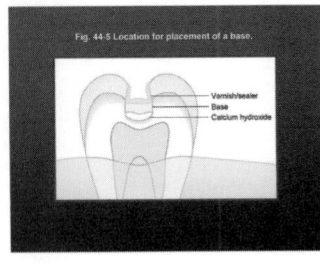

- This diagram shows the proper order of placement of the base over the liner.

- The varnish or sealer is then placed over the base.

- A bonding agent would be placed over the base (after etching), if composite resin was to be placed.

Slide 21

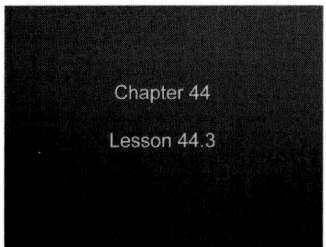

Slide 22

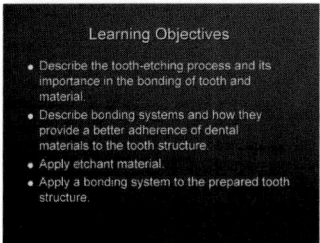

Slide 23

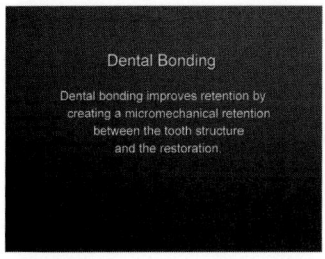

- Bonding agents allow for the removal of less tooth structure before definitive restoration placement as minimal retentive features are needed.

- Direct bonding to the tooth is achieved by removal of the smear layer with etchant.

- The use of a light helps the operator control the set time of the material.

Slide 24

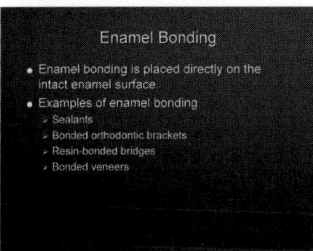

- Sealant material is held in place also by occlusal developmental grooves.

- Bonded veneers are an example of an esthetic option available to a person who wishes to change the shape, size, and color of the teeth. A very small layer of the facial enamel is removed, followed by an impression that allows the dental laboratory to fabricate a new facial surface in porcelain; this surface is bonded permanently to the prepared teeth.

Bird/Robinson

Slide 25

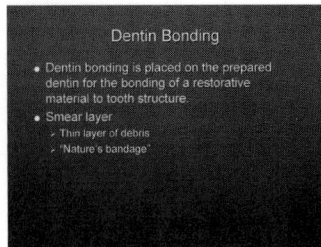

- Preparing the tooth surface properly with acid etch for removal of the smear layer before bonding allows for more exposed microscopic surface area, and thus micromechanical retention is also achieved.

Slide 26

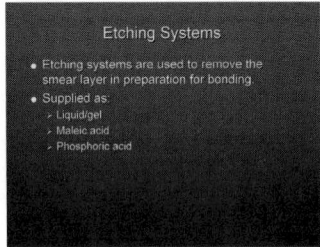

- Proper isolation of the teeth to be treated is necessary because contact with skin or soft tissues in the mouth will cause a burn and/or irritation.

- The acid etch is usually 35% phosphoric acid gel, colored (for example, blue) so that it is easier to see where it is placed and whether it has been completely washed off.

Slide 27

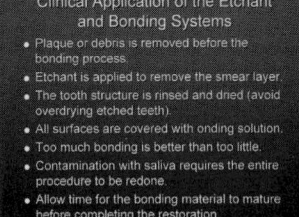

- How is plaque removed before bonding?

- Note: the fluoride usually found in prophy paste may interfere with proper bonding.

- The bonding agent is usually light-cured.

- Some practitioners, as well as manufacturers, advocate the application of multiple layers of bonding agent.

Slide 28

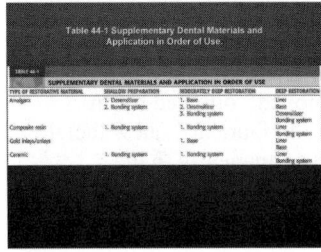

- This table is a simplified guide to how some of the materials discussed may be used in clinical practice.

- The treatment plan often changes once a tooth is actually opened up and evaluated.

- As research in the field of restorative dentistry continues to progress, the methods and materials used will change.

Bird/Robinson

TEACHING FOCUS

This chapter will introduce the student to topics related to dental cements. The student will become acquainted with the classification of dental cements, the variables affecting final cementation, types of cements, and cement removal. Mixing various types of cements, including zinc oxide-eugenol, zinc phosphate, polycarboxylate, glass ionomer, and composite resin will be discussed. The student will have the opportunity to put this information into context by participating in classroom activities and discussions.

MATERIALS AND RESOURCES

- ☐ applicators (Lesson 45.2)
- ☐ basic setup (Lesson 45.2)
- ☐ bonding system (Lesson 45.2)
- ☐ computer and PowerPoint projector (all Lessons)
- ☐ cotton pellets (Lesson 45.2)
- ☐ dental floss (Lesson 45.2)
- ☐ etching system (Lesson 45.2)
- ☐ eugenol liquid and dropper (Lesson 45.2)
- ☐ gauze pads, 2 in. by 2 in. (all Lessons)
- ☐ glass ionomer liquid and dropper (Lesson 45.2)
- ☐ glass ionomer powder and dispenser (Lesson 45.2)
- ☐ glass slab (Lesson 45.2)
- ☐ mixing pad (Lesson 45.2)
- ☐ paper mixing pad (Lesson 45.2)

- ☐ polycarbonate liquid (in plastic squeeze bottle or calibrated syringe) (Lesson 45.2)
- ☐ polycarbonate powder and dispenser (Lesson 45.2)
- ☐ resin cement (Lesson 45.2)
- ☐ spatula (flexible stainless steel) (all Lessons)
- ☐ spoon evacuator (Lesson 45.2)
- ☐ treated paper pad (all Lessons)
- ☐ zinc oxide powder and dispenser (Lesson 45.2)
- ☐ zinc phosphate liquid and dropper (Lesson 45.2)
- ☐ zinc phosphate powder and dispenser (Lesson 45.2)
- ☐ ZOE accelerator paste (Lesson 45.2)
- ☐ ZOE eugenol catalyst paste (Lesson 45.2)

LESSON CHECKLIST

Preparations for this lesson include:

- lecture
- evaluation of student knowledge and skills needed to perform all entry-level activities related to dental cements, including:
  - ○ understanding the classification of dental cements
  - ○ noting the variables affecting final cementation
  - ○ mixing and preparing zinc oxide-eugenol for temporary and permanent cementation
  - ○ mixing and preparing zinc phosphate, polycarboxylate, glass ionomer, and composite resin for cementation
  - ○ removing cement

KEY TERMS

dissipate (p. 730)
exothermic (p. 723)
luting agent (p. 722)

provisional (p. 722)
retard (p. 730)
spatulate (p. 730)

ADDITIONAL RESOURCES

PowerPoint slides (Evolve): 1-39
Multimedia Procedures DVD:
    Mixing Zinc Phosphate for Permanent Cementation
    Removing Cement

Legend

CTQ
Critical
Thinking
Question

DVD
Multimedia
Procedures
Videos and
Animations

ESLR
EVOLVE
Student
Learning
Resources

IDO
Interactive
Dental
Office
CD-ROM

SW
Student
Workbook

TB
Test Bank
on the
TEACH
CD-ROM

PPT
PowerPoint
Slides

Class Activities are indicated in ***bold italic***.

ELSEVIER

Torres and Ehrlich Modern Dental Assisting, 9th ed.

Bird/Robinson

LESSON 45.1

PRETEST

1. What are temporary cements primarily used for?
   a. veneers
   b. crowns
   c. denture repairs
   d. provisional temporaries

2. What is the term used to describe the releasing of heat from a chemical reaction?
   a. setting time
   b. exothermic
   c. hypothermic
   d. retard

3. What ingredient has a soothing effect on the pulp?
   a. polyacrylic acid
   b. phosphoric acid
   c. eugenol
   d. water

4. What is the normal mixing time for zinc oxide-eugenol?
   a. 10 to 30 seconds
   b. 30 to 60 seconds
   c. 1 to 2 minutes
   d. 3 to 5 minutes

5. Zinc oxide-eugenol is mixed on a(n)
   a. oil-resistant pad.
   b. paper pad.
   c. glass slab.
   d. metal slab.

6. What is type I glass ionomer cement used for?
   a. a liner and dentin bonding agent
   b. restoring areas of erosion near the gingiva
   c. cementation of metal restorations and direct-bonded orthodontic brackets
   d. cementation of veneers

7. How is zinc phosphate dispensed?
   a. powder/liquid form
   b. capsules
   c. gel
   d. pastes

8. When mixing zinc phosphate, what is the ideal temperature of the glass slab?
   a. 60°
   b. 65°
   c. 68°
   d. 74°

9. Premeasured capsules are commonly used with cements because they
   a. are inexpensive.
   b. are convenient.
   c. have a longer working time.
   d. can be reused.

10. What type of cement is used for veneers?
    a. composite resin
    b. ZOE
    c. zinc phosphate
    d. polycarboxylate

Answers

1. d	3. c	5. a	7. a	9. b
2. b	4. b	6. c	8. c	10. a

Bird/Robinson

BACKGROUND ASSESSMENT

Question: What does the term *luting* mean?

Answer: Luting means to "glue" two items together. It describes the adhesion of an indirect restoration to the tooth structure. Luting agents can be manufactured for permanent or temporary adhesion.

Question: What are the proper procedural steps for mixing zinc phosphate for permanent cementation?

Answer: The first step is to read the manufacturer's directions on the amounts of powder and liquid to be used for a permanent restoration. Next, dispense the appropriate amounts of powder and liquid onto a cooled glass slab, and divide the powder into increments as directed by the manufacturer. To start the mixing procedure, add one increment at a time to the liquid and mix over a large area on the glass slab. Figure-eight motions are suggested to help dissipate the heat that is generated during the spatulation. Continue to add increments of powder until the desired consistency has been reached. The material should string up about 1 inch from the glass slab. Approximate mixing time from start to finish is 1 to 2 minutes.

CRITICAL THINKING QUESTION

A woman comes to the office to have a gold crown on tooth #3 placed permanently. However, she mentions that she has been experiencing a dull ache and temperature sensitivity in that area for the past five days. After the dentist examines the area, he informs the dental assistant that he will cement the gold crown on tooth #3 with temporary cement. Why is this change in cementation needed?

Guidelines: Because the woman is experiencing pain in the area of tooth #3, the dentist may want to wait to cement the restoration permanently in case the restoration needs to be removed. For example, if tooth #3 is diagnosed for root canal therapy because of the pain the woman is experiencing, it will be easier to remove the restoration if it is cemented temporarily than if it is cemented permanently. Using temporary cement also decreases the chance of damaging the restoration upon removal.

OBJECTIVES	CONTENT	TEACHING RESOURCES
Pronounce, define, and spell the Key Terms.	■ Key terms (p. 721)	*e* ESLR Electronic Flashcards SW Fill in the Blank questions 1-6 (p. 359) ▸ Discuss each of the key terms in Chapter 45, focusing on the definition, pronunciation, and spelling of each term. ***Class Activity Have students use each key term in a sentence.***
Describe luting cements and differentiate between permanent and temporary cements.	■ Classification of dental cements (p. 722) ☐ Permanent cements (p. 722) ☐ Temporary cementation (p. 722)	PPT 5-9 TB questions 1-2 SW Short-Answer Questions 1; Fill in the Blank questions 3-4, 6; Multiple Choice questions 1-2; Case Study question 1 (pp. 359-360) Figure 45-1 Casting ready to be cemented (p. 723) Recall questions 1-2 (p. 723) CTQ 2 (p. 733) ▸ Discuss the three classes of dental cements. ▸ Discuss permanent and temporary cements and the uses of each.

Torres and Ehrlich Modern Dental Assisting, 9th ed.

Bird/Robinson

OBJECTIVES	CONTENT	TEACHING RESOURCES
		Class Activity Ask students to identify and provide a rationale for the appropriate use of permanent or temporary cement in the following situations: – *Full gold crown; no symptoms* – *PFM; major discomfort* – *Provisional restoration*
Discuss the factors that influence luting cements.	■ Variables affecting final cementation (p. 722) □ Mixing time (p. 722) – Guidelines for mixing dental cements (p. 722) □ Humidity (p. 723) □ Powder-to-liquid ratio (p. 723) □ Temperature (p. 723)	⊠▪ PPT 10-11 TB questions 3-4 SW Short-Answer Questions 2; Fill in the Blank question 2; Multiple Choice question 3; Case Study questions 2-4 (pp. 359-361) Figure 45-2 Hold the bottle upright when dispensing the liquid of a cement (p. 723) Recall question 3 (p. 723) CTQ 1, 4 (p. 733) ▸ Discuss mixing time, and outline guidelines for mixing dental cements. ▸ Discuss the effect of humidity on the water content of the cement. Emphasize the need to dispense the powder first and then the liquid, to minimize evaporation. ▸ Discuss the powder-to-liquid ratio and note the need to fluff the powder in the bottle before dispensing it. ▸ Discuss temperature and describe ways to manage cements with an exothermic reaction. *Class Activity Lead a group discussion on how to correct errors that were caused by certain factors, such as humidity and temperature, which affect cements.*

Torres and Ehrlich Modern Dental Assisting, 9th ed.

Bird/Robinson

45.1 Homework/Assignments:

45.1 Instructor's Notes/Student Feedback:

LESSON 45.2

CRITICAL THINKING QUESTION

A patient is in the office for permanent cementation of a porcelain crown on tooth #30. After reading the manufacturer's directions, the assistant prepares a mixture of polycarboxylate cement for the crown. The dentist seats the crown and asks the patient to bite down on a cotton roll. The procedure goes without incident. What is the next step that must be completed before the patient is excused?

Guidelines: Once the polycarboxylate cement has completed its initial setting, an explorer will be used to ensure the cement is at the proper stage. With a stable fulcrum, the dentist (or dental assistant in states that allow expanded functions) will use the edge of the explorer to carefully move the excess material away from the tooth in a horizontal direction. Overlapping strokes will remove the bulk of the cement from tooth #30. The next step is to check the margins of the restoration for any remaining cement. The dentist or dental assistant should pass a knotted floss through the mesial and distal contact areas to remove any excess cement. Postoperative home care instructions must be given to the patient before dismissal.

OBJECTIVES	CONTENT	TEACHING RESOURCES
List the five cements discussed in the chapter and identify their similarities and differences.	■ Types of cements (p. 723) □ Glass ionomer cement (p. 724) – Chemical makeup of glass ionomer cement (p. 724) – Application (p. 724)	PPT 15-20 TB question 9 SW Short-Answer Questions 3; Multiple Choice questions 13-14 (pp. 359-360) Examples of Commercial Glass Ionomer (p. 724) Figure 45-3 Premeasured capsules of glass ionomer permanent cement (p. 724) Recall questions 4-5 (p. 746) ▸ Discuss the three types of glass ionomer cement and the uses of each. ▸ Discuss the benefits of glass ionomer cement. ▸ Discuss the different forms of glass ionomer cement and note the advantages of the capsule form. *Class Activity Have students make a chart for glass ionomer cement that includes the following information:* *– Mixing time* *– Liquid/powder ratio (if applicable)* *– Temperature* *– What it is mixed on* *– Mixing method* *– Setting time*
Mix and prepare glass ionomer for cementation.	– Application (p. 724) Procedure 45-1 Mixing glass ionomer cement for permanent cementation (p. 746) (SW/ESLR Competency 45-1, p. 363)	SW/ESLR Competency 45-1 Mixing Glass Ionomer for Permanent Cementation (p. 363) ▸ Discuss the procedural steps involved in mixing glass ionomer. *Class Activity Demonstrate to the class the appropriate mixing method for glass ionomer cement.*

Torres and Ehrlich Modern Dental Assisting, 9th ed.

Bird/Robinson

OBJECTIVES	CONTENT	TEACHING RESOURCES
List the five cements discussed in the chapter and identify their similarities and differences.	☐ Composite resin cement (p. 724) – Chemical makeup of composite resin cement (p. 724) – Application (p. 725)	PPT 21-24 TB questions 10-11 SW Short-Answer Questions 3; Multiple Choice question 15 (pp. 359-360) Recall questions 6-7 (p. 725) Commercial Resin Cements (p. 725) Figure 45-4 Examples of composite resin cements supplied in variable systems (p. 725) CTQ 5 (p. 733) ▸ Discuss the indications for use of composite resin cement. ▸ Discuss the forms in which composite resin is supplied. *Class Activity **Have students make a chart for composite resin cement that includes the following information:*** 　– *Mixing time* 　– *Liquid/powder ratio (if applicable)* 　– *Temperature* 　– *What it is mixed on* 　– *Mixing method* 　– *Setting time*
Mix and prepare composite resin for cementation.	– Application (p. 725) **Procedure** 45-2 Mixing composite resin cement for permanent cementation (p. 726) (SW/ ESLR Competency 45-2, p. 365)	SW/ ESLR Competency 45-2 Mixing Composite Resin for Permanent Cementation (p. 365) ▸ Discuss the procedural steps involved in mixing composite resin for permanent cementation. ▸ Discuss the importance of removing all plaque and debris and other preparatory steps before cementation, using composite resin. *Class Activity **Demonstrate to the class the appropriate mixing method for composite resin cement.***
List the five cements discussed in the chapter and identify their similarities and differences.	☐ Zinc oxide-eugenol cement (p. 725) – Chemical makeup of zinc oxide-eugenol cement (p. 726) – Application (p. 726)	PPT 25-29 TB questions 5-6 SW Short-Answer Questions 3; Multiple Choice question 4 (pp. 359-360) Examples of Commercial ZOE Cement (p. 727) Figure 45-5 ZOE type I cement for temporary cementation (p. 726) Figure 45-6 ZOE type II cement for permanent cementation (p. 727)

Torres and Ehrlich Modern Dental Assisting, 9th ed.

Bird/Robinson

OBJECTIVES	CONTENT	TEACHING RESOURCES
		Recall questions 8-10 (p. 727)
		CTQ 3 (p. 733)
		▶ Discuss the five types of cements covered by the chapter, and note circumstances under which each might be used.
		▶ Discuss the difference between ZOE type I and ZOE type II.
		▶ Discuss precautions necessary when using ZOE.
		Class Activity Have students make a chart for zinc oxide-eugenol cement that displays the following information:
		– *Mixing time*
		– *Liquid/powder ratio (if applicable)*
		– *Temperature*
		– *What it is mixed on*
		– *Mixing method*
		– *Setting time*
Mix and prepare two-paste zinc oxide-eugenol (Tempbond) for temporary cementation.	– Application (p. 726) [Procedure] 45-3 Mixing zinc oxide-eugenol for temporary cementation (p. 727) (SW/ESLR Competency 45-3, p. 367)	SW Multiple Choice question 6 (p. 360) SW/ESLR Competency 45-3 Mixing Zinc Oxide-Eugenol for Temporary Cementation (p. 367) ▶ Discuss the procedural steps involved in mixing ZOE for temporary cementation. Note the need to fill the provisional rather than line it. *Class Activity Have students manipulate the two-paste zinc oxide-eugenol for cementation.*
Mix and prepare zinc oxide-eugenol for cementation.	– Application (p. 726) [Procedure] 45-4 Mixing zinc oxide-eugenol for permanent cementation (p. 728) (SW/ESLR Competency 45-4, p. 369)	SW Multiple Choice question 5 (p. 360) SW/ESLR Competency 45-4 Mixing Zinc Oxide-Eugenol for Permanent Cementation (p. 369) ▶ Discuss the mixing time and setting time of ZOE. ▶ Discuss the procedural steps involved in mixing ZOE for permanent cementation. *Class Activity Demonstrate to the class the appropriate mixing method for zinc oxide-eugenol.*

ELSEVIER

OBJECTIVES	CONTENT	TEACHING RESOURCES

List the five cements discussed in the chapter and identify their similarities and differences.	☐ Polycarboxylate cement (p. 727)
	
	– Chemical makeup of polycarboxylate cement (p. 728)
	
	– Application (p. 728)
		☒ PPT 30-33
		
		TB questions 7-8
		
		SW Short-Answer Questions 3; Fill in the Blank questions 1, 5; Multiple Choice questions 9-12; Case Study questions 1-5 (pp. 359-360)
		
		Figure 45-7 Powder and calibrated syringe of polycarbonate cement (p. 728)
		
		Recall questions 11-12 (p. 729)
		
		Class Activity **Have students make a chart for polycarboxylate cement that includes the following information:**
		
		  – *Mixing time*
		
		  – *Liquid/powder ratio (if applicable)*
		
		  – *Temperature*
		
		  – *What it is mixed on*
		
		  – *Mixing method*
		
		  – *Setting time*

Mix and prepare polycarboxylate for cementation.	– Application (p. 728) Procedure 45-5 Mixing polycarboxylate for permanent cementation (p. 729) (SW/ESLR Competency 45-5, p. 371)	SW/ESLR Competency 45-5 Mixing Polycarboxylate for Permanent Cementation (p. 371) ▶ Discuss the procedural steps involved in the application of polycarboxylate. *Class Activity* **Demonstrate to the class the appropriate mixing method for polycarboxylate cement.**
List the five cements discussed in the chapter and identify their similarities and differences.	☐ Zinc phosphate cement (p. 729) – Chemical makeup of zinc phosphate cement (p. 730) – Application (p. 730) Procedure 45-6 Mixing zinc phosphate for permanent cementation (p. 731) (SW/ESLR Competency 45-6, pp. 373-374)	☒ PPT 34-37 Multimedia Procedures DVD: Mixing Zinc Phosphate for Permanent Cementation TB questions 7-8 SW Short-Answer Questions 3; Fill in the Blank questions 1, 5; Multiple Choice questions 7-10; Case Study questions 1-5 (pp. 359-360) SW/ESLR Competency 45-6 Mixing Zinc Phosphate for Permanent Cementation (pp. 373-374) Figure 45-8 Zinc phosphate type I cement for permanent cementation (p. 729) Recall questions 13-16 (p. 730) ▶ Discuss the difference between type I and type II zinc phosphate.

Torres and Ehrlich Modern Dental Assisting, 9th ed.

Bird/Robinson

OBJECTIVES	CONTENT	TEACHING RESOURCES
		▸ Discuss the irritating properties of zinc phosphate, and emphasize the need to use a liner, sealer, or desensitizer.
		▸ Discuss the procedural steps involved in the application of zinc phosphate.
		Class Activity Have students make a chart for zinc phosphate cement that includes the following information:
		– Mixing time
		– Liquid/powder ratio (if applicable)
		– Temperature
		– What it is mixed on
		– Mixing method
		– Setting time
Remove cement from permanent and temporary cementations.	■ Cement removal (p. 730) [*Procedure*] 45-7 Removing cement from permanent or temporary cementation (expanded function) (p. 732)	PPT 38-39 Multimedia Procedures DVD: Removing Cement TB question 12 SW Case Study question 5 (p. 361) SW/ESLR Competency 45-7 Removing Cement from Permanent or Temporary Cementation (Expanded Function) (pp. 375) Figure 45-9 Excess cement must be removed after setting process (p. 730) Patient Education (p. 731) Legal and Ethical Implications (p. 733) Eye to the Future (p. 733) ▸ Discuss the need to remove excess cement from around the gingival margin and sulcus of the tooth. ▸ Discuss whether cement removal is an expanded option in your state. ▸ Discuss patient education points necessary for cementation procedures. *Class Activity Demonstrate to the class how to remove permanent and temporary cement from a typodont. Then have students practice removing permanent and temporary cement from the typodont.*

Bird/Robinson

OBJECTIVES	CONTENT	TEACHING RESOURCES
Performance Evaluation		🖥️ TB
		📖 SW questions (pp. 359-360)
		📖 SW Case Study (pp. 360-361)
		🎥 Multimedia Procedures DVD: Mixing Zinc Phosphate for Permanent Cementation
		🎥 Multimedia Procedures DVD: Removing Cement
		📖 𝑒 SW/ ESLR Competency 45-1 Mixing Glass Ionomer for Permanent Cementation (p. 363)
		📖 𝑒 SW/ ESLR Competency 45-2 Mixing Composite Resin for Permanent Cementation (p. 365)
		📖 𝑒 SW/ ESLR Competency 45-3 Mixing Zinc Oxide-Eugenol (ZOE) for Temporary Cementation (p. 367)
		📖 𝑒 SW/ ESLR Competency 45-4 Mixing Zinc Oxide-Eugenol (ZOE) for Permanent Cementation (p. 369)
		📖 𝑒 SW/ ESLR Competency 45-5 Mixing Polycarboxylate for Permanent Cementation (p. 371)
		📖 𝑒 SW/ ESLR Competency 45-6 Mixing Zinc Phosphate for Permanent Cementation (pp. 373-374)
		📖 𝑒 SW/ESLR Competency 45-7 Removing Cement from Permanent or Temporary Cementation (Expanded Function) (pp. 375)
		𝑒 ESLR Electronic Flashcards
		𝑒 ESLR Practice Quiz
		Recall questions (pp. 723-730)
		💡 CTQ 1-5 (p. 733)

45.2 Homework/Assignments:

45.2 Instructor's Notes/Student Feedback:

Slide 1

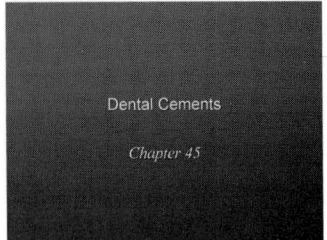

Slide 2

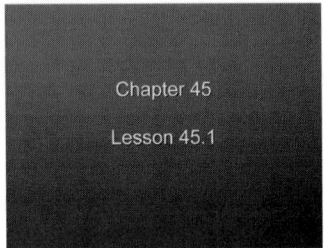

Slide 3

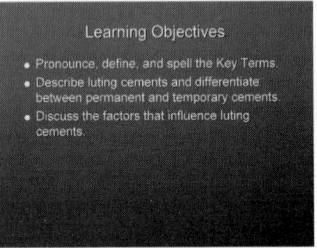

Slide 4

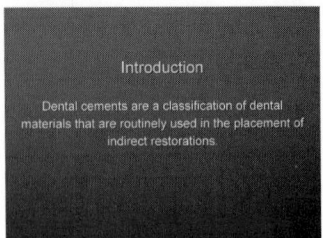

- What are examples of indirect restorations?

Torres and Ehrlich Modern Dental Assisting, 9th ed.

Bird/Robinson

Slide 5

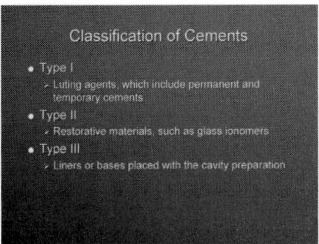

- What is a luting agent?

Slide 6

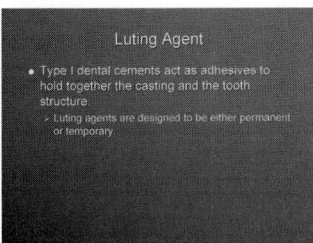

- What type of restoration can be permanently cemented?
- Why would a dentist temporarily cement a restoration?

Slide 7

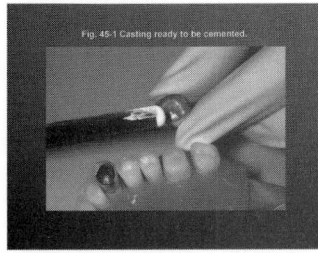

- What type of restoration is being cemented?
- What tooth number is involved?

Slide 8

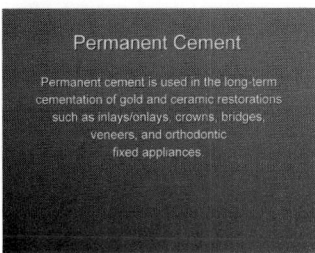

- Most restorations are cemented permanently once they are fabricated in the laboratory.

Bird/Robinson

Slide 9

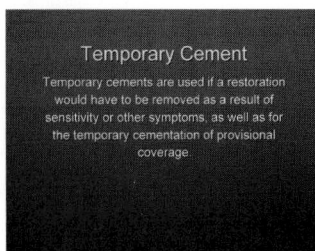

- What is provisional coverage?

Slide 10

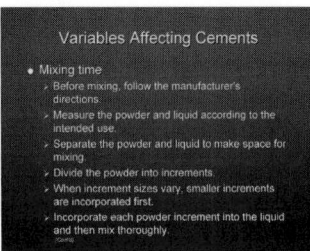

- Each type of cement has its own mixing time.

Slide 11

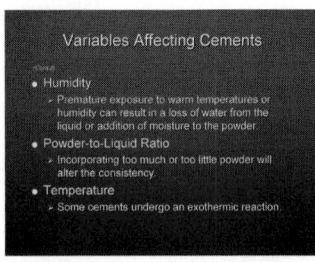

- Always dispense the powder first, then the liquid, to minimize the loss of water from evaporation.
- Always wait to dispense powder and liquid until you are ready to mix.

Slide 12

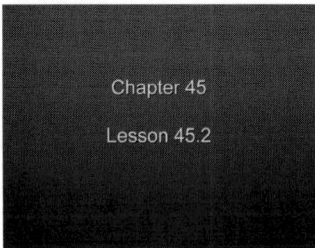

Slide 13

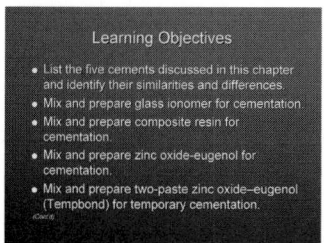

Slide 14

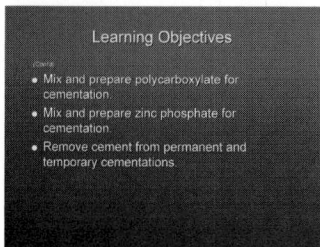

Slide 15

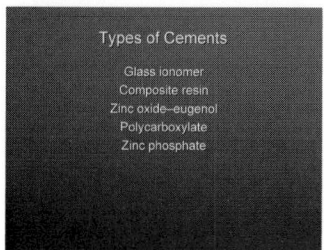

- Zinc oxide-eugenol is often referred to as ZOE.

Slide 16

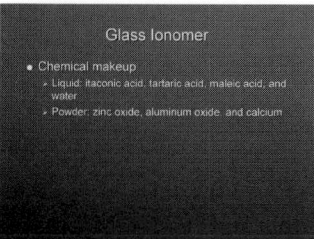

- Adheres to enamel, dentin, and metallic materials.

Slide 17

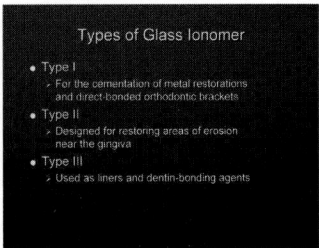

- Available in self-curing and light-curing formulas.

Slide 18

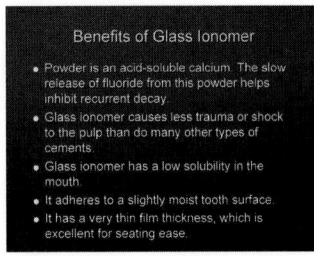

- If light-cured, what additional equipment will need to be used?

Slide 19

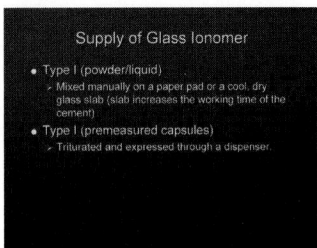

- Will a cool glass slab decrease or increase the working time?

Slide 20

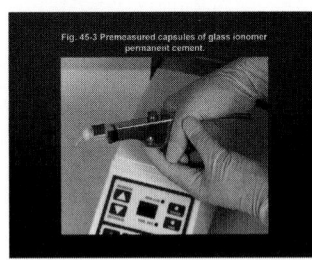

- Advantages of capsules:
  - convenience
  - decreased mixing time
  - consistent mixes because of controlled ratios
- What additional equipment will need to be used for capsules?

Slide 21

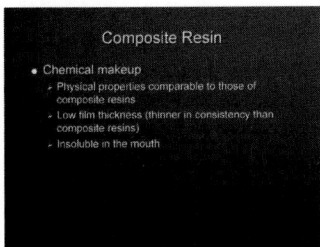

- What does *insoluble* mean?
- Tooth must be free of plaque and debris before etching.

Slide 22

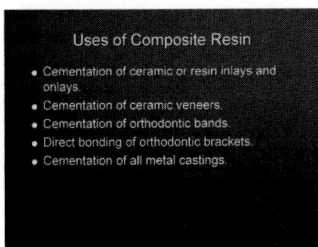

- Is etch necessary?

Slide 23

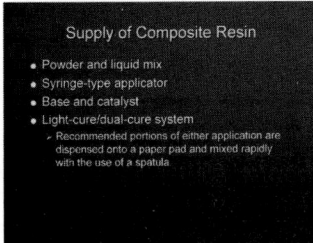

- Composite resin is used for veneers.

Slide 24

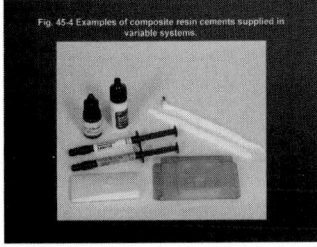

Slide 25

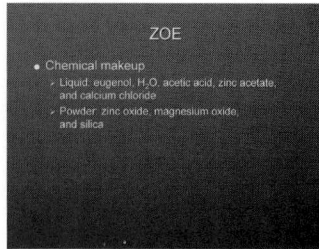

- What effect does eugenol have on the pulp?
- ZOE has a pH level close to 7.0, making it less acidic than other cements.
- Smells like cloves.

Slide 26

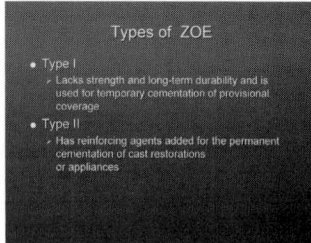

- What is provisional coverage?

Slide 27

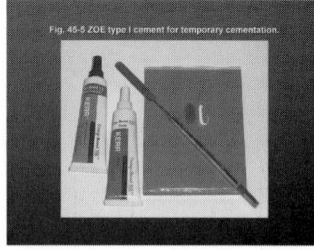

- This photo is an example of two-paste system.
- Dispense equal amounts from each tube, but leave room on the paper pad to mix them together.

Slide 28

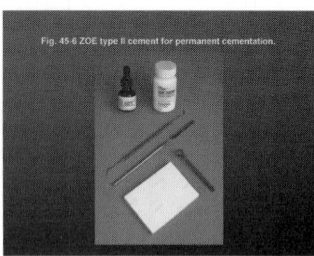

- This is an example of a powder/liquid system.
- Dispense powder on one side and liquid on the other side of the paper pad or glass slab.
- Be sure to follow the manufacturer's instructions for measurement and mixing.

Bird/Robinson

Slide 29

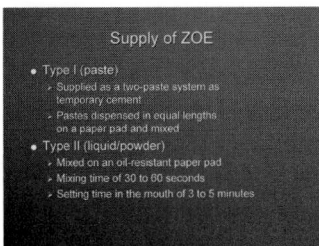

- Both systems are mixed on an oil-resistant paper pad, so the pad will not absorb the liquid.
- When a slower set is required, a glass slab is used.

Slide 30

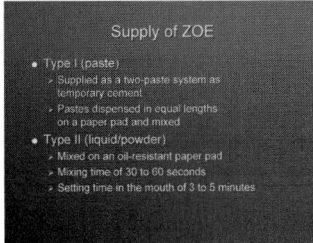

- Polycarboxylate cement is also known as polyacrylic cement.
- Can be used as a nonirritating base under composite and resin restorations.

Slide 31

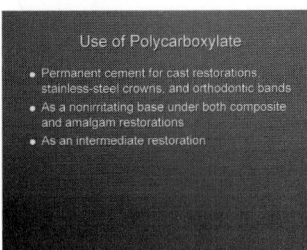

- Polycarboxylate is less irritating to tooth pulp than zinc phosphate cement.

Slide 32

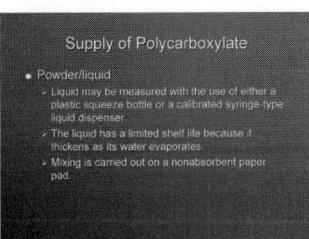

- What would be used if the working time needed to be increased?

Slide 33

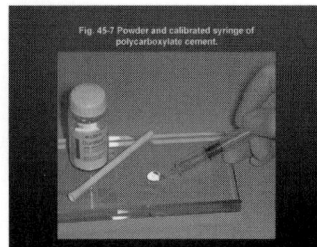

- This product is usually mixed on a paper pad.
- The liquid part of the product comes in a syringe.
- Do not dispense liquid until you are ready to mix the cement.
- Could you mix the cement on a glass slab? Why would you do this?

Slide 34

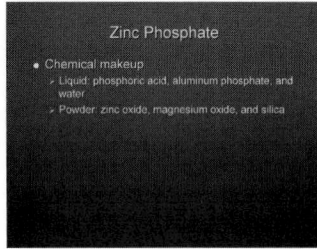

- Zinc phosphate is the oldest cement used in dentistry.
- Is zinc phosphate a permanent or temporary cement?

Slide 35

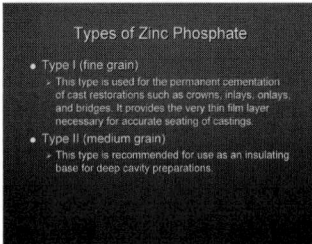

- Phosphoric acid can be irritating to the tooth pulp.

Slide 36

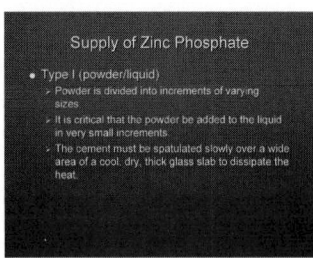

- What does *dissipate* mean?
- Powder and liquid should be dispensed just before mixing.

Slide 37

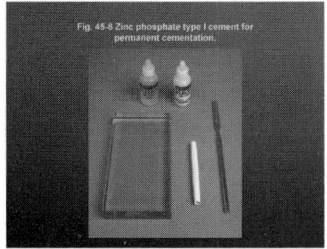

- Dispense powder at one end of the slab and liquid on the other; mix in the middle.
- Is the mixing process (1) add powder to liquid or (2) add liquid to powder?

Slide 38

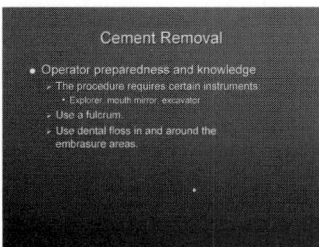

- If excess cement is not removed, what could happen to the gum tissue?
- The floss is usually knotted.

Slide 39

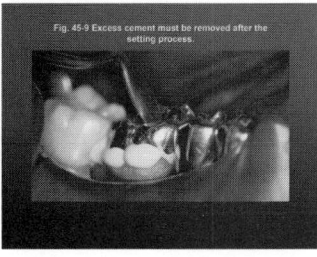

- Wait to remove cement after the initial setting is complete.
- Who can remove cement from a permanent restoration?

46 Lesson Plan
Impression Materials

TEACHING FOCUS

This chapter introduces the student to topics related to impression materials. The student will become acquainted with classification of impressions, impression trays, hydrocolloid materials, elastomeric materials, and occlusal registration. Mixing impression materials and taking impressions will be emphasized. The student will have the opportunity to put this information into context by participating in classroom activities and discussions.

MATERIALS AND RESOURCES

- ☐ alginate (Lesson 46.1)
- ☐ alginate measure scoop (provided by manufacturer) (Lesson 46.1)
- ☐ alginate powder (Lesson 46.1)
- ☐ baseplate wax (Lesson 46.2)
- ☐ beavertail-shaped wide-blade spatula (Lesson 46.1)
- ☐ bite tray (all Lessons)
- ☐ cartridge of bite registration material (base and catalyst) (Lesson 46.2)
- ☐ cartridge of heavy-bodied material (Lesson 46.2)
- ☐ cartridge of light-bodied material (Lesson 46.2)
- ☐ computer and projector for PowerPoint (all Lessons)
- ☐ extruder mixing tips (2) (Lesson 46.2)
- ☐ extruder units (2) (Lesson 46.2)
- ☐ gauze pads, 2 in. by 2 in. (Lesson 46.2)
- ☐ heat source (warm water, Bunsen burner, or torch) (Lesson 46.2)
- ☐ heavy spatula (Lesson 46.2)
- ☐ heavy-bodied base and catalyst (Lesson 46.2)
- ☐ impression syringe with sterile tip (Lesson 46.2)
- ☐ index cards (Lesson 46.1)
- ☐ laboratory knife (Lesson 46.2)
- ☐ large paper pads (2) (Lesson 46.2)
- ☐ large, stiff, tapered spatulas (2) (Lesson 46.2)
- ☐ light-bodied base and catalyst (Lesson 46.2)
- ☐ light-bodied mixing tip (Lesson 46.2)
- ☐ maxillary tray (Lesson 46.1)
- ☐ medium-size rubber bowl (Lesson 46.1)
- ☐ mixing pad (Lesson 46.2)
- ☐ mixing tip (Lesson 46.2)
- ☐ polysiloxane bite registration (Lesson 46.2)
- ☐ powder measure (Lesson 46.1)
- ☐ precaution (biohazard) bag (Lesson 46.1)
- ☐ room-temperature water (Lesson 46.1)
- ☐ saliva ejector (Lesson 46.1)
- ☐ sterile impression trays (Lesson 46.1)
- ☐ stock or custom tray with appropriate adhesive (all Lessons)
- ☐ tray (all Lessons)
- ☐ tray adhesive (used on nonperforated trays) (Lesson 46.1)
- ☐ typodont (Lesson 46.1)
- ☐ utility wax (Lesson 46.1)
- ☐ water measure (Lesson 46.1)
- ☐ wax bit registration (Lesson 46.2)
- ☐ wide-blade spatula (Lesson 46.1)
- ☐ ZOE bite registration material (Lesson 46.2)

LESSON CHECKLIST

Preparations for this lesson include:

- lecture
- guest speaker: dental assistant (optional)
- evaluation of student knowledge and skills needed to perform all entry-level activities related to the use of impression materials, including:
  - understanding the types of impression trays
  - discussing hydrocolloidal impression materials and their uses, mixing techniques, and application
  - discussing elastometric impression materials and their uses, mixing techniques, and application
  - understanding the use of occlusal registration
  - preparing impression materials
  - taking maxillary and mandibular preliminary impressions
  - taking a wax bite
  - preparing and assisting in a closed bite registration procedure

ELSEVIER

KEY TERMS

agar (p. 742)
alginate (p. 738)
base (p. 745)
border molding (p. 740)
catalyst (p. 745)
centric (p. 750)
colloid (p. 738)
elastomeric (p. 744)

extrude (p. 747)
hydro- (p. 738)
imbibition (p. 738)
occlusal registration (p. 750)
syneresis (p. 738)
tempering (p. 744)
viscous, viscosity (p. 744)

ADDITIONAL RESOURCES

PowerPoint slides (Evolve): 1-59
Multimedia Procedures DVD:
    Mixing alginate and taking preliminary impressions

Legend

CTQ
Critical
Thinking
Question

DVD
Multimedia
Procedures
Videos and
Animations

ESLR
EVOLVE
Student
Learning
Resources

IDO
Interactive
Dental
Office
CD-ROM

SW
Student
Workbook

TB
Test Bank
on the
TEACH
CD-ROM

PPT
PowerPoint
Slides

Class Activities are indicated in ***bold italic.***

Torres and Ehrlich Modern Dental Assisting, 9th ed.

Bird/Robinson

LESSON 46.1

PRETEST

1. What is the purpose of a bite registration?
   a. to show the anatomy of the maxillary teeth
   b. to show the anatomy of the mandibular teeth
   c. to show the relationship of the maxillary and mandibular teeth
   d. to identify any missing teeth in the oral cavity

2. What type of wax is added to the periphery of an impression tray to add length?
   a. sticky wax
   b. utility wax
   c. inlay wax
   d. bite registration wax

3. How long should tray adhesive be applied before use?
   a. immediately
   b. 5 minutes
   c. 10 minutes
   d. 15 minutes

4. What is the shelf-life of alginate impression material?
   a. 3 months
   b. 6 months
   c. 1 year
   d. indefinite

5. What is the working time of normal-set alginate?
   a. 30 seconds
   b. 1 minute
   c. 2 minutes
   d. 3 minutes

6. What is the term used to describe a closer adaptation of impression edges to the mucobuccal fold?
   a. impression
   b. border molding
   c. extrude
   d. syneresis

7. When loading a maxillary alginate impression, where is the bulk of material placed?
   a. anterior portion
   b. posterior portion
   c. palatal portion
   d. all over the tray

8. Which type of elastomeric impression material is used to flow in and around the details of a prepared tooth?
   a. light-bodied
   b. regular-bodied
   c. heavy-bodied
   d. extra-heavy-bodied

9. Which elastomeric impression material can have a body modifier added to the mix?
   a. silicone
   b. polysiloxane
   c. polysulfide
   d. polyether

10. What tray is used when taking a polysiloxane bite registration?
    a. an anterior tray
    b. a maxillary tray
    c. a mandibular tray
    d. a triple -tray

Answers

| 1. c | 3. d | 5. c | 7. a | 9. d |
| 2. b | 4. c | 6. b | 8. a | 10. d |

BACKGROUND ASSESSMENT

Question: What are preliminary impressions used for?

Answer: Preliminary impressions are taken to obtain diagnostic models of a patient's teeth to help design a specific dental treatment plan. These impressions are also taken to construct provisional restorations during crown and bridge preparations and to make custom trays used in partial denture and denture fabrication. Preliminary impressions are also used to fabricate orthodontic appliances and to document pretreatment and posttreatment records.

Question: What are the specific criteria required before an alginate impression can be accepted?

Answer: Despite the many reasons why alginate impressions are used, they all must meet specific criteria before use. Acceptable alginate impressions should be centered over the central and lateral incisors; and the retromolar area, lingual frenum, tongue space, and mylohyoid ridge should be reproduced. The alginate impression should be seated far enough on the areas that are to be reproduced—but not over-seated to expose areas of the impression tray. All alginate impressions should have sharp details of the area being reproduced, and should be free of tears and voids that would distort the reproduction. The hard-palate, tuberosities, and the vestibular areas should also be seen on the alginate impressions.

CRITICAL THINKING QUESTION

A 36-year-old man came to the office to have impressions taken of his teeth and mouth as study models for possible orthodontic treatment. Before the procedure began, he explained that he has a severe gag reflex, and he worries about the impression trays that will be placed in his mouth. What could the dental assistant tell him to suppress his anxiety, and what modifications will need to be made with the impression material?

Guidelines: The dental assistant should first explain to the man that this procedure is quick and can be virtually painless. The impression material will feel cold at first but does not taste unpleasant. The patient should be instructed to breath through his nose to help avoid gagging during the procedure. A fast-set alginate should be used on the patient because of his sensitive gag reflex. The fast-set alginate will set within 1 minute versus the regular alginate, which takes about 2 minutes to set. It is also important to obtain an accurate impression on the first try to avoid retakes, which might stimulate the patient's gag reflex to a more aggressive stage.

OBJECTIVES	CONTENT	TEACHING RESOURCES
Pronounce, define, and spell the Key Terms.	■ Key terms (p. 734)	SW Fill In the Blank questions 1-15 (pp. 375-376) ESLR Electronic Flashcards ▶ Discuss each of the key terms in Chapter 46, focusing on the definition, pronunciation, and spelling of each term. *Class Activity Have the students make flash cards of the key terms with the terms on one side and the definitions on the reverse. Then, have the students quiz each other with the cards. Correct their pronunciation as needed.*
List the three types of impressions taken in a dental office.	■ Classification of impressions (p. 735) ☐ Preliminary impressions (p. 735) ☐ Final impressions (p. 735) ☐ Bite registrations (p. 735)	PPT 5-10 TB questions 1-4, 12 SW Short-Answer Questions 1; Multiple Choice questions 1-3 (pp. 375-376) Recall questions 1-3 (p. 735) ▶ Discuss the factors a dentist considered in selecting the dental material used for an impression.

OBJECTIVES	CONTENT	TEACHING RESOURCES
		▶ Discuss the difference between preliminary impressions and final impressions. Explain why final impressions must be performed by the dentist. *Class Activity Divide the class into groups. Have each group discuss the various impressions and which to use during the following situtions:* — *Study models for orthodontic work* — *Crown prep impression* — *Provisional restoration* *Then have each group share its findings with the class.*
Describe the types of impression trays and their characteristics of use.	■ Impression trays (p. 736) □ Stock trays (p. 736) — Selection (p. 736) — Characteristics (p. 737) — Adaptation (p. 737) □ Custom trays (p. 737) □ Tray adhesives (p. 737)	⊠▤ PPT 11-16 ▤ TB questions 5-6, 10-11 ▥ SW Short-Answer Questions 2; Multiple Choice questions 4-6 (pp. 375-376) Figure 46-1 Types of stock trays (p. 736) Figure 46-2 Examples of quadrant, section, and full-arch impression trays (p. 737) Figure 46-3 Extending impression tray with utility wax (p. 737) Figure 46-4 Impression tray with adhesive applied (p. 737) Recall questions 4-7 (p. 737) ♀ CTQ 1-2 (p. 753) ▶ Discuss the goals that will be met by the selection of the correct tray. ▶ Discuss types of custom trays and note the circumstances under which each type would be selected. ▶ Discuss considerations for use of an adhesive. *Class Activity Bring several sample impression trays to class. Have each student find the correct tray that fits his or her mouth.*
Discuss hydrocolloid impression materials and their uses, mixing techniques, and application.	■ Hydrocolloid materials (p. 738) □ Irreversible hydrocolloid: alginate (p. 738) — Composition and chemistry (p. 738) — Physical phases (p. 738)	⊠▤ PPT 17-24 ▤ TB questions 7-8 ▥ SW Short-Answer Questions 3; Multiple Choice questions 8, 11-12 (pp. 375-377) ▥ SW Case Study question 1 (p. 378) Figure 46-5 Packaging of alginate (p. 738) Recall questions 8-9, 11 (p. 742)

Bird/Robinson

OBJECTIVES	CONTENT	TEACHING RESOURCES
	– Strength (p. 738) – Packaging and storage (p. 738) – Types of setting (p. 738) – Altering Setting Time (p. 739) – Water-to-powder ratio (p. 739) – Taking an alginate impression (p. 739) – Explain procedure to patient (p. 739) – Evaluating alginate impression (p. 739) – Impressions of edentulous arches (p. 740)	▸ Discuss alginate. Describe alginate's composition, chemistry, physical phases, strength, packaging, and storage. ▸ Discuss syneresis and imbibition. Define the terms and how they apply to storage of an alginate impression. ▸ Discuss normal-setting and fast-setting alginate and when each would be used. ***Class Activity Divide the class into groups. Assign each group one of the following factors about the properties of hydrocolloid materials (reversible versus irreversible):*** – ***Physical factors*** – ***Chemical factors*** – ***Thermal factors*** ***Have each group summarize its findings for the class.***
Mix alginate impression material at a competent level.	☐ Irreversible hydrocolloid: alginate (p. 738) – Composition and chemistry (p. 738) – Physical phases (p. 738) – Strength (p. 738) – Packaging and storage (p. 738) – Types of setting (p. 738) – Altering setting time (p. 739) – Water-to-powder ratio (p. 739) – Taking an alginate impression (p. 739) – Explain procedure to patient (p. 739) – Evaluating alginate impression (p. 739) – Impressions of edentulous arches (p. 740)	⊠ PPT 25-31 🎥 Multimedia Procedures DVD: Mixing Alginate and Taking Preliminary Impressions 💻 TB question 13 📖 SW Multiple Choice questions 9-10, 13 (pp. 376-377) 📖 SW Case Study questions 2-3 (p. 378) 📖 *e* SW/ESLR Competency 46-1 Mixing Alginate Impression Material (p. 379) Figure 46-6 A plastic scoop and plastic cylinder are supplied with alginate (p. 739) Recall question 10 (p. 742) ▸ Discuss normal-setting and fast-setting alginate and the timing involved with each. Note the circumstances under which each would be selected. ▸ Discuss the steps involved in mixing alginate impression material. ▸ Discuss the water/powder ratio. Note the importance of accurate measurement and describe differences based on whether the impression is maxillary or mandibular. ***Class Activity Demonstrate the mixing method of normal-set alginate and fast-set alginate.***

ELSEVIER

Torres and Ehrlich Modern Dental Assisting, 9th ed.

Bird/Robinson

OBJECTIVES	CONTENT	TEACHING RESOURCES
	Procedure 46-1 Mixing alginate impression material (p. 740) (SW/ESLR Competency 46-1, p. 379)	
Take a maxillary and mandibular preliminary impression at competency level.	☐ Irreversible hydrocolloid: alginate (p. 738) – Composition and chemistry (p. 738) – Physical phases (p. 738) – Strength (p. 738) – Packaging and storage (p. 738) – Types of setting (p. 738) – Altering setting time (p. 739) – Water-to-powder ratio (p. 739) – Taking an alginate impression (p. 739) – Explain procedure to patient (p. 739) – Evaluating alginate impression (p. 739) – Impressions of edentulous arches (p. 740) ☐ Reversible hydrocolloid (p. 742) – Tray material (p. 744) – Syringe material (p. 744) – Application of Reversible Hydrocolloid Impression Material (p. 744) Procedure 46-2 Taking a mandibular preliminary impression	PPT 32-36 TB question 9 SW Multiple Choice questions 7, 14 (pp. 376-377) SW Case Study questions 4-5 (p. 378) SW/ESLR Competencies 46-2 and 46-3 Taking a Mandibular or a Maxillary Preliminary Impression (Expanded Function) (pp. 381-384) Figure 46-7 How an impression must appear (p. 739) Figure 46-8 Conditioning bath for reversible hydrocolloid (p. 744) Figure 46-9 Reversible hydrocolloid tray material (p. 744) Recall questions 12-14 (p. 744) ▸ Discuss the important topics to cover during patient education before taking a preliminary impression. ▸ Discuss the criteria used to evaluate an alginate impression. ▸ Discuss the steps involved in taking mandibular or maxillary preliminary impressions. ▸ Discuss the steps involved in applying a reversible hydrocolloid impression material. Note the special properties that must be considered when using this material. ***Class Activity Demonstrate and have students manipulate alginate impressions on a typodont.***

OBJECTIVES	CONTENT	TEACHING RESOURCES
	(expanded function) (pp. 741-742) (SW/ESLR Competencies 46-2 and 46-3, pp. 381-384)	
	[Procedure] 46-3 Taking a maxillary preliminary impression (expanded function) (p. 743) (SW/ESLR Competencies 46-2 and 46-3, pp. 381-384)	

46.1 Homework/Assignments:

46.1 Instructor's Notes/Student Feedback:

LESSON 46.2

CRITICAL THINKING QUESTION

A wax-bite registration was taken from a patient and sent to the dental laboratory along with the patient's final impression, for fabrication of a three-unit bridge. The dental laboratory technician called and said the wax-bite registration that was sent was damaged during delivery. The technician needs a new bite registration from the patient. What other material can be used to ensure the bite registration will not be damaged during delivery?

Guidelines: There are other materials that can be used for bite registration, but one could question why the bite registration arrived damaged. You will need to contact the patient to schedule another bite registration appointment and explain the situation to the patient. A polysiloxane bite registration paste can be used to obtain a new bite registration, as it is more durable for delivery to the dental laboratory. Zinc oxide eugenol bite registration paste can also be used because of its durability.

OBJECTIVES	CONTENT	TEACHING RESOURCES
Discuss elastomeric impression materials and their uses, mixing techniques, and application.	■ Elastomeric materials (p. 744) ☐ Characteristics (p. 745) ☐ Form of materials (p. 745) – Light-bodied material (p. 745) – Regular and heavy-bodied material (p. 745) ☐ Curing stages and types (p. 745) – Initial set (p. 745) – Final set (p. 745) – Final cure (p. 745)	⊠ PPT 40-44 TB questions 14-15 SW Short-Answer Questions 4; Multiple Choice questions 15-17, 19 (pp. 375, 377) Figure 46-10 Example of a final impression (p. 745) Figure 46-11 Mixing unit for final impression material (p. 748) Recall questions 15-19 (pp. 749, 750) CTQ 4 (p. 754) ▸ Discuss the purpose and uses of elastomeric materials. Describe light-bodied, regular, and heavy-bodied materials and note when each is used. ▸ Discuss the three curing stages. Explain the changes that occur during each stage. *Class Activity Divide the class into groups. Assign each group one of the following elastomeric materials:* – *Polysulfide* – *Polyether* – *Silicone* – *Polysiloxane* *Have each group discuss the advantages and disadvantages of its assigned material and present its findings to the class. Write them on the board as each material is presented.*

OBJECTIVES	CONTENT	TEACHING RESOURCES
Competently mix a paste final impression material.	☐ Mixing of materials (p. 745) – Paste system (p. 745) – Automix system (p. 745) – Mixing unit system (p. 745) – Putty system (p. 745) – Basic impression technique (p. 748) ☐ Types of elastomeric materials (p. 749) Procedure 46-4 Mixing a two-paste final impression material (pp. 746-747) (SW/ESLR Competency 46-4, pp. 385-386)	⊠ PPT 45 TB questions 16-17 SW Multiple Choice question 20 (p. 377) SW/ESLR Competency 46-4 Mixing a Two-Paste Final Impression Material (pp. 385-386) Recall question 20 (p. 750) CTQ 3 (p. 754) ▸ Discuss the importance of timing when using the paste system. Describe the precautions a dental assistant might take to ensure proper timing. ▸ Discuss the steps involved in mixing a two-paste final impression material. *Class Activity Demonstrate and have students manipulate a paste material for a final impression.*
Competently prepare an automix impression material.	☐ Mixing of materials (p. 745) – Paste system (p. 745) – Automix system (p. 745) – Mixing unit system (p. 745) – Putty system (p. 745) – Basic impression technique (p. 748) ☐ Types of elastomeric materials (p. 749) – Polysulfide (p. 749) – Polyether (p. 749) – Silicone (p. 750) – Polysiloxane (p. 750) Procedure 46-5 Preparing an automix final impression material (pp. 747-748) (SW/ESLR Competency 46-5, p. 387)	⊠ PPT 46-54 SW Multiple Choice question 18 (p. 377) SW/ESLR Competency 46-5 Preparing an Automix Final Impression Material (p. 387) Figure 46-12 Polysulfide material (p. 749) Figure 46-13 Polyether material (p. 749) Figure 46-14 Silicone material (p. 750) Figure 46-15 Polysiloxane (polyvinyl siloxane) material (p. 750) ▸ Discuss the steps involved in preparing an automix final impression material. ▸ Discuss types of elastomeric materials. Note the importance of dimensional stability, deformation, and permanent deformation. ▸ Discuss guidelines for mixing polysulfide, polyether, silicone, and polysiloxane impression materials. *Class Activity Demonstrate and have students manipulate the automix system.*

OBJECTIVES	CONTENT	TEACHING RESOURCES
Describe the importance of an occlusal registration and its use in a procedure.	■ Occlusal (bite) registration (p. 750) □ Wax=bite registration (p. 750) □ Polysiloxane bite registration paste (p. 751)	PPT 55-59 TB question 18 SW Short-Answer Questions 5; Multiple Choice questions 21, 23 (pp. 375, 377) Figure 46-16 Example of a bite registration (p. 752) Figure 46-17 Wax-bite registration (p. 752) Recall questions 21, 23 (p. 753) CTQ 5 (p. 754) ▸ Discuss the different materials that may be chosen for a bite registration. Note the circumstances under which each material might be chosen. ▸ Discuss the advantages of using polysiloxane for a bite registration. ***Class Activity Demonstrate two methods of obtaining bite registrations: a wax-bite registration and a polysiloxane bite registration. Then have the students practice on the typodont or each other.***
Take a wax bite.	□ Wax bite registration (p. 750) *Procedure* 46-6 Taking a wax bite registration (p. 751) (SW/ESLR Competency 46-6, p. 389)	SW/ESLR Competency 46-6 Taking a Wax-Bite Registration (p. 389) ▸ Discuss the steps involved in taking a wax- bite registration. Note any patient instructions that should be given. ***Class Activity Demonstrate the wax bite registration and have the students practice on a typodont.***
Prepare and assist in a closed bite registration procedure.	□ Polysiloxane bite registration paste (p. 751) □ Zinc oxide-eugenol bite registration paste (p. 753) *Procedure* 46-7 Mixing polysiloxane material for a bite registration (p. 752) (SW/ESLR Competency 46-7, p. 391) *Procedure* 46-8 Mixing zinc oxide-eugenol bite registration material (p. 753) (SW/ESLR Competency 46-8, p. 393)	SW Multiple Choice questions 22, 24-25 (p. 377) SW/ESLR Competency 46-7 Mixing Polysiloxane Material for a Bite Registration (p. 391) SW/ESLR Competency 46-8 Mixing Zinc Oxide-Eugenol Registration Material (p. 393) Recall question 22 (p. 753) Patient Education (p. 753) Legal and Ethical Implications (p. 753) Eye to the Future (p. 753) ▸ Discuss the steps involved in mixing and applying polysiloxane for a bite registration. Note any patient instructions that should be given. ▸ Discuss the steps involved in mixing and applying zinc oxide-eugenol for a bite registration. Note any patient instructions that should be given.

Bird/Robinson

OBJECTIVES	CONTENT	TEACHING RESOURCES
		‣ Discuss patient education issues, and highlight teaching points to cover. Note concerns and discomfort of patients having an impression and describe communication skills that are important for the dental assistant when explaining the procedure. ***Class Activity** Have students manipulate polysiloxane bite registration material on the typodont.*
Performance Evaluation		🖥️ TB 📗 SW questions (pp. 375-377) 📗 SW Case Study (p. 378) 📗 *e* SW/ESLR Competency 46-1 Mixing Alginate Impression Material (p. 379) 📗 *e* SW/ESLR Competencies 46-2 and 46-3 Taking a Mandibular or a Maxillary Preliminary Impression (Expanded Function) (pp. 381-384) 📗 *e* SW/ESLR Competency 46-4 Mixing a Two-Paste Final Impression Material (pp. 385-386) 📗 *e* SW/ESLR Competency 46-5 Preparing an Automix Final Impression Material (p. 387) 📗 *e* SW/ESRL Competency 46-6 Taking a Wax-Bite Registration (p. 389) 📗 *e* SW/ESLR Competency 46-7 Mixing Polysiloxane Material for a Bite Registration (p. 391) 📗 *e* SW/ESLR Competency 46-8 Mixing Zinc Oxide-Eugenol Registration Material (p. 393) *e* ESLR Electronic Flashcards *e* ESLR Practice Quiz Recall questions (pp. 735-753) 💡 CTQ (pp. 753-754)

46.2 Homework/Assignments:

46.2 Instructor's Notes/Student Feedback:

Slide 1

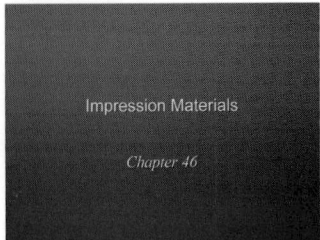

Impression Materials

Chapter 46

Slide 2

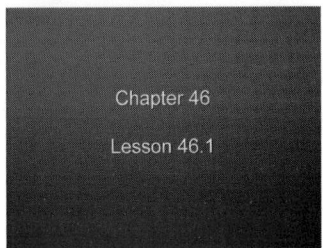

Chapter 46

Lesson 46.1

Slide 3

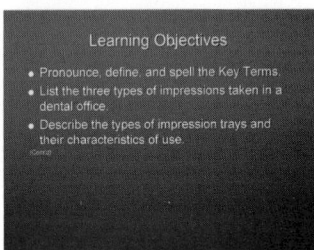

Learning Objectives

- Pronounce, define, and spell the Key Terms.
- List the three types of impressions taken in a dental office.
- Describe the types of impression trays and their characteristics of use.

(Cont'd)

Slide 4

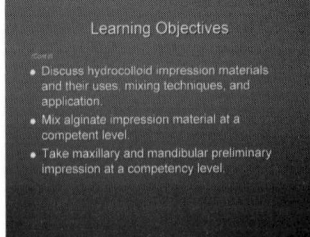

Learning Objectives

(Cont'd)

- Discuss hydrocolloid impression materials and their uses, mixing techniques, and application.
- Mix alginate impression material at a competent level.
- Take maxillary and mandibular preliminary impression at a competency level.

Torres and Ehrlich Modern Dental Assisting, 9th ed.

Bird/Robinson

Slide 5

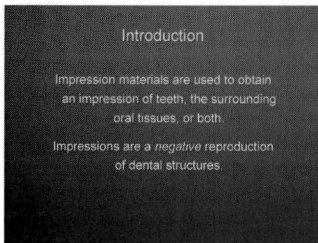

- How many students have had impressions taken?
- For what reason?

Slide 6

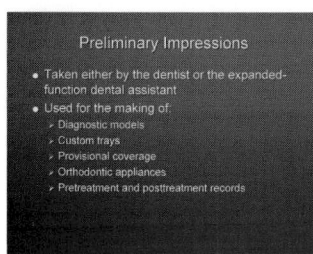

- Preliminary impressions are almost always taken by a competent dental assistant.
- What are diagnostic models used for?
- What are custom trays used for?
- What is provisional coverage?
- What types of orthodontic appliances can be made?

Slide 7

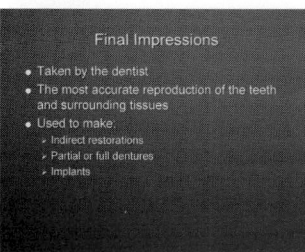

- Final impressions are never taken by the dental assistant.
- What are examples of indirect restorations?

Slide 8

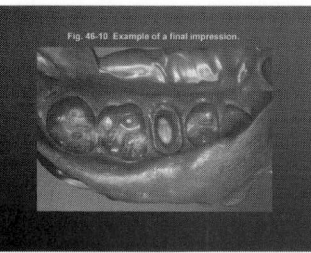

- Which tooth is involved in this impression?

Bird/Robinson

Slide 9

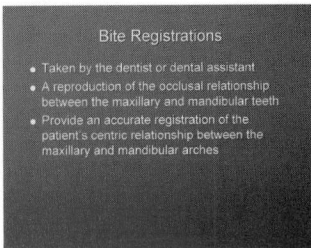

- Why are bite registrations important in fabricating indirect restorations?

Slide 10

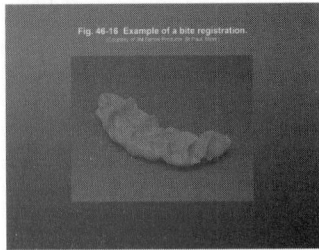

- Example of a polysiloxane bite registration.
- What arch is this?

Slide 11

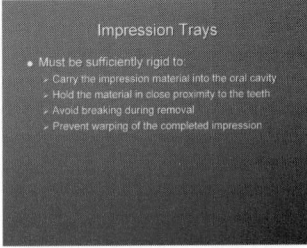

- Are impressions a positive or negative reproduction?

Slide 12

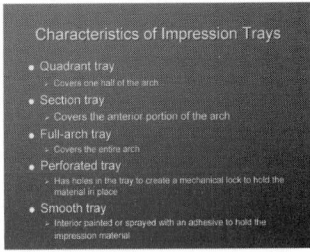

- Are impression trays metal or plastic?

Slide 13

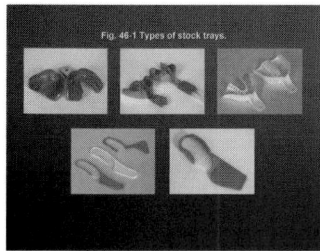

- What is a triple tray?
- What are the advantages of using a triple tray?
- Which of these impression trays needs an adhesive applied?

Slide 14

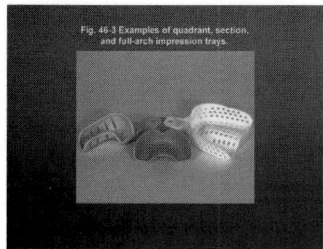

Slide 15

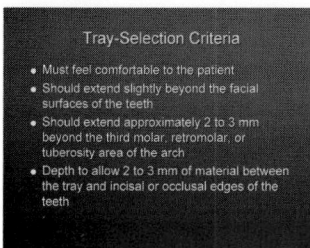

- Try on the tray in the patient's mouth before mixing material.
- Explain the procedure to the patient.

Slide 16

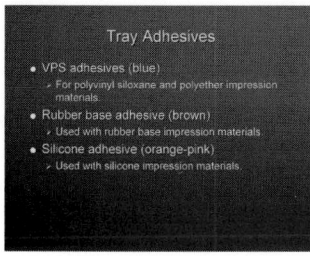

- Tray adhesives should be applied *after* the tray has been tried in the patient's mouth.
- How long should the tray adhesive be applied to the tray before adding the impression material?

Bird/Robinson

Slide 17

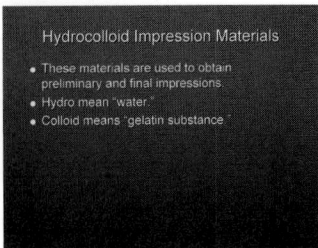

Slide 18

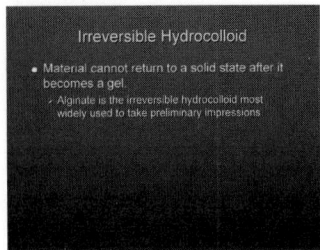

- What can alginate impressions be used for?

Slide 19

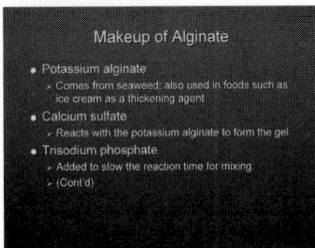

- No taste.
- Flavors are available. (Cherry is the most common.)
- Odorless.

Slide 20

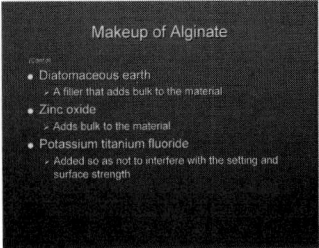

Slide 21

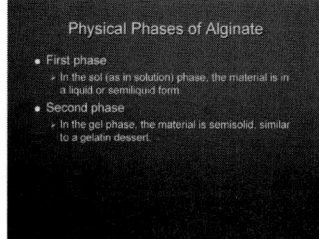

- Upon completion of both phases, alginate is susceptible to tearing and stretching.

Slide 22

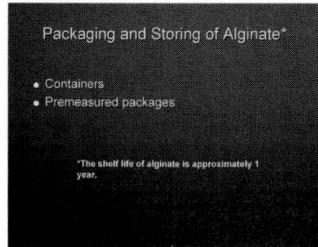

- Should be stored at room temperature.

Slide 23

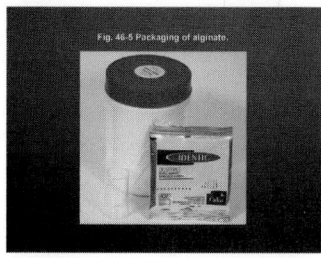

- Alginate impression materials come in a reusable tub with a measuring scoop. This is the most common form of alginate.
- Premeasured foil packets are also available at a slightly higher cost.

Slide 24

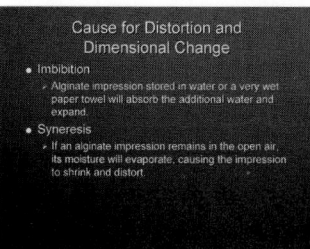

- How long after the impression is obtained should we proceed to the pouring?
- Storing impression in a plastic baggie can help prevent distortion.

Torres and Ehrlich Modern Dental Assisting, 9th ed.

Bird/Robinson

Slide 25

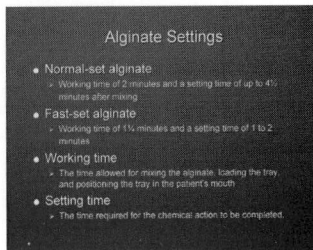

- Which setting time would be preferred for a patient who has a gag reflex?

Slide 26

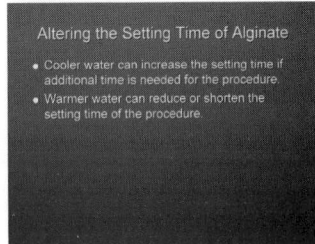

- Which water temperature would be preferred for a patient who has a gag reflex? Why?

Slide 27

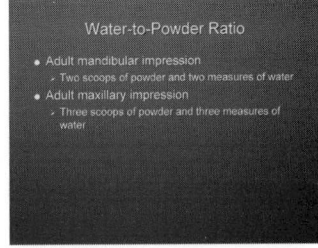

- These ratios are only guidelines for measurement.
- Check manufacturers directions before measuring.
- May need to adjust measurements as not all patients are the same.

Slide 28

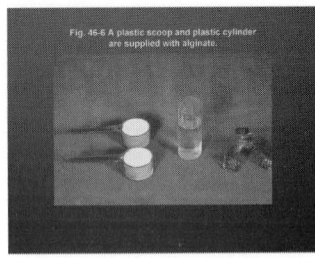

- Do not pack powder into scoops.
- Use spatula to even off top of scoop.

Slide 29

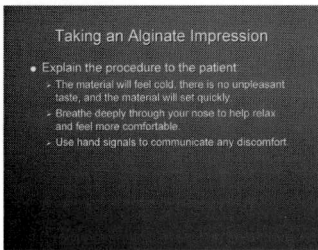

- Never leave the patient alone during this procedure.
- Would we ask the patient if he or she has a gag reflex? Why or why not?

Slide 30

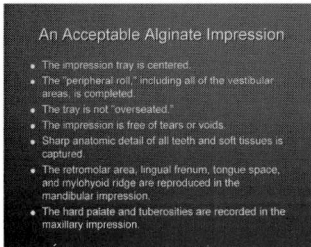

- If criteria are not met, you must retake the impression.

Slide 31

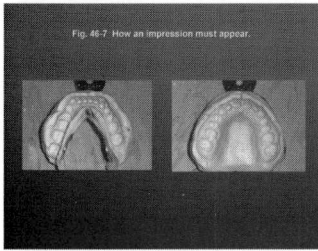

Slide 32

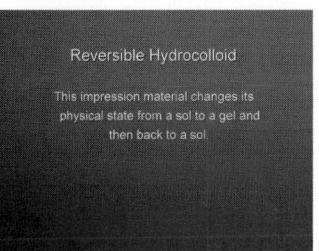

- Not commonly used in dental offices.

Slide 33

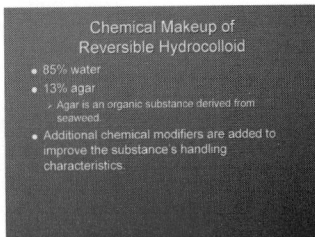

- Requires additional equipment to obtain impression.

Slide 34

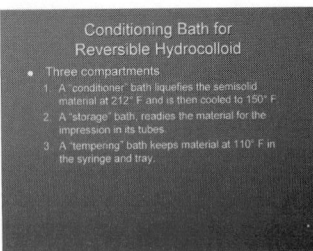

- Longer steps are required to obtain this type of impression.

Slide 35

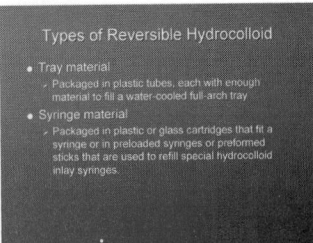

Slide 36

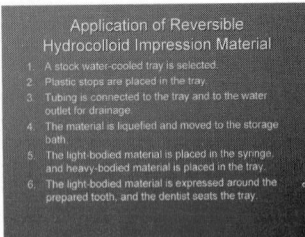

- Is this type of material used for preliminary or final impressions?

Torres and Ehrlich Modern Dental Assisting, 9th ed.
Bird/Robinson

Slide 37

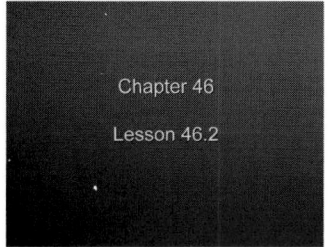

Slide 38

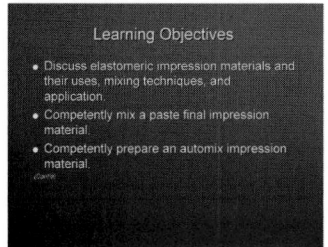

Slide 39

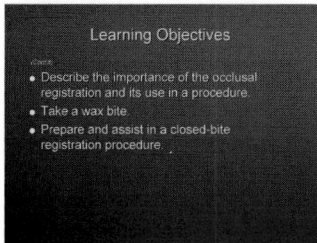

Slide 40

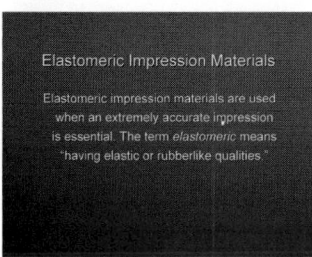

- Commonly used in dental offices.
- Easier to use than reversible hydrocolloids.

Slide 41

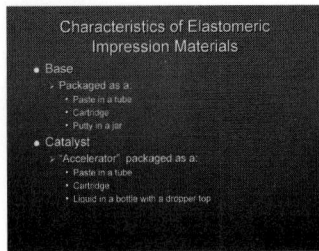

- Very accurate impressions are obtained using this material.

Slide 42

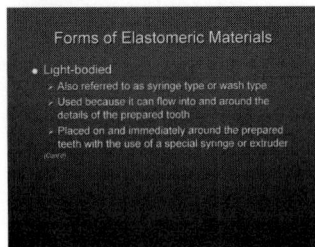

- Syringe can be disposable or sterilized and reused.
- Extruder tips are disposed of after each use.

Slide 43

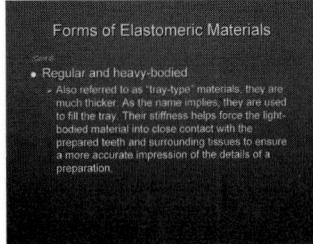

- Would this material be used to define details of the prepared tooth?

Slide 44

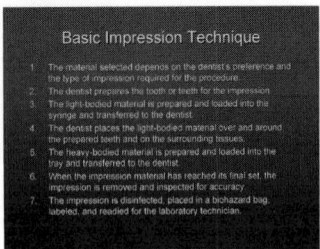

- What is the process for tray selection?

Slide 45

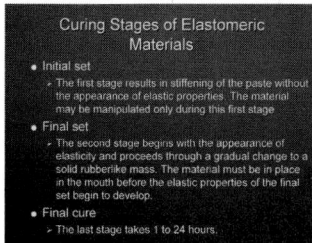

- Must these impressions be disinfected before delivery to the dental laboratory?

Slide 46

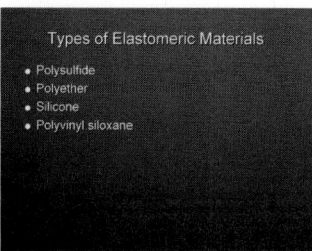

- All of these materials are very similar products; all provide the same outcome.
- Dimensional stability is a main concern.

Slide 47

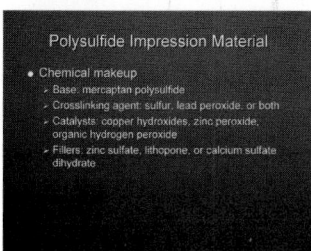

- Also known as rubber base.
- Has strong odor.
- Can stain clothing.

Slide 48

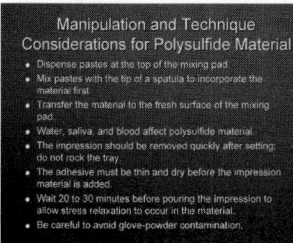

- Has a long working time.
- Has a long setting time.
- Would this material be used on a patient with a gag reflex?

Slide 49

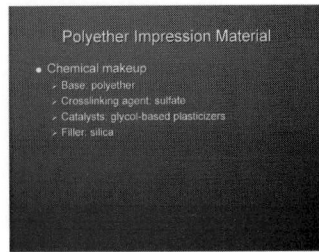

- A thinner can be used with this material.
- What is a thinner used for?

Slide 50

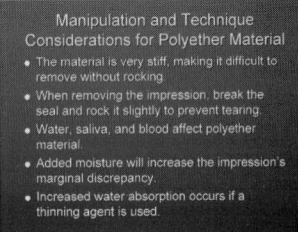

- Supplied in a two-paste system or cartridge system.

Slide 51

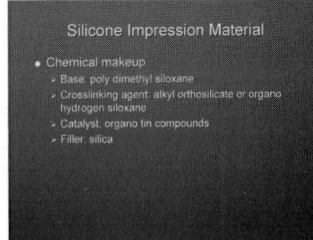

- Odorless
- Does not stain.
- Very good dimensional stability.

Slide 52

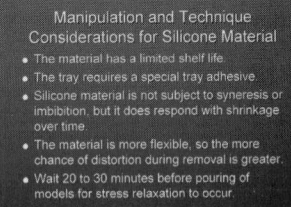

- Supplied in a tube for the base and a bottle or smaller tube for the catalyst.

Bird/Robinson

Slide 53

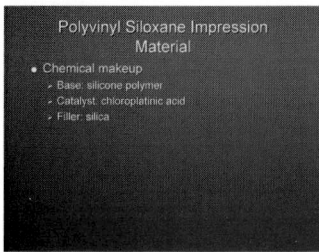

- Also known as polysiloxane.
- High dimensional stability.
- Low tear resistance.

Slide 54

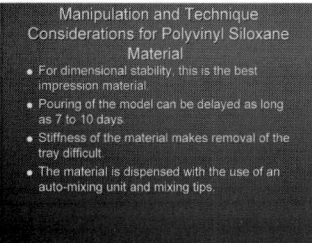

- Most commonly used impression material.
- No odor.
- Tasteless.
- Available in light, regular, and heavy bodied forms.
- Supplied in cartridges or putty form.

Slide 55

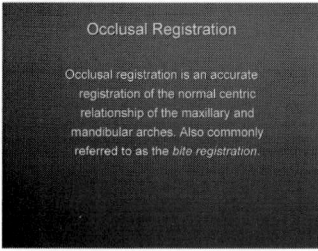

- What is centric occlusion?

Slide 56

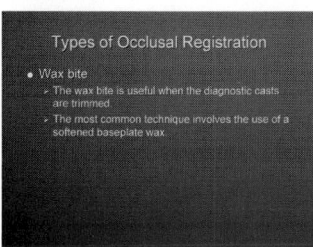

- Equipment needed: laboratory knife and heat source.
- What type of heat source is used?

Torres and Ehrlich Modern Dental Assisting, 9th ed.

Bird/Robinson

Slide 57

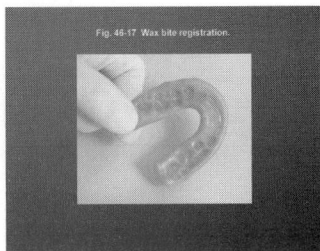

- How long should the wax bite registration stay in the patient's mouth?
- Does this impression need to be disinfected?

Slide 58

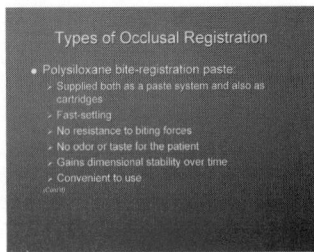

- Widely used.
- Does not require a heat source.

Slide 59

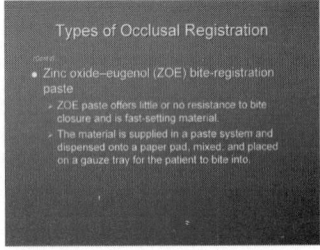

Torres and Ehrlich Modern Dental Assisting, 9th ed.

TEACHING FOCUS

This chapter gives the student an opportunity to learn about laboratory materials and procedures. Safety in the dental laboratory will be discussed. The student will also have an opportunity to understand the materials and skills needed to pour preliminary impressions, trim and finish diagnostic models, prepare custom trays, and polish indirect prosthesis.

MATERIALS AND RESOURCES

- ☐ barrier coating (Lesson 47.2)
- ☐ baseplate wax (Lesson 47.2)
- ☐ computer and PowerPoint projector (all Lessons)
- ☐ crown and bridge scissors (Lesson 47.2)
- ☐ diagnostic model (Lesson 47.2)
- ☐ flexible rubber mixing bowl (clean and dry) (Lesson 47.1)
- ☐ glass jar with lid or smooth surface paper cup (Lesson 47.2)
- ☐ glass slab or tile (Lesson 47.1)
- ☐ heat source (Lesson 47.2)
- ☐ laboratory knife and cutters (all Lessons)
- ☐ laboratory spatula (Lesson 47.2)
- ☐ light-curing system (Lesson 47.2)
- ☐ maxillary and mandibular impression (Lesson 47.1)
- ☐ measures for liquid and powder (Lesson 47.2)
- ☐ metal spatula (Lesson 47.1)
- ☐ model trimmer (Lesson 47.1)
- ☐ pencil (all Lessons)
- ☐ petroleum jelly (Lesson 47.2)
- ☐ plaster-150 g (additional is needed for the base) (Lesson 47.1)
- ☐ poured stone maxillary and mandibular dental model (Lesson 47.1)
- ☐ prefabricated tray model (Lesson 47.2)
- ☐ room-temperature water (Lesson 47.1)
- ☐ ruler (Lesson 47.1)
- ☐ scale (Lesson 47.1)
- ☐ scalpel or laboratory knife (Lesson 47.2)
- ☐ separating medium with brush (Lesson 47.2)
- ☐ thermoplastic resin model (Lesson 47.2)
- ☐ tongue blade (Lesson 47.2)
- ☐ tray resin (Lesson 47.2)
- ☐ vacuum former (Lesson 47.2)
- ☐ vibrator with a disposable cover (Lesson 47.1)
- ☐ water-60 ml (additional water is needed for the base) (Lesson 47.1)
- ☐ water-measuring device (Lesson 47.1)
- ☐ wax-bite registration (Lesson 47.1)
- ☐ wax spatula #7 (Lesson 47.2)

LESSON CHECKLIST

Preparations for this lesson include:

- lecture
- evaluation of student knowledge and skills needed to perform all entry-level activities related to laboratory materials and procedures, including:
  - ○ custom impression trays
  - ○ dental laboratory equipment
  - ○ dental models
  - ○ dental waxes
  - ○ safety in the dental laboratory

KEY TERMS

anatomic portion (p. 760)
articulator (p. 758)
crystallization (p. 760)
die (p. 760)
dihydrate (p. 760)
dimensionally stable (p. 766)
facebow (p. 758)
gypsum (p. 759)

hemihydrate (p. 760)
homogeneous (p. 767)
lathe (p. 759)
model (p. 758)
monomer (p. 766)
polymer (p. 766)
slurry (p. 765)
volatile (p. 766)

ADDITIONAL RESOURCES

PowerPoint slides (Evolve): 1-42
Multimedia Procedures DVD:
    Pouring Dental Models Using Inverted-Pour Method
    Constructing a Vacuum-Formed Tray

Legend

 CTQ Critical Thinking Question

 DVD Multimedia Procedures Videos and Animations

 ESLR EVOLVE Student Learning Resources

 IDO Interactive Dental Office CD-ROM

 SW Student Workbook

 TB Test Bank on the TEACH CD-ROM

 PPT PowerPoint Slides

Class Activities are indicated in ***bold italic***.

ELSEVIER

Torres and Ehrlich Modern Dental Assisting, 9th ed.

Bird/Robinson

LESSON 47.1

PRETEST

1. What piece of equipment is used to remove air from the mix of gypsum products?
   - a. vacuum former
   - b. vibrator
   - c. articulator
   - d. spatula

2. What piece of equipment is used to polish dentures?
   - a. slow-speed hand piece
   - b. high-speed hand piece
   - c. lathe
   - d. model trimmer

3. Which type of gypsum is commonly referred to as plaster of Paris?
   - a. model plaster
   - b. dental stone
   - c. high strength stone
   - d. densite

4. Which type of stone is used as a working model for making dentures?
   - a. model plaster
   - b. dental stone
   - c. high-strength stone
   - d. densite

5. What is the recommended water/powder ratio for high-strength stone?
   - a. 100 g powder/45-50 ml water
   - b. 100 g powder/30-32 ml water
   - c. 100 g powder/19-24 ml water
   - d. 100 g powder/10-18 ml water

6. During the pouring procedure, where should the gypsum material be placed to flow to all areas of the impression?
   - a. anterior portion
   - b. canine area
   - c. most posterior tooth
   - d. palatal area

7. What is the term used to describe something that evaporates easily and is very explosive?
   - a. volatile
   - b. monomer
   - c. polymer
   - d. galvanic

8. What type of wax is used to form a wall around a preliminary impression?
   - a. sticky wax
   - b. rope wax
   - c. utility wax
   - d. boxing wax

9. What type of inlay casting wax is used for indirect wax patterns?
   - a. type A
   - b. type B
   - c. type C
   - d. type D

10. Which type of wax is used to cover orthodontic brackets?
    - a. boxing wax
    - b. utility wax
    - c. sticky wax
    - d. baseplate wax

Answers

1. b	3. a	5. c	7. a	9. a
2. c	4. b	6. c	8. d	10. b

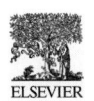

Torres and Ehrlich Modern Dental Assisting, 9th ed.

Bird/Robinson

BACKGROUND ASSESSMENT

Question: What is a model trimmer used for in the dental laboratory?

Answer: A model trimmer is used to trim stone or plaster models. The trimmer has a large, circular grinding wheel that spins at high speeds to remove the stone or plaster from models poured from the patient's impressions. The wheel stones have several different abrasive levels, and they should be cleaned often with a brush to keep the cutting edges working effectively. The model trimmer also has a waterspout that puts a constant stream of water on the models being trimmed. This is done to reduce the levels of dust that can be expelled during trimming.

Question: What is the purpose of a spacer when fabricating a custom impression tray?

Answer: Placing the spacer over the cast in which the custom impression tray is to be fabricated creates room for the impression material. The spacer can be made of baseplate wax, a moist paper towel, or a commercial nonstick molding material. If a spacer is not used, the impression material will not have enough room when seating the tray in the patient's mouth, and will eventually spill over the sides of the custom impression tray.

CRITICAL THINKING QUESTION

The dentist has prescribed maxillary and mandibular alginate impressions for a patient. The dental assistant follows the dentist's orders and obtains both impressions. In the laboratory the dental assistant begins to pour up the models using model plaster and mistakenly adds too much water, making the mix too runny. The dental assistant decides to add more powder to the mix to make it thicker. Why is this the wrong thing to do, and what can the dental assistant do to the mix to correct it?

Guidelines: It's extremely important that the measurements used in all gypsum products are exact. For model plaster, the correct measurement is 100 g powder/45 to 50 ml water. A scale should be used to measure the powder, while the water should be measured with a large syringe or a milliliter-graduated cylinder. Because more powder was added to the mix to make it thicker, the dental assistant has created a model that will be significantly weaker and more susceptible to breaking during separation from the impression tray or during trimming of the model. If the model should break, the patient would have to return for new impressions. The mix should be disposed of and the dental assistant should start over using the correct measurements.

OBJECTIVES	CONTENT	TEACHING RESOURCES
Pronounce, define, and spell the Key Terms.	■ Key terms (pp. 755-756)	*e* ESLR Electronic Flashcards ▶ Discuss each of the key terms, focusing on the definition, pronunciation, and spelling of each term. ***Class Activity** Have students make flash cards of the key terms with the terms on one side and the definitions on the other. Then have the students quiz each other with the flash cards; correct their pronunciation as needed.*
Discuss the safety precautions that should be taken in the dental laboratory.	■ Safety in the dental laboratory (p. 756) ☐ Laboratory Rules (p. 756) ☐ Physical safety (p. 757) ☐ Chemical safety (p. 757) ☐ Biohazards (p. 757)	PPT 5-8 TB question 1 SW Short-Answer Questions 1; Multiple Choice questions 1-3 (pp. 395-396) Figure 47-1 Commercial dental laboratory (p. 756) Recall questions 1-3 (p. 757) ▶ Discuss physical safety precautions that should be taken in the dental laboratory. ▶ Discuss chemical safety precautions that should be taken in the dental laboratory.

Bird/Robinson

OBJECTIVES	CONTENT	TEACHING RESOURCES
		▸ Discuss biohazards in the dental laboratory. *Class Activity **Lead a group discussion stressing the need to follow these laboratory rules:*** – *No eating, drinking, smoking* – *No cosmetics* – *Wear PPE at all times* – *Keep hair back* – *Report all accidents immediately* – *Follow all manufacturer's directions* – *Clean work area before and after each procedure*
List the types of equipment found in a dental laboratory and their uses.	■ Dental laboratory equipment (p. 757) ☐ Heat sources (p. 757) ☐ Model trimmer (p. 757) ☐ Vacuum former (p. 757) ☐ Vibrator (p. 758) ☐ Laboratory handpiece (p. 758) ☐ Sandblaster (p. 758) ☐ Articulator (p. 758) ☐ Dental lathe (p. 759) ☐ Specialized spatulas and bowls (p. 759) – Wax spatulas (p. 759) – Mixing spatulas (p. 759) – Rubber bowls (p. 759)	⊞ PPT 9 ▦ TB question 2 📖 SW Short-Answer Questions 2; Fill in the Blank questions 2, 7, 11, 13; Multiple Choice questions 4-6 (pp. 395-396) Figure 47-2 Dental laboratory within a dental office (p. 757) Figure 47-3 Model trimmer (p. 758) Figure 47-4 Vacuum former (p. 758) Figure 47-5 Vibrator (p. 758) Figure 47-6 Articulator (p. 759) Recall questions 4-6 (p. 759) ▸ Discuss the use of equipment that is found in the dental laboratory. *Class Activity **Demonstrate the equipment found in a dental lab:*** – *Heat sources* – *Model trimmer* – *Vacuum former* – *Vibrator* – *Laboratory handpiece* – *Sandblaster* – *Articulator* – *Dental lathe* *Encourage students to observe closely and ask questions.*
Describe dental models and how they are used in dentistry.	■ Dental models (p. 759)	⊞ PPT 10-12 📖 SW Short-Answer Questions 3; Multiple Choice question 7 (pp. 395-396)

OBJECTIVES	CONTENT	TEACHING RESOURCES
		Figure 47-7 Dental models (p. 759)
		Recall questions 7-8 (p. 760)
		▸ Discuss the uses for dental models.
		Class Activity **Divide the class into small groups, and have each group discuss why dental models are used for several procedures. Then have each group report its findings to the class.**
Discuss gypsum products and their role in making dental models.	☐ Gypsum products (p. 759) – Chemical properties (p. 760) – Setting reactions (p. 760) – Forms (p. 760)	⊠▤ PPT 13-15 ▤ TB questions 3-4 ▤ SW Short-Answer Questions 4; Fill in the Blank questions 3, 5, 10; Multiple Choice questions 8-12 (pp. 396-397) Recall questions 9-12 (p. 760) ♀ CTQ 1-2 (p. 772) ▸ Discuss the chemical properties, setting reactions, and forms of gypsum products. *Class Activity* **Demonstrate and have students manipulate the three types of gypsum material in the laboratory:** – **Model plaster** – **Dental stone** – **High-strength stone**
Mix dental stone.	– Water-to-powder ratio (p. 760) *Procedure* 47-1 Mixing dental plaster (p. 761) (SW/ESLR Competency 47-1, p. 399)	⊠▤ PPT 16 ▤ SW Multiple Choice question 14 (p. 397) ▤ ℮ SW/ESLR Competency 47-1 Mixing Dental Plaster (p. 399) ▸ Discuss the water/powder ratio of gypsum products. ▸ Discuss the proper technique to mix dental stone. *Class Activity* **Divide the class into small groups, and have each group practice mixing dental plaster.**
Pour a set of dental models using the inverted-pour method.	■ Pouring dental models (p. 760) ☐ Double-pour method (p. 760) ☐ Box-and-pour method (p. 762) ☐ Inverted-pour method (p. 762)	⊠▤ PPT 17-20 🎥 Multimedia Procedures DVD: Pouring Dental Models Using Inverted-Pour Method ▤ TB questions 5-6 ▤ SW Fill in the Blank question 9; Multiple Choice question 15 (pp. 396-397) ▤ SW Case Study questions 1-5 (p. 398)

Bird/Robinson

OBJECTIVES	CONTENT	TEACHING RESOURCES

	Procedure 47-2 Pouring dental models using inverted-pour method (pp. 762-763) (SW/ESLR Competency 47-2, pp. 401-403)	SW/ESLR Competency 47-2 Pouring Dental Models Using the Inverted-Pour Method (pp. 401-403)
		
		Recall questions 13-15 (p. 764)
		
		CTQ 3 (p. 772)
		
		▸ Discuss the three different pouring methods to crease the base portion of dental models.
		
		▸ Discuss the techniques used in the inverted-pour method to create dental models.
		
		Class Activity Conduct a group discussion on the uses of dental models in dentistry. Consider each of these topics:
		
		  – *Diagnosis for prosthesis*
		
		  – *Diagnosis of orthodontic work*
		
		  – *Visual presentation of dental treatment*
		
		  – *Custom trays*
		
		  – *Orthodontic appliances*
		
		  – *Provisional coverage*
		
		  – *Mouth guards*

Trim and finish a set of dental models.	☐ Trimming and finishing dental models (p. 764)
	
	  – Anatomic and art portions (p. 764)
	
	  – Polishing plaster models (p. 764)
	
	Procedure 47-3 Trimming and finishing dental models (pp. 764-765) (SW/ESLR Competency 47-3, pp. 405-406)
		PPT 21-23
		
		TB question 7
		
		SW Fill in the Blank questions 12-15; Multiple Choice questions 13, 16-18 (pp. 396-397)
		
		SW/ESLR Competency 47-3 Trimming and Finishing Dental Models (pp. 405-406)
		
		Figure 47-8 Anatomic and art portions of a dental model (p. 761)
		
		Figure 47-9 Examples of pouring methods (p. 761)
		
		Recall questions 16-18 (p. 764)
		
		CTQ 4 (p. 772)
		
		▸ Discuss the techniques used to trim and finish dental models.
		
		▸ Discuss the importance of trimming and finishing dental models.
		
		Class Activity Divide the class into small groups, and have students practice trimming and finishing dental models. Have students provide feedback on one another's work.

ELSEVIER

47.1 Homework/Assignments:

47.1 Instructor's Notes/Student Feedback:

LESSON 47.2

CRITICAL THINKING QUESTION

Maxillary and mandibular alginate impressions must be taken on a patient for bleach trays. What type of gypsum should be used for this procedure? What type of custom impression material will be used to fabricate the bleach trays?

Guidelines: The dental assistant should use dental stone to pour up the models. Dental stone is used because it is more durable and stronger than the other gypsum products. A vacuum-formed thermoplastic resin material should be used to fabricate the bleach trays. A lighter gauge plastic will be "melted" on the models using a vacuum former. Once the material has cooled, it can be removed from the models and trimmed with scissors to remove sharp edges that might cause the patient discomfort.

OBJECTIVES	CONTENT	TEACHING RESOURCES

Describe the three types of custom impression trays and their use in dentistry.	■ Custom impression trays (p. 764)
	
	☐ Criteria for creating custom impression trays (p. 764)
	
	☐ Guidelines and terminology for creating a custom impression tray (p. 766)
		⊠▤ PPT 26-32
		
		💻 TB question 10
		
		SW Short-Answer Questions 5; Fill in the Blank questions 4, 6, 8, 14; Multiple Choice questions 19-20 (pp. 395-397)
		
		💡 CTQ 5 (p. 772)
		
		▸ Discuss the primary materials used to construct custom trays: self-curing acrylic resin, light-cured resin, and thermoplastic material.
		
		▸ Discuss the elements and guidelines for creating a custom impression tray.
		
		Class Activity Demonstrate and have students manipulate the three types of custom impression material:
		
		   – ***Acrylic resin tray***
		
		   – ***Light-cured resin tray***
		
		   – ***Vacuum-formed thermoplastic***

Construct an acrylic resin custom tray.	☐ Acrylic resin tray materials (p. 766) ⎡Procedure⎤ 47-4 Constructing an acrylic resin custom tray (pp. 767-768) (SW/ESLR Competency 47-4, pp. 407-408)	⊠▤ PPT 33 SW Multiple Choice question 20 (p. 397) SW/ESLR Competency 47-4 Constructing an Acrylic Resin Custom Tray (pp. 407-408) ▸ Discuss the technique used in constructing an acrylic resin custom tray. ▸ Discuss the procedural steps in constructing an acrylic resin custom tray. ***Class Activity Divide the class into small groups, and have each group practice constructing an acrylic resin custom tray.***

Torres and Ehrlich Modern Dental Assisting, 9th ed.
Bird/Robinson

OBJECTIVES	CONTENT	TEACHING RESOURCES
Construct a light-cured custom tray.	☐ Light-cured resin tray materials (p. 766) Procedure 47-5 Creating a light-cured custom tray (p. 768) (SW/ESLR Competency 47-5, pp. 409-410)	PPT 34 SW Multiple Choice questions 19-20 (p. 397) SW/ESLR Competency 47-5 Creating a Light-Cured Custom Tray (pp. 409-410) ▸ Discuss the technique to construct a light-cured custom tray. ▸ Discuss the procedural steps in constructing a light-cured custom tray. *Class Activity Divide the class into small groups, and have each group practice creating a light-cured custom tray.*
Construct a vacuum-formed custom tray.	☐ Vacuum-formed thermoplastic resin (p. 766) Procedure 47-6 Constructing a Vacuum-formed custom tray (p. 770) (SW/ESLR Competency 47-6, pp. 411-412)	PPT 35 Multimedia Procedures DVD: Constructing a Vacuum-Formed Tray TB question 8 SW Multiple Choice questions 19-21 (p. 397) SW/ESLR Competency 47-6 Constructing a Vacuum-Formed Custom Tray (pp. 411-412) Recall questions 19-24 (p. 769) ▸ Discuss the technique used to construct a vacuum-formed custom tray. ▸ Discuss the procedural steps in constructing a vacuum-formed custom tray. *Class Activity Divide the class into small groups, and have each group practice constructing a vacuum-formed custom tray.*
Describe the types of dental waxes and their use in dentistry.	■ Dental waxes (p. 769) ☐ Boxing wax (p. 769) ☐ Utility wax (p. 769) ☐ Sticky wax (p. 769) ☐ Inlay casting wax (p. 769) ☐ Casting wax (p. 771) ☐ Baseplate wax (p. 771) ☐ Bite-registration wax (p. 771)	PPT 36-42 TB question 9 SW Short-Answer Questions 6; Multiple Choice questions 22-25 (pp. 395, 397) Figure 47-10 Boxing wax (p. 769) Figure 47-11 Utility wax (p. 769) Figure 47-12 Inlay casting wax (p. 771) Figure 47-13 Baseplate wax (p. 771) Figure 47-24 Bite-registration wax (p. 771) Recall questions 25-28 (p. 771) Patient Education (p. 771)

OBJECTIVES	CONTENT	TEACHING RESOURCES
		Legal and Ethical Implications (p. 771)
		Eye to the Future (p. 772)
		▶ Discuss the uses for the following types of dental waxes: boxing wax, utility wax, sticky wax, inlay casting wax, casting wax, baseplate wax, and bite-registration wax.
		*Class Activity **Demonstrate and have students manipulate the following types of dental waxes:***
		– *Boxing wax*
		– *Utility wax*
		– *Sticky wax*
		– *Inlay casting wax*
		– *Casting wax*
		– *Baseplate wax*
		– *Bite-registration wax*
Performance Evaluation		🖥 TB
		📘 SW questions (pp. 395-397)
		📘 SW Case Study (p. 398)
		📘 *e* SW/ESLR Competency 47-1 Mixing Dental Plaster (p. 399)
		📘 *e* SW/ESLR Competency 47-2 Pouring Dental Models Using the Inverted-Pour Method (pp. 401-403)
		📘 *e* SW/ESLR Competency 47-3 Trimming and Finishing Dental Models (pp. 405-406)
		📘 *e* SW/ESLR Competency 47-4 Constructing an Acrylic Resin Custom Tray (pp. 407-408)
		📘 *e* SW/ESLR Competency 47-5 Creating a Light-Cured Custom Tray (pp. 409-410)
		📘 *e* SW/ESLR Competency 47-6 Constructing a Vacuum-Formed Custom Tray (pp. 411-412)
		e ESLR Electronic Flashcards
		e ESLR Practice Quiz
		Recall questions (pp. 757-771)
		💡 CTQ (p. 772)

ELSEVIER

Torres and Ehrlich Modern Dental Assisting, 9th ed.

     Bird/Robinson

47.2 Homework/Assignments:

47.2 Instructor's Notes/Student Feedback:

47 Laboratory Materials and Procedures

Slide 1

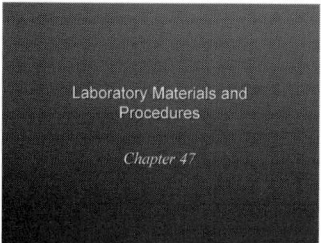

Laboratory Materials and Procedures

Chapter 47

Slide 2

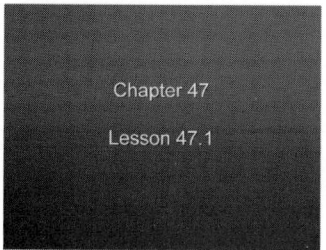

Chapter 47

Lesson 47.1

Slide 3

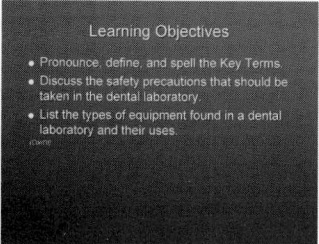

Learning Objectives

- Pronounce, define, and spell the Key Terms.
- Discuss the safety precautions that should be taken in the dental laboratory.
- List the types of equipment found in a dental laboratory and their uses.

Slide 4

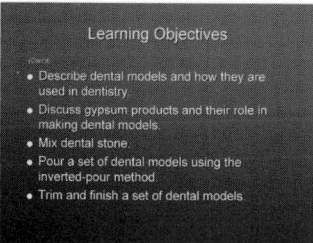

Learning Objectives

- Describe dental models and how they are used in dentistry.
- Discuss gypsum products and their role in making dental models.
- Mix dental stone.
- Pour a set of dental models using the inverted-pour method.
- Trim and finish a set of dental models.

Slide 5

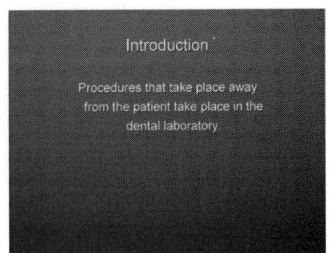

- Where is the in-house dental laboratory located?
- Discuss the distinctions between the in-house and outsourced dental laboratory.

Slide 6

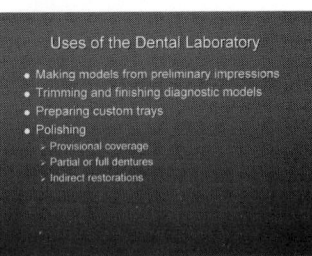

- What are preliminary impressions used for?
- What are diagnostic models used for?
- What are custom trays used for?
- What is provisional coverage?
- What is an indirect restoration?

Slide 7

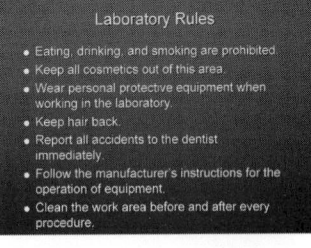

- These rules should be followed in the laboratory on campus as well.

Slide 8

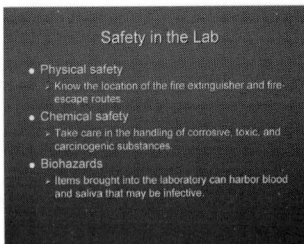

- Do you know the correct procedure for a fire?
- What is an MSDS sheet?
- How is biohazardous material labeled?

Torres and Ehrlich Modern Dental Assisting, 9th ed.

Bird/Robinson

Slide 9

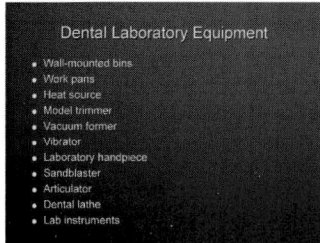

- What is the purpose of each piece of equipment in the dental laboratory?

Slide 10

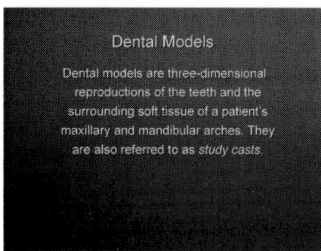

- Dental models are also known as study models or diagnostic casts.

Slide 11

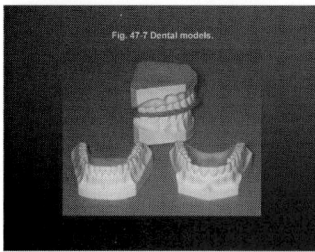

- What type of impression material is used to obtain these study models?
- Models should be free of voids and errors before presentation.

Slide 12

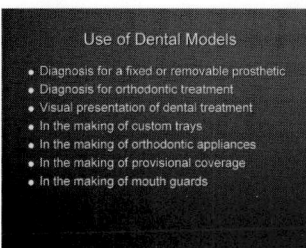

- How many students have had study models made?
- For what reasons?
- What is an example of a fixed or removable prosthetic?

Slide 13

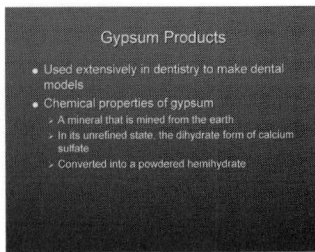

- The differences in hemihydrate crystals determine the water/powder ratios for all three different types of gypsum.
- What are the three types of gypsum?

Slide 14

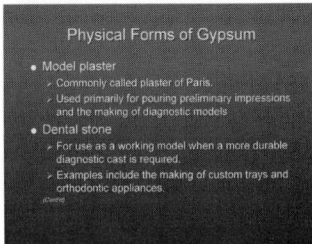

- Model plaster is white..
- What are diagnostic models used for?
- What is the correct water-to-powder ratio?

Slide 15

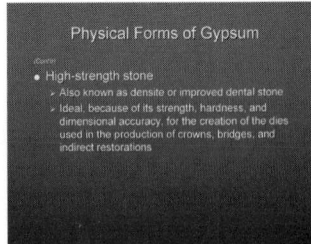

- Densite is blue..
- Mostly used by dental laboratory technicians.
- What is the appropriate water/powder ratio?

Slide 16

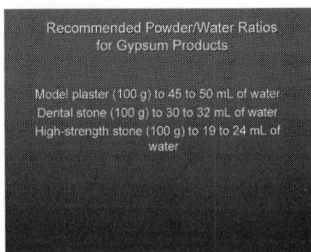

- Dental stone is yellow-gold..
- What are working models used for?
- What is the appropriate water/powder ratio?

Torres and Ehrlich Modern Dental Assisting, 9th ed.

Bird/Robinson

Slide 17

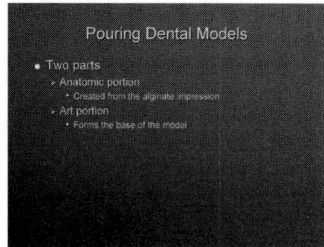

- Strict measurements must be followed.
- Mix should be smooth and creamy.

Slide 18

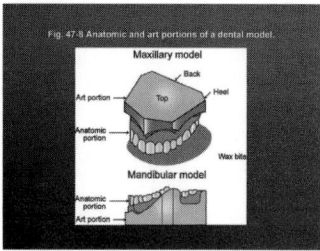

Slide 19

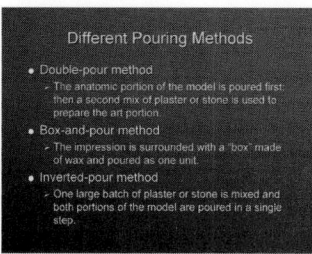

- The double-pour method is the easiest to use in the learning stages; two mixes are used.
- The box-and-pour method is not commonly used in the dental office.
- The inverted-pour method uses measurements of water/powder that must be exact and must have enough mix for both the anatomic and art portion.
- What happens if powder is added to a thin, runny mix?
- What happens if water is added to a thicker mix?

Slide 20

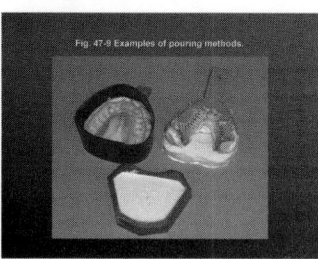

- Which is the box-and-pour?
- What is used around the impression for the box-and-pour?
- Rubber bases can be used to eliminate trimming.

Slide 21

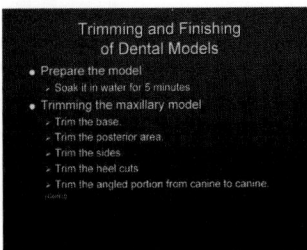

- Why soak models before trimming them? *(To make trimming easier.)*
- Follow the guidelines to obtain an even appearance.

Slide 22

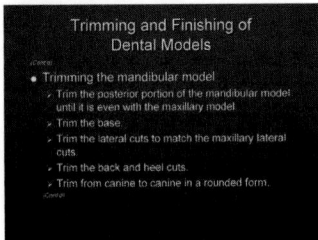

Slide 23

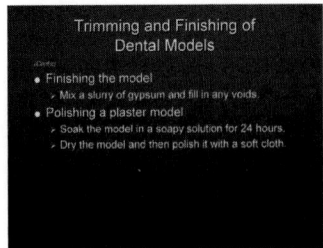

- What is slurry?
- Why polish a model?

Slide 24

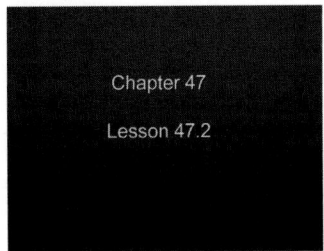

Bird/Robinson

Slide 25

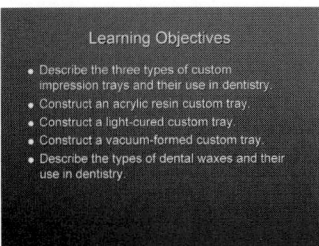

Slide 26

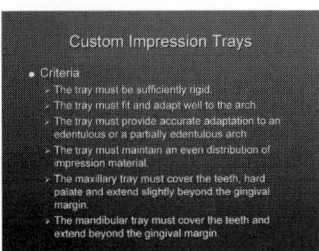

- For whom are custom trays made?
- For what procedures are custom trays used?

Slide 27

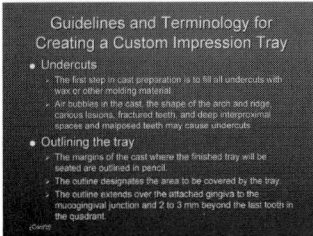

Slide 28

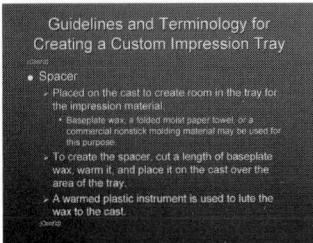

Torres and Ehrlich Modern Dental Assisting, 9th ed.

Bird/Robinson

Slide 29

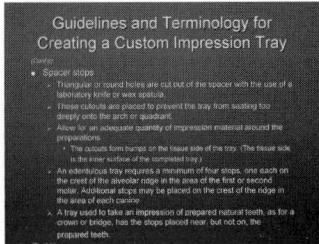

Slide 30

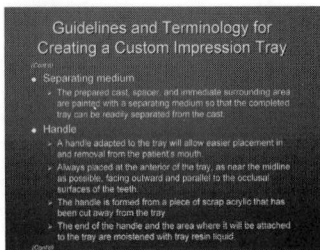

Slide 31

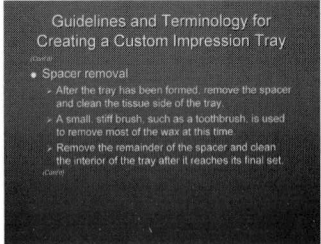

Slide 32

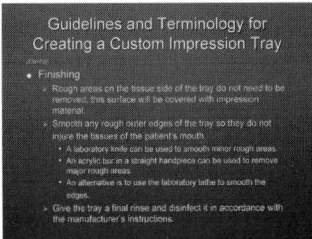

Torres and Ehrlich Modern Dental Assisting, 9th ed.

Bird/Robinson

Slide 33

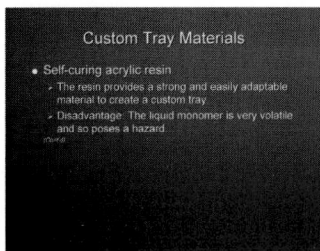

- Work area must be well ventilated
- PPE must be worn.
- Self-curing acrylic resin may irritate the skin.
- What does volatile mean?

Slide 34

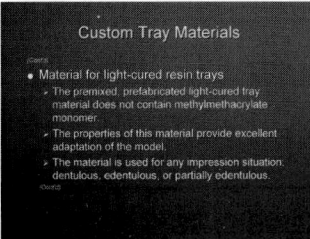

- Light-cured resin requires special light to cure the material.
- This method and material provides low shrinkage.
- Using these materials for models takes longer to make than a self-curing resin material would take.

Slide 35

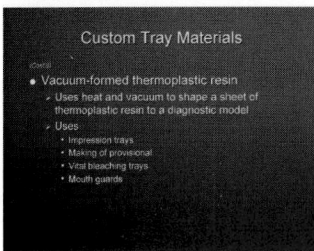

- Different gauges of plastic are available and are chosen based on their intended use.
- A vacuum former melts the plastic, and then the vacuum is turned on and the material is "sucked" onto the cast.

Slide 36

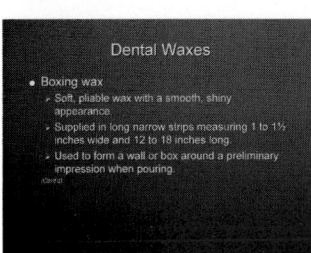

- For which pouring method would the boxing wax be used?
- Boxing wax is not often used in dental offices.

Torres and Ehrlich Modern Dental Assisting, 9th ed.

Bird/Robinson

Slide 37

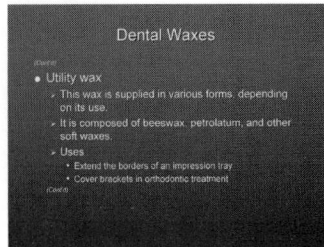

- Utility wax appears clear-to-white or red..
- It is most often supplied in long ropes.
- It is easy to apply and remove.

Slide 38

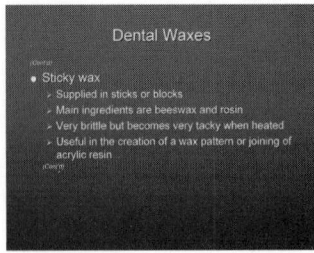

- Sticky wax can be used in the dental laboratory to fix a broken tooth on a dental cast.

Slide 39

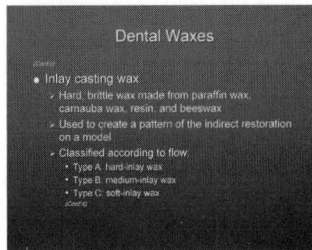

- Inlay casting wax is mostly used by the dental laboratory technician.
- For what processes are the different classifications of inlay wax used?

Slide 40

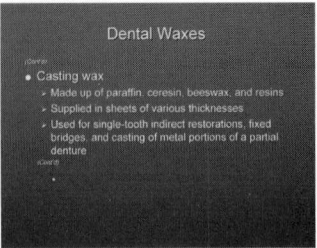

- For what processes is casting wax used?

Torres and Ehrlich Modern Dental Assisting, 9th ed.

Bird/Robinson

Slide 41

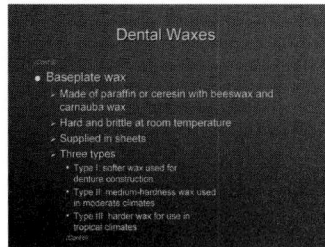

- Baseplate wax is pink.
- What else can baseplate wax be used for? *(Bite registration.)*

Slide 42

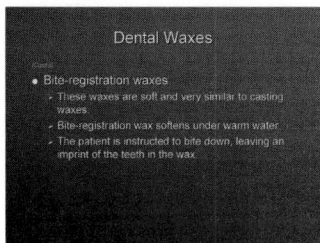

- Bite registration waxes are supplied in wafer form.
- What is the purpose of a bite registration?

TEACHING FOCUS

This chapter will give students an opportunity to understand restorative and esthetic dentistry, along with the dental assistant's role in providing this type of care. Students will also have an opportunity to learn about cavity preparation, permanent restorations, complex restorations, veneers, and tooth whitening.

MATERIALS AND RESOURCES

- ☐ abrasive strips (Lesson 48.1)
- ☐ articulating paper (all Lessons)
- ☐ basic setup (Lesson 48.2)
- ☐ burs, assorted (dentist's choice) (all Lessons)
- ☐ composite material (all Lessons)
- ☐ composite shade guide (all Lessons)
- ☐ computer and PowerPoint projector (all Lessons)
- ☐ condenser (Lesson 48.2)
- ☐ cotton pellet (Lesson 48.2)
- ☐ cotton pellets, cotton rolls, 2 x 2 inch gauze (Lesson 48.1)
- ☐ curing light with protective shield (all Lessons)
- ☐ dental dam setup (Lesson 48.1)
- ☐ dental dam setup (cervical clamp) (Lesson 48.1)
- ☐ dental liners, base, sealers, bonding agents (all Lessons)
- ☐ dental floss (all Lessons)
- ☐ discoid/cleoid carver (Lesson 48.2)
- ☐ finishing burs and diamonds (all Lessons)
- ☐ high-speed and low-speed handpieces (all Lessons)
- ☐ high-volume oral evacuator (HVE) tip (all Lessons)

- ☐ intermediate restoration material (IRM) setup (material, treated pad, spatula) (Lesson 48.2)
- ☐ local anesthetic setup (all Lessons)
- ☐ matrix setup (Lesson 48.1)
- ☐ Mylar matrix setup (all Lessons)
- ☐ permanent restorative material (composite or amalgam) (Lesson 48.1)
- ☐ polishing kit (disc and mandrel) (Lesson 48.1)
- ☐ plastic instrument (Lesson 48.2)
- ☐ polishing paste (all Lessons)
- ☐ premeasured amalgam capsules (Lesson 48.1)
- ☐ restorative tray (basic setup, hand cutting instruments, composite placement instrument, amalgam carrier, condensers, burnishers, carvers, articulating paper holder) (all Lessons)
- ☐ retracting cord and packer (Lesson 48.1)
- ☐ saliva ejector (all Lessons)
- ☐ Tofflemire matrix retainer (for class II) (Lesson 48.2)
- ☐ wedge (for classes II, III, and IV) (Lesson 48.2)

LESSON CHECKLIST

Preparations for this lesson include:

- lecture
- evaluation of student knowledge and skills needed to perform all entry-level activities related to general dentistry, including:
  - ○ cavity preparation
  - ○ permanent restorations
  - ○ complex restorations
  - ○ retention pins
  - ○ veneers
  - ○ tooth whitening

KEY TERMS

axial wall (p. 776)
cavity (p. 775)
cavity preparation (p. 775)
cavity wall (p. 776)
convenience form (p. 776)
diastema (p. 789)
esthetic dentistry (p. 775)
line angle (p. 776)
operative dentistry (p. 775)

outline form (p. 775)
pulpal wall (p. 776)
resistance form (p. 776)
restoration (p. 775)
restorative dentistry (p. 775)
retention form (p. 776)
retention (retentive) pin (p. 784)
veneer (p. 789)

ADDITIONAL RESOURCES

PowerPoint slides (Evolve): 1-40
The Interactive Dental Office CD-ROM: Crystal Malone
Multimedia Procedures DVD: Placing an Intermediate Restoration

---

Legend

CTQ
Critical
Thinking
Question

DVD
Multimedia
Procedures
Videos and
Animations

ESLR
EVOLVE
Student
Learning
Resources

IDO
Interactive
Dental
Office
CD-ROM

SW
Student
Workbook

TB
Test Bank
on the
TEACH
CD-ROM

PPT
PowerPoint
Slides

Class Activities are indicated in ***bold italic.***

ELSEVIER

Torres and Ehrlich Modern Dental Assisting, 9th ed.

Bird/Robinson

LESSON 48.1

PRETEST

1. The internal surface of the tooth that is prepared for a restoration is the
   a. cavity wall.
   b. internal wall.
   c. external wall.
   d. axial wall.

2. Which classification of restoration involves the interproximal surface of a posterior tooth?
   a. Class I
   b. Class II
   c. Class III
   d. Class IV

3. To check the occlusion of a Class I restoration, one should use
   a. dental floss.
   b. articulating paper.
   c. the matrix system.
   d. an abrasive strip.

4. Which classification of restoration requires the use of a Mylar matrix system?
   a. Class I
   b. Class II
   c. Class III
   d. Class V

5. Which classification of restoration is also referred to as a smooth surface restoration?
   a. Class II
   b. Class III
   c. Class IV
   d. Class V

6. What type of dental material is used for an intermediate restoration?
   a. amalgam
   b. composite
   c. veneer
   d. IRM

7. A space between two teeth is called
   a. diastema.
   b. proximal.
   c. interproximal.
   d. intermediate restoration.

8. On which tooth surface is a veneer placed?
   a. facial
   b. buccal
   c. lingual
   d. occlusal

9. Veneers which are directly applied to the tooth surface are
   a. permanent cement
   b. temporary cement
   c. bonded
   d. adhesive strips

10. Whitening systems can last for
    a. up to 6 months.
    b. 1 to 2 years.
    c. 2 to 4 years.
    d. 3 to 5 years.

Answers

1. a	3. b	5. d	7. a	9. c
2. b	4. c	6. d	8. a	10. d

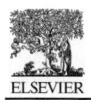

Torres and Ehrlich Modern Dental Assisting, 9th ed.

Bird/Robinson

BACKGROUND ASSESSMENT

Question: What is restorative dentistry?

Answer: Restorative dentistry, also known as operative dentistry, includes procedures such as amalgam restorations, composite resin restorations, intermediate restorations, resin veneers, and tooth-whitening procedures. It is performed when teeth must be restored to their usual structure and function through use of direct and indirect restorative materials. Amalgam and composite are most commonly used to restore the tooth to its normal function. Reasons for restoration include initial or recurrent decay, replacement of failed restorations, and abrasion or erosion of tooth structure.

Question: Why are retention pins used in complex restorations?

Answer: Retention pins are used when tooth decay extends beyond a normal size or shape to help retain the restoration and provide added strength. They are placed inside the cavity preparation, and the restorative material is placed around the pin. Retention pins are commonly used in complex restorations when grooves and the bonding material would be deemed insufficient.

CRITICAL THINKING QUESTION

During preparation for an MODL amalgam on tooth #4 the dentist notices that the decay extends well beyond his initial assessment and is very close to the pulpal chamber. He informs the patient that the treatment plan must be altered to see how the tooth will react now that the decay has been removed. What changes will need to be made in the setup?

Guidelines: Because the decay is close to the pulp chamber, the tooth must be monitored for the next few weeks to determine the health and extent of decay of the affected tooth. The dental assistant will need to set up for an intermediate restoration that will consist of the IRM material. In many states, placement of an immediate restoration can be performed by certified dental assistants permitted to do expanded functions.

OBJECTIVES	CONTENT	TEACHING RESOURCES
Define, spell, and pronounce the Key Terms.	■ Key terms (p. 774)	TB questions 1-2 SW Fill in the Blank question 10; Multiple Choice question 1 (p. 414) ESLR Electronic Flashcards ▶ Discuss each of the key terms in chapter 48, focusing on the definition, pronunciation, and spelling of each term. *Class Activity Go around the room and have each student use one of the key terms in a clinically relevant sentence in order to define the term. Continue until all terms have been used; if students get stuck, have the rest of the class offer suggestions.*
Describe the process and principles of cavity preparation.	■ Cavity preparation (p. 775) ☐ Terminology (p. 775) ☐ Initial preparation (p. 775) ☐ Final preparation (p. 776)	PPT 4-9 TB question 3 SW Short-Answer Questions 1; Fill in the Blank questions 2-3, 6-9, 11-12; Multiple Choice questions 2-4 (pp. 413-414) Box 48-1 Terminology Related to Cavity Preparation (p. 776) Figure 48-1 Outline form of a cavity preparation (p. 776) Figure 48-2 Resistance form of a cavity preparation (p. 776) Figure 48-3 Retention form placed in the cavity preparation (p. 776)

Torres and Ehrlich Modern Dental Assisting, 9th ed.

Bird/Robinson

OBJECTIVES	CONTENT	TEACHING RESOURCES
		Figure 48-4 Convenience form is used for easy access to tooth decay (p. 777)
		Recall questions 1-4 (p. 777)
		‣ Discuss the initial preparation required for cavity preparation.
		‣ Discuss the final preparation required for cavity preparation.
		Class Activity Divide the class into groups. Have each group outline the steps involved in preparing a tooth for restorative procedures. What are the dentist's roles, and what are the dental assistant's roles? Have groups share their findings with the class for discussion.

Discuss the differences in assisting with an amalgam versus assisting with a composite restoration.	■ Permanent restorations (p. 777)
	
	☐ Standardized format of a restorative procedure (p. 777)
	
	☐ Dental assistant's responsibility in a restorative procedure (p. 777)
	
	☐ Class I restorations (p. 777)
	  – Tooth preparation (p. 778)
	  – Special considerations (p. 778)
	
	☐ Class II restorations (p. 778)
	  – Tooth preparation (p. 778)
	  – Special considerations (p. 778)
	
	☐ Class III and IV restorations (p. 780)
	  – Tooth preparation (p. 780)
	  – Special considerations (p. 780)
	
	☐ Class V restorations (p. 780)
		⊠▤ PPT 10-21
		
		▤ TB questions 4-7
		
		▨ SW Short-Answer Questions 2; Fill in the Blank questions 1, 4; Multiple Choice questions 5-10, 18-20 (pp. 413-415)
		
		▨ SW Case Study questions 1-5 (p. 415)
		
		Figure 48-5 Class I restorations (p. 777)
		
		Figure 48-6 (A) Class I tooth preparation for amalgam on maxillary premolar; (B) Tooth preparation walls (p. 778)
		
		Figure 48-7 Class II restorations (p. 778)
		
		Figure 48-8 (A) Class II MO conventional tooth preparation for amalgam on maxillary; (B) Tooth preparation walls: molar (p. 780)
		
		Figure 48-9 Class III composite restoration (p. 780)
		
		Figure 48-10 Class IV composite restoration (p. 780)
		
		Figure 48-11 (A) Class III conventional tooth preparation on maxillary central incisor; (B) Tooth preparation walls (p. 783)
		
		Figure 48-12 (A) Class IV conventional tooth preparation of maxillary canine; (B) Tooth preparation walls (p. 783)
		
		Figure 48-13 (A) Class V conventional tooth preparation; (B) Tooth preparation (p. 784)
		
		Recall questions 5-10 (p. 784)
		
		‣ Discuss the steps involved in a restorative procedure.
		
		‣ Discuss the characteristics of Class I, II, III, IV, and V restorations.
		
		‣ Discuss the differences in assisting with an amalgam versus a composite restoration.

OBJECTIVES	CONTENT	TEACHING RESOURCES
	– Tooth preparation (p. 784) – Special considerations (p. 784)	***Class Activity** Make two lists on the board; label one side **Amalgam Restoration** and the other **Composite Restoration**. Have students compare and contrast the two types of procedures and ask student volunteers to record responses in the diagram.*
Prepare the setup and assist in a Class I restoration.	☐ Class I restorations (p. 777) – Tooth preparation (p. 778) – Special considerations (p. 778) Procedure 48-1 Assisting in a class I restoration (p. 779) (SW/ESLR Competencies 48-1and 48-2, pp. 417-418)	PPT 13-14 SW Multiple Choice questions 5, 18-20 (pp. 414-415) SW/IDO Patient Case Exercise questions 1-3 (p. 416) (The Interactive Dental Office CD-ROM) SW/ESLR Competencies 48-1 and 48-2 Assisting in an Amalgam Restoration (pp. 417-418) CTQ 5 (p. 794) ▸ Discuss the procedures used to assist with a Class I restoration. ***Class Activity** Divide the class into groups. Have each group outline the preparatory steps to be performed by the dental assistant before a permanent restoration is performed. Have students share their answers with the class for discussion.*
Prepare the setup and assist in a Class II restoration.	☐ Class II restorations (p. 778) – Tooth preparation (p. 778) – Special considerations (p. 778) Procedure 48-2 Assisting in a Class II amalgam restoration (pp. 781-783) (SW/ESLR Competencies 48-1 and 48-2, pp. 417-418)	PPT 15-16 TB question 5 SW Multiple Choice questions 6-7, 18-20 (pp. 414-415) SW/IDO Patient Case Exercise questions 1-3 (p. 416) (The Interactive Dental Office CD-ROM) SW/ESLR Competencies 48-1 and 48-2 Assisting in an Amalgam Restoration (pp. 417-418) CTQ 1 (p. 794) ▸ Discuss the procedures used to assist with a Class II restoration. ***Class Activity** Lead a class discussion about Class II lesions and ask students to differentiate between conservative and comprehensive restorations. Why is it difficult for the dentist to restore this type of cavity? Record student responses on the board for comparison.*
Prepare the setup and assist in a Class III restoration.	☐ Class III and IV restorations (p. 780) – Tooth preparation (p. 780)	PPT 17-18 SW Multiple Choice questions 9, 18-20 (pp. 414-415)

Bird/Robinson

OBJECTIVES	CONTENT	TEACHING RESOURCES
	– Special considerations (p. 780) Procedure 48-3 Assisting in a Class III or Class IV restoration (pp. 785-786) (SW/ESLR Competencies 48-3 and 48-4, pp. 419-420)	SW/IDO Patient Case Exercise questions 1-3 (p. 416) (The Interactive Dental Office CD-ROM) SW/ESLR Competencies 48-3 and 48-4 Assisting in a Composite Restoration (pp. 419-420) ▸ Discuss the procedures used to assist with a Class III restoration. *Class Activity Divide the class into groups. Have each group outline preparatory procedures and special considerations to take when restoring Class III and Class IV lesions, and identify three jobs of the dental assistant during these procedures. Have groups share their findings with the class for discussion.*
Prepare the setup and assist in a Class IV restoration.	☐ Class III and IV restorations (p. 780) – Tooth preparation (p. 780) – Special considerations (p. 780) Procedure 48-3 Assisting in a class III or IV restoration (pp. 785-786) (SW/ESLR Competencies 48-3 and 48-4, pp. 419-420)	PPT 17, 19 TB question 6 SW Multiple Choice questions 8, 9, 18-20 (pp. 414-415) SW/IDO Patient Case Exercise questions 1-3 (p. 416) (The Interactive Dental Office CD-ROM) SW/ESLR Competencies 48-3 and 48-4 Assisting in a Composite Restoration (pp. 419-420) ▸ Discuss the procedures used to assist with a Class IV restoration. *Class Activity Lead a class discussion about Class III and Class IV lesions and ask students to differentiate between the two classes. How does one determine if a lesion is Class III or Class IV? Record student responses on the board for comparison.*
Prepare the setup and assist in a Class V restoration.	☐ Class V restorations (p. 780) – Tooth preparation (p. 784) – Special considerations (p. 784) Procedure 48-4 Assisting in a Class V restoration (p. 787) (SW/ESLR Competencies 48-3 and 48-4, pp. 419-420)	PPT 20-21 TB question 7 SW Multiple Choice questions 10, 18-20 (pp. 414-415) SW/ESLR Competencies 48-3 and 48-4 Assisting in a Composite Restoration (pp. 419-420) ▸ Discuss the procedures used to assist with a Class V restoration. *Class Activity Lead a class discussion about Class V restorations and ask students to explain why this type of lesion affects the root of the tooth in older adults. What are some ways these lesions could be prevented? Record student responses on the board for comparison.*

Bird/Robinson

48.1 Homework/Assignments:

48.1 Instructor's Notes/Student Feedback:

LESSON 48.2

CRITICAL THINKING QUESTION

A patient is self-conscious about coffee stains on his maxillary anterior teeth and asks the dental assistant about tooth whiteners. He says that he has tried over-the-counter whitening strips and found that they are not as effective as he would like. He also travels frequently and is not in town very often. What information can the dental assistant provide about other bleaching options?

Guidelines: Because the patient's stains are extrinsic, he would be a good candidate for either an in-office or at-home bleaching treatment. The dental assistant should explain to the patient that the in-office treatment can be accomplished in less than an hour, but, depending on how much coffee he consumes, he may require additional treatments. At-home bleaching systems use a bleaching tray whenever it is convenient for the patient. This system would be a good choice for the patient because of his frequent travel; however he needs to be told that appointments must be scheduled with the dentist to observe for signs of abuse from bleaching.

OBJECTIVES	CONTENT	TEACHING RESOURCES
Discuss why retention pins would be selected for a complex restorative procedure.	■ Complex restorations (p. 784) ☐ Retention pins (p. 784)	PPT 24-25 TB question 8 SW Short-Answer Questions 3 (p. 413) SW/IDO Patient Case Exercise question 5 (p. 416) (The Interactive Dental Office CD-ROM) Figure 48-14 Retention (retentive) pins placed in tooth structure for retaining and supporting a restoration (p. 786) ▸ Discuss when a complex restoration is needed. ▸ Discuss when it is necessary to use retention pins for a complex restoration. ***Class Activity** Lead a class discussion about complex restorations. Ask students to identify the indications for a complex restoration and discuss when and why retention pins are used. What are the advantages and disadvantages of using retention pins? Record student responses on the board for discussion.*
Describe the need for placement of an intermediate restoration.	■ Intermediate restorations (p. 784)	PPT 26-27 SW Short-Answer Questions 4; Multiple Choice question 11 (pp. 413-414) Recall questions 11-12 (p. 789) ▸ Discuss the reasons for performing intermediate restorations. ▸ Discuss the process of placing and carving an intermediate restoration. ***Class Activity** Divide the class into groups. Have each group discuss the expanded functions of certified dental assistants, explain what those functions are, and identify three other expanded functions. Have groups share their findings with the class for discussion.*

Torres and Ehrlich Modern Dental Assisting, 9th ed.

Bird/Robinson

OBJECTIVES	CONTENT	TEACHING RESOURCES
Prepare the setup and place and carve an intermediate restoration (expanded function).	Procedure 48-5 Placing and carving an intermediate restoration (expanded function) (pp. 788-789) (SW/ESLR Competency 48-5, pp. 421-422)	🎥 Multimedia Procedures DVD: Placing an Intermediate Restoration 📖 SW Short-Answer Questions 4; Multiple Choice question 11 (pp. 413-414) 📖 *e* SW/ESLR Competency 48-5 Placing and Carving an Intermediate Restoration (Expanded Function) (pp. 421-422) ▸ Discuss the procedure used to set up, carve, and place an intermediate restoration. *Class Activity **Divide the class into groups. Have each group compare and contrast the procedures for applying permanent and intermediate restorations and outline the role of the dental assistant in each. Have groups share their findings with the class for discussion.***
Describe the procedure of composite veneers.	■ Veneers (p. 789) Procedure 48-6 Assisting in the placement of a veneer (pp. 791-792) (SW/ESLR Competency 48-6, p. 423)	📊 PPT 28-30 💻 TB question 9 📖 SW Short-Answer Questions 5; Fill in the Blank question 5; Multiple Choice questions 6, 13 (pp. 413-414) 📖 *e* SW/ESLR Competency 48-6 Assisting in the Placement of a Veneer (p. 423) Figure 48-15 Veneers placed on teeth 8 and 9 to reduce discoloration and cover stain (p. 790) Figure 48-16 Veneers placed to close diastema (p. 790) Recall questions 13-14 (p. 790) ▸ Discuss the reasons that veneers are used. ▸ Discuss the procedure involved in placing a veneer. *Class Activity **Divide the class into groups. Have each group identify five patient teaching points to be provided to a patient receiving veneers and then present its list to the class.***
Describe tooth-whitening procedures and the role of the dental assistant.	■ Tooth whitening (p. 790) ☐ Treatment options (p. 790) – In-office treatment (p. 790) – At-home treatment (p. 792) – Over-the-counter options (p. 792)	📊 PPT 31-40 💻 TB question 10 📖 SW Short-Answer Questions 6; Multiple Choice questions 14-17 (pp. 413, 415) Figure 48-17 Before and after photos of tooth whitening used for extrinsic stains (p. 790) Figure 48-18 Before and after photos of tooth whitening used for intrinsic stains (p. 792)

ELSEVIER

Torres and Ehrlich Modern Dental Assisting, 9th ed.

Bird/Robinson

OBJECTIVES	CONTENT	TEACHING RESOURCES
	☐ Abuse of whitening products (p. 793)	Figure 48-19 Custom-fitted tray for bleaching procedure (p. 792)
	☐ Adverse effects of tooth whitening (p. 793)	Recall questions 15-18 (p. 793)
	– Thermal hypersensitivity (p. 793)	💡 CTQ 3 (p. 794)
		▸ Discuss the differences between extrinsic and intrinsic stains.
	– Tissue irritation (p. 793)	▸ Discuss the various types of tooth-whitening procedures: in-office treatment, at-home treatment, and over-the-counter options.
	☐ Assistant's role in tooth whitening (p. 793)	▸ Discuss the dental assistant's role in tooth whitening, along with the instructions an assistant would give to the patient.
	☐ Patient instructions in tooth whitening (p. 793)	***Class Activity** Have students research five different over-the-counter tooth-whitening products and present their findings to the class. They should include price information, instructions, effectiveness, and special considerations. (For students to prepare for this activity, see Homework/Assignments #1.)*
Performance Evaluation		🖥 TB
		📓 SW questions (pp. 413-415)
		📓 SW Case Study (p. 415)
		📓💿 SW/IDO Patient Case Exercise (p. 416) (The Interactive Dental Office CD-ROM)
		📓 *e* SW/ESLR Competencies 48-1 and 48-2 Assisting in an Amalgam Restoration (pp. 417-418)
		📓 *e* SW/ESLR Competencies 48-3 and 48-4 Assisting in a Composite Restoration (pp. 419-420)
		📓 *e* SW/ESLR Competency 48-5 Placing and Carving an Intermediate Restoration (Expanded Function) (pp. 421-422)
		📓 *e* SW/ESLR Competency 48-6 Assisting in the Placement of a Veneer (pp. 423)
		e ESLR Electronic Flashcards
		e ESLR Practice Quiz
		Recall questions (pp. 777-793)
		💡 CTQ (p. 794)

48.2 Homework/Assignments:

1. Have students research five different over-the-counter tooth-whitening products and present their findings to the class. They should include price information, instructions, effectiveness, and special considerations.

48.2 Instructor's Notes/Student Feedback:

Slide 1

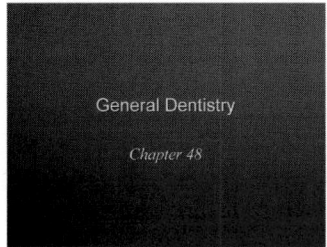

Slide 2

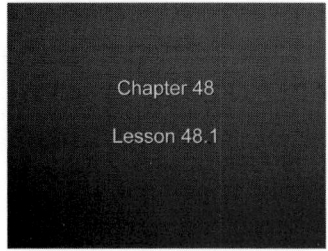

Slide 3

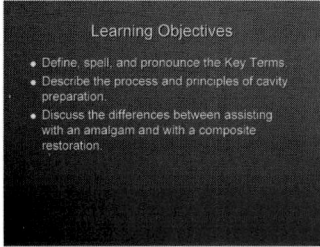

Slide 4

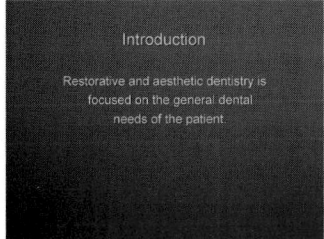

- Restorative dentistry is also called operative dentistry.

Bird/Robinson

Slide 5

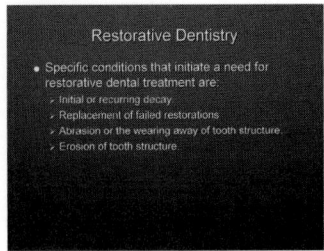

- What type of materials would be used for restorative dentistry?

Slide 6

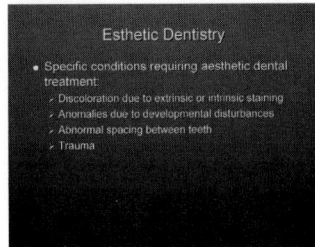

- What type of materials would be used for esthetic dentistry?
- Why are esthetics important?

Slide 7

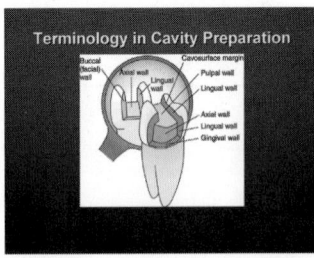

- Understanding the terminology will help dental assistants prepare the correct instruments for a procedure.

Slide 8

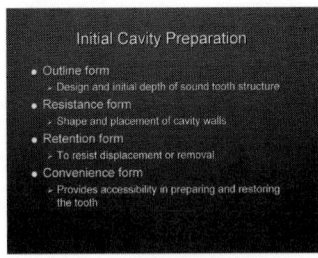

- Initial cavity preparation is the first of two stages of cavity preparation and has a set number of steps that the dentist follows in an exact order.
- This process is done to gain access to the decay or defect.

Slide 9

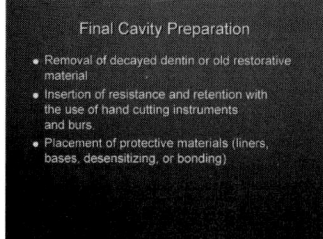

- Final cavity preparation is the second stage of cavity preparation.
- This procedure is followed after the steps in the initial cavity preparation have been completed.

Slide 10

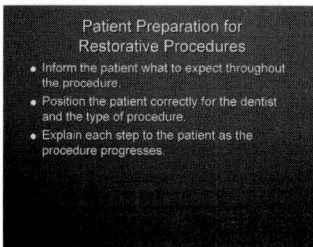

- What is the correct position of a patient during the procedure?
- How would the dental assistant explain the procedure to the patient?

Slide 11

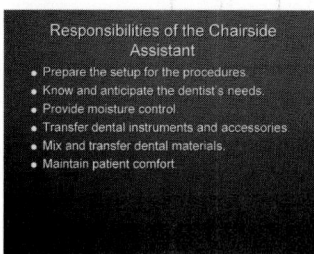

- What are the appropriate setup items needed for an amalgam restoration?
- What are the appropriate setup items needed for a composite restoration?
- How can the dental assistant provide moisture control?

Slide 12

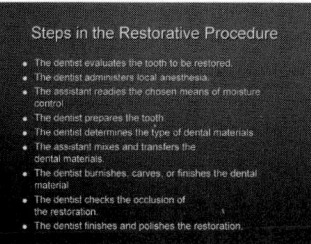

Bird/Robinson

Slide 13

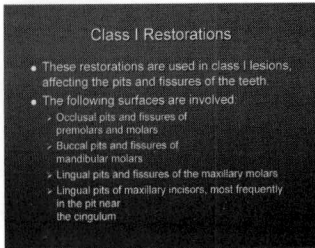

- Why are Class I restorations so common?
- What are pits and fissures?
- Where are they located?

Slide 14

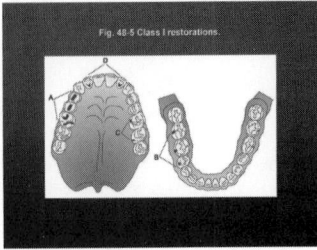

- Which anterior teeth would have a Class I restoration?

Slide 15

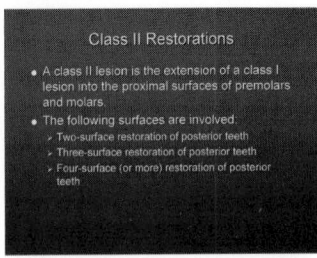

- What accessory items would be needed for Class II restorations? *(Matrix system.)*
- Why would this be needed?

Slide 16

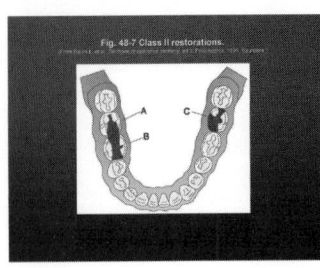

- Which teeth are involved in this example?
- Which surfaces are involved in this example?

Slide 17

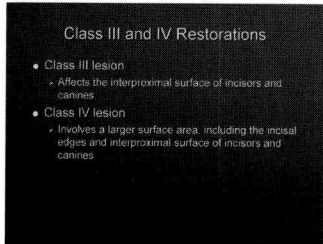

- What accessory items would be needed for a Class III and Class IV restoration? *(Mylar strip matrix system.)*
- Why is this needed?
- Can a metal matrix system be used?

Slide 18

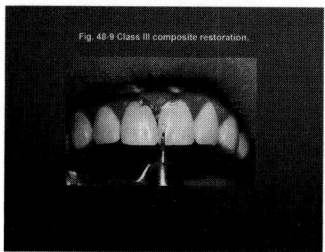

- Which teeth are involved in this example?
- What surfaces are involved in this example?
- Why would a dental dam be needed in this procedure?

Slide 19

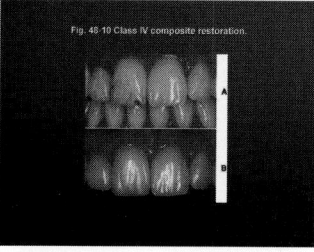

- How does a Class IV restoration differ from a Class III restoration?
- Why would a dental dam be used?

Slide 20

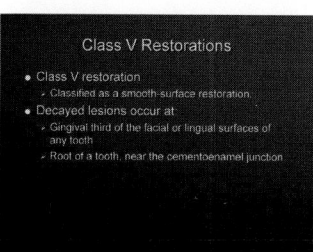

- Class V lesions tend to occur in older patients.
- Why are the elderly more susceptible to this type of decay?
- What material is generally used for this type of restoration?

Slide 21

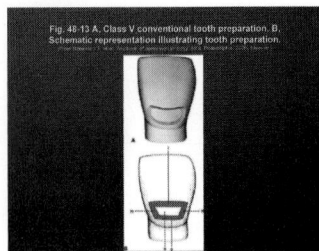

● What could be used to help deflect the tissue from the preparation?

Slide 22

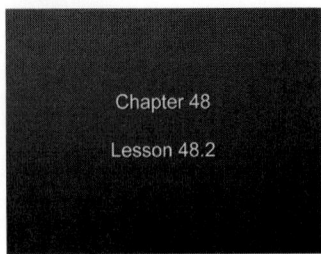

Slide 23

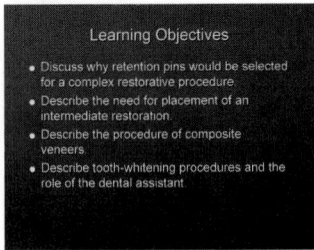

Slide 24

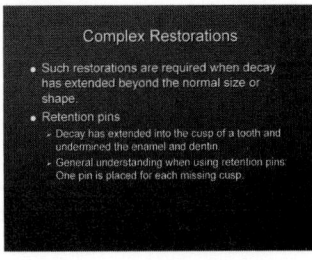

● Retention pins are commonly used in a tooth to retain and support a restoration.

● One tooth may have multiple pins placed.

● Pins are available in different widths and are supplied in a kit.

Torres and Ehrlich Modern Dental Assisting, 9th ed.

Bird/Robinson

Slide 25

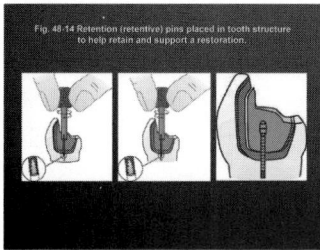

Fig. 48-14 Retention (retentive) pins placed in tooth structure to help retain and support a restoration.

- A "drill" is used to place the pin in a prepared tooth.
- No cementation of the pin is required.
- The extended portion of the retention pin is open to adhere to the restorative material that is to be placed.
- Why is it important to use a dental dam when preparing and placing pins? *(Because the pins are so small, they are easily dropped or misplaced.)*

Slide 26

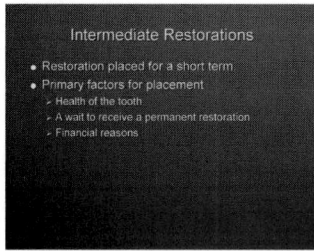

Intermediate Restorations
- Restoration placed for a short term
- Primary factors for placement
  - Health of the tooth
  - A wait to receive a permanent restoration
  - Financial reasons

- Intermediate restorations are not meant to be permanent.
- An intermediate restoration is a preliminary step before a final restoration is placed.
- Why has this procedure been approved as an expanded function of the dental assistant?

Slide 27

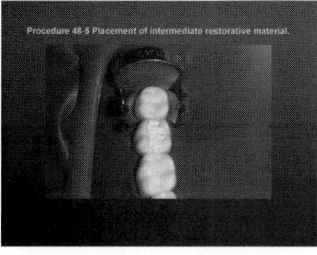

Procedure 48-5 Placement of intermediate restorative material.

- What is the appropriate consistency of the IRM?

Slide 28

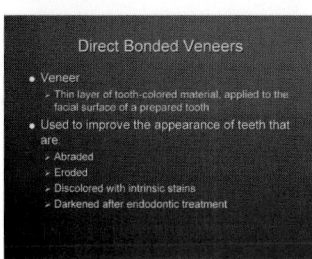

Direct Bonded Veneers
- Veneer
  - Thin layer of tooth-colored material, applied to the facial surface of a prepared tooth
- Used to improve the appearance of teeth that are:
  - Abraded
  - Eroded
  - Discolored with intrinsic stains
  - Darkened after endodontic treatment

- Direct veneers are not fabricated by the dental laboratory technician.
- Direct veneers are made of a resin composite material.
- What are examples of intrinsic stains?

ELSEVIER

Torres and Ehrlich Modern Dental Assisting, 9th ed.

Bird/Robinson

Slide 29

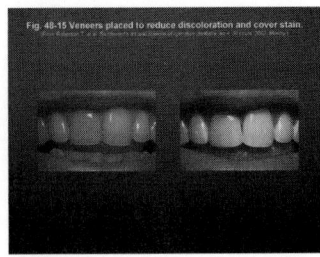

- Which teeth may have been involved in this procedure?
- Do posterior teeth receive veneers? Why or why not?

Slide 30

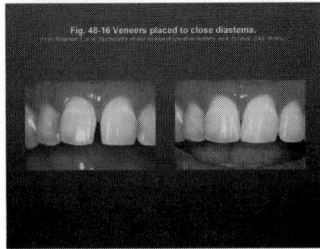

- What is a diastema?

Slide 31

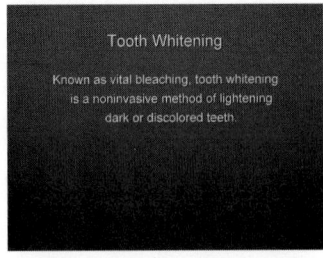

- How many students know someone who is currently using a bleaching system?
- What does the term "vital" mean?

Slide 32

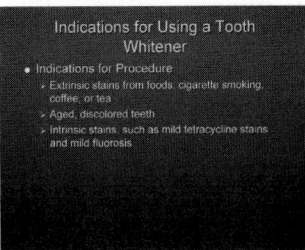

- Patients should be advised that bleaching is neither guaranteed nor permanent.

Bird/Robinson

Slide 33

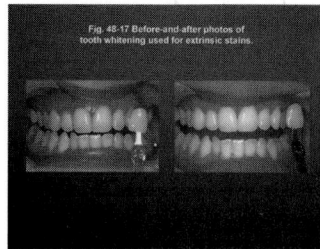

- How long do the effects of most whitening systems last? *(Three to five years.)*

Slide 34

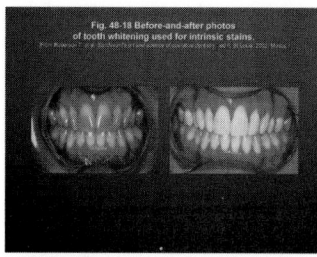

- What causes intrinsic stains?
- Intrinsic stains are harder to bleach.

Slide 35

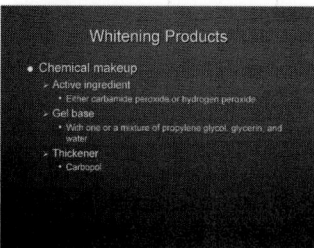

- Whitening product is applied only to the facial surfaces of the tooth.

Slide 36

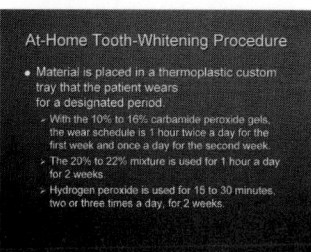

- What type of impression is taken?
- What symptoms would patients experience if they wore the bleach tray longer than recommended?
- Many patients do not see the effects of bleaching if they do the maxillary and mandibular arch at the same time.

Slide 37

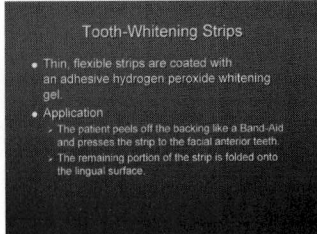

- Extra-strength whitening strips are dispensed by a dental office only.

Slide 38

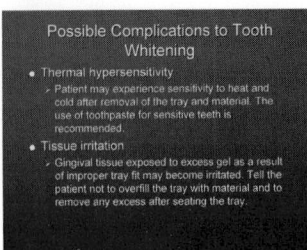

- Why do patients undergoing whitening of teeth need to schedule follow-up dental appointments?

Slide 39

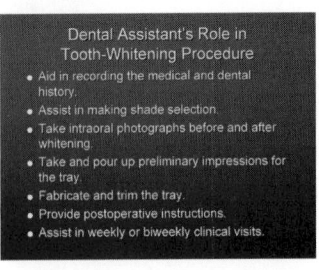

- What is the purpose of taking a preshade?
- Why are photographs taken before and after the tooth-whitening process?

Slide 40

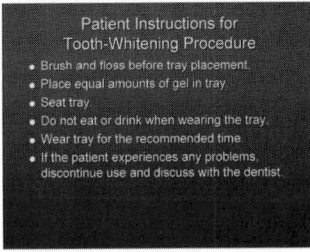

- Why should patients not eat or drink while wearing the bleaching trays?
- What sorts of problems may a patient experience during tooth whitening?

Torres and Ehrlich Modern Dental Assisting, 9th ed.

Bird/Robinson

TEACHING FOCUS

This chapter introduces students to key terms relating to matrix systems for restorative dentistry and how a matrix system is used in Class II, III, and IV restorations. Students have the opportunity to describe the type of matrices used for posterior and anterior restorations and to discuss the purpose and use of a wedge. The chapter also covers alternative methods of matrix systems. Students have the opportunity to assemble a universal retainer and matrix band and to place and remove a matrix band and wedge for Class II, Class III, and Class IV restorations.

MATERIALS AND RESOURCES

- ☐ computer and PowerPoint projector (Lesson 49.1)
- ☐ examples of alternative matrix systems: automatrix system, sectional matrix system, and matrix systems for primary teeth (Lesson 49.1)
- ☐ typodont (Lesson 49.1)

LESSON CHECKLIST

Preparations for this lesson include:

- lecture
- evaluation of student knowledge and skills needed to perform all entry-level activities related to the comprehension and application of matrix systems for restorative dentistry, including:
  - ○ Class II, III, and IV restorations
  - ○ functions of the matrix system in restorations
  - ○ buccal surface, lingual surface, occlusal, gingival, and proximal walls
  - ○ patient education

ELSEVIER

KEY TERMS

AutoMatrix (p. 802)
celluloid strip (p. 799)
cupping (p. 799)
matrix (p. 796)
Mylar (p. 797)

overhang (p. 799)
Palodent (p. 803)
universal retainer (p. 796)
wedge (p. 799)

ADDITIONAL RESOURCES

PowerPoint slides (Evolve): 1-23
The Interactive Dental Office CD-ROM: Miguel Ricardo
Multimedia Procedures DVD: Assembling and Placing a Matrix Band and Universal Retainer

---

Legend

CTQ
Critical
Thinking
Question

DVD
Multimedia
Procedures
Videos and
Animations

ESLR
EVOLVE
Student
Learning
Resources

IDO
Interactive
Dental
Office
CD-ROM

SW
Student
Workbook

TB
Test Bank
on the
TEACH
CD-ROM

PPT
PowerPoint
Slides

Class Activities are indicated in ***bold italic.***

LESSON 49.1

PRETEST

1. What is another term for a universal retainer?
   a. T-band
   b. spot-welded
   c. Tofflemire
   d. buccal

2. The larger circumference of the matrix band is always placed toward which surface?
   a. buccal
   b. lingual
   c. occlusal
   d. gingival

3. On the universal retainer, which area is used to increase or decrease the size of the band loop?
   a. outer knob
   b. inner knob
   c. spindle
   d. outer guide slots

4. What is used to position the matrix band firmly against the gingival margin of the preparation?
   a. spindle
   b. Tofflemire
   c. floss
   d. wedge

5. What is used to contour the bands?
   a. Howe pliers
   b. explorer
   c. burnisher
   d. mirror

6. For which classification of restoration is a celluloid strip used?
   a. Class I
   b. Class II
   c. Class III
   d. Class VI

7. For which teeth are T-band matrices used?
   a. permanent anterior
   b. permanent posterior
   c. deciduous anterior
   d. deciduous posterior

8. How many wedges will be needed for an MOD amalgam restoration?
   a. one
   b. two
   c. three
   d. none

9. What is a term for a small, oval-shaped matrix made of stainless steel used interproximally?
   a. palodent
   b. Mylar
   c. T-band
   d. Tofflemire

10. Where is the diagonal slot on a universal retainer always positioned?
    a. toward the incisal
    b. toward the occlusal
    c. toward the gingiva
    d. on the lingual

Answers

| 1. c | 3. b | 5. c | 7. d | 9. a |
| 2. c | 4. d | 6. c | 8. b | 10. c |

Bird/Robinson

BACKGROUND ASSESSMENT

Question: What is the purpose of a matrix system?
Answer: A matrix system is used if the interproximal surfaces are involved in a tooth preparation. The purpose of a matrix system is to create a temporary wall for the restorative material. Matrix systems enable the dentist to manipulate the material to resemble closely the contours of a natural tooth and create a smooth external surface for patient comfort and easy cleaning.

Question: Why is it necessary to use a wedge with a matrix system?
Answer: Certain tooth preparations involve the interproximal surfaces, and a matrix system would be used to create a temporary wall during the restorative phase. A wedge is inserted into the lingual embrasure area to position the matrix band firmly against the marginal wall. Using a wedge also eliminates overhangs during the restorative phase. Wedges come in different sizes and are made of wood or plastic.

CRITICAL THINKING QUESTION

The patient comes to the office for an occlusal amalgam on tooth #15 and a DI/resin on tooth #8. During the procedure the dentist notices that #15 also has distal caries, but the dental assistant has set up the procedure only for a resin matrix system. Can a resin system be used for a posterior tooth amalgam preparation? What items are needed?

Guidelines: A celluloid or Mylar strip is used only for anterior composite or resin restorations because it is clear and is able to let the curing light penetrate to the composite or resin material. A celluloid or Mylar strip is not used on posterior teeth. Instead, a thin, flexible stainless steel matrix band would be used for tooth #15. The appropriate armamentarium for this procedure would include a universal retainer, metal band, and a burnisher to contour the band.

OBJECTIVES	CONTENT	TEACHING RESOURCES
Pronounce, define, and spell the Key Terms.	■ Key terms (p. 795)	🖝 ESLR Electronic Flashcards *Class Activity Have students make flash cards of the key terms with the terms on one side and the definitions on the reverse. Then have students quiz each other with the flash cards. Correct pronunciation as needed.*
Describe the use of a matrix system in Class II, III, and IV restorations.	■ Introduction (p. 796)	▣ PPT 5 🖳 TB question 1 📖 SW Short-Answer Questions 1; Fill in the Blank question 5; Multiple Choice questions 1-2 (pp. 425-426) 📖 SW/IDO Patient Case Exercise questions 1-5 (p. 427) 📖 SW Case Study questions 1, 5 (pp. 426-427) ▸ Discuss the purposes of using a matrix system in restorative dentistry. *Class Activity Conduct a group discussion on how to appropriately identify the use of a matrix system for Class I, II, III, IV, V, and VI restorations.*
Describe the type of matrices used for posterior restorations.	■ Posterior matrix systems (p. 796) ☐ Universal retainer (p. 796)	▣ PPT 6-9 🖳 TB questions 2-4, 7, 8, 10 📖 SW Short-Answer Questions 2; Fill in the Blank

OBJECTIVES	CONTENT	TEACHING RESOURCES

	☐ Matrix band (p. 796)
	
	– Contouring (p. 797)
	
	☐ Criteria for Placing the Posterior Matrix Retainer and Band (p. 799)
		questions 2-4, 8; Multiple Choice questions 3-5 (pp. 425-426)
		
		Figure 49-1 Tooth preparation with mesial and distal proximal walls missing (p. 796)
		
		Figure 49-2 Most commonly used posterior matrix bands (p. 496)
		
		Components of Universal Retainer (p. 797)
		
		Figure 49-3 Contouring the band assists in the restoration process (p. 797)
		
		Recall questions 1-5 (p. 797)
		
		▸ Discuss how to position the matrix retainer and band in a Class II restoration.
		
		Class Activity Ask students how to appropriately identify the use of a matrix system on posterior teeth for:
		
		  – *#8—MO/Amalgam*
		
		  – *#5—DOB/Resin*
		
		  – *#30—MODBL/Amalgam*

Assemble a universal retainer and matrix band.	☐ Universal retainer (p. 796) ☐ Matrix band (p. 796) – Contouring (p. 797) Procedure 49-1 Assembling a matrix band and universal retainer (p. 798) (SW/ESLR Competency 49-1, p. 429)	Multimedia Procedures DVD: Assembling and Placing a Matrix Band and Universal Retainer SW/ESLR Competency 49-1 Assembling the Matrix Band and Universal Retainer (p. 429) *Class Activity Have students correctly identify the parts of the universal retainer and describe their uses.*
Describe the purpose and use of a wedge.	☐ Wedges (p. 799)	PPT 10-11 TB question 9 SW Short-Answer Questions 4; Multiple Choice questions 6-7 (pp. 425-426) SW Case Study question 4 (p. 427) Figure 49-4 Wedge correctly positioned interproximally (p. 799) Figure 49-5 Assortment of precontoured wedges (p. 799) Figure 49-6 The type of wedge placed is determined by the depth of the preparation (p. 800) Recall questions 6-7 (p. 799) CTQ 1 (p. 805) ▸ Discuss how to select the correct wedge for the specific situation during a restoration.

Torres and Ehrlich Modern Dental Assisting, 9th ed.

Bird/Robinson

OBJECTIVES	CONTENT	TEACHING RESOURCES
		Class Activity Demonstrate the correct placement of wedge on a typodont. Have students take turns manipulating placement. Then invite students to ask questions and share what they learned.
Place and remove a matrix band and wedge for a Class II restoration.	☐ Wedges (p. 799) Procedure 49-2 Placing and removing a matrix band and wedge for a Class II restoration (expanded function) (pp. 800-801) (SW/ESLR Competency 49-2, pp. 431-432)	SW/ESLR Competency 49-2 Placement and Removal of a Matrix Band and Wedge for a Class II Procedure (pp. 431-432)

Describe the type of matrices used for anterior restorations.	■ Anterior matrix systems (p. 799)	PPT 12-14
		
		 TB question 5
		
		 SW Short-Answer Questions 3; Fill in the Blank question 1; Multiple Choice questions 9-10 (pp. 425-426)
		
		 Figure 49-7 A clear matrix system (p. 802)
		
		 Figure 49-8 Contouring a plastic matrix band (p. 802)
		
		 Recall questions 8-9 (p. 802)
		
		 ▸ Discuss why clear plastic matrices are used with anterior restorations.
		
		 Class Activity Lead a discussion in which students explain how to appropriately identify the use of a matrix system on anterior teeth for:
		
		   – *#7—I/Resin*
		
		   – *#10—MIDL/Resin*
		
		   – *#2—DI/Resin*

Place and remove a matrix and wedge for a Class III restoration.	■ Anterior matrix systems (p. 799) Procedure 49-3 Placing a plastic matrix for a class III or IV restoration (expanded function) (p. 803) (SW/ESLR Competency 49-3, p. 433)	SW/ESLR Competency 49-3 Placement and Removal of a Plastic Matrix (p. 433) *Class Activity Demonstrate the placement and removal of a matrix and wedge for a Class III restoration.*
Discuss alternative methods of matrix systems used in restorative dentistry.	■ Alternative matrix systems (p. 802) ☐ AutoMatrix system (p. 802) ☐ Sectional matrices (p. 802)	PPT 15-23 TB question 6 SW Short-Answer Questions 5; Fill in the Blank questions 6-7; Multiple Choice question 8 (pp. 425-426) Figure 49-9 AutoMatrix system (p. 802)

OBJECTIVES	CONTENT	TEACHING RESOURCES
	☐ Matrix systems for primary teeth (p. 803) – T-band (p. 804) – Spot-welded band (p. 804)	Figure 49-10 Sectional matrix system (p. 803) Figure 49-11 Copper T-band used for primary molars (p. 804) Figure 49-12 Spot-welder used for primary molars (p. 804) Recall questions 10-12 (p. 804) ▶ Discuss the advantage of an automatrix system over the universal retainer. ***Class Activity Demonstrate the assembly of a matrix system and correct placement of matrix systems on a typodont. Have students manipulate the systems on the typodont.*** – ***Universal retainer*** – ***Automatrix system*** – ***Sectional matrices*** – ***T-band***
Performance Evaluation		🖥 TB 📖 SW questions (pp. 425-426) 📖 SW Case Study (pp. 426-427) 📖 *e* SW/ESLR Competency 49-1 Assembling the Matrix Band and Universal Retainer (p. 429) 📖 *e* SW/ESLR Competency 49-2 Placement and Removal of a Matrix Band and Wedge for a Class II Procedure (p. 431-432) 📖 *e* SW/ESLR Competency 49-3 Placement and Removal of a Plastic Matrix (p. 433) *e* ESLR Electronic Flashcards *e* ESLR Practice Quiz Recall questions (pp. 797-804) 💡 CTQ (p. 805)

49.1 Homework/Assignments:

49.1 Instructor's Notes/Student Feedback:

Slide 1

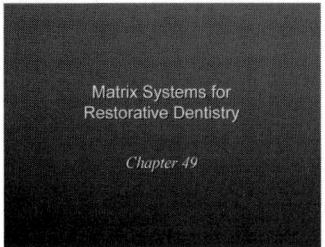

Slide 2

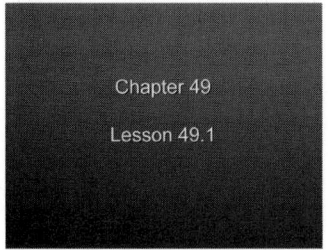

Slide 3

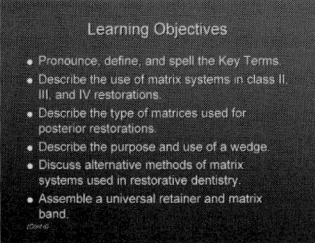

Slide 4

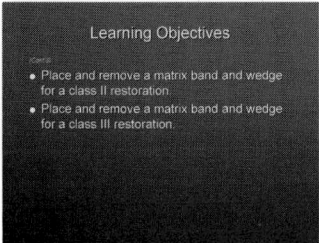

Bird/Robinson

Slide 5

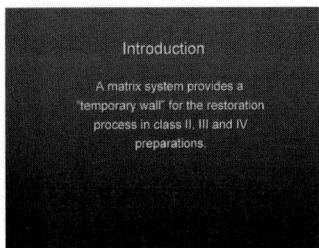

- What are Class II, III, and IV preparations? Which teeth do they involve? *(Class II: proximal surface of molars and premolars; Class III: proximal surface of incisors and canines; Class IV proximal surface of incisors and canines that include the incisal edge.)*

- "Matrices" is the plural term for "matrix."

- There are different systems for posterior and anterior teeth.

Slide 6

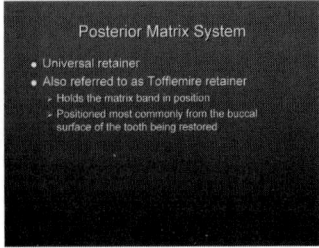

- Usually assembled before the start of restoration process.

- How does the posterior matrix system create a temporary wall during the restorative phase?

- Why is the universal retainer placed from the buccal position?

Slide 7

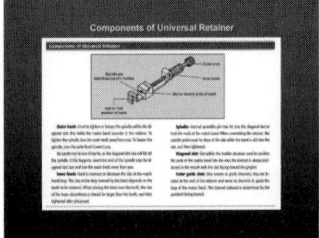

Slide 8

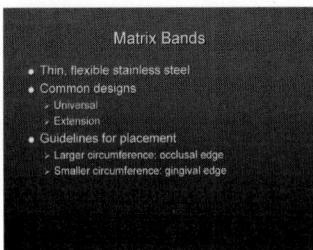

- Extension bands are used for Class II preparations where a universal band could not reach the height of the tooth.

- What instrument would be needed to contour a band?

Bird/Robinson

Slide 9

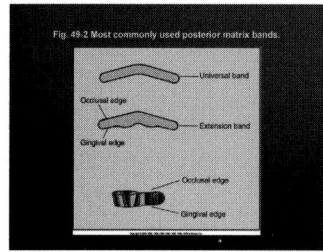

- Top photo: universal band.

- Middle photo: extension band.

- The larger circumference is placed toward which surface?

- The smaller circumference is placed toward which surface?

- Bands must be contoured to make proper contact with the adjacent teeth.

- What instrument is used to contour bands?

Slide 10

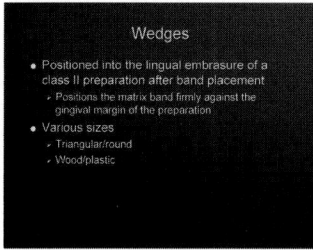

- What is an embrasure? *(V-shaped space in a gingival direction between the proximal surfaces of two adjoining teeth in contact.)*

- Used to add pressure to the interproximal area during the restorative phase.

- Used to prevent overhangs.

- What is an overhang?

Slide 11

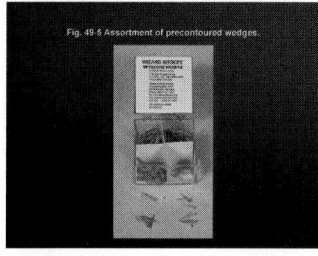

- During transfer, ask the dentist what size wedge would be appropriate.

- Wedges are transferred and applied with cotton pliers or 110 pliers.

- How many wedges are used in an MOD/amalgam preparation?

- How many wedges are used in a DI/resin preparation?

Slide 12

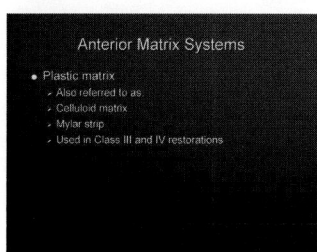

- Metal bands are not used because the resin/composite material can be scratched or marked by the stainless steel.

- No retainers are used.

- Why are clear strips used in resin/composite restorations?

Torres and Ehrlich Modern Dental Assisting, 9th ed.

Bird/Robinson

Slide 13

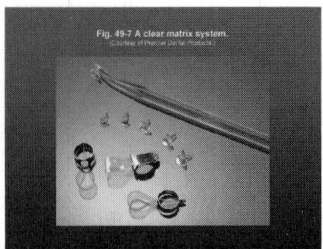

- Examples of clear matrix systems.

Slide 14

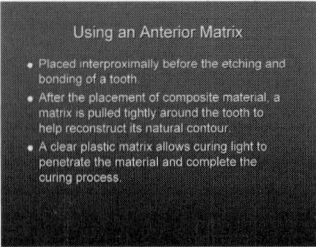

- Anterior matrices can be contoured using the end of a mouth mirror.
- Why would the matrix be placed before etching or bonding?
- Why would a wedge be used with a celluloid or Mylar strip?

Slide 15

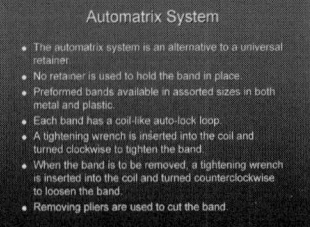

- Wedges are still used with this system.
- The tightening wrench and removing pliers are sterilized after each use.
- The band is removed and placed in the sharps container.

Slide 16

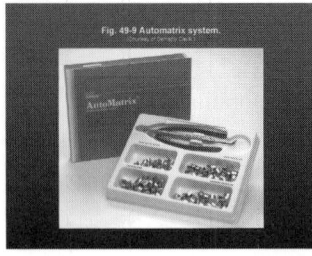

- The blue-handled instrument is the removing pliers. It has cover to "catch" the cut piece of band for easy removal.
- The tightening wrench is the small "wand" in the box.

Bird/Robinson

Slide 17

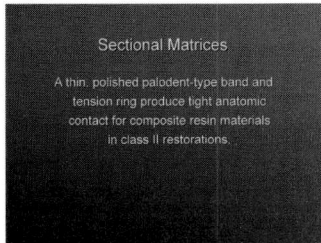

- These are not commonly used.
- They are small, oval-shaped, and made of stainless steel.
- The tension ring is the "retainer."

Slide 18

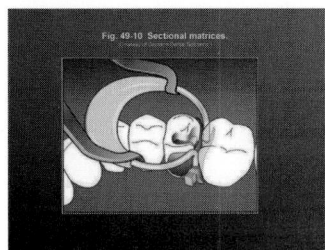

- Used on posterior teeth only.
- Why would a sectional matrix be used instead of a universal retainer?
- How many rings would be used on a DO restoration?

Slide 19

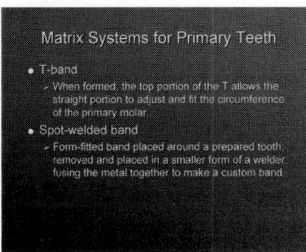

- A T-band is made of copper and adjusted to fit a primary tooth.
- A spot-welded band requires premeasuring stainless steel matrix material; requires more prep time.
- Why would a universal retainer NOT be used on primary teeth?

Slide 20

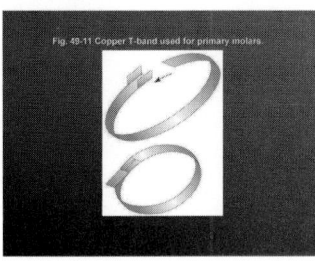

- After placing the end of the band through the "wings" of the other end, secure the wings around.
- Why would this system NOT be used on permanent teeth?

Bird/Robinson

Slide 21

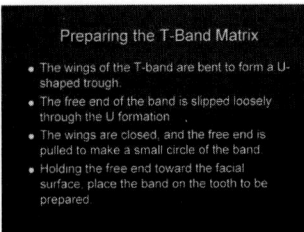

Preparing the T-Band Matrix
- The wings of the T-band are bent to form a U-shaped trough.
- The free end of the band is slipped loosely through the U formation.
- The wings are closed, and the free end is pulled to make a small circle of the band.
- Holding the free end toward the facial surface, place the band on the tooth to be prepared.

- Wedges are still used with the T-band matrices.

Slide 22

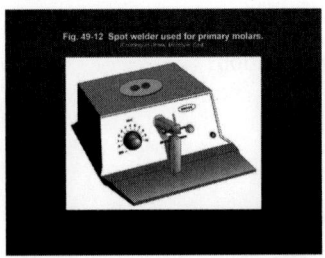

Fig. 49-12 Spot welder used for primary molars.

- A spot-welder is used for the spot-welded bands.

Slide 23

Preparing a Spot-Welded Matrix Band
- Measure ¾ to 1 inch of stainless-steel matrix material.
- Fit the matrix band around the prepared tooth.
- Adapt the band, making sure that the ends of the matrix material are at the facial surface for the sake of visibility and control.
- Using Howe pliers, hold the ends tightly and remove the band in an occlusal direction.
- Place the band in the spot welder.
- Spot-weld the matrix at three positions.

- This requires use of a spot welder.
- The process requires additional preparation time.
- The spot-welded band is form-fitted around the tooth.
- What size pliers are usually used?

Torres and Ehrlich Modern Dental Assisting, 9th ed.

Bird/Robinson

50 Fixed Prosthodontics

TEACHING FOCUS

This chapter gives students the opportunity to learn about the preparation, making, and placement of indirect restorations, including crowns, inlays, onlays, veneers, and bridges. Students will learn how to identify the indications and contraindications for fixed dental prosthodontics, the components of a fixed bridge, the steps for a diagnostic workup, and the role of the laboratory technician. The uses of core buildups, pins, and posts in crown retention and the function of provisional coverage for a crown or fixed bridge will be discussed. Students will also have the opportunity to demonstrate the placement and removal of a gingival retraction cord and assist in the preparation and cementation procedures of an indirect restoration.

MATERIALS AND RESOURCES

- ☐ computer and PowerPoint projector (all Lessons)
- ☐ examples of crowns and bridges (all Lessons)
- ☐ examples of equipment and supplies used in a restoration procedure (Lesson 50.2)

- ☐ index cards (Lesson 50.1)
- ☐ several types of retraction cords (Lesson 50.2)
- ☐ shade guide (Lesson 50.1)
- ☐ typodont (Lesson 50.2)

LESSON CHECKLIST

Preparations for this lesson include:

- lecture
- guest speaker: laboratory technician
- evaluation of student knowledge and skills needed to perform all entry-level activities related to fixed prosthodontics, including:
  - ○ the dental assistant's role in evaluating a patient's dental condition before treatment is initiated
  - ○ the dental assistant's role in the restoration procedure
  - ○ the role of the laboratory technician in dental restorations

ELSEVIER

Torres and Ehrlich Modern Dental Assisting, 9th ed.

Bird/Robinson

KEY TERMS

abutment (p. 810)
articulator (p. 811)
bevel (p. 813)
cast post (p. 814)
chamfer (p. 813)
core (p. 813)
die (p. 811)
fixed bridge (p. 810)
full crown (p. 809)
gingival retraction (p. 814)
hypertrophied (p. 815)
infuser (p. 815)
inlay (p. 808)

investment material (p. 811)
master cast (p. 811)
onlay (p. 808)
opaquer (p. 809)
pontic (p. 810)
porcelain-fused-to-metal (PFM) crown (p. 810)
prosthesis (p. 807)
resin-bonded bridge (p. 811)
shade guide (p. 813)
shoulder (p. 813)
three-quarter crown (p. 809)
unit (p. 810)
veneer (p. 809)

ADDITIONAL RESOURCES

PowerPoint slides (Evolve): 1-29
The Interactive Dental Office CD-ROM: Jessica Brooks
Multimedia Procedures DVD: Placing and Removing Retraction Cord

---

Legend

CTQ
Critical
Thinking
Question

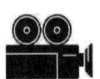

DVD
Multimedia
Procedures
Videos and
Animations

ESLR
EVOLVE
Student
Learning
Resources

IDO
Interactive
Dental
Office
CD-ROM

SW
Student
Workbook

TB
Test Bank
on the
TEACH
CD-ROM

PPT
PowerPoint
Slides

Class Activities are indicated in ***bold italic.***

Bird/Robinson

LESSON 50.1

PRETEST

1. What is another term for a tooth, root, or implant used for the retention of a fixed prosthesis?
   a. abutment
   b. pontic
   c. articulator
   d. inlay

2. Which cast restoration is designed to fit snugly inside the tooth and involves the proximal surface and most or all of the occlusal surface?
   a. inlay
   b. onlay
   c. amalgam
   d. veneer

3. Which cast restoration is designed to fit snugly inside the tooth and involves the proximal surface and only part of the occlusal surface?
   a. inlay
   b. onlay
   c. amalgam
   d. veneer

4. What is another term to describe the number of teeth involved in a fixed prosthesis?
   a. length
   b. bridge
   c. crown
   d. unit

5. What are prefabricated posts made of?
   a. stainless steel
   b. copper
   c. titanium
   d. gold

6. Which instrument should be used to pack the retraction cord into the gingival sulcus?
   a. explorer
   b. spoon excavator
   c. cotton pliers
   d. cord-packing instrument

7. What is another term for an exact replica of the prepared portion of the tooth?
   a. die
   b. articulator
   c. impression
   d. final impression

8. What type of lighting is preferred when selecting a shade?
   a. natural sunlight
   b. fluorescent light
   c. flashlight
   d. light-curing unit

9. How many appointments does it take to complete a single cast restoration?
   a. only one
   b. minimum of two
   c. minimum of three
   d. minimum of four

10. What home-care aid would a patient need to thoroughly clean underneath a three-unit bridge?
    a. toothbrush
    b. bridge threader
    c. mouth rinse
    d. fluoride

Answers

1. a	3. a	5. c	7. a	9. b
2. b	4. d	6. d	8. a	10. b

Bird/Robinson

BACKGROUND ASSESSMENT

Question: How do you define fixed prosthodontics?

Answer: Fixed prosthodontics is a specialized area of dentistry that deals with replacing missing teeth. The term *fixed* refers to a prosthetic appliance that is cemented permanently in the oral cavity. Examples include single crowns, bridges, onlays, inlays, and veneers.

Question: Why is gingival retraction important when preparing a tooth for a fixed prosthesis?

Answer: Gingival retraction is accomplished by temporarily displacing the gingival tissue away from the tooth that is being prepared and widening the gingival sulcus so the impression material will flow around all parts of the prepared tooth. Gingival retraction takes place after the tooth has been prepared and just before the final impression is taken. The dental laboratory technician will need an accurate impression showing the marginal preparation of the tooth to ensure that the permanent fixed prosthetic will match the prepared tooth. Gingival retraction cords are available in a variety of sizes (thicknesses) and are available twisted, untwisted (plain), or braided. The dentist will choose the appropriate retraction cord for the preparation.

CRITICAL THINKING QUESTION

A patient is in the office for a dental examination and has expressed concern over his gold crown on tooth #28. Although the tooth is not causing any problems for the patient, he has said that he does not like the way it looks when he smiles. He had the gold crown placed many years ago and didn't realize at the time how much it would affect his appearance. What type of fixed prosthesis could the dental assistant recommend to the patient for the replacement of the gold crown on tooth #28?

Guidelines: The patient is a good candidate for a porcelain-fused-to-metal (PFM) crown. Dental laboratory technicians construct PFM crowns by adding a thin layer of porcelain over a metal crown. This type of crown is very durable and can withstand the forces of mastication. The PFM crown can be shaded to match the patient's natural teeth, making it an esthetically appealing choice for the patient.

OBJECTIVES	CONTENT	TEACHING RESOURCES
Pronounce, define, and spell the Key Terms.	■ Key terms (p. 806)	*e* ESLR Electronic Flashcards ▸ Discuss each of the key terms in Chapter 50, focusing on the definition, pronunciation, and spelling of each term. *Class Activity Have students make flash cards of the key terms by writing the terms on one side of an index card and the definitions on the reverse. Then have the students quiz each other with the flash cards. Correct their pronunciation as needed.*
List indications and contraindications for a fixed prosthesis.	■ Introduction (p. 807) ■ Plan of care (p. 807) ☐ Indications and contraindications for fixed dental prosthodontics (p. 807) – Indications (p. 807) – Contraindications (p. 807)	PPT 4-6 TB question 1 SW Short-Answer Questions 1; Multiple Choice questions 1-2 (pp. 435-437) SW Case Study question 1 (p. 438) Recall questions 1-2 (p. 808) CTQ 5 (p. 821) ▸ Discuss how to talk with a patient who is contraindicated for fixed dental prosthodontics. *Class Activity Conduct a group discussion on how to appropriately identify the indications and contraindications for fixed prosthetics in the circumstances below.*

Bird/Robinson

OBJECTIVES	CONTENT	TEACHING RESOURCES
		1. Patient comes in with tooth #12 missing; #11 and #13 are stable; wants space "filled in."
		2. Patient comes in with teeth #27 and #28 missing; has poor oral health conditions; wants to replace teeth, but cost is an issue.
		3. Patient comes in with tooth #25 missing; good oral health care; does not want a removable appliance.
Identify the steps for a diagnostic workup.	■ Plan of care (p. 807) □ Indications and contraindications for fixed dental prosthodontics (p. 807) – Indications (p. 807) – Contraindications (p. 807)	SW Short-Answer Questions 2 (p. 435) SW Case Study question 1 (p. 438) SW/IDO Patient Case Exercise question 1 (p. 439) (The Interactive Dental Office CD-ROM) Recall question 2 (p. 808) ▶ Discuss why a diagnostic workup is important before fixed prosthodontics are undertaken. *Class Activity Have the students set up a mock diagnostic workup in the dental operatory according to infection-control protocol.*
Describe the differences among full crowns, inlays, onlays, and veneer crowns.	■ Indirect restorations (p. 808) □ Inlays and onlays (p. 808) – Computer assisted restorations (p. 808) □ Veneers (p. 809) – Porcelain veneers (p. 809) □ Crowns (p. 809)	PPT 7-12 TB questions 2-4 SW Short-Answer Questions 4; Fill in the Blank questions 8-9, 16, 19 (pp. 435-437) Figure 50-1 Inlay cast restoration (p. 808) Figure 50-2 Onlay cast restoration (p. 808) Figure 50-3 Onlay fabricated from porcelain to match tooth color (p. 808) Figure 50-4 CAD/CAM system is computer-driven software that controls the milling device (p. 808) Figure 50-5 A ceramic block is used in the milling device to prepare the inlay or onlay restoration (p. 809) Figure 50-6 (A) and (B) Porcelain veneers placed to cover hypocalcification defects (p. 809) Figure 50-7 Posterior gold crown (p. 809) Figure 50-8 Anterior porcelain-fused-to-metal (PFM) crown (p. 810) ▶ Discuss the reasons to use various materials in making crowns, inlays, onlays, and veneer crowns. *Class Activity Have each student write a brief paper defining the differences among full crowns, inlays, onlays, and veneer crowns, and the indications and contraindications of all categories. Read a few of the completed papers to the class.*

Bird/Robinson

OBJECTIVES	CONTENT	TEACHING RESOURCES
Describe the uses of porcelain for fixed prosthodontics.	■ Indirect restorations (p. 808) □ Inlays and onlays (p. 808) – Computer-assisted restorations (p. 808) □ Veneers (p. 809) – Porcelain veneers (p. 809) □ Crowns (p. 809)	▣▦ PPT 13 📖 SW Short-Answer Questions 6; Fill in the Blank questions 14-15, 18 (pp. 435-437) 📖💿 SW/IDO Patient Case Exercise questions 2, 4 (p. 439) (The Interactive Dental Office CD-ROM) Figure 50-9 Four-unit PFM anterior fixed bridge (p. 810) Recall question 3 (p. 811) 💡 CTQ 4 (p. 821) ▸ Discuss situations in which porcelain would be chosen over other materials in fixed prosthodontics. *Class Activity* **Divide the class into student pairs. Have each pair take turns making shade selections for each other.**
Identify the components of a fixed bridge.	□ Fixed bridge (p. 810) – Components of a fixed bridge (p. 810) – Resin-bonded bridge (p. 811)	▣▦ PPT 14-15 🖥 TB questions 5-6 📖 SW Short-Answer Questions 5; Fill in the Blank questions 4, 6, 13, 17, 20 (pp. 435-437) 📖 SW Case Study questions 2-3 (p. 438) Figure 50-8 Three-unit PFM bridge (p. 810) Figure 50-9 Resin-bonded bridge (p. 811) Recall questions 3-4 (p. 811) 💡 CTQ 1 (p. 821) ▸ Discuss the meaning of the term *abutment* as it applies to the fixed bridge. *Class Activity* **Show the class examples of the fixed bridges listed below. Divide the class into small groups, and have them discuss the components of each bridge. Have the groups share their findings with the class.** – **Three-unit bridge** – **Cantilever bridge** – **Maryland bridge**

Bird/Robinson

50.1 Homework/Assignments:

50.1 Instructor's Notes/Student Feedback:

Bird/Robinson

LESSON 50.2

CRITICAL THINKING QUESTION

A patient is in the dental office to begin a preparation for veneers on teeth #6, #7, #8, #9, and #10. The dental assistant has set up the operatory for the procedure and has all the correct armamentarium ready to start the preparation. After reviewing the patient's medical history, the dental assistant notices that the patient has had four heart surgeries. What changes should be made in the setup of this procedure, and why?

Guidelines: Some gingival retraction cords are impregnated, meaning they contain an astringent vasoconstrictor that controls bleeding and causes the desired provisional shrinkage of the tissues next to the prepared tooth. A vasoconstrictor may cause strain on the heart as it is absorbed into the body. Vasoconstrictors are not used on patients who have a history of unstable angina, recent myocardial infarction, recent coronary artery bypass surgery, untreated or uncontrolled severe hypertension, and untreated or uncontrolled congestive heart failure. A gingival retraction cord that is impregnated with aluminum chloride should be used instead.

OBJECTIVES	CONTENT	TEACHING RESOURCES
Identify the role of the laboratory technician.	■ Role of the dental laboratory technician (p. 811) ☐ Laboratory prescription (p. 811) ☐ Laboratory working days (p. 812)	PPT 29 TB question 10 SW Short-Answer Questions 3; Fill in the Blank questions 3, 5, 11-12; Multiple Choice questions 9-10, 15 (pp. 435-438) Laboratory Steps in Creating Indirect Restoration (p. 811) Figure 50-12 Laboratory prescription (p. 812) Recall questions 5-7 (p. 812) Patient Education (p. 821) Legal and Ethical Implications (p. 821) Eye to the Future (p. 821) ▶ Discuss how to write a prescription to a laboratory technician. Refer to Figure 50-12. *Class Activity Invite a laboratory technician to speak to the class about his or her role in cast restoration. Have the students prepare questions in advance for the technician.*
Describe the preparation and placement of a cast crown.	■ Overview of a crown procedure (p. 813) ☐ Shade selection (p. 813) ☐ Preparation (p. 813)	PPT 19-20 TB question 7 SW Short-Answer Questions 7; Multiple Choice question 3 (pp. 435, 437) Figure 50-13 Shade guide, used to match the exact color of teeth (p. 813) Figure 50-14 Prepared tooth structure showing height and contour (p. 813)

OBJECTIVES	CONTENT	TEACHING RESOURCES
		Figure 50-15 Prepared tooth structures showing different designs of the margin (p. 814)
		⚲ CTQ 2-4 (p. 821)
		▸ Discuss various methods of gingival retraction used in preparing the placement of a crown.
		*Class Activity **Have students set up a mock preparation and mock placement of a cast crown in the dental operatory according to infection-control protocol.***
Discuss the uses of core buildups, pins, and posts in crown retention.	☐ Retention aids for crowns (p. 813) – Core buildup (p. 813) – Retention pins (p. 814) – Post and core (p. 814)	🖥 PPT 21 🖥 TB question 8 📀 SW Short-Answer Questions 8; Fill in the Blank questions 1-2; Multiple Choice question 4 (pp. 435-437) 📀💿 SW/IDO Patient Case Exercise question 3 (p. 439) (The Interactive Dental Office CD-ROM) Figure 50-16 An existing amalgam restoration is prepared for the core buildup designed to support the crown (p. 814) Figure 50-17 An abutment for a fixed partial denture was restored using a cast post and core (p. 815) Recall questions 8-11 (p. 818) ▸ Discuss when a core buildup, retention pins, or post and core would be necessary in a restoration. *Class Activity **Divide the class into three groups and assign one type of retention aid (core buildup, pins, or posts) to each group. Have each group discuss the uses of its assigned retention aid. Then, have each group present its findings to the class.***
Describe the use of retraction cord before taking a final impression.	☐ Gingival retraction and tissue management (p. 814) – Gingival retraction cord (p. 815) – Retraction cord packing (p. 815)	🖥 PPT 22-23 🖥 TB question 9 📀 SW Short-Answer Questions 9; Fill in the Blank question 7; Multiple Choice questions 5-6 (pp. 435-437) Figure 50-18 Different types of gingival retraction cords (p. 815) Recall questions 12-13 (p. 818) ⚲ CTQ 2 (p. 821) ▸ Discuss the different types of gingival retraction cord. *Class Activity **Divide the class into small groups. Assign each group a different type of retraction cord. Have each group discuss the indications and contraindications of its assigned retraction cord. Have each group present its findings to the class.***

Torres and Ehrlich Modern Dental Assisting, 9th ed.

Bird/Robinson

OBJECTIVES	CONTENT	TEACHING RESOURCES
Demonstrate the placement and removal of gingival retraction cord.	*Procedure* 50-1 Placing and removing gingival retraction cord (pp. 816-817) (SW/ESLR Competency 50-1, pp. 441-442)	Multimedia Procedures DVD: Placing and Removing Retraction Cord SW Case Study question 5 (p. 438) SW/ESLR Competency 50-1 Placing and Removing Gingival Retraction Cord (pp. 441-442)
Describe the use of retraction cord before taking a final impression.	– Surgical retraction (p. 815) – Mechanical retraction (p. 817)	SW Fill in the Blank question 10; Multiple Choice question 7 (pp. 436-437) Recall question 14 ▸ Discuss the procedure for removing a gingival retraction cord. ***Class Activity** Demonstrate to the class the placement and removal of the retraction cord on a typodont. Then, have the students perform the retraction cord placement and removal on a typodont.*

Describe the function of provisional coverage for a crown or fixed bridge.	☐ Final impression and bite registration (p. 817)
	
	☐ Provisional coverage (p. 817)
		PPT 24-26
		
		SW Short-Answer Questions 10; Multiple Choice questions 8, 11 (pp. 435, 437)
		
		SW Case Study question 4 (p. 438)
		
		Recall questions 15-16 (p. 818)
		
		▸ Discuss the dental assistant's role in a crown or bridge restoration.
		
		***Class Activity** List on the blackboard the following types of provisional coverage used in prosthetic preparation procedures. Ask the students to call out the function of each. Write their responses on the blackboard.*
		
		   *– **Stainless Steel***
		
		   *– **Preformed Acrylic***
		
		   *– **Custom Acrylic***

Assist in the preparation procedure of an indirect restoration.	*Procedure* 50-2 Assisting in a crown and bridge restoration (p. 819) (SW/ESLR Competency 50-2, p. 443)	SW/ESLR Competency 50-2 Assisting in a Crown and a Bridge Preparation (p. 443)
Describe the function of provisional coverage for a crown or fixed bridge.	☐ Delivery appointment (p. 818) ☐ Provisional placement of a permanent casting (p. 818)	PPT 27 Recall questions 16-17 (p. 818) ▸ Discuss the dental assistant's role during the preparation procedure of an indirect restoration.

OBJECTIVES	CONTENT	TEACHING RESOURCES
		Class Activity Divide the class into small groups. Have each group list both the dentist's role during the preparation procedure of an indirect restoration and the dental assistant's role in assisting with the procedure. Have the groups exchange their completed lists and discuss any differences among the listed items.
Assist in the cementation procedure of an indirect restoration.	■ Overview of a bridge procedure (p. 818) ☐ Preparation appointment (p. 818) ☐ Try-in and cementation appointment (p. 818) Procedure 50-3 Assisting in delivery and cementation of a cast restoration (p. 819) (SW/ESLR Competency 50-3, p. 445)	TB question 11 SW Multiple Choice questions 12-13 (pp. 437-438) SW/ESLR Competency 50-3 Assisting in the Delivery and Cementation of a Cast Restoration (p. 445) Figure 50-19 Bridge cemented in place (p. 821) ▶ Discuss what the dental assistant is legally allowed to do in your state during the cementation procedure of an indirect restoration. *Class Activity Make a list on the blackboard of procedures the dental assistant is allowed to perform in the cementation of an indirect restoration and procedures that are the dentist's sole responsibility. Have students call out which procedures are not to be performed by the dental assistant.*
Identify home care instructions for a permanent fixed prosthesis.	■ Patient instructions (p. 818)	PPT 28 SW Short-Answer Questions 11; Multiple Choice question 14 (pp. 435, 438) SW/IDO Patient Case Exercise question 5 (p. 438) (The Interactive Dental Office CD-ROM) Recall questions 18-20 (p. 821) ▶ Discuss the importance of maintenance by the patient on a fixed prosthesis. *Class Activity Divide the class into student pairs. Have the student pairs take turns role-playing an assistant giving verbal home care instructions for fixed prosthetics to a patient.*
Performance Evaluation		TB SW questions (pp. 435-438) SW Case Study (p. 438) SW/IDO Patient Case Exercise (pp. 438-439) (The Interactive Dental Office CD-ROM) SW/ESLR Competency 50-1 Placing and Removing Gingival Retraction Cord (pp. 441-442)

Bird/Robinson

OBJECTIVES	CONTENT	TEACHING RESOURCES
		SW/ESLR Competency 50-2 Assisting in a Crown and a Bridge Preparation (p. 443)
		SW/ESLR Competency 50-3 Assisting in the Delivery and Cementation of a Cast Restoration (p. 445)
		ESLR Electronic Flashcards
		ESLR Practice Quiz
		Recall questions (pp. 808-821)
		CTQ (p. 821)

50.2 Homework/Assignments:

50.2 Instructor's Notes/Student Feedback:

Torres and Ehrlich Modern Dental Assisting, 9th ed.

Bird/Robinson

Slide 1

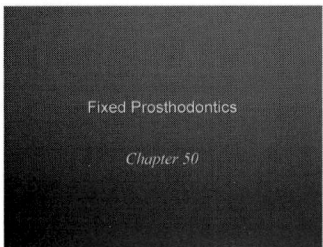

Slide 2

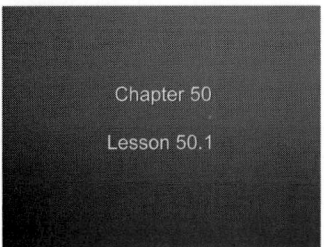

Slide 3

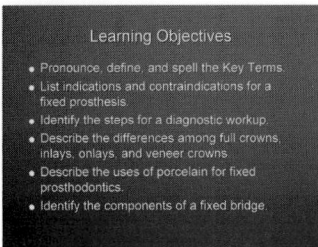

Slide 4

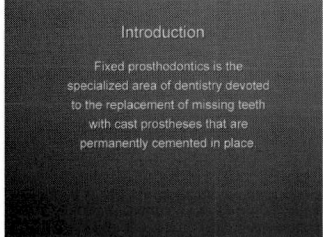

- A prosthodontist is a dentist with an additional three years of specialized training.

Bird/Robinson

Slide 5

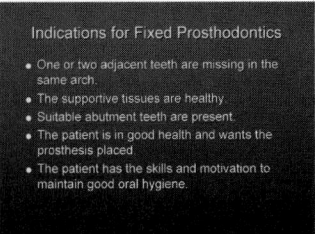

Indications for Fixed Prosthodontics

- One or two adjacent teeth are missing in the same arch.
- The supportive tissues are healthy.
- Suitable abutment teeth are present.
- The patient is in good health and wants the prosthesis placed.
- The patient has the skills and motivation to maintain good oral hygiene.

- Fixed prosthodontics is also known as "crown and bridge."
- Fixed prosthetics require good home care by the patient.
- Supportive tissues must be healthy because they will be supporting the bridge.

Slide 6

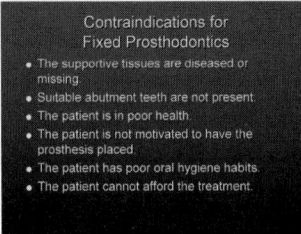

Contraindications for Fixed Prosthodontics

- The supportive tissues are diseased or missing.
- Suitable abutment teeth are not present.
- The patient is in poor health.
- The patient is not motivated to have the prosthesis placed.
- The patient has poor oral hygiene habits.
- The patient cannot afford the treatment.

- Would patients with severe periodontal disease be good candidates for fixed prostheses? Why or why not?
- If suitable abutment teeth are not present, what would be another option for the patient? *(Removable prosthesis or implants.)*

Slide 7

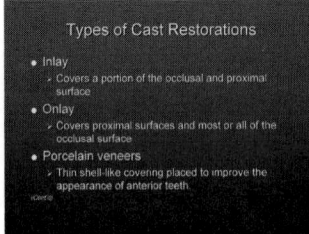

Types of Cast Restorations

- Inlay
  - Covers a portion of the occlusal and proximal surface
- Onlay
  - Covers proximal surfaces and most or all of the occlusal surface
- Porcelain veneers
  - Thin shell-like covering placed to improve the appearance of anterior teeth

- Cast restorations are also known as "indirect restorations."
- They are fabricated outside the patient's mouth in a dental laboratory.
- Where is the proximal surface?
- Why can't veneers be placed on posterior teeth?

Slide 8

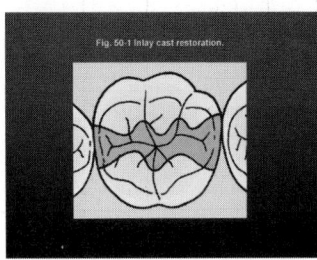

Fig. 50-1 Inlay cast restoration.

- An inlay involves the proximal surface and only a portion of the occlusal surface.

Slide 9

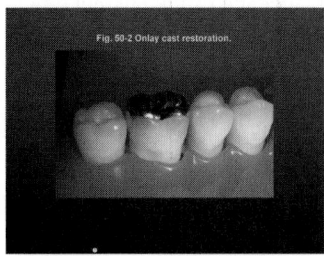

- An onlay involves the proximal surface and most, or all, of the occlusal surface.
- Cusp tips are involved.

Slide 10

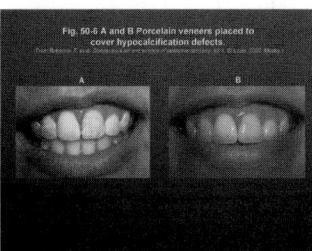

- Veneers are placed to cover defects, such as hypocalcification and intrinsic stains.
- What is an intrinsic stain? *(A stain that comes from the inside.)*
- An opaquer may be used to block out any underlying color or structural defects.
- Cement used for veneers may also be shaded to enhance the color match.
- What is the best lighting for shade selection?

Slide 11

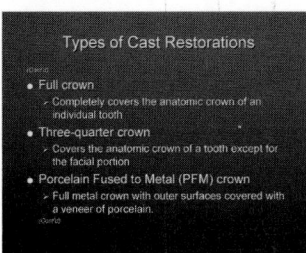

- Full crowns are used when a tooth has decay so severe that reconstruction cannot be performed with a direct restoration.
- The facial surface is not involved in the preparation of three-quarter crowns; this technique is not commonly used.
- With a PFM, porcelain is added for esthetic reasons and matched to natural teeth.

Slide 12

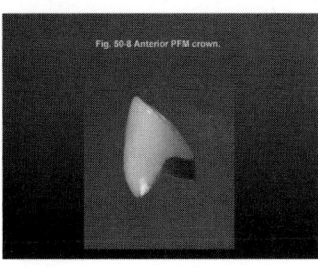

- Which anterior tooth might this be? *(Canine.)*
- Metal "ring" is healthier for the gum tissue because it is not as "bulky" as the porcelain fused to metal.

ELSEVIER

Torres and Ehrlich Modern Dental Assisting, 9th ed.

Bird/Robinson

Slide 13

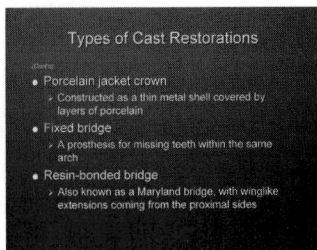

- A porcelain jacket crown is a very thin metal shell covered by layers of porcelain to resemble the shading and translucence of the enamel of a natural tooth.

- A fixed bridge contains a series of two or more units and is cemented permanently in place.

- Winglike extensions of the resin-bonded bridge are bonded onto the lingual surfaces of the teeth adjacent to the missing tooth.

Slide 14

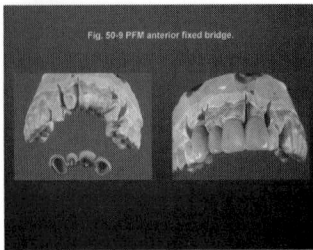

- How many units are involved with this bridge?

- What are the components of the bridge? (*two pontics, two abutments.*)

- Which teeth are being replaced?

Slide 15

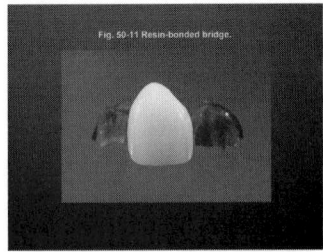

- This is an example of a Maryland bridge.

- Wings are bonded onto the lingual surface of the adjacent teeth.

- Would a Maryland bridge be placed on the posterior teeth? Why or why not?

Slide 16

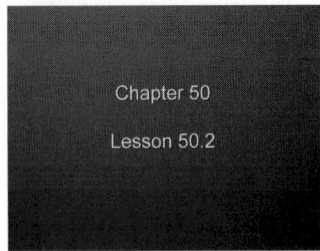

Slide 17

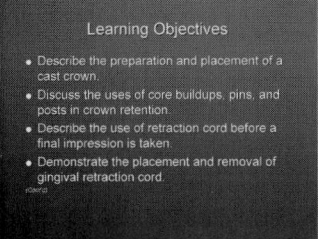

Slide 18

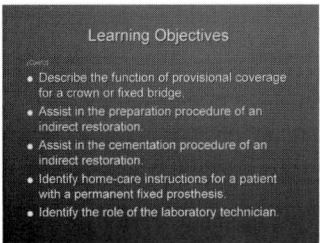

Slide 19

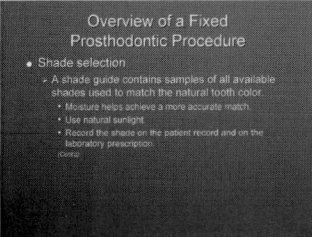

- Shade selection should be done *before* anesthetic is administered.

- Unfortunately, there are times when the initial shade selection does not match at the final appointment. The shade will have to be reselected.

- Some dental labs have the patient come to the lab for a "custom" shade.

Slide 20

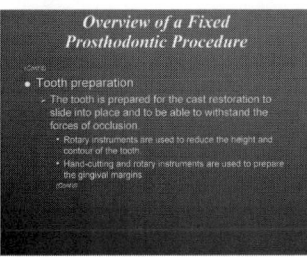

- Gingival margins are designed to provide a smooth junction of the edge of the restoration to the tooth.

- What is a bevel?

- What is a chamfer?

- What is a shoulder?

Slide 21

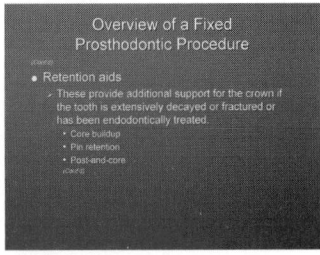

- Pins are placed before the core buildup.
- Post and core can be used only on teeth that have been endodontically treated.
- A cast post is made from an acrylic pattern and fabricated by a dental lab technician.
- Not all teeth require pin retention for a core buildup.
- What material is used for a core buildup?
- What is a prefabricated post made of? *(Titanium and titanium alloys.)*

Slide 22

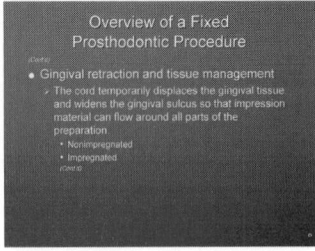

- Gingival retraction cords come in a variety of sizes (thicknesses). They are available twisted, untwisted, or braided.
- Impregnated cords contain a vasoconstrictor.
- What is a vasoconstrictor?
- What medical conditions would contraindicate the use of retraction cords that are impregnated?
- A hemostatic solution is used to control bleeding.

Slide 23

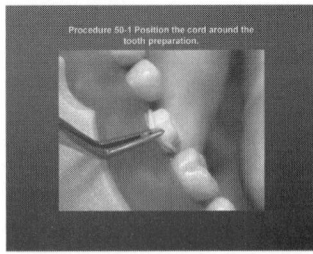

- Retraction cord is positioned around the prepared tooth.
- Transfer is done with cotton pliers.
- Packing is easier if the tissues are dry.
- Typically, hemostatic solution would be placed *after* the cord has been successfully packed, but sometimes bleeding must be controlled before placement of the cord or while the cord is being placed.
- Some cords are presoaked in a hemostatic agent.

Slide 24

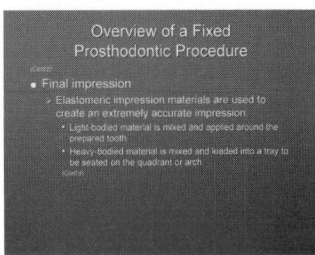

- The final impression MUST be accurate to prevent the dental laboratory technicians from fabricating the restoration according to the inaccurate impression (requiring additional appointments for the patient).
- Always ask the dentist which type of elastomeric material will be used for the final impression. Dentists usually use one to three different types of material (one to two for crown and bridge impressions; one for denture impressions).

ELSEVIER

Torres and Ehrlich Modern Dental Assisting, 9th ed.

Bird/Robinson

Slide 25

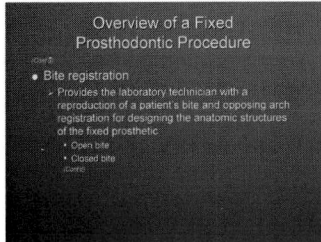

- Why is it necessary to obtain a bite registration? *(To show the dental laboratory technicians the relationship between both arches.)*

Slide 26

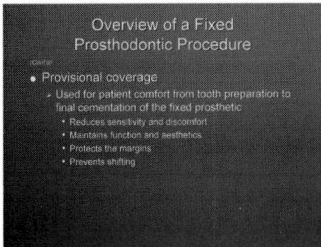

- The temporary is made to last long enough for the dental laboratory technicians to fabricate the permanent restoration.

- Good contact and occlusion are important when fabricating the provisional restoration.

- What might happen if the provisional temporary does not have good contacts with the adjacent teeth? *(Drifting.)*

- What are the postoperative instructions for care of the provisional temporary?

Slide 27

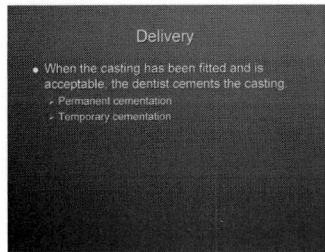

- The shade should be checked before cementation.

- The cement is placed on the inside of the restoration and transferred to the dentist for placement.

- What types of cement would be used?

- Why would the restoration be cemented temporarily?

Slide 28

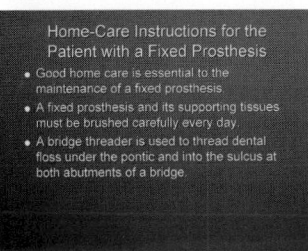

- Fixed prosthetics must be taken care of just like normal teeth.

- If symptoms do not subside, the patient should be instructed to contact the office immediately.

- Is it normal for a patient to have slight temperature sensitivity after the crown has been placed?

Bird/Robinson

Slide 29

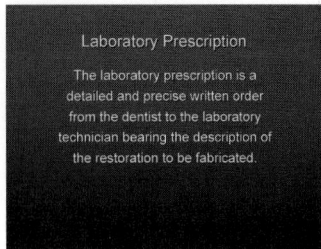

- Lab slips can be filled out by the dental assistant.
- Always have the dentist check the slip before sending it out to the dental laboratory.
- The slip should be completely filled out.

TEACHING FOCUS

This chapter introduces the student to topics related to provisional coverage, including indications for a crown or fixed-bridge preparation and types of provisional coverage. Custom provisional coverage, preformed polymer and polycarbonate crowns, and aluminum crowns are discussed. The student has the opportunity to become acquainted with procedures for expanded functions, such as fabricating and cementing a custom acrylic provisional crown or bridge, fabricating and cementing a preformed provisional crown, and fitting and cementing a preformed polycarbonate crown. The student also has the opportunity to learn about patient education relating to provisional coverage.

MATERIALS AND RESOURCES

☐ computer and PowerPoint projector (Lesson 51.1)

LESSON CHECKLIST

Preparations for this lesson include:

- lecture
- evaluation of student knowledge and skills needed to perform all entry-level activities related to provisional coverage, including:
  - indications for and types of provisional coverage, including custom provisional coverage, preformed polymer and polycarbonate crowns, and aluminum crowns
  - fabricate and cement a custom acrylic provisional crown or bridge
  - fabricate and cement a preformed provisional crown
  - fit and cement a preformed polycarbonate crown
  - provide appropriate patient education relating to provisional coverage

Torres and Ehrlich Modern Dental Assisting, 9th ed.

Bird/Robinson

KEY TERMS

custom provisional (p. 823)
polycarbonate crown (p. 823)
polymer crown (p. 823)

preformed (p. 823)
provisional (p. 823)
stainless steel crown (p. 823)

ADDITIONAL RESOURCES

PowerPoint slides (Evolve): 1-14
The Interactive Dental Office CD-ROM: Chester Higgins
Multimedia Procedures DVD: Fabricating a Custom Acrylic Provisional Crown

Legend

CTQ
Critical
Thinking
Question

DVD
Multimedia
Procedures
Videos and
Animations

ESLR
EVOLVE
Student
Learning
Resources

IDO
Interactive
Dental
Office
CD-ROM

SW
Student
Workbook

TB
Test Bank
on the
TEACH
CD-ROM

PPT
PowerPoint
Slides

Class Activities are indicated in **_bold italic_**.

ELSEVIER

LESSON 51.1

PRETEST

1. Which type of provisional coverage is used for a single anterior tooth?
   a. aluminum
   b. laboratory fabricated
   c. gold
   d. preformed polycarbonate

2. When is a laboratory provisional coverage used?
   a. single tooth; posterior
   b. single tooth; anterior
   c. primary tooth
   d. multiple teeth; long-span bridge

3. What can be completed to avoid trauma to the prepared tooth?
   a. take provisional coverage out of occlusion
   b. do not place a provisional restoration
   c. cement provisional coverage permanently
   d. cement provisional coverage temporarily

4. What is the most common type of material used for provisional coverage?
   a. alginate
   b. self-curing acrylic
   c. light-cured acrylic
   d. IRM

5. How long does the initial set take with a self-curing resin?
   a. less than 30 seconds
   b. 1 minute
   c. 2 minutes
   d. 3 minutes

6. What is used to trim the custom provisional?
   a. acrylic bur
   b. #557
   c. #3 round bur
   d. polishing wheel

7. What is the purpose of using petroleum jelly?
   a. dilutes the taste of acrylic.
   b. facilitates faster setting times.
   c. facilitates easy removal of provisional coverage
   d. gives a gloss to provisional coverage

8. What is used to check the occlusion of provisional crown?
   a. floss
   b. articulating paper
   c. matrix system
   d. abrasive strip

9. What type of temporary cement is most commonly used on a provisional temporary?
   a. zinc oxide eugenol
   b. zinc phosphate
   c. glass ionomer
   d. polycarboxylate

10. What instrument is used to remove excess cement from a provisional temporary?
    a. chisel
    b. curette
    c. explorer
    d. crown and bridge scissor

Answers

| 1. d | 3. a | 5. d | 7. c | 9. a |
| 2. d | 4. b | 6. a | 8. b | 10. c |

BACKGROUND ASSESSMENT

Question: What is the importance of using provisional coverage?
Answer: Provisional coverage is necessary after a tooth or teeth have been prepared for a crown or bridge. It covers the prepared tooth to avoid any discomfort because of temperature sensitivity. Provisional coverage also gives function back to the prepared tooth while the permanent restoration is fabricated by the dental laboratory, which can take up to two weeks. Provisional coverage also protects the margins of the tooth preparation and prevents drifting of adjacent or opposing teeth.

ELSEVIER

Bird/Robinson

Question: Why would a dental assistant take an alginate impression before preparing a tooth for indirect restoration?

Answer: An alginate impression is taken so the dental assistant has an exact replica of the tooth before tooth preparation. Having an alginate impression eliminates the need to use a preformed polymer or preformed polycarbonate crown. Because the alginate impression gives a replica of the tooth before preparation, very little adjustment will need to be made to the acrylic temporary. This can save a lot of chair time for the patient and the dental assistant.

CRITICAL THINKING QUESTION

A patient comes to the office with a loose temporary, which fell off tooth #13 while she was eating. Her permanent restoration has not yet been completed by the dental laboratory. What should the dental assistant do for this temporary? What instructions should be reviewed with the patient to avoid loosening the temporary again?

Guidelines: Temporaries are placed on prepared teeth to protect them from sensitivity and to avoid any damage to the already prepared tooth. The dental assistant will clean out the temporary and remove any old cement from the temporary, then set up the IRM to mix for recementation. The patient should be instructed to avoid foods such as caramel, gum, and taffy, which can loosen a temporary. She should also be instructed to avoid crunchy foods such as tortilla chips to avoid breaking the temporary. The dental assistant should instruct the patient to use good toothbrushing techniques and to floss around the temporary to help keep the gum tissues from becoming irritated. The floss should be pulled through the contact areas, instead of "popped," to avoid loosening the temporary.

OBJECTIVES	CONTENT	TEACHING RESOURCES
Pronounce, define, and spell the Key Terms.	■ Key terms (p. 822)	🖉 ESLR Electronic Flashcards 📖 SW Fill in the Blank questions 1-5 (p. 439) *Class Activity Create a matching exercise in which students match each key term with its description.*
Discuss the indications for provisional coverage for a crown or fixed-bridge preparation.	■ Introduction (p. 823)	🖼 PPT 4 🖥 TB question 1 📖 SW Short-Answer Questions 1; Multiple Choice questions 1-2 (pp. 447-448) Recall questions 1-2 (p. 824) ▸ Discuss the concept of provisional coverage. What are the indications for provisional coverage for a crown or fixed-bridge preparation? *Class Activity Conduct a group discussion on how to evaluate which provisional coverage should be used for each of the following:* — *#2* — *#30* — *#8* — *#23-25 three-unit bridge*

Torres and Ehrlich Modern Dental Assisting, 9th ed.

Bird/Robinson

OBJECTIVES	CONTENT	TEACHING RESOURCES

Describe the types of provisional coverage.	■ Types of provisional coverage (p. 823)
	
	☐ Custom provisional (p. 823)
	
	☐ Prefabricated crowns (p. 823)
	
	■ Criteria for provisional fabrication (p. 824)
	
	■ Custom provisional coverage (p. 824)
		⊠▤ PPT 5-8
		
		▦ TB questions 2-6
		
		▨ SW Short-Answer Questions 2; Multiple Choice questions 3-5 (pp. 447-448)
		
		Recall questions 3-5 (p. 824)
		
		Figure 51-1 Custom provisional coverage (p. 823)
		
		Figure 51-2 Preformed polymer crown (p. 823)
		
		Figure 51-3 Preformed polycarbonate crowns (p. 823)
		
		Figure 51-4 Stainless steel crown (p. 824)
		
		Figure 51-5 Acrylic resin in powder/liquid form (p. 824)
		
		▽ CTQ 1 (p. 831)
		
		▸ Discuss the criteria for provisional fabrication.
		
		▸ Discuss the materials used for custom provisional coverage.
		
		Class Activity Demonstrate the fabrication of provisional coverage for each of the following:
		
		  – Custom
		
		  – Preformed crowns
		
		  – Preformed polycarbonate crowns
		
		  – Aluminum crowns

Discuss the dental assistant's role in making a provisional crown or bridge.	Procedure 51-1 Fabricating and cementing a custom acrylic provisional crown (expanded function) (pp. 825-826) (SW/ESLR Competencies 51-1 to 51-3, pp. 451-452) Procedure 51-2 Fabricating and cementing a custom acrylic provisional bridge (expanded function) (pp. 827-828) (SW/ESLR Competencies 51-1 to 51-3, pp. 451-452) ■ Preformed crowns (p. 828)	⊠▤ PPT 9-13 🎥 Multimedia Procedures DVD: Fabricating a Custom Acrylic Provisional Crown ▦ TB questions 7-8 ▨ SW Short-Answer Questions 3; Multiple Choice questions 6-10 (pp. 447-448) ▨ SW Case Study (p. 448) ▨ ✐ SW/ESLR Competencies 51-1 to 51-3 Fabricating and Cementing an Acrylic and Preformed Provisional Crown or Bridge (Expanded Function) (pp. 451-452) Recall questions 6-10 (p. 828) ▽ CTQ 2-4 (p. 831) ▸ Discuss and compare the nature and use of preformed polymer and polycarbonate crowns and aluminum crowns.

OBJECTIVES	CONTENT	TEACHING RESOURCES
	Procedure 51-3 Fabricating and cementing a preformed provisional crown (expanded function) (p. 829) (SW/ESLR Competencies 51-1 to 51-3, pp. 451-452) ■ Trouble-shooting when making a provisional (p. 830)	*Class Activity Divide the class into groups, and assign each group one of the following types of provisional coverage: crown, preformed crown, preformed polycarbonate crown, and aluminum crown. Give the groups appropriate materials and have them manipulate the materials. Ask each group to describe to the class the dental assistant's role in making a provisional crown or bridge. Ask students to share what they learned.*
Identify home care instructions for provisional coverage.	■ Home care instructions (p. 830) ■ Removal of temporary crowns (p. 830)	PPT 14 TB questions 9-10 SW Short-Answer Questions 4 (p. 447) SW/IDO Patient Case Exercise questions 1-5 (p. 449) (The Interactive Dental Office CD-ROM) Figure 51-6 Provisional crown-removing forceps (p. 830) Patient Education (p. 830) Legal and Ethical Implications (p. 830) Eye to the Future (p. 830) ▶ Discuss patient education relating to provisional coverage. Why is it important? What are some of the key instructions to communicate? ▶ Discuss legal considerations relating to an expanded-functions dental assistant (EFDA). What are the state rulings and regulations regarding expanded functions for dental assistants? *Class Activity Have pairs of students take turns role-playing a dental assistant explaining to a patient how to care for a provisional coverage while waiting for the permanent crown or bridge. Pairs should emphasize key points and explain why the procedures are necessary. Ask volunteer pairs to present to the class and ask students to share what they learned.*
Performance Evaluation		TB SW questions (pp. 447-448) SW Case Study (p. 448) SW/IDO Patient Case Exercise questions 1-5 (p. 449) (The Interactive Dental Office CD-ROM) SW/ESLR Competencies 51-1 to 51-3 Fabricating and Cementing an Acrylic and Preformed Provisional

ELSEVIER

Bird/Robinson

OBJECTIVES	CONTENT	TEACHING RESOURCES
		Crown or Bridge (Expanded Function) (pp. 451-452)
		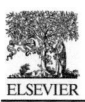 ESLR Electronic Flashcards
		ESLR Practice Quiz
		Recall questions (pp. 824-828)
		CTQ (p. 831)

51.1 Homework/Assignments:

51.1 Instructor's Notes/Student Feedback:

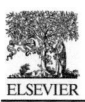

Slide 1

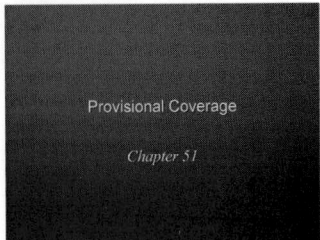

Slide 2

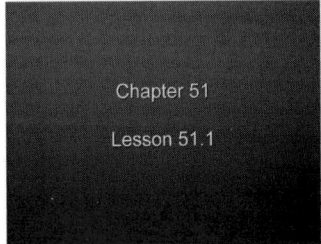

Slide 3

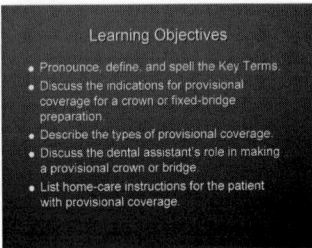

Slide 4

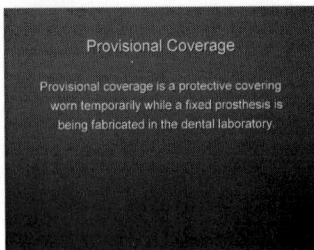

- What does the term provisional mean?
- How long can a provisional last?
- What is an example of a fixed prosthesis?

Slide 5

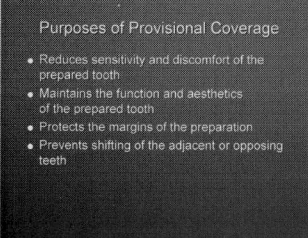

- It is important for the dental assistant to know the normal anatomy of each tooth.
- What is a term used to describe the shifting of opposing teeth? (*Supereruption.*)

Slide 6

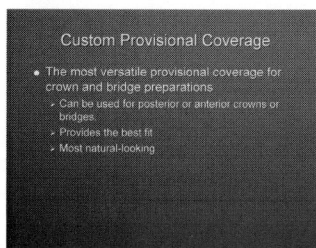

- Custom provisionals are designed specifically for the needs of each patient.
- Different shades of acrylic are available.
- Which teeth would benefit most from the shaded acrylic? Why?

Slide 7

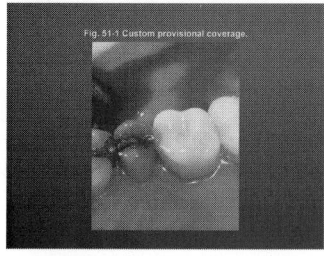

- Which tooth is involved?
- Notice the anatomy that has been trimmed into the temporary.

Slide 8

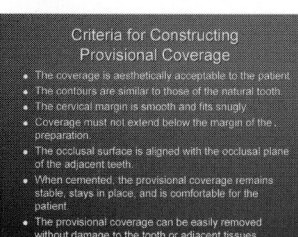

- What does the margin look like on a prepared tooth?
- Why are esthetics important considerations for the patient?
- What is the provisional cemented with?

Torres and Ehrlich Modern Dental Assisting, 9th ed.
Bird/Robinson

Slide 9

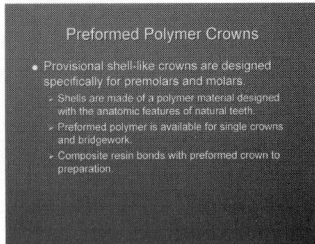

- Does this type of provisional require a preliminary impression?
- Can shaded acrylic be used? Why or why not?

Slide 10

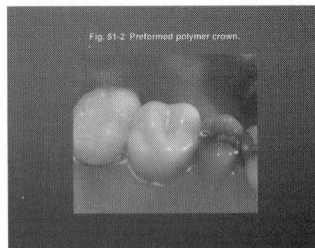

- Notice that the anatomy of this temporary was preformed.
- Little adjusting is necessary to add anatomic details.

Slide 11

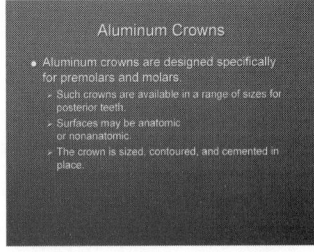

- Why would aluminum crowns not be used on anterior teeth?
- These can be lined with acrylic for a more customized fit.

Slide 12

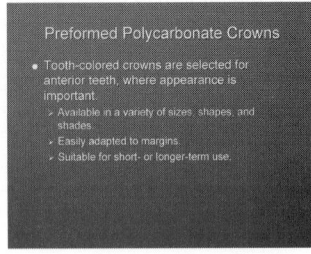

- Preformed polycarbonate crowns are commonly used when an anterior tooth is fractured.
- A preliminary impression cannot be taken because of the missing tooth structure.
- These have easy-grab tabs and can be readily adjusted.
- They can be lined with acrylic for a better fit.

Torres and Ehrlich Modern Dental Assisting, 9th ed.
Bird/Robinson

Slide 13

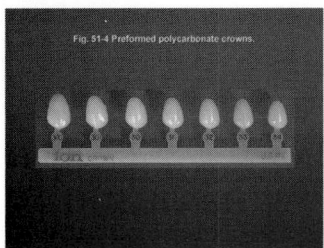

- Can try-in several options.
- Can a preformed polycarbonate crown be disinfected after try-in?

Slide 14

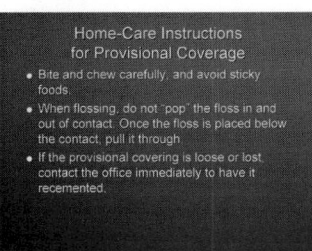

- What are examples of sticky foods? The dental assistant should always give examples of foods the patient should avoid.
- Give oral and written directions to patient.

52 Lesson Plan
Removable Prosthodontics

TEACHING FOCUS

This chapter introduces the student to topics related to removable prosthodontics, including both partial and full dentures. The student will have the opportunity to learn about procedures for assisting in the delivery of a partial or full denture, procedures for assisting in a wax denture try-in, and patient education relating to removable partial and full dentures. Immediate dentures, overdentures, and denture relining and repairs will be discussed.

MATERIALS AND RESOURCES

- ☐ blank cards for flash cards (Lesson 52.1)
- ☐ computer and PowerPoint projector (all Lessons)
- ☐ photocopies of Figure 52-2 (Lesson 52.2)

LESSON CHECKLIST

Preparations for this lesson include:

- lecture
- guest speaker: removable prosthodontist and dental laboratory technician
- evaluation of student knowledge and skills needed to perform all entry-level activities related to removable prosthodontics, including:
  - ○ factors influencing the choice of a removable prosthesis and the indications and contraindications for removable partial and full dentures
  - ○ how to assist in the delivery of a partial or full denture
  - ○ how to assist in a wax denture try-in
  - ○ appropriate patient education relating to removable partial and full dentures

KEY TERMS

alveoplasty (p. 835)
articulator (p. 841)
baseplate (p. 841)
border molding (p. 841)
centric relation (p. 842)
connector (p. 836)
coping (p. 845)
edentulous (p. 840)
festooning (p. 842)
flange (p. 840)
framework (p. 836)
full denture (p. 833)
immediate denture (p. 844)
lateral excursion (p. 842)
mastication (p. 835)

occlusal rim (p. 841)
overdenture (p. 845)
partial denture (p. 833)
post dam (p. 840)
pressure points (p. 835)
protrusion (p. 842)
rebasing (p. 845)
relining (p. 845)
resorption (p. 835)
rest (p. 837)
retainer (p. 836)
retrusion (p. 842)
template (p. 845)
tori (p. 835)
tuberosity (p. 840)

ADDITIONAL RESOURCES

PowerPoint slides (Evolve): 1-40
The Interactive Dental Office CD-ROM: Jose Escobar

Legend

CTQ
Critical
Thinking
Question

DVD
Multimedia
Procedures
Videos and
Animations

ESLR
EVOLVE
Student
Learning
Resources

IDO
Interactive
Dental
Office
CD-ROM

SW
Student
Workbook

TB
Test Bank
on the
TEACH
CD-ROM

PPT
PowerPoint
Slides

Class Activities are indicated in **bold italic**.

ELSEVIER

Torres and Ehrlich Modern Dental Assisting, 9th ed.

Bird/Robinson

LESSON 52.1

PRETEST

1. Which is an example of the extraoral factors influencing the choice of a removable prosthesis?
   a. musculature
   b. physical health
   c. salivary flow
   d. oral mucosa

2. Which is an example of the intraoral factors influencing the choice of a removable prosthesis?
   a. residual alveolar ridge
   b. mental health
   c. patient motivation
   d. dietary habits

3. What is the term used to describe abnormal growths of bone in a specific area of the mouth?
   a. alveolar bone
   b. bone spurs
   c. tori
   d. tuberosity

4. What is the term used to describe chewing?
   a. occlusion
   b. occlusal surface
   c. masticatory surface
   d. mastication

5. Which component of the partial denture is known as a clasp?
   a. framework
   b. connector
   c. retainer
   d. stress breaker

6. Which teeth are not included on a full denture?
   a. first molars
   b. third molars
   c. first premolars
   d. second premolars

7. What type of impression tray is used to take the preliminary impression for a full denture?
   a. anterior quadrant
   b. quadrant
   c. full-mouth tray
   d. edentulous tray

8. What is the term for a prosthesis that is placed just after extractions?
   a. immediate denture
   b. replacement denture
   c. intermediate denture
   d. healing denture

9. What is the term for placing a new layer of denture resin over the tissue surface of the prosthesis?
   a. rebasing
   b. recontouring
   c. reconditioning
   d. relining

10. What is the term for the replacement of a denture base?
    a. rebasing
    b. recontouring
    c. reconditioning
    d. relining

Answers

| 1. b | 3. c | 5. c | 7. d | 9. d |
| 2. a | 4. d | 6. b | 8. a | 10. a |

BACKGROUND ASSESSMENT

Question: What are the differences between a partial denture and a full denture?

Answer: A removable partial denture is used when one or more teeth are missing in an arch, while a full denture is used when all the teeth in one arch are missing. Many factors influence whether a patient should wear a partial denture or a full denture; thus a complete examination must be performed before diagnosis.

Question: How does a patient's salivary flow affect the choice of a removable prosthesis?

Answer: Some patients may be taking certain medications that slow the salivary flow in the oral cavity. This can make wearing the prosthesis very uncomfortable. On the other hand, placing anything in the oral cavity

Bird/Robinson

will accelerate the flow of saliva. When the patient wears the prosthesis, the salivary flow can be excessive at first, but will normally subside after the patient has become accustomed to the new appliance.

CRITICAL THINKING QUESTION

During an examination, a male patient has questions about the replacement of his missing teeth. The dentist finds that he is missing several teeth in the mandibular arch. The dentist also notes that the existing teeth have rampant decay, and the patient has severe periodontal disease that is affecting his entire oral cavity. What options does the patient have to replace the missing teeth in the mandibular arch?

Guidelines: The patient seems to be very motivated to replace his missing teeth; however, present conditions must be addressed before the dentist will place a prosthesis. The rampant decay of his teeth and periodontal disease have affected the remaining teeth in the mandibular arch, making them unsuitable to retain a partial denture. The patient would probably benefit from having the remaining teeth extracted and having an immediate denture placed to help with the healing process. If he is not concerned with his appearance after the extractions have been completed, a full denture could be constructed 6 to 8 months after the extraction sites have completely healed.

OBJECTIVES	CONTENT	TEACHING RESOURCES
Pronounce, define, and spell the Key Terms.	■ Key terms (pp. 832-833)	SW Fill in the Blank questions 1-20 (pp. 455-456) ESLR Electronic Flashcards ▸ Discuss each of the key terms in Chapter 52, focusing on the definition, pronunciation, and spelling of each term. **Class Activity *Have students make flash cards of the key terms with the terms on one side and the definitions on the reverse. Then have the students quiz one another with the flash cards. Correct their pronunciation as needed.***
Differentiate between a partial and a full denture.	■ Introduction (p. 833)	PPT 4-6 TB question 1 SW Short-Answer Questions 1; Multiple Choice question 1 (pp. 455, 457) Figure 52-1 Partial denture (p. 834) Figure 52-2 Full denture (p. 834) Recall question 1 (p. 835) ▸ Discuss the differences between a partial and a full denture. **Class Activity *Invite a removable prosthodontist and dental laboratory technician to speak to the class and explain the features of partial and full dentures and the differences between them. Have students prepare questions beforehand.***
Identify indications and contraindications for removable	■ Factors influencing the choice of a removable prosthesis (p. 833)	PPT 7-10 TB questions 2-3

OBJECTIVES	CONTENT	TEACHING RESOURCES
partial and full dentures.	☐ Extraoral factors (p. 833) – Physical health (p. 833) – Mental health (p. 833) – Patient motivation (p. 834) – Age (p. 834) – Dietary habits (p. 834) – Social and economic factors (p. 834) – Occupation (p. 834) ☐ Intraoral factors (p. 835) – Musculature (p. 835) – Salivary flow (p. 835) – Residual alveolar ridge (p. 835) – Oral mucosa (p. 835) – Oral habits (p. 835) – Tori (p. 835) ■ Removable partial denture (p. 835) ☐ Indications and contraindications (p. 835)	SW Short-Answer Questions 2; Multiple Choice questions 2-5; Case Study (pp. 455, 457-458) Recall questions 2-5 (p. 834) ▸ Discuss the extraoral and intraoral factors influencing the choice of a removable prosthesis. ▸ Discuss the indications and contraindications for a removable partial denture. What is required for this type of prosthesis to be successful? *Class Activity Divide the class into four groups and assign each group one of the following situations. Have each group identify the indications and contraindications for a partial denture for the patient.* *Chris: missing six maxillary teeth, has good oral hygiene, concerned with esthetics* *Joel: missing eight mandibular teeth, active periodontal disease, remaining teeth are in bad condition* *Jack: missing four maxillary anteriors, rampant decay detected, does not have esthetic concerns* *Lisa: missing four maxillary teeth, active periodontal disease, concerned with esthetics* *Have each group present its findings to the class, and ask the class to provide feedback.*
List the components of a partial denture.	☐ Components of a partial denture (p. 836) – Framework (p. 836) – Connectors (p. 836)	PPT 11-13 TB questions 4-5 SW Short-Answer Questions 3; Multiple Choice questions 6-8 (pp. 455, 457) Figure 52-3 Components of a partial denture (p. 836)

Torres and Ehrlich Modern Dental Assisting, 9th ed.
Bird/Robinson

OBJECTIVES	CONTENT	TEACHING RESOURCES
	– Retainer (p. 836) – Rest (p. 837) – Artificial teeth (p. 837)	Figure 52-4 Different types of clasps (p. 836) Figure 52-5 Artificial teeth (p. 837) Recall questions 6-8 (p. 839) ▸ Discuss the components of a partial denture, including the framework, connectors, retainers, denture base, artificial teeth, and rests. *Class Activity Give students a handout depicting an unlabeled partial denture, such as Figure 52-1 on p. 849. Ask students to identify the basic components of a partial denture in the figure by using arrows and labels. Ask volunteers to share their work with the class.*
Describe the steps in the construction of a removable partial denture.	☐ Appointment sequencing for a partial denture (p. 837) – Appointment one: records (p. 837) – Appointment two: preparation (p. 837) – Appointment three: try-in (p. 837) – Appointment four: delivery (p. 838) Procedure 52-1: Assisting in the delivery of a partial denture (p. 839) (SW/ESLR Competencies 52-1 to 52-3, pp. 461-462) – Appointment five: postdelivery check (p. 839)	▦ PPT 14-18 ▤ SW Short-Answer Questions 5; Multiple Choice questions 9-10 (p. 455, 457) ▤ ⓔ SW/ ESLR Competencies 52-1 to 52-3 Assisting in the Delivery of the Partial and Complete Denture (pp. 461-462) Figure 52-6 Laboratory prescription (p. 838) Recall questions 9-10 (p. 839) ▾ CTQ 1 (p. 847) ▸ Discuss the appointment sequencing for a partial denture. How would you present this in patient education? *Class Activity Divide the class into groups and have each group develop a timeline that outlines the scheduling and construction of a removable partial denture. Have groups present their timelines to the class for discussion.*
Identify home care instructions for removable partial and full dentures.	☐ Home care instructions (p. 841)	▦ PPT 19 ▸ Discuss the appropriate home-care instructions relating to a removable partial denture. ▸ Discuss the role and importance of patient education with regard to removable prostheses. How would you handle a patient who is dissatisfied with a new removable prosthesis?

Torres and Ehrlich Modern Dental Assisting, 9th ed.

Bird/Robinson

OBJECTIVES	CONTENT	TEACHING RESOURCES
		Class Activity Have student pairs take turns role-playing a patient and a dental assistant having a conversation in which the dental assistant gives home-care instructions to the patient who has just received a removable partial denture. After each student has played both roles, have the pairs share their exchanges with the class.

52.1 Homework/Assignments:

52.1 Instructor's Notes/Student Feedback:

Torres and Ehrlich Modern Dental Assisting, 9th ed.

Bird/Robinson

LESSON 52.2

CRITICAL THINKING QUESTION

A man returns to the office for a recall examination. Eight months previously, he completed full extractions of the maxillary arch and had an immediate denture placed. He states that he is very happy with the appearance of his new denture, but that it is falling out of his mouth and doesn't fit as well as it did a few months ago. The patient wants to know whether he will have to continue using an over-the-counter adhesive material to help retain the denture in the oral cavity or whether a permanent solution is available. What information can you give him regarding his retention problem?
Guidelines: An immediate denture serves as a bandage to protect the surgical area and compresses the surgical area to help with the healing process. After any type of extraction, resorption can occur in the alveolar area, which ultimately changes the overall shape of the alveolar bone and alters the fit of the immediate denture. The patient would benefit from a relining of the immediate denture. A reline is accomplished by placing a new layer of denture resin over the tissue surface of the appliance. This may help the patient with his retention problems, but if problems continue to occur, a rebase procedure to replace the entire denture base might be necessary.

OBJECTIVES	CONTENT	TEACHING RESOURCES
Identify indications and contraindications for removable partial and full dentures.	■ Full (complete) denture (p. 840) ☐ Indications and contraindications (p. 840)	🖼 PPT 23-24 ▸ Discuss the indications and contraindications for a removable full denture. What is required for this type of prosthesis to be successful? *Class Activity **Make two lists on the board, one for Indications for Removable Full Dentures and the other for Contraindications for Removable Full Dentures. Ask students to call out items to include on the lists. Then discuss each item with the class.***
List the components of a full denture.	☐ Components of a full denture (p. 840) – Base (p. 840) – Flange (p. 840) – Post dam (p. 840) – Artificial teeth (p. 840)	🖼 PPT 25-26 📖 TB question 6 💾 SW Short-Answer Questions 4; Multiple Choice questions 11-12 (pp. 455, 457) Figure 52-7 Components of a full denture (p. 840) Recall questions 11-12 (p. 844) ▸ Discuss the basic components of a full denture, including the base, post dam, artificial teeth, and flange. *Class Activity **Give students a handout depicting an unlabeled full denture, such as Figure 52-2 on p. 850. Ask students to identify the basic components of a full denture in the figure by using arrows and labels. Ask volunteers to share their work with the class.***
Describe the steps in construction of a full denture.	☐ Appointment sequencing for a full denture (p. 840) – Appointment one: records (p. 840) – Appointment two:	🖼 PPT 27-33 📖 TB question 7 💾 SW Short-Answer Questions 6; Multiple Choice questions 13-15 (pp. 455, 457)

Bird/Robinson

OBJECTIVES	CONTENT	TEACHING RESOURCES
	final impression (p. 841) – Appointment three: try-in of baseplate and occlusal rim (p. 841) – Artificial teeth (p. 841) – Occlusal registration (p. 842) – Functionally generated path technique (p. 842) – Appointment four: try-in (p. 842) Procedure 52-2 Assisting in a wax denture try-in (p. 843) (SW/ ESLR Competencies 52-1 to 52-3, pp. 461-462) – Appointment five: delivery (p. 843) – Appointment six: postdelivery (p. 843) Procedure 52-3 Assisting in the delivery of a full denture (p. 844) (SW/ ESLR Competencies 52-1 to 52-3, pp. 461-462)	SW/ESLR Competencies 52-1 to 52-3 Assisting in the Delivery of the Partial and Complete Denture (pp. 461-462) Essentials of a Final Impression for Dentures (p. 841) Figure 52-8 Final impression for a full denture (p. 841) Figure 52-9 Recording made from the baseplate-occlusal rim assembly (p. 841) Figure 52-10 Wax setup within the articulated cast (p. 842) Recall questions 13-15 (p. 844) CTQ 2, 3, 5 (p. 847) ▸ Discuss the appointment sequencing for a full denture. How would you present this in patient education? *Class Activity Draw a two-column table on the board and label one column Partial Denture and the other Full Denture. Have the class compare and contrast the steps in construction and the appointment scheduling for each. Ask student volunteers to record responses in the appropriate column of the table.*
Identify home-care instructions for removable partial and full dentures.	☐ Home-care instructions (p. 843)	PPT 34 SW Short-Answer Questions 8 (p. 447) Figure 52-11 Denture and denture brush (p. 843) Patient Education (p. 846) Legal and Ethical Implications (p. 846) ▸ Discuss the appropriate home-care instructions relating to a full denture. *Class Activity After lecturing on home care, have students write down all postoperative home-care procedures and how they will encourage the patient to continue with follow-up visits.*

Torres and Ehrlich Modern Dental Assisting, 9th ed.

Bird/Robinson

OBJECTIVES	CONTENT	TEACHING RESOURCES

Discuss the construction of an overdenture and an immediate denture.	■ Immediate dentures (p. 844)
	
	  □ Construction (p. 844)
	
	  □ Surgical template (p. 845)
	
	  □ Placement (p. 845)
	
	■ Overdentures (p. 845)
	
	■ Denture relining (p. 845)
	
	  □ Tissue conditioners (p. 845)
	
	  □ Impression (p. 845)
	
	  □ Delivery (p. 846)
		⊠ PPT 35-36
		
		TB question 8
		
		SW Short-Answer Questions 7; Multiple Choice questions 16-18 (pp. 455, 457-458)
		
		Recall questions 16-18 (pp. 845-846)
		
		Eye to the Future (p. 847)
		
		CTQ 4 (p. 847)
		
		▸ Discuss the function of an immediate denture. What patient education is needed before such a prosthesis?
		
		▸ Discuss the function of an overdenture. How does it compare with a normal denture?
		
		*Class Activity **Have student pairs take turns role-playing a conversation in which the dental assistant gives home-care instructions to a patient who received an immediate denture. After each student has played both roles, have the pairs share with the class any difficulties they had.***

Identify the process of relining or repairing a partial or full denture.	■ Denture repairs (p. 846) ■ Denture duplication (p. 846)	⊠ PPT 37-40 TB questions 9-10 SW Short-Answer Questions 9; Multiple Choice questions 19-20 (pp. 455, 458) SW/IDO Patient Case Exercise questions 1-5 (pp. 458-459) (The Interactive Dental Office CD-ROM) Recall questions 19-20 (p. 846) Figure 52-12 Broken denture (p. 846) ▸ Discuss the process of denture relining. What are the indications for this process? ▸ Discuss denture repairs and denture duplication. What would you tell a patient who asks about a duplicate denture? *Class Activity **Divide the class into four groups and assign each group one of the following clinical findings: loose or ill-fitting denture, loss of vertical dimension, presence of inflammatory hyperplasia, presence of traumatic ulcers. After group discussions, have each group present to the class an explanation of its clinical finding and how it indicates a reline procedure.***
Performance Evaluation		TB SW questions (pp. 455-458)

Torres and Ehrlich Modern Dental Assisting, 9th ed.

Bird/Robinson

OBJECTIVES	CONTENT	TEACHING RESOURCES
		SW Case Study (p. 458)
		SW/IDO Patient Case Exercise (pp. 458-459) (The Interactive Dental Office CD-ROM)
		SW/ESLR Competencies 52-1 to 52-3 Assisting in the Delivery of the Partial and Complete Denture (pp. 461-462)
		ESLR Electronic Flashcards
		ESLR Practice Quiz
		Recall questions (pp. 835-846)
		CTQ (p. 847)

52.2 Homework/Assignments:

52.2 Instructor's Notes/Student Feedback:

ELSEVIER

Torres and Ehrlich Modern Dental Assisting, 9th ed.

Bird/Robinson

Slide 1

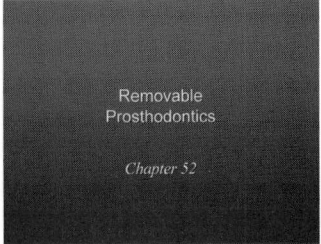

Slide 2

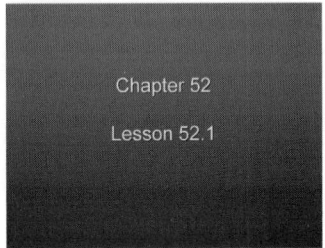

Slide 3

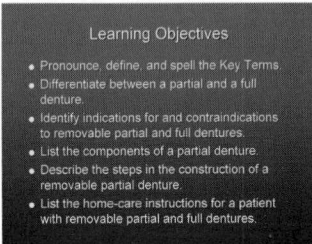

Slide 4

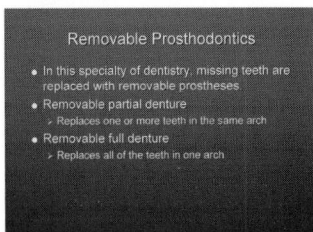

- The removable partial denture is also known as a partial.

- The removable full denture is also know as a denture; older patients may refer to it as a plate.

- Can a general dentist perform procedures related to removable prosthetics?

Torres and Ehrlich Modern Dental Assisting, 9th ed.

Bird/Robinson

Slide 5

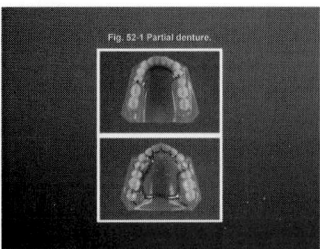

- Which teeth are replaced in the top photograph?
- Which teeth are replaced in the bottom photograph?

Slide 6

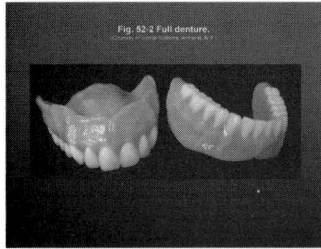

- Which teeth are not placed in a full denture?
- Why not?

Slide 7

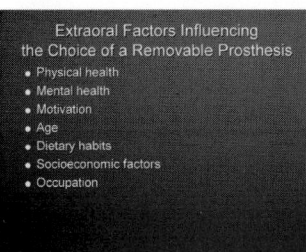

- What physical health factors may make the patient a poor candidate for a removable prosthesis? *(Diabetes, patients who have poor overall health.)*
- Why is the patient's mental health important for the dentist to consider?
- Why would a patient's dietary habits affect his or her candidacy for a removable prosthesis?
- What types of jobs would cause people to be especially anxious about a changed physical appearance? *(Those in jobs that involve meeting the public.)*

Slide 8

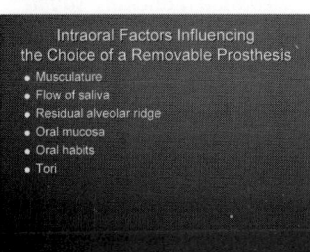

- Mucosa covering the residual ridge can be irritated by prosthesis.
- Tori are abnormal growths of bone that can affect a patient's ability to wear a prosthesis.
- What oral habits must be considered when planning a removable prosthodontic treatment? *(Jaw clenching, teeth grinding, mouth breathing.)*
- How do the facial muscles contribute to the ability to use a prosthesis?
- What are characteristics of an alveolar ridge that supports the prosthesis? *(High and evenly contoured.)*

Bird/Robinson

Slide 9

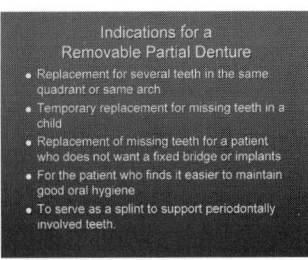

- Are children good candidates for removable prostheses?
- Why would a child benefit from a removable prosthesis?

Slide 10

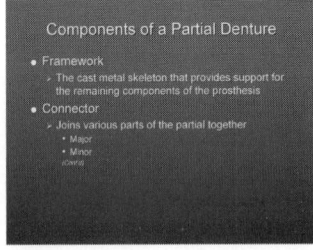

Slide 11

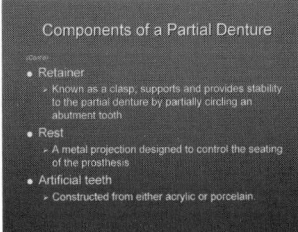

- The framework is covered with acrylic resin so that it resembles the gingiva.
- What are the functions of the major connector? *(Joins the right-and-left-quadrant framework and helps support remaining teeth.)*
- What is the stress-breaker? The minor connector?

Slide 12

- Which connector is used for the clasps and rests?
- What are the drawbacks of porcelain teeth? *(Produce a clicking sound and fracture easily.)*
- Acrylic teeth are more commonly used. What are the drawbacks of acrylic teeth? *(Wear faster and are susceptible to stains.)*

Bird/Robinson

Slide 13

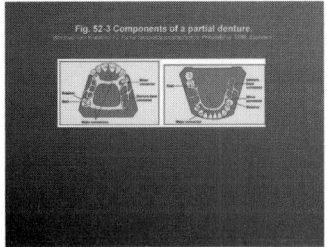

- Identify the components of the partial denture. Include the framework, connectors, retainer, rest, and artificial teeth.

Slide 14

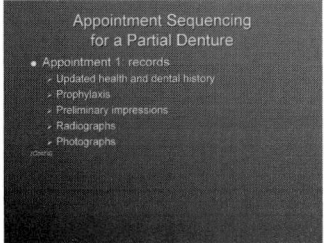

- Patients should know the treatment length. *(Approximately five to six appointments.)*
- Answer any questions before starting procedures.
- What types of radiographs would be obtained and why?
- What types of photographs would be obtained?

Slide 15

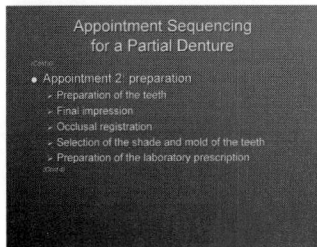

- Why would teeth need to be prepared?
- What type of material is used to take the final impression? *(An elastomeric material.)*
- What factors influence the choice of tooth shade and mold?

Slide 16

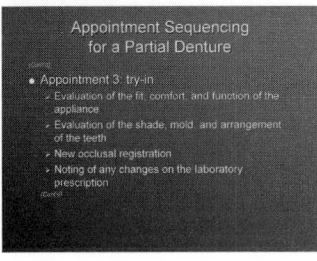

- At this point, what does the appliance consist of? *(Cast framework and teeth set in wax.)*
- Patient acceptance is important in this appointment.
- Should this wax setup be disinfected before sending it to the dental laboratory?

Slide 17

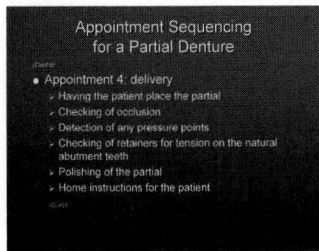

- What are pressure points?
- How can they be relieved?
- How is the partial polished?

Slide 18

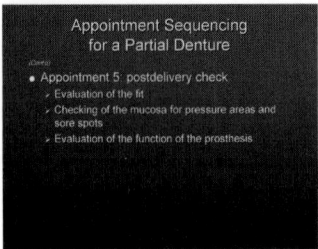

- This is generally scheduled a few days after delivery of the partial.

Slide 19

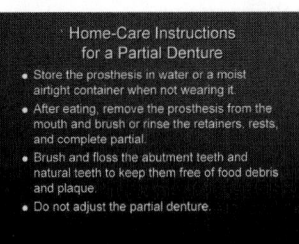

- Patient should be instructed to contact the dental office if any adjustments need to be made.
- Mouthwash may be used to rinse partial to improve its taste.

Slide 20

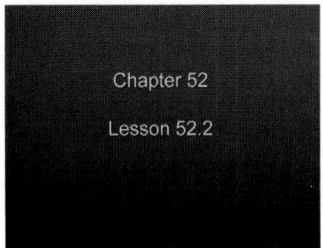

Torres and Ehrlich Modern Dental Assisting, 9th ed.

Bird/Robinson

Slide 21

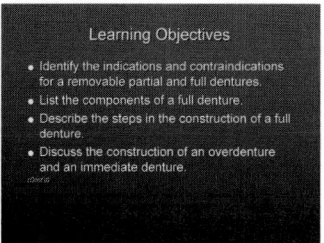

Slide 22

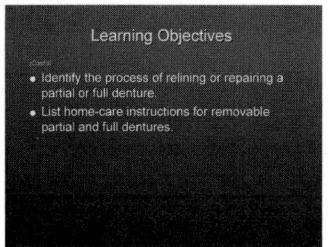

Slide 23

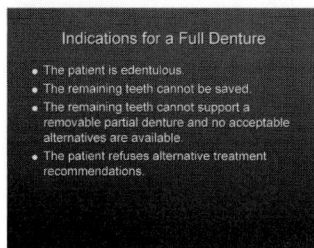

- What does *edentulous* mean?
- If remaining teeth cannot support a partial, what must be done to them? *(Extract.)*

Slide 24

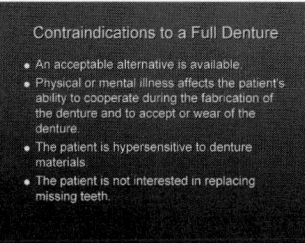

- Hypoallergenic denture material is available.

Slide 25

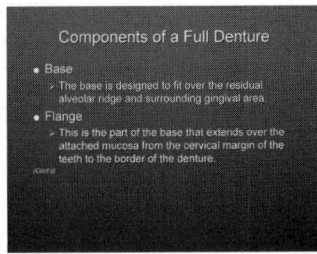

- Base is usually made of acrylic, but can have mesh embedded in acrylic. Fibers make it look like natural gum tissue.
- Where is the flange located on a mandibular denture?
- Where is the flange located on a maxillary denture?

Slide 26

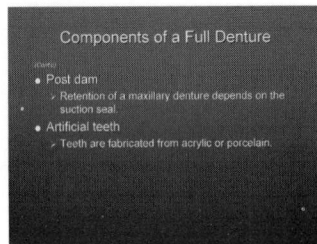

- Why is the post dam important? Where is the post-dam area?
- How many teeth per arch does a full denture have? *(14.)*

Slide 27

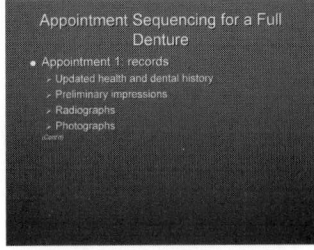

- What type of radiographs would be obtained? *(Panoramic.)*
- What type of photographs would be obtained? *(Intraoral and extraoral.)*
- What is border molding?

Slide 28

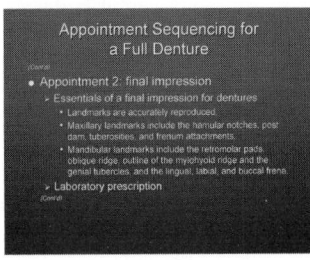

- What type of impression material is used to take the final impression? *(Elastomeric.)*
- What type of tray is used when taking the impression?

Bird/Robinson

Slide 29

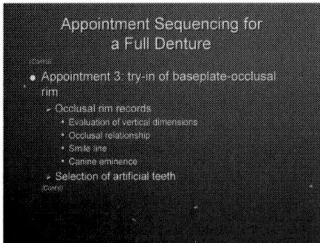

- What does vertical dimension refer to?
- What is the smile line? *(Teeth visible when the patient smiles.)*
- Where is the canine eminence located?

Slide 30

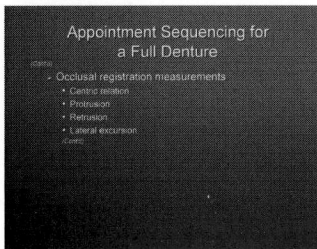

- What is the centric relation?
- What is protrusion?
- What is retrusion?
- What is lateral excursion?

Slide 31

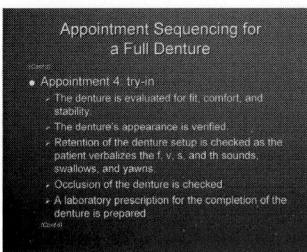

- Festooning is the shaping of the wax to resemble normal tissue grooves, contours, and eminences.
- More than one wax-try-in visit may be necessary.
- Which teeth are excluded on a full denture? Why?

Slide 32

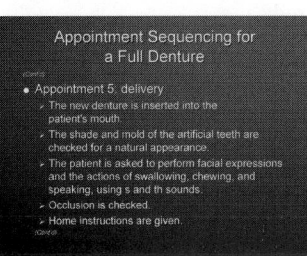

- Patient acceptance is critical.
- Dentures must be disinfected before they are placed in the mouth.

Slide 33

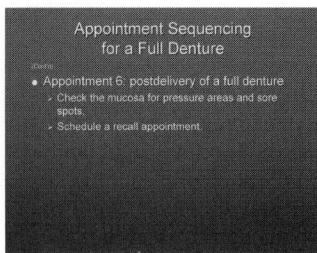

- Scheduled two to three days after initial delivery.

Slide 34

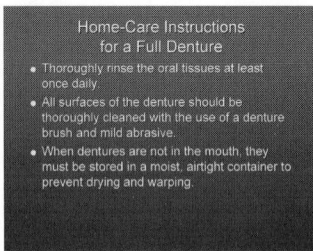

- What types of liquids can damage the appliance? *(Hot liquids, undiluted bleach.)*
- Have the patient read out loud at home to help adjust to denture.
- Do patients who have full dentures need to visit the dentist regularly?

Slide 35

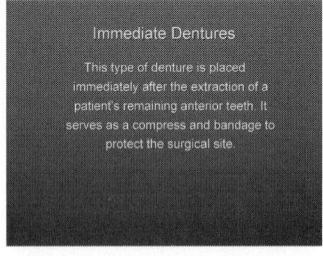

- Why would a patient have immediate dentures placed?
- It can be used on maxillary or mandibular arch.

Slide 36

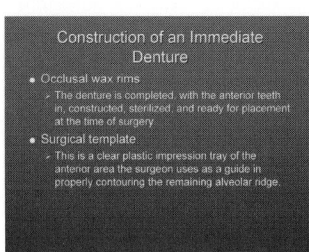

- The laboratory technician constructs the immediate denture.
- Why must the immediate denture be sterilized?
- Six months after placement, immediate denture would need to be replaced.

Bird/Robinson

Slide 37

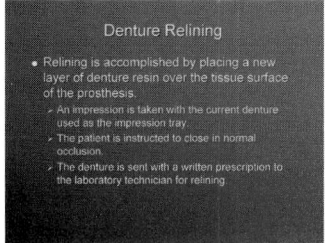

- What are the reasons why a denture would need to be relined?

- What is the difference between relining and rebasing? *(Relining resurfaces the prosthesis, and rebasing replaces the denture base.)*

- What are tissue conditioners used for? *(Restore unhealthy supporting tissues to health.)*

Slide 38

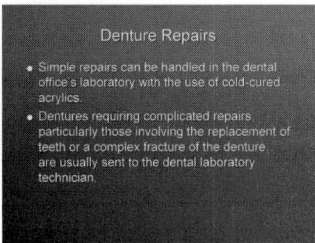

- How can a denture break?

- Ventilation is important when using acrylics.

Slide 39

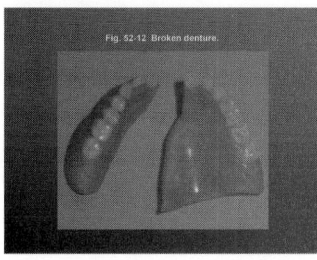

- Patient would drop off denture in the morning and come back in the afternoon for delivery.

Slide 40

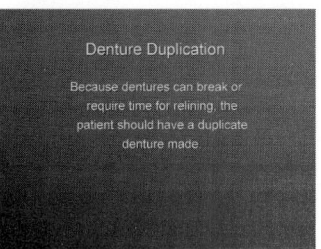

- Not a common procedure.

Torres and Ehrlich Modern Dental Assisting, 9th ed.

Bird/Robinson

TEACHING FOCUS

This chapter will introduce the student to topics related to dental implants. The student will become acquainted with indications and contraindications to implants as well as the psychological evaluation, dental examination, medical history, and evaluation of the dental implant patient. Specialized radiographs, diagnostic casts, surgical stents, and the types of dental implants will also be discussed. The chapter will cover preparation for implant surgery and proper follow-up care. The student will have the opportunity to put this information into context by participating in classroom activities and discussions.

MATERIALS AND RESOURCES

- ☐ basic setup (Lesson 53.1)
- ☐ computer and Powerpoint projector (Lesson 53.1)
- ☐ electrosurgical unit and tips (Lesson 53.1)
- ☐ hydrogen peroxide (3%) with syringe (Lesson 53.1)
- ☐ implant instrument kit (Lesson 53.1)
- ☐ implant kit (Lesson 53.1)
- ☐ inserting mallet (Lesson 53.1)
- ☐ local anesthetic (Lesson 53.1)
- ☐ low-speed handpiece with contra-angle attachment (Lesson 53.1)
- ☐ periosteal elevator (Lesson 53.1)
- ☐ scalpel (Lesson 53.1)
- ☐ sterile cotton pellets (Lesson 53.1)
- ☐ sterile 2x2 inch gauze sponges (Lesson 53.1)
- ☐ sterile saline solution (Lesson 53.1)
- ☐ sterile surgical drilling unit (Lesson 53.1)
- ☐ sterile surgical gloves (Lesson 53.1)
- ☐ surgical irrigation tip (Lesson 53.1)
- ☐ suture setup (Lesson 53.1)

LESSON CHECKLIST

Preparations for this lesson include:

- lecture
- evaluation of student knowledge and skills needed to perform all entry-level activities related to dental implants, including:
  - ○ home-care procedures
  - ○ indications and contraindications for dental implants
  - ○ patient selection
  - ○ role of the dental assistant in implant surgery
  - ○ surgical procedures for implantation
  - ○ types of dental implants

KEY TERMS

circumoral (p. 851)
endosteal (p. 851)
implant (p. 849)
osseointegration (p. 851)

stent (p. 850)
subperiosteal (p. 852)
titanium (p. 851)
transosteal (p. 852)

ADDITIONAL RESOURCES

PowerPoint slides (Evolve): 1-22
The Interactive Dental Office CD-ROM: Greggory Brooks

Legend

CTQ
Critical
Thinking
Question

DVD
Multimedia
Procedures
Videos and
Animations

ESLR
EVOLVE
Student
Learning
Resources

IDO
Interactive
Dental
Office
CD-ROM

SW
Student
Workbook

TB
Test Bank
on the
TEACH
CD-ROM

PPT
PowerPoint
Slides

Class Activities are indicated in ***bold italic***.

Torres and Ehrlich Modern Dental Assisting, 9th ed.

Bird/Robinson

LESSON 53.1

PRETEST

1. What is the term used to describe artificial teeth that have been surgically embedded in the bone?
    - a. stent
    - b. implant
    - c. partial denture
    - d. full denture

2. A _____ evaluation is used to assess a patient's attitude, ability to cooperate, and overall outlook on implants.
    - a. dental
    - b. medical history
    - c. psychological
    - d. radiographic

3. What is the term used for surrounding the mouth?
    - a. intraoral
    - b. extraoral
    - c. circumference
    - d. circumoral

4. Informed consent for implant surgery should include which of the following?
    - a. possible complications
    - b. cost
    - c. other treatment options
    - d. guarantees

5. The process in which a dental implant becomes attached to healthy bone is called
    - a. orthognathic.
    - b. alveoplasty.
    - c. osseointegration.
    - d. a stent.

6. The osseointegration period is generally _____ long
    - a. 1 to 3 months
    - b. 3 to 6 months
    - c. 6 to 9 months
    - d. 9 to 2 months

7. What is the most common type of material used for implants?
    - a. aluminum
    - b. steel
    - c. gold
    - d. titanium

8. What is the term used to describe a metal frame that is placed on top of the bone?
    - a. subgingival
    - b. subperiosteal
    - c. supragingival
    - d. supraperiosteal

9. What is the term used to describe an implant that is inserted through the inferior border of the mandible?
    - a. transosteal
    - b. endosteal
    - c. peri-implant
    - d. subperiosteal

10. A(n) _____ is used as a guide during surgery to place the implants in the proper position.
    - a. alginate impression
    - b. stent
    - c. diagnostic cast
    - d. surgical dressing

Answers

1. b	3. d	5. c	7. d	9. a
2. c	4. a	6. b	8. b	10. b

BACKGROUND ASSESSMENT

Question: What is a dental implant?

Answer: Implants are artificial teeth attached to anchors that have been surgically embedded into the bone. An implant is a natural-looking replacement for missing teeth that incorporates principles from both fixed and removable prosthodontics with the use of bone-anchored implants.

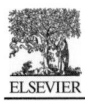

Question: What are the contraindications of implants?

Answer: Several components will make up the contraindication list for implants. Those patients who have diseases of the cardiovascular, respiratory, and gastrointestinal systems may not be good candidates to have implants placed. Those who have compromised immune systems and other chronic conditions that hinder healing may also not qualify as good candidates. Patients should be aware that an implant procedure requires a commitment on their part, because the treatment can be quite lengthy. Patients may choose not to have an implant procedure done because of the large financial investment required.

CRITICAL THINKING QUESTION

A healthy 40-year-old man comes to the office with an ill-fitting lower partial denture. His partial denture is replacing four teeth in the lower right quadrant; the other teeth in the lower arch are in good, stable condition. He tells the dentist that the partial denture does not stay in place as it once used to. He is finding that it falls out during eating and sometimes while he is talking. He has become more self-conscious of his partial denture and does not smile or talk as much as he used to. He has expressed interest in having dental implants placed. What information could you give him?

Guidelines: Implants do improve the patient's confidence level, leading to better overall psychological health. It would need to be explained that implants require a commitment from the patient: regularly scheduled recall appointments and good home care are essential to the success of the implants. The patient would have to undergo an oral, radiographic, psychological, and medical history evaluation to find out whether he is a good candidate for implants. Depending on the type of implant that would be used, the implants would help with the retention of a partial denture or possibly replace the partial denture completely. He could be qualified to receive edosteal implants to replace the four teeth that are missing in the lower right quadrant. Because the remaining teeth in the quadrant are in good health, the patient would not be a good candidate for a subperiosteal implant. If cared for appropriately, implants can last as long as 20 years. Good care would constitute regularly scheduled visits to the office for cleanings and radiographs to ensure the implants are stable. Good home care can be established by brushing and flossing after each meal, and also by using such items as single-tufted toothbrushes, interproximal brushes, and dental implant floss.

OBJECTIVES	CONTENT	TEACHING RESOURCES
Pronounce, define, and spell the Key Terms.	■ Key terms (p. 848)	SW Fill in the Blank questions 1-9 (pp. 463-464) ESLR Electronic Flashcards ▶ Discuss each of the key terms, focusing on the definition, pronunciation, and spelling of each term. *Class Activity Have students make flash cards of the key terms with the terms on one side and the definitions on the reverse. Then divide the class into student pairs and have the students take turns quizzing each other with the flash cards. Correct their pronunciation as needed.*
Discuss the indications and contraindications for dental implants.	■ Introduction (p. 849) ■ Indications for implants (p. 849) ■ Contraindications to implants (p. 849)	PPT 5-8 TB questions 1- 2 SW Short-Answer Questions 1; Fill in the Blank question 8; Multiple Choice questions 1-5 (pp. 463-464) SW Case Study questions 1-2 (p. 465) Figure 53-1 Dental implant (p. 849) Recall questions 1-5 (pp. 849-850) CTQ 5 (p. 856)

OBJECTIVES	CONTENT	TEACHING RESOURCES
		▶ Discuss the major indications for dental implants. Note that when properly placed, dental implants have a success rate of more than 90%.
		▶ Discuss the major contraindications to dental implants. Note the need for proper and thorough screening of patients.
		Class Activity *Divide the class into small groups and have each group identify the indications and contraindications for implants with the following patients:*
		Bob: six anterior teeth missing from the maxillary arch; has good alveolar bone levels; is concerned with comfort level of existing partial; is very motivated for new treatment options
		Mary: is edentulous on mandibular arch; has existing lower full denture; medical history states patient is HIV-positive and has been hospitalized for respiratory infections twice over the past 12 months; has financial concerns over treatment options
		Clark: missing teeth numbers 17-22; does not have prosthetic in place today; interested in permanent solution; is in good health; finances are not a concern; moving to another state in five months
		Have each group present its findings to the class.
Describe the selection of patients to receive dental implants.	■ The dental implant patient (p. 850) □ Psychological evaluation (p. 850) □ Dental examination (p. 850) □ Medical history and evaluation (p. 850) □ Specialized radiographs (p. 850) □ Diagnostic casts and surgical stents (p. 850) ■ Preparation for implants (p. 850) □ Informed consent (p. 850) □ Surgical preparation (p. 850)	⊠▤ PPT 9-10 ▥ TB questions 3-4 ▤ SW Short-Answer Questions 2; Fill in the Blank questions 4, 7; Multiple Choice questions 6-7, 15 (pp. 463-465) ▤ SW Case Study question 4 (p. 455) Recall questions 6-7 (p. 850) Figure 53-2 Custom stent used to aid the dentist in placing an implant (p. 850) ♀ CTQ 3-4 (p. 856) ▶ Discuss the importance of the psychological evaluation of the dental implant patient. Emphasize the need for the patient to cooperate and maintain realistic expectations. ▶ Discuss the steps involved in the surgical preparation of a patient undergoing implant surgery. **Class Activity** *Lead the class in a discussion on the patient selection process for the following implant procedures:* – *Endosteal* – *Subperiosteal* – *Transosteal* *List the selection criteria on the board, and have the class discuss the similarities and differences.*

Bird/Robinson

OBJECTIVES	CONTENT	TEACHING RESOURCES
Identify the types of dental implants.	■ Types of dental implants (p. 851) □ Endosteal implant (p. 851) □ Subperiosteal implant (p. 852) □ Transosteal implant (p. 852)	⊞ PPT 11-19 ▣ TB questions 5-7, 9 📖 SW Short-Answer Questions 3; Fill in the Blank questions 1-3, 5, 9; Multiple Choice questions 8-11 (pp. 463-464) Figure 53-3 Second stage surgery (p. 851) 💡 CTQ 2 (p. 856) ▸ Discuss endosteal implants. Describe the implant, noting its three components, and where it is placed. ▸ Discuss subperiosteal implants. Describe the implant and where it is placed. Note for which patients these implants are indicated. ▸ Discuss transosteal implants. Describe the implant and where it is placed. Note for which patients these implants are indicated. *Class Activity **Before class, have students research on the Internet new implant systems as well as the success rate and failure rate of current systems. Have student volunteers present their findings to the class.** (For students to prepare for this activity, see Homework/Assignments #1.)*
Describe the surgical procedures for implantation.	■ Types of dental implants (p. 851) □ Endosteal implant (p. 851) □ Subperiosteal implant (p. 852) □ Transosteal implant (p. 852)	⊞ PPT 11-19 ▣ TB question 8 📖 SW Short-Answer Questions 4; Multiple Choice question 14 (pp. 463, 465) 📖 SW Case Study question 3 (p. 465) *Class Activity **Divide the class into two groups. Have one group create teaching plans for the two surgical procedures required to place endosteal implants. Have the other group create teaching plans for the two surgical procedures required to place subperiosteal implants. Have the groups share their plans with the class.***
Assist in implant surgery.	■ Types of dental implants (p. 851) □ Endosteal implant (p. 851) Procedure 53-1 Assisting in an endosteal implant surgery (pp. 853-855) (SW/ESLR Competency 53-1, p. 467)	📖 🄮 SW/ESLR Competency 53-1 Assisting in Endosteal Implant Surgery (p. 467) Figure 53-4 Panoramic radiograph of a subperiosteal implant (p. 852) Figure 53-5 Subperiosteal implant (p. 852) Recall questions 8-11 (p. 852) 💡 CTQ 1 (p. 856)

ELSEVIER

Torres and Ehrlich Modern Dental Assisting, 9th ed.

Bird/Robinson

OBJECTIVES	CONTENT	TEACHING RESOURCES
	☐ Subperiosteal implant (p. 852)	▸ Discuss the dental assistant responsibilities that are legally allowed in your state regarding assisting with dental implant surgery.
	☐ Transosteal implant (p. 852)	*Class Activity As a class, discuss the role and responsibilities of the dental assistant during implant surgery.*
Give home-care procedures and follow-up visits required after receiving dental implants.	■ Maintenance of dental implants (p. 852) ☐ Home care (p. 855) ☐ Routine office visits (p. 856)	PPT 20-22 TB question 10 SW Short-Answer Questions 5; Fill in the Blank question 6; Multiple Choice questions 12-13 (pp. 463-464) SW Case Study question 5 (p. 455) SW/IDO Patient Case Exercise questions 1-5 (p. 465) (The Interactive Dental Office CD-ROM) Figure 53-6 Instruments used to remove calculus from a dental implant (p. 855) Recall questions 12-13 (p. 856) Patient Education (p. 856) Legal and Ethical Implications (p. 856) Eye to the Future (p. 856) ▸ Discuss the devices that are essential for plaque removal for implant patients. ▸ Discuss the purpose of routine office visits following implant surgery. *Class Activity Divide the class into small groups. Have each group develop patient education materials on the importance of the health of the peri-implant tissue following implant surgery. Have each group share its materials with the class.*
Performance Evaluation		TB SW questions (pp. 463-465) SW Case Study (p. 465) SW/IDO Patient Case Exercise (p. 465) (The Interactive Dental Office CD-ROM) SW/ESLR Competency 53-1 Assisting in Endosteal Implant Surgery (p. 467) ESLR Electronic Flashcards ESLR Practice Quiz Recall questions (pp. 849-856) CTQ (p. 856)

53.1 Homework/Assignments:

1. Have the students research on the Internet new implant systems as well as the success rate and the failure rate of current systems.

53.1 Instructor's Notes/Student Feedback:

Slide 1

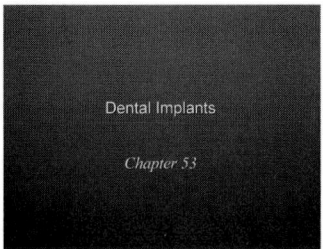

Slide 2

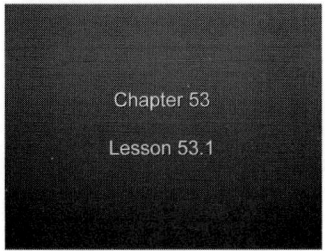

Slide 3

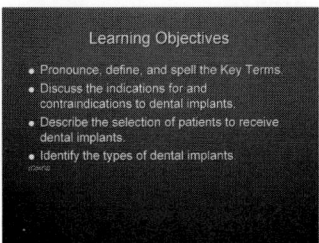

Slide 4

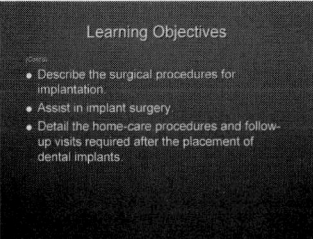

Slide 5

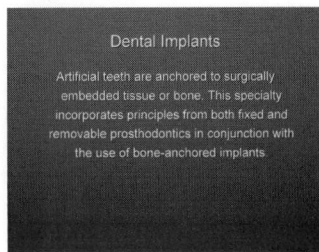

- Natural-looking replacement for missing teeth.
- Expensive treatment option.

Slide 6

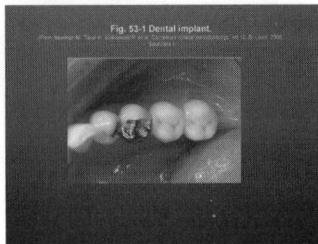

- Can you see the implant?
- Which tooth may be involved with an implant?
- Does the shade of the implant match the rest of the dentition?

Slide 7

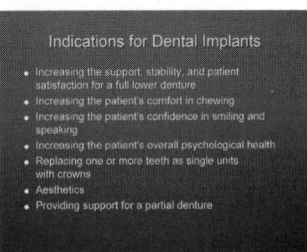

- Most patients find that having a full lower denture can be a "mouth-full" and that implants are a good option.
- Implants have a 90% success rate.
- Requires heavy commitment on the patient's part.
- Is a large financial responsibility for the patient.
- If a patient is missing only tooth #19 in the lower arch, would the patient be better suited for an implant or a fixed bridge?

Slide 8

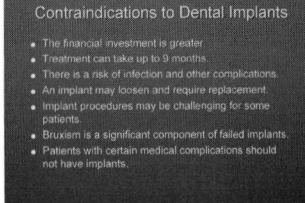

- The risk for infection is much greater for an implant than a fixed bridge.
- Patients with diseases of the cardiovascular, respiratory, and gastrointestinal systems would not be good candidates for implants.
- Patients with seriously compromised immune systems and other diseases that might slow down the healing process would not be good candidates.
- Would a patient who is HIV-positive be a good candidate for implants? *(No.)*
- Would a patient who is undergoing chemotherapy be a good candidate for implants? *(No.)*

Bird/Robinson

Slide 9

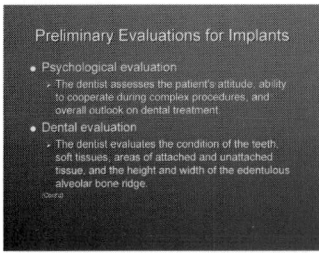

- Psychological Evaluation: Is the patient ready for this involved procedure? Does the patient have a realistic expectation of the implants?
- Dental Evaluation: It is important for the dentist to evaluate the supportive tissues; is it in good condition to support an implant?
- Would a patient who is looking for a "quick fix" be a good candidate for an implant?
- Would a patient who has severe periodontal disease be a good candidate for an implant?

Slide 10

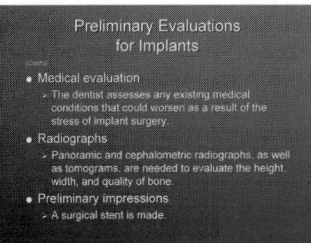

- A medical evaluation should be done on all patients, regardless of the procedure.
- What is a panoramic radiograph? *(Shows entire dentition in one radiograph.)*
- What is a cephalometric radiograph? *(Used to study the bone and tissue structure of the head.)*
- What is a tomogram? *(Imaging of one section of the body, while blurring images from structures in another plane.)*
- Surgical stent: made of clear plastic; used as a guide for the dentist to place the implant in the correct area.

Slide 11

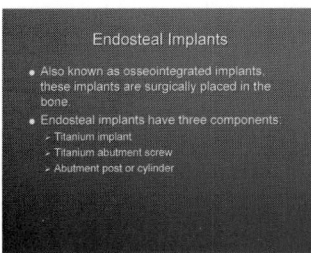

- Osseo = bone.
- Titanium implant is placed into the bone during the first stage of the procedure.
- Titanium abutment screw is screwed onto the implant during the second stage of the procedure. Osseointegration must be complete.
- Abutment attaches to the tooth or the denture.
- Titanium is very strong and is a compatible material for the oral cavity.
- Informed consent must be obtained before starting treatment.

Slide 12

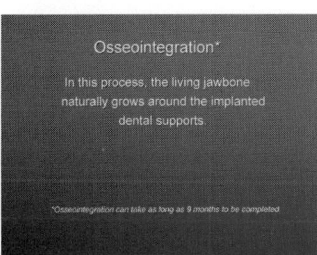

- The bond between living bone and the dental implant.
- How long is the osseointegration process? *(Three to six months.)*
- Used to support removable dentures, fixed bridges, and single-tooth implants.

Bird/Robinson

Slide 13

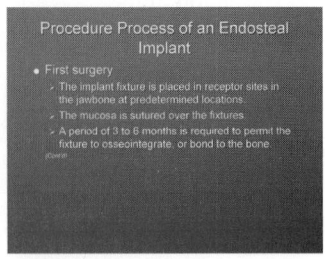

- Patient must be extremely careful during this stage not to cause any trauma to the mucosa area.
- Strict sterile conditions are enforced during this procedure.
- What would the surgical area be irrigated with? *(Sterile saline solution.)*
- Implants to be placed should be sterilized before placement.
- Be sure patient has signed informed consent before starting procedure.
- Surgical techniques may vary from patient to patient.

Slide 14

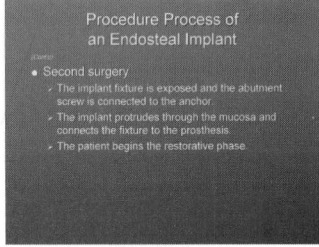

- Fixture is exposed; tissue is reflected away from the implant.
- What is the time frame between the first surgery and the second surgery?
- Strict sterile conditions are enforced during procedure.
- What would the surgical area be irrigated with? *(Sterile saline solution.)*
- Surgical techniques may vary from patient to patient.
- Restorative phase: placement of final crown, bridge, partial or full denture.

Slide 15

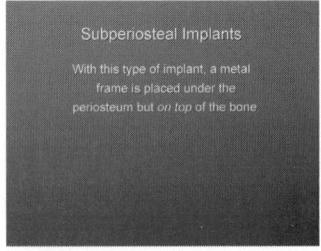

- Not placed in the bone like an endosteal implant.
- Most commonly used for patients with insufficient alveolar ridges.
- Most commonly used on the mandibular arch.
- Why wouldn't this type of implant be used on the maxillary arch? *(Easier to replicate the alveolar bone on the mandible vs. the maxilla.)*

Slide 16

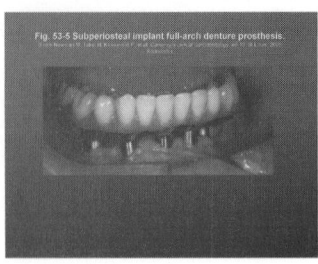

- Requires a two-step surgical procedure; may vary from patient to patient.
- What are these subperiosteal implants supporting?
- Would a surgical stent have be used in this procedure?

Slide 17

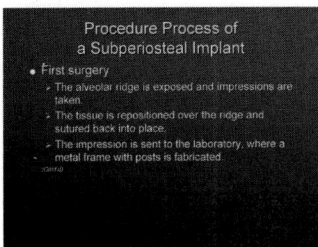

- Which patients would be good candidates for subperiosteal implants? *(Those with insufficient alveolar ridges.)*
- Sterile surgical conditions are enforced during procedure.

Slide 18

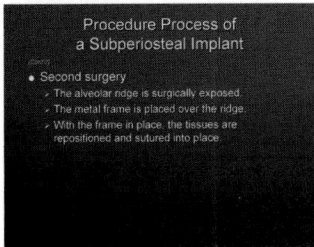

- Requires 3 to 6 months of healing time between first and second surgery.
- Sterile surgical conditions are enforced during procedure.

Slide 19

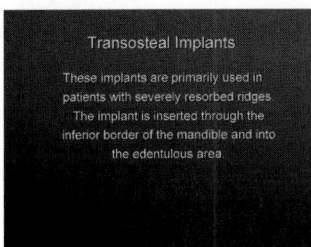

- Most common type is the transmandibular staple implant.
- It is used when there are no other options for the patient.

Slide 20

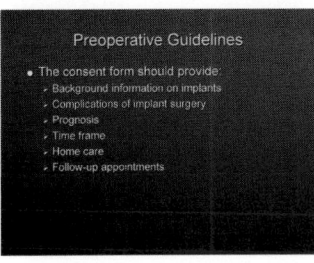

- What background information would you give to the patient? *(Can be 90% successful if patient is cooperative.)*
- What complications can arise from having implants placed? *(Greater risk of infection.)*
- What is the prognosis? *(It can be 90% successful if patient is cooperative and there are no complications.)*
- What is the time frame? *(Up to 9 months of treatment.)*
- What is the appropriate home care? *(Use of aids specifically designed for implants.)*

Slide 21

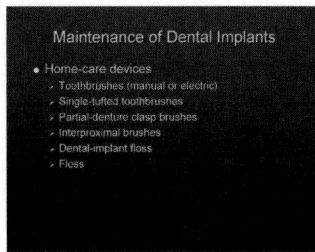

- Success of implants depends on good home care.
- Complete instruction on home-care devices is important.
- Patients should keep up their regular recall visits.

Slide 22

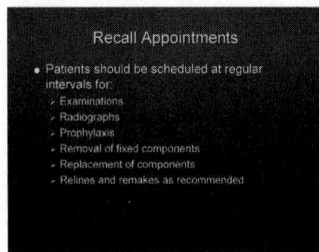

- Success of implants depends on regular recall appointments.
- Patients should understand that these implants must be cleaned thoroughly, the way they clean their natural teeth.

Torres and Ehrlich Modern Dental Assisting, 9th ed.

Bird/Robinson

TEACHING FOCUS

This chapter will introduce the student to topics related to endodontics. The student will become acquainted with the causes and symptoms of pulpal damage, endodontic diagnosis, endodontic procedures, and root canal therapy. The student will have the opportunity to put this information into context by participating in classroom activities and discussions.

MATERIALS AND RESOURCES

- ☐ basic setup (Lesson 54.2)
- ☐ broaches and Hedstrom/K-type files (assorted sizes and lengths) (Lesson 54.2)
- ☐ computer and PowerPoint projector (all Lessons)
- ☐ dental dam setup (Lesson 54.2)
- ☐ electric pulp tester (Lesson 54.1)
- ☐ electric pulp testing kit (Lesson 54.1)
- ☐ endodontic explorer (Lesson 54.2)
- ☐ endodontic sealer supplies (Lesson 54.2)
- ☐ endodontic spoon excavator (Lesson 54.2)
- ☐ Glick Number 1 (Lesson 54.2)
- ☐ gutta-percha points (Lesson 54.2)
- ☐ hemostat (Lesson 54.2)
- ☐ high-speed handpiece with burs (Lesson 54.2)
- ☐ high-volume oral excavator (HVE) tip (Lesson 54.2)
- ☐ lentulo spiral (Lesson 54.2)
- ☐ local anesthetic agent setup (Lesson 54.2)
- ☐ locking cotton pliers (Lesson 54.2)
- ☐ low-speed handpiece with latch attachment (Lesson 54.2)
- ☐ millimeter rule (Lesson 54.2)
- ☐ paper points (Lesson 54.2)
- ☐ rubber instrument stops (Lesson 54.2)
- ☐ sodium hydrochloride solution (Lesson 54.2)
- ☐ syringe (5ml to 6ml) with 27-gauge needle (Lesson 54.2)
- ☐ toothpaste (Lesson 54.1)

LESSON CHECKLIST

Preparations for this lesson include:

- lecture
- guest speaker: dental assistant (optional)
- evaluation of student knowledge and skills needed to perform all entry-level activities related to endodontics, including:
  - ○ application of root canal therapy procedures
  - ○ diagnostic conclusions for endodontic therapy
  - ○ diagnostic testing performed for endodontic diagnosis
  - ○ medicaments and dental materials used in endodontics
  - ○ proper circumstances and use of surgical endodontic techniques
  - ○ types of endodontic procedures

Torres and Ehrlich Modern Dental Assisting, 9th ed.

Bird/Robinson

KEY TERMS

abscess (p. 858)
acute (p. 862)
apical curettage (p. 868)
apicoectomy (p. 868)
chronic (p. 862)
control tooth (p. 859)
debridement (p. 868)
endodontist (p. 858)
gutta-percha (p. 860)
hemisection (p. 871)
indirect pulp cap (p. 862)
irreversible pulpitis (p. 862)
nonvital (p. 860)
obturation (p. 863)
palpation (p. 860)

percussion (p. 859)
perforation (p. 865)
periodontal abscess (p. 862)
periradicular (p. 858)
periradicular abscess (p. 862)
periradicular cyst (p. 862)
pulp cap (p. 862)
pulpectomy (p. 863)
pulpitis (p. 862)
pulpotomy (p. 863)
retrograde restoration (p. 868)
reversible pulpitis (p. 862)
root amputation (p. 868)
root canal therapy (p. 858)

ADDITIONAL RESOURCES

PowerPoint slides (Evolve): 1-41
The Interactive Dental Office CD-ROM: Antonio DeAngelis

Legend

CTQ
Critical
Thinking
Question

DVD
Multimedia
Procedures
Videos and
Animations

ESLR
EVOLVE
Student
Learning
Resources

IDO
Interactive
Dental
Office
CD-ROM

SW
Student
Workbook

TB
Test Bank
on the
TEACH
CD-ROM

PPT
PowerPoint
Slides

Class Activities are indicated in ***bold italic.***

ELSEVIER

Torres and Ehrlich Modern Dental Assisting, 9th ed.

Bird/Robinson

LESSON 54.1

PRETEST

1. What is the term used to describe a localized area of pus?
   a. fistula
   b. abscess
   c. pulpitis
   d. pimple

2. A subjective examination of a patient would include which of the following?
   a. extent of decay
   b. swelling or discoloration
   c. chief complaint
   d. tooth mobility

3. What is the term used to describe inflammation of pulpal tissues that can be eliminated once the irritant is removed?
   a. normal pulp
   b. reversible pulpitis
   c. irreversible pulpitis
   d. necrosis

4. Which procedure involves removal of the coronal portion of an exposed vital pulp?
   a. root canal
   b. pulpectomy
   c. pulpotomy
   d. pulp capping

5. Which term describes the actual filling of the canal?
   a. obturation
   b. plugger
   c. gutta percha
   d. debridement

6. Which type of medicament is most commonly used as a sealer for a pulpotomy of a deciduous tooth?
   a. hydrogen peroxide
   b. saline solution
   c. sodium hypochlorite
   d. formocresol

7. What is the main purpose of debridement?
   a. to remove bacteria and necrotic tissue
   b. to smooth canal walls
   c. to gain access into the canal
   d. to find the appropriate working length

8. What is the main purpose of paper points?
   a. to measure the length of the canal
   b. to place a sealer
   c. to dry the canal
   d. to sterilize the canal

9. What is the term used to describe removal of the soft tissue around the apex of the tooth?
   a. retrograde restoration
   b. root canal therapy
   c. apicoectomy
   d. apical curretage

10. What is the term used to describe symptoms that persist over a long period?
    a. chronic
    b. acute
    c. generalized
    d. nonvital

Answers

1. b	3. b	5. a	7. a	9. d
2. c	4. c	6. d	8. c	10. a

BACKGROUND ASSESSMENT

Question: What are the causes of pulpal damage?

Answer: There are two sources of pulpal damage. The first is caused by physical irritation. Physical irritation is most often caused by bacteria or decay that has moved into the pulp. Once this occurs, the bacteria can attack the pulpal tissues and can ultimately cause an abscess to the tooth. Root canal therapy is inevitable when this happens because the pulpal tissues are diseased because of the bacteria invasion. The second cause would be trauma. Trauma to the oral cavity can occur from a blow to the jaw or blunt force trauma to the face. It is very common for a tooth to become necrotic after a traumatic accident.

Question: What is the importance of obtaining an estimated working length during the root canal procedure?

Answer: Many problems can occur as a result of a tooth that did not have an estimated working length before filling the canal. Such an error may cause a perforation of the apex, over-instrumentation or under-instrumentation of the canal, over-filling or under-filling of the canal, and postoperative pain for the patient. Since apex locations vary from patient to patient, a working length is estimated by using a reference point on the tooth and a millimeter ruler used to measure the files that are inserted into the canal. These estimated working length measurements should always be documented in the patient's chart.

CRITICAL THINKING QUESTION

A patient comes to the dental office with a swollen left cheek and pressure discomfort in the same area. She states that one specific tooth is very sensitive to temperature and she is having difficulty eating on that side of her mouth. She also says that the discomfort started six days ago, and the swollen cheek appeared yesterday. What procedures are required to diagnose the problem?

Guidelines: After discussing the problems that the patient has been having for the past week, the dentist will need to evaluate the tooth. A visual examination would include evaluating any intraoral swelling, tooth mobility, or tissue discoloration. The dentist would also check the upper left quadrant using the percussion and palpation evaluation. Percussion evaluation requires the use of a mouth mirror that is tapped on the tooth in question. The palpation evaluation would involve applying firm pressure to the apex of the tooth. Any positive response from the patient would be noted in the patient's chart. Thermal sensitivity can also be done by applying ice to the cervical area of the tooth in question and also on a control tooth. A necrotic tooth will not respond to the ice, but a tooth with irreversible pulpitis may initiate a lingering pain. An electronic pulp tester can also be used to assess the vitality of a tooth by delivering small electrical stimuli to the tooth. The final tool used to assist in the diagnosis would be radiographs. Periapicals should be taken of the tooth in question, making sure to obtain the apex of that specific tooth.

OBJECTIVES	CONTENT	TEACHING RESOURCES
Pronounce, define, and spell the Key Terms.	■ Key terms (p. 858)	*e* ESLR Electronic Flashcards ▸ Discuss each of the key terms in Chapter 54, focusing on the definition, pronunciation, and spelling of each term. *Class Activity Have students make flash cards of the key terms, with the terms on one side and the definitions on the reverse. Then divide the class into student pairs, and have the students quiz each other with the flash cards. Correct their pronunciation as needed.*
Describe the diagnostic testing performed for endodontic diagnosis.	■ Introduction (p. 858) ■ Causes of pulpal damage (p. 858) ■ Symptoms of pulpal damage (p. 859) ■ Endodontic diagnosis (p. 859)	PPT 4-10 TB questions 1-4 SW Short-Answer Questions 1; Fill in the Blank questions 2-3, 12, 15, 19; Multiple Choice questions 1-5 (pp. 469-471) SW Case Study questions 1-4 (p. 472)

OBJECTIVES	CONTENT	TEACHING RESOURCES
		⬛🔵 SW/IDO Patient Case Exercise question 1 (p. 472) (The Interactive Dental Office CD-ROM)
		Figure 54-1 Radiograph showing extensive decay into the pulp (p. 858)
		Figure 54-2 Radiograph of a necrotic tooth resulting from trauma (p. 859)
		Recall questions 1-3 (p. 859)
		▸ Discuss the subjective examination. Note that the examination includes an evaluation of problems experienced by the patient, including the chief complaint, the character and duration of pain, painful stimuli, and sensitivity to biting and pressure.
		▸ Discuss the objective examination. Note the factors evaluated by the endodontist during the objective examination.
		Class Activity Divide the class into small groups, and have the groups discuss the causes and the four most common signs of pulpal nerve damage. Have each group present its findings to the class.
List the conclusions of the subjective and objective tests in the endodontic diagnosis.	⬛ Endodontic diagnosis (p. 859) ☐ Percussion and palpation (p. 859) ☐ Thermal sensitivity (p. 860) ☐ Electric pulp testing (p. 860) ☐ Radiographs (p. 860) ☐ Electronic apex locator (p. 861)	🖼 PPT 11-21 💻 TB question 5 ⬛ SW Short-Answer Questions 2; Fill in the Blank questions 4-5, 8, 10; Multiple Choice questions 6-7 (pp. 469-471) Figure 54-3 Percussion test (p. 859) Figure 54-4 Palpation test (p. 860) Figure 54-5 Ice used for testing thermal sensitivity (p. 860) Requirements of Endodontic Films (p. 861) Figure 54-6 Good-quality radiographs are necessary for endodontic evaluation (p. 862) Figure 54-7 Electronic apex locator (p. 862) Recall questions 4-7 (p. 861) 💡 CTQ 4-5 (p. 872) ▸ Discuss the difference between the percussion test and the palpation test. ▸ Discuss tests related to thermal sensitivity. Explain that thermal stimuli are never placed on a metallic restoration or the gingival tissue. Describe the performance of the cold test and the heat test. Class Activity Divide the class into small groups, and have each group identify the subjective and objective tests in the endodontic diagnosis procedure in the following situations:

OBJECTIVES	CONTENT	TEACHING RESOURCES
		– *Patient # 1 complains of sensitivity to hot and cold of lower right quadrant; has had dull ache for one month; informed dentist that she missed her appointment for a cavity filling on tooth #30 months ago.* – *Patient # 2 hit his front teeth on handlebars during a bicycle accident last night; cannot bite into anything; is in pain, but no temperature sensitivity is noted.* – *Patient # 3 has a swollen jaw on the left side; teeth #19 and #20 are mobile; patient is unable to chew on that side of mouth; fistula is present on buccal of #19.*
Assist in electric pulp vitality test.	Procedure 54-1 Assisting in electric pulp vitality test (p. 861) (SW/ESLR Competency 54-1, p. 473)	SW/IDO Patient Case Exercise question 2 (p. 472) (The Interactive Dental Office CD-ROM) SW/ESLR Competency 54-1 Assisting in an Electric Pulp Vitality Test (p. 473) ▶ Discuss electric pulp testing. List the factors that influence the reliability of the pulp tester. ▶ Discuss radiographs. List the films required to diagnose and complete endodontic treatment. *Class Activity Divide the class into small groups. Have each group prepare educational materials explaining the procedural steps involved in the electric pulp vitality test and the dental assistant's role.*
Describe diagnostic conclusions for endodontic therapy.	■ Diagnostic conclusions (p. 862)	PPT 22-28 TB question 6 SW Short-Answer Questions 3; Fill in the Blank questions 17, 20; Multiple Choice questions 8-9 (pp. 469-471) Recall questions 8-9 (p. 862) ▶ Discuss the difference between reversible and irreversible pulpitis. Explain differences in treatment. *Class Activity Divide the class into two groups to discuss the possible diagnostic conclusions of the subjective and objective tests. Have one group describe the diagnoses of normal pulp, pulpitis, and periradicular abscess. Have the other group describe periodontal abscess, periradicular cyst, and necrosis. Have each group report its findings to the class.*

54.1 Homework/Assignments:

54.1 Instructor's Notes/Student Feedback:

LESSON 54.2

CRITICAL THINKING QUESTION

A patient comes into the office with a persistent infection around tooth #4. A root canal was performed approximately nine months ago and the infection around the tooth has not subsided, even with continual antibiotic treatment. The patient has stated that he does not want to lose the tooth and is willing to try another treatment option. What would his treatment options be?

Guidelines: Root canal therapy is 90% to 95% successful, but this patient's case falls into that small percentage of those that fail. The dentist may want to first take a biopsy of the area, because the infection has been persistent over the past nine months, and determine the type of infection. Tooth #4 has obviously failed because of the infection, but a perforation of the canal, fractured roots, pulp stones, or accessory canals could have contributed to the failure of the root canal. Exploratory surgery may be necessary to determine exactly why this root canal failed. If all those procedures have been performed, the patient may be a good candidate for an apicoectomy, apical curettage, and retrograde restoration. The procedure would involve surgically removing the apex of tooth #4, removing the pathological tissue around the apex of the tooth, and finally, sealing the apex of tooth #4 with material such as gutta-percha, amalgam, or composite.

OBJECTIVES	CONTENT	TEACHING RESOURCES

List the types of endodontic procedures.	■ Endodontic procedures (p. 862)
	
	□ Pulp capping (p. 862)
	
	□ Pulpotomy (p. 863)
	
	□ Pulpectomy (p. 863)
		PPT 31-33
		
		TB question 7
		
		SW Short-Answer Questions 4; Fill in the Blank questions 7, 13, 16; Multiple Choice questions 10-11 (pp. 469-471)
		
		Recall questions 10-11 (p. 863)
		
		▸ Discuss the difference between an indirect pulp cap and a direct pulp cap. Describe the circumstances in which each is used.
		
		▸ Discuss the difference between a pulpotomy and a pulpectomy, and explain when each procedure is indicated.
		
		Class Activity Divide the class into small groups, and have each group prepare patient teaching materials on the following types of endodontic procedures and the steps required to complete each:
		
		   – Pulp capping
		
		   – Direct vs. indirect pulp cap
		
		   – Pulpotomy
		
		   – Root canal therapy
		
		   – Apicoectomy
		
		   – Apical curettage
		
		   – Root amputation
		
		   – Hemisection
		
		Have the groups present their materials to the class for discussion.

OBJECTIVES	CONTENT	TEACHING RESOURCES
Discuss the medicaments and dental materials used in endodontics.	■ Instruments and accessories (p. 863) ☐ Hand instruments (p. 863) – Explorer (p. 863) – Endodontic spoon excavator (p. 863) – Spreaders and pluggers (p. 863) – Glick Number 1 (p. 863) ☐ Hand-operated files (p. 864) – Broaches (p. 864) – K-type file (p. 864) – Hedstrom file (p. 864) – Reamer file (p. 864) ☐ Rotary-operated files (p. 865) ☐ Ancillary instruments (p. 865) – Rubber stops (p. 865) – Paper points (p. 865) ■ Medicaments and dental materials in endodontics (p. 866) ☐ Irrigation solutions (p. 866) ☐ Root canal filling materials (p. 866) ☐ Root canal sealers (p. 867)	⊠≣ PPT 34-36 ▣ TB questions 8-9 SW Short-Answer Questions 5; Fill in the Blank question 14; Multiple Choice questions 12-16 (pp. 469-471) Figure 54-8 Endodontic explorer (p. 863) Figure 54-9 Endodontic spoon excavator (p. 863) Figure 54-10 Spreader and plugger used to obturate the canal (p. 863) Figure 54-11 Glick Number 1 (p. 863) Table 54-1 Color Coding and Sizing of Hand-Operated Files (p. 864) Figure 54-12 Dental broach (p. 864) Figure 54-13 K-type files (p. 864) Figure 54-14 Hedstrom files (p. 864) Figure 54-15 Reamer files (p. 864) Figure 54-16 Rotary handpiece used for endodontics (p. 865) Figure 54-17 Gates-Glidden burs (p. 865) Figure 54-18 Rubber stops (p. 865) Figure 54-19 Paper points (p. 866) Recall questions 12-16 (p. 866) Figure 54-20 Materials needed for preparing and obturating the pulpal canal (p. 866) Figure 54-21 The Touch 'N Heat is used to warm gutta-percha for obturation (p. 867) Recall question 17 (p. 867) ▸ Discuss instruments for pulp preparation. Describe the uses of hand-operated files, finger-operated files, rotary files, and instruments attached to the low-speed handpiece. ▸ Discuss the uses of irrigation solutions, root canal filling materials, and root canal sealers. ***Class Activity Display all the endodontic instruments on a table, and have the students identify each and explain their use in endodontic therapy.***

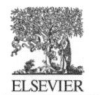

OBJECTIVES	CONTENT	TEACHING RESOURCES
Provide an overview of root canal therapy.	■ Overview of root canal therapy (p. 867) ☐ Anesthesia and pain control (p. 867) ☐ Isolation and disinfection of the operating field (p. 867) ☐ Access preparation (p. 867) – Estimated working length (p. 867) ☐ Debridement and shaping the canal (p. 868) ☐ Obturation (p. 868)	⊠ PPT 37 TB questions 10-11 SW Short-Answer Questions 6; Fill in the Blank question 9; Multiple Choice questions 17-19 (pp. 469-471) SW Case Study question 5 (p. 472) Figure 54-22 Two types of stop setting and measuring devices (p. 868) Recall questions 18-20 (p. 868) CTQ 1-3 (p. 872) ▶ Discuss the use of the dental dam in isolation and disinfection of the operating field. ▶ Discuss the need to accurately measure the length of the completed canal preparation. Note the problems that result from inaccurate measurement. *Class Activity Divide the class into small groups to discuss anesthesia and pain control in root canal therapy. Have each group describe the anesthesia techniques of choice for endodontic treatment and explain the circumstances under which each is used. Have the groups report their findings to the class.*
Assist in root canal therapy.	Procedure 54-2 Assisting in root canal therapy (pp. 869-871) (SW/ESLR Competency 54-2, pp. 475-476)	SW/IDO Patient Case Exercise questions 3-5 (p. 472) (The Interactive Dental Office CD-ROM) SW/ESLR Competency 54-2 Assisting in Root Canal Therapy (pp. 475-476) ▶ Discuss the procedural steps involved in root canal therapy. ▶ Discuss patient education. List general post-treatment instructions and follow-up information that should be provided by the dental assistant. *Class Activity Divide the class into small groups, and have each group create a teaching plan on the dental assistant's role in root canal therapy. Have the groups present their plans to the class.*
Describe surgical endodontics and how it affects treatment.	■ Surgical endodontics (p. 868) ☐ Apicoectomy and apical curettage (p. 868) ☐ Retrograde restoration (p. 868)	⊠ PPT 38-41 SW Short-Answer Questions 7; Fill in the Blank questions 1, 6, 11, 18; Multiple Choice question 20 (pp. 469-471) Figure 54-23 The apex of this mesiofacial root has been surgically removed (p. 868)

OBJECTIVES	CONTENT	TEACHING RESOURCES
	☐ Root amputation and hemisection (p. 868)	Figure 54-24 Root end filling is completed on a central incisor (p. 871)
		Figure 54-25 (A) Periodontal loss involving the mesial root; (B) Root amputation; (C) Hemisection (p. 872)
		Recall questions 21-22 (p. 871)
		Patient Education (p. 871)
		Legal and Ethical Implications (p. 872)
		Eye to the Future (p. 872)
		▸ Discuss the difference between root canal therapy and surgical endodontics. List three indications for surgical intervention.
		▸ Discuss pain experienced by the patient. Describe communication skills that can help a dental assistant provide appropriate care to a patient, and offer suggestions for appropriate and inappropriate statements.
		Class Activity Divide the class into small groups to discuss different surgical endodontic techniques. Have the groups describe the purpose of apicoectomy, apical curettage, retrograde restoration, root amputation, and hemisection, and the circumstances under which each technique is used. Have the groups report their findings to the class.
Performance Evaluation		▦ TB
		▤ SW questions (pp. 469-471)
		▤ SW Case Study (p. 472)
		⊙ SW CD-ROM Patient Case Exercise (p. 472) (The Interactive Dental Office CD-ROM)
		▤ 🅮 SW/ESLR Competency 54-1 Assisting in an Electric Pulp Vitality Test (p. 473)
		▤ 🅮 SW/ESLR Competency 54-2 Assisting in Root Canal Therapy (pp. 475-476)
		🅮 ESLR Electronic Flashcards
		🅮 ESLR Practice Quiz
		Recall questions (pp. 859-871)
		♀ CTQ (p. 872)

Torres and Ehrlich Modern Dental Assisting, 9th ed.

Bird/Robinson

54.2 Homework/Assignments:

54.2 Instructor's Notes/Student Feedback:

ELSEVIER

Torres and Ehrlich Modern Dental Assisting, 9th ed.

Slide 1

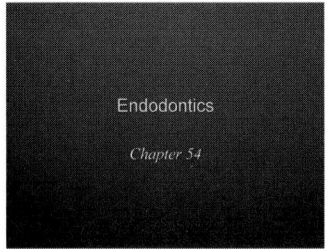

Slide 2

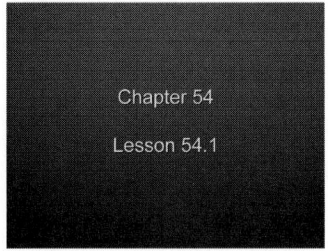

Slide 3

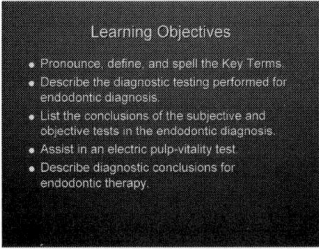

Slide 4

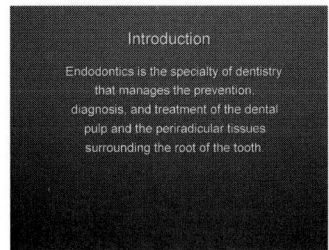

- General dentists are able to perform endodontic treatment.

- Endodontists have three years of continued training in endodontics.

- What is another name for endodontics?

- What is the name of the specialist that deals with the diseases of the pulp?

Slide 5

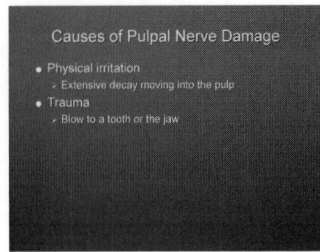

- Symptoms: pain on occlusion, pain during mastication, sensitive to temperature, and facial swelling
- Who has had a root canal?
- What was the source of the nerve damage?
- What were the symptoms?

Slide 6

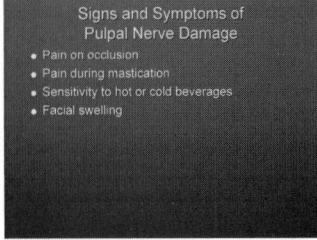

- Symptoms differ from patient to patient.
- Other symptoms include a dull ache in a tooth that lasts over a period of time.
- How would we put these symptoms in layman's terms?

Slide 7

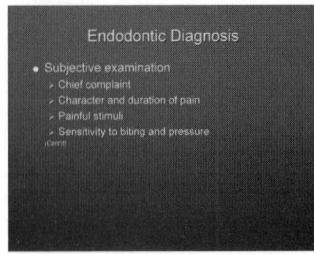

- The subjective examination includes an evaluation of all symptoms the patient describes.
- All symptoms should be documented in the patient's chart.
- What may be a patient's chief complaint?

Slide 8

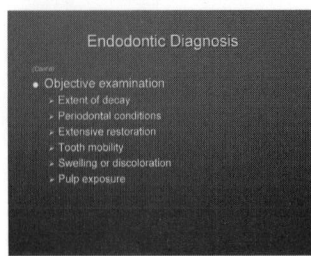

- The objective examination includes all findings by the dentist in the oral cavity.
- All findings must be documented in the patient's chart.
- Control tooth:
  - What is it?
  - How is it selected?
  - Students: If tooth #14 is hurting, which tooth would be the control tooth?

Torres and Ehrlich Modern Dental Assisting, 9th ed.

Bird/Robinson

Slide 9

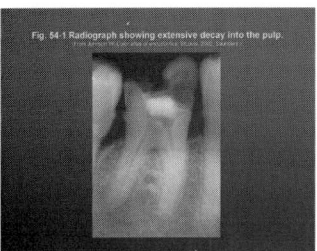

Slide 10

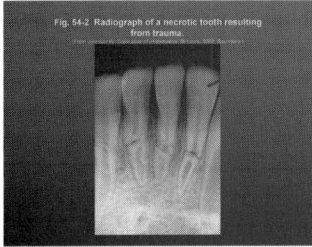

- What can we see on this radiograph?
- Which teeth are involved?
- What was the probable cause of pulpal damage?
- What may be the number one symptom this patient is experiencing?

Slide 11

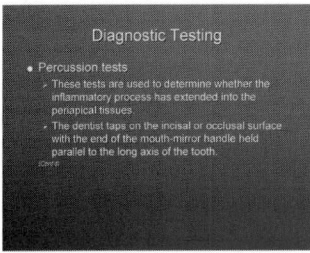

- All findings should be documented in the patient's chart.
- Where are the periapical tissues?

Slide 12

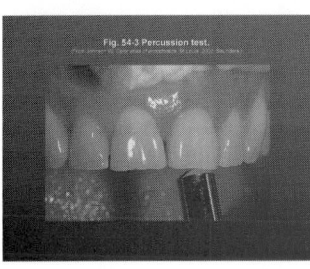

- Which tooth is the dentist testing?
- Which tooth would be the control tooth?

ELSEVIER

Torres and Ehrlich Modern Dental Assisting, 9th ed.

Bird/Robinson

Slide 13

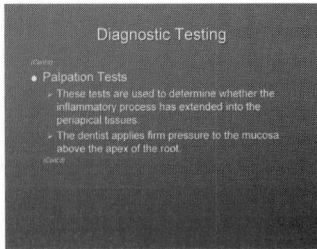

- All findings should be documented in the patient's chart.
- Dentist uses fingertips to palpate the mucosa.

Slide 14

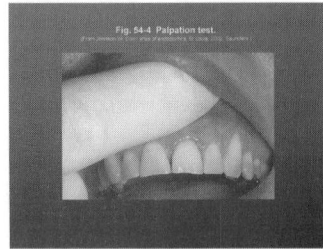

- Which area is the dentist palpating?
- What is the dentist looking for?

Slide 15

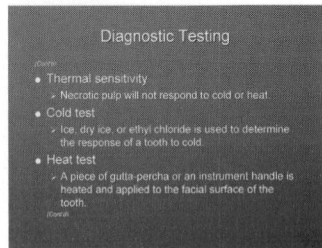

- Thermal stimuli are never placed on a metallic restoration or the gingival tissue. Why?
- Control tooth is used.
- Heat test is not used very often.
- Cold relieves pain = irreversible pulpitis
- Pain in teeth lingers = irreversible pulpitis
- What is pulpitis?
- What does "necrotic" mean?

Slide 16

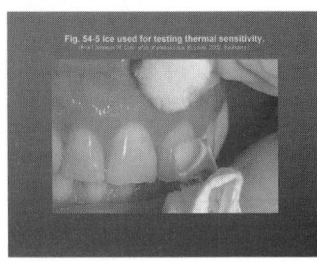

- Ice is applied to the cervical area of tooth only.
- What would be the control tooth for this photograph?
- All findings must be documented in the patient's chart.

Torres and Ehrlich Modern Dental Assisting, 9th ed.

Bird/Robinson

Slide 17

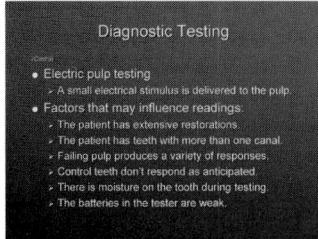

- Electric pulp testing is used to determine if tooth is vital or nonvital.
- The test can produce a false-positive or false-negative response.
- Would this type of diagnostic testing be used alone or in conjunction with another test?

Slide 18

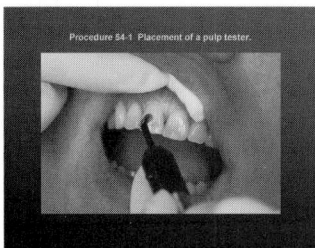

- All findings must be documented in the patient's chart.
- Explain to patient that he or she may feel a tingling or warm sensation during this test.
- Toothpaste is used as a conductor.
- Testing should only be done on the facial surface of the cervical third of tooth.

Slide 19

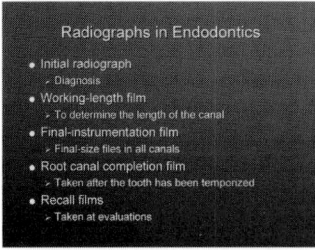

- Initial radiograph should be of diagnostic quality; the dental assistant must see the apex of tooth or teeth in question.
- Working-length film is taken once pulp is accessed.
- Final film: Radiograph shows files in place in canal.
- Completed film: Root canal procedure is completed.
- Recall films: Taken at prophylaxis appointments or as needed to check status of tooth.
- What type of film should be taken?

Slide 20

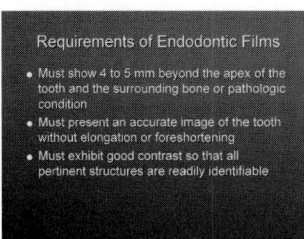

- What type of film would be taken?
- What if we didn't get the apex of the tooth? What would we need to do?

Slide 21

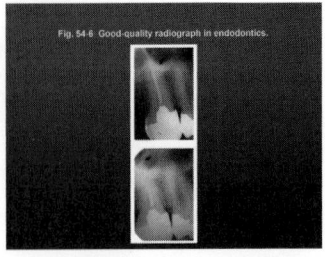

- Top radiograph: Shows at least 4 mm beyond the apex; apex is not distorted; good contrast

- Bottom radiograph: Does not show at least 4 mm beyond apex; apex is distorted; poor contrast is evident

- What would we need to do to make the bottom radiograph of diagnostic quality?

Slide 22

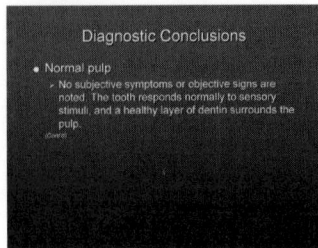

- If tooth is "normal," what could be the cause of the pain for the patient?

Slide 23

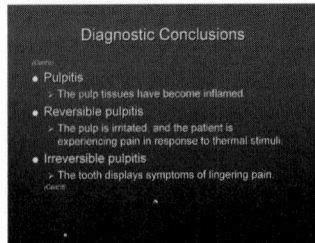

- *itis* = inflammation

- Reversible pulpitis: When irritant is removed, tooth can be saved from root canal treatment.

- What could be the irritant?

- Irreversible pulpitis: Pulp is incapable of healing.

- If root canal therapy does not improve the situation, extraction of tooth would be the next option.

Slide 24

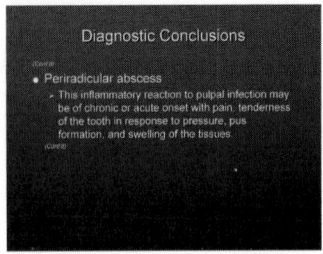

- What is another term for pus? *(Exudate)*

- Odor/Smell/Color

- Chronic periradicular abscess: presence of a draining sinus tract

- Acute periradicular abscess: pain, tenderness, swelling as a result of the necrosis

Slide 25

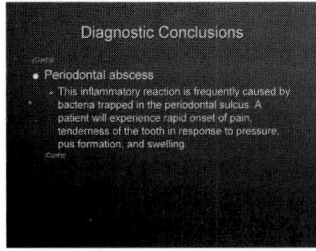

- Odor/Smell/Color
- Where is the sulcus located?
- If the patient has a periodontal abscess, does that always indicate root canal therapy is needed?

Slide 26

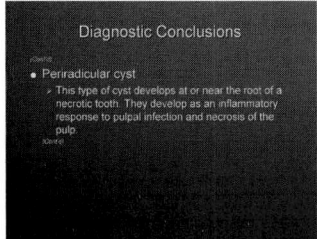

- Not very common.

Slide 27

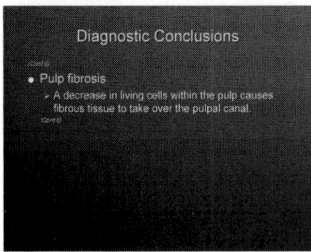

- Mostly seen in older patients
- Patients with recent trauma to tooth may be susceptible.

Slide 28

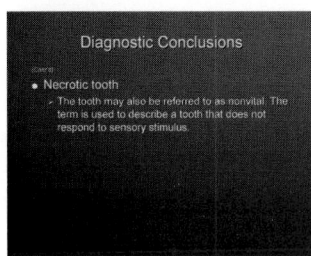

- What is another term for necrotic?
- Tooth is still attached to the alveolus by way of the cementum and periodontal ligaments.
- If the tooth is necrotic, will it fall out on its own?

Slide 29

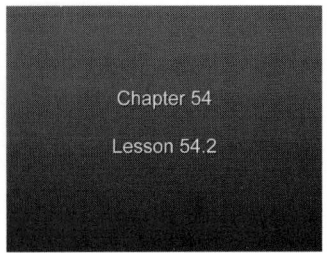

Chapter 54

Lesson 54.2

Slide 30

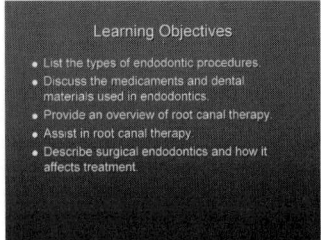

Learning Objectives
- List the types of endodontic procedures.
- Discuss the medicaments and dental materials used in endodontics.
- Provide an overview of root canal therapy.
- Assist in root canal therapy.
- Describe surgical endodontics and how it affects treatment.

Slide 31

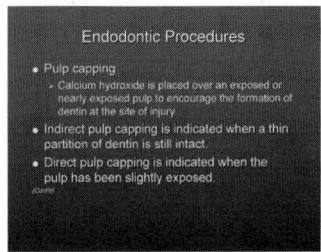

Endodontic Procedures
- Pulp capping
  - Calcium hydroxide is placed over an exposed or nearly exposed pulp to encourage the formation of dentin at the site of injury
  - Indirect pulp capping is indicated when a thin partition of dentin is still intact.
  - Direct pulp capping is indicated when the pulp has been slightly exposed.
  (Cont'd)

- Can be used as an attempt to save the pulp.
- Mostly used when bacteria has come very close to infecting the pulp.
- Goals: to promote pulpal healing and to stimulate production of reparative dentin.
- Most commonly referred to as IPC or DPC.
- Dentist must inform the patient that this procedure may not be a long-term solution.

Slide 32

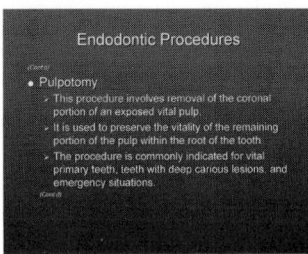

Endodontic Procedures
(Cont'd)
- Pulpotomy
  - This procedure involves removal of the coronal portion of an exposed vital pulp.
  - It is used to preserve the vitality of the remaining portion of the pulp within the root of the tooth
  - The procedure is commonly indicated for vital primary teeth, teeth with deep carious lesions, and emergency situations.
  (Cont'd)

- Where is the coronal portion of the tooth?
- Most commonly done on deciduous teeth.
- Why wouldn't root canal therapy be done on a deciduous tooth?

Torres and Ehrlich Modern Dental Assisting, 9th ed.

Bird/Robinson

Slide 33

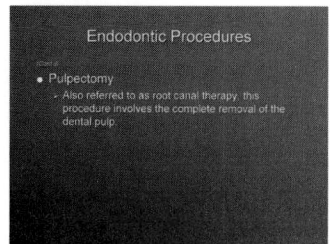

Slide 34

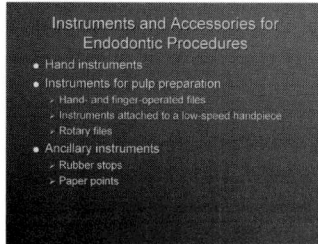

- Most root canal instruments are slim in design to fit inside the canals of the tooth and flexible enough to adapt to the curves of the canals.

- Hand Instruments: endodontic explorer, endodontic spoon excavator, spreaders, pluggers, Glick Number 1

- Finger files: broaches, K-type files, Hedstrom files

- Rotary files: Gates-Glidden burs, Pesso reamers

- Ancillary instruments: rubber stops, paper points

Slide 35

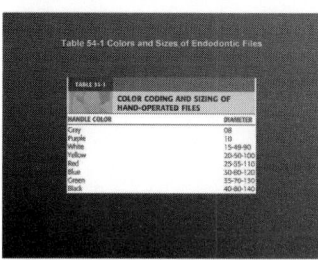

- Universal color-coded system.

- For example, a white file can be at a diameter of 15, 49, or 90.

- Most manufacturers place the number on the handle of the file.

Slide 36

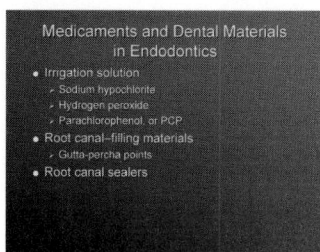

- Irrigation solutions help remove debris, bleach and deodorize canal, and control hemorrhaging. Sodium hypochlorite is the most commonly used.

- HVE must be used at all times when irrigating. Why would this be important?

- Filling materials: Gutta-percha is solid at room temperature, but a heat source is needed during filling.

- Variety of sizes; first gutta-percha point in canal is referred to as the "master cone." Size should be documented in patient's chart.

- What does "obturation" mean?

Slide 37

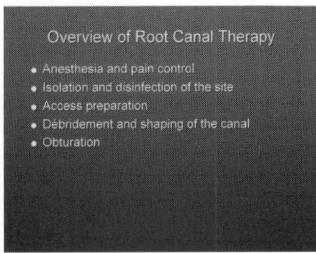

- Local anesthetic is most commonly used.
- Infiltration for maxillary teeth; nerve blocks for mandibular teeth.
- Sedatives may also be used to alleviate apprehension.
- Rubber dams are always used during root canal procedures.
- Why is the use of a rubber dam important?
- What is debridement?
- What problems could occur if the working length is incorrect?

Slide 38

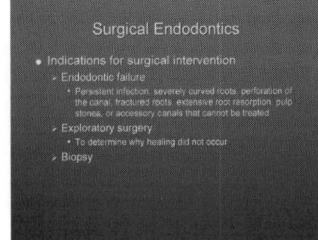

- Root canals have a 10% to 15% chance of failure.
- Used to save tooth from extraction.

Slide 39

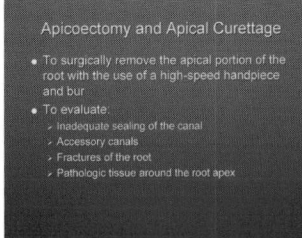

- Invasive procedure.
- A flap is made on buccal mucosa to gain access to apex.
- Endodontists generally perform this procedure.

Slide 40

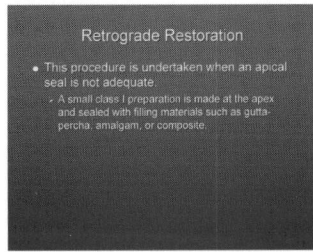

- Used in conjunction with apicoectomy and/or apical curettage.
- Commonly referred to as "root end filling."
- Amalgam is most commonly used filling material.
- Why would this procedure be done by an endodontist rather than a general dentist?

Bird/Robinson

Slide 41

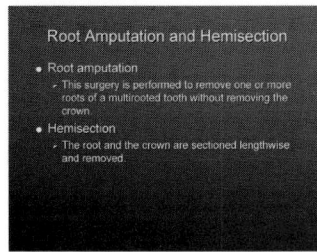

- A root amputation occurs at the furcation.

- What is furcation?

- Hemisections are most commonly performed on mandibular molars.

- Why wouldn't hemisections be performed on maxillary molars?

TEACHING FOCUS

This chapter introduces the student to topics related to periodontics. The student will become acquainted with the periodontal examination, periodontal instruments, surgical and nonsurgical periodontal treatment, and scaling and root planing. Procedural steps involved in assisting with a dental prophylaxis; gingivectomy; gingivoplasty; and the preparation, placement, and removal of periodontal dressings will also be discussed. The student will have the opportunity to put this information into context by participating in classroom activities and discussions.

MATERIALS AND RESOURCES

- ☐ basic instrument setup (Lesson 55.1)
- ☐ computer and PowerPoint projector (all Lessons)
- ☐ computer-generated periodontal chart (Lesson 55.1)

LESSON CHECKLIST

Preparations for this lesson include:

- lecture
- guest speakers: dentist and periodontist
- evaluation of student knowledge and skills needed to perform all entry-level activities related to periodontics, including:
  - ○ explaining the procedures necessary for a comprehensive periodontal examination
  - ○ identifying and describing the instruments used in periodontal therapy
  - ○ describing the types of nonsurgical and surgical periodontal therapy
  - ○ assisting with a dental prophylaxis procedure
  - ○ demonstrating periodontal charting
  - ○ assisting with gingivectomy
  - ○ assisting with gingivoplasty
  - ○ preparing, placing, and removing surgical dressings

Torres and Ehrlich Modern Dental Assisting, 9th ed.

Bird/Robinson

KEY TERMS

bleeding index (p. 876)
bone augmentation (p. 888)
chisel scaler (p. 879)
crown lengthening (p. 889)
curette (p. 880)
file (p. 880)
gingivectomy (p. 885)
gingivoplasty (p. 885)
Gracey curette (p. 880)
hoe scaler (p. 879)
Kirkland knife (p. 880)
laser (p. 893)
mobility (p. 876)
occlusal trauma (p. 878)
Orban knife (p. 880)
osseous surgery (p. 888)

ostectomy (p. 888)
osteoplasty (p. 888)
periodontal charting (p. 875)
periodontal dressing (Perio Pak) (p. 889)
periodontal explorer (p. 879)
periodontal flap surgery (flap surgery) (p. 888)
periodontal plastic surgery (p. 891)
periodontal pocket (p. 876)
periodontal probe (p. 876)
periodontics (p. 875)
periodontist (p. 875)
root planing (p. 884)
scaling (p. 884)
sickle scaler (p. 879)
ultrasonic scaler (p. 881)
universal curette (p. 880)

ADDITIONAL RESOURCES

PowerPoint slides (Evolve): 1-78
The Interactive Dental Office CD-ROM: Mrs. Louisa Van Doren
Multimedia Procedures Videos and Animations DVD:
   Noneugenol Periodontal Dressing
   Removing a Periodontal Dressing

Legend

CTQ
Critical
Thinking
Question

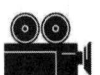

DVD
Multimedia
Procedures
Videos and
Animations

ESLR
EVOLVE
Student
Learning
Resources

IDO
Interactive
Dental
Office
CD-ROM

SW
Student
Workbook

TB
Test Bank
on the
TEACH
CD-ROM

PPT
PowerPoint
Slides

Class Activities are indicated in ***bold italic.***

ELSEVIER

Bird/Robinson

LESSON 55.1

PRETEST

1. What would a periodontist use to record the depth of periodontal pockets, furcation involvement, and tooth mobility?
   a. radiographs
   b. prophylaxis
   c. periodontal charting
   d. impressions

2. What is the depth of a normal sulcus?
   a. 0 to 3 mm
   b. 3 to 4 mm
   c. 4 to 5 mm
   d. greater than 5 mm

3. What instrument is used to locate deposits of calculus?
   a. scaler
   b. curette
   c. periodontal explorer
   d. surgical knife

4. What is the main difference between a scaler and a curette?
   a. A curette is always single ended.
   b. A scaler is always double ended.
   c. A curette has a pointed end.
   d. A scaler has a pointed end.

5. The instrument that provides rapid calculus removal is a(n)
   a. prophylaxis.
   b. ultrasonic scaler.
   c. surgical knife.
   d. Gracey curette.

6. Which of the following antibiotic therapies is most effective in treating periodontal disease?
   a. penicillin
   b. fluoride rinse
   c. chlorhexidine rinse
   d. tetracycline

7. The surgical periodontal treatment that involves the surgical reshaping and recontouring of gingival tissues is
   a. gingivoplasty.
   b. gingivectomy.
   c. incisional surgery.
   d. osseous surgery.

8. What is most commonly placed over the surgical site to assist in the healing process?
   a. ZOE dressing
   b. noneugenol dressing
   c. sutures
   d. gauze squares

9. The purpose of using a laser in periodontics is to
   a. remove calculus.
   b. make an incision.
   c. measure periodontal pockets.
   d. remove tumors and lesions.

10. How much additional time should a patient with periodontal disease spend on daily home care?
    a. 10 minutes
    b. 15 to 30 minutes
    c. 1 hour
    d. 2 hours

Answers

1. c	3. c	5. b	7. a	9. d
2. a	4. d	6. d	8. b	10. b

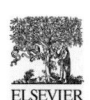

Bird/Robinson

BACKGROUND ASSESSMENT

Question: Why are periodontal pockets a contributing factor to periodontal disease?

Answer: The normal depth of a gingival sulcus is 3 mm or less. A periodontal pocket forms when disease causes the sulcus to become deeper than normal. When periodontal pockets are present, it is nearly impossible for the patient to properly clean these areas to free them of debris and bacteria. The bacteria will multiply and the periodontal disease will ultimately worsen until the tooth is lost. Therefore, periodontal measurements should be taken at each recall appointment to ensure the patient's gingival sulcus is normal.

Question: What are the advantages of incisional periodontal surgery?

Guidelines: Incisional surgery is indicated when the tissues involved in periodontal disease do not need to be removed. Incisional surgery, also known as flap surgery, is performed by pushing the tissue away from the teeth and away from the alveolar bone. With the tissue deflected from the teeth and the alveolar bone, the dentist is able to complete a thorough scaling and root planing of the exposed surfaces of the root and can recontour the underlying bone structure to remove any existing abnormalities. The advantages of this type of surgery may include lower costs, shorter time, and lower levels of discomfort.

CRITICAL THINKING QUESTION

An adult man has returned to the office for a recall examination. The dentist has prescribed bite-wing radiographs to evaluate the patient's periodontal disease. The patient is refusing radiographs, stating that the ones he had taken a year ago should be sufficient. What information could the dentist give this patient to convince him that new radiographs are necessary to correctly identify periodontal disease?

Guidelines: The dentist should explain to this patient that a correct diagnosis of existing periodontal disease cannot be detected by the naked eye alone. New radiographs are used as a comparison to the ones obtained a year ago. Making this comparison will help determine whether periodontal disease has worsened. Radiographs are used to detect any interproximal bone loss and locate any furcation involvement that may be present. Finally, the dentist should explain to this patient that early diagnosis of periodontal disease is essential in the treatment phase.

OBJECTIVES	CONTENT	TEACHING RESOURCES
Pronounce, define, and spell the Key Terms.	■ Key terms (pp. 873-874)	SW Fill in the Blank questions 1-14 (pp. 477-478) ESLR Electronic Flashcards ▶ Discuss each of the key terms in the chapter, focusing on the definition, pronunciation, and spelling of each term. ▶ Discuss the difference between the various periodontal instruments. *Class Activity Divide the class into pairs. Have each pair create flash cards of the key terms in the chapter, with the term on one side and the definition on the other, and quiz each other on the terms. Correct the students' pronunciation as needed.*
Describe the role of the dental assistant in a periodontal practice.	■ The periodontal practice (p. 875)	PPT 4-5 SW Short-Answer Questions 1; Fill in the Blank question 1; Multiple Choice question 1 (pp. 477-478) Recall question 1 (p. 878) CTQ 1 (p. 895) ▶ Discuss the typical responsibilities of the dental assistant in a periodontal practice.

Torres and Ehrlich Modern Dental Assisting, 9th ed.

Bird/Robinson

OBJECTIVES	CONTENT	TEACHING RESOURCES
		Class Activity Have students go to www.ada.org on the Internet and research their respective states' dental practice acts. In class, have students discuss the stipulations these acts place on the role of a dental assistant in a periodontal office. (For students to prepare for this activity, see Homework/Assignments #1.)
Explain the procedures necessary for a comprehensive periodontal examination.	■ The periodontal examination (p. 875) □ Medical and dental history (p. 875) □ Dental examination (p. 876) – Mobility (p. 876) – Oral tissues and supporting structures (p. 876) – Periodontal probing (p. 876) – Bleeding index (p. 876) – Occlusal adjustment (p. 876) – Radiographic analysis (p. 878)	⊠ PPT 6-21 TB questions 1-2 SW Short-Answer Questions 2, 5; Fill in the Blank questions 2-3, 5-6; Multiple Choice questions 2-5 (pp. 477-478) Early Signs of Periodontal Disease (p. 876) Figure 55-1 Computerized diagram showing periodontal parameters (p. 875) Table 55-1 Dental conditions that contribute to periodontal disease (p. 876) Figure 55-2 A periodontal chart on a computer screen (p. 876) Figure 55-3 Mobility is detected with the blunt ends of two instruments (p. 877) Table 55-2 Periodontal examination of gingiva and supporting tissues (p. 877) Figure 55-4 Cross-section of a tooth, gingiva, and bone (p. 877) Figure 55-5 Diagram showing probing of the periodontal pocket depth (p. 878) Figure 55-6 Six probing depths are taken for each tooth (p. 878) Recall questions 2-5 (p. 878) ▸ Discuss early signs of periodontal disease. Note conditions that can contribute to periodontal disease. ▸ Discuss the categories that are assessed during periodontal examination of gingiva and supporting tissues. Note the role of the dental assistant in the assessment of each category. *Class Activity Have student pairs take turns role-playing a dental assistant and a patient in a periodontist's office. Have the dental assistant do a medical and dental history on the patient, focusing on gathering information on conditions that can indicate periodontal disease. Students should discuss their assessments with the rest of the class.*

Bird/Robinson

OBJECTIVES	CONTENT	TEACHING RESOURCES
Demonstrate periodontal charting.	■ The periodontal examination (p. 875) □ Medical and dental history (p. 875) □ Dental examination (p. 876) – Mobility (p. 876) – Oral tissues and supporting structures (p. 876) – Periodontal probing (p. 876) – Bleeding index (p. 876) – Occlusal adjustment (p. 876) – Radiographic analysis (p. 878)	⊠▤ PPT 7-8 Figure 55-1 Computerized diagram showing periodontal parameters (p. 875) Figure 55-2 A periodontal chart on a computer screen (p. 876) ▸ Discuss the information that is charted for each periodontal exam. ▸ Discuss the format of the periodontal chart and note how this format assists in efficient and thorough charting. *Class Activity **Bring a computer-generated periodontal chart to class and give each student a copy. After students review the chart, discuss the different types of information recorded on the chart and how this information leads to clinical findings.***
Describe the role of radiographs in periodontal treatment.	– Radiographic analysis (p. 878)	⊠▤ PPT 19-20 ▤ TB question 3 SW Short-Answer Questions 6; Multiple Choice question 6 (pp. 477-478) SW/IDO Patient Case Exercise question 5 (p. 480) (The Interactive Dental Office CD-ROM) Figure 55-7 Bone loss in periodontal disease (p. 878) Recall question 6 (p. 878) Figure 55-8 Molar and premolar bite-wings (p. 879) ▸ Discuss radiographic analysis, noting the value of the bite-wing radiograph. Describe the role of the dental assistant in radiographic analysis. *Class Activity **Call on students and have them correctly identify when vertical bite-wings should be used and when horizontal bite-wings should be used.***
Identify and describe the instruments used in periodontal therapy.	■ Periodontal instruments (p. 878) □ Explorers (p. 879) □ Scalers and files (p. 879) □ Curettes (p. 880)	⊠▤ PPT 22-35 SW Short-Answer Questions 3; Fill in the Blank question 7; Multiple Choice questions 7-11 (pp. 477-479) SW/IDO Patient Case Exercise question 6 (p. 480) (The Interactive Dental Office CD-ROM) Figure 55-9 Working end of a periodontal probe (p. 879)

ELSEVIER

Bird/Robinson

OBJECTIVES	CONTENT	TEACHING RESOURCES
	☐ Surgical knives (p. 880) ☐ Pocket markers (p. 880)	Figure 55-10 Various styles of periodontal explorers (p. 879) Figure 55-11 Anterior and posterior curettes (p. 880) Figure 55-12 Comparison of the end of a scaler (pointed) and the end of a curette (rounded) (p. 880) Figure 55-13 Universal curette (p. 881) Figure 55-14 Assorted Gracey curettes (p. 881) Figure 55-15 Kirkland and Orban interdental knives (p. 881) Figure 55-16 Periodontal pocket marker (p. 881) Recall questions 7-11 (p. 880) ▸ Discuss the purpose of periodontal explorers. Note how their shape differs from explorers used for caries detection. ▸ Discuss the purpose and use of the pocket marker. *Class Activity **Bring a basic instrument setup to class. Have students correctly identify each instrument, discussing their uses in periodontal therapy.***
Describe the indications and contraindications for the use of the ultrasonic scaler.	☐ Ultrasonic scaler (p. 881) ☐ Indications and contraindications (p. 881) ☐ Precautions for children (p. 882)	PPT 36-41 TB question 4 SW Short-Answer Questions 7; Fill in the Blank question 8; Multiple Choice questions 12-14 (pp. 477-479) SW/IDO Patient Case Exercise questions 1, 4 (p. 480) (The Interactive Dental Office CD-ROM) Figure 55-17 A series of ultrasonic tips (p. 882) Figure 55-18 (A) Positioning of the ultrasonic scaler; (B) Ultrasonic scaler with water source turned on (p. 882) Hand scaling versus ultrasonic scaling (p. 883) Recall questions 12-14 (p. 882) CTQ 2 (p. 895) ▸ Discuss the purpose of the ultrasonic scaler and describe how it works. Note its advantages and disadvantages. ▸ Discuss the contraindications for use of an ultrasonic scaler. Note that the use of ultrasonic scalers is contraindicated on primary and newly erupted permanent teeth. *Class Activity **Conduct a group discussion on how to appropriately determine when ultrasonic scalers should be used in the following situations:***

Bird/Robinson

OBJECTIVES	CONTENT	TEACHING RESOURCES
		1. Patient has had orthodontic brackets removed
		2. Patient is HIV-positive
		3. Patient is scheduled to have periodontal surgery

55.1 Homework/Assignments:

1. Have students go to www.ada.org on the Internet and research the state's dental practice act. In class, have students discuss the stipulations the act places on the role of a dental assistant in a periodontal office.

55.1 Instructor's Notes/Student Feedback:

LESSON 55.2

CRITICAL THINKING QUESTION

An adult patient comes to the office to see about an ill-fitting denture. He complains of discomfort in his palate. Upon examination, the dentist notes that a bony growth is present. What procedure might the dentist recommend?

Guidelines: The bony growth is interfering with the comfort level of the patient's full denture. He would benefit from an ostectomy procedure, which involves removing the bony growth from his palate by means of surgery. Once the bony growth has been removed, the patient may benefit from a denture reline to help adapt the denture to the newly contoured tissues.

OBJECTIVES	CONTENT	TEACHING RESOURCES
Describe the goals of nonsurgical periodontal therapy.	■ Nonsurgical periodontal treatment (p. 883) ☐ Dental prophylaxis (p. 883) ☐ Scaling and root planing (p. 884) ☐ Gingival curettage (p. 884) ☐ Antimicrobial and antibiotic agents (p. 884) ☐ Locally delivered antibiotics (p. 884)	PPT 44-50 TB question 5 SW Multiple Choice questions 15-16 (p. 479) Recall questions 15-18 (p. 884) ▸ Discuss the dental prophylaxis procedure. Note that it is commonly referred to as a "cleaning." *Class Activity Have students correctly identify the goals of the different types of nonsurgical periodontal therapy:* *1. prophylaxis* *2. scaling and root planing* *3. gingival curettage* *4. antimicrobial and antibiotic therapy* *5. locally delivered antibiotics*
Assist with a dental prophylaxis procedure.	■ Nonsurgical periodontal treatment (p. 883) ☐ Dental prophylaxis (p. 883) Procedure 55-1 Assisting with a dental prophylaxis (p. 883) (SW/ESLR Competency 55-1, p. 481) ☐ Scaling and root planing (p. 884) ☐ Gingival curettage (p. 884) ☐ Antimicrobial and antibiotic agents (p. 884) ☐ Locally delivered antibiotics (p. 884)	SW/ESLR Competency 55-1 Assisting with a Dental Prophylaxis (p. 481) ▸ Discuss the role of the dental assistant in a dental prophylaxis procedure. ▸ Discuss the procedural steps involved in assisting with a dental prophylaxis procedure. *Class Activity Ask students to think about their own experiences when receiving a dental prophylaxis. Have students discuss their impressions—both positive and negative—and how these impressions might affect the way they assist with a dental prophylaxis.*

OBJECTIVES	CONTENT	TEACHING RESOURCES
Describe the types of nonsurgical periodontal therapy.	☐ Dental prophylaxis (p. 883) ☐ Scaling and root planing (p. 884) ☐ Gingival curettage (p. 884) ☐ Antimicrobial and antibiotic agents (p. 884) ☐ Locally delivered antibiotics (p. 884)	⊠☰ PPT 44-50 ▣ TB question 6 ▣ SW Short-Answer Questions 8; Multiple Choice question 18 (pp. 477, 479) Figure 55-19 A Gracey curette is used during scaling and root planing (p. 884) Figure 55-20 Irrigator (p. 885) Recall questions 17-18 (p. 900) ▸ Discuss the goal of debridement. ▸ Describe the patient circumstances that would require gingival curettage. *Class Activity Divide the class into four groups and assign each group one of the four antimicrobial or antibiotic agents on p. 899 of the textbook. Using a drug reference, have each group create a fact sheet on each agent, including the advantages and disadvantages and side effects of each one. Have the groups present their findings to the class. (For students to prepare for this activity, see Homework/Assignments #1.)*
Describe the types of surgical periodontal therapy.	■ Surgical periodontal treatment (p. 850) ☐ Advantages and disadvantages (p. 885) ☐ Remaining bone (p. 885) ☐ Excisional surgery (p. 885) – Gingivectomy (p. 885) – Gingivoplasty (p. 885) ☐ Incisional surgery (p. 888) ☐ Osseous surgery (p. 888) – Osteoplasty (p. 888) – Ostectomy (p. 888) ☐ Crown lengthening (p. 889)	⊠☰ PPT 51-64 ▣ SW Short-Answer Questions 9; Multiple Choice question 17 (pp. 477, 479) ▣ ℮ SW/IDO Patient Case Exercise question 2 (p. 479) (The Interactive Dental Office CD-ROM) Figure 55-21 Prognosis based on amount of bone loss (p. 885) Recall questions 19-22 (p. 889) ▸ Discuss the advantages and disadvantages of surgical periodontal treatment. ▸ Discuss the assessment of remaining bone in deciding whether and when to proceed with surgical treatment. *Class Activity Discuss the patient conditions that would indicate the following types of surgical treatment:* *– gingivectomy* *– gingivoplasty* *– flap surgery* *– osteoplasty* *– ostectomy*

ELSEVIER

Torres and Ehrlich Modern Dental Assisting, 9th ed.

Bird/Robinson

OBJECTIVES	CONTENT	TEACHING RESOURCES
	☐ Soft tissue grafts (p. 889)	
	– Pedicle graft (p. 889)	
	– Free gingival soft tissue graft (p. 889)	
	☐ Postsurgical patient instructions (p. 889)	
Assist with gingivectomy and gingivoplasty.	☐ Excisional surgery (p. 885)	⊠▪ PPT 51-64
	– Gingivectomy (p. 885)	💻 TB questions 7-8
	– Gingivoplasty (p. 885)	SW Fill in the Blank questions 10-11 (p. 478)
	☐ Incisional surgery (p. 888)	SW Case Study questions 1-3 (pp. 479-480)
	☐ Osseous surgery (p. 888)	SW ℰ SW/ESLR Competency 55-2 Assisting with a Gingivectomy and a Gingivoplasty (p. 483)
	– Osteoplasty (p. 888)	Figure 55-22 Gingivectomy surgery to treat gingival enlargement (p. 887)
	– Ostectomy (p. 888)	Figure 55-23 Instruments often used in osseous surgery (p. 888)
	☐ Crown lengthening (p. 889)	Figure 55-24 Reduction of bony ledges by osteoplasty (p. 889)
	☐ Soft tissue grafts (p. 889)	Figure 55-25 Surgical crown lengthening (p. 890)
	– Pedicle graft (p. 889)	Figure 55-26 Before and after soft tissue graft (p. 891)
	– Free gingival soft tissue graft (p. 889)	Recall questions 19-22 (p. 889)
	☐ Postsurgical patient instructions (p. 889)	Patient instructions after periodontal surgery (p. 890)
	Procedure 55-2 Assisting with gingivectomy and gingivoplasty (pp. 886-887) (SW/ESLR Competency 55-2, p. 483)	💡 CTQ 3 (p. 895)
		▸ Discuss the procedural steps involved in assisting with a gingivectomy or gingivoplasty.
		▸ Discuss important patient instructions after periodontal surgery.
		***Class Activity** Invite a dentist and periodontist to speak to the class about the dental assistant's role in a gingivectomy or gingivoplasty procedure. Have the dentist discuss common mistakes assistants make during these sorts of procedures and how they can help make the procedure as smooth as possible for both the patient and the dentist.*

55.2 Homework/Assignments:

1. Divide the class into four groups and assign each group one of the four antimicrobial or antibiotic agents on p. 899 of the textbook. Using a drug reference, have each group create a fact sheet on each agent, including the advantages and disadvantage and side effects of each one. Have the groups present their findings to the class.

55.2 Instructor's Notes/Student Feedback:

Bird/Robinson

LESSON 55.3

CRITICAL THINKING QUESTION

An adult patient returns to the office two days after she received periodontal surgery. She complains of soreness and a burning sensation in the gum tissues. After reviewing the patient's chart, it is noted that a zinc oxide-eugenol (ZOE) periodontal dressing was initially placed. What is this patient experiencing? What can be done to treat her problems?

Guidelines: The dentist determined that the patient is likely experiencing an allergic reaction to the eugenol in the periodontal dressing. The dressing would need to be removed immediately with a spoon excavator inserted under the margin of the dressing with lateral pressure. Care should be taken during removal, as the tissues have been traumatized from the allergic reaction. Floss should be used to remove the material from the interproximal areas. A mix of noneugenol periodontal dressing should then be mixed and placed over the surgical site to protect the area from trauma and to promote the healing process. The allergic reaction should be noted in the patient's chart.

OBJECTIVES	CONTENT	TEACHING RESOURCES
Identify the indications for placement of periodontal surgical dressings, and describe the technique for proper placement.	☐ Periodontal surgical dressings (p. 889) – Zinc oxide-eugenol dressing (p. 890) – Noneugenol dressing (p. 891)	⊞ PPT 67-72 TB question 9 SW Short-Answer Questions 4; Fill in the Blank question 4 (p. 477-478) SW Case Study question 4 (p. 480) SW/IDO Patient Case Exercise question 3 (p. 480) (The Interactive Dental Office CD-ROM) Recall questions 23-24 (p. 891) Figure 55-27 Zinc oxide powder and liquid eugenol are mixed in advance (p. 891) Figure 55-28 Paste for noneugenol dressing is ready to be mixed (p. 891) ▶ Discuss the purposes of periodontal surgical dressings. ▶ Discuss the differences between ZOE and noneugenol dressing. Note the circumstances under which each would be used. ***Class Activity** Have students research ZOE, using the Internet and health references. Have students create a fact sheet on ZOE that includes general information, consumer uses, classification, physical data, properties, and any other information relative to its use in periodontal surgical dressings. (For students to prepare for this activity, see Homework/Assignments #1.)*
Prepare and place noneugenol periodontal dressings (expanded function).	☐ Periodontal surgical dressings (p. 889) – Zinc oxide-eugenol dressing (p. 890)	⊞ PPT 67-72 Multimedia Procedures DVD: Noneugenol Periodontal Dressing SW/ESLR Competency 55-3 Preparing and Placing

OBJECTIVES	CONTENT	TEACHING RESOURCES
	– Noneugenol dressing (p. 891) Procedure 55-3 Preparing and placing noneugenol periodontal dressing (p. 892) (SW/ESLR Competency 55-3, pp. 485-486)	Noneugenol Periodontal Dressing (pp. 485-486) ▸ Discuss the procedural steps involved in preparing and placing noneugenol periodontal dressings. *Class Activity Have student pairs take turns role-playing a dental assistant giving a patient postsurgery instructions. Ask students what tools they could use to make this process as effective as possible for the patient, including written take-home instructions, follow-up calls, and so on.*
Remove a periodontal surgical dressing (expanded function).	☐ Periodontal surgical dressings (p. 889) – Zinc oxide-eugenol dressing (p. 890) – Noneugenol dressing (p. 891) Procedure 55-4 Removing a periodontal dressing (p. 893) (SW/ESLR Competency 55-4, p. 487)	Multimedia Procedures DVD: Removing a Periodontal Dressing SW/ESLR Competency 55-4 Removing a Periodontal Dressing (p. 487) ▸ Discuss the procedural steps involved in removing a periodontal dressing. *Class Activity, Write down on the board some of the precautions that should be taken during the removal of a periodontal surgical dressing. Discuss the purpose of each one with the class. Have students document the results.*
Describe the types of surgical periodontal therapy.	☐ Esthetic and plastic periodontal surgery (p. 891) ■ Lasers in periodontics (p. 893) ☐ Advantages of laser surgery (p. 894) ☐ Laser safety (p. 894)	PPT 73-78 TB question 10 SW Short-Answer Questions 9; Fill in the Blank question 14 (pp. 477-478) Types of Periodontal Plastic Surgery (p. 893) Figure 55-29 (A and B) Presurgical recession of gingival tissues; (C and D) Healed tissues after gingival graft surgery (p. 894) Figure 55-30 Laser unit (p. 894) Figure 55-31 Post warning signs to prevent injury to the eyes of persons who are not wearing special light filter glasses. Recall question 25 (p. 895) Patient Education (p. 895 Legal and Ethical Implications (p. 895) Eye to the Future (p. 895) ▸ Discuss the advantages and disadvantages of laser surgery. *Class Activity Divide the class into small groups. Have each group develop a thorough home care plan for a patient who has neglected his or her dental health. Have*

OBJECTIVES	CONTENT	TEACHING RESOURCES
		each group share its plan with the rest of the class. Discuss why some patients with periodontal disease require more complex home-care instructions than others.
Performance Evaluation		TB TB
		SW questions (pp. 477-479)
		SW Case Study (pp. 479-480)
		SW/IDO Patient Case Exercise (p. 480) (The Interactive Dental Office CD-ROM)
		SW/ESLR Competency 55-1 Assisting with a Dental Prophylaxis (p. 481)
		SW/ESLR Competency 55-2 Assisting with a Gingivectomy and a Gingivoplasty (p. 483)
		SW/ESLR Competency 55-3 Preparing and Placing a Noneugenol Periodontal Dressing (pp. 485-486)
		SW/ESLR Competency 55-4 Removing a Periodontal Dressing (p. 487)
		ESLR Electronic Flashcards
		ESLR Practice Quiz
		Recall questions (pp. 878-895)
		CTQ (p. 895)

55.3 Homework/Assignments:

1. Have students research ZOE, using the Internet and health references. Have students create a fact sheet on ZOE that includes general information, consumer uses, classification, physical data, properties, and any other information relative to its use in periodontal surgical dressings.

55.3 Instructor's Notes/Student Feedback:

Bird/Robinson

Slide 1

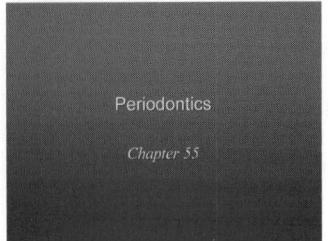

Periodontics

Chapter 55

Slide 2

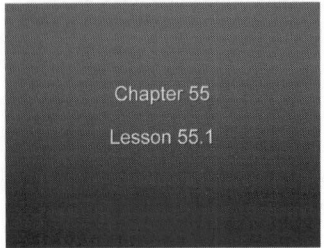

Chapter 55

Lesson 55.1

Slide 3

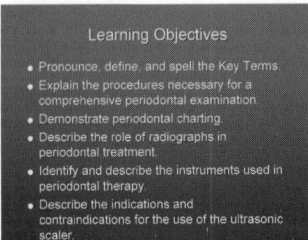

Learning Objectives

- Pronounce, define, and spell the Key Terms.
- Explain the procedures necessary for a comprehensive periodontal examination.
- Demonstrate periodontal charting.
- Describe the role of radiographs in periodontal treatment.
- Identify and describe the instruments used in periodontal therapy.
- Describe the indications and contraindications for the use of the ultrasonic scaler.

Slide 4

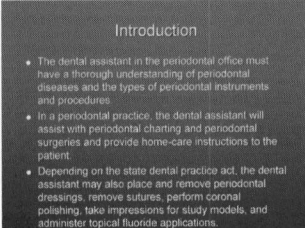

Introduction

- The dental assistant in the periodontal office must have a thorough understanding of periodontal diseases and the types of periodontal instruments and procedures.
- In a periodontal practice, the dental assistant will assist with periodontal charting and periodontal surgeries and provide home-care instructions to the patient.
- Depending on the state dental practice act, the dental assistant may also place and remove periodontal dressings, remove sutures, perform coronal polishing, take impressions for study models, and administer topical fluoride applications.

- What is periodontal disease?

Bird/Robinson

Slide 5

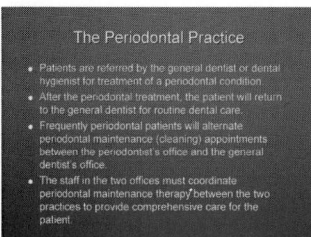

- Some general dentists will perform in-office periodontal surgery.
- Maintenance appointments are critical.

Slide 6

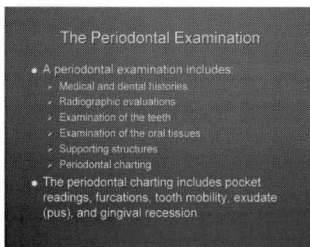

- Discuss what the radiographs will help to evaluate.
- When examining the oral tissues, what is the dentist looking for?
- Where is the furcation? (The point at which the roots of a multirooted tooth diverge.)

Slide 7

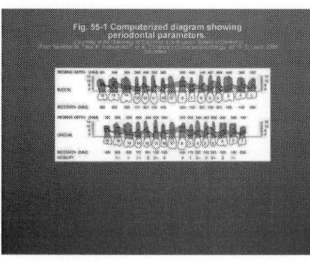

- What information does periodontal charting provide?
  (Periodontal pocket readings, furcations, tooth mobility, exudate, gingival recession.)

Slide 8

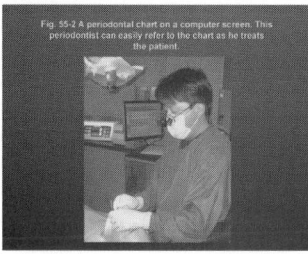

- Information is recorded either manually by dental assistant or by a computer program.

Torres and Ehrlich Modern Dental Assisting, 9th ed.
Bird/Robinson

Slide 9

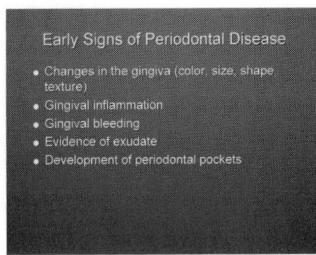

- What instrument is used to measure periodontal pockets? *(Periodontal probes.)*

Slide 10

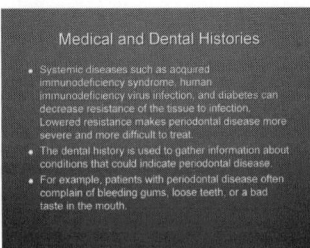

- Ask the patient if he or she has experienced any changes since the last visit, and make a record of them.

Slide 11

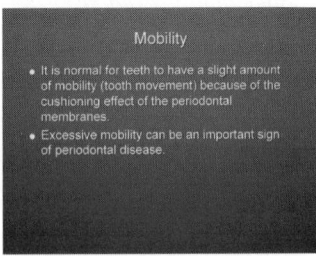

- Mobility is recorded using the following scale:
  - 0 = normal
  - 1 = slight mobility
  - 2 = moderate mobility
  - 3 = extreme mobility

Slide 12

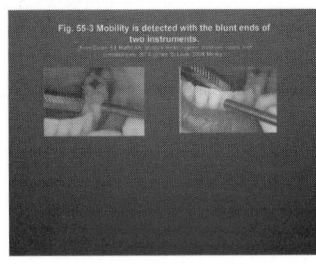

- What type of instrument is used to measure mobility?
- All findings should be documented in the patient's chart.

Slide 13

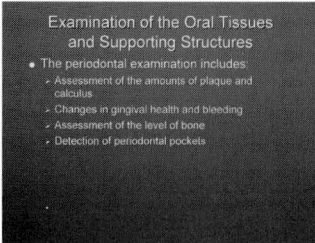

- What instrument is used to detect any calculus that has formed on the teeth?
- What changes in the gingiva would indicate the early signs of periodontal disease?

Slide 14

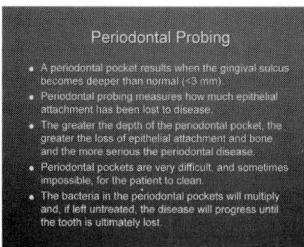

- What instrument is used to measure the depth of the sulcus? *(Periodontal probe.)*

Slide 15

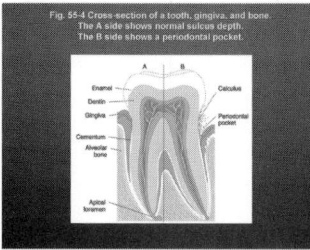

- Where is the epithelial attachment?
- What happens to the epithelial attachment if periodontal disease is present?

Slide 16

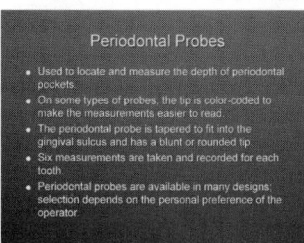

- Periodontal probes can be metal or plastic.
- Periodontal probes can be rounded or flat.
- What is the unit of measurement of a periodontal probe?

Slide 17

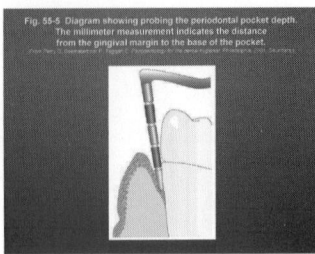

Fig. 55-5 Diagram showing probing the periodontal pocket depth. The millimeter measurement indicates the distance from the gingival margin to the base of the pocket.

- What measurements does the periodontal probe take? *(Six: distobuccal, buccal, mesiobuccal, distolingual, lingual, and mesiolingual.)*
- How deep is the sulcus in the above figure?

Slide 18

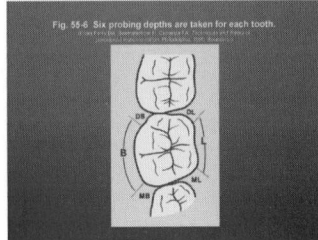

Fig. 55-6 Six probing depths are taken for each tooth.

- What surfaces are involved in periodontal probing?
- Who is able to perform periodontal probing?

Slide 19

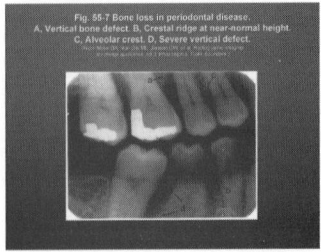

Fig. 55-7 Bone loss in periodontal disease. A, Vertical bone defect. B, Crestal ridge at near-normal height. C, Alveolar crest. D, Severe vertical defect.

- What type of radiograph is shown?

Slide 20

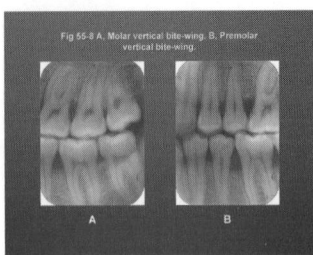

Fig 55-8 A, Molar vertical bite-wing. B, Premolar vertical bite-wing.

- The benefit of taking bite-wings vertically instead of horizontally is that the bone height along the root surface can be accurately depicted.

Bird/Robinson

Slide 21

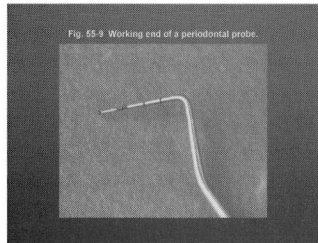

- Where is the periodontal probe placed?
- If bleeding occurs during periodontal probing, how is it noted in the patient's chart?

Slide 22

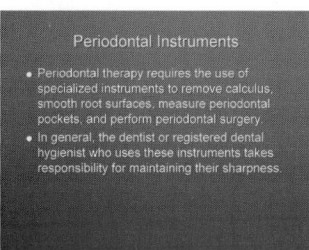

- What is calculus? *(Hard, mineralized plaque.)*

Slide 23

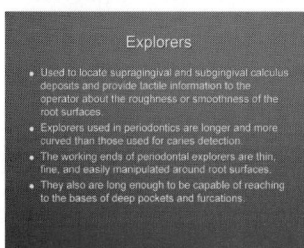

- What is supragingival? *(Above the gums.)*
- What is subgingival? *(Beneath the gums.)*

Slide 24

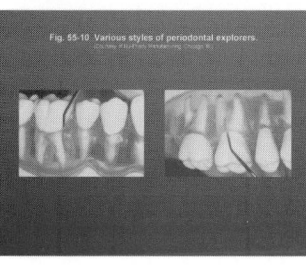

- The explorer on the left allows access to periodontal pockets that are deeper than 5 mm. The explorer on the right has a longer design, which is useful for exploring the furcation area.

Bird/Robinson

Slide 25

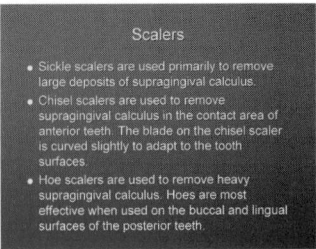

- Which of these scalers is more commonly used in periodontal procedures? *(Sickle.)*

- What is a contra-angle sickle scaler? *(A sickle scaler angled at the shank, which is designed to remove calculus from the posterior teeth.)*

- What is the design of the tip of a scaler? *(Pointed.)*

Slide 26

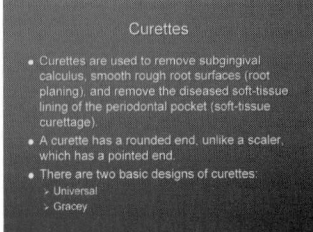

- Universal: designed to adapt to all tooth surfaces There are two cutting edges.

- Gracey: one cutting edge, used for a specific area The dental assistant may need several different ones for a procedure.

Slide 27

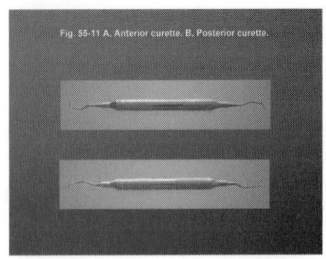

- What is the main difference between a curette and a scaler? *(Scalers remove supragingival calculus; curettes remove subgingival calculus.)*

Slide 28

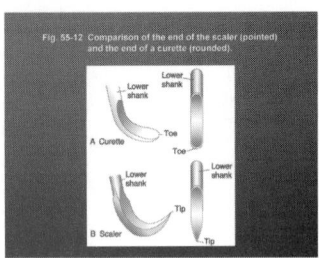

- Which instrument resembles a spoon excavator? *(Universal curette.)*

Torres and Ehrlich Modern Dental Assisting, 9th ed.

Bird/Robinson

Slide 29

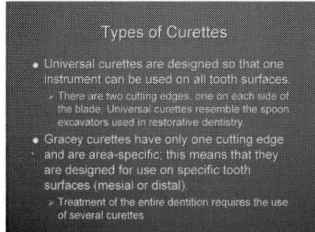

- What is the tip design of a curette? *(Rounded.)*

Slide 30

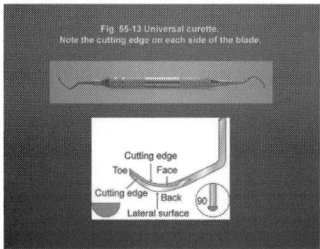

Slide 31

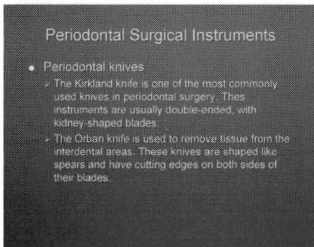

- What is the definition of interdental? *(Intended for use between the teeth.)*

Slide 32

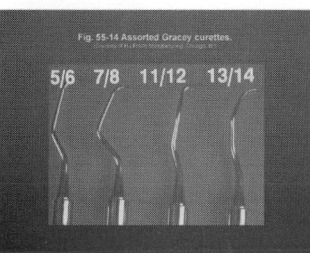

- These instruments are most commonly referred to by number.
- Several Gracey curettes are needed for a patient's whole set of teeth.

Bird/Robinson

Slide 33

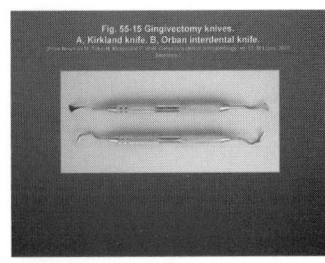

- Which surgical knife is kidney shaped? *(Kirkland.)*
- Which surgical knife is spear shaped? *(Orban.)*

Slide 34

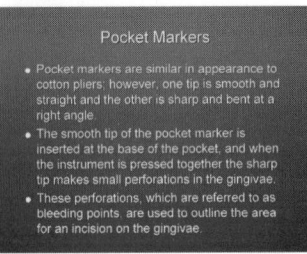

- Can pocket markers be used to measure the depth of the sulcus?

Slide 35

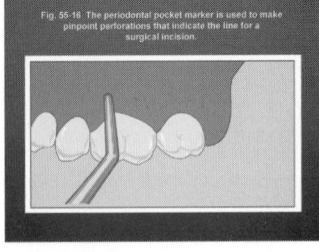

- The areas of perforation are referred to as "bleeding points."

Slide 36

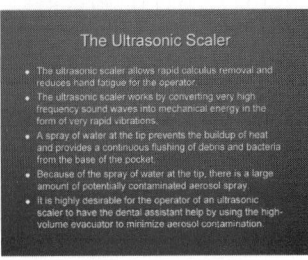

- A high-volume evacuator (HVE) use is critical. Why?

Bird/Robinson

Slide 37

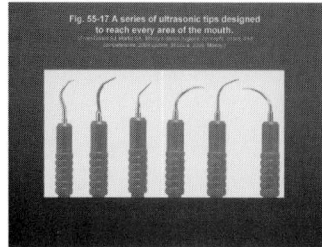

- These instruments can be sterilized.
- Ultrasonic scalers are being used more and more in periodontist's offices. Why? *(Reduced hand fatigue for the operator and better access to subgingival pockets.)*

Slide 38

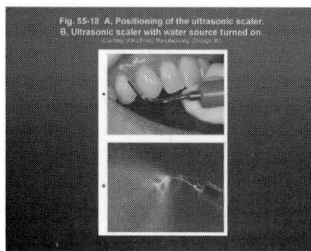

- What are the advantages of using ultrasonic scaling in contrast to hand scaling?

Slide 39

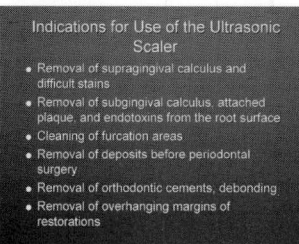

- What type of stain would be removed with the ultrasonic scaler? *(Extrinsic.)*

Slide 40

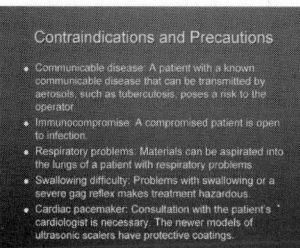

- Why would a severe gag reflex in a patient contraindicate the use of an ultrasonic scaler?
- What PPE should be worn during ultrasonic scaling?

Bird/Robinson

Slide 41

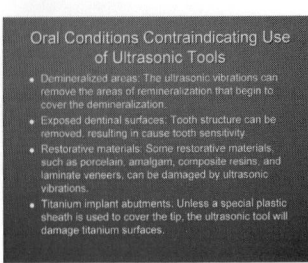

- Not commonly used on children, since it can cause damage to newer tissues and teeth.
- When might an anesthetic be used in ultrasonic scaling procedures?

Slide 42

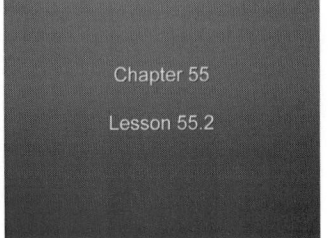

Slide 43

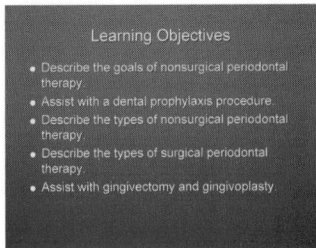

Slide 44

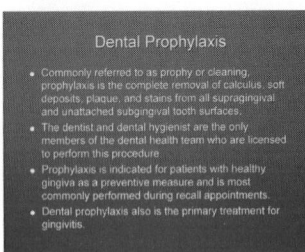

- What is gingivitis?
- How often is a dental prophylaxis completed?

Slide 45

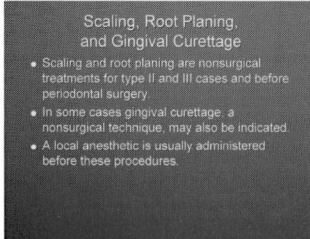

Scaling, Root Planing, and Gingival Curettage
- Scaling and root planing are nonsurgical treatments for type II and III cases and before periodontal surgery.
- In some cases gingival curettage, a nonsurgical technique, may also be indicated.
- A local anesthetic is usually administered before these procedures.

- Define necrotic.
- What is one of the health benefits of root planing for the patient?

Slide 46

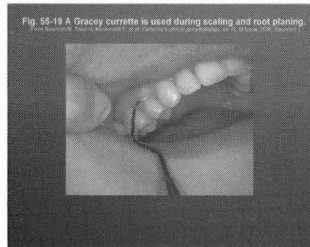

Fig. 55-19 A Gracey curette is used during scaling and root planing.

- These procedures are necessary for dental health, because they help return the tissues to a healthy state.

Slide 47

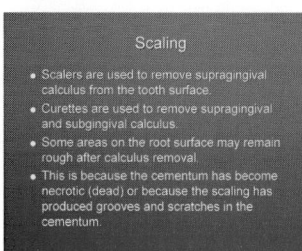

Scaling
- Scalers are used to remove supragingival calculus from the tooth surface.
- Curettes are used to remove supragingival and subgingival calculus.
- Some areas on the root surface may remain rough after calculus removal.
- This is because the cementum has become necrotic (dead) or because the scaling has produced grooves and scratches in the cementum.

- Which scaler is the most commonly used?
- What is cementum?

Slide 48

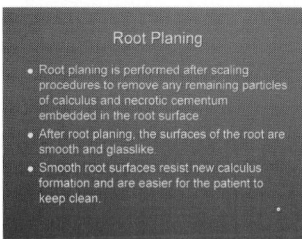

Root Planing
- Root planing is performed after scaling procedures to remove any remaining particles of calculus and necrotic cementum embedded in the root surface
- After root planing, the surfaces of the root are smooth and glasslike.
- Smooth root surfaces resist new calculus formation and are easier for the patient to keep clean.

- Why would anesthetic usually be required in this procedure?
- What instruments are used in the root planing procedure?

Slide 49

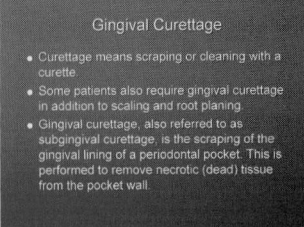

- What are the two main types of curettes?

Slide 50

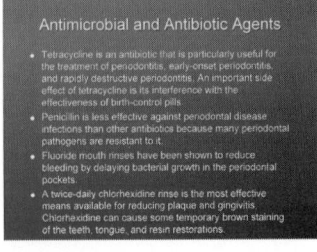

- If a woman patient is taking an oral contraceptive, inform her that some antibiotic therapies interfere with the contraceptive's effectiveness.

- Always ask patients whether they have any allergies to medications when taking the medical history.

Slide 51

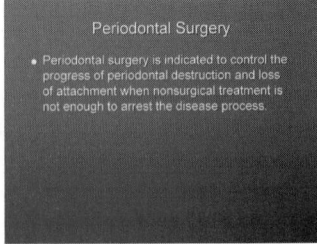

- Surgery is recommended when nonsurgical intervention has failed.

Slide 52

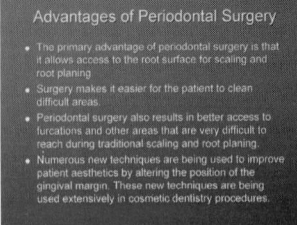

- Periodontal surgery requires the same standard of care as other types of oral surfaces require.

Torres and Ehrlich Modern Dental Assisting, 9th ed.

Bird/Robinson

Slide 53

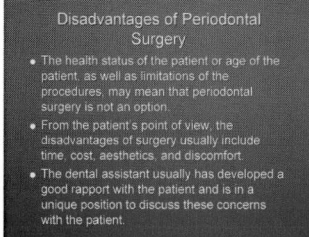

- What health conditions would contraindicate periodontal surgery?

Slide 54

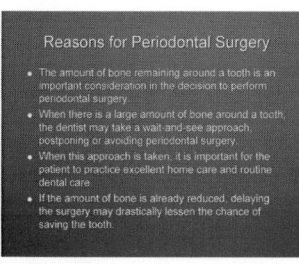

- The following items help the dentist detect the amount of remaining bone around the teeth:
  - Periodontal probes
  - Radiographs
  - Periodontal charting

Slide 55

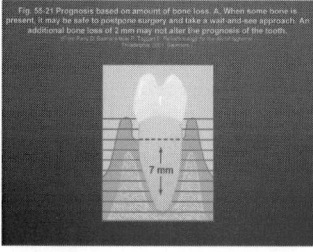

- When is surgery usually necessary?

Slide 56

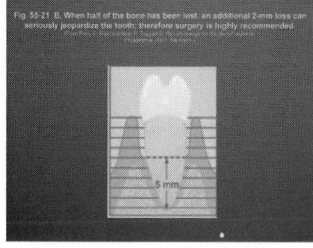

Torres and Ehrlich Modern Dental Assisting, 9th ed.

Bird/Robinson

Slide 57

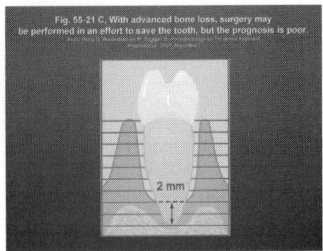

- What are basic measures a patient can take to prevent this type of bone loss?
  - *Regular dental checkups and professional cleanings.*
  - *Brushing teeth well twice a day.*
  - *Daily cleaning between the teeth (flossing).*
  - *Eating a well-balanced diet.*

Slide 58

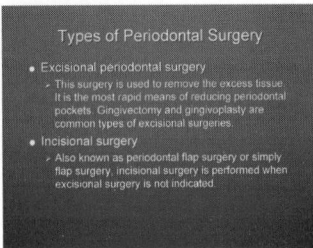

- Excisional: gingivectomy, gingivoplasty.
- What does *ectomy* mean?

Slide 59

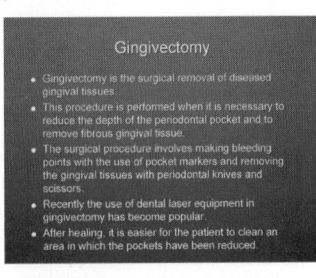

- Excisional surgery is the surgical method in reduction of periodontal pockets.
- What instruments would be used to remove the gingiva?

Slide 60

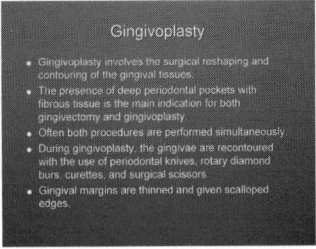

Slide 61

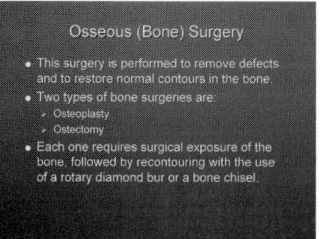

Slide 62

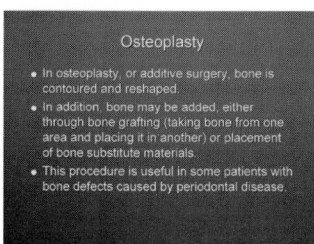

- Sutures are placed following surgery.
- What is the dental assistant's role regarding sutures?

Slide 63

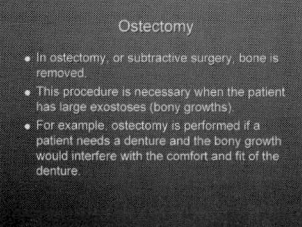

- What is a term for a bony growth?
- *Extoses* is another term for bony growths.

Slide 64

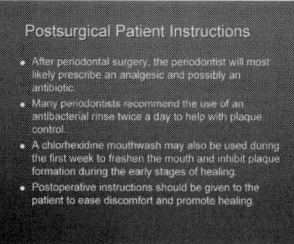

- A dental assistant provides postoperative instructions to the patient for the patient's well-being and to comply with all legal and ethical requirements.

Bird/Robinson

Slide 65

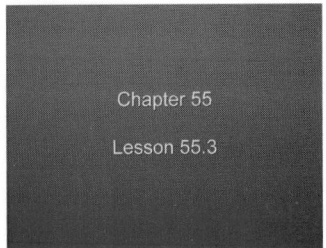

Chapter 55

Lesson 55.3

Slide 66

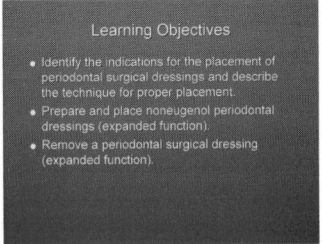

Learning Objectives

- Identify the indications for the placement of periodontal surgical dressings and describe the technique for proper placement.
- Prepare and place noneugenol periodontal dressings (expanded function).
- Remove a periodontal surgical dressing (expanded function).

Slide 67

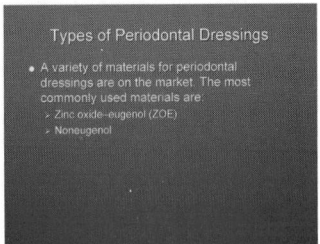

Periodontal Surgical Dressings

- A periodontal surgical dressing is much like a bandage over the surgical site. Periodontal dressings, also known as periopacks, are used to:
  - Hold the flaps in place
  - Protect the newly forming tissues
  - Minimize postoperative pain, infection, and hemorrhage
  - Protect the surgical site from trauma during eating and drinking
  - Support mobile teeth during the healing process

- Home-care instructions given to a patient with a surgical dressing include:
  - Brush the top of the dressing lightly with a soft toothbrush.
  - Rinse gently with a prescribed medicated mouthwash or with warm salt water.
  - Do not smoke or drink alcohol.

Slide 68

Types of Periodontal Dressings

- A variety of materials for periodontal dressings are on the market. The most commonly used materials are:
  - Zinc oxide–eugenol (ZOE)
  - Noneugenol

- Which type of dressing is more commonly used?

Torres and Ehrlich Modern Dental Assisting, 9th ed.

Bird/Robinson

Slide 69

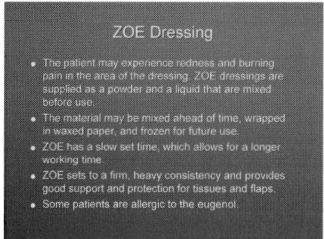

- A ZOE dressing is generally mixed at time of appointment.

Slide 70

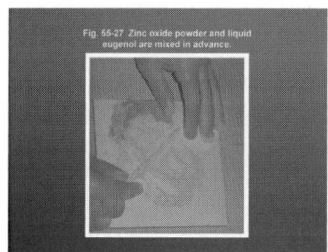

Slide 71

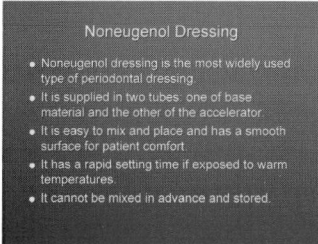

- It usually takes 2 to 3 minutes to mix the pastes.

Slide 72

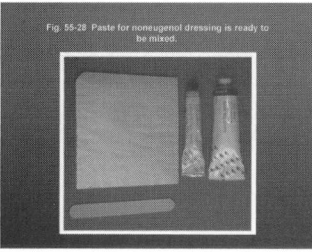

- The following equipment and supplies are used:
  - Paper mixing pad
  - Wooden tongue depressor
  - Noneugenol dressing (base and accelerator)
  - Paper cup filled with room-temperature water
  - Saline solution
  - Plastic-type filing instrument
- Where is the embrasure area?

Slide 73

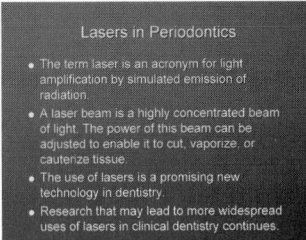

- Laser technology used widely in other areas of medicine.

- Lasers are being marketed for a number of dental procedures that involve both hard and soft tissues.

Slide 74

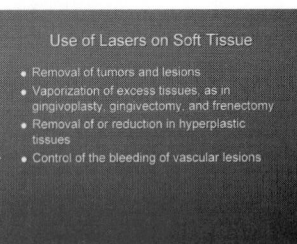

- Frenectomy is an excision of the frenulum, or a connecting fold of membrane serving to support or restrain a part (as the tongue).

Slide 75

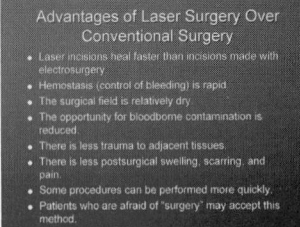

Slide 76

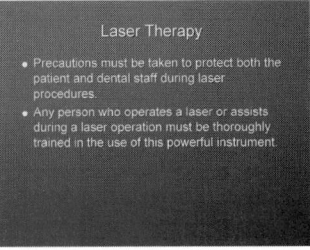

Slide 77

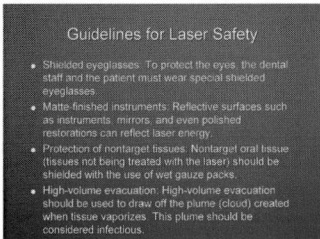

Slide 78

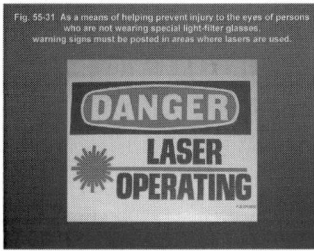

Fig. 55-31 As a means of helping prevent injury to the eyes of persons who are not wearing special light-filter glasses, warning signs must be posted in areas where lasers are used.

- Who may operate a laser?
- In some states both the dentist and dental hygienist may operate lasers after completing a special certification course.

Torres and Ehrlich Modern Dental Assisting, 9th ed.

Bird/Robinson

56 Oral and Maxillofacial Surgery

TEACHING FOCUS

This chapter will introduce the student to topics related to oral and maxillofacial surgery. The student will become acquainted with the surgical setting, specialized instruments and accessories, surgical asepsis, surgical preparation, surgical procedures, sutures, postoperative care, and postsurgical complications. The procedural steps involved in assisting with numerous activities, including preparing a sterile field, performing a surgical scrub, performing sterile gloving, forceps extraction, removing an impacted tooth, suture placement, suture removal, and alveolitis treatment, will also be discussed. The student will also have the opportunity to put this information into context by participating in classroom activities and discussions.

MATERIALS AND RESOURCES

- ☐ antimicrobial soap (Lesson 56.1)
- ☐ basic setup (Lessons 56.2 and 56.3)
- ☐ bone file (Lesson 56.2)
- ☐ computer and PowerPoint projector (all Lessons)
- ☐ conventional high-speed handpiece with surgical bur or mallet and chisel (Lesson 56.2)
- ☐ copies of state dental practice act (Lesson 56.1)
- ☐ cotton tip applicator (Lesson 56.3)
- ☐ curettes (Lesson 56.2)
- ☐ elevator (Lesson 56.2)
- ☐ forceps (Lesson 56.2)
- ☐ forceps extraction setup (Lesson 56.2)
- ☐ hemostats (Lesson 56.3)
- ☐ high-volume evacuator (HVE) tip (Lesson 56.3)
- ☐ index cards (Lesson 56.1)
- ☐ iodoform gauze (Lesson 56.3)
- ☐ irrigating syringe (Lessons 56.2 and 56.3)
- ☐ local anesthetic setup (Lesson 56.2)
- ☐ medicated dressing (Lesson 56.3)

- ☐ needle holder or hemostat (Lessons 56.2 and 56.3)
- ☐ orange stick (Lesson 56.1)
- ☐ periosteal elevator (Lesson 56.2)
- ☐ rongeur (Lesson 56.2)
- ☐ root tip picks (Lesson 56.2)
- ☐ scalpel (Lesson 56.2)
- ☐ scalpel, #15 blade and handle (Lesson 56.2)
- ☐ scissors (Lesson 56.3)
- ☐ sterile cotton gauze (Lesson 56.3)
- ☐ sterile disposable towels (Lesson 56.1)
- ☐ sterile gauze sponges (Lessons 56.2 and 56.3)
- ☐ sterile saline solution (Lesson 56.2)
- ☐ sterile surgical gloves (Lesson 56.1)
- ☐ sterile surgical scrub brush (Lesson 56.1)
- ☐ surgical aspirator tip (Lesson 56.2)
- ☐ surgical curette (Lesson 56.2)
- ☐ surgical scissors (Lessons 56.2 and 56.3)
- ☐ suture material and needle (Lessons 56.2 and 56.3)
- ☐ suture scissors (Lessons 56.2 and 56.3)
- ☐ warm saline solution (Lesson 56.3)

LESSON CHECKLIST

Preparations for this lesson include:

- lecture
- evaluation of student knowledge and skills needed to perform all entry-level activities related to oral and maxillofacial surgery, including:
  - o identifying specialized instruments
  - o describing surgical procedures
  - o preparing a sterile field
  - o performing a surgical scrub and a sterile gloving
  - o assisting in a simple extraction, a multiple extraction with alveoplasty, the removal of an impacted tooth, and suture placement
  - o performing suture removal
  - o assisting in the treatment of alveolitis

KEY TERMS

alveolitis (p. 918)
alveoplasty (p. 908)
bone file (p. 901)
chisel (p. 902)
curette (p. 899)
donning (p. 905)
elevator (p. 899)
excisional biopsy (p. 909)
exfoliative biopsy (p. 909)
forceps (p. 899)
hard tissue impaction (p. 908)
hemostat (p. 901)
impacted tooth (p. 908)

incisional biopsy (p. 908)
luxate (p. 899)
mallet (p. 903)
needle holder (p. 902)
oral and maxillofacial surgeon (OMFS) (p. 898)
oral and maxillofacial surgery (p. 897)
outpatient (p. 898)
retractor (p. 902)
rongeur (p. 899)
root tip picks (p. 899)
scalpel (p. 901)
soft tissue impaction (p. 908)

ADDITIONAL RESOURCES

PowerPoint slides (Evolve): 1-46
The Interactive Dental Office CD-ROM: Lee Wong
Multimedia Procedures DVD: Suture Removal

Legend

CTQ
Critical
Thinking
Question

DVD
Multimedia
Procedures
Videos and
Animations

ESLR
EVOLVE
Student
Learning
Resources

IDO
Interactive
Dental
Office
CD-ROM

SW
Student
Workbook

TB
Test Bank
on the
TEACH
CD-ROM

PPT
PowerPoint
Slides

Class Activities are indicated in **bold italic.**

Bird/Robinson

LESSON 56.1

PRETEST

1. How many additional years of postgraduate training does an oral and maxillofacial surgeon receive?
   a. 1
   b. 2
   c. 3
   d. 4 to 6

2. What instrument is used to remove fragments that have broken off during the extraction procedure?
   a. rongeur
   b. root tip pick
   c. scalpel
   d. bone file

3. Which instrument is used in a push-and-pull motion to smooth the surface of the bone?
   a. hemostat
   b. elevator
   c. forceps
   d. bone file

4. Which instrument is used with a mallet for splitting teeth?
   a. bi-beveled chisel
   b. single-beveled chisel
   c. root tip pick
   d. surgical curette

5. What is the recommended length of time for a surgical scrub?
   a. 1 minute
   b. 2 minutes
   c. 5 minutes
   d. 7 minutes

6. What type of procedure is performed on a tooth that is fully erupted?
   a. forceps extraction
   b. complex extraction
   c. full bony extraction
   d. partial bony extraction

7. Which type of biopsy involves the removal of the entire lesion?
   a. incisional biopsy
   b. excisional biopsy
   c. exfoliative biopsy
   d. smear biopsy

8. Which type of suture material is nonabsorbable?
   a. nylon
   b. chromic catgut
   c. vicryl
   d. plain catgut

9. What medication may the dentist prescribe to prevent and control swelling?
   a. aspirin
   b. pain medication
   c. ibuprofen
   d. antianxiety medication

10. What is another term for alveolitis?
    a. dry socket
    b. wet socket
    c. inflammation
    d. infiltration

Answers

1. d	3. d	5. d	7. b	9. c
2. b	4. a	6. a	8. a	10. a

BACKGROUND ASSESSMENT

Question: What procedures are performed by an oral and maxillofacial surgeon?

Answer: The most common procedure performed by an oral and maxillofacial surgeon is extraction of impacted teeth. The oral and maxillofacial surgeon performs tooth extractions for other reasons, including removal of teeth for orthodontic treatment, removal of nonvital teeth, recontouring of alveolar bone, and removing root fragments that may have been left behind. Most general dentists do not want to perform these procedures because of the complexity involved. The oral and maxillofacial surgeon works with fractures of the maxilla and mandible because of traumatic injury and also the alteration of the maxilla and mandible because of congenital defects. The surgeon can also perform biopsies and, in some cases, remove cysts or tumors that have been defined by the biopsies.

Question: What types of biopsies are performed by an oral and maxillofacial surgeon?

Answer: Three distinct types of biopsies can be performed, depending on the size of the lesion. An incisional biopsy is diagnosed when the lesion is larger than 1 cm in all dimensions. This type of biopsy is accomplished by cutting a wedge of the lesion and part of the normal tissue that surrounds it. An excisional biopsy requires complete removal of the lesion and a portion of the normal tissue that surrounds the lesion. The exfoliative biopsy is a noninvasive procedure that entails swabbing the lesion with a sterile, flat-ended brush to gather the surface cells of the lesion.

CRITICAL THINKING QUESTION

A new dental assistant has joined the oral surgery practice and is ready to start assisting in her first surgical procedure. The new dental assistant washes her hands, and an experienced dental assistant notices that she lathers for only about 45 seconds and does not use the appropriate soap. What information should the experienced dental assistant give to the new assistant regarding her hand-washing technique?

Guidelines: The experienced dental assistant should approach the new assistant immediately, because the procedure for hand washing in a surgical setting is different from that in a general dental setting. First, the experienced assistant should explain that it is important to follow the steps of a surgical scrub to lessen the chance of infection. A surgical scrub requires the use of an orange stick, antimicrobial soap, scrub brush, and disposable towels. The new assistant should first don the appropriate protective wear and remove all jewelry. The orange stick should be used first to clean under the fingernails. The new assistant should then wet her hands and forearms and lather the antimicrobial soap for 7 minutes. During this time, the surgical brush should be used to scrub the hands and forearms. The arms should be rinsed with warm water and the hands held above the waist level so the water runs off the elbow area. This surgical scrub should be repeated, and, after rinsing, the hands and forearms should be dried using a sterile towel.

OBJECTIVES	CONTENT	TEACHING RESOURCES
Pronounce, define, and spell the Key Terms.	■ Key terms (pp. 896-897)	SW Fill in the Blank questions 1-20 (pp. 489-490) ESLR Electronic Flashcards ▸ Discuss each of the key terms in Chapter 56, focusing on the definition, pronunciation, and spelling of each term. ***Class Activity** Have students make flash cards of the key terms by writing each term on one side of an index card and the definition on the reverse. Then have the students quiz each other with the flash cards. Correct their pronunciation as needed.*

Bird/Robinson

OBJECTIVES	CONTENT	TEACHING RESOURCES
Describe the specialty of oral and maxillofacial surgery.	■ Indications for oral and maxillofacial surgery (p. 897) ■ The oral surgeon (p. 897)	PPT 5-7 TB question 1 SW Short-Answer Questions 1; Fill in the Blank questions 16-17; Multiple Choice questions 1-2 (pp. 489-490) Recall question 1 (p. 898) ▶ Discuss the indications for oral and maxillofacial surgery. ▶ Discuss the specialized training of the oral surgeon. ***Class Activity** Ask students to call out procedures that are performed by an oral and maxillofacial surgeon. Write their responses on the blackboard.*
Discuss the role of an oral surgery assistant.	■ The surgical assistant (p. 898) ■ The surgical setting (p. 898) ☐ Private practice (p. 898) ☐ Operating room (p. 898)	PPT 8-9 TB question 2 SW Short-Answer Questions 2; Fill in the Blank question 18; Multiple Choice questions 3-4 (pp. 489-490) Figure 56-1 The operating room (p. 898) Recall questions 2-4 (p. 898) CTQ 4-5 (p. 918) ▶ Discuss the surgical assistant's role in oral surgery. Note responsibilities related to treatment room and patient preparation, as well as during and after the surgery. ▶ Discuss the role of the surgical assistant with regard to patient education. Note the communication skills and behaviors necessary for responding to patient questions and concerns. ***Class Activity** Distribute copies of the state dental practice act to the class. Ask the students to find the stipulations of the role of a dental assistant in an oral and maxillofacial surgery office.*
Identify specialized instruments used for basic surgical procedures.	■ Specialized instruments and accessories (p. 898) ☐ Elevators (p. 899) ☐ Forceps (p. 899) ☐ Surgical curette (p. 899) ☐ Rongeur (p. 899) ☐ Bone file (p. 901) ☐ Scalpel (p. 901)	PPT 10-25 TB questions 3-4 SW Fill in the Blank questions 1-2, 4-5, 7, 10, 14-15, 19-20; Multiple Choice questions 5-9 (pp. 489-491) Figure 56-2 Periosteal elevators (p. 899) Figure 56-3 Straight elevator (p. 899) Figure 56-4 Root tip picks (p. 899) Figure 56-5 A-E Types of extraction forceps (p. 900) Figure 56-6 Surgical curettes (p. 901)

ELSEVIER

Torres and Ehrlich Modern Dental Assisting, 9th ed.

OBJECTIVES	CONTENT	TEACHING RESOURCES
	☐ Hemostat (p. 901) ☐ Needle holder (p. 902) ☐ Surgical and suture scissors (p. 902) ☐ Retractors (p. 902) ☐ Mouth props (p. 902) ☐ Chisel and mallet (p. 902) ☐ Surgical burs (p. 903)	Figure 56-7 Rongeurs (p. 901) Figure 56-8 Bone files (p. 901) Figure 56-9 Scalpel handles and blades (p. 902) Figure 56-10 Hemostats (p. 902) Figure 56-11 Needle holders (p. 903) Figure 56-12 Surgical scissors (p. 903) Figure 56-13 Tissue retractors (p. 904) Figure 56-14 Cheek and tongue retractor (p. 904) Figure 56-15 Mouth props (p. 904) Figure 56-16 Chisel and mallet (p. 904) Figure 56-17 Surgical handpiece (p. 905) Recall questions 5-10 (p. 903) ▸ Discuss the purposes, identifying features, and uses of instruments and accessories used in oral and maxillofacial surgery. ▸ Discuss the different purposes and uses of periosteal elevators and straight elevators. *Class Activity Divide the class into groups. Assign each group one of the instruments used in oral and maxillofacial surgery. Have each group discuss its assigned instrument and write a short description of its use. Then have the groups share their descriptions with the class.*
Discuss the importance of the chain of asepsis during a surgical procedure.	■ Surgical asepsis (p. 904)	⊠ PPT 26-27 TB question 5 SW Short-Answer Questions 3 (p. 499) SW/IDO Patient Case Exercise question 3 (p. 492) (The Interactive Dental Office CD-ROM) ▸ Discuss the role of surgical asepsis and how it expands beyond the standard infection-control practices in a dental office. ▸ Discuss the chain of asepsis and how it is established and maintained. *Class Activity Have each student write a short paper discussing the differences in infection-control procedures between an oral surgery office and a general dental office. Ask for student volunteers to read their papers to the class.*

Bird/Robinson

OBJECTIVES	CONTENT	TEACHING RESOURCES
Prepare a sterile field.	☐ Sterile field (p. 905) [*Procedure*] 56-1 Preparing a sterile field for instruments and supplies (p. 905) (SW/ESLR Competency 56-1, p. 493)	PPT 27 SW/ESLR Competency 56-1 Preparing a Sterile Field for Instruments and Supplies (p. 493) CTQ 1 (p. 918) ▸ Discuss the procedural steps involved in preparing a sterile field. ▸ Discuss the timing involved in establishing a sterile field. ***Class Activity** Demonstrate how to prepare a mock sterile field in the dental operatory according to infection-control protocol. Then ask for student volunteers to perform the same demonstration.*
Perform a surgical scrub.	☐ Surgical scrub (p. 905) [*Procedure*] 56-2 Performing a surgical scrub (pp. 906-907) (SW/ESLR Competency 56-2, p. 495)	SW Multiple Choice question 10 (p. 491) SW/ESLR Competency 56-2 Performing a Surgical Scrub (p. 495) Recall question 11 (p. 905) ▸ Discuss the procedural steps involved in performing a surgical scrub. ▸ Discuss the need for a surgical scrub. Note that a scrub must be performed even though gloves are used. ***Class Activity** Demonstrate how to perform a surgical scrub. Then ask for student volunteers to perform the same demonstration.*
Perform sterile gloving.	☐ Proper gloving (p. 905) [*Procedure*] 56-3 Performing sterile gloving (pp. 907-908) (SW/ESLR Competency 56-3, p. 497) ■ Surgical preparation (p. 908)	PPT 28-32 TB question 6 SW Fill in the Blank question 11; Multiple Choice question 11 (pp. 490-491) SW/ESLR Competency 56-3 Performing Sterile Gloving (p. 497) Recall question 12 (p. 905) Surgical Assistant's Role in Oral Surgery (p. 909) ▸ Discuss the procedural steps involved in performing sterile gloving. ▸ Discuss the surgical assistant's role in advance preparation, treatment preparation, and patient preparation. ***Class Activity** Divide the class into pairs. Have one student from each pair read the procedural steps for sterile gloving to the other student, while the other student performs the procedure.*

56.1 Homework/Assignments:

56.1 Instructor's Notes/Student Feedback:

LESSON 56.2

CRITICAL THINKING QUESTION

A patient is in the office for extraction of tooth #32. The tooth is partially erupted, and the surgical assistant has prepared all of the equipment necessary for the surgeon to complete the procedure. During the extraction process, the assistant hears a quick "snap" and the surgeon removes tooth #32. Upon removal, the surgeon notes that one of the root tips is missing. What happened to the root tip? What additional instrument(s) will the surgeon need?

Guidelines: The roots of tooth #32 were probably curved, and as the surgeon removed the tooth, the tip of the root was retained in the alveolar bone. This can be a common occurrence, depending on how the tooth is positioned in the alveolar bone or how curved the roots are. The surgeon will need a root tip pick or a small surgical curette to remove the retained root tip.

OBJECTIVES	CONTENT	TEACHING RESOURCES
Describe surgical procedures typically performed in a general practice.	■ Surgical procedures (p. 908) ☐ Forceps extraction (p. 908) ☐ Multiple extractions and alveoplasty (p. 908) ☐ Removal of impacted teeth (p. 908) ☐ Biopsy (p. 908) – Incisional biopsy (p. 908) – Excisional biopsy (p. 909) – Exfoliative biopsy (p. 909) – Biopsy results (p. 909)	⊠ PPT 35-38 TB questions 7-9 SW Short-Answer Questions 5; Fill in the Blank questions 3, 6, 8-9, 12-13; Multiple Choice questions 12-14 (pp. 489-491) SW Case Study questions 1-4 (p. 492) SW/IDO Patient Case Exercise questions 1-2 (p. 492) (The Interactive Dental Office CD-ROM) Surgical Assistant's Role in Oral Surgery (p. 909) Figure 56-18 Brush used to gather surface cells (p. 911) Recall questions 13-15 (p. 911) ▶ Discuss simple and multiple extractions, and note when each type of extraction is indicated. ▶ Discuss the differences between an incisional biopsy, an excisional biopsy, and an exfoliative biopsy. Note when each type of biopsy is indicated. ***Class Activity** Conduct a group discussion on how to appropriately identify the following types of surgical procedures:* *– Forceps extraction* *– Multiple extractions and alveoloplasty* *– Impacted teeth extractions*
Assist in a simple extraction.	☐ Forceps extraction (p. 908) Procedure 56-4 Assisting in forceps extraction (pp. 910-911) (SW/ESLR Competencies 56-4 to 56-6, pp. 499-500)	SW Short-Answer Questions 4 (p. 489) SW/ESLR Competencies 56-4 to 56-6 Assisting in a Surgical Extraction (pp. 499-500) CTQ 3 (p. 918) ▶ Discuss the procedural steps involved in a forceps extraction.

ELSEVIER

Torres and Ehrlich Modern Dental Assisting, 9th ed.

OBJECTIVES	CONTENT	TEACHING RESOURCES
	☐ Multiple extractions and alveoplasty (p. 908) ☐ Removal of impacted teeth (p. 908) ☐ Biopsy (p. 908) – Incisional biopsy (p. 908) – Excisional biopsy (p. 909) – Exfoliative biopsy (p. 909) – Biopsy results (p. 909)	▸ Discuss the instruments needed for this procedure. *Class Activity* **Have students set up a mock simple extraction procedure in the dental operatory according to infection control protocol.**
Assist in a multiple extraction procedure with alveoplasty.	☐ Multiple extractions and alveoplasty (p. 924) ☐ Removal of impacted teeth (p. 908) Procedure 56-5 Assisting in multiple extraction and alveoplasty (p. 912) (SW/ESLR Competencies 56-4 to 56-6, pp. 499-500) ☐ Biopsy (p. 908) – Incisional biopsy (p. 908) – Excisional biopsy (p. 909) – Exfoliative biopsy (p. 909) – Biopsy results (p. 909)	SW Case Study question 1 (p. 492) SW/ESLR Competencies 56-4 to 56-6 Assisting in a Surgical Extraction (pp. 499-500) CTQ 2 (p. 918) ▸ Discuss the procedural steps involved in a multiple extraction with alveoplasty. ▸ Discuss the instruments needed for this procedure. *Class Activity* **Have students set up a mock multiple extraction with alveoloplasty procedure in the dental operatory according to infection-control protocol.**
Assist in removal of an impacted tooth.	☐ Removal of impacted teeth (p. 908) Procedure 56-6 Assisting in removal of an impacted tooth (p. 913) (SW/ESLR Competencies 56-4 to 56-6, pp. 499-500) ☐ Biopsy (p. 908)	SW/ESLR Competencies 56-4 to 56-6 Assisting in a Surgical Extraction (pp. 499-500) ▸ Discuss the procedural steps involved in removal of an impacted tooth. ▸ Discuss the instruments needed for this procedure. *Class Activity* **Have students set up a mock impacted tooth extraction procedure in the dental operatory according to infection-control protocol.**

Torres and Ehrlich Modern Dental Assisting, 9ᵗʰ ed.

OBJECTIVES	CONTENT	TEACHING RESOURCES
	– Incisional biopsy (p. 908)	
	– Excisional biopsy (p. 909)	
	– Exfoliative biopsy (p. 909)	
	– Biopsy results (p. 909)	

56.2 Homework/Assignments:

56.2 Instructor's Notes/Student Feedback:

Torres and Ehrlich Modern Dental Assisting, 9th ed.

Bird/Robinson

LESSON 56.3

CRITICAL THINKING QUESTION

A man comes to the office two days after removal of his four third molars. He complains of severe pain in the lower left side of his mouth and says that taking Ibuprofen doesn't ease the discomfort. He feels that he followed the post-operative instructions that were given to him at the extraction appointment. What is this patient experiencing? What is the cause?

Guidelines: The dentist determined that the patient is most likely experiencing discomfort associated with alveolitis. Alveolitis, more commonly known as dry socket, generally occurs when the blood clot has become dislodged from the socket or a blood clot was never formed in the first place. Unfortunately, because it cannot be predicted, the risk of alveolitis cannot be completely avoided. A dry socket can also result from trauma to the extraction site or an infection that has developed inside the socket. Alveolitis can be treated with special medicated gauze strips or squares placed inside the extraction site. This medication contains a topical anesthetic to soothe the nerve endings in the exposed bone. Packing the material into the socket helps prevent any food or debris from becoming lodged in the extraction site.

OBJECTIVES	CONTENT	TEACHING RESOURCES
Assist in suture placement.	■ Sutures (p. 914) □ Suture placement (p. 914) ⎡Procedure⎤ 56-7 Assisting in suture placement (p. 915) (SW/ESLR Competency 56-7, p. 501)	PPT 41-42 SW Multiple Choice questions 15-16 (p. 491) SW/IDO Patient Case Exercise question 4 (p. 492) (The Interactive Dental Office CD-ROM) SW Competency 56-7 Assisting in Suture Placement (p. 501) Figure 56-19 Types of suture material labeled according to size, type, length, and type of needle (p. 914) Recall questions 16-17 (p. 914) ▶ Discuss the types of suture materials that are available. Describe the difference between absorbable and nonabsorbable materials and when each might be used. ▶ Discuss the procedural steps and instruments involved in suture placement. ***Class Activity Demonstrate the correct transfer method of a suture needle, needle holder, and suture scissors. Then ask for student volunteers to perform the same demonstration.***
Perform suture removal.	□ Suture removal (p. 914) ⎡Procedure⎤ 56-8 Performing suture removal (expanded function) (p. 916) (SW/ESLR Competency 56-8, p. 503)	PPT 43 Multimedia Procedures DVD: Suture Removal TB question 10 SW Multiple Choice question 17 (p. 491) SW/ESLR Competency 56-8 Performing Suture Removal (Expanded Function) (p. 503) Recall question 18 (p. 914)

Torres and Ehrlich Modern Dental Assisting, 9th ed.

Bird/Robinson

OBJECTIVES	CONTENT	TEACHING RESOURCES
		▸ Discuss the procedural steps and instruments involved in suture removal.
		▸ Discuss whether suture removal is an expanded function in your state.
		Class Activity Divide the class into groups, and have each group make a list of the instruments needed for suture removal. Then have the groups discuss how each instrument is used in the procedure.
Describe postoperative care given to a patient after a surgical procedure.	■ Postoperative care (p. 914) □ Control of bleeding (p. 914) □ Control of swelling (p. 914)	⊠ PPT 44-45 TB question 11 SW Short-Answer Questions 6; Multiple Choice questions 18-20 (pp. 489, 491) Surgical Assistant's Role in Oral Surgery (p. 909) Recall questions 19-21 (p. 918) ▸ Discuss the surgical assistant's role after surgery. Note that postoperative care instructions cover immediate care following the procedure as well as the home care required. ▸ Discuss instructions given to the patient with regard to control of bleeding and swelling. *Class Activity Divide the class into pairs. Have each pair of students take turns role-playing a surgical assistant giving postoperative care instructions to a patient who has had a surgical procedure.*
Discuss possible complications from surgery.	■ Postsurgical complications (p. 918) □ Alveolitis (p. 918)	⊠ PPT 46 TB question 12 SW Short-Answer Questions 7; Case Study questions 2-4 (pp. 489, 492) SW/IDO Patient Case Exercise question 5 (p. 492) (The Interactive Dental Office CD-ROM) ▸ Discuss the possible causes of alveolitis. *Class Activity Conduct a group discussion on the following possible complications from surgery and how the patient can help prevent such complications:* *– Bleeding* *– Swelling* *– Alveolitis*

ELSEVIER

OBJECTIVES	CONTENT	TEACHING RESOURCES
Assist in the treatment of alveolitis (dry socket).	☐ Alveolitis (p. 918) Procedure 56-9 Assisting in the treatment of alveolitis (p. 917) (SW/ESLR Competency 56-9, p. 505)	SW/ESLR Competency 56-9 Assisting in the Treatment of Alveolitis (p. 505) Patient Education (p. 918) Legal and Ethical Implications (p. 918) Eye to the Future (p. 918) ▸ Discuss the procedural steps and instruments involved in the treatment of alveolitis. ▸ Discuss informed consent with regard to oral and maxillofacial surgery. Note the elements that are necessary for informed consent. *Class Activity Have students set up a mock treatment of alveolitis procedure in the dental operatory according to infection-control protocol.*
Performance Evaluation		TB SW questions (pp. 489-491) SW Case Study (p. 492) SW/IDO Patient Case Exercise (p. 492) (The Interactive Dental Office CD-ROM) SW/ESLR Competency 56-1 Preparing a Sterile Field for Instruments and Supplies (p. 493) SW/ESLR Competency 56-2 Performing a Surgical Scrub (p. 495) SW/ESLR Competency 56-3 Performing Sterile Gloving (p. 497) SW/ESLR Competencies 56-4 to 56-6 Assisting in a Surgical Extraction (pp. 499-500) SW/ESLR Competency 56-7 Assisting in Suture Placement (p. 501) SW/ESLR Competency 56-8 Performing Suture Removal (Expanded Function) (p. 503) SW/ESLR Competency 56-9 Assisting in the Treatment of Alveolitis (p. 505) ESLR Electronic Flashcards ESLR Practice Quiz Recall questions (pp. 898-918) CTQ (p. 918)

56.3 Homework/Assignments:

56.3 Instructor's Notes/Student Feedback:

ELSEVIER

Torres and Ehrlich Modern Dental Assisting, 9th ed.

Bird/Robinson

Slide 1

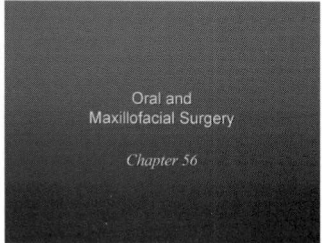

Oral and
Maxillofacial Surgery

Chapter 56

Slide 2

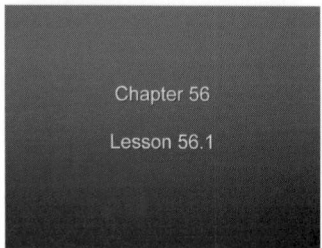

Chapter 56

Lesson 56.1

Slide 3

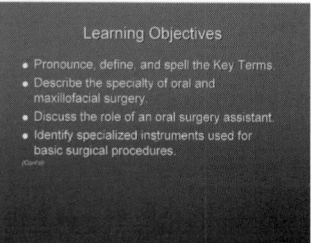

Learning Objectives

- Pronounce, define, and spell the Key Terms.
- Describe the specialty of oral and maxillofacial surgery.
- Discuss the role of an oral surgery assistant.
- Identify specialized instruments used for basic surgical procedures.

Slide 4

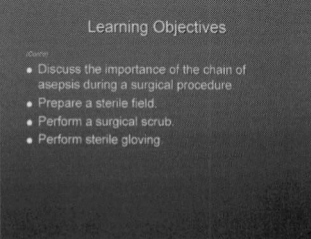

Learning Objectives

- Discuss the importance of the chain of asepsis during a surgical procedure.
- Prepare a sterile field.
- Perform a surgical scrub.
- Perform sterile gloving.

Slide 5

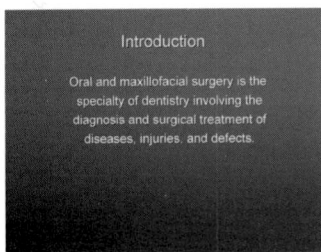

- An oral and maxillofacial surgeon is a dentist with four to six additional years of postgraduate training.

Slide 6

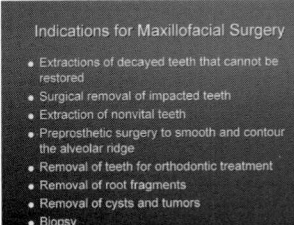

- Some general dentists are competent to perform these procedures in their offices.

Slide 7

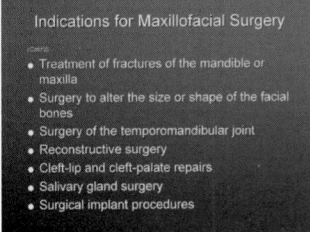

Slide 8

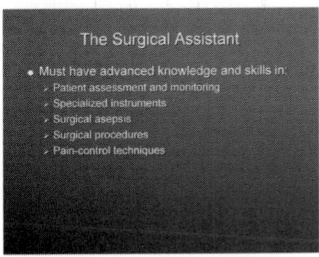

- What should be monitored on a patient during a surgical procedure?
- Assistants can attend an Oral and Maxillofacial Anesthesia Assisting Program (OMAAP). These programs include four to six months of study with a board-certified OMFS and a test.

Torres and Ehrlich Modern Dental Assisting, 9th ed.

Bird/Robinson

Slide 9

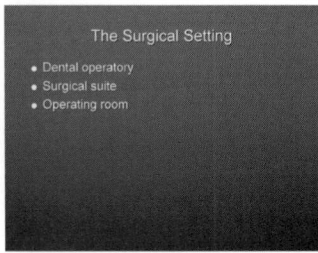

- A dental operatory is an in-office operatory.
- A surgical suite is generally located in the office and has specialized equipment used for certain procedures.

Slide 10

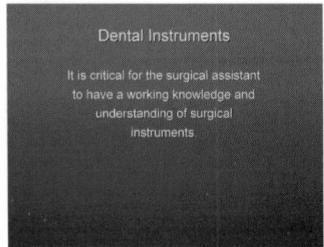

- Each instrument has a specific purpose.
- How are these instruments disinfected or sterilized?

Slide 11

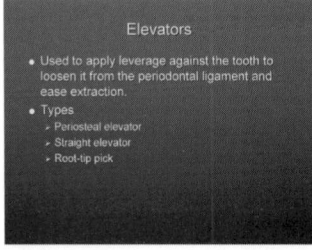

- Bulbous handle.
- Single-ended.

Slide 12

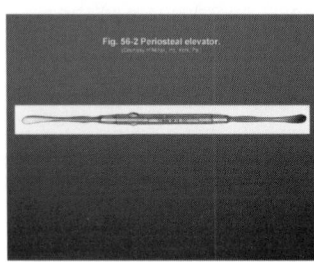

- Double-ended.
- What is this instrument used to reflect?
- First instrument used in a surgical procedure.

Bird/Robinson

Slide 13

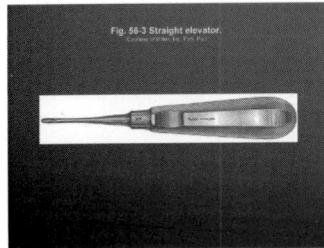

- Note the bulbous handle.
- Single-ended.
- What is this instrument used for?
- The working end resembles a spoon.

Slide 14

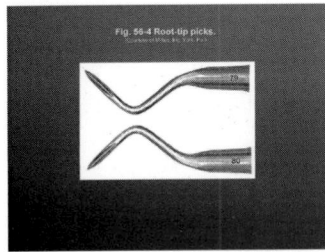

- Single-ended.
- Can have a bulbous or slim handle.
- Smaller working end.
- What is this instrument used for?

Slide 15

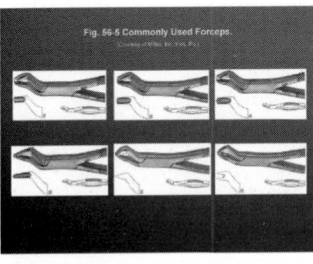

- The working ends are available in a variety of shapes and sizes.
- Some handles are curved to fit into the palm of the dentist's hand.
- What is this instrument used for?
- What does a universal forceps mean?
- Photographs are of maxillary forceps.

Slide 16

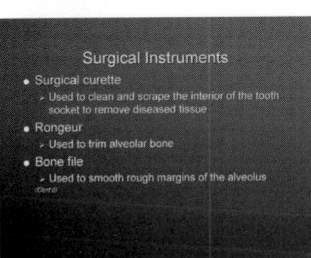

- Instruments commonly used after the tooth has been removed from the socket.
- Rongeur: hinged instrument, similar to a fingernail clipper. During a procedure sharp edges must be kept clean with gauze squares.

ELSEVIER

Torres and Ehrlich Modern Dental Assisting, 9th ed.
Bird/Robinson

Slide 17

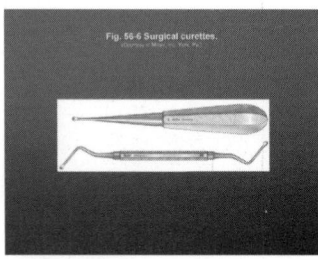

- Double-ended is most commonly used.
- Smaller working end.
- What instrument does it resemble?
- What is it used for?

Slide 18

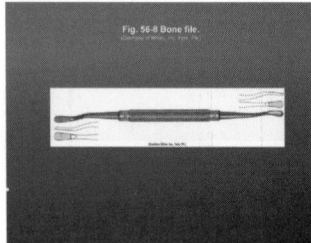

- Used in a push-and-pull motion.
- Grated.
- What is the use of this instrument?
- Watch terminology used in patient's presence.

Slide 19

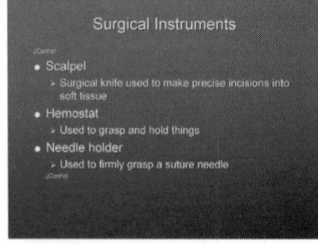

- Depending on treatment plan, these instruments may not be needed.
- Sutures are not placed on all extraction sites.
- What type of extraction would require an incision to be made?

Slide 20

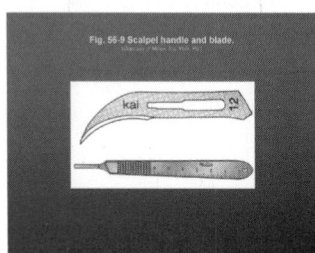

- Different-sized blades are available.
- Commonly referred to as a Bard Parker.
- The scalpel can be one piece (blade and handle together, one-time use, disposed of).
- How is the used blade disposed of?

Torres and Ehrlich Modern Dental Assisting, 9th ed.

Slide 21

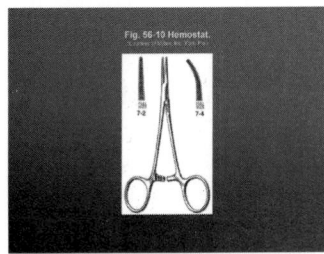

- Locking handle.
- Curved or straight beaks available.
- Serrated edges.
- What is the use of a hemostat in a surgical procedure?

Slide 22

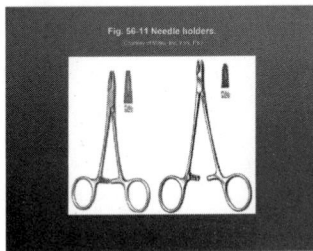

- What instrument does a needle holder resemble?
- How would a dental assistant transfer this instrument?

Slide 23

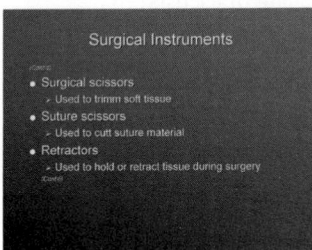

- These are accessory instruments.
- Retractors: tissue and tongue.
- Tissue retractor: fork-like prongs.
- Tongue retractor: larger, curved instrument.

Slide 24

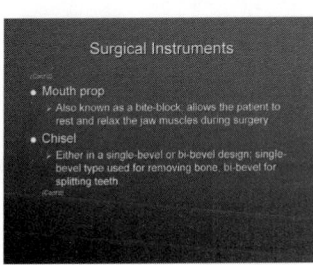

- Be guarded about terminology used in patient's presence. Patients may become anxious when they hear the word "chisel."
- Chisel is used with a mallet.
- When would a mouth prop be used?

Slide 25

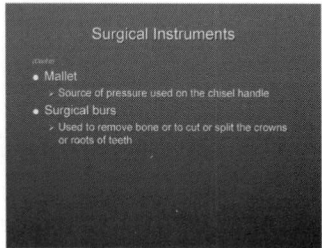

- Mallet is like a hammer and is used with a chisel.
- Can use high-speed handpiece or a surgical handpiece for surgical burs.
- Surgical burs are disposed of in the sharps container after each use.
- What item must be used when a surgical bur is used?

Slide 26

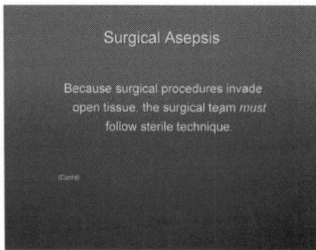

- What does the term *asepsis* mean?

Slide 27

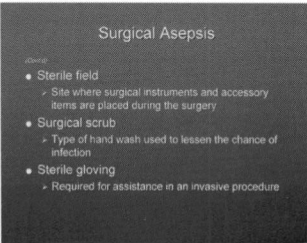

- Who are we protecting by maintaining the chain of asepsis?
- How is a sterile field prepared?
- How is a surgical scrub different from a non-surgical scrub?

Slide 28

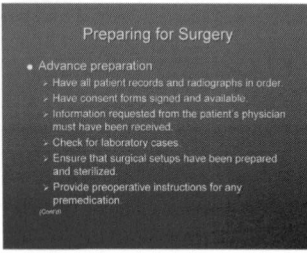

- What type of radiographs are used in a surgical procedure?
- Why should consent forms be completed before starting the surgical procedure?

Bird/Robinson

Slide 29

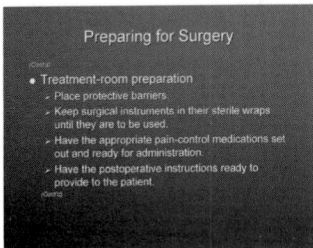

- Where are protective barriers placed?
- When should we give a patient postoperative instructions?

Slide 30

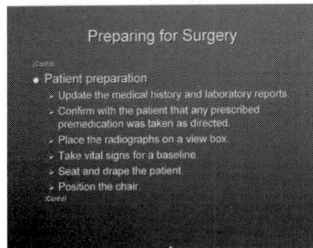

- What type of premedication could the patient take before a surgical procedure?
- What vital signs must be obtained before starting the procedure?
- What is the correct positioning of the patient?

Slide 31

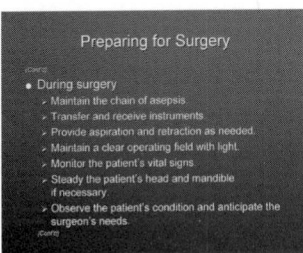

- Surgical HVE tip should be used (smaller head to fit into the socket).
- How would the assistant support the patient's head during a surgical procedure?

Slide 32

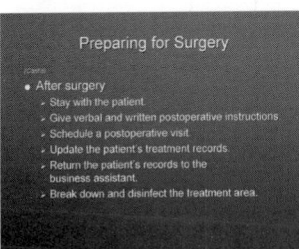

- Why is it important to stay with the patient?
- Why would we give postoperative instructions *before* the surgical procedure?

Slide 33

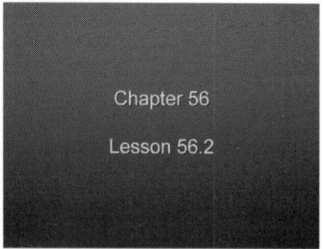

Slide 34

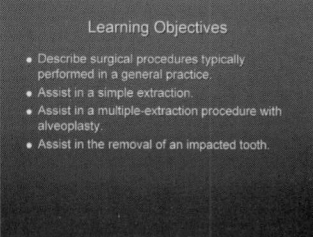

Slide 35

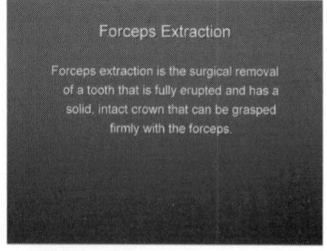

- Does not require that sutures be placed.
- Commonly referred to as a simple or routine extraction.

Slide 36

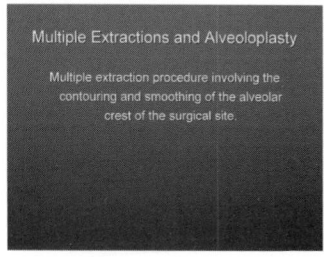

- Most commonly done when a partial or denture is being constructed.
- Can be multiple extractions in different arches; would not need alveoplasty.
- Same procedure as a forceps extraction.
- Why would the alveolar bone need to be contoured and smoothed?

Slide 37

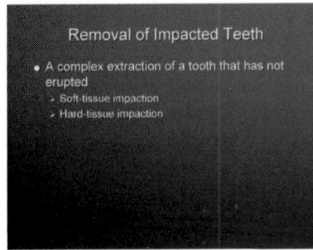

- Sutures are placed.
- May need to use surgical burs to access tooth below the bone level.
- Scalpel would be used to make incision to gain access.

Slide 38

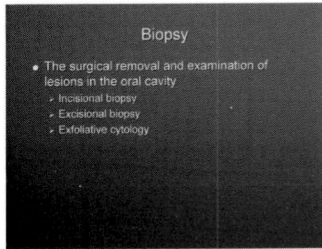

- What is a malignancy?
- An incisional biopsy is done on lesions larger than 1 cm; cut wedge of lesion along with normal tissue.
- Exfoliative cytology is also known as a smear biopsy; brush lesion and spread on slide.

Slide 39

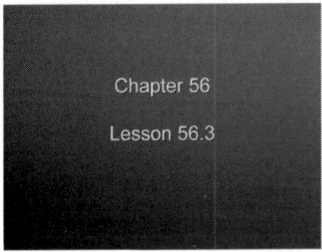

Slide 40

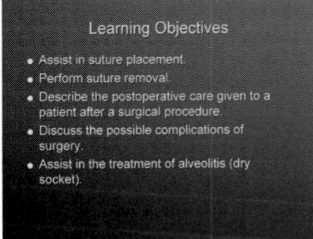

Slide 41

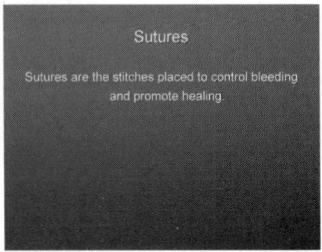

- Sutures are not placed for all procedures and are an important part of the healing process.
- When would sutures need to be placed?

Slide 42

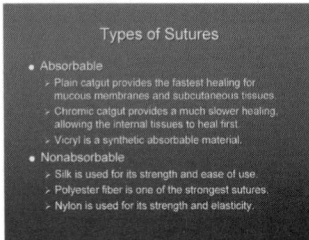

- Dentist preference determines the type of suture material used.
- Usually supplied with the needle already attached to the suture material.
- What does the term *absorbable* mean?
- What does the term *non-absorbable* mean?
- What will need to be done for non-absorbable sutures?

Slide 43

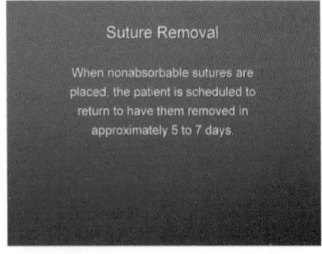

- What instruments are needed for suture removal procedure?
- Who is allowed to remove sutures?

Slide 44

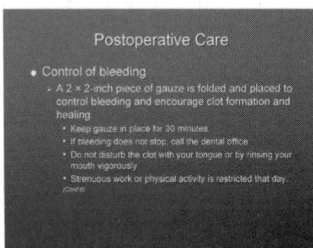

- Frequently remind patient how to care for extraction sites.
- Advise patient to keep head elevated, sleep with an extra pillow.
- Should a patient be given postoperative instructions even though the patient received the instructions preoperatively?
- Are postoperative instructions given orally or written?

Slide 45

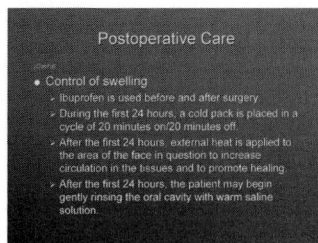

- Advice for patient:
  - Eat and drink cool, smooth things (ice cream, pudding, yogurt)
  - No spicy food
  - No straws
  - No sucking motion
  - No smoking or chewing tobacco
  - No alcohol

Slide 46

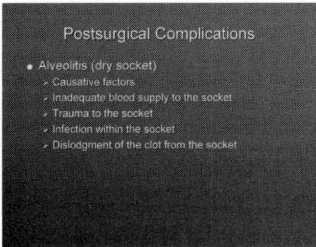

- How can the clot become dislodged from the socket?
- What is the purpose of the medicated dressing or squares?
- Will the patient need to return for evaluation?

Torres and Ehrlich Modern Dental Assisting, 9th ed.

Bird/Robinson

57 Lesson Plan
Pediatric Dentistry

TEACHING FOCUS

This chapter introduces students to the specialty of pediatric dentistry, including the stages of childhood and behavior management. Students have an opportunity to understand diagnosis and treatment planning, preventive dentistry, and pediatric procedures. The chapter also discusses patients with special needs, dental trauma, and signs of child abuse.

MATERIALS AND RESOURCES

- ☐ articulating paper and holder (Lesson 57.2)
- ☐ basic setup (Lesson 57.2)
- ☐ dental dam setup (Lesson 57.2)
- ☐ cementation setup (Lesson 57.2)
- ☐ computer and PowerPoint projector (all Lessons)
- ☐ contouring and crimping pliers (Lesson 57.2)
- ☐ cotton rolls (Lesson 57.2)
- ☐ crown and bridge scissors (Lesson 57.2)
- ☐ dental floss (Lesson 57.2)
- ☐ final restorative material and instrument for placement (Lesson 57.2)
- ☐ finishing and polishing discs (Lesson 57.2)
- ☐ formocresol (Lesson 57.2)
- ☐ friction grip burs (Lesson 57.2)
- ☐ high-volume oral evacuator (HVE) tip (Lesson 57.2)

- ☐ local anesthetic agent setup (Lesson 57.2)
- ☐ low-speed handpiece (Lesson 57.2)
- ☐ low-speed and high-speed handpieces (Lesson 57.2)
- ☐ mandrel (Lesson 57.2)
- ☐ mounted green stones (Lesson 57.2)
- ☐ round burs (Lesson 57.2)
- ☐ office decorating/supply catalogs (Lesson 57.1)
- ☐ pediatric dental exam sheets (Lesson 57.1)
- ☐ selection of stainless steel crowns (Lesson 57.2)
- ☐ spoon excavators (Lesson 57.2)
- ☐ sterile cotton pellets (Lesson 57.2)
- ☐ zinc oxide-eugenol (ZOE) base (Lesson 57.2)

LESSON CHECKLIST

Preparations for this lesson include:
- lecture
- demonstration
- guest speakers: pediatric dentist or dental assistant
- evaluation of student knowledge and skills needed to perform all entry-level activities related to pediatric dentistry, including:
  - ○ pediatric dental office
  - ○ stages of childhood and behavior management
  - ○ patients with special needs
  - ○ diagnosis and treatment planning
  - ○ preventive dentistry for children
  - ○ pediatric procedures
  - ○ dental trauma
  - ○ child abuse

Bird/Robinson

KEY TERMS

analogy (p. 925)
athetosis (p. 924)
autonomy (p. 922)
avulsed (p. 933)
cerebral palsy (p. 924)
chronologic age (p. 921)
contour (p. 930)
crossbite (p. 926)
Down syndrome (p. 924)
emotional age (p. 921)
extrusion (p. 933)
festooning (p. 930)
Frankl scale (p. 922)

intrusion (p. 932)
luxation (p. 933)
mental age (p. 921)
mental retardation (p. 923)
neural (p. 924)
open bay (p. 921)
papoose board (p. 923)
pediatric dentistry (p. 920)
postnatal (p. 924)
prenatal (p. 924)
pulpotomy (p. 929)
spasticity (p. 924)
T-band (p. 929)

ADDITIONAL RESOURCES

PowerPoint slides (Evolve): 1-35
The Interactive Dental Office CD-ROM: Raul Ortega Jr.

Legend

CTQ
Critical
Thinking
Question

DVD
Multimedia
Procedures
Videos and
Animations

ESLR
EVOLVE
Student
Learning
Resources

IDO
Interactive
Dental
Office
CD-ROM

SW
Student
Workbook

TB
Test Bank
on the
TEACH
CD-ROM

PPT
PowerPoint
Slides

Class Activities are indicated in **_bold italic._**

ELSEVIER

Torres and Ehrlich Modern Dental Assisting, 9th ed.

Bird/Robinson

LESSON 57.1

PRETEST

1. What is placed on an avulsed permanent anterior incisor to keep the tooth stable after replantation?
   a. nothing
   b. removable appliance
   c. mouthguard
   d. splint

2. What instrument is used to crimp a stainless steel crown prior to seating it?
   a. crown and bridge scissors
   b. explorer
   c. contouring pliers
   d. cotton pliers

3. During a pulpotomy on a primary tooth, what medicament is usually used?
   a. polycarboxylate cement
   b. formocresol
   c. fluoride varnish
   d. calcium hydroxide

4. What is the term used to describe a tooth that has been forcibly driven into the alveolus?
   a. intrusion
   b. extrusion
   c. luxation
   d. avulsion

5. What is sometimes used to restrain a child during dental treatment?
   a. papoose board
   b. handcuffs
   c. blanket
   d. nothing

6. Underdeveloped nasal and maxillary bones, flattened back of the head, and almond-shaped eyes are characteristics of individuals who have
   a. mental retardation.
   b. cerebral palsy.
   c. Down syndrome.
   d. multiple sclerosis.

7. The most commonly injured teeth due to trauma in children are
   a. posterior teeth.
   b. all teeth.
   c. anterior teeth.
   d. mandibular teeth.

8. The development of autonomy and taking initiative are important during which stage of childhood development?
   a. birth through 2 years
   b. age 3 through 5 years
   c. age 6 through 11 years
   d. age 12 through 17 years

9. What type of instrument is commonly used to help restore a class II preparation in a primary posterior tooth?
   a. #2 tofflemire band
   b. plastic strip
   c. periosteal elevator
   d. T-band matrix

10. Unexplained chipped or injured teeth, bruises or swelling around the face, head, or neck, tears of the labial frenum, and injuries in various stages of healing on a child could indicate
    a. a high sugar diet.
    b. physical abuse.
    c. a vitamin deficiency.
    d. an infection.

Answers

1. d	3. b	5. a	7. c	9. d
2. c	4. a	6. c	8. b	10. b

ELSEVIER

BACKGROUND ASSESSMENT

Question: What is the main goal of pediatric dentistry? What knowledge and skills should the dental assistant have to help put patients of different ages at ease and facilitate treatment?

Answer: Pediatric dentistry focuses on providing dental care and prevention to children from infancy through adolescence. In addition, pediatric dental teams often provide dental care for patients of all ages who have special needs. One of the dental assistant's main roles is to provide a warm and friendly environment and to help patients remain comfortable during treatment. An initial positive experience will make subsequent treatments easier. Little efforts, such as asking about a child's special nickname or a favorite toy, can help put the child at ease. The dental assistant should understand the chronological ages of childhood and that emotional and mental ages do not always correspond to the chronological age. The dental assistant should adapt to each child's age range and developmental level. For example, 3- to 5-year-olds begin to develop autonomy and like control over their environment, so the patient should be allowed to make appropriate choices, such as the flavor of toothpaste. The ability to explain procedures patiently using the tell-show-do method is an essential skill for the pediatric dental assistant. The assistant also must understand that some patients are premedicated, sedated, or restrained for their own safety and for immediate and long-term dental health, so the assistant must be competent in skills such as securing a patient to a papoose board.

Question: What skills must the dental assistant have that require modifications of adult procedures for pediatric patients?

Answer: One of the pediatric dental assistant's roles is to educate patients and families about preventive dentistry and to assist with the procedures. These procedures may include professional and home fluoride treatments, space maintenance, sealant placement, diet counseling, oral hygiene education, and fabrication of sports guards. Additional procedures more common in a pediatric practice involve treatments for trauma, especially to the front teeth. The dental assistant needs to be competent in taking radiographs and photographs, in addition to setting up for splinting. The dental assistant also must understand how materials, set-up, and procedural steps for a pulpotomy differ from the adult's corresponding root canal. The same is true for final restoration of an endodontically treated posterior tooth, which usually involves placement of a stainless steel crown for a child instead of an indirect laboratory fabricated crown. With respect to basic restoration, although procedures are similar, most instruments for children are smaller. A pediatric example that the assistant should be familiar with is the proper folding of a T-band, which is used more often when re-establishing interproximal contacts in posterior teeth, compared to that used for an adult.

CRITICAL THINKING QUESTION

The dental office receives a call from a mother about how to treat her son who tripped and knocked out a front tooth just moments ago. The mother reports that her son is a 10-year-old boy who is mentally challenged and now hysterical. The mother wants to know if she should attempt to replace the tooth. What instructions should the dental assistant provide over the telephone? When the patient arrives at the office, how should the dental assistant be prepared to respond?

Guidelines: The dental assistant should tell the mother that, especially because the child is upset, replanting the tooth in the controlled environment of the dental office is preferable to replacing it at the accident site. Ask the mother to keep the avulsed tooth in clean moist gauze and bring it with the child to the dental office immediately, because the sooner replantation takes place, the greater the likelihood of a positive outcome. Encourage the mother to try to soothe the child and explain that he will soon get help. When the patient arrives, the assistant should introduce herself right away. This is important because it is the assistant who will spend the most time with him, and having a familiar face helps calm fears. Ask the parent to stay with the boy during the emergency exam to help keep him calm and provide an opportunity to become familiar with his needs, temperament, and mental and emotional age. The dental assistant should understand that the child's reactions and behaviors may be extreme or unpredictable and should be ready to respond appropriately. Be ready to hold his hand and have alternative restraints such as a papoose board available. Be prepared to expose radiographs and have anesthesia and surgical and splinting materials ready for use. Be prepared to explain as much as possible, using the tell-show-do method. Because emergency visits occur between regularly scheduled patients, the dental assistant may be instrumental in coordinating timely treatment of all patients. When the emergency treatment is complete, the dentist will review post-treatment home care and the dental assistant will schedule follow-up visits.

Torres and Ehrlich Modern Dental Assisting, 9th ed.

Bird/Robinson

OBJECTIVES	CONTENT	TEACHING RESOURCES
Pronounce, define, and spell the Key Terms.	■ Key terms (pp. 919-920)	PPT 5 SW Fill in the Blank question 17 (p. 508) ESLR Electronic Flashcards ▸ Discuss each of the key terms, focusing on the definition, pronunciation, and spelling of each term. *Class Activity Divide the class into pairs, and assign each pair three or four key terms. Ask the pairs to role-play a dentist-dental assistant interaction or a dental assistant-patient interaction using their assigned terms. Then ask pairs to present their role-play to the class for discussion.*
Describe the appearance and setting of a pediatric dental office.	■ The pediatric dentist (p. 920) ■ The pediatric dental assistant (p. 920) ■ The pediatric dental office (p. 921)	PPT 6-7 TB question 1 SW Short-Answer Questions 1; Fill in the Blank question 17; Multiple Choice questions 2-3 (pp. 507-508) Figure 57-1 Patient at a pediatric dental office (p. 920) Figure 57-2 Example of pleasing, patient-friendly reception area (p. 921) Figure 57-3 Clinical assistants should dress professionally but in a non-threatening manner (p. 921) Recall questions 1-3 (p. 921) ▸ Discuss characteristics of a successful pediatric dental office. ▸ Discuss the benefits of the "open bay" concept. *Class Activity Divide the class into small groups, and ask them to design the ideal pediatric dental office. Encourage the groups to pick a mission statement and a theme for their office that considers the needs of patients, family, dentist, and other office staff. The groups should create a floor plan, decorating theme, furniture, instruments, supplies, apparel, and waiting room materials and toys. Provide students with various dental supply catalogues for materials, instruments, furniture, apparel, goodies for children of various ages, and so on. Then have groups present their designs to the class for feedback and evaluation.*
Give the stages of childhood from birth through adolescence.	■ The pediatric patient (p. 921) ☐ Stages of childhood (p. 921) – Birth through age 2 years (p. 921)	PPT 8-11 TB questions 2-3 SW Short-Answer Questions 2; Fill in the Blank questions 2-3, 11-12; Multiple Choice questions 1, 4-6 (pp. 507-508)

OBJECTIVES	CONTENT	TEACHING RESOURCES
	– Ages 3 through 5 years (p. 922) – Ages 6 through 11 years (p. 922)	Examples of Including a Young Child in a Procedure (p. 922) Recall questions 4-5 (p. 923) ▸ Discuss the three stages of childhood. ▸ Discuss chronologic age, mental age, and emotional age. *Class Activity Divide the class into groups of three, and have them take on the roles of pediatric patient, dentist, and dental assistant within each group. Encourage the students to select a range of ages for their pediatric patients, from preschool through early adolescence. Ask each group to develop a short skit in which the pediatric patient visits the dentist for a routine exam. The pediatric patient should behave age appropriately. Then ask groups to present their skits to the class for feedback and discussion.*
Discuss the specific behavior techniques that work as positive reinforcement when treating children.	☐ Behavior management (p. 922) – Guidelines for child behavior (p. 922) – The challenging patient (p. 923)	⊞ PPT 12-13 🖥 TB question 4 📖 SW Short-Answer Questions 3; Fill in the Blank question 18; Multiple Choice question 7 (pp. 507-509) Table 57-1 Frankl Scale for Pediatric Dental Patient Behavior (p. 922) Figure 57-4 Papoose board is a form of restraint used to prevent pediatric patients from hurting themselves (p. 923) Recall questions 6-7 (p. 923) 💡 CTQ 1-2 (p. 935) ▸ Discuss the procedural guidelines in behavior confidence. ▸ Discuss the Frankl scale to measure a pediatric patient's behavior. *Class Activity Divide the class into small groups, and give each a card on which one of the following dental procedures is listed:* – *Initial clinical exam with radiographs* – *Filling a cavity* – *Fluoride varnish (Vivadent)* – *Pulpotomy* *Have each pair create a tell-show-do narrative for performing the assigned procedure in a pediatric dental office. Have groups exchange narratives with another group, which acts out the narrative. Have students*

OBJECTIVES	CONTENT	TEACHING RESOURCES
		include child-friendly terms for various instruments, materials, and procedures with which a child may not be familiar. Have students provide feedback on each other's presentation. What were effective positive reinforcement techniques? Were anxieties soothed? Did the child cooperate?
Describe why children and adults with special needs are treated in a pediatric practice.	■ Patients with special needs (p. 923) □ Mental retardation (p. 923) □ Down syndrome (p. 924) □ Cerebral palsy (p. 924)	⊠ PPT 14-16 TB question 5 SW Short-Answer Questions 4; Fill in the Blank questions 1, 5-6, 14-16, 20; Multiple Choice questions 8-10 (pp. 507-509) Recall questions 8-10 (p. 924) CTQ 4 (p. 935) ▸ Discuss the various kinds of special needs patients who are treated in a pediatric dental office. *Class Activity Invite a pediatric dentist or dental assistant to discuss practical considerations involved in treating special needs patients of different types. What adjustments or modifications are necessary? What technical and interpersonal skills are important for the dental assistant to have? Have students prepare questions in advance.*

57.1 Homework/Assignments:

57.1 Instructor's Notes/Student Feedback:

Bird/Robinson

LESSON 57.2

CRITICAL THINKING QUESTION

The dental assistant is setting up the treatment room for tomorrow's first patient, a 7-year-old girl who is having a pulpotomy on tooth #K (lower left primary second molar). What materials should the dental assistant have ready?

Guidelines: The dental assistant should set up local and topical anesthesia and should have available a current radiograph of tooth #K. An appropriately pre-punctured rubber dam corresponding to tooth #K, coupled with the clamp and clamp forceps, floss, and rubber dam holder should be set up. A mouth prop may be helpful. A basic instrument set-up, including high- and slow-speed handpieces with burs (access bur for high speed and round burs for the actual removal of pulpal tissue), will be required. The dental assistant also should have ready spoon excavators, sterile cotton pellets, formocresol, and zinc oxide-eugenol. A final restorative material with the corresponding instruments for placement should also be set up.

OBJECTIVES	CONTENT	TEACHING RESOURCES

Describe what is involved in the diagnosis and treatment planning of a pediatric patient.	■ Diagnosis and treatment planning (p. 924)
	
	☐ Medical and dental history (p. 925)
	
	☐ Initial clinical exam (p. 925)
	
	  – Radiographic exam (p. 925)
	
	  – Extraoral exam (p. 925)
	
	  – Intraoral soft tissue exam (p. 925)
	
	  – Examination and charting of teeth (p. 925)
		PPT 20-22
		
		TB questions 6-7
		
		SW Short-Answer Questions 5; Multiple Choice questions 11-12 (pp. 507, 509)
		
		Specific Information Noted in the Pediatric Medical and Dental History (p. 925)
		
		Recall questions 11-12 (p. 925)
		
		CTQ 3, 5 (p. 935)
		
		▸ Discuss what is involved in taking a medical and dental history for a pediatric patient.
		
		▸ Discuss the procedures involved in the initial clinical exam.
		
		Class Activity Distribute a different pediatric dental exam sheet that has a missing or inadequate element to each student. Patient charts may be for an initial comprehensive exam or for a periodic oral exam for a child with:
		
		  – All primary teeth
		
		  – Mixed dentition
		
		  – Permanent dentition
		
		Ask students to identify where information is missing or inadequate and what a correct or complete entry would be. Have students present their findings to the class for a discussion of different types of dentition.

Discuss the importance of preventive dentistry in pediatrics.	■ Preventive dentistry for children (p. 925) ☐ Oral hygiene (p. 926) ☐ Fluorides (p. 926)	PPT 22-24 TB question 8 SW Short-Answer Questions 6; Multiple Choice questions 13-16 (pp. 507, 509)

ELSEVIER

Bird/Robinson

OBJECTIVES	CONTENT	TEACHING RESOURCES
	– Fluoride varnish (p. 926)	▣ SW Case Study questions 1-5 (p. 500)
	☐ Diet (p. 926)	Figure 57-5 Example of a dental report card used for recall appointments (p. 927)
	☐ Sealants (p. 926)	Figure 57-6 Fluoride varnish (Vivadent) is a new fluoride system (p. 928)
	☐ Orofacial development (p. 926)	Figure 57-7 Space maintainer used to "reserve" the space until permanent tooth erupts (p. 928)
	☐ Sports safety (p. 926)	Figure 57-8 Example of a fixed appliance to discourage thumb sucking (p. 928)
		Figure 58-9 Example of a fixed appliance to correct crossbite (p. 928)
		Figure 57-10 Palatal expansion appliance used to widen the maxillary arch (p. 928)
		Recall questions 13-16 (p. 928)
		Sports Requiring Mouth Protection (p. 929)
		▸ Discuss the following aspects of preventive dentistry for children: oral hygiene, fluorides, diet, sealants, and sports safety.
		Class Activity Divide the class into groups, and ask them to design educational materials encouraging preventive dental health practices. The materials should be:
		– Posters aimed at children for display in the pediatric dental office
		– Companion brochures designed for parents and children
		Topics may include oral hygiene, fluoride, diet, sealants, periodic exams including radiographs, and sports safety. The materials may include indications, guidelines, recommendations, benefits, frequently asked questions and answers, and brief descriptions of procedures. Then have groups present their materials to the class for evaluation.
Give the types of procedures for the pediatric patient compared with the treatment of patients with permanent teeth.	■ Pediatric procedures (p. 928)	▣ PPT 25
	☐ Restorative procedures (p. 929)	▣ TB questions 9-11
	– Instrument size (p. 929)	▣ SW Short-Answer Questions 7; Fill in the Blank questions 4, 7-10, 19; Multiple Choice questions 18-25 (pp. 507-510)
	– Matrix system (p. 929)	Figure 57-11 A deep calcium hydroxide pulpotomy completed on central incisor (p. 929)
	☐ Endodontic procedures (p. 929)	Recall questions 17-19 (p. 930)

ELSEVIER

OBJECTIVES	CONTENT	TEACHING RESOURCES
	– Pulp therapy (p. 929)	▸ Discuss restorative, endodontic, and prosthodontic procedures for pediatric patients.
	– Pulpotomy (p. 929)	*Class Activity Bring various dental instruments and materials to class that are relevant to modifications of adult procedures performed on a child. Examples:*
	☐ Prosthodontic procedures (p. 929)	*1. tofflemire matrix band and holder versus a T-band matrix*
	– Stainless steel crown (p. 929)	*2. laboratory fabricated porcelain fused to metal crown versus a stainless steel crown*
	– Types of crowns (p. 930)	*3. root canal therapy materials versus those used for pulpotomies*
		4. adult rubber dam clamps versus pediatric-sized clamps
		Demonstrate the differences in use for each item for a child as opposed to those used for an adult, and then have students manipulate and explore the variations.
Assist in a pulpotomy of a primary tooth.	Procedure 57-1 Assisting in pulpotomy of a primary tooth (p. 930) (SW/ESLR Competency 57-1, p. 511)	⊠ PPT 25 SW Fill in the Blank question 19; Multiple Choice question 18 (pp. 508-509) SW/ESLR Competency 57-1 Assisting in the Pulpotomy of a Primary Tooth (p. 511) ▸ Discuss the procedure to assist in the pulpotomy of a primary tooth. *Class Activity Demonstrate a pulpotomy on a pediatric dental typodont, and have students take turns assisting. Ask students to refer to SW/ESLR Competency 57-1, p. 511.*
Assist in the placement of a stainless steel crown.	Procedure 57-2 Assisting in placement of a stainless steel crown (pp. 931-932) (SW/ESLR Competency 57-2, p. 513)	⊠ PPT 25 TB question 9 SW Multiple Choice question 19 (p. 509) SW/IDO Patient Case Exercise questions 1-5 (p. 510) (The Interactive Dental Office CD-ROM) SW/ESLR Competency 57-2 Assisting in the Placement of a Stainless Steel Crown (p. 513) ▸ Discuss the procedure to assist in the placement of a stainless steel crown. *Class Activity Demonstrate placement of a stainless steel crown on a pediatric dental typodont, and have students take turns assisting. Ask students to refer to SW/ESLR Competency 57-2, p. 513.*

OBJECTIVES	CONTENT	TEACHING RESOURCES

Give the types of procedures for the pediatric patient compared with the treatment of patients with permanent teeth.	■ Dental trauma (p. 930)
	
	☐ Fractured anterior teeth (p. 932)
	
	☐ Traumatic intrusion (p. 932)
	
	☐ Extrusion and lateral luxation injuries (p. 933)
	
	☐ Avulsed teeth (p. 933)
	
	– Replanting an avulsed tooth (p. 934)
	
	■ Child abuse (p. 934)
		PPT 26-35
		
		SW Case Study questions 1-5 (p. 510)
		
		Figure 57-12 Traumatized maxillary incisor (p. 932)
		
		Figure 57-13 Flyer on actions to take in a dental emergency distributed to school personnel (p. 933)
		
		Figure 57-14 Fracture of an anterior tooth (p. 933)
		
		Figure 57-15 Avulsion of maxillary central incisors (p. 933)
		
		Recall questions 20-25 (p. 934)
		
		Patient Education (p. 934)
		
		Legal and Ethical Implications (p. 935)
		
		Eye to the Future (p. 935)
		
		▸ Discuss types of dental trauma, including fractured anterior teeth, traumatic intrusion, extrusion and lateral luxation injuries, extrusion and lateral luxation injuries, and avulsed teeth.
		
		▸ Discuss signs of child abuse that may present in the pediatric dental office and how the dental assistant should respond.
		
		Class Activity Have students develop a flow chart explaining what to do for primary and permanent dentition if the following traumas occur:
		
		   – ***Fractured anterior teeth***
		
		   – ***Traumatic intrusion***
		
		   – ***Traumatic extrusion***
		
		   – ***Lateral luxation***
		
		   – ***Avulsed teeth***
		
		Target the information to adults who respond to emergencies at home, school, camp, or during sports activities. Have students include a lay person's definition of the dental terms and a brief description of what may happen at the dental office.

Performance Evaluation		TB SW questions (pp. 507-510) SW Case Study (p. 510) SW/IDO Patient Case Exercise questions (p. 510) (The Interactive Dental Office CD-ROM)

OBJECTIVES	CONTENT	TEACHING RESOURCES
		SW/ESLR Competency 57-1 Assisting in the Pulpotomy of a Primary Tooth (p. 511)
		SW/ESLR Competency 57-2 Assisting in the Placement of a Stainless Steel Crown (p. 513)
		ESLR Electronic Flashcards
		ESLR Practice Quiz
		Recall questions (pp. 921-934)
		CTQ (p. 935)

57.2 Homework/Assignments:

57.2 Instructor's Notes/Student Feedback:

Slide 1

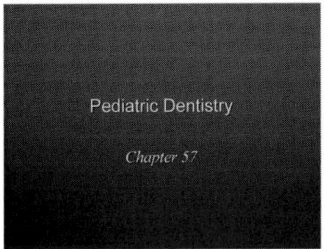

Pediatric Dentistry

Chapter 57

Slide 2

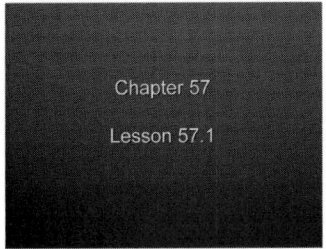

Chapter 57

Lesson 57.1

Slide 3

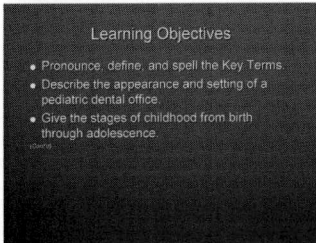

Learning Objectives

- Pronounce, define, and spell the Key Terms.
- Describe the appearance and setting of a pediatric dental office.
- Give the stages of childhood from birth through adolescence.

Slide 4

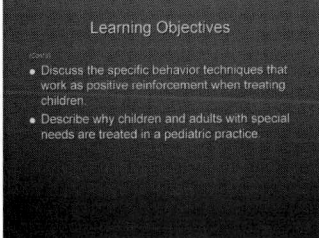

Learning Objectives

- Discuss the specific behavior techniques that work as positive reinforcement when treating children.
- Describe why children and adults with special needs are treated in a pediatric practice.

Slide 5

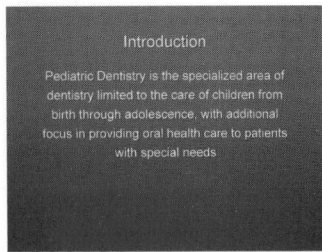

- Children are treated in pediatric dental settings and in general dental offices.
- What are the pros and cons of treating pediatric and special needs patients at a specialized practice versus treating them within a general dental practice?

Slide 6

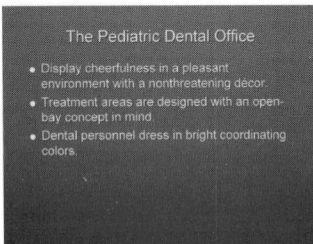

- What is an open bay concept?
- How can a general dental practice adapt its facilities to appeal to pediatric patients and still consider the needs of adult patients?

Slide 7

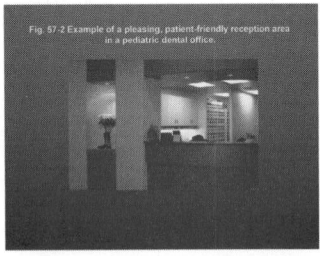

- What features of this pediatric dental office welcome children and put them at ease?
- What features appeal to parents and staff?

Slide 8

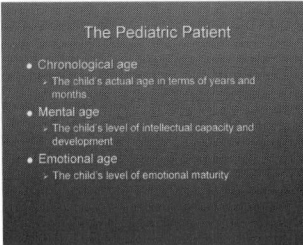

- A child's *dental age* may vary by a year or two from the chronological age.
- The dental assistant may encounter physical, mental, emotional, and behavioral differences between boys and girls and between children of different cultures and socioeconomic backgrounds.
- With so many variables in pediatric patients, what skills should the dental assistant develop?

Slide 9

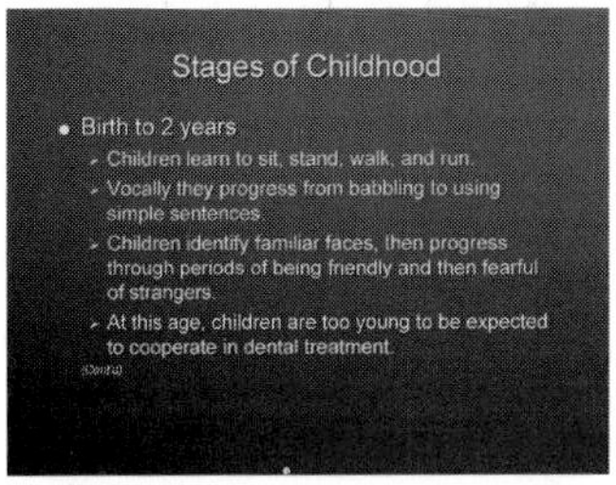

- What fairly common dental or oral conditions require dental care at this age?
- A child's entire primary dentition, consisting of 20 teeth, erupts by about age 3.
- What other conditions may require initial evaluation by a pediatric dentist?

Slide 10

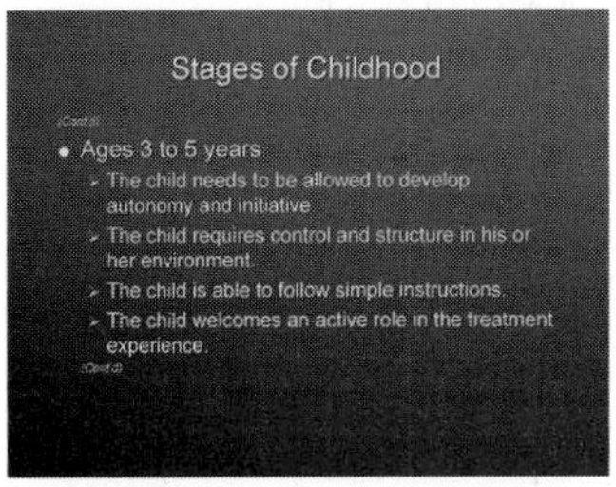

- Child-friendly names for instruments and procedures also help reduce anxiety.
- Children may need a parent during all or part of the treatment.
- Why do dental office policies vary regarding the presence of a parent?

Slide 11

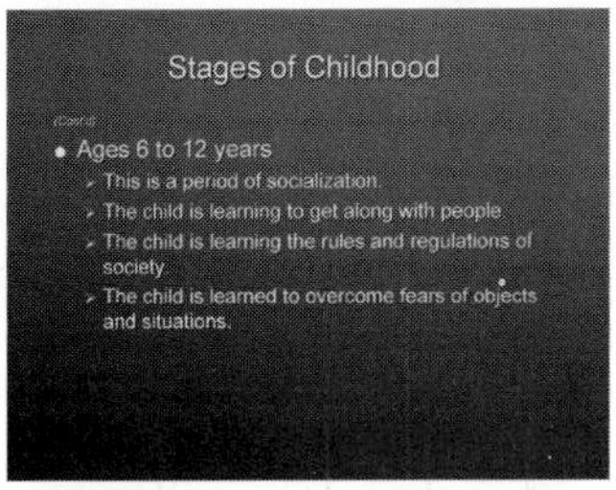

- Treatment is usually performed without parent or guardian present.
- Children may present with memories, positive or negative, of past dental treatment, and also may have misconceptions.
- How should the dental assistant respond?

Slide 12

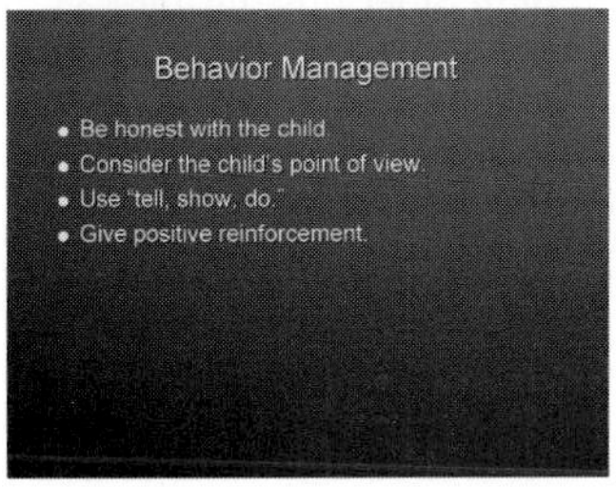

- Dental offices differ in the amount of interaction a dental assistant has with pediatric patients. Often, it is the assistant's role to provide a welcoming environment and to orient the patient to instruments, materials, and procedures.
- It is important to listen to the child and to provide him or her ways of communicating any anxieties or discomfort. Why?
- Tell-show-do is very important at this age to prepare the child and for appropriate cooperation.

Slide 13

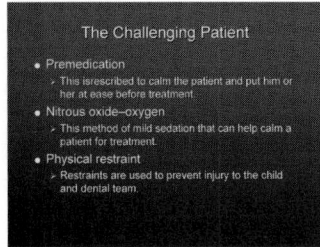

- It is important that children who are treated pharmcologically for conditions such as ADD or ADHD take medication as usual before dental treatment.

- Nitrous oxide is an inhaled sedative that helps calm the patient during treatment and wears off quickly. Local anesthesia also may be used.

- Under what conditions would physical restraints, ranging from hand-holding to a papoose board, be required?

Slide 14

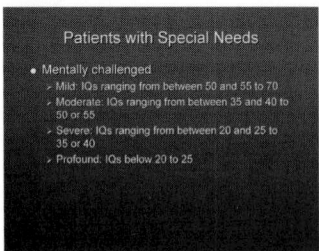

- Severely to profoundly mentally challenged children and adults typically receive dental treatment under general anesthesia in the operating room of a hospital.

- Moderately mentally challenged patients may require sedation or treatment under general anesthesia.

- What is the role of the dental assistant in treating patients with special needs?

Slide 15

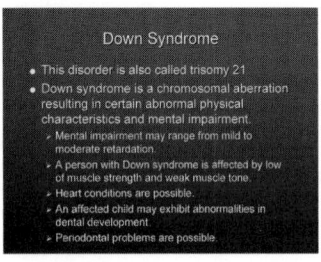

- These patients are usually pleasant, warm and friendly but will likely require undivided attention, patience, and encouragement.

- What dental and periodontal issues are commonly seen in patients who have Down syndrome? What special procedures may be required for treatment?

- How can the dental assistant help make the dental office experience a positive one?

Slide 16

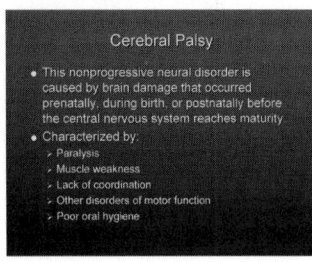

- If not combined with other disorders, children who have cerebral palsy have normal intelligence. It is imperative to remember this during treatment.

- Why might oral hygiene be problem at home for patients who have cerebral palsy? What home care aids are available?

- How can the dental assistant help in patient education?

Torres and Ehrlich Modern Dental Assisting, 9th ed.

Bird/Robinson

Slide 17

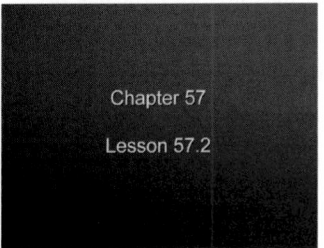

Slide 18

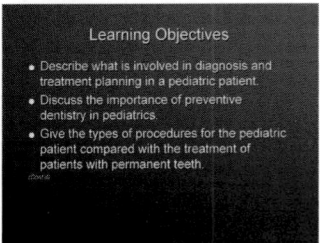

Slide 19

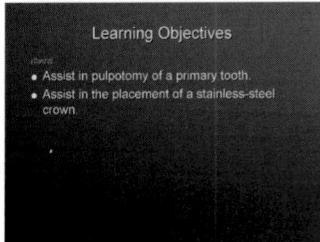

Slide 20

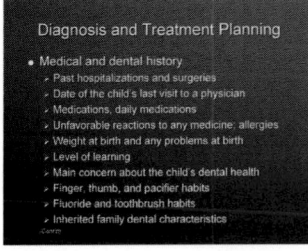

- Ask about and record regular or as needed medications, such as asthma inhalers, vitamins, or antibiotics. Parents may forget to mention all medications.

- What are the implications for dental care if a child has an allergic reactions to medication?

- Why should the type of water the child was raised on and consumes now be documented?

Slide 21

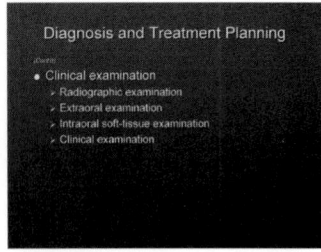

- The radiographic examination may include a combination of radiographs, a single radiograph, or none if they are not indicated or the child does not cooperate.

- What may the extraoral examination include?

- What soft tissues are evaluated and documented?

- What will the intraoral examination of hard tissues include?

Slide 22

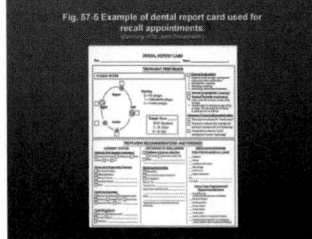

- This is an example of a form that may be used at a periodic oral examination as a report card.

- What information is included on the dental report card?

- Why is the report card useful?

Slide 23

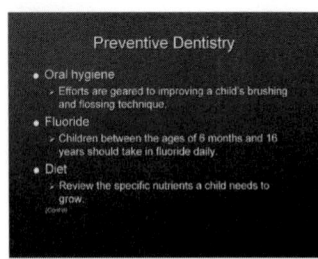

- Demonstrate proper flossing and brushing during the office visit. Provide constructive feedback.

- Depending on water type, fluoride supplements or fluoride toothpaste should be recommended.

- How does insufficient nutrition contribute to caries, staining, halitosis, and chemical erosion?

Slide 24

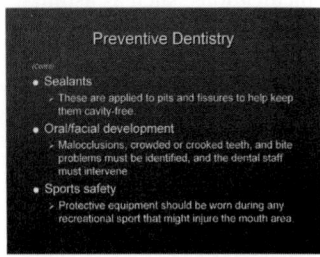

- Sealants are frequently applied to prevent occlusal caries resulting from food debris and bacterial entrapment in newly erupted, permanent posterior teeth (most often molars).

- Why is early evaluation of oral and facial development important?

Bird/Robinson

Slide 25

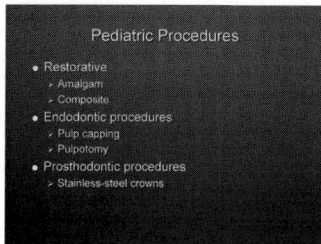

- Why is an alternative matrix band used in restorative dentistry for children, instead of the standard adult matrix band?

- What is the difference between a pulpotomy and a root canal?

- Following a pulpotomy or root canal of a primary molar, how do pediatric and adult crowns differ?

Slide 26

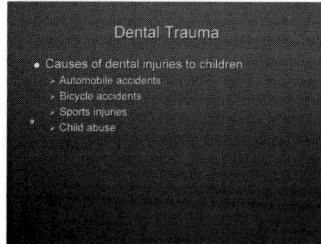

- Why would surrounding or supporting hard and soft tissues require different treatments?

- In addition the above most common causes of dental trauma, what else can cause dental and facial trauma?

Slide 27

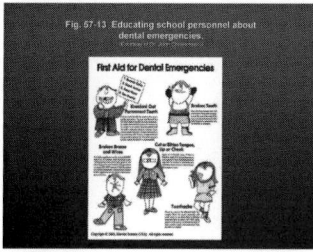

- What should supervising adults be familiar with on this poster?

- In what ways can appropriate immediate care result in a more favorable outcome?

Slide 28

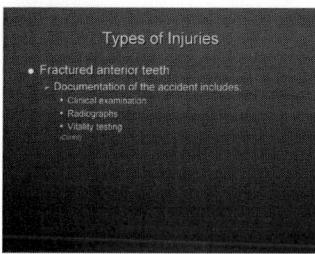

- Anterior teeth are the most commonly fractured teeth in children.

- Why is proper documentation of dental injuries important?

- What factors determine how fractured anterior teeth are treated?

Bird/Robinson

Slide 29

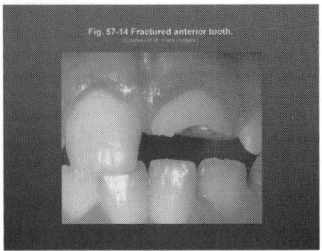

- If the above tooth is salvageable, it will require root canal therapy (if the pulp is involved) followed by a post and core buildup, and finally a crown.

- What is an example of a fracture in which the tooth cannot be saved? What is the treatment?

- Why is it important to evaluate the teeth adjacent to and opposing the fractured tooth?

Slide 30

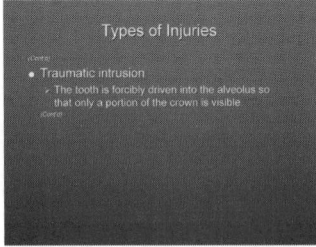

- For a primary tooth, the dentist treats the symptoms and a tooth may be allowed to reerupt. The tooth is treated according to clinical and radiographic findings.

- Why do these teeth often need root canal therapy?

Slide 31

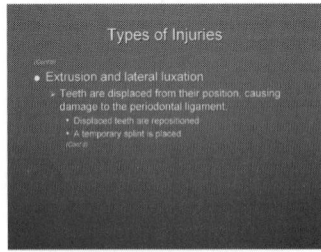

- What is the difference between extrusion and lateral luxation?

- How are displaced teeth typically treated?

Slide 32

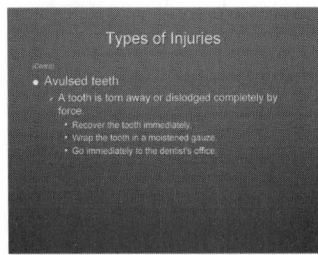

- Primary teeth are not usually replanted. Sound permanent teeth avulsed without root fracture are commonly replanted.

- What treatment will most likely take place in the dental office?

- Why is immediate replantation advisable?

Torres and Ehrlich Modern Dental Assisting, 9th ed.

Bird/Robinson

Slide 33

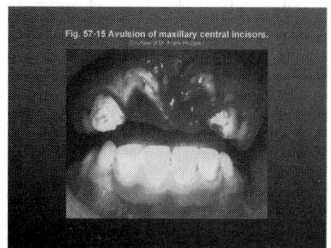

- This is an intraoral view of a child's mouth missing permanent teeth #8 and #9, most likely due to traumatic avulsion.

- If the teeth and the situation are suitable for replantation, teeth will be held in place with a splint and will require root canal therapy in the future.

- Antibiotics will most likely also be prescribed.

Slide 34

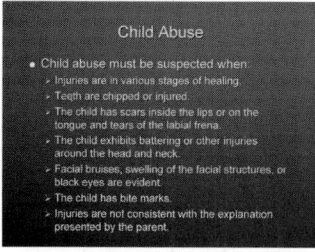

- Unless a state has mandated reporter requirement for health care professionals, the dental assistant has no legal obligation to report suspected child abuse. This is the responsibility of the dentist or dental hygienist. However, the assistant may serve as an important witness.

- Suspicion may also be warranted with intraoral palatal bruising, lacerations, or petechiae, as well as various extraoral bruises in the same area but in different stages of healing.

- What should the dental assistant do if he or she suspects abuse?

Slide 35

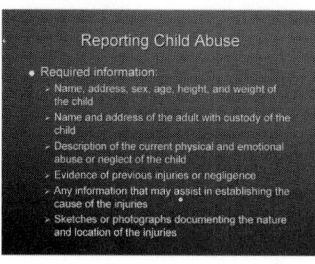

- Proper documentation including photographs is crucial in documenting physical evidence.

- This information should be kept confidential and reported in a professional manner.

- Why is it important also to address and report child neglect?

Bird/Robinson

TEACHING FOCUS

This chapter will give the student an opportunity to understand the differences between coronal polishing and a prophylaxis. The indications, contraindications, and techniques for coronal polishing will be discussed. The student will have an opportunity to learn about types of dental stains and the methods to remove them. Handpieces and attachments for coronal polishing, along with abrasives, will be covered.

MATERIALS AND RESOURCES

- ☐ air-water syringe and sterile tip (Lesson 58.2)
- ☐ bridge threader (Lesson 58.2)
- ☐ bristle brush, snap-on or screw-on (Lesson 58.2)
- ☐ computer and PowerPoint projector (all Lessons)
- ☐ cotton-tipped applicator (if disclosing solution is used) (Lesson 58.2)
- ☐ dental floss (Lesson 58.2)
- ☐ dental tape (Lesson 58.2)
- ☐ disclosing agent (tablets, gel, or solution) (Lesson 58.2)
- ☐ HVE tip or saliva ejector (Lesson 58.2)
- ☐ instruments for demonstrating coronal polishing (Lesson 58.2)

- ☐ manufacturer information inserts that accompany materials that are indicated for polishing composite resin restorations (Lesson 58.2)
- ☐ mounted extracted teeth containing both direct and indirect restorations (Lesson 58.2)
- ☐ photographs or slides of dental staining due to endogenous or exogenous factors (Lesson 58.1)
- ☐ polishing cup accessory, snap-on or screw-on (Lesson 58.2)
- ☐ prophy angle, sterile or disposable (Lesson 58.2)
- ☐ prophy paste or other abrasive in slurry (Lesson 58.2)
- ☐ scientific material and clinical research papers about polishing porcelain restorations (Lesson 58.2)

LESSON CHECKLIST

Preparations for this lesson include:

- lecture
- evaluation of student knowledge and skills needed to perform all entry-level activities related to coronal polishing, including:
  - ○ selective polishing
  - ○ understanding dental stains
  - ○ using handpieces and attachments for coronal polishing
  - ○ using abrasives
  - ○ using prophylaxis angle and handpiece
  - ○ coronal polishing steps
  - ○ understanding the sequence of polishing
  - ○ flossing after polishing

Bird/Robinson

KEY TERMS

calculus (p. 937)
clinical crown (p. 937)
coronal polishing (p. 937)
endogenous stains (p. 938)
exogenous stains (p. 938)
extrinsic stains (p. 938)

fulcrum (p. 944)
intrinsic stains (p. 938)
oral prophylaxis (p. 937)
prophy paste (p. 941)
rubber cup polishing (p. 941)

ADDITIONAL RESOURCES

PowerPoint slides (Evolve): 1-65
Multimedia Procedures DVD: Coronal Polishing

Legend

CTQ
Critical
Thinking
Question

DVD
Multimedia
Procedures
Videos and
Animations

ESLR
EVOLVE
Student
Learning
Resources

IDO
Interactive
Dental
Office
CD-ROM

SW
Student
Workbook

TB
Test Bank
on the
TEACH
CD-ROM

PPT
PowerPoint
Slides

Class Activities are indicated in **bold italic**.

Torres and Ehrlich Modern Dental Assisting, 9th ed.

Bird/Robinson

LESSON 58.1

PRETEST

1. A rubber polishing cup with abrasives is used to remove
   a. plaque from the interproximal contact areas.
   b. plaque and debris from the tongue.
   c. extrinsic plaque and stain from the clinical crown.
   d. intrinsic amalgam staining.

2. Before etching and bonding of orthodontic brackets on enamel, teeth may be polished using a
   a. whitening toothpaste.
   b. fluoridated prophylaxis paste.
   c. diamond polishing paste.
   d. fine pumice.

3. Proper positioning of the patient and right-handed operator for coronal polishing of the maxilla involves
   a. positioning of the patient's mandible parallel to the floor.
   b. the operator seated at the 3 o'clock position.
   c. having the operator sit with legs crossed.
   d. the operator seated at the 9 o'clock position.

4. What is recommended when polishing?
   a. Always polish at 20,000 rpm.
   b. Polish from incisal third towards the gingival third.
   c. Begin with the distal surface of most posterior tooth.
   d. Always use the finer grit before the most abrasive.

5. To avoid the abrasive effects, what is the recommended amount of time to spend polishing each tooth?
   a. 3 to 5 seconds
   b. 30 to 45 seconds
   c. 1 to 2 minutes
   d. 3 to 5 minutes

6. What is another term used to describe the finger rest used to stabilize the handpiece during polishing?
   a. fulcrum
   b. rheostat
   c. index area
   d. pressure point

7. What is recommended for polishing of porcelain indirect restorations?
   a. diamond paste
   b. aluminum oxide paste
   c. course grit slurry
   d. medium grit pumice

8. The term "mottled enamel" is an endogenous stain that is also known as
   a. dental plaque.
   b. dental fluorosis.
   c. green stain.
   d. dental caries.

9. Endogenous stains on teeth may be due to
   a. drinking coffee and tea.
   b. smoking tobacco.
   c. tetracycline usage during tooth development.
   d. drinking red wine.

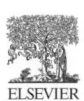

10. Coronal polishing is limited to removal of plaque and stains from which part of the tooth?
    a. the root
    b. the crown below the gingiva
    c. the crown and the root
    d. the clinical crown only

Answers

1. c	3. d	5. a	7. a	9. c
2. d	4. c	6. a	8. b	10. d

BACKGROUND ASSESSMENT

Question: What is coronal polishing? What are its indications and contraindications?

Answer: Coronal polishing is the removal of stain and plaque from only the clinical crowns of teeth. Coronal polishing is indicated before placement of dental sealants, before the placement of the rubber dam, and before cementation of orthodontic bands and brackets. Coronal polishing is also very important before etching of enamel required for bonding of composite resins as well as before the cementation of crowns and bridges. In these cases, a nonfluoridated abrasive such as pumice is indicated. Selective coronal polishing may also be an important service following a dental prophylaxis. Coronal polishing is not advised in the absence of stain or plaque, in areas of thin demineralized enamel, on sensitive teeth, or on newly erupted teeth,because mineralization may still be inadequate.

Question: What are endogenous stains? What are exogenous stains? What is the difference between extrinsic and intrinsic staining, and what are examples of each?

Answer: Endogenous stains originate within the tooth. Tetracycline staining is an example of endogenous staining, which may not be removed via coronal polishing. If this antibiotic is taken by a pregnant mother during fetal tooth development or by an infant during tooth formation, a stain—varying in color from light green to dark yellow to a gray brown—may result. Exogenous stains are those that originate outside of the tooth, some of which may be removed with coronal polishing. An extrinsic exogenous stain may eventually become incorporated endogenously, at which point coronal polishing will no longer help. Stain from smoking tobacco is an example of an exogenous, extrinsic stain that may become intrinsic over time.

CRITICAL THINKING QUESTION

A dental assistant qualified to perform coronal polishing is preparing for the next patient, a 50-year-old smoker who has had a moderate amount of direct composite resin and indirect porcelain posterior restorations placed. Following the patient's adult prophylaxis by the hygienist, the dental assistant is asked to do selective polishing. What instruments and materials will be required?

Guidelines: Although tobacco smoking contributes to exogenous extrinsic stain on the dentition, over time the stain may become incorporated intrinsically and thus can no longer be removed completely with coronal polishing alone. Personal protective devices should be ready for both the dental assistant and the patient. The treatment room should have a slow-speed handpiece, dental mouth mirror, prophy angle (sterile or disposable), polishing cup and bristle brush, high-speed evacuator, saliva ejector, and an air-water syringe. Cotton-tipped applicators will be important for application of the disclosing agent before and following the polishing if tablets are not used. Dental tape and floss should be available as well as a bridge floss threader, if applicable. The polishing should begin with the use of a diamond paste for any surfaces restored with porcelain, and an aluminum oxide paste for surfaces restored with composite resin. Fluoride prophylaxis pastes of various grits should be available for polishing the natural crowns of teeth that require coronal polishing to remove stain and plaque. If, during the coronal polishing, the assistant detects calculus that was not removed during the prophylaxis, it is important that the assistant ask the treating hygienist or dentist to remove it before polishing.

OBJECTIVES	CONTENT	TEACHING RESOURCES
Pronounce, define, and spell the Key Terms.	■ Key terms (p. 936)	*e* ESLR Electronic Flashcards ▸ Discuss each of the key terms in Chapter 58, focusing on the definition, pronunciation, and spelling of each term. ***Class Activity** Have student pairs take turns role-playing a patient asking an assistant questions that require the assistant to properly pronounce and define all the key*

ELSEVIER

Bird/Robinson

OBJECTIVES	CONTENT	TEACHING RESOURCES
		terms.,Encourage students to use creative props such as dental instruments, materials, and clinical photos as they are available to help in communication. Then have students discuss what they learned from the activity.
Explain the difference between a prophylaxis and coronal polishing.	■ Introduction (p. 937) ■ Selective polishing (p. 938)	PPT 4-7 TB questions 1, 3 SW Short-Answer Questions 1; Fill in the Blank questions 1-3; Multiple Choice questions 1-3 (pp. 515-516) SW Case Study questions 2, 5 (pp. 516-517) Figure 58-1 (A) Bristle brush; (B) Rubber polishing cup; (C) Reusable prophy angle; (D) Disposable prophy angle (p. 937) Recall questions 1-5 (p. 939) ▸ Discuss what an oral prophylaxis cleaning accomplishes. ▸ Discuss what a coronal polishing accomplishes. *Class Activity Have students work in small groups to design a patient information brochure that explains the difference between a prophylaxis and coronal polishing. The brochure should explain why a coronal polish is not a substitute for an oral prophylaxis and also should identify who is qualified to perform each of these procedures. Then have each group present its brochure to the class.*
Explain the indications for and contraindications to a coronal polish.	■ Introduction (p. 937) ■ Selective polishing (p. 938)	TB question 2 SW Short-Answer Questions 2 (p. 515) SW Case Study questions 3-4 (p. 517) Box 58-1 Indications and Contraindications to Coronal Polishing (p. 937) Box 58-2 Possible Damaging Effects of Coronal Polishing (p. 938) Benefits of Coronal Polishing (p. 938) ▸ Discuss the indications and contraindications to a coronal polishing. ▸ Discuss the possible damaging effects that can occur with coronal polishing. *Class Activity Divide the class into small groups, and have each group create a chart that lists the indications and contraindications for coronal polishing. Then have groups present their charts to the class for feedback.*

Torres and Ehrlich Modern Dental Assisting, 9th ed.

Bird/Robinson

OBJECTIVES	CONTENT	TEACHING RESOURCES
Name and describe the types of extrinsic stains.	■ Dental stains (p. 938) □ Types of stains (p. 938) □ Methods of removing plaque and stains (p. 941) – Air-powder polishing (p. 941) – Rubber cup polishing (p. 941)	⊠ PPT 8-11 TB question 5 SW Short-Answer Questions 3; Fill in the Blank question 5; Multiple Choice question 4 (pp. 515-516) Table 58-1 Extrinsic stains (p. 940) Patient Education (p. 949) ▸ Discuss how endogenous stains originate. ▸ Discuss the types of extrinsic stains, and the appearance and cause of each type. ***Class Activity Divide the class into small groups. Ask students to design posters for display in a dental office that inform patients about foods and other substances that can stain teeth over short and prolonged periods. Encourage use of photographs from magazines or product advertisements as well as clinical photos or sketches that display teeth before and after coronal polishing. The poster should also outline stains that begin as extrinsic but might become intrinsic, as well as endogenous stains that might not be removed with polishing but require additional procedures. (For students to prepare for this activity, see Homework/Assignments #1.)***
Name and describe the two categories of intrinsic stains.	■ Dental stains (p. 938) □ Types of stains (p. 938) □ Methods of removing plaque and stains (p. 941) – Air-powder polishing (p. 941) – Rubber cup polishing (p. 941)	⊠ PPT 12-17 TB questions 4, 6, 8-9 SW Short-Answer Questions 4; Fill in the Blank question 4; Multiple Choice question 5 (pp. 515-516) Figure 58-2 Endogenous development stain: tetracycline (p. 939) Figure 58-3 Endogenous developmental stain: enamel hypoplasia (p. 939) Figure 58-4 Endogenous development stain: dental fluorosis (p. 939) Figure 58-5 Endogenous developmental stain: secondary caries (p. 939) Figure 58-6 Endogenous stain: amalgam restoration (p. 939) Table 58-2 Intrinsic Stains (p. 940) CTQ question 1 (p. 949) ▸ Discuss the types of intrinsic stains, and the appearance and cause of each type.

ELSEVIER

Bird/Robinson

OBJECTIVES	CONTENT	TEACHING RESOURCES
		Class Activity Display photographs or slides of dental staining due to endogenous or exogenous factors, including intrinsic and extrinsic factors. Ask students to categorize the type of staining and its source, determine whether coronal polishing would remove the stain, and, if not, suggest another procedure that would remove it. If possible display before-and-after photos of stain removal by means of various clinical methods.
Describe types of abrasives used for polishing the teeth.	■ Handpieces and attachments for coronal polishing (p. 941) □ Polishing cups (p. 941) □ Bristle brushes (p. 941) – Bristle brush polishing stroke (p. 941) ■ Polishing agents (p. 941)	⊠▪ PPT 18-22 TB. TB questions 8-9, 12-14 SW Short-Answer Questions 5 (p. 515) Table 58-3 Commonly Used Abrasives (p. 942) Figure 58-7 Prophy pastes and equipment (p. 942) Factors that Influence the Rate of Abrasion (p. 942) Polishing Tips (p. 942) ▶ Discuss the polishing cups and bristle brushes used in coronal polishing. ▶ Discuss commonly used abrasives for coronal polishing. ▶ Discuss the factors that influence the amount of abrasion in coronal polishing. *Class Activity Call out a type of abrasive agent and ask students to respond with a description of the agent's action. Then state the action of an abrasive agent and ask students to identify the abrasive agent that is associated with the stated action.*

Bird/Robinson

58.1 Homework/Assignments:

1. Ask students to design posters for display in a dental office that inform patients about foods and other substances that can stain teeth over short and prolonged periods of time. Encourage use of photographs from magazines or product advertisements as well as clinical photos or sketches that display teeth before and after coronal polishing. The posters should also outline stains that begin as extrinsic but might become intrinsic, as well as endogenous stains that might not be removed with polishing but might require other procedures.

58.1 Instructor's Notes/Student Feedback:

CRITICAL THINKING QUESTION

An experienced dental assistant is training a right-handed dental assistant who is a recent graduate. The next patient on the schedule is a 15-year-old boy who will require coronal polishing before placement of his bands and brackets. The experienced assistant has already helped the trainee set up the required instruments and materials. What are some useful tips that should be provided to the new dental assistant?

Guidelines: The new assistant should be advised to adjust the treatment chair to a comfortable height after the patient is seated, parallel to the floor, with the back slightly raised and the headrest adjusted for the comfort of both the patient and the operator. While working on the maxilla, the patient chin should be tilted upward so that the maxilla is more visible and easier to illuminate with lighting. Polishing the mandible may require that the headset and the back of the chair be adjusted so that the arch is positioned parallel to the floor. The assistant should adjust her own chair so that she can rest her feet flat on the floor while gaining easy access to the rheostat. The new assistant should be able to move freely beside and under the back of the patient's chair, and the instruments should be within reach. As a right-handed operator, the new assistant should be reminded that she will probably begin at the eight o'clock or nine o'clock position. The assistant should be encouraged to use a finger fulcrum to support the instruments she is using. The assistant should verify that she and the patient are situated so that light may be directed to the surfaces being worked on directly, or indirectly by way of reflection in the dental mouth mirror. Retraction of the cheek and tongue for access to the posterior areas is important. The assistant should be encouraged to develop a set order of instrumentation so that no surfaces that need polishing will be left untreated. Completing one arch before beginning the next is advised, as is completing all buccal or lingual surfaces of a quadrant or sextant before moving on.

OBJECTIVES	CONTENT	TEACHING RESOURCES
Describe the types of abrasives used for porcelain esthetic restorations.	■ Polishing esthetic restorations (p. 941)	PPT 26-27
		SW Short-Answer Questions 6 (p. 515)
		Figure 58-8 It can be difficult to detect esthetic restorations (p. 943)
		▸ Discuss the issues to consider when performing coronal polishing on patients who have undergone esthetic dentistry.
		▸ Discuss the types of abrasives that should be used when polishing porcelain esthetic restorations.
		Class Activity Divide the class into small groups, and provide them with scientific material and clinical research papers about polishing porcelain restorations (crowns, inlays, onlays, veneers). Have them highlight important points with respect to techniques and materials. Then ask the groups to summarize their findings for the class.
Name materials to avoid when polishing esthetic restorations.	■ Polishing esthetic restorations (p. 941)	SW Short-Answer Questions 6 (p. 515)
		Recall question 9 (p. 944)
		▸ Discuss the materials that should be avoided when polishing porcelain esthetic restorations.

ELSEVIER

Torres and Ehrlich Modern Dental Assisting, 9th ed.

Bird/Robinson

OBJECTIVES	CONTENT	TEACHING RESOURCES
		Class Activity Provide students with the manufacturer information inserts that accompany materials that are indicated for polishing composite resin restorations. Provide other inserts from products contraindicated for polishing esthetic restorations. Ask students to highlight and compare the ingredients of the various products and their indications. Help students locate the information and provide feedback and clinical advice.
Describe the technique for polishing esthetic restorations.	■ Polishing esthetic restorations (p. 941)	Recall question 9 (p. 944) ▸ Discuss the polishing stroke used for esthetic restoration. *Class Activity Using mounted extracted teeth that have both direct and indirect restorations in place, describe how restorations are polished. If appropriate materials are available, demonstrate how restorations are polished using the correct instruments, materials, and technique, including the amount of polish, proper finger movement and rests, control of the rheostat, time involved and pressure applied, techniques applied, etc. Allow volunteers to perform the exercise. Critique the students' techniques. Inform students that extracted teeth are dehydrated and will most likely have much intrinsic stain, and that defective restorations will not allow for stain removal.*
Demonstrate the handpiece grasp and positioning for the prophy angle.	■ Prophylaxis angle and handpiece (p. 943) ☐ Grasping the handpiece (p. 943) ☐ Handpiece operation (p. 943)	⊠▤ PPT 29, 36-38 ▸ Discuss the handpiece grasp and positioning for the prophy angle. *Class Activity Have students work in pairs and use a pen or pencil to practice the handpiece grasp, pretending that the writing end is the prophy cup end. Have partners provide feedback to each other as each student demonstrates the grasp. Next, have students practice the handpiece grasp with the actual handpiece, prophy angle, and cup. Have students practice flaring and adapting the cup on one another's fingernails.*
Demonstrate the fulcrum or finger rest used in each quadrant during a coronal polish procedure.	☐ The fulcrum and finger rest (p. 944)	⊠▤ PPT 39 ▥ TB question 15 ▨ SW Fill in the Blank question 6; Multiple Choice question 8 (pp. 515-516) ▸ Discuss the fulcrum or finger rest used in each quadrant during a coronal polish procedure. *Class Activity Demonstrate the fulcrum or finger rest used in each quadrant during a coronal polishing. Then divide the class into groups of three. Have students practice the handpiece grasp and positioning for the*

Torres and Ehrlich Modern Dental Assisting, 9th ed.

Bird/Robinson

OBJECTIVES	CONTENT	TEACHING RESOURCES
		prophy angle extraorally, integrating proper use of a fulcrum. Ask one partner to randomly select a specific tooth and surface to polish. Ask the other partner to provide a verbal explanation for the corresponding fulcrum area using visualization only. Ask the third student to provide constructive feedback as an observer. Have students switch roles.
Demonstrate the proper seating positions for the operator and the assistant during a coronal polish procedure.	■ Coronal polishing steps (p. 944) □ Polishing stroke (p. 944) □ Positioning the patient and operator (p. 945) – Positioning the patient (p. 945) – Positioning the operator (p. 945)	PPT 28, 30-35, 40 ▶ Discuss the proper seating positions for the operator and the assistant during a coronal polish procedure. *Class Activity Divide the class into groups of four. Assign the roles of (1) operator, (2) patient, (3) instructor, and (4) position caller. With the proper materials and equipment in a student operatory or mock environment, ask the position caller to first assign an area and surfaces to be polished. Then have the operator check that the chair, light, patient, headrest, and the operator are properly positioned for the assigned area of the mouth. Have the position caller provide feedback to the other students during the role-play for proper instrument grasp and hand positioning, including a fulcrum. One minute before a switch in roles, call out a new area. See which group is able to set up first.*
Demonstrate safety precautions during coronal polish.	■ Coronal polishing steps (p. 944) □ Polishing stroke (p. 944) □ Positioning the patient and operator (p. 945) – Positioning the patient (p. 945) – Positioning the operator (p. 945)	SW Multiple Choice questions 10, 12 (p. 516) ▶ Discuss the necessary safety precautions that should be observed during coronal polishing. *Class Activity Have students observe the instructor setting up and performing coronal polishing on a volunteer. Intentionally omit a safety precaution and proceed. Have students interrupt the demonstration to correct the process by identifying the missing or incorrect step. Examples of lapses in safety may include: omission of review of the medical history, forgetting to wear protective glasses as an operator or for the patient, cross-contamination, polishing at too high a speed, polishing a surface for too long, and not using adequate suction or rinses.*
In states where it is legal, demonstrate coronal polishing technique.	┌Procedure┐ 58-1 Rubber cup coronal polishing (pp. 946-949) (SW/ESLR Competency 58-1, p. 519)	Multimedia Procedures DVD: Coronal Polishing TB questions 6-7 SW Fill in the Blank questions 6-7; Multiple Choice questions 6-7, 10-11 (pp. 515-516) SW Case Study questions 1-2, 5 (pp. 515-516) SW/ESLR Competency 58-1 Rubber Cup Coronal Polishing (p. 519)

OBJECTIVES	CONTENT	TEACHING RESOURCES
		Figure 58-9 Close-up of hand with handpiece and proper grasp (p. 943)
		Figure 58-10 Use overlapping strokes to ensure complete coverage of the tooth (p. 944)
		Figure 58-11 Stroke from the gingival third with just enough pressure to cause the cup to flare (p. 944)
		Figure 58-12 For the mandibular arch, the patient's head is positioned so that the lower jaw is parallel to the floor with the mouth open (p. 945)
		Figure 58-13 For access to the maxillary arch, position the patient's head with the chin up (p. 945)
		Figure 58-14 The right-handed operator is seated at the nine o'clock position (p. 945)
		Recall questions 6-8, 10-12 (pp. 944, 946)
		♀ CTQ questions 2-3 (p. 949)
		▸ Discuss the proper technique for coronal polishing.
		▸ Discuss the proper positioning of both patient and operator during coronal polishing.
		Class Activity Demonstrate coronal polishing on a student volunteer. Then divide the class into pairs. Provide each pair with the necessary instruments and setting to practice supervised coronal polishing on each other, including proper positioning corresponding to each arch and surface. Ask students to provide a self-evaluation on positioning and technique before delivering professional feedback.
Complete coronal polishing without causing tissue trauma.	■ Sequence of polishing (p. 946) ■ Flossing after polishing (p. 946)	▦ PPT 41-63
		♀ CTQ questions 2-3 (p. 949)
		▸ Discuss how to complete a coronal polish without causing tissue trauma.
		▸ Discuss the correct sequence of steps during coronal polishing.
		Class Activity Divide the class into groups according to the number of operatories and instruments available for use. Ask students to practice polishing one another's teeth. Have an additional group member available for feedback on overall positioning, illumination, control of the handpiece, and removal of coronal plaque by use of disclosing solution. Call out areas in the mouth to practice polishing. Concentrate on the maxillary arch, then the mandibular arch. Allow each student ample time to complete a partner's entire dentition.

OBJECTIVES	CONTENT	TEACHING RESOURCES
Be able to determine that the teeth are free from stains and plaque.	■ Evaluation of polishing (p. 946)	⊠▤ PPT 64-65
		💻 TB question 7
		Patient Education (p. 949)
		Legal and Ethical Implications (p. 949)
		▸ Discuss how to determine if the teeth are free from stains and plaque.
		Class Activity Divide the class into pairs. Have students chew disclosing tablets, allowing students to record which teeth and surfaces on a partner show plaque. Ask students to brush and floss their teeth and then redisclose with the tablets. Have students evaluate and identify which surfaces on their partners and themselves were not efficiently cleaned of plaque by flossing and brushing alone. Lead a class discussion of the techniques that showed the most success in plaque removal.
Performance Evaluation		💻 TB
		📖 SW questions (pp. 515-516)
		📖 SW Case Study (pp. 516-517)
		📖 ℮ SW/ESLR Competency 58-1 Rubber Cup Coronal Polishing (p. 519)
		℮ ESLR Electronic Flashcards
		℮ ESLR Practice Quiz
		Recall questions (pp. 939-946)
		💡 CTQ (p. 949)

58.2 Homework/Assignments:

58.2 Instructor's Notes/Student Feedback:

Bird/Robinson

Slide 1

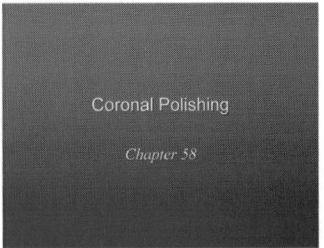

Slide 2

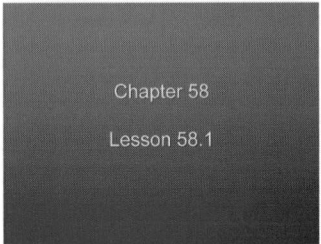

Slide 3

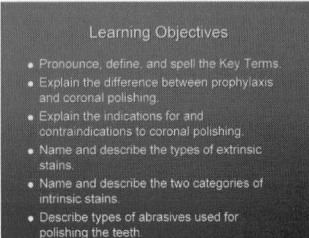

Slide 4

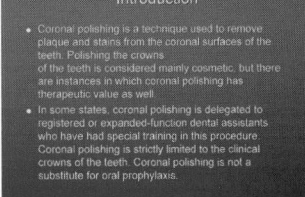

- Even if an assistant is not required to perform coronal polishing, the assistant should become familiar with it because it is likely he or she will have to set up for and assist with such a procedure.

- Removal of coronal plaque following a prophylaxis helps reinforce to patients what their teeth should feel like after proper brushing and flossing, and brushing of the tongue.

Torres and Ehrlich Modern Dental Assisting, 9th ed.

Bird/Robinson

Slide 5

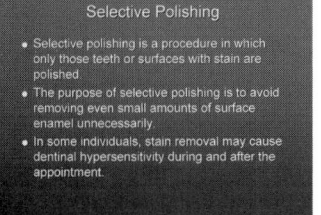

- Discuss with the dentist what should and should not be polished so that you are in agreement.

Slide 6

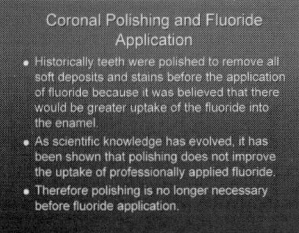

Slide 7

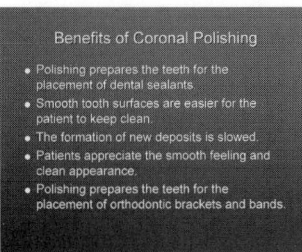

- Polishing with pumice, a nonfluoridated abrasive, is important before sealant placement.

Slide 8

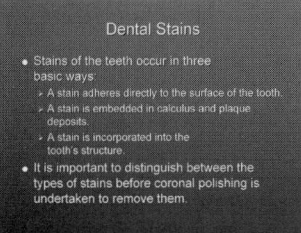

- Only exogenous, extrinsic stains may be removed by coronal polishing. Endogenous or intrinsically incorporated exogenous stains are not removed.

Torres and Ehrlich Modern Dental Assisting, 9th ed.
Bird/Robinson

Slide 9

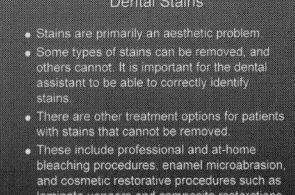

- Before veneer placement, a patient is often instructed to do at-home bleaching so that the other areas of the teeth are adequately brightened to match the new color chosen for the veneers.

- Some endogenous or intrinsic stains are found in conjunction with surface alterations in the enamel, and bleaching alone will not remove them.

Slide 10

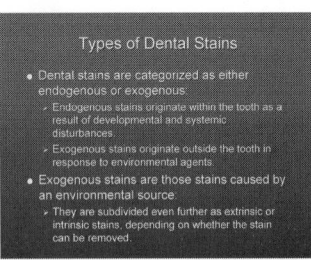

- What are some examples of causes of exogenous stains?

- What are some examples of causes of endogenous stains?

Slide 11

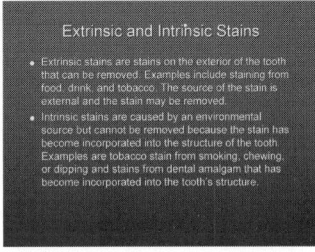

Slide 12

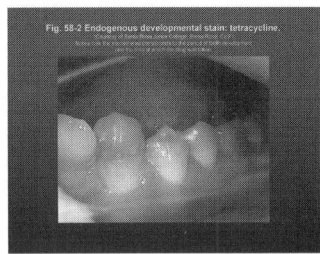

- Notice the light green to dark yellow or gray-brown endogenous stain in teeth systemically exposed to tetracycline antibiotics during their development.

Bird/Robinson

Slide 13

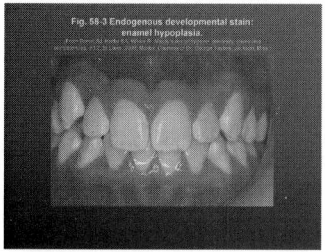

- This photograph shows incisal areas that have diffuse white opaque enamel when compared with the rest of the clinical crown. Pitting or grooving are also seen, in combination with a partial or total lack of enamel.

- Enamel hypoplasia is developmental, frequently found in individuals with a wide range of congenital abnormalities that may also involve other mineralization defects.

Slide 14

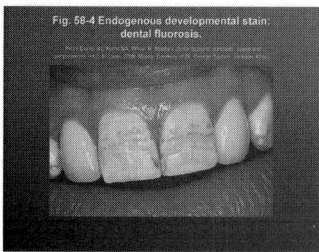

- This staining pattern is called "dental fluorosis" and may also be termed "mottled enamel." It occurs when fluoride consumption, combined from all sources (water, fluoride supplements, food sources, toothpaste consumption) is thought to exceed 1 part per million.

- Cosmetic procedures may involve veneers, or crowns.

Slide 15

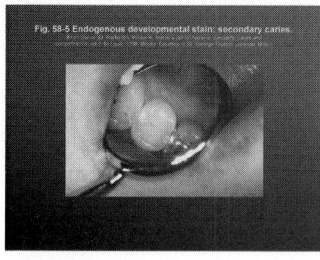

- This photograph displays teeth being reflected by indirect vision in a dental mouth mirror.

- The centrally located tooth is a second permanent premolar and is next to a first molar with an amalgam restoration over the occlusal and distal.

- Secondary or recurrent decay is visible on the interproximal aspect of the premolar with the amalgam because of the altered, more opaque color of the enamel.

Slide 16

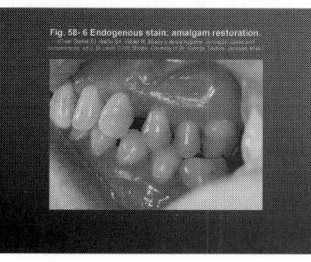

- This photograph shows multiple teeth (a maxillary molar and two premolars, etc.) that have had amalgam restorations placed in the past.

- This is an example of an endogenous source of stain that has been incorporated intrinsically into the tooth.

Bird/Robinson

Slide 17

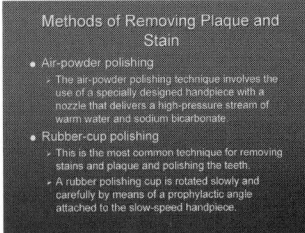

- Using air-powder polishing can be an efficient way to remove stain fast and thoroughly. The operator can control the flow rate; this leads to differences in abrasion.

- The rate at which appropriately chosen stain and plaque are removed depends on the abrasiveness of the polishing paste, the pressure applied to the rubber cup against the tooth, the length of time for polishing, and the technique used to polish.

Slide 18

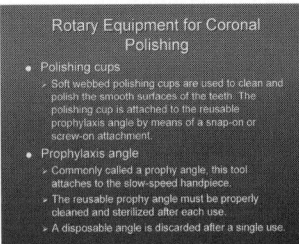

- Polishing cups either come already attached to a disposable prophy angle or they must be newly attached to the reusable resterilized prophy angle heads for each use.

- Disposable prophy angles with attached cups come in a variety of shapes, colors, sizes, and materials.

Slide 19

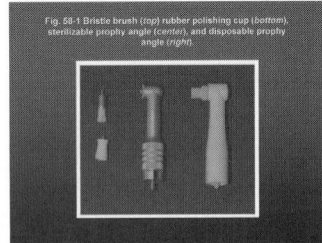

- This photograph shows the bristle brush on the top left and the rubber polishing cup on the bottom left that must be attached as appropriate to the reusable prophy head..

- On the right, a disposable prophy head (white) with the polishing cup (green) already attached is shown.

Slide 20

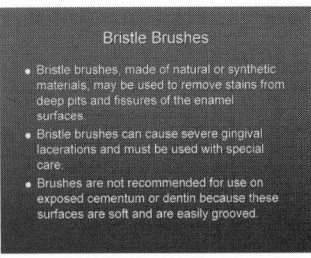

- Always make sure that the patient's cheeks and lips are properly retracted so they are not traumatized by the revolving bristle brush.

- Bristle brushes should be used only on sound enamel.

Bird/Robinson

Slide 21

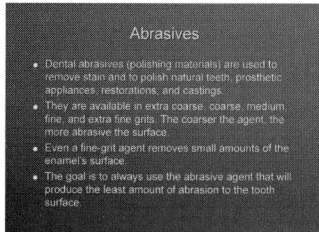

- When choosing the appropriate abrasive, the dental assistant must try to choose the one least harmful to the enamel or restorative surface while still providing enough abrasion to satisfactorily remove the stain and plaque.

Slide 22

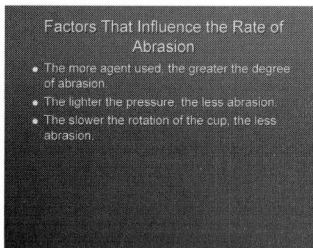

- Using a fulcrum on a nearby tooth will help the operator control the amount of pressure used.

- Rheostats have varying sensitivities. First test the sensitivity of the rheostat that controls the handpiece speed outside of the mouth and away from the patient.

Slide 23

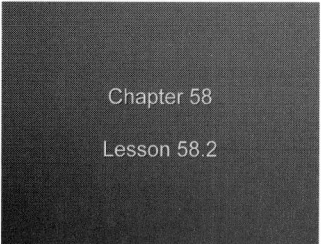

Slide 24

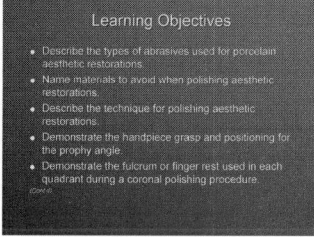

Slide 25

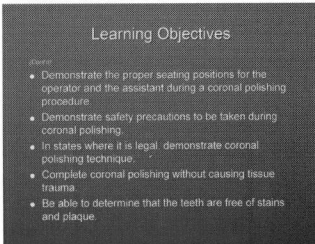

Slide 26

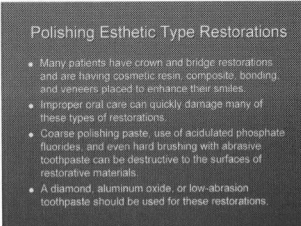

- Should indirect and direct esthetic restorations be polished first? If yes, why?

- Some exogenous sources of staining as well as plaque may not be effectively removed from these restorations via polishing.

Slide 27

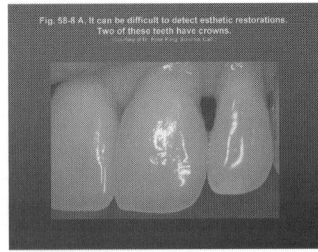

- Teeth #8, #9, and #10 show moderate gingival recession. Avoid polishing the exposed root cementum.

- Although well disguised, now that gingival recession has occurred, it is more noticeable that #8 and #9 have esthetic restorations that should be polished with a low-abrasive polish.

Slide 28

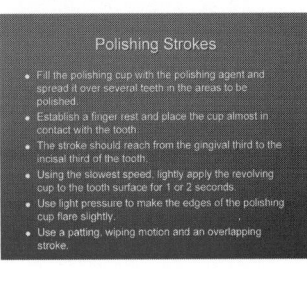

- For better control of the handpiece it is very important to place the fulcrum finger close to the tooth on which the dental assistant is working..

- The cup should be flared to adapt to contours, especially in the interproximal areas where most plaque and stain tends to build up.

Bird/Robinson

Slide 29

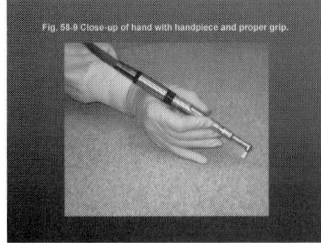

Fig. 58-9 Close-up of hand with handpiece and proper grip.

- Notice that proper infection control is being used, which includes covering the cuffs of the laboratory coat with the gloves.
- What type of prophy angle is shown in this photograph?

Slide 30

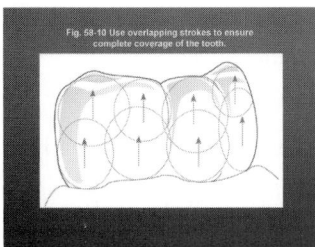

Fig. 58-10 Use overlapping strokes to ensure complete coverage of the tooth.

- This diagram of a molar demonstrates multiple overlapping strokes, always initiated gingivally and directed in the occlusal direction.

Slide 31

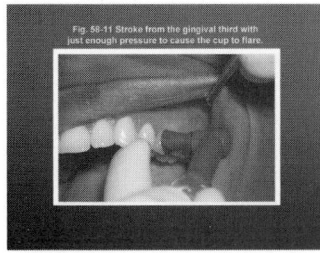

Fig. 58-11 Stroke from the gingival third with just enough pressure to cause the cup to flare.

- This photograph demonstrates proper flaring of the prophy cup.
- Remnants of disclosing solution may be seen on the maxillary labial mucosa.
- What is being used to retract the cheek? *(Dental mouth mirror.)*
- What tooth is the fulcrum on? *(The canine.)*

Slide 32

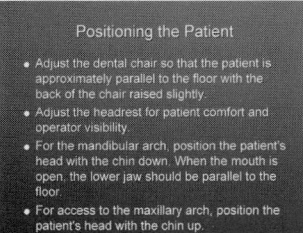

Positioning the Patient

- Adjust the dental chair so that the patient is approximately parallel to the floor with the back of the chair raised slightly.
- Adjust the headrest for patient comfort and operator visibility.
- For the mandibular arch, position the patient's head with the chin down. When the mouth is open, the lower jaw should be parallel to the floor.
- For access to the maxillary arch, position the patient's head with the chin up.

- Positioning the mandibular arch parallel to the floor when open for instrumentation purposes allows for better placement of the light and for direct vision in some areas.
- Positioning the maxillary arch for instrumentation with the chin up places the maxilla almost perpendicular to the floor, allowing for better light placement and access for instrumentation.

ELSEVIER

Torres and Ehrlich Modern Dental Assisting, 9th ed.
Bird/Robinson

Slide 33

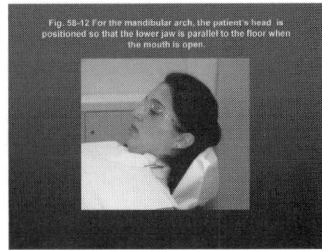

- This photograph displays the recommended placement of the head when polishing the maxillary arch.

- Notice that the chin is directed upwards, and the maxilla is almost perpendicular to the floor.

- Notice that the patient is wearing safety glasses to protect her from any potential splatter from the polishing agent. There is also a headrest covering.

Slide 34

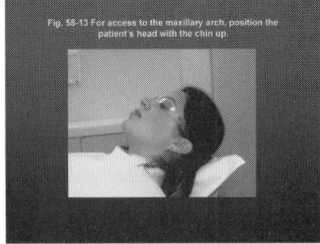

- Polishing of what arch requires this head positioning? *(Mandibular arch.)*

- Notice that the mandible has been placed parallel to the floor.

- This allows for ideal instrumentation and illumination.

- A patient napkin is present to protect the patient's clothes from debris.

Slide 35

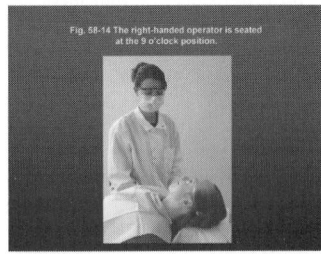

- Remember that the operator may rotate from the 8 o'clock through the 12 o'clock positions as appropriate for treatment.

- What position would the left-handed operator take?

- Notice that the operator has placed the patient at waist level.

Slide 36

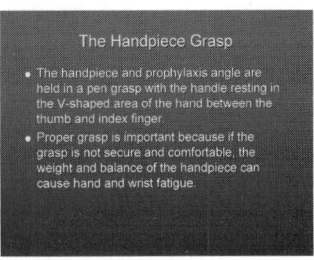

- A proper hand grasp is important for control of the handpiece and the pressure that is exerted on each tooth.

- Ask students to practice this pen grasp with a fulcrum with the pens they are using to take notes in class.

Torres and Ehrlich Modern Dental Assisting, 9th ed.

Bird/Robinson

Slide 37

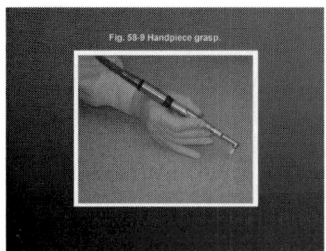

- This is a photograph of the proper hand grasp for a right-handed operator.

Slide 38

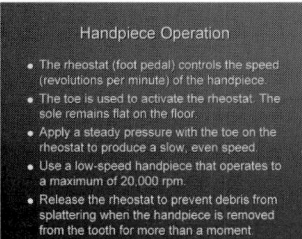

- Make sure that the rheostat is placed conveniently close so it can be reached with the foot. If the rheostat is placed too far away, the operator must strain to reach it.

- Release the rheostat between teeth to insure that the revolving prophy cup or brush tip is not caught on a patient's intraoral soft tissues.

Slide 39

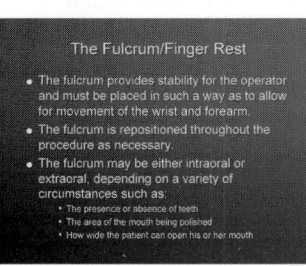

- The operator should always attempt to position the fulcrum close to the tooth being worked on.

- The operator should be sure to change the fulcrum position correspondingly with each tooth in order not to strain his or her fingers and to provide the best support possible to the handpiece.

Slide 40

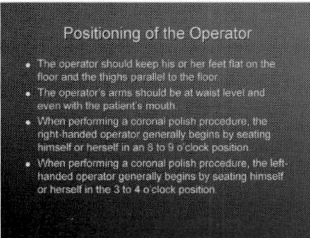

Slide 41

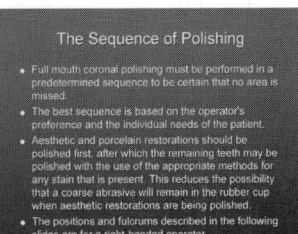

- It is best if possible to complete one arch before the other because of the different head-rest adjustments needed.
- It is also recommended that all buccal or lingual surfaces of one quadrant or sextant are polished before advancing to the next surface because all surfaces require different positioning.
- Remember to polish the esthetic restorations first with the finer polishing agent before completing the rest of the mouth.

Slide 42

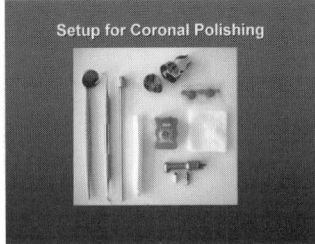

- This photograph illustrates some of the disposable materials that should be available for coronal polishing.
- What is shown in this photograph?
- What are some of the other materials that would be desirable for this procedure?

Slide 43

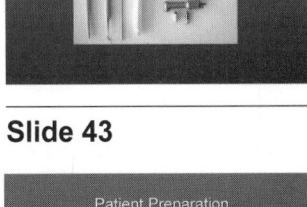

- If a patient is wearing a removable denture or partial, this may be a good time to offer a complimentary cleaning of the prosthesis and placing it in the ultrasonic.
- "Always inform before you perform." The dental assistant should report any suspicious intraoral lesions to the dentist. Some lesions may need further follow-up, while others may contraindicate a coronal polishing at that time.

Slide 44

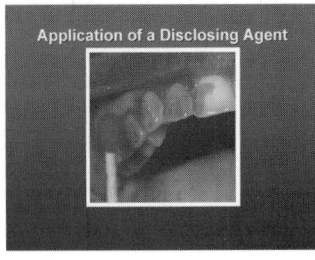

- Once this solution is rinsed off, tooth surfaces with plaque will remain stained for better visibility of areas needing attention.
- This also serves as a tool for patient education by having patients look in a hand mirror while showing them the areas with plaque buildup that should receive more attention during home care.

Slide 45

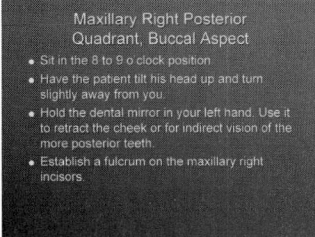

- The following slides follow Procedure 58-1 in the textbook and offer one example of a sequence that may be used for systematic coronal polishing by the right-handed operator.

- The mirror is used for cheek retraction because the buccal surfaces of the right maxilla can usually be seen via direct vision.

- The dental assistant should be positioned for best comfort, control and visibility.

Slide 46

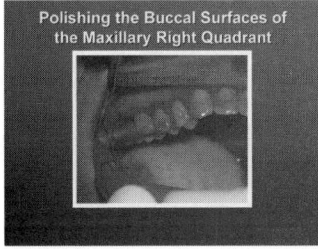

- Notice the disclosing agent that remains, highlighting areas of plaque or tooth structure that naturally attract plaque or stain.

- Be sure to warn the patient if you will use a disclosing agent. Some patients may not wish it to be used as the pink solution may stain other oral tissues for a few hours after the appointment, which may not be socially desirable for their daily activities.

Slide 47

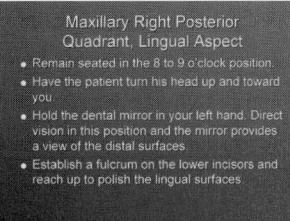

- Only slight adjustments are needed to transfer next to the maxillary right posterior lingual surfaces.

- The patient should be asked to turn his or her head toward the operator.

- Use of the mirror will help with indirect vision, especially of the posterior surfaces. The operator may need to redirect the light source as well.

Slide 48

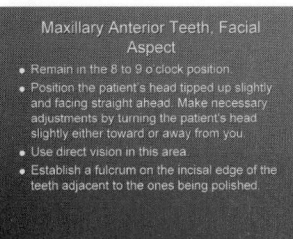

- The operator should remember to add more polishing agent as needed and to be careful not to harm the gingiva.

- Some operators may wish to operate from the 11 o'clock to the 12 o'clock position for this area.

Slide 49

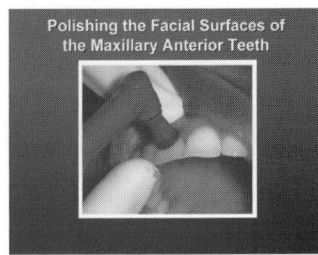

- Notice that the operator has established a fulcrum on an adjacent incisor.
- Notice remnants of the disclosing solution.

Slide 50

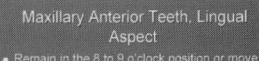

- The most noticeable difference for the lingual aspect of the maxillary teeth is that indirect vision with the mirror is needed.
- The operator should be aware of a variety of developmental lingual pits in the cingulum areas of these teeth that tend to trap much stain and plaque.

Slide 51

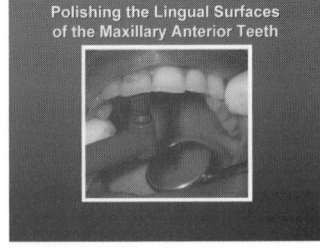

- Notice the use of the mirror for indirect vision.
- Notice the fulcrum on the upper right first premolar.
- Light should be redirected for optimal illumination.

Slide 52

- The patient's head should be tipped slightly toward the operator when the operator is polishing surfaces that are located opposite the operator.
- The patient's napkin should be secured to adequately cover his or her shirt during polishing to avoid unnecessary staining of the patient's clothing.

Slide 53

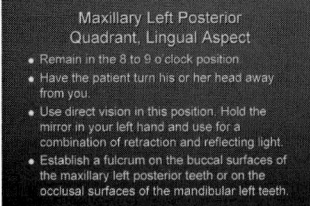

- The patient should turn away from the right-handed operator when the operator polishes surfaces that face the operator.

- What are all of the posterior surfaces that face a right-handed operator when the operator is seated in the 9 o'clock position?

- What are all of the posterior surfaces that face away from a right-handed operator when the operator is seated in the 9 o'clock position?

Slide 54

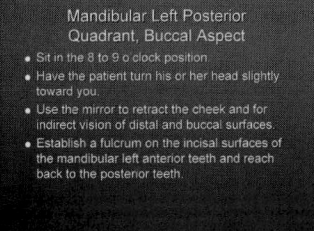

- How would positioning of both operator and patient change for a left-handed operator polishing these surfaces?

Slide 55

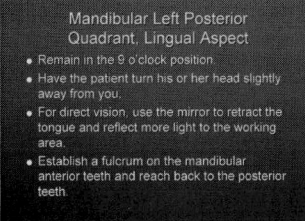

- When polishing the mandibular lingual surfaces, the operator may wish to place a saliva ejector in the area. Saliva tends to pool in these areas during polishing and dilutes the polishing agent or makes the area too slippery to polish.

- The operator may also wish to polish the most posterior teeth first, immediately after suctioning the area, moving anteriorly thereafter.

Slide 56

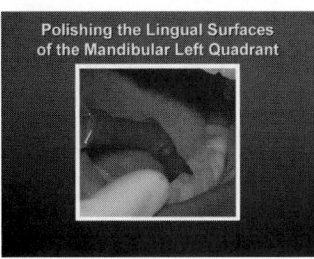

- This operator has chosen a fulcrum position on the mandibular left lateral incisor area.

Bird/Robinson

Slide 57

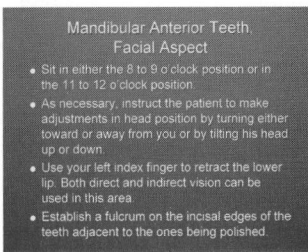

- The operator can retract the lower lip using a square piece of gauze.
- Be sure to establish a stable fulcrum and modify as necessary.

Slide 58

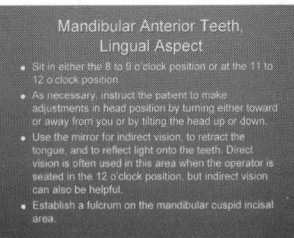

- Depending on the lingual inclination of a patient's mandibular anterior teeth, direct vision may not be possible even with the operator seated at the 12 o'clock position.
- This is a common area of the mouth that tends to accumulate much stain and plaque.

Slide 59

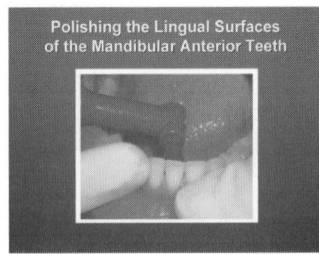

- Notice that a fulcrum is placed on the adjacent teeth for stability, while a finger from the opposite hand helps to retract the lower lip.
- Retraction of the lower lip also helps with transillumination of the tooth.

Slide 60

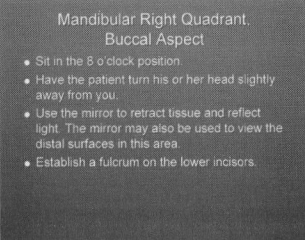

- A right-handed operator should remember to have the patient turn his or her head slightly away for better visibility and access.
- What will change in the positioning of an operator and the positioning of the patient when the operator completes these surfaces and prepares to polish the lingual surfaces?

Torres and Ehrlich Modern Dental Assisting, 9th ed.

Bird/Robinson

Slide 61

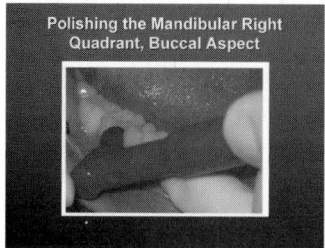

Polishing the Mandibular Right Quadrant, Buccal Aspect

- A fulcrum is placed more anteriorly.
- The mirror is being used for retraction of the cheek.

Slide 62

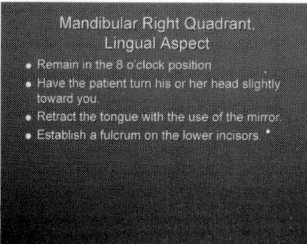

Mandibular Right Quadrant, Lingual Aspect
- Remain in the 8 o'clock position
- Have the patient turn his or her head slightly toward you.
- Retract the tongue with the use of the mirror.
- Establish a fulcrum on the lower incisors.

- Suction may be required when polishing the mandibular lingual surfaces because much saliva tends to accumulate in this area.
- A high-speed suction may be used to simultaneously retract the tongue and provide suction if the mirror is not needed for indirect vision.

Slide 63

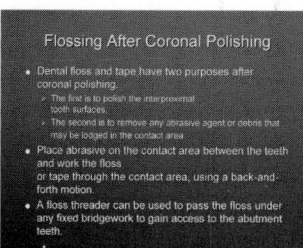

Flossing After Coronal Polishing
- Dental floss and tape have two purposes after coronal polishing.
  - The first is to polish the interproximal tooth surfaces.
  - The second is to remove any abrasive agent or debris that may be lodged in the contact area
- Place abrasive on the contact area between the teeth and work the floss or tape through the contact area, using a back-and-forth motion.
- A floss threader can be used to pass the floss under any fixed bridgework to gain access to the abutment teeth.

- Be sure to ask patients if they can feel any remaining polish between their teeth.
- If a patient had a tremendous amount of plaque between teeth, this may be a good time to review proper use of floss.

Slide 64

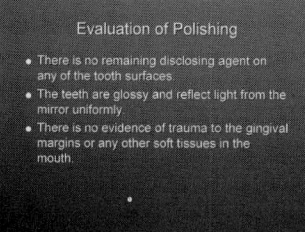

Evaluation of Polishing
- There is no remaining disclosing agent on any of the tooth surfaces.
- The teeth are glossy and reflect light from the mirror uniformly.
- There is no evidence of trauma to the gingival margins or any other soft tissues in the mouth.

- Some operators wish to reapply the disclosing agent after polishing to see if any plaque remains that might require additional polishing before the patient is dismised.
- Ask the patient to run his or her tongue over the surfaces of the teeth to feel the difference after polishing.

Bird/Robinson

Slide 65

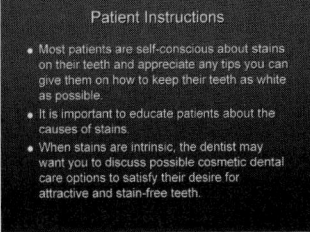

- For the esthetically conscious patient, have the dentist discuss other alternatives, such as at-home vital bleaching, that may help the patient achieve whiter teeth.

- Many patients do not realize how some foods, drinks, and tobacco contribute to initial extrinsic tooth staining. Educate the patient about these issues.

Bird/Robinson

TEACHING FOCUS

This chapter provides students the opportunity to learn about dental sealants, including the clinical indications and contraindications for dental sealants and the rationales for filled and unfilled sealant materials. Students also have the opportunity to describe the two types of polymerization, explain the most important factor in sealant retention, and demonstrate the steps in the application of dental sealants. Finally, students have the opportunity to describe and demonstrate the steps necessary for the patient and operator during sealant placement.

MATERIALS AND RESOURCES

- ☐ applicator syringe or device (Lesson 59.1)
- ☐ articulating paper and holder (Lesson 59.1)
- ☐ basic setup (Lesson 59.1)
- ☐ computer and PowerPoint projector (Lesson 59.1)
- ☐ cotton rolls or rubber dam setup (Lesson 59.1)
- ☐ curing light and appropriate shield (Lesson 59.1)
- ☐ dental floss (Lesson 59.1)
- ☐ dental model (Lesson 59.1)
- ☐ etching agent (liquid or gel) (Lesson 59.1)
- ☐ high-volume oral evacuator (Lesson 59.1)
- ☐ low-speed dental handpiece with contra-angle attachment (Lesson 59.1)
- ☐ materials for occlusal adjustment (Lesson 59.1)
- ☐ prophy brush (Lesson 59.1)
- ☐ pumice and water (Lesson 59.1)
- ☐ round white stone (latch type) (Lesson 59.1)

LESSON CHECKLIST

Preparations for this lesson include:

- lecture
- evaluation of student knowledge and skills needed to perform all entry-level activities related to dental sealants, including:
  - ○ common types of caries seen in schoolchildren
  - ○ pits and fissures, and the accumulation of acid-producing bacteria
  - ○ use of dental sealants
  - ○ dental assistant's role in the application of dental sealants

Torres and Ehrlich Modern Dental Assisting, 9th ed.
Bird/Robinson

KEY TERMS

acrylate (p. 956)
dental sealant (p. 951)
filled resin (p. 953)
light-cured (p. 953)
microleakage (p. 953)

polymerization (p. 952)
sealant retention (p. 956)
self-cured (p. 952)
unfilled resin (p. 953)

ADDITIONAL RESOURCES

PowerPoint slides (Evolve): 1-30
The Interactive Dental Office CD-ROM:
    Todd Ledbetter
    Christopher Brooks
Multimedia Procedures DVD: Applying Dental Sealants

Legend

CTQ
Critical
Thinking
Question

DVD
Multimedia
Procedures
Videos and
Animations

ESLR
EVOLVE
Student
Learning
Resources

IDO
Interactive
Dental
Office
CD-ROM

SW
Student
Workbook

TB
Test Bank
on the
TEACH
CD-ROM

PPT
PowerPoint
Slides

Class Activities are indicated in ***bold italic.***

LESSON 59.1

PRETEST

1. What does the term *polymerization* mean?
   a. changing of a simple chemical into another substance containing the same element
   b. leakage at the margin of the tooth structure and dental sealant material
   c. hardening of a dental material by exposure to ultraviolet light
   d. dental sealant material having the ability to slowly release fluoride

2. Bacteria cannot survive under a properly placed sealant because bacteria need
   a. light in order to live.
   b. a supply of carbohydrates as a nutrient supply in order to live.
   c. a moist environment in order to live.
   d. exposure to new bacterial growth in order to live.

3. What type of procedure is the placement of a dental sealant?
   a. restorative
   b. surgical
   c. preventive invasive
   d. preventive noninvasive

4. What is placed in sealant material to reduce occlusal wear?
   a. color
   b. polymer
   c. filler resin
   d. fluoride

5. What common allergen in dental sealants could cause an allergic reaction if the person already has sensitivity present?
   a. acrylate resin
   b. phosphoric acid
   c. fluoride
   d. bis-GMA

6. What is the primary cause of failure of sealant retention?
   a. preparation of the tooth surface
   b. moisture contamination
   c. curing technique
   d. occlusal height

7. For how many seconds should etchant be in contact with the enamel surface?
   a. 5 to 10 seconds
   b. 10 to 15 seconds
   c. 15 to 60 seconds
   d. 75 to 90 seconds

8. The purpose of the dental floss during dental sealant placement is to
   a. help flow the material into the pits and fissures.
   b. remove excess materials from the occlusal surfaces.
   c. remove excess materials from interproximal surfaces.
   d. remove bacteria that may have come in contact with the enamel surface.

9. What is the time of exposure needed to cure each surface of the dental sealant with the ultraviolet light?
   a. 20 seconds
   b. 40 seconds
   c. 60 seconds
   d. 90 seconds

ELSEVIER

Torres and Ehrlich Modern Dental Assisting, 9th ed.

Bird/Robinson

10. What is the recommended instrument used to check the occlusion of the sealant after placement?
    a. explorer
    b. prophy angle
    c. articulation paper and holder
    d. dental mirror

Answers

1. a	3. d	5. a	7. c	9. a
2. b	4. c	6. b	8. c	10. c

BACKGROUND ASSESSMENT

Question: What tooth surfaces are most susceptible to the development of dental caries? What dental caries preventive agents are recommended for these surfaces? What is the dental material of choice for this preventive agent?

Answer: Smooth surfaces and pits and fissures are all susceptible to dental caries, but natural saliva and regular toothbrushing with a fluoride toothpaste can remove decay-causing bacteria more easily from smooth surfaces. The more vulnerable surfaces are the lingual pit on the maxillary lingual surfaces around the cusps, buccal surfaces of mandibular molars, and lingual surfaces of maxillary incisors. Fissured occlusal surfaces of posterior teeth also are susceptible to developing dental caries. Pit and fissure caries account for at least 88 % of total caries in school-age children in the United States. The recommended dental caries preventive agent for pitted and fissured areas is the dental sealant. Dental sealants are made from acrylate resins.

Question: Are dental sealants recommended for every patient? When are dental sealants contraindicated?

Answer: Sealants are placed primarily in children's teeth, but in certain circumstances adults also can benefit from their use. Dental sealants are especially useful through the caries-active period (ages 6 to 15) to prevent caries formation. Patients who have special needs and limited dexterity also benefit from dental sealant placement. Other people at risk for dental caries (those who undergo head and neck radiation therapy, take medications that cause xerostomia, and children who live in nonfluoridated environments) also would benefit from dental sealants. Sealants are contraindicated if there is a lack of deep fissures and pits; dental decay is obvious; there is proximal surface decay; teeth are insufficiently erupted; the tooth in question is going to be lost soon; or the patient does not cooperate in the dental chair.

CRITICAL THINKING QUESTION

The patient, a 12-year-old boy, shows several areas of tooth decay: #3 mesial, #12 occlusal, #20 occlusal, and #30 on the occlusal and buccal surfaces. His mother expresses concern about the amount of decay and asks the dental assistant what can be done to prevent more problems. How should the dental assistant respond?

Guidelines: The dental assistant should explain that the dentist will treat the cavities appropriately in the office. The dentist will also evaluate the risk for dental caries based on the amount of pitted and fissured areas present in the boy's teeth. Regarding reducing the risk for more decay, the dental assistant should explain that fluoride is the best agent for preventing caries from forming on smooth surfaces of teeth. Many community water supplies contain fluoride. Many toothpastes, gels, and mouth rinses also contain fluoride. At home, the boy should brush and floss his teeth at least twice a day and eat a balanced diet. In addition, a sealant to prevent caries from forming in pitted and fissured areas of the teeth, which can lead to decay of the kind presented at this visit, can be applied in the dental office. The dental assistant should explain that applying a sealant prevents the accumulation of acid-producing bacteria in pitted and fissured (or grooved) areas of the teeth, where saliva is not as effective in removing food particles. Even toothbrush bristles are too large to thoroughly clean these areas. The sealant forms a physical barrier against bacteria and dietary carbohydrates that produce acid, causing caries. The dental assistant can tell the patient and his mother that placing the sealant is a noninvasive procedure that can help preserve tooth structure and prevent tooth decay. For the procedure to be effective, the dental assistant should emphasize that it is important for the patient to remain still so that proper placement and adhesion can occur.

Bird/Robinson

OBJECTIVES	CONTENT	TEACHING RESOURCES
Pronounce, define, and spell the Key Terms.	■ Key terms (p. 950)	*e* ESLR Electronic Flashcards ▸ Discuss each of the key terms in the chapter, focusing on definition, pronunciation, and spelling of each term. ***Class Activity** Have students make flash cards with the key term on one side and the definition on the other side, and then quiz each other. As a class, have students use each key term correctly in a sentence.*
Describe the purpose of dental sealants.	■ Introduction (p. 951) ■ How sealants work (p. 951) ■ Dental caries and sealants (p. 951)	PPT 5-6 TB question 1 SW Short-Answer Questions 1; Multiple Choice questions 1-2 (pp. 521-522) Figure 59-1 Scanning electron micrograph (SEM) of occlusal pits and fissures (p. 951) Figure 59-2 Micrograph showing toothbrush bristle in a groove (p. 951) Figure 59-3 Molar with a properly placed sealant (p. 951) Recall questions 1-2 (p. 951) ▸ Discuss how fluorides affect the pits and fissures of teeth. ***Class Activity** Divide the class into groups and ask each group to identify the purpose of placing dental sealants. Groups also should describe three situations in which application of dental sealants would be recommended. Have groups share their findings with the class.*
Describe the clinical indications for dental sealants.	■ Indications for sealants (p. 952)	PPT 7-11 TB questions 2, 9 SW Short-Answer Questions 2; Multiple Choice question 3 (pp. 521-522) SW Case Study questions 1, 5 (pp. 522-523) Indications for Sealant Placement (p. 952) Recall question 3 (p. 953) CTQ 1, 3 (p. 957) ▸ Discuss the components of a preventive program for children, including the role of dental sealants. ***Class Activity** Present the following clinical situations to the class and have students determine if a dental sealant is appropriate or contraindicated. Ask students to explain their reasons.*

OBJECTIVES	CONTENT	TEACHING RESOURCES
		– *Composite restoration, anterior teeth, 55-year-old man*
		– *Mandibular molars have deep pits, school-age girl*
		– *Small cavity in 47-year-old woman who has had few dental problems*
		– *Severe decay in several teeth of HIV-positive man*
		– *Elderly stroke patient who has limited arm movement and who takes medication that produces dry mouth*
Describe the contraindications for dental sealants.	■ Contraindications to sealants (p. 952)	PPT 12 TB question 3 SW Short-Answer Questions 3; Multiple Choice question 3 (pp. 521-522) Contraindications of Sealant Placement (p. 952) Recall question 3 (p. 953) CTQ 2-3 (p. 957) ▸ Discuss why the cooperation of the patient during dental sealant placement is important. What is the role dental sealants play in a preventive program? *Class Activity Ask the class to describe contraindications for dental sealants and write student responses on the board. Write on the board two column headings: Harmful and Unsuccessful. Ask students which column the contraindication belongs in and why.*
Describe the two types of polymerization.	■ Types of sealant materials (p. 952) ☐ Method of polymerization (p. 952) ☐ Color (p. 953)	PPT 13-16 TB questions 7-8 SW Short-Answer Questions 5; Fill in the Blank questions 3-4; Multiple Choice question 4 (pp. 521-522) Figure 59-4 Helioseal Clear sealant material (p. 952) Recall questions 4-5 (p. 953) ▸ Discuss the advantages of light-cured dental sealants compared to self-cured dental sealants. *Class Activity Divide the class into groups and assign each group a filled resin or an unfilled resin dental sealant to study. Students may research their topics outside of class. Ask each group to make a presentation about the properties of the assigned resin. As a class compare and contrast filled and unfilled resins. For what procedures are each commonly used? (For students to prepare for this activity, see Homework/Assignments #1.)*

OBJECTIVES	CONTENT	TEACHING RESOURCES
Discuss the rationale for filled and unfilled sealant materials.	☐ Fillers (p. 953) ☐ Working time (p. 953) ☐ Placement technique (p. 953) ☐ Fluoride release (p. 953)	PPT 17-18 TB questions 4, 12-13 SW Short-Answer Questions 4; Fill in the Blank questions 5-6; Multiple Choice question 6 (pp. 521-522) Recall questions 6-7 (pp. 953, 956) ▸ Discuss the difference in microleakage between filled and unfilled resins, and compare their rates of retention. ***Class Activity** Ask for student volunteers to participate in a debate in which one side argues for filled sealant materials and the other side argues for unfilled sealant materials. Each side should describe how its sealant works, its composition, address microleakage, and present rationales for its position. Have the rest of the class evaluate the arguments for accuracy, clarity, and completeness.*
Demonstrate the steps in the application of dental sealants.	■ Storage and use (p. 956) ■ Precautions for dental personnel and patients (p. 956) ☐ Etchant precautions (p. 956) ☐ Sealant precautions (p. 956) ■ Factors in sealant retention (p. 956) Procedure 59-1 Application of dental sealants (pp. 955-956) (SW/ESLR Competency 59-1, p. 525)	PPT 19-30 Multimedia Procedures DVD: Applying Dental Sealants TB questions 6, 10-11, 14 SW Short-Answer Questions 6; Multiple Choice questions 7, 9 (521-522) SW Case Study (pp. 522-523) SW/IDO Patient Case Exercise: Ledbetter questions 1-3 (p. 523) (The Interactive Dental Office CD-ROM) SW/ESLR Competency 59-1 Application of Dental Sealants (p. 525) Manufacturer's Instructions (p. 956) Recall questions 8-9 (p. 956) ▸ Discuss the basic equipment and supplies needed to apply dental sealants. ▸ Discuss how moisture control can affect sealant retention. What are appropriate moisture control procedures and isolation techniques for dental sealant application? ***Class Activity** Demonstrate the steps used in the application of dental sealants. Then have students practice working with the materials using a typodont.*

ELSEVIER

Bird/Robinson

OBJECTIVES	CONTENT	TEACHING RESOURCES
Describe and demonstrate the safety steps necessary for the patient and operator during sealant placement.	■ Precautions for dental personnel and patients (p. 956) □ Etchant precautions (p. 956) □ Sealant precautions (p. 956) ■ Factors in sealant retention (p. 956)	⊠▤ PPT 20-22 ▤ SW Short-Answer Questions 7; Multiple Choice questions 9 (pp. 521-522) ▤● SW/IDO Patient Case Exercise: Brooks questions 1-4 (p. 523) (The Interactive Dental Office CD-ROM) Recall question 9 (p. 956) ▸ Discuss why protective eyewear should be worn when using etchants and sealants containing acrylate resins. ***Class Activity As a class describe the safety procedures necessary for patient and operator when dental sealant is placed on teeth. Demonstrate the steps and then have students practice in pairs using a typodont. Ask student volunteers to demonstrate the safety techniques on the typodont, explaining the steps and the reasons for each one to the class. What would happen if the safety measures were not followed?***
Explain the most important factor in sealant retention.	■ Factors in sealant retention (p. 956)	⊠▤ PPT 23 ▤ SW Short-Answer Questions 8; Multiple Choice question 10 (pp. 521-522) Recall question 10 (p. 956) 💡 CTQ 2 (p. 957) ***Class Activity Lead a discussion in which students describe the main factors affecting how long sealant remains on the tooth. What specific steps in the sealant application procedure are designed to ensure sealant retention?***
Performance Evaluation		🖥 TB ▤ SW questions (pp. 521-522) ▤ SW Case Study (pp. 522-523) ▤● SW/IDO Patient Case Exercise (p. 523) (The Interactive Dental Office CD-ROM) ▤✎ SW/ESLR Competency 59-1 Application of Dental Sealants (p. 525) ✎ ESLR Electronic Flashcards ✎ ESLR Practice Quiz questions Recall questions (pp. 951-956) 💡 CTQ (p. 957)

Torres and Ehrlich Modern Dental Assisting, 9th ed.

Bird/Robinson

59.1 Homework/Assignments:

1. Divide the class into groups and assign each group a filled resin or an unfilled resin dental sealant to study. Students may research their topics outside of class. Ask each group to make a presentation about the properties of the assigned resin. As a class compare and contrast filled and unfilled resins. For what procedures are they commonly used?

59.1 Instructor's Notes/Student Feedback:

Bird/Robinson

Slide 1

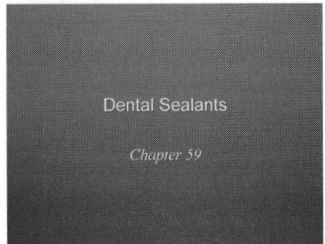

Dental Sealants

Chapter 59

Slide 2

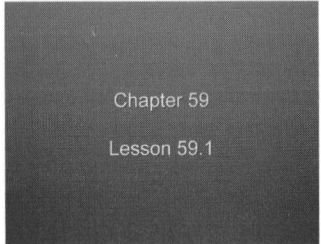

Chapter 59

Lesson 59.1

Slide 3

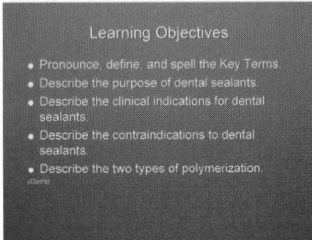

Learning Objectives

- Pronounce, define, and spell the Key Terms.
- Describe the purpose of dental sealants.
- Describe the clinical indications for dental sealants.
- Describe the contraindications to dental sealants.
- Describe the two types of polymerization.

Slide 4

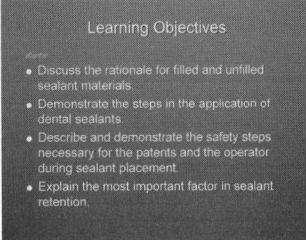

Learning Objectives

- Discuss the rationale for filled and unfilled sealant materials.
- Demonstrate the steps in the application of dental sealants.
- Describe and demonstrate the safety steps necessary for the patents and the operator during sealant placement.
- Explain the most important factor in sealant retention.

Bird/Robinson

Slide 5

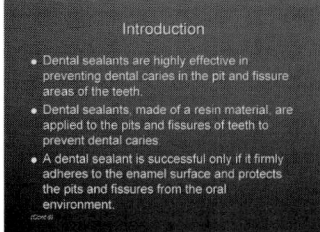

- As part of a complete prevention program, dental sealants, sometimes called pit and fissure sealants, are indicated for selected patients.
- Which dental caries preventive agent protects smooth surfaces best? (*Topical fluoride.*)
- What dental caries preventive agent protects the pits and fissures found on occlusal surfaces and pits on buccal and lingual surfaces best? (*Dental sealants.*)

Slide 6

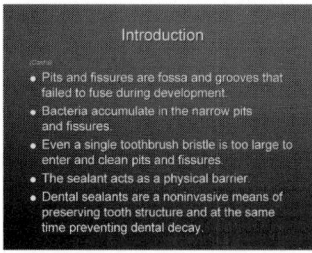

- Why are dental sealants the best defense against occlusal caries formation?
- A barrier must be created between the vulnerable pits and fissures of the tooth and the oral environment.

Slide 7

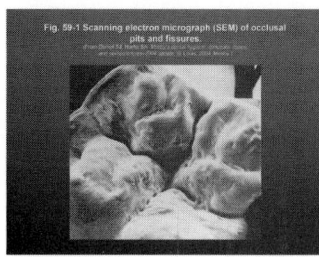

- Notice the crevice-type appearance of fissures and pits viewed on this occlusal surface.
- Sealants are recommended for primary and permanent teeth that have pits and fissures.
- Where on the teeth surfaces are pits and fissures located?

Slide 8

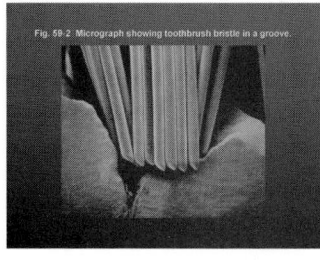

- Even though toothbrush bristles are thin and fine, access into the minute pits and fissures is impossible.
- Areas that cannot be accessed during toothbrushing and dental flossing to remove harmful microorganisms are vulnerable to the formation of caries.

Torres and Ehrlich Modern Dental Assisting, 9th ed.
Bird/Robinson

Slide 9

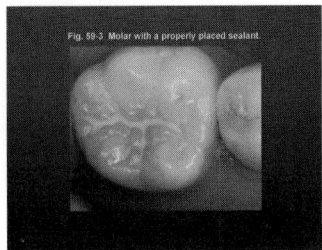

Fig. 59-3 Molar with a properly placed sealant.

- Notice that the deep, vulnerable pits and fissures viewed on the previous slides now are sealed and smooth for easier cleaning and removal of harmful microorganisms by toothbrush bristles.

- The dental sealant material used on the molar pictured on the slide is an opaque, or white-colored, material; opaque dental materials are often referred to as "tooth-colored" materials.

- Dental sealants are made of a resin material; currently, most sealants are made of Bis-GMA.

Slide 10

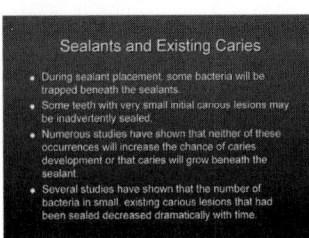

Sealants and Existing Caries

- During sealant placement, some bacteria will be trapped beneath the sealants.
- Some teeth with very small initial carious lesions may be inadvertently sealed.
- Numerous studies have shown that neither of these occurrences will increase the chance of caries development or that caries will grow beneath the sealant.
- Several studies have shown that the number of bacteria in small, existing carious lesions that had been sealed decreased dramatically with time.

- What is the most common microorganism responsible for the formation of dental caries? *(Streptococcus mutans.)*

- What type of bacteria is a *S. mutans*? *(Aerobic.)*

- If the microorganisms are cut off from oxygen after dental sealant placement, will they survive? Why or why not? *(No, because they need oxygen to survive.)*

Slide 11

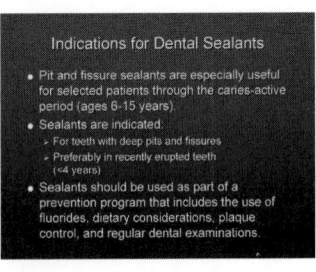

Indications for Dental Sealants

- Pit and fissure sealants are especially useful for selected patients through the caries-active period (ages 6-15 years).
- Sealants are indicated:
  - For teeth with deep pits and fissures
  - Preferably in recently erupted teeth (<4 years)
- Sealants should be used as part of a prevention program that includes the use of fluorides, dietary considerations, plaque control, and regular dental examinations.

- When current caries lesions and previous restored teeth exist, newly erupted teeth should be treated promptly with dental sealants..

- Which other patients would benefit from the placement of dental sealants as part of a dental caries prevention program?

Slide 12

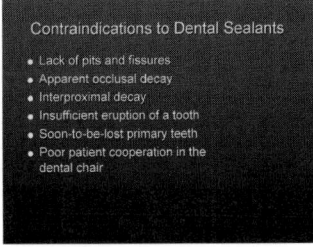

Contraindications to Dental Sealants

- Lack of pits and fissures
- Apparent occlusal decay
- Interproximal decay
- Insufficient eruption of a tooth
- Soon-to-be-lost primary teeth
- Poor patient cooperation in the dental chair

- What tools or methods can be used to determine if contraindications to dental sealants exists?

- Who can determine whether an area viewed clinically or radiographically may have dental caries or is susceptible to dental caries formation?

- Who can diagnose dental caries and determine which teeth should or should not be sealed? *(The dentist.)*

Bird/Robinson

Slide 13

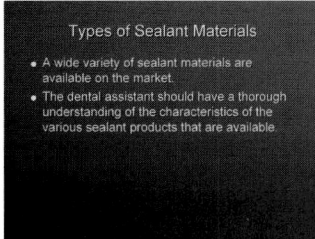

- Sealants are classified by their method of polymerization, their sealant content, and their color.

- What does the term "polymerization" mean? (*Process of changing a simple chemical into another substance containing the same elements.*)

Slide 14

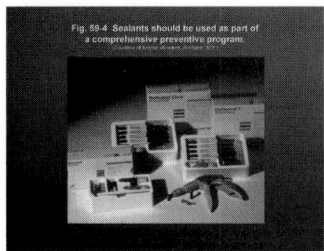

- Pictured on this slide is *Helioseal Clear* sealant material.

- Sealant kits contain all the dental materials needed to place the sealant; additional disposable equipment may be included.

- Accessory materials and instruments may be needed as well, including: cotton roll, gauze, saliva ejector, dental mirror, cotton forceps/pliers, explorer, dental floss, disposable prophy angle, and articulating paper.

Slide 15

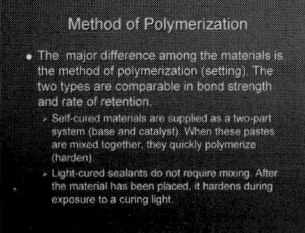

- Self-cured materials usually set within 1 minute. It is important to place the material before the initial stage of hardening or curing begins.

- Light-cured materials are available in a one-step delivery system in which the material is provided in a light-protected preloaded syringe and is ready for direct application to the tooth.

- What is an advantage to using light-cured sealant material?

Slide 16

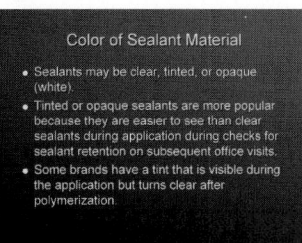

- Why are clear sealant materials still used even though tinted or opaque materials are easier for the clinician to use and identify later?

- Does the color of the sealant affect retention?

Bird/Robinson

Slide 17

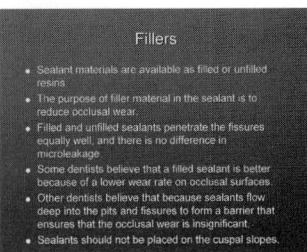

- What is microleakage? (*Leakage between the tooth surface and the sealant material.*)
- Unfilled sealants are recommended for use in school-based sealant programs because there is no—or limited—access to a dentist's handpiece.

Slide 18

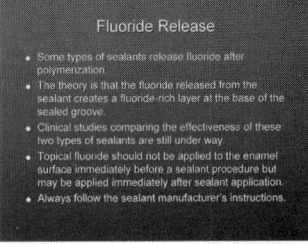

- What type of material is a fluoride-releasing sealant made of? (*Glass ionomer, because it ionomer contains slow-release fluoride.*)
- What is a disadvantage of using glass ionomer sealant materials? (*Glass ionomer sealants may crack readily when placed and show high occlusal wear.*)

Slide 19

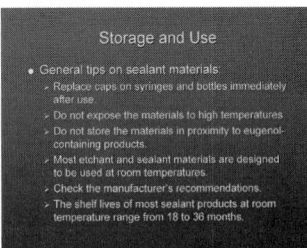

- Why is it important to read and follow instruction specifications for the brand being used?
- Storage of some sealant materials in a cool, dry place such as a refrigerator will increase shelf life.

Slide 20

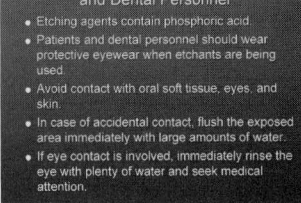

- Why is acid etchant used during the dental sealant placement procedure?
- Etchant is usually in a gel form that can be painted on with a small brush or delivered in a preloaded syringe.
- It is important to avoid touching the etched enamel surface with an instrument after etching has taken place to avoid smoothing the micropores.

Slide 21

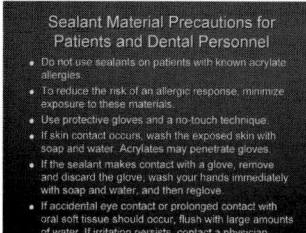

- What are signs and symptoms of an allergic reaction? *(Skin irritation, rash, burning sensation of the area exposed to the allergen, swelling of the mucosa, breathing difficulty, dyspnea, cyanosis, sweating, dilation of pupils, and cardiovascular involvement.)*

Slide 22

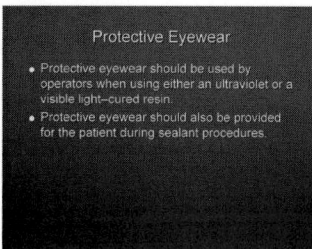

- Many light-curing wands also have an ultraviolet light shield near the tip of the light wand to protect the operator's and the dental assistant's eyes from exposure to the ultraviolet light.

Slide 23

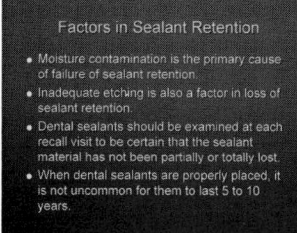

- Moisture control techniques enhance the retention success of the sealant.

- What are some isolation moisture control techniques used during dental sealant placement?

Slide 24

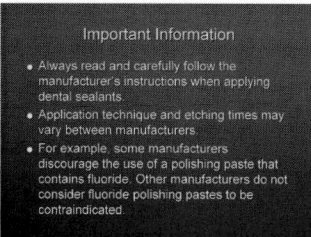

- Why is it important to read and follow manufacturer's guidelines when using dental sealant materials and products?

Slide 25

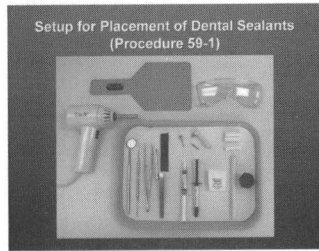

- The tray contains examination instruments, articulating paper and holder, sealant material (etch and sealant), dental floss to check the contact areas after sealant placement, disposable prophy angle to prepare the tooth, moisture control items (cotton rolls and HVE), and a dappen dish to hold liquid materials such as the pumice.

Slide 26

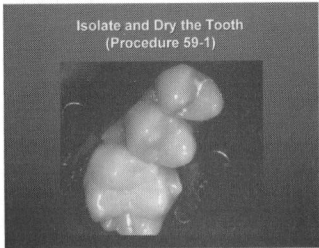

- Remember, moisture contamination during sealant placement can cause the sealant to fail.

- What isolation technique is shown in the slide? *(Dental dam.)*

Slide 27

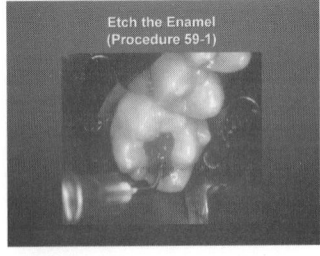

- Apply a generous amount of etchant to all enamel surfaces to be sealed, extending slightly beyond the anticipated margin of the sealant.

- Etchant is usually placed for a minimum of 15 seconds but no longer than 60 seconds.

- What is a consequence of incomplete etching of the enamel surface? *(Decreased retention of the sealant.)*

Slide 28

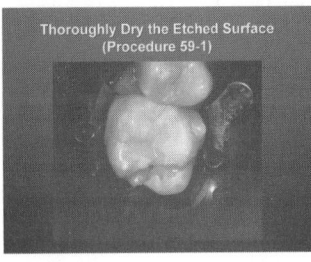

- After the allotted time for exposure of the enamel to the etchant, rinse the etched teeth thoroughly.

- Dry the surfaces with the air-water syringe.

- When the surface of the enamel is etched, the dried etched surface will appear as matte frosty white.

- What if the matte frosty white enamel surface is not evident? *(Repeat the etch step.)*

Bird/Robinson

Slide 29

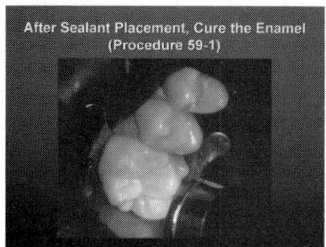

After Sealant Placement, Cure the Enamel (Procedure 59-1)

- Place the sealant using the delivery method recommended by the manufacturer.
- Slowly introduce the sealant material to the pits and fissures to avoid damaging the micropores and to avoid the formation of air bubbles.
- Next, cure the sealant using the ultraviolet light.

Slide 30

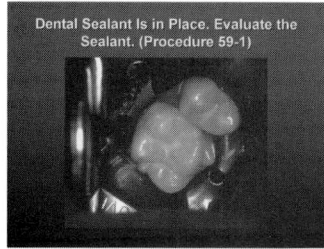

Dental Sealant Is in Place. Evaluate the Sealant. (Procedure 59-1)

- Always evaluate the sealant after placement:
  - Use an explorer to ensure that all margins are sealed and no microleakage can occur.
  - Floss the contacts to ensure that no excess sealant materials have flowed into the interproximal areas.
  - Check the occlusion with articulating paper to ensure the patient is comfortable when biting on the newly placed sealant.

TEACHING FOCUS

This chapter gives students the opportunity to learn key terms relating to orthodontics and learn how to describe the environment of an orthodontic practice. The students will also have the opportunity to describe the types of malocclusion, discuss corrective orthodontics, describe the types of treatment involved, and become familiar with the types of diagnostic records used to assess orthodontic problems. The components of the fixed appliance, the use and function of headgear, and the ways to convey the importance of dietary and oral hygiene habits in orthodontics will be discussed. How to place and remove brass wire separators, steel-separating springs, and elastomeric ring separators will also be described. Students will also have the opportunity to assist in the fitting and cementation of orthodontic bands, assist in the direct bonding of orthodontic brackets, place an arch wire, and place and remove ligature ties and elastomeric ties.

MATERIALS AND RESOURCES

- ☐ computer and PowerPoint projector (all Lessons)
- ☐ examples of headgear and retainers (Lesson 60.2)
- ☐ examples of orthodontic records (Lesson 60.1)
- ☐ examples of specialized tools used in orthodontics (Lesson 60.2)
- ☐ fixed appliances: brackets, bands, ligature ties, arch wires, headgear tubes, separators, edgewise tubes, labial hooks, and lingual arch attachments (Lesson 60.2)
- ☐ materials and equipment to demonstrate bracket bonding (Lesson 60.2)
- ☐ study model, brass wire separator, and instruments for placement and removal (Lesson 60.2)
- ☐ study models with different malocclusions (Lesson 60.1)

- ☐ study models, elastic ring separators, and instruments for placement and removal (Lesson 60.2)
- ☐ study models, instruments for fitting and placement of an arch wire, and a variety of arch wires (Lesson 60.2)
- ☐ study models, materials, and instruments for placement and removal of elastomeric ties (Lesson 60.2)
- ☐ study models, materials, and instruments for the placement and removal of ligature ties (Lesson 60.2)
- ☐ study models, orthodontic bands, instruments for filing and cementation of orthodontic bands, cement, spatulas, and glass slab (Lesson 60.2)
- ☐ study models, steel-separating springs, and instruments for placement and removal (Lesson 60.2)
- ☐ typodonts showing different types of occlusion (Lesson 60.1)

LESSON CHECKLIST

Preparations for this lesson include:

- lecture
- evaluation of student knowledge and skills needed to perform all entry-level activities related to orthodontics, including:
  - o identifying other dentists with whom orthodontists work
  - o understanding the education required to be an orthodontist
  - o understanding causes of occlusion
  - o performing basic procedures in orthodontic treatment

Bird/Robinson

KEY TERMS

arch wire (p. 969)
auxiliary (p. 969)
band (p. 970)
braces (p. 969)
bracket (p. 973)
cephalometric radiograph (p. 964)
crossbite (p. 962)
crowding (p. 962)
dentofacial (p. 959)
distoclusion (p. 961)
fetal molding (p. 960)
headgear (p. 978)

ligature tie (p. 978)
malocclusion (p. 961)
mesioclusion (p. 961)
occlusion (p. 960)
open bite (p. 962)
orthodontics (p. 959)
overbite (p. 962)
overjet (p. 962)
positioner (p. 981)
retainer (p. 981)
separator (p. 970)

ADDITIONAL RESOURCES

PowerPoint slides (Evolve): 1-59
The Interactive Dental Office CD-ROM: Kevin McClelland

Legend

CTQ	**DVD**	**ESLR**	**IDO**	**SW**	**TB**	**PPT**
Critical Thinking Question	Multimedia Procedures Videos and Animations	EVOLVE Student Learning Resources	Interactive Dental Office CD-ROM	Student Workbook	Test Bank on the TEACH CD-ROM	PowerPoint Slides

Class Activities are indicated in ***bold italic.***

Torres and Ehrlich Modern Dental Assisting, 9th ed.

Bird/Robinson

LESSON 60.1

PRETEST

1. Orthodontic appliances can move teeth because
   a. bone is elastic.
   b. roots dissolve.
   c. bone resorbs under pressure.
   d. new bone forms under tension and dissolves under pressure.

2. When is a Hawley retainer used?
   a. during the active phase of treatment to align the teeth
   b. when fixed appliances cannot fit because of movement of the teeth
   c. in conjunction with headgear
   d. after fixed appliances have been removed during the retention phase of the orthodontic treatment

3. What facial profile is associated with Class I occlusion?
   a. retrognathic
   b. mesognathic
   c. distognathic
   d. prognathic

4. What occlusion is known as *mesioocclusion*?
   a. Class I
   b. Class II, division 1
   c. Class II, division 2
   d. Class III

5. An excessive protrusion of the maxillary incisors that causes space or distance between the facial surface of the mandibular incisors and the lingual surface of the maxillary incisors is known as
   a. crossbite.
   b. open bite.
   c. overjet.
   d. crowding.

6. The degree of cooperativeness of the patient is evaluated during
   a. social and behavior evaluation.
   b. dental and medical history evaluation.
   c. clinical evaluation.
   d. collection of the diagnostic record.

7. How many standard extraoral photographs are taken during the diagnostic record collection step?
   a. one
   b. two
   c. three
   d. four

8. What radiograph is used for orthodontic treatment?
   a. full mouth series
   b. bite-wing x-rays
   c. cephalometric radiograph
   d. panoramic radiograph

9. What orthodontic instrument is used to help seat a molar band for a fixed appliance?
   a. orthodontic scaler
   b. orthodontic plugger
   c. orthodontic tweezer
   d. bird-beak pliers

10. What must be placed before orthodontic bands can be seated?
    a. bracket
    b. ligature
    c. arch wire
    d. separator

Answers

1. d	3. b	5. c	7. b	9. b
2. d	4. d	6. a	8. c	10. d

BACKGROUND ASSESSMENT

Question: What is orthodontics? What is an orthodontist? How does the environment of an orthodontic office differ from that of a general dental practice?

Answer: Orthodontics is the specialty of dentistry concerned with the supervision, guidance, and correction of the growing and mature dentofacial structures. The emphasis of the orthodontist is orofacial growth and development. Orthodontists work with pediatric and general dentists to provide an opportunity to change a person's smile. Orthodontists are specialists who have at least two years additional education beyond their dental degree. Most accredited orthodontic programs are three years long. The orthodontic office is designed to accommodate many patients at a time. Because very little equipment is required in orthodontic procedures, most orthodontic offices use an "open bay" concept. The patient care area of the office is sectioned off to serve three functions: (1) to obtain records and create a more private setting, (2) to take radiographs, and (3) to provide patient care for all stages of treatment.

Question: What is malocclusion? How is malocclusion classified? What causes malocclusion?

Answer: Malocclusion is the abnormal or malpositioned relationship of the maxillary teeth to the mandibular teeth when occluded. Angle's classification of malocclusion covers three different categories or classifications. Class I malocclusion of neutroclusion is considered normal occlusion with a few possible variations of crowding in the anterior teeth, protruded or retruded anterior teeth, and crossbites or slight mesial drifting of teeth. In Class II malocclusion or distoclusion the body of the mandible is in an abnormal distal relationship to the maxilla. Class II is further divided into two divisions. In division one, the mandible is retruded and the maxillary incisors are protruded; in division two, both mandibular and maxillary anterior teeth are retruded. In Class III malocclusion, or mesioclusion, the mandibular teeth are anterior to the normal position in relation to maxillary teeth. Malocclusion problems of most people come from an interaction of developmental, genetic, environmental, and functional influences.

CRITICAL THINKING QUESTION

An experienced dental assistant is instructed by the orthodontist to train the new assistant so that she can be an effective member of the orthodontic team. What background information should an orthodontic assistant understand about malocclusion and its causes? What aspects of the patient and the patient record relate to treatment and appointment procedures?

Guidelines: To understand malocclusion, it is important to understand the variations among individuals in the size and shape of the jaws and in the occlusions, and why some teeth become crowded. Generally malocclusion and other dentofacial deformities result from moderate distortions of normal development. The orthodontic problems of most patients come from the interaction of developmental, genetic, environmental, and functional influences. Disturbances in development usually include congenitally missing teeth, malformed teeth, supernumerary teeth, eruption interruption, and ectopic eruption. Genetic causes are responsible for malocclusion when there are discrepancies in the size of the jaw or the teeth. Environmental causes include birth injuries during fetal development or delivery and traumatic injury throughout life. Functional or oral habits involving sucking the thumb, lip, tongue, or fingers can all influence malalignment of teeth. The dental assistant must also be able to evaluate the patient and the patient records. The first step to determine what should be prepared for each appointment is to learn about the patient's orthodontic condition. Careful review of the medical and dental histories to understand the physical condition of the patient is important. A physical growth evaluation should also be reviewed to understand the current stage of treatment. Social and behavioral evaluation will tell the dental assistant what motivates the patient in terms of his or her orthodontic care and how cooperative the patient will be during the appointment. The clinical evaluation is reviewed and updated to determine changes that might have occurred with the facial aspects, the occlusal relationship, and functional characteristics. Review of the diagnostic records, including the radiographs, photographs, and study models, will guide the dental assistant in determining the overall goal of the treatment—what has been achieved, and what has not yet been completed.

Bird/Robinson

OBJECTIVES	CONTENT	TEACHING RESOURCES
Pronounce, define, and spell the Key Terms.	■ Key terms (pp. 958-959)	*e* ESLR Electronic Flashcards ***Class Activity** Have students make flash cards of each term with the key term on one side and the definition on the other. Then, have the students quiz one another with the flash cards.*
Describe the environment of an orthodontic practice.	■ Introduction (p. 959) ■ The orthodontist (p. 959) ■ The orthodontic assistant (p. 960) ■ The orthodontic office (p. 960)	⊠■ PPT 4 SW Short-Answer Questions 1; Fill in the Blank question 16 (pp. 527-528) Recall question 1 (p. 961) ▸ Discuss the various functions of the orthodontic office. ***Class Activity** Before class, have each student research an orthodontic office floor plan and layout. Have each student download or print photos, pictures, and/or floor plans of the office he or she researches. Then ask students to present their findings in class, including a description of the strengths and weaknesses of the floor plan. (For students to prepare for this activity, see Homework/Assignments #1.)*
Describe the types of malocclusion.	■ Understanding occlusion (p. 960) ☐ Developmental causes (p. 960) ☐ Genetic causes (p. 960) ☐ Environmental causes (p. 960) – Birth injuries (p. 960) – Injury throughout life (p. 960) ☐ Habits (p. 960) ■ Occlusion (p. 961) ☐ Malocclusion (p. 961) – Class II malocclusion (p. 961) – Class III malocclusion (p. 961) ☐ Malaligned teeth (p. 962)	⊠■ PPT 5-16 TB TB questions 1-3 SW Short-Answer Questions 2; Fill in the Blank questions 8-9, 11, 14-15, 19; Multiple Choice questions 2-3, 5-6 (pp. 527-529) Recall question 2 (p. 961) Table 60-1 Habits Affecting the Dentition (p. 961) Figure 60-1 Class I occlusion (p. 961) Figure 60-2 Class II malocclusion (p. 961) Figure 60-3 Class III malocclusion (p. 962) Figure 60-4 Crowding of teeth in the mandibular arch (p. 962) Figure 60-5 Excessive protrusion of the maxillary incisors creates an overjet (p. 962) Figure 60-6 Overbite (p. 962) Figure 60-7 An open bite is created when patient's anterior teeth make an opening (p. 963) Figure 60-8 An example of a crossbite showing an improper alignment of the maxillary and mandibular canines (p. 963) Recall questions 3-6 (p. 963)

Torres and Ehrlich Modern Dental Assisting, 9th ed.

Bird/Robinson

OBJECTIVES	CONTENT	TEACHING RESOURCES
		▶ Discuss the meanings of the words occlusion and malocclusion.
		Class Activity Divide the class into small groups. Have each group examine a variety of study models in class and discuss the different malocclusions of the models. Then have groups describe to the class where the maxillary teeth occlude with the mandibular teeth in each classification.
Discuss corrective orthodontics and describe what type of treatment is involved.	■ Benefits of orthodontic treatment (p. 962) ☐ Psychosocial problems (p. 963) ☐ Oral malfunction (p. 963) ☐ Dental disease (p. 963) ■ Management of orthodontic problems (p. 963) ☐ Corrective orthodontics (p. 963)	PPT 17-18 TB question 4 SW Short-Answer Questions 3 (p. 527) SW Case Study question 2 (p. 530) CTQ 4-5 (p. 983) ▶ Discuss the different areas of corrective orthodontics. *Class Activity Before class have each student research a patient case and the orthodontic treatment the patient completed. Have students characterize the results of the treatment and discuss other approaches that could have been taken to treat the condition. Then have students present their information to the class. (For students to prepare for this activity, see Homework/Assignments #2.)*
List the types of diagnostic records used to assess orthodontic problems.	■ Orthodontic records and treatment planning (p. 963) ☐ Medical and dental history (p. 964) ☐ Physical growth evaluation (p. 964) ☐ School and behavioral evaluation (p. 964) ☐ Clinical examination (p. 964) – Evaluation of facial esthetics (p. 964) – Evaluation of oral health (p. 964) – Evaluation of jaw and occlusal function (p. 964) ☐ Diagnostic records (p. 964)	PPT 19-26 TB questions 5-7 SW Short-Answer Questions 4; Fill in the Blank question 10; Multiple Choice questions 8-10 (pp. 527-529) SW Case Study question 1 (p. 530) Figure 60-9 Standard extraoral photographs (p. 965) Figure 60-10 (A) Intraoral photographs showing a patient's front view in occlusion; (B) Maxillary occlusal view; (C) Right buccal view (p. 965) Figure 60-11 (A) Cephalometric radiograph; (B) Cephalometric analysis (p. 966) Figure 60-12 Diagnostic model (p. 966) Cephalometric Landmarks and Points (p. 966) Recall questions 7-10 (p. 966) CTQ 1 (p. 983) ▶ Discuss what should be done with original radiographs when they are requested by a patient.

Torres and Ehrlich Modern Dental Assisting, 9th ed.

OBJECTIVES	CONTENT	TEACHING RESOURCES
	– Photographs (p. 964) – Radiographs (p. 964) – Cephalometric analysis (p. 965) – Diagnostic models (p. 965) ■ Case presentation (p. 966) □ Financial arrangements (p. 967)	***Class Activity** Divide the class into seven groups, and assign each group one of the seven components needed for orthodontic record and treatment planning: medical and dental history, physical growth evaluation, social and behavioral evaluation, clinical examination, photographs, radiographs, and diagnostic models. Have each group list the importance and reasons for use of its assigned component in the assessment of orthodontic problems. Then, have each group present its information to the class.*

60.1 Homework/Assignments:

1. Have each student research an orthodontic office floor plan and layout. Have each student download or print photos, pictures, and/or floor plans of the office he or she researches.

2. Have each student research a patient case and the orthodontic treatment the patient completed. Have students characterize the results of the treatment and discuss other approaches that could have been taken to treat the condition. The students will present their information to the class.

60.1 Instructor's Notes/Student Feedback:

ELSEVIER

LESSON 60.2

CRITICAL THINKING QUESTION

The third patient of the day is scheduled for a long appointment. The dental assistant reads in the chart that all initial patient assessment and data have been collected and a treatment plan has been designed by the orthodontist and approved by the patient. The patient's last appointment was ten days ago, during which separators were placed between the patient's posterior teeth. Today's appointment will include placement of the fixed orthodontic appliances. What components of the fixed orthodontic appliance will need to be set up? What orthodontic instruments will be used during today's appointment? What postoperative directions should be given to the patient before dismissal?

Guidelines: Before patient arrives the treatment area should be prepared with the necessary fixed appliances and auxiliaries. Orthodontic bands are selected based on the size of the teeth viewed in the patient's study model. Brackets are chosen based on the size of teeth and area of placement. Glass ionomer cement, glass slab, a cement spatula, and dental mirror are needed to cement the bands. A bonding setup and material is used to seat the brackets. Auxiliary supplies, including headgear tubes, edgewise tubes, labial hooks, and lingual attachments, should be available. A nickel titanium arch wire is used because it is recommended for initial movement of malaligned teeth. Ligature ties are set up to secure the arch wire to the bands and brackets. Specialized instruments are needed during this appointment. The orthodontic scaler is used to remove the separators. The instruments for band placement include the band pusher, band seater, band remover, and contouring pliers. Bracket placement requires using the bracket placement tweezers and orthodontic scaler. The preformed arch wire is placed using Weingart pliers, bird-beak pliers, torquing pliers, and a distal wire cutter. The ligature ties are fastened using a ligature director, hemostat, and ligature cutter. Before dismissal the patient should be instructed about the care and maintenance of the orthodontic appliance. Proper toothbrushing and flossing instructions must be given to the patient, who also must understand the importance of healthy eating during the orthodontic treatment.

OBJECTIVES	CONTENT	TEACHING RESOURCES
Describe the components of the fixed appliance.	■ Specialized instruments and accessories (p. 967) ☐ Intraoral instruments (p. 967) ☐ Pliers (p. 967) ■ Orthodontic treatment (p. 969) ☐ Fixed appliances (p. 969)	🖼 PPT 30-39 💻 TB questions 8-10 📖 SW Short-Answer Questions 5; Fill in the Blank questions 1-7; Multiple Choice questions 14, 16-18, 20 (pp. 527-529) 📖💿 SW/IDO Patient Case Exercise question 3 (p. 531) (The Interactive Dental Office CD-ROM) Figure 60-13 Intraoral instruments (pp. 967-968) Figure 60-14 Pliers (p. 969) Recall questions 11-13 (p. 967) Figure 60-15 Full braces (p. 970) Figure 60-16 Molar band ready for cementation (p. 970) Figure 60-17 The band pusher is used to seat the band interproximally (p. 973) Figure 60-18 Bracket placement (p. 973) Figure 60-19 Auxiliary attachment on a molar band (p. 974) Figure 60-20 An assortment of arch wires (p. 977)

ELSEVIER

Torres and Ehrlich Modern Dental Assisting, 9th ed.

Bird/Robinson

OBJECTIVES	CONTENT	TEACHING RESOURCES
		Figure 60-21 A ligature tie can be placed around one bracket or placed in a figure-eight pattern to create a chain around several brackets (p. 978)
		Figure 60-22 The Kobyashi hook has a welded hook at the end of a ligature tie that is used to hold auxiliaries (p. 978)
		Recall questions 14, 16-17, 20 (p. 978)
		▶ Discuss and list the components of braces. Also discuss what effect braces are designed to achieve in terms of tooth movement.
		Class Activity Display the fixed appliances (brackets, bands, ligature ties, arch wires, headgear tubes, separators, edgewise tubes, labial hooks, and lingual arch attachments) and ask students to identify and describe the use and function of each one.
Place and remove brass wire separators.	■ Orthodontic treatment (p. 969) □ Fixed appliances (p. 969) □ Separators (p. 970) **Procedure** 60-1 Placing and removing brass wire separators (p. 971) (SW/ESLR Competencies 60-1 to 60-3, p. 533)	PPT 40 SW Short-Answer Questions 5; Fill in the Blank question 7; Multiple Choice question 14 (pp. 527-529) SW Case Study question 3 (p. 530) SW/ESLR Competencies 60-1 to 60-3 Placing Separators (p. 533) CTQ 2 (p. 983) ▶ Discuss the instruments used to place and remove brass wire separators. ***Class Activity Discuss the purpose of separating teeth before fitting bands, and ask students to describe the three methods of separation used for posterior teeth. Then ask each student to demonstrate on a study model the placement and removal of the brass wire separator using the proper instruments.***
Place and remove steel separating springs.	■ Orthodontic treatment (p. 969) □ Fixed appliances (p. 969) □ Separators (p. 970) **Procedure** 60-2 Placing and removing steel separating springs (pp. 972-973) (SW/ESLR Competencies 60-1 to 60-3, p. 533)	SW Short-Answer Questions 5; Fill in the Blank question 7 (pp. 527-528) SW Case Study question 3 (p. 530) SW/ESLR Competencies 60-1 to 60-3 Placing Separators (p. 533) CTQ 2 (p. 983) ▶ Discuss the instruments used to place and remove steel separating springs. ***Class Activity Discuss the procedural steps for placing and removing steel separating springs. Then ask each student to demonstrate on a study model the placement and removal of steel separating springs using the proper instruments.***

ELSEVIER

Bird/Robinson

OBJECTIVES	CONTENT	TEACHING RESOURCES
Place and remove elastomeric ring separators.	■ Orthodontic treatment (p. 969) ☐ Fixed appliances (p. 969) ☐ Separators (p. 970) Procedure 60-3 Placing and removing elastomeric ring separators (p. 974) (SW/ESLR Competencies 60-1 to 60-3, p. 533)	SW Short-Answer Questions 5; Fill in the Blank question 7; Multiple Choice question 14 (pp. 527-529) SW Case Study question 3 (p. 530) SW/ESLR Competencies 60-1 to 60-3 Placing Separators (p. 533) CTQ 2 (p. 983) ▸ Discuss the instruments used to place and remove elastomeric ring separators. *Class Activity Lead a class discussion to compare and contrast the three methods used to separate teeth. Then ask each student to demonstrate on a study model the placement and removal of elastic ring separators using the proper instruments.*
Assist in the fitting and cementation of orthodontic bands.	☐ Orthodontic bands (p. 970) – Fitting molar bands (p. 970) – Cementation of orthodontic bands (p. 970) Procedure 60-4 Assisting in the fitting and cementation of orthodontic bands (p. 975) (SW/ESLR Competency 60-4, p. 534)	PPT 41-42 SW Short-Answer Questions 5; Fill in the Blank question 1; Multiple Choice questions 11, 15 (pp. 527, 529) SW Case Study question 4 (p. 530) SW/IDO Patient Case Exercise question 1 (p. 531) (The Interactive Dental Office CD-ROM) SW/ESLR Competency 60-4 Assisting in the Fitting and Cementation of Orthodontic Bands (p. 534) Recall question 15 (p. 978) ▸ Discuss the instruments used in fitting and cementing orthodontic bands. *Class Activity Lead a class discussion about the divisions of bands into maxillary and mandibular and the purpose of this division. What is the most common location for band placement? Then ask each student to demonstrate on a study model the proper way to select the size of the band, fit the band, and cement the band.*
Assist in the direct bonding of orthodontic brackets.	☐ Bonded brackets (p. 973) Procedure 60-5 Assisting in the direct bonding of orthodontic brackets (p. 976) (SW/ESLR Competency 60-5, p. 537)	PPT 43-44 SW Short-Answer Questions 5; Fill in the Blank question 3; Multiple Choice questions 12, 16 (pp. 527-529) SW Case Study question 5 (p. 530) SW/ESLR Competency 60-5 Assisting in the Direct Bonding of Orthodontic Brackets (p. 537)

Torres and Ehrlich Modern Dental Assisting, 9th ed.

Bird/Robinson

OBJECTIVES	CONTENT	TEACHING RESOURCES
		Recall question 16 (p. 978) ▸ Discuss the instruments used in direct bonding of orthodontic brackets. ***Class Activity Have each student demonstrate the procedure for assisting the orthodontist when bracket bonding is to be completed. Have each student set up for the procedure and describe the various materials and equipment needed.***
Place an arch wire.	☐ Auxiliary attachments (p. 973) ☐ Arch wire (p. 974) – Types of arch wire (p. 977) – Shapes of arch wire (p. 977) Procedure 60-6 Placing arch wires (p. 977) (SW/ESLR Competencies 60-6 to 60-8, pp. 539-540)	PPT 45-49 SW Short-Answer Questions 5; Fill in the Blank question 6; Multiple Choice questions 18-20 (pp. 527-529) SW Case Study question 5 (p. 530) SW/ESLR Competencies 60-6 to 60-8 Placing and Removing Ligature Wires and Elastomeric Ties (pp. 539-540) Recall questions 18-19 (p. 978) ▸ Discuss the instruments used to place an arch wire. ***Class Activity Ask each student to demonstrate on a study model the proper fitting and placement of a preformed arch wire. Have students identify the various arch wire materials used and under what conditions each of the arch wire types would be recommended.***
Place and remove ligature ties.	☐ Ligating the arch wire (p. 978) Procedure 60-7 Placing and removing ligature ties (p. 979) (SW/ESLR Competencies 60-6 to 60-8, pp. 539-540)	PPT 50 TB question 10 SW Short-Answer Questions 5; Fill in the Blank question 4; Multiple Choice question 20 (pp. 527-529) SW Case Study question 5 (p. 530) SW/IDO Patient Case Exercise question 2 (p. 531) (The Interactive Dental Office CD-ROM) SW/ESLR Competencies 60-6 to 60-8 Placing and Removing Ligature Wires and Elastomeric Ties (pp. 539-540) Figure 60-21 A ligature tie can be placed around one bracket or placed in a figure-eight pattern to create a chain around several brackets. (p. 978) Figure 60-22 The Kobyashi hook has a welded hook at the end of a ligature tie that is used to hold auxiliaries (p. 978) Recall question 20 (p. 978)

Bird/Robinson

OBJECTIVES	CONTENT	TEACHING RESOURCES
		▸ Discuss the instruments used to place and remove ligature ties.
		Class Activity Lead a class discussion about the purpose of ligating the arch wire. Identify the two ways in which ligature ties are used to tie the arch wires. Then ask each student to demonstrate on a study model the placement and removal of ligature ties using the proper instruments.
Place and remove elastomeric ties.	☐ Ligating the arch wire (p. 978) Procedure 60-8 Placing and removing elastomeric ties (p. 980) (SW/ESLR Competencies 60-6 to 60-8, pp. 539-540) ☐ Power products (p. 978)	PPT 51-53 TB question 10 SW Short-Answer Questions 5; Fill in the Blank question 4; Multiple Choice question 20 (pp. 527-529) SW Case Study question 5 (p. 530) SW/ESLR Competencies 60-6 to 60-8 Placing and Removing Ligature Wires and Elastomeric Ties (pp. 539-540) ▸ Discuss instruments used to place and remove elastomeric ties. *Class Activity Ask each student to demonstrate on a study model the placement and removal of elastomeric ties using the proper instruments.*
Describe the use and function of headgear.	■ Headgear (p. 978) ☐ Facebow (p. 978) ☐ Traction devices (p. 978) ■ Adjustment visits (p. 978) ☐ Checking the appliance (p. 980)	PPT 54-55 SW Short-Answer Questions 6; Fill in the Blank question 12; Multiple Choice question 21 (pp. 527-528, 530) Figure 60-23 (A) High-pull headgear; (B) Cervical traction; (C) Combination headgear; (D) Chin cap (p. 981) Recall question 21 (p. 980) ▸ Discuss different types of headgear used in orthodontics. *Class Activity Assign each student one of the four types of headgear described in the text. Have the students research their assigned orthodontic headgear and its function, uses, and purpose. Also have students find one patient case with before-and-after photos showing the effectiveness of the headgear. Then have each student present his or her findings to the class. (For students to prepare for this activity, see Homework/Assignments #1.)*

Torres and Ehrlich Modern Dental Assisting, 9th ed.

Bird/Robinson

OBJECTIVES	CONTENT	TEACHING RESOURCES

Describe ways to convey the importance of good dietary and oral hygiene habits in the treatment of orthodontics.	■ Oral hygiene and dietary instructions (p. 980)
	
	 ■ Completed treatment (p. 981)
	
	   □ Retention (p. 981)
	
	     – Orthodontic positioner (p. 981)
	
	     – Hawley retainer (p. 981)
	
	     – Lingual retainer (p. 982)
	
	 ■ Treatment options (p. 982)
		⊠▤ PPT 56-59
		
		 💻 TB questions 11-12
		
		 📖 SW Short-Answer Questions 7; Multiple Choice questions 22-23 (pp. 527, 530)
		
		 📀 SW/IDO Patient Case Exercise questions 4-5 (p. 531) (The Interactive Dental Office CD-ROM)
		
		 Toothbrushing Instructions (p. 980)
		
		 Figure 60-24 An orthodontic positioner (p. 982)
		
		 Figure 60-25 Examples of Hawley retainers (p. 982)
		
		 Recall questions 22-23 (p. 980)
		
		 Table 60-2 Dietary Habits and Orthodontics (p. 981)
		
		 Recall questions 24-25 (p. 982)
		
		 ▸ Discuss how oral hygiene and good dietary habits can help orthodontic treatment to be successful.
		
		 Class Activity Have student pairs take turns role-playing an assistant teaching an orthodontic patient about oral hygiene and good eating habits. Have the pairs create a variety of situations, including occlusion, type of appliance, patient compliance and attitude, current homecare practices, and identify modifications that should be made in current practices. Then, have the pairs make presentations to the class, including the oral hygiene aids they are recommending, dietary recommendations, and the rationale underlying their recommendations.

Performance Evaluation		💻 TB 📖 SW questions (pp. 527-530) 📖 SW Case Study (p. 530) 📀 SW/IDO Patient Case Exercise (pp. 530-531) (The Interactive Dental Office CD-ROM) 📖 *e* SW/ESLR Competencies 60-1 to 60-3 Placing Separators (p. 533) 📖 *e* SW/ESLR Competency 60-4 Assisting in the Fitting and Cementation of Orthodontic Bands (p. 535) 📖 *e* SW/ESLR Competency 60-5 Assisting in the Direct Bonding of Orthodontic Brackets (p. 537) 📖 *e* SW/ESLR Competencies 60-6 to 60-8 Placing and Removing Ligature Wires and Elastomeric Ties (pp. 539-540)

Torres and Ehrlich Modern Dental Assisting, 9th ed.

OBJECTIVES	CONTENT	TEACHING RESOURCES
		e ESLR Electronic Flashcards
		e ESLR Practice Quiz
		Recall questions (pp. 961-983)
		💡 CTQ (p. 983)

60.2 Homework/Assignments:

1. Assign each student one of the four types of headgear described in the text. Have the students research their assigned orthodontic headgear and its function, uses, and purpose. Ask students to also find one patient case and present before-and-after photos demonstrating the effectiveness of the headgear.

60.2 Instructor's Notes/Student Feedback:

Bird/Robinson

Slide 1

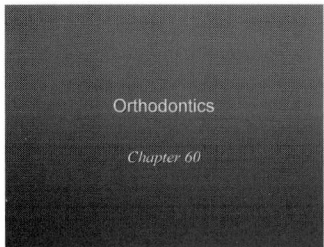

Slide 2

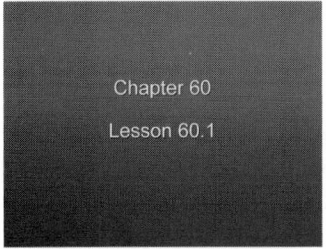

Slide 3

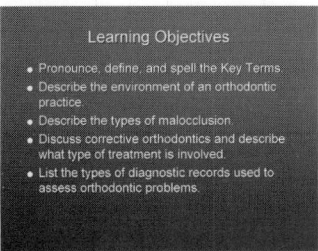

Slide 4

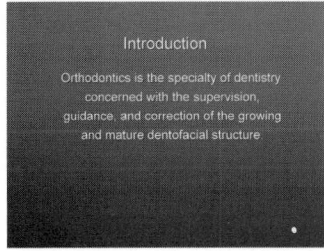

- An orthodontist must receive at least two additional years of formal education in an accredited university after attaining a dental degree. To become a board-certified orthodontist, he or she must pass an examination by the American Association of Orthodontists.

- In many states, the expanded functions dental assistant (EFDA) is allowed to perform many of the tasks involved, such as sizing and placing bands and placing ligature ties and separators.

Bird/Robinson

Slide 5

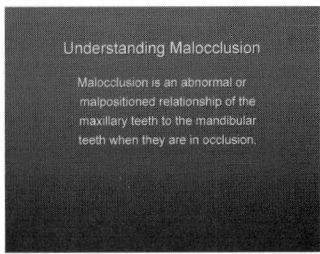

- Malocclusion is occlusion that deviates from a Class I normal occlusion because of irregularities, such as in the positions of teeth and in bite relationships.

- What causes or influences malocclusion?

Slide 6

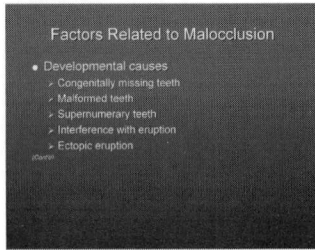

- Congenitally missing teeth result when tooth bud formation was interrupted or never occurred.

- What are malformed teeth?

- What are supernumerary teeth?

- What is an ectopic eruption?

Slide 7

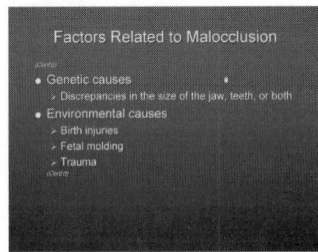

- Genetic: The patient usually has a small jaw from one parent and larger teeth from the other parent, or congenitally missing teeth.

- What is fetal molding?

Slide 8

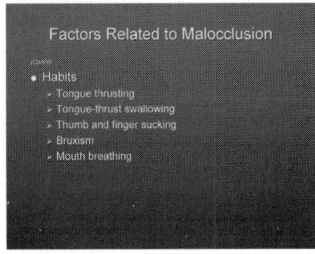

- The orthodontist corrects oral habits that cause malalignment.

- Thumb and finger sucking beyond age 5 will affect facial structure development and growth.

- What is bruxism?

Torres and Ehrlich Modern Dental Assisting, 9th ed.

Bird/Robinson

Slide 9

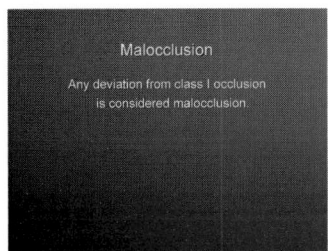

- In 1899 Dr. Edward Angle introduced a classification of malocclusion based on the relationship of the maxillary and mandibular first permanent molars.
- What is this system known as? *(Angle's Classification of Malocclusion.)*

Slide 10

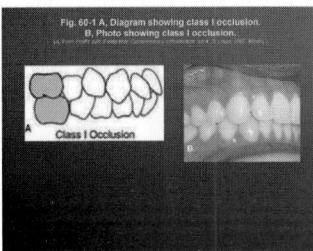

- Class I malocclusion is also known as neutroclusion. The facial profile is known as mesognathic.
- What should be used as a guide if one or both of the first molars are missing from the side that is being classified?

Slide 11

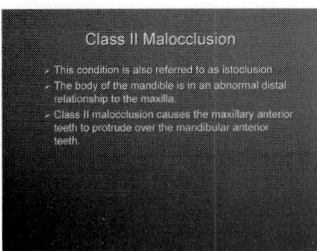

- The facial profile is known as retrognathic.
- The maxilla protrudes.
- The lower lip is full and often rests between the maxillary and mandibular incisors.
- The mandible appears retruded or weak.

Slide 12

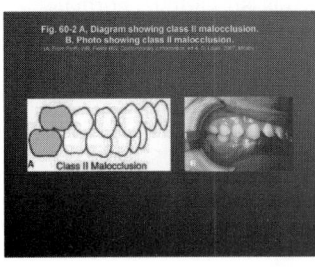

- Molar relation: The buccal groove of the mandibular first molar is distal to the mesiobuccal cusp of the maxillary first molar by at least one width of a premolar.
- Canine relation: The distal surface of the mandibular canine is distal to the mesial surface of the maxillary canine by at least one width of a premolar.

Torres and Ehrlich Modern Dental Assisting, 9th ed.
Bird/Robinson

Slide 13

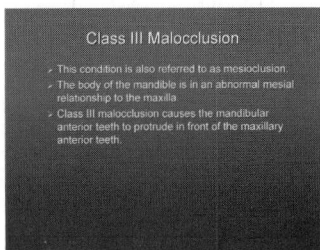

- Facial profile is known as prognathic.
- The lower lip and mandible are prominent.

Slide 14

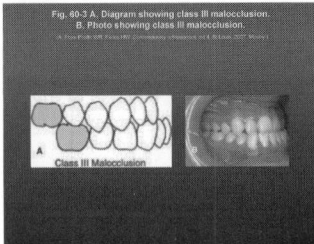

- Molar relation: The buccal groove of the mandibular first molar is mesial to the mesiobuccal cusp of the maxillary first permanent molar by at least the width of a premolar.
- Canine relation: The distal surface of the mandibular canine is mesial to the mesial surface of the maxillary canine by at least the width of a premolar.

Slide 15

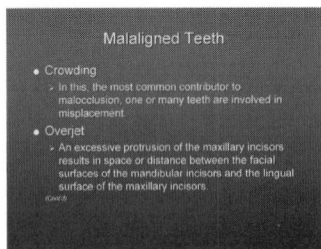

- Crowding or overlapping makes oral hygiene (toothbrushing and flossing) more of a challenge for the patient.
- Overjet is the horizontal distance between the labioincisal surfaces on the mandibular incisors and the linguoincisal surfaces of the maxillary incisors.
- What instrument would you use to measure an overjet? *(Probe.)*

Slide 16

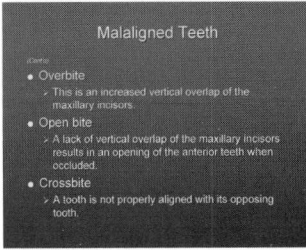

- Overbite is the vertical distance by which the maxillary incisors overlap the mandibular incisors. It has three classifications: normal, moderate, and deep/severe.
- Crossbites occur when the maxillary or mandibular teeth are either facial or lingual to their normal position.
- What is the condition called when the mandibular anterior teeth occlude anteriorly or facially to the maxillary anterior teeth? *(Underjet.)*

Bird/Robinson

Slide 17

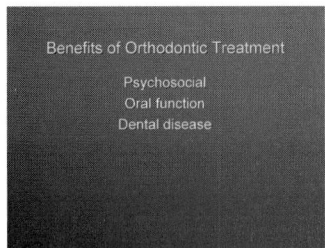

- Severe malocclusion and dental facial deformities can be social handicaps.
- Oral function is influenced when malocclusion compromises chewing, jaw movement, speech, and temporomandibular joint (TMJ) function.
- What could be affected if the oral functional needs of the patient are not met?
- What could be affected if the need to have a healthy and sound dentition are not achieved?

Slide 18

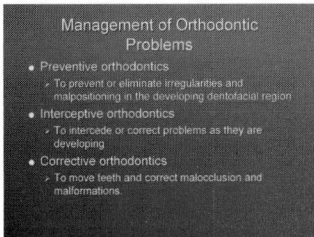

- Corrective orthodontics include fixed appliances, removable appliances, or orthognathic surgery.

Slide 19

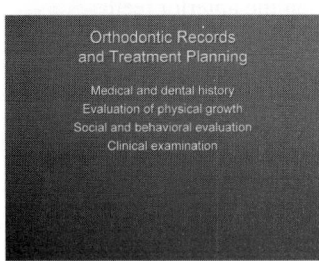

- What could the medical and dental history reveal about a patient's orthodontic condition or needs?
- Why is a physical growth evaluation necessary?
- Why is a social and behavioral evaluation necessary?
- Clinical evaluation includes evaluation of facial esthetics, oral health, and jaw and occlusal function.

Slide 20

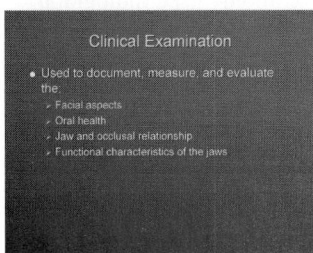

- Facial symmetry is assessed, including a frontal evaluation and a profile evaluation.
- The jaw and the occlusal relationship between the teeth and jaws are key to determining the orthodontic treatment and strategies.
- Functional characteristics of the jaws are also inspected. Lateral or anterior shifts of the mandible on closure are of special interest.

Bird/Robinson

Slide 21

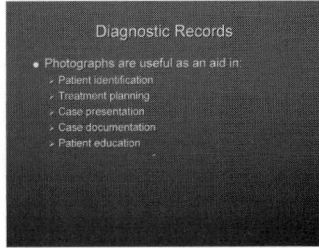

- Two standard extraoral photographs are taken: frontal view and profile view.

- Three standard intraoral photographs are required: full direct view, maxillary occlusal view, and right buccal view.

Slide 22

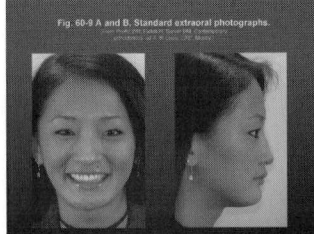

- The photo on the left is the profile view.

- The photo on the right is the frontal view.

- What visual aspects are noted on these photographs? (*Jaw size, jaw shape, and jaw symmetry.*)

Slide 23

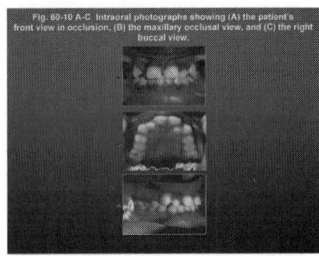

- A: Front view shows the relationship between the anterior teeth including the overjet, overbite, and whether an open bite exists.

- B: Occlusal view of the maxillary arch shows crowding and or overlapping, occlusal wear, and malalignment of teeth.

- C: Right buccal view will show crossbites, openbites, and molar and canine relationship.

Slide 24

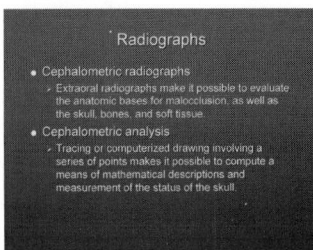

- The cephalometric radiograph is the most commonly used radiograph in orthodontic evaluation.

- The analysis of the radiograph is completed by marking cephalometric landmarks at a series of points to determine skull size and shape.

- These measurements will determine skull growth patterns, which will determine the type of orthodontic treatment necessary.

Slide 25

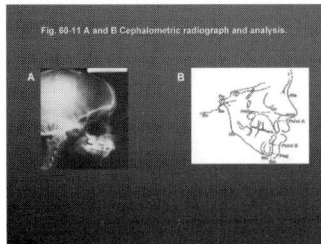

- The cephalometric radiograph is a profile or lateral view. It is taken at different intervals: before, during, and after orthodontic treatment.

- The radiographs can be superimposed to demonstrate jaw growth.

Slide 26

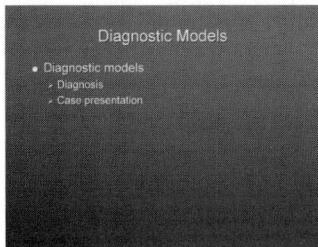

- Diagnostic models are also called study models. Diagnostic models are used for the diagnosis and case presentation of the orthodontic patient.

- Diagnostic models are made from plaster after taking an alginate impression of the patient's mouth. Models are often fabricated before orthodontic treatment and after the treatment is completed.

Slide 27

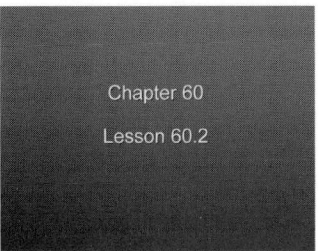

Slide 28

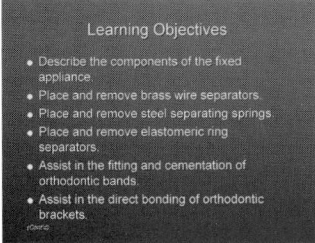

Slide 29

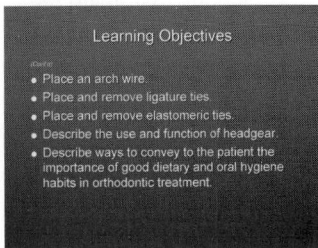

Slide 30

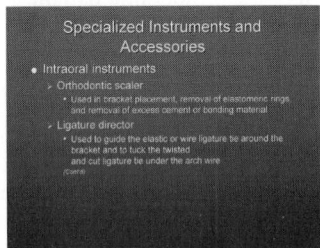

- Numerous intraoral instruments are used, including orthodonic scalers, ligature directors, band plugger and bite stick, bracket-placement tweezers, and pliers.

- Ligature director is used with a push stroke to place the ligature where needed around brackets and bands.

Slide 31

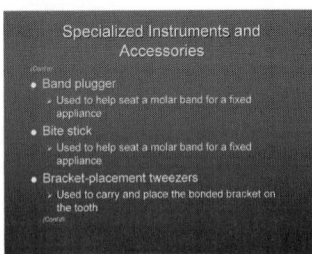

- Band plugger is the instrument that seats molar brackets into place. This instrument is important because bands fit snugly and would be difficult to seat by simply pressing them down with a finger.

- An instrument known as a bite stick also helps to seat bands. The patient occludes on the bite stick, which also helps to seat the snugly fitting molar bands by gently using occlusal forces.

Slide 32

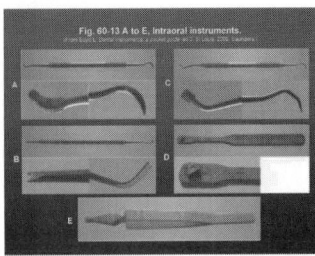

- Care must be taken when sterilizing hinged instruments, such as the bracket tweezer.

- What is the most common result when hinged instruments are sterilized incorrectly? (*Corrosion or rust around the hinged area.*)

Torres and Ehrlich Modern Dental Assisting, 9th ed.

Bird/Robinson

Slide 33

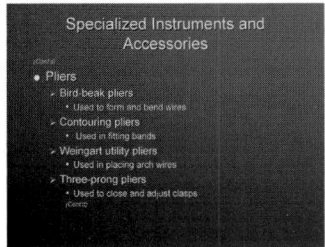

- Bird-beak pliers bend wires for both removable and fixed appliances.

- Contouring pliers have a bent beak. The bent beak of the contouring pliers aids in placement of molar or posterior bands.

- What are Weingart utility pliers?

Slide 34

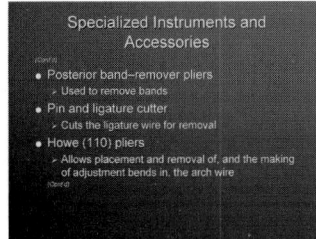

- Pin and ligature cutters cut the ligature wire once it has been ligated around the bracket.

- Howe (110) pliers are versatile because of their instrument design. They have a round, flat, wide tip, making them suitable for holding orthodontic materials and appliances intraorally.

Slide 35

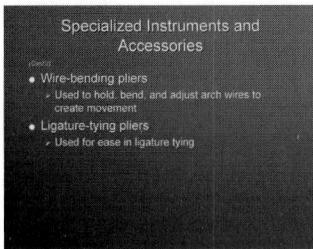

- Wire bending pliers have notched areas throughout the beak to allow ease of wire bending while the wire is held securely in the pliers.

- Ligature–tying pliers have finely serrated narrow beaks to allow ease in ligature tying.

Slide 36

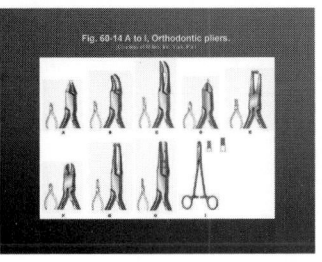

- Top row: (A) Bird-beak pliers; (B) Contouring pliers; (C) Weingart utility pliers; (D) Three-prong pliers; (E) Posterior band remover.

- Bottom row: (F) Ligature pin and ligature cutter; (G) Howe (110) pliers; (H) Wire bending pliers; (I) Ligature-tying pliers.

Bird/Robinson

Slide 37

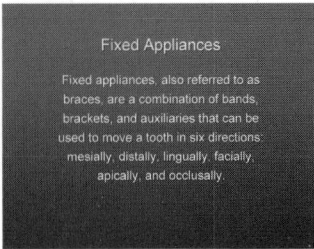

Fixed Appliances

Fixed appliances, also referred to as braces, are a combination of bands, brackets, and auxiliaries that can be used to move a tooth in six directions: mesially, distally, lingually, facially, apically, and occlusally.

- Fixed appliances are cemented to the teeth and cannot be removed by the patient.

- Auxiliaries, such as hooks and tubes, are also attached to brackets and bands.

- The arch wire is attached to all brackets and places opposing forces on the teeth to cause them to move.

Slide 38

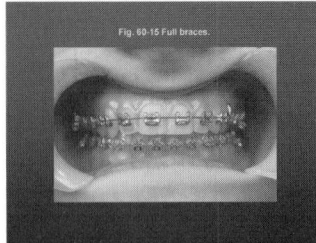

Fig. 60-15 Full braces.

- Can you name the pieces of the fixed appliances viewed on this slide?

- What will become an increased daily challenge to this patient?

Slide 39

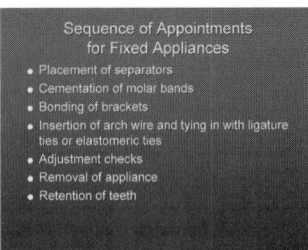

Sequence of Appointments for Fixed Appliances
- Placement of separators
- Cementation of molar bands
- Bonding of brackets
- Insertion of arch wire and tying in with ligature ties or elastomeric ties
- Adjustment checks
- Removal of appliance
- Retention of teeth

- The sequence of events in each orthodontic treatment plan may vary slightly from patient to patient.

- After the data has been collected, diagnostic records have been assembled, and clinical evaluation is complete, the orthodontist will outline the treatment sequence, including how and when the orthodontic appliances will be placed in the patient's mouth and when they wll later be removed.

Slide 40

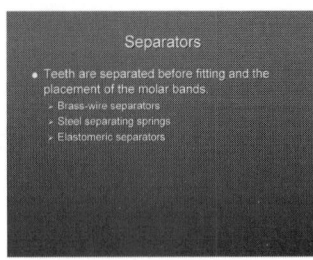

Separators
- Teeth are separated before fitting and the placement of the molar bands.
  › Brass-wire separators
  › Steel separating springs
  › Elastomeric separators

- How do you place the separator?

- Who places the separator?

- How do you remove the separator?

- Who removes the separator?

Slide 41

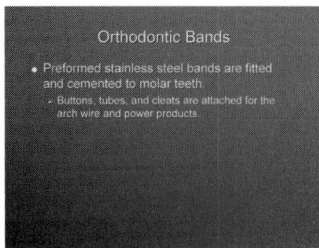

Orthodontic Bands

- Preformed stainless steel bands are fitted and cemented to molar teeth.
  - Buttons, tubes, and cleats are attached for the arch wire and power products.

- How is an orthodontic band placed?
- Who places the band?

Slide 42

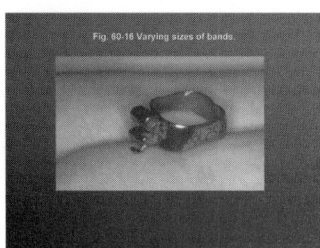

Fig. 60-16 Varying sizes of bands.

- Orthodontic bands come in a variety of sizes.
- Bands are most commonly placed on molars.
- The occlusal aspect of the band is slightly rolled or contoured.
- The gingival aspect of the band is straight and smooth.

Slide 43

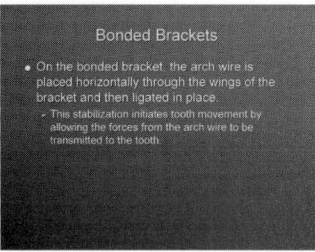

Bonded Brackets

- On the bonded bracket, the arch wire is placed horizontally through the wings of the bracket and then ligated in place.
  - This stabilization initiates tooth movement by allowing the forces from the arch wire to be transmitted to the tooth.

- The bonded bracket is the most common type of attachment for fixed appliances.
- Brackets are placed in a number of ways depending on the teeth.

Slide 44

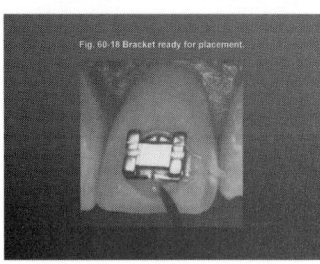

Fig. 60-18 Bracket ready for placement.

- Brackets vary in size according to the teeth to which they will be bonded.
- Notice the four tie wings on each of the brackets.
- What is the purpose of the tie wings?

ELSEVIER

Bird/Robinson

Slide 45

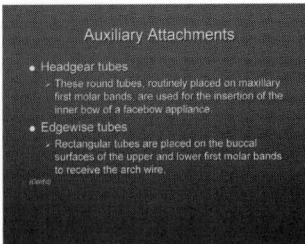

- Headgear is usually a removable appliance inserted and removed by the patient as recommended by the orthodontist.
- Edgewise tubes are an integral part of contemporary orthodontic procedures.
- Edgewise tubes are rectangular in shape and hold the arch wire securely.

Slide 46

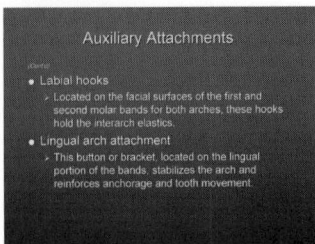

- In addition to arch wires and ligatures for providing forces to encourage teeth movement, elastics are also used.
- Elastics extend to and from various hooks attached to the facial surfaces of bands and brackets.

Slide 47

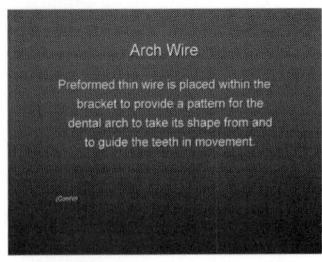

- The arch wire fits into a horizontal slot in the brackets or slides into the buccal tubes on molar teeth.
- Arch wires come in a variety of diameters, which affect the magnitude of the force that is applied to the teeth.

Slide 48

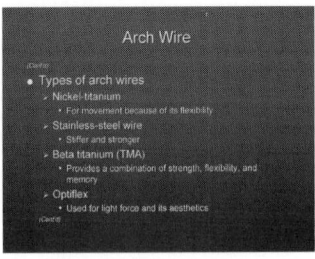

- Nickel titanium wire is used during initial stages of tooth movement for malaligned or crowded teeth.
- Stainless steel wire is used to apply more force and give better stability to control the teeth. Stainless steel can withstand greater forces and is known as the working arch wire.
- Optiflex wire is a newer type of arch wire made from composite materials with a top coating of optical glass fibers.

Bird/Robinson

Slide 49

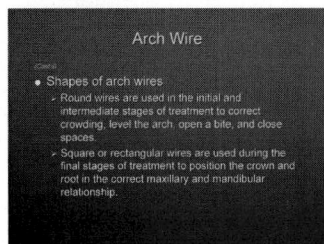

- The shape of the arch wire used is determined by the treatment and movement needed during each stage of the orthodontic procedures.
- The shape of the arch wire is also determined by the current phase of the treatment.

Slide 50

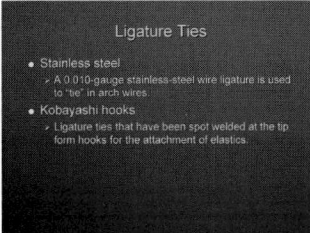

- Arch wires are anchored into the brackets by ligature ties.
- Ligature ties can be made of thin wire or tiny elastic bands.
- The orthodontist can assign individual brackets to be tied with individual ligatures or an entire quadrant or sextant tied with one ligature.

Slide 51

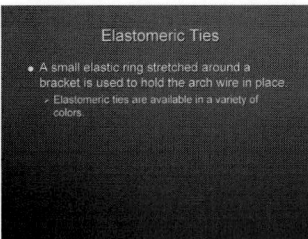

- Elastic ties are also used to secure the arch wire to the brackets.
- Young patients like the elastic ties because they come in a variety of colors.

Slide 52

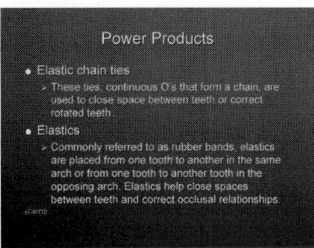

- Power products are accessory items made of elastic materials that help in tooth movement.
- These power products are attached to the fixed appliances by placing them over the brackets or attaching them to labial hooks or lingual arch attachments.

Slide 53

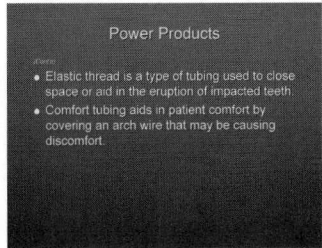

- It is important to avoid using power products containing latex materials because of an increase of latex sensitivity experienced by operators, dental assistants, and patients in the dental office.

- Instruments used to place elastic power products include the Hemostat and Orthodontic scaler.

Slide 54

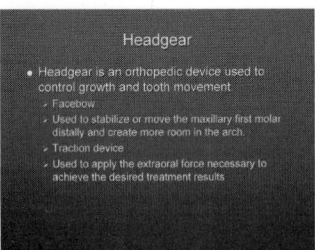

- Headgear is made up of two parts: (1) The facebow is inserted into headgear tubes, which are attached to the buccal aspect of molar orthodontic bands; (2) The traction device can be designed in a variety of styles, depending on the force needed to move the maxillary arch.

Slide 55

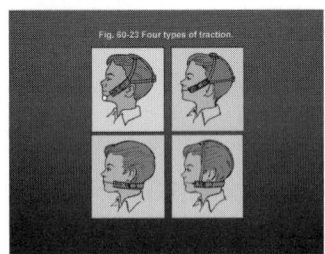

- *Upper left:* Chin cap traction device is a combination of a high-pull strap and chin cup to help control the growth of the mandible in patients with Class III malocclusion.

- *Lower right:* Combination headgear traction device is a combination of a high-pull and cervical traction device. It exerts a force along the occlusal plane and upward.

- What is headgear in upper right?

- What is headgear in lower left?

Slide 56

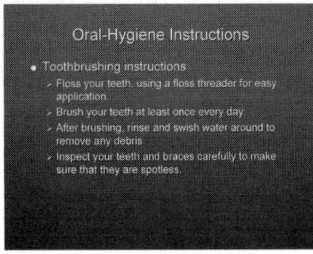

- The biggest day-to-day challenge faced by a patient with full-mouth fixed orthodontic appliances is plaque control and maintaining a healthy mouth.

- Orthodontic appliances offer areas for food and plaque to be trapped and hidden.

- What will result from poor oral hygiene?

Bird/Robinson

Slide 57

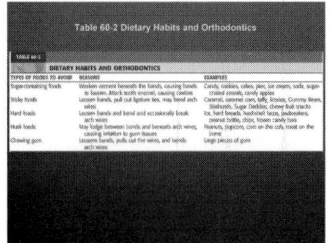

- Besides good oral hygiene habits, the orthodontic patient must also develop good eating habits.

- Healthy foods and good eating habits will help to maintain healthy teeth and gingiva and will also prevent damage to the orthodontic appliances.

Slide 58

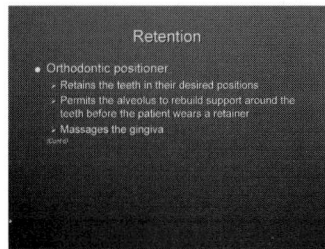

- After the fixed appliances have been removed, the orthodontic treatment is not yet complete.

- The orthodontic positioner is a custom-made appliance made of rubber or pliable acrylic that fits over the patient's dentition after orthodontic therapy.

Slide 59

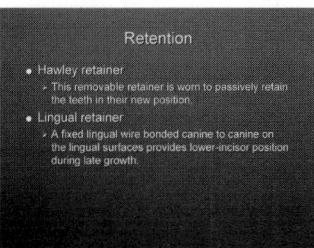

- The Hawley retainer is the most commonly used removable retainer.

- The Hawley retainer is made of a clear, self-polymerizing acrylic that is designed to hold wire clasps on molar teeth.

Bird/Robinson

61 Communication in the Dental Office

TEACHING FOCUS

This chapter will introduce students to topics related to communication in the dental office, including verbal, nonverbal, and written forms of communication. Patient needs and ways to meet them will be discussed, along with the skills of answering the phone, courtesy, and taking messages. Students will also become acquainted with written communications, such as business letters and the marketing of a dental practice. The importance of teamwork and ways to reduce stress in the dental office will be presented as well.

MATERIALS AND RESOURCES

☐ computer and PowerPoint projector (all Lessons)

LESSON CHECKLIST

Preparations for this lesson include:

- lecture
- evaluation of student knowledge and skills needed to perform all entry-level activities related to communication in the dental office, including:
  - ○ understanding the importance of,achieving good communication in the dental office and the various means of achieving it
  - ○ achieving patient satisfaction by meeting patient needs
  - ○ using the phone with courtesy and effectiveness
  - ○ writing business letters and other communications to support the dental practice
  - ○ marketing the dental practice
  - ○ fostering teamwork and reducing stress in the dental office

ELSEVIER

KEY TERMS

copier (p. 996)
fax machine (p. 996)
HIPAA (p. 1000)
human behavior (p. 987)
letterhead (p. 997)
marketing (p. 999)

nonverbal communication (p. 989)
salutation (p. 997)
socialization (p. 987)
verbal communication (p. 988)
word-processing software (p. 997)

ADDITIONAL RESOURCES

PowerPoint slides (Evolve): 1-26

Legend

CTQ	**DVD**	**ESLR**	**IDO**	**SW**	**TB**	**PPT**
Critical Thinking Question	Multimedia Procedures Videos and Animations	EVOLVE Student Learning Resources	Interactive Dental Office CD-ROM	Student Workbook	Test Bank on the TEACH CD-ROM	PowerPoint Slides

Class Activities are indicated in ***bold italic.***

LESSON 61.1

PRETEST

1. The Health Insurance Portability and Accountability Act (HIPAA) specifies
   a. recommendations with which dental offices should comply.
   b. federal regulations ensuring privacy of a patient's healthcare information.
   c. safety rules and regulations with which dental offices must comply.
   d. COBRA insurance regulations.

2. The backbone of a well-run organization is
   a. good communication.
   b. rules and regulations.
   c. excellent salary and benefits.
   d. a large client list.

3. One of the most important traits to everyday social and business relationships is
   a. honesty.
   b. mutual respect.
   c. interpersonal communication.
   d. problem-solving skills.

4. Communication can be defined as
   a. explanations.
   b. statement proper.
   c. words we use.
   d. sending of a message and receipt of the same message by another.

5. Words are
   a. statement proper.
   b. verbal symbols used to represent an object or a meaning.
   c. explanations.
   d. messages.

6. What accounts for one-third of the impact of the total message?
   a. words
   b. statement proper and voice quality
   c. voice quality
   d. explanations

7. Close-ended questions are those that
   a. can be answered with either *yes* or *no*.
   b. require more than *yes* or *no* for an answer.
   c. are best used to obtain information.
   d. maintain control of the conversation.

8. Open-ended questions are those that
   a. can be answered with either *yes* or *no*.
   b. begin with *is, do,,has, have, can,* or *will*.
   c. require more than *yes* or *no* for an answer.
   d. are best used to confirm information.

9. What approximate percentage of all spoken words is never heard?
   a. 10%
   b. 30%
   c. 50%
   d. 90%

Torres and Ehrlich Modern Dental Assisting, 9th ed.
Bird/Robinson

10. Objective fears are
   a. learned fears.
   b. subjective fears.
   c. anecdotal fears.
   d. acquired fears.

Answers

| 1. b | 3. c | 5. b | 7. a | 9. d |
| 2. a | 4. d | 6. c | 8. c | 10. a |

BACKGROUND ASSESSMENT

Question: In terms of communication with the patient, how can the dental team meet patient needs?
Answer: Some of the methods the dental team can use to meet patient needs are creating a positive atmosphere, being sincere, showing respect, respecting the patient's time, resolving complaints and misunderstandings, remaining approachable, and respecting patient confidentiality.
Question: What are the three pathways of communication?
Answer: The three pathways of communication are verbal communication, nonverbal communication, and listening skills. Verbal communication is made up of the words we use, voice quality, and asking questions. Nonverbal communication is conveyed by our body language. Posture, attitude, and movements transmit major messages. Listening skills require a person to concentrate entirely on the message being communicated by another.

CRITICAL THINKING QUESTION

A dental assistant answers the phone at a busy dental practice. The caller is a longtime patient and asks to speak to the dentist. The dental assistant informs the patient that this is not possible. The patient continues to demand to speak to the dentist. How should the dental assistant handle this phone call?
Guidelines: In general, the dentist should not be interrupted at chairside to come to the phone. Phone interruptions can reduce productivity, are inconsiderate to the current seated patient, and make it difficult to maintain infection control. It is the responsibility of the dental assistant to know what the dentist's policy is for handling phone interruptions. If the call does not meet the dentist's specified criteria for interruption, be tactful and polite. A statement, such as "The doctor is with a patient. How may I help you?" would be an appropriate response.

OBJECTIVES	CONTENT	TEACHING RESOURCES
Pronounce, define, and spell the Key Terms.	■ Key terms (p. 986)	*e* ESLR Electronic Flashcards ▶ Discuss each of the key terms in Chapter 61, focusing on the definition, pronunciation, and spelling of each term. *Class Activity Have students develop a crossword puzzle using key terms. They can use a Web site, such as www.puzzlemaker.com, or create a puzzle on their own. Have students exchange their puzzles with a classmate to solve them.*
Discuss human behavior, cultural diversity and their effect on oral communication, and identify the differences between verbal and nonverbal communications.	■ Understanding human behavior (p. 987) □ Significant people in psychology (p. 987) □ Social attitudes (p. 987) □ Peer pressure (p. 987) ■ Cultural diversity (p. 988)	⊠ PPT 5-9 TB questions 1-2 SW Short-Answer Questions 2; Fill in the Blank questions 2, 6; Multiple Choice questions 1-4 (pp. 541-542) Figure 61-1 Maslow's Hierarchy of Needs (p. 988) Basic Dental Terms in Spanish (p. 988) Recall questions 1-3 (p. 988) Box 61-1 Effective Words (p. 989)

ELSEVIER

Torres and Ehrlich Modern Dental Assisting, 9th ed.

Bird/Robinson

OBJECTIVES	CONTENT	TEACHING RESOURCES
	■ Communication pathways (p. 988) □ Verbal communication (p. 988) – Words are important (p. 988) – Voice quality (p. 989) – Asking questions (p. 989) □ Nonverbal communication (p. 989) □ Listening skills (p. 989)	Table 61-1 Nonverbal Communication (p. 990) Recall questions 4-7 (p. 990) ▶ Discuss why social diversity is an important factor for a professional to consider. What are some ways a dental office can improve understanding and communication with culturally diverse patients? ▶ Discuss verbal and nonverbal communications. Why is it important to pay attention to both forms of communication? ▶ Discuss the importance of listening well. What are some important guidelines to remember? *Class Activity Present the following words to the class, and have students determine whether each is considered an effective communication:* – *Pain* – *Remove* – *False teeth* – *Reception area*
Discuss the team concept for bettering communication.	■ Communicating with colleagues (p. 990)	⊠▪ PPT 10-11 TB question 12 SW Short-Answer Questions 7; Multiple Choice questions 17, 19 (pp. 541, 543) Figure 61-2 Team meeting (p. 990) Recall question 8 (p. 991) ▶ Discuss ways to foster teamwork in the dental office. *Class Activity Divide the class into small groups. Have each group discuss and develop an example of the team concept for bettering communication. Then have each group share its example with the class.*
Discuss stress in the dental practice.	□ Stress in the dental office (p. 990) – Causes (p. 990) – Methods of stress reduction (p. 991)	⊠▪ PPT 12-13 TB questions 13-14 SW Short-Answer Questions 6; Multiple Choice question 18 (pp. 541, 543) Recall question 9 (p. 991) ▶ Discuss some of the causes of stress in the dental office. What are some ways to control or reduce stress? *Class Activity Present the following information to the class. Ask the class to determine whether the items presented can be a cause of stress.*

Bird/Robinson

OBJECTIVES	CONTENT	TEACHING RESOURCES
		– Lack of sufficient staff
		– Lack of good communication
		– Good pay
		– Plenty of job advancement opportunities
		– Job satisfaction
Describe the type of relationship the patient and dental team should have.	■ Communicating with patients (p. 991) □ Patient needs (p. 991) – Psychologic needs (p. 991) – Anxiety and fear of pain (p. 991) – Dental phobic patients (p. 992) – Patient's responses (p. 992) – Physical and mental needs (p. 992) – Financial needs (p. 992) □ Meeting patient needs (p. 992) – Positive atmosphere (p. 992) – Sincerity (p. 992) – Showing respect (p. 992) – Respecting the patient's time (p. 992) – Resolving complaints and misunderstandings (p. 993) – Remaining approachable (p. 993) – Respecting patient confidentiality (p. 993)	⊠▤ PPT 14-16 ▦ TB questions 3-4 ▨ SW Short-Answer Questions 1; Multiple Choice questions 5-7 (pp. 541-542) Figure 61-3 Communication is the most important tool in a practice (p. 991) Recall questions 10-12 (p. 993) ▽ CTQ 3 (p. 1000) ▸ Discuss basic patient needs. What common patient fears should the dental assistant be aware of, and how might they be addressed? ▸ Discuss ways to meet patient needs. How could a dental assistant deal with an irate or unhappy patient? Why is it important to convey a sense of approachability? *Class Activity Divide the class into two groups. One group will be an audience for role-play performed by student pairs formed in the other group. Have each pair role-play a dental assistant responding to an angry or unhappy patient. Then lead a class discussion on how the dental assistant should handle such a situation.*

OBJECTIVES	CONTENT	TEACHING RESOURCES
Describe good phone courtesy.	■ Phone skills (p. 993) ☐ Courtesy (p. 993)	⊠▤ PPT 17 ▥ TB question 5 ▤ SW Short-Answer Questions 3; Multiple Choice questions 8-10 (pp. 541-542) Figure 61-4 The business assistant answers the phone (p. 993) Recall question 13 (p. 996) ♀ CTQ 2 (p. 1000) ▸ Discuss why the phone is such an important tool in the dental office. ▸ Discuss the essential guidelines for courtesy on the phone. ***Class Activity Divide the class into small groups. Ask each group to discuss and describe good phone courtesy. Have each group share with the class one example of good phone courtesy and one example of poor phone courtesy.***
Describe and compare the handling of different types of phone calls.	☐ Incoming calls (p. 993) ☐ Placing a caller on hold (p. 994) – On-hold message systems (p. 994) ☐ Callers wanting to speak to the dentist (p. 994) ☐ Taking messages (p. 994) *Procedure* 61-1 Answering the phone (p. 995) (SW/ESLR Competency 61-1, p. 545) ☐ Phone message systems (p. 994) – Answering service (p. 994) – Answering machine (p. 995) – Voice mail (p. 995) ☐ Phone equipment (p. 995)	⊠▤ PPT 18 ▥ TB questions 6-8 ▤ SW Short-Answer Questions 4; Fill in the Blank question 5; Multiple Choice question 11 (pp. 541-542) ▤ 𝑒 SW/ESLR Competency 61-1 Answering the Phone (p. 545) Figure 61-5 An example of a printed form for taking messages (p. 994) Figure 61-6 A multipurpose phone system with multiple lines and answering machine (p. 995) Figure 61-7 A facsimile (fax) machine (p. 996) Recall questions 14-16 (p. 996) ▸ Discuss the best way to answer incoming phone calls. How should you place a caller on hold? ▸ Discuss how to handle callers who want to speak to the dentist. ***Class Activity Divide the class into small groups. Assign each group a type of phone call. Ask each group to discuss and determine how it would handle its type of phone call. Then have each group share its findings with the class.***

Torres and Ehrlich Modern Dental Assisting, 9th ed.

Bird/Robinson

OBJECTIVES	CONTENT	TEACHING RESOURCES
	– Headsets (p. 995)	
	– Pager (p. 996)	
	– Facsimile ("fax") machine (p. 996)	

61.1 Homework/Assignments:

61.1 Instructor's Notes/Student Feedback:

Torres and Ehrlich Modern Dental Assisting, 9th ed.

Bird/Robinson

LESSON 61.2

CRITICAL THINKING QUESTION

A dental practice wants to publish a quarterly newsletter. The dentists in the practice ask the rest of the dental team to help them decide what information to include in the newsletter. What suggestions might the dental team give?

Guidelines: The dental team must remember that a newsletter represents a valuable communication tool for the practice. Examples of information to include in the newsletter are technology and treatment advances, dental team profiles, a contest for patients to enter, patient education, and announcements of any changes that have taken place. The above examples are a few ways to help the dental practice develop a quality quarterly newsletter for internal marketing purposes.

OBJECTIVES	CONTENT	TEACHING RESOURCES

Describe external and internal marketing.	■ Written communications (p. 996)
	
	□ Equipment (p. 996)
	
	□ Business letters (p. 997)
	
	  – Parts of a letter (p. 997)
	
	Procedure 61-2 Composing a business letter (p. 999) (SW/ESLR Competency 61-2, p. 547)
	
	□ Types of business letters (p. 997)
	
	  – Letters to colleagues (p. 997)
	
	  – Letters to insurance carriers (p. 997)
	
	■ Marketing your dental practice (p. 999)
	
	□ Goals of practice marketing (p. 999)
	
	□ Logistics of marketing (p. 999)
	
	  – The plan (p. 999)
	
	  – Marketing budget (p. 999)
	
	  – Tracking responses (p. 999)
	
	□ Types of practice marketing (p. 999)
		☒▤ PPT 21-26
		
		▦ TB questions 9-11
		
		✎ SW Short-Answer Questions 5; Fill in the Blank questions 1, 3-4, 7-8; Multiple Choice questions 12-16 (pp. 541-543)
		
		✎ SW Activity (p. 543)
		
		✎ *e* SW/ESLR Competency 61-2 Composing a Business Letter (p. 547)
		
		Figure 61-8 Business equipment is set up within the office management area (p. 996)
		
		Figure 61-9 A desktop computer system used in the office (p. 996)
		
		Figure 61-10 Copier, printer, scanner, and fax machine all in one (p. 997)
		
		Figure 61-11 A business letter (p. 998)
		
		Recall questions 17-18, 19-21 (pp. 998, 1000)
		
		💡 CTQ 1 (p. 1000)
		
		▸ Discuss the characteristics of a good business letter. Why are these important?
		
		▸ Discuss the goals, logistics, and types of practice marketing. Why is it important to track responses to marketing?
		
		Class Activity Present the following examples of marketing to the class, and have students determine whether each is an example of external or internal marketing:
		
		  – Publishing a practice newsletter
		
		  – A health fair
		
		  – Presentations to school groups
		
		  – Sending cards to patients on special occasions

ELSEVIER

OBJECTIVES	CONTENT	TEACHING RESOURCES
	– Practice newsletter (p. 1000)	
	– Patient education materials (p. 1000)	
Performance Evaluation		TB
		SW questions (pp. 541-543)
		SW/ESLR Competency 61-1 Answering the Phone (p. 545)
		SW/ESLR Competency 61-2 Composing a Business Letter (p. 547)
		ESLR Electronic Flashcards
		ESLR Practice Quiz
		Recall questions (pp. 988-1000)
		CTQ (p. 1000)

61.2 Homework/Assignments:

61.2 Instructor's Notes/Student Feedback:

Torres and Ehrlich Modern Dental Assisting, 9th ed.

Bird/Robinson

Slide 1

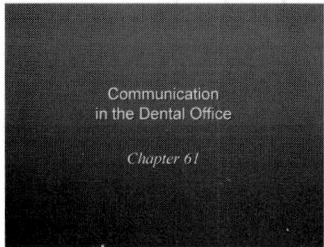

Communication
in the Dental Office

Chapter 61

Slide 2

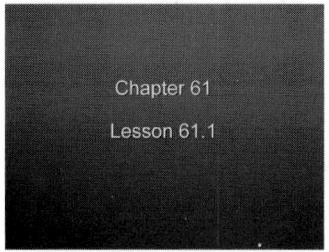

Chapter 61

Lesson 61.1

Slide 3

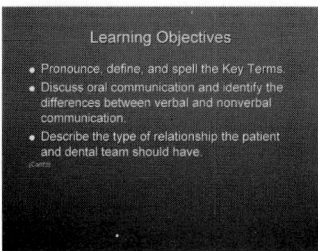

Learning Objectives

- Pronounce, define, and spell the Key Terms.
- Discuss oral communication and identify the differences between verbal and nonverbal communication.
- Describe the type of relationship the patient and dental team should have.
(Cont'd)

Slide 4

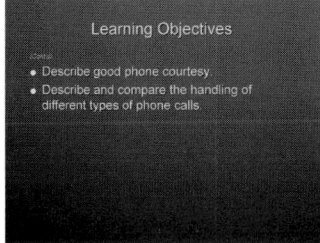

Learning Objectives

(Cont'd)
- Describe good phone courtesy.
- Describe and compare the handling of different types of phone calls.

ELSEVIER

Bird/Robinson

Slide 5

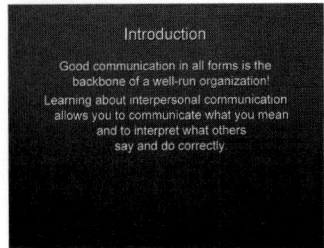

- What are some different forms of communication?

Slide 6

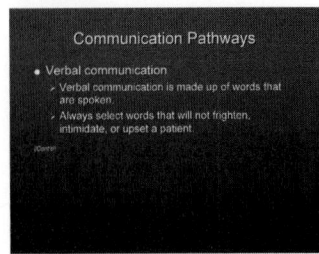

- Clarity in speaking is also important. Ask students to say the following sentences three times each as quickly as possible while fully enunciating each word:
  - Success seeds success.
  - Bigger business isn't better business but better business brings bigger rewards.
  - Ensuring excellence isn't easy.

Slide 7

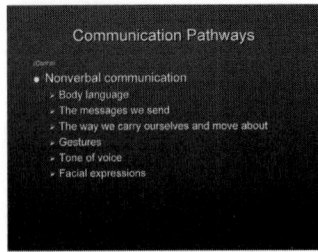

- Always remember that patients are the key to your success.
- Why is eye contact important? *(It helps regulate the flow of communication.)*

Slide 8

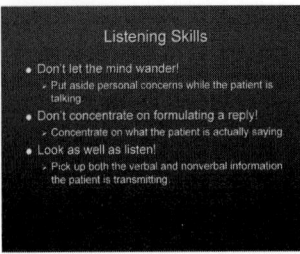

- Lack of communication is the major reason why patients leave a practice.
- Listening requires a great deal of self-control and concentration.

ELSEVIER

Torres and Ehrlich Modern Dental Assisting, 9th ed.

Bird/Robinson

Slide 9

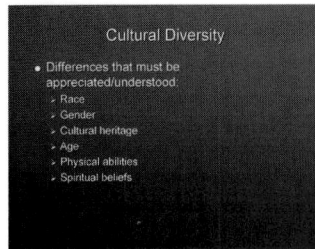

- What is ethnogeriatrics? *(The branch of geriatrics that focuses on how race, culture, and ethnicity influence the health and well-being of the elderly.)*

Slide 10

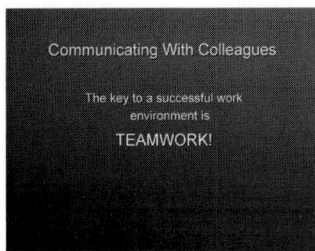

- Remember that a patient is able to determine instantly what kind of working environment exists in the practice.

Slide 11

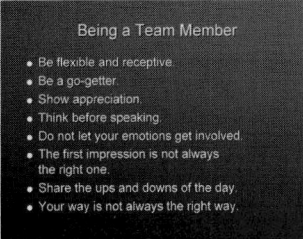

- What other qualities and actions does being a team member involve?

Slide 12

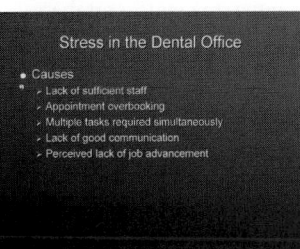

- What are some other causes of stress in the work environment?

Slide 13

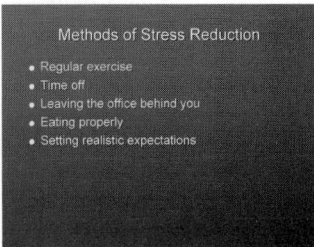

- What are some other ways to reduce stress?

Slide 14

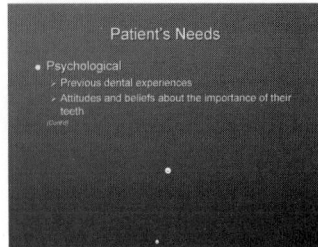

- How could the dental assistant better empathize with patients?
  (Try to see the issue from the patient's point of view.)

Slide 15

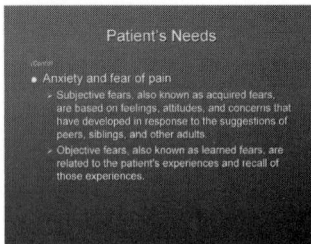

- What are some examples of acquired and learned fears about dental visits?

Slide 16

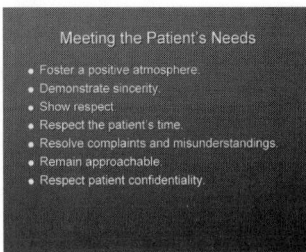

- The dental team should ask itself three questions:
  - What do patients most like about the dentist, the staff, and the practice in general?
  - What do they most dislike?
  - Why do some patients switch to other practices in the area?

Bird/Robinson

Slide 17

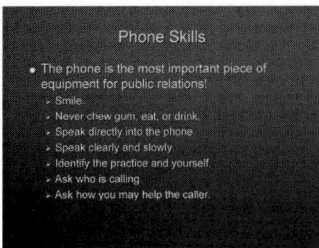

- Smiles are often contagious. What types of feelings are transmitted by a smile? *(Happiness, friendliness, warmth, affection, affiliation, etc.)*
- Can you tell if someone is smiling when they are speaking on the phone? *(Generally, yes.)* Experiment with this when talking to a friend on the phone sometime.

Slide 18

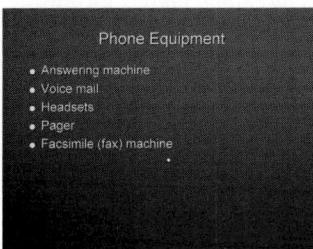

- How does voice mail differ from an answering machine? What are the advantages and disadvantages of each?

Slide 19

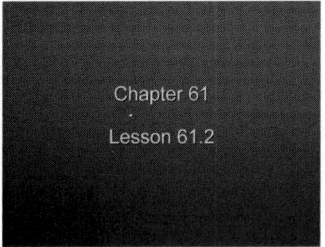

Slide 20

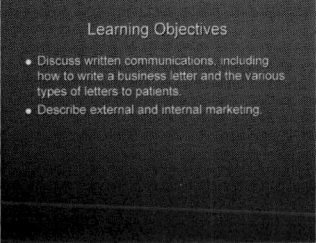

Slide 21

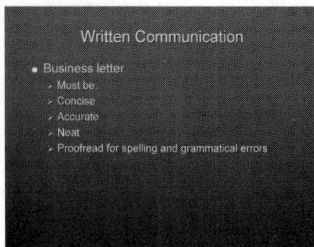

- What kinds of things should be avoided when writing?
  (Slang words, abbreviations, symbols, clichés.)

Slide 22

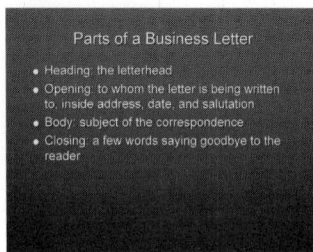

- Some professionals break a business letter into six parts. What might these six parts be? *(Heading, inside address, greeting, body, closing, signature line.)*

Slide 23

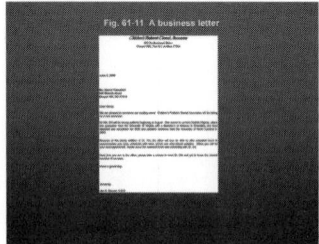

- Ask students to break this letter into four and six parts.

Slide 24

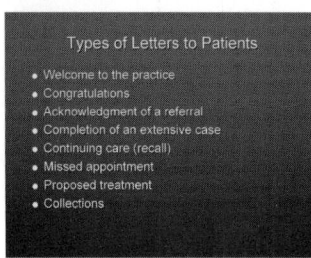

- Letters are also used to communicate with other professionals and with insurance carriers.

- How do these types of letters compare to letters used to communicate with patients?

Bird/Robinson

Slide 25

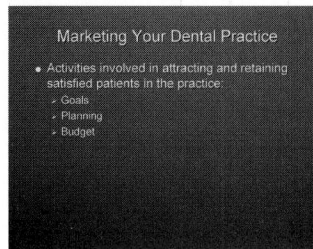

- What are some methods of advertising a dental practice?
  (Web site, online and print dental directories, newsletters, promotional materials, thank-you notes, office open house, giveaways, direct mail.)

Slide 26

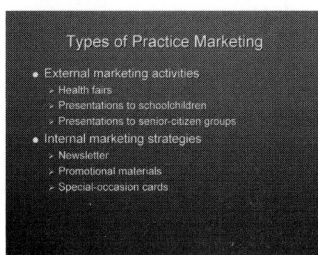

- Are patient education materials external or internal marketing strategies?

ELSEVIER

Torres and Ehrlich Modern Dental Assisting, 9th ed.

Bird/Robinson

TEACHING FOCUS

This chapter introduces the student to topics related to business operating systems, including record-keeping, filing, appointment scheduling, and inventory management. Types of filing systems and guidelines to efficient filing will be discussed. The student will also have the opportunity to become acquainted with effective procedures for scheduling appointments as well as preventive recall programs. This chapter also includes information on procedures for managing inventory and ordering dental supplies and equipment. Furthermore, the student will have the opportunity to learn how to handle equipment repairs.

MATERIALS AND RESOURCES

☐ computer and PowerPoint projector (all Lessons)

LESSON CHECKLIST

Preparations for this lesson include:

- lecture
- guest speaker: business assistant from a dental office
- evaluation of student knowledge and skills needed to perform all entry-level activities related to business operating systems, including:
  - maintaining adequate patient and practice records
  - organizing and implementing an efficient filing system
  - scheduling appointments effectively and implementing a preventive recall program
  - organizing and implementing an efficient inventory management system
  - handling equipment repairs

Bird/Robinson

KEY TERMS

active files (p. 1008)
buffer time (p. 1010)
call list (p. 1013)
chronologic file (p. 1008)
cross-reference file (pp. 1007-1008)
daily schedule (p. 1014)
downtime (p. 1012)
file guides (p. 1006)
filing (p. 1006)
inactive files (p. 1008)
lead time (p. 1017)

ledger (p. 1005)
outguide (p. 1006)
patient of record (p. 1012)
purchase order (p. 1018)
rate of use (p. 1017)
requisition (p. 1018)
reorder tags (p. 1017)
shelf life (p. 1017)
units of time (p. 1010)
want list (p. 1017)
warranty (p. 1018)

ADDITIONAL RESOURCES

PowerPoint slides (Evolve): 1-43

Legend

CTQ
Critical
Thinking
Question

DVD
Multimedia
Procedures
Videos and
Animations

ESLR
EVOLVE
Student
Learning
Resources

IDO
Interactive
Dental
Office
CD-ROM

SW
Student
Workbook

TB
Test Bank
on the
TEACH
CD-ROM

PPT
PowerPoint
Slides

Class Activities are indicated in ***bold italic.***

Torres and Ehrlich Modern Dental Assisting, 9th ed.

Bird/Robinson

LESSON 62.1

PRETEST

1. The procedure manual should include
   a. pay periods.
   b. working hours.
   c. information concerning employee benefits.
   d. OSHA and infection-control policies.

2. The personnel manual should include
   a. emergency procedures.
   b. office communications.
   c. information concerning employee benefits.
   d. professional organizations.

3. Dental practice tasks have been improved by
   a. computer applications.
   b. procedure manuals.
   c. personnel manuals.
   d. HIPAA.

4. What is one of the most important organizational responsibilities of the business assistant?
   a. preparing business letters
   b. maintaining adequate records
   c. scheduling appointments
   d. employee benefits

5. When filing, how many inches of working space should be available?
   a. 1 inch
   b. 2 inches
   c. 3 inches
   d. 4 inches

6. What is an outguide?
   a. a hanging file folder
   b. a bookmark for the filing system
   c. policy manual for scheduling
   d. explanation of benefits

7. Which filing system is the easiest and most commonly used?
   a. alphabetic by last name
   b. color-coding
   c. chronologic
   d. numeric

8. Active files are files of patients who have been seen within the past
   a. 1 to 2 weeks.
   b. 2 to 3 months.
   c. 2 to 3 years.
   d. 5 to 6 years.

9. Inactive files are records of patients who have not been seen in the last
   a. 3 months.
   b. 1 year.
   c. 3 years.
   d. 5 years.

10. The recall system is designed to
    a. notify patients of new products.
    b. notify patients of defective products.
    c. help patients keep their appointments.
    d. help patients return for regular preventive care.

Answers

1. d	3. a	5. d	7. a	9. c
2. c	4. b	6. b	8. c	10. d

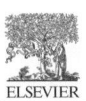
ELSEVIER

Torres and Ehrlich Modern Dental Assisting, 9th ed.

Bird/Robinson

BACKGROUND ASSESSMENT

Question: What are the four basic elements to be outlined in the appointment book?
Answer: The four basic elements to be outlined are office hours, buffer time, meetings, and holidays.

Question: What is the purpose of buffer time?
Answer: Buffer time is an allotment of time reserved each day for emergency patients. It is usually scheduled in the late morning or in the afternoon. If the time is not needed for emergency patients, last-minute appointments can be scheduled.

CRITICAL THINKING QUESTION

The business assistant at a dental office is given the task of reviewing the office operating procedure manual for compliance with the Health Insurance Portability and Accountability Act of 1996 (HIPAA). What specific areas must be included in the office operating procedure manual to be compliant with HIPAA?

Guidelines: HIPAA was adopted to enhance and protect the rights of patients. The dental office must be educated on its state's medical privacy laws. In addition, the dental staff must be trained on privacy policies and procedures. This training must be documented. A privacy officer must also be appointed and a contact person identified who can receive complaints. Dental offices must also adopt or develop the required forms to put into the privacy policies and procedures. Patients must be notified of the new policies by posting and distributing a Notice of Privacy Practice, and obtain written permission by the patient's Acknowledgement of Receipt of Notice of Privacy Practice. Lastly, the business assistant should make sure the policies are current and fully implemented. For further assistance, the business assistant could contact the American Dental Association and request its HIPAA Privacy Kit.

OBJECTIVES	CONTENT	TEACHING RESOURCES
Pronounce, define, and spell the Key Terms.	■ Key terms (p. 1001)	📀 ESLR Electronic Flashcards ▶ Discuss each of the key terms in Chapter 62, focusing on the definition, pronunciation, and spelling of each term. *Class Activity **Divide the class into small groups. Assign each group several key terms. Have the groups practice pronouncing, defining, and spelling the assigned key terms.***
Discuss the role of the office manager/business assistant in the dental office.	■ Introduction (p. 1002) ■ Operating procedure manual (p. 1002) □ HIPAA compliance (p. 1002) – HIPAA privacy compliance list (p. 1003) □ Personnel manual (p. 1003) ■ Computer applications in the dental office (p. 1003) □ Characteristics of the computer (p. 1003)	🖥 PPT 4-8 💻 TB questions 4 📝 SW Short-Answer Questions 1; Fill in the Blank questions 1-20; Multiple Choice questions 1-3 (pp. 549-551) Figure 62-1 Components of a computer (p. 1004) Recall questions 1-3 (p. 1003) ▶ Discuss the essential elements of an operating procedure manual. What topics related to personnel might be included? ▶ Discuss HIPAA compliance and how it applies to a dental practice. *Class Activity **Present the following roles of the business assistant in the dental office. Facilitate a class discussion on each of these roles:***

ELSEVIER

Bird/Robinson

OBJECTIVES	CONTENT	TEACHING RESOURCES
		– *Scheduling patients*
		– *Answering telephones*
		– *Managing payroll*
		– *Maintaining patient records*

Identify types of practice records and files.	■ Record-keeping (p. 1003)
	
	□ Types of records and files (p. 1005)
	
	  – Patient dental records (p. 1005)
	
	  – Patient financial records (p. 1005)
	
	  – Practice business records (p. 1005)
		PPT 9-12
		
		TB questions 5-6
		
		SW Short-Answer Questions 2; Multiple Choice question 4 (pp. 549, 551)
		
		Figure 62-2 Patient ledger (p. 1020)
		
		Figure 62-3 Computerized patient account summary (p. 1020)
		
		Recall question 4 (p. 1006)
		
		Legal and Ethical Implications (p. 1019)
		
		▸ Discuss the three basic types of records that are important to a dental practice.
		
		Class Activity *Divide the class into three groups. Assign each group one of the types of practice records and files. Have each group discuss the characteristics of its assigned type. Then have each group share information about its assigned type of practice record and files with the class.*

Identify how to use these filing systems: alphabetic, numeric, cross-reference, chronologic, and subject.	■ Guidelines to efficient filing (p. 1006)
	
	□ Basic filing systems (p. 1007)
	
	  – Alphabetic (p. 1007)
	
	  – Color-coding (p. 1007)
	
	  – Numeric (p. 1007)
	
	  – Chronologic (p. 1008)
	
	  – Electronic (p. 1008)
	
	□ Active and inactive files (p. 1008)
	
	□ Purge tabs (p. 1008)
	
	□ Record protection
		PPT 13-18
		
		TB questions 7-9
		
		SW Short-Answer Questions 3; Multiple Choice questions 5-8 (pp. 549, 551)
		
		Figure 62-4 Keep filing systems simple (p. 1006)
		
		Figure 62-5 Label drawers (p. 1006)
		
		Figure 62-6 Use an outguide (p. 1006)
		
		Table 62-1 Indexing Rules for Alphabetic Filing (p. 1007)
		
		Figure 62-7 A variety of coding systems is used for filing patient records (p. 1007)
		
		Recall questions 5-8 (p. 1008)
		
		CTQ 1, 5 (p. 1019)
		
		▸ Discuss the advantages and disadvantages of the five basic filing systems. How are purge tabs used?
		
		▸ Discuss record protection and confidentiality for both a paper and an electronic filing system. What are HIPAA requirements in this regard?

OBJECTIVES	CONTENT	TEACHING RESOURCES
	and confidentiality (p. 1008) – HIPAA safeguards (p. 1008) – Protecting electronic files (p. 1008) – Protecting paper files (p. 1008)	*Class Activity Divide class into four groups. Assign each group one of the filing systems. Ask each group to discuss how to use its assigned filing system. Then have each group demonstrate to the class how to use its filing system.*
Describe the function of computerized practice management systems and manual bookkeeping systems.	■ Appointment scheduling (p. 1008) ☐ Efficient appointment scheduling (p. 1009) ☐ Computerized or manual scheduling (p. 1009) ☐ The appointment book (p. 1009)	SW Short-Answer Questions 6 (p. 549) ▸ Discuss manual appointment books and electronic appointment systems and the advantages and disadvantages of each. *Class Activity Divide the class into two groups. Ask each group to discuss one function of computerized practice management systems and manual bookkeeping systems. Then have each group share its function with the class.*
Describe the process of scheduling appointments for maximum productivity.	■ Appointment scheduling (p. 1008) ☐ Efficient appointment scheduling (p. 1009) ☐ Computerized or manual scheduling (p. 1009) ☐ The appointment book (p. 1009) ☐ Guidelines for scheduling (p. 1010) – Units of time (p. 1010) – Columns per day (p. 1010) ☐ Outlining the appointment schedule (p. 1010) – Office hours (p. 1010)	PPT 19-30 TB questions 10-18 SW Short-Answer Questions 4; Multiple Choice questions 9-11 (pp. 549, 551) Figure 62-8 Computerized schedules (p. 1009) Figure 62-9 A typical daily format for scheduling (p. 1011) Figure 62-10 An appointment card is completed (p. 1011) Figure 62-11 A daily schedule (p. 1014) Recall questions 9-11 (p. 1014) CTQ 2-4 (p. 1019) ▸ Discuss the goals of efficient appointment scheduling. What is the purpose of outlining the appointment book and how is this accomplished? ▸ Discuss some of the special considerations for scheduling. How would you handle a new patient or an emergency patient? *Class Activity Invite a business assistant in a dental office to speak to the class. Have the speaker discuss the process of scheduling appointments for maximum productivity. Encourage feedback and discussion from the class.*

OBJECTIVES	CONTENT	TEACHING RESOURCES
	– Buffer time (p. 1010)	
	– Meetings (p. 1010)	
	– Holidays (p. 1010)	
	☐ Making appointment book and appointment card entries (p. 1010)	
	☐ Special considerations for scheduling (p. 1011)	
	– Daily scheduling rules (p. 1012)	
	– New patients (p. 1012)	
	– Scheduling for the dental hygienist (p. 1012)	
	– Recall patients (p. 1012)	
	– Children (p. 1012)	
	– Emergency patients (p. 1012)	
	– Scheduling an appointment series (p. 1013)	
	– Scheduling for an expanded-functions dental assistant (p. 1013)	
	☐ Confirmation of appointments (p. 1013)	
	☐ Patient circumstances (p. 1013)	

OBJECTIVES	CONTENT	TEACHING RESOURCES
	– Late patients (p. 1013)	
	– Canceled appointments (p. 1013)	
	– Short-notice appointments (p. 1013)	
	☐ Daily treatment area schedule (p. 1014)	
	– Prior appointment preparations (p. 1014)	
	– Daily meeting (p. 1014)	

62.1 Homework/Assignments:

62.1 Instructor's Notes/Student Feedback:

Torres and Ehrlich Modern Dental Assisting, 9th ed.

Bird/Robinson

LESSON 62.2

CRITICAL THINKING QUESTION

A dental assistant working in a busy dental office has been assigned the task of ordering supplies that are low according to the office inventory system. The supplies that need to be ordered include disposable needles, local anesthetic solutions, radiographic film, laboratory supplies, and business office supplies. What information will the dental assistant need to reorder various products?
Guidelines: The inventory system should include the following information for ordering: full brand name of product, descriptive information of product, reorder point of product, purchase source (including name, address, and telephone number of supplier), catalog number for product, along with quantity purchase rates and reorder quantity. Having all of the above information will allow for proper ordering of dental supplies.

OBJECTIVES	CONTENT	TEACHING RESOURCES
Identify three types of preventive recall systems and state the benefits of each.	■ Preventive recall programs (p. 1014) ☐ Types of recall systems (p. 1015) – Continuing appointment system (p. 1015) – Written recall notification (p. 1015) – Recall by telephone (p. 1015)	PPT 33-34 TB questions 19-20 SW Short-Answer Questions 5; Multiple Choice questions 12-13 (pp. 549, 551) Box 62-1 Calculating 6-Month Recall Time (p. 1015) Figure 62-12 Recall postcards are mailed (p. 1015) Recall questions 12-13 (p. 1015) ▸ Discuss the goal and function of a preventive recall program. What types of systems are there and how do they compare? ***Class Activity** Divide the class into three groups. Assign each group one of the three types of preventive recall systems. Have each group discuss its assigned preventive recall system. Then have each group share with the class the benefits of its assigned preventive recall system.*
Discuss the management of inventory systems.	■ Inventory management (p. 1015) ☐ Computerized inventory system (p. 1016) ☐ Guidelines for ordering dental supplies (p. 1016) – When ordering supplies (p. 1017) – Reorder point (p. 1017) – Marking the reorder point (p. 1017) – Automatic shipments (p. 1017)	PPT 35-43 TB questions 21-25 SW Short-Answer Questions 7; Multiple Choice questions 14-20 (pp. 549, 551) Figure 62-13 An example of a computerized inventory management system (p. 1016) Recall questions 14-18 (p. 1018) Eye to the Future (p. 1019) ▸ Discuss the importance of an effective inventory management system. What are some important elements of a good system? ▸ Discuss the basic categories of a dental supply budget. What factors would you use in deciding which category an item belongs to?

ELSEVIER

Torres and Ehrlich Modern Dental Assisting, 9th ed.

Bird/Robinson

OBJECTIVES	CONTENT	TEACHING RESOURCES
	– Quantity purchase rate (p. 1017)	*Class Activity* **Present the following information to the class. Ask the class to determine whether the information is part of the management of inventory systems.**
	– Reorder quantity (p. 1017)	– **Barcode reorder system**
	– Backorders (p. 1017)	– **Reorder point**
	– Order exchange, return, or replacement (p. 1017)	– **Patient charge for equipment**
	– Requisitions and purchase orders (p. 1018)	– **Recruiting patients**
	☐ Dental supply budget (p. 1018)	
	– Consumables and disposables (p. 1018)	
	– Expendables (p. 1018)	
	– Nonexpendables (p. 1018)	
	– Major equipment (p. 1018)	
	■ Equipment repairs (p. 1018)	
	☐ Equipment records (p. 1018)	
	– Service contracts (p. 1018)	
	– Service call (p. 1019)	
Performance Evaluation		**TB** TB **SW** SW questions (pp. 549-552) **SW** SW Topics for discussion (p. 552) **e** ESLR Electronic Flashcards **e** ESLR Practice Quiz Recall questions (pp. 1003-1018) CTQ (p. 1019)

62.2 Homework/Assignments:

62.2 Instructor's Notes/Student Feedback:

Slide 1

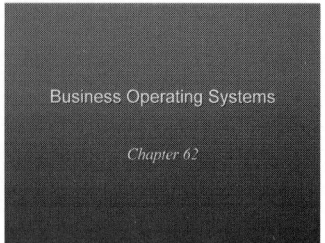

Slide 2

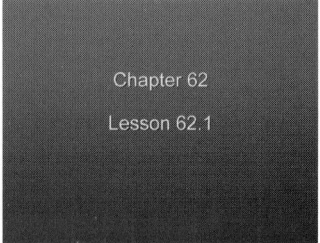

Slide 3

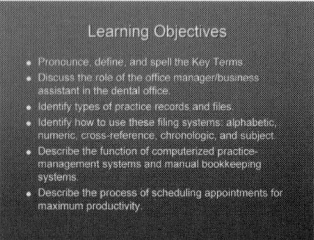

Slide 4

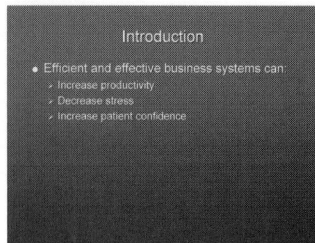

- What component is necessary to achieve organizational goals, satisfied employees working in teams, and financial success? *(Effective management.)*

Torres and Ehrlich Modern Dental Assisting, 9th ed.

Bird/Robinson

Slide 5

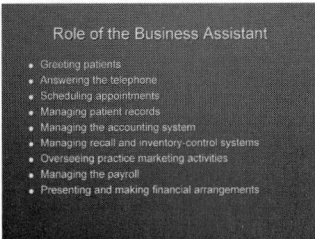

- What plays a crucial role in a successful dental practice under normal economic conditions? *(Patient retention.)*

Slide 6

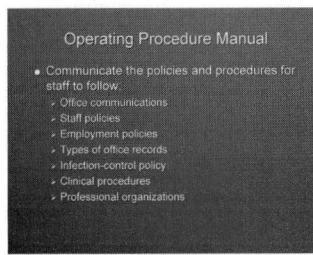

- Why is the operating procedure manual important? *(It contains the policies and procedures of the practice that the dentist wants the staff to follow.)*

Slide 7

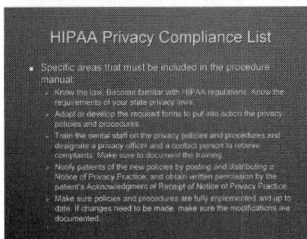

- Why is it important to incorporate HIPAA provisions in a useful procedures manual?

Slide 8

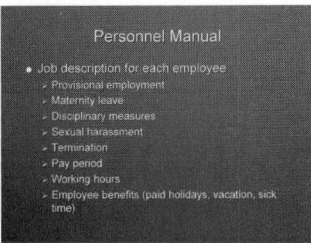

- A good personnel manual is an essential business tool that benefits everyone in the company.

Torres and Ehrlich Modern Dental Assisting, 9th ed.

Bird/Robinson

Slide 9

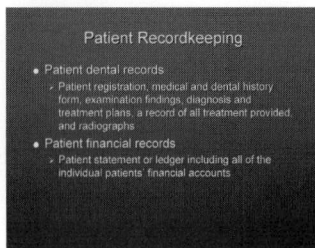

- Why should records be kept indefinitely? *(They are vital for supporting diagnostic and treatment decisions and preventing payment problems in cases where dental benefit plans apply.)*

Slide 10

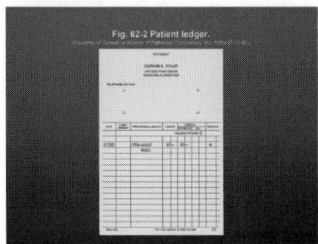

- What information is included on the patient ledger? *(All the financial information, date, name, description of service, charges, payments, and balance.)*

Slide 11

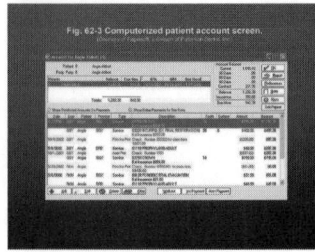

- The business assistant can access the patient account screen and review or enter information on all aspects of financial charges, payments, and insurance transactions.

Slide 12

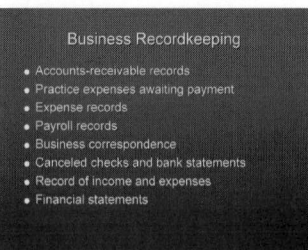

- How are business records kept? *(They are filed according to a subject system: e.g., "laboratory expenses.")*

Slide 13

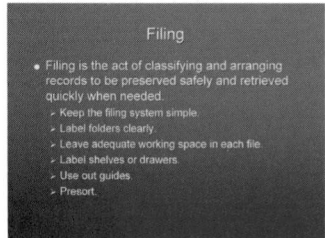

- What is a file guide?

Slide 14

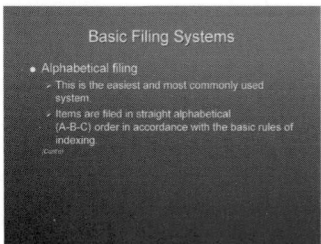

- Under what part of the patient name is a record filed?

Slide 15

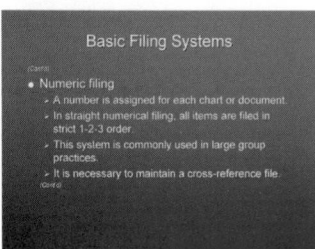

- Why is it necessary to cross-reference a numerical list?

Slide 16

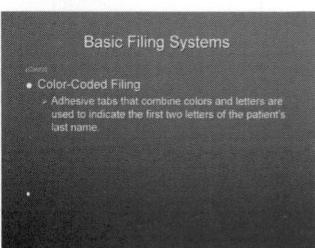

- What is the purpose of color-coded filing?

Slide 17

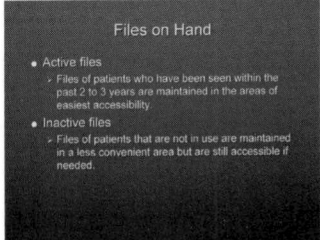

• Why are files split between active and inactive patients?

Slide 18

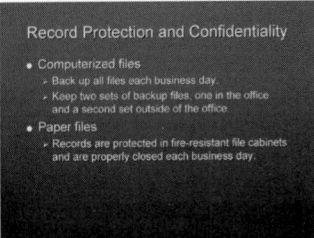

• Why is it necessary to maintain duplicate sets of files?

Slide 19

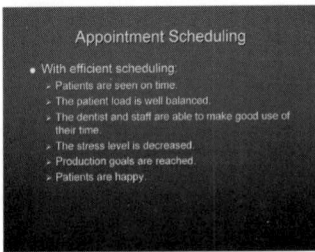

• Why is it important in a dental practice to schedule appointments efficiently and effectively?

Slide 20

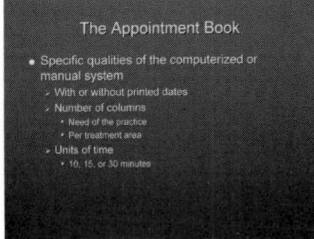

• These basic components are necessary in the system used: format, outlined days, and effective scheduling.

Torres and Ehrlich Modern Dental Assisting, 9th ed.

Bird/Robinson

Slide 21

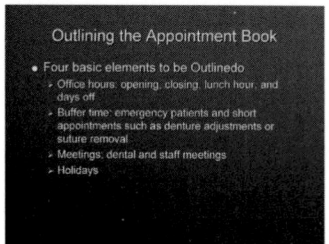

- When should the book be outlined?

Slide 22

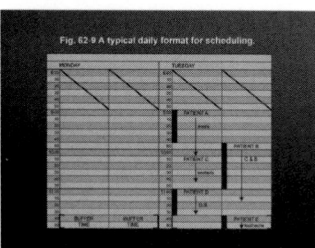

- What is one of the benefits of computer scheduling?

Slide 23

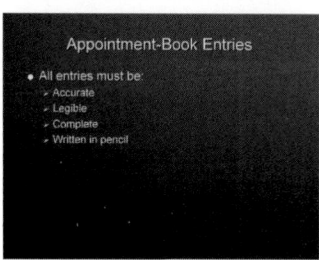

- Why is it important to make certain that appointment book entries are accurate, legible, complete, and in pencil?

Slide 24

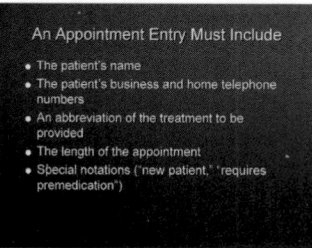

- What is the proper sequence of recording entries?

Slide 25

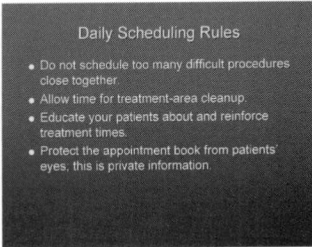

- Why should the business assistant not schedule too many difficult procedures close together?
- What is the best time of day for lengthy and difficult procedures? *(Early morning.)*

Slide 26

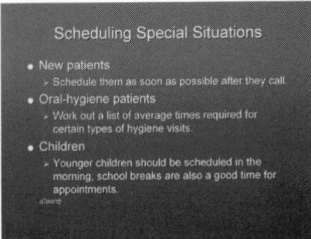

- Some practices reserve a block of time each day for new patients.
- In some cases the dental hygienist performs 90% of the work.
- Why should procedures with younger children be done in the morning?

Slide 27

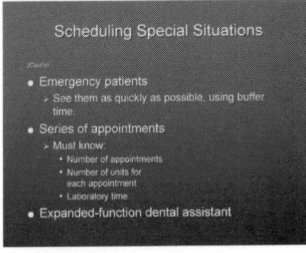

- A patient who is in pain and has been seen before in the practice is known by what name? *(Patient of record.)*
- It is important to promptly schedule an appointment for a patient of record who calls with an apparent emergency so that the dentist is not open to charges of abandonment.

Slide 28

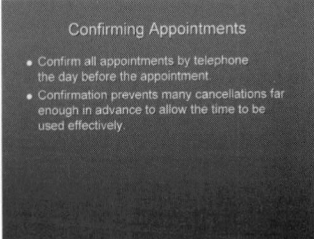

- What is the role of confirming appointments in a successful practice?

Torres and Ehrlich Modern Dental Assisting, 9th ed.

Bird/Robinson

Slide 29

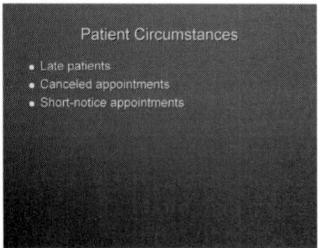

- How should the above circumstances be handled?

Slide 30

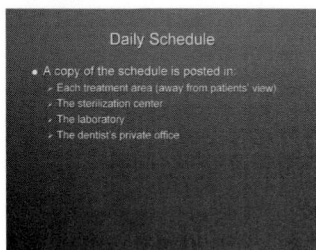

- Why would a dental office want to post a copy of the schedule in these areas?

Slide 31

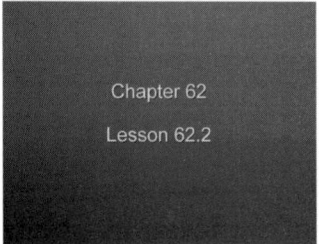

Slide 32

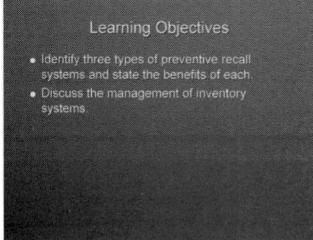

Slide 33

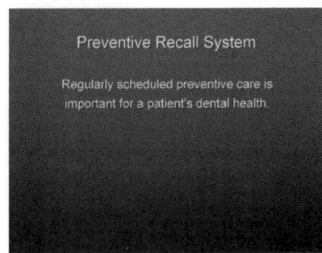

- Discuss the relationship between preventive and corrective dental care.

Slide 34

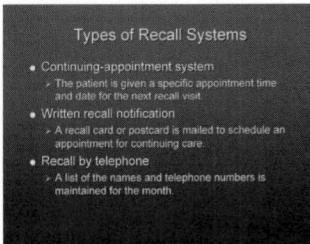

- What are the advantages of these recall systems in dental practice? Why?

Slide 35

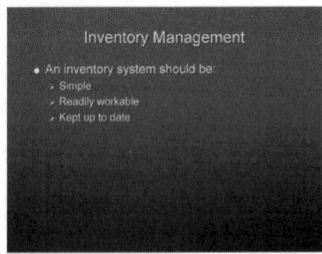

- Discuss the role each requirement plays within a workable inventory system.

Slide 36

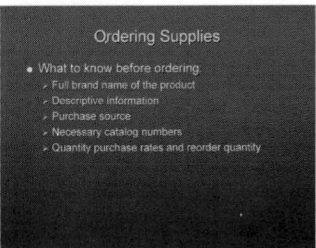

- Have students review sample supply information from a catalog.

Slide 37

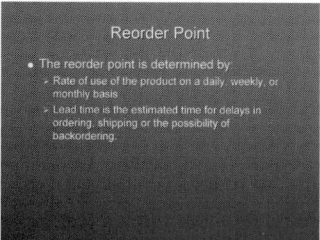

- Discuss several difficulties in establishing a reorder point.

Slide 38

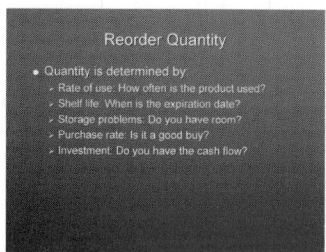

- Provide some guidelines for obtaining precise information about the five factors listed here.

Slide 39

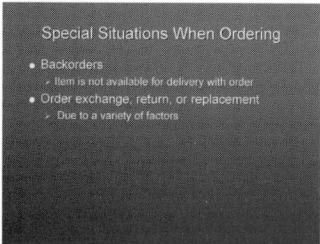

- What is the best way to handle the situations listed?

Slide 40

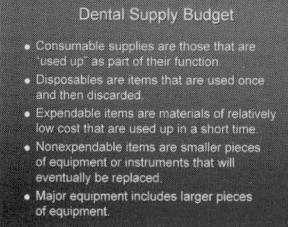

- Review copies of the dental supply budget of several dental offices. Compare the differences based on the size of the dental practice.

Torres and Ehrlich Modern Dental Assisting, 9th ed.

Bird/Robinson

Slide 41

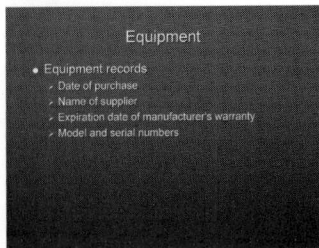

- Why is it important to maintain equipment records for the dental practice?

Slide 42

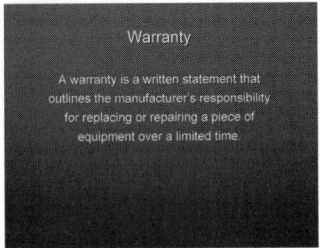

- Discuss examples of warranties.

Slide 43

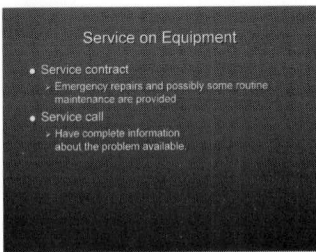

- Name some specific areas of the dental practice that service contracts and calls must cover.

Bird/Robinson

TEACHING FOCUS

This chapter introduces students to topics related to financial management in the dental office. Students will have the opportunity to become acquainted with preventive account management, accounts receivable, accounts payable, writing checks, and payroll. Topics related to dental insurance, including types of prepaid dental programs, eligibility and benefits determination, dental procedure codes, and claim forms are covered. In addition, students have the opportunity to learn about HIPAA provisions, electronic transactions, claim processing, payments from insurance carriers, handling overpayments, and insurance fraud.

MATERIALS AND RESOURCES

- ☐ blank dental claim form (Lesson 63.3)
- ☐ blank patient registration form (Lesson 63.1)
- ☐ blank sample checks (Lesson 63.2)
- ☐ computer and PowerPoint projector (all Lessons)

LESSON CHECKLIST

Preparations for this lesson include:

- lecture
- guest speaker: business manager of a dental office
- evaluation of student knowledge and skills needed to perform all entry-level activities related to financial management in the dental office, including:
  - ○ description of manual and computerized bookkeeping systems
  - ○ collections management, including accounts receivable and accounts payable
  - ○ process of check writing
  - ○ purpose of business summaries
  - ○ common payroll deductions
  - ○ purpose of dental insurance
  - ○ types of prepaid dental programs
  - ○ basic dental insurance terminology
  - ○ identification of dental procedures and coding
  - ○ description of claims form processing and follow-up
  - ○ identification of insurance fraud

KEY TERMS

accounting (p. 1021)
accounts payable (p. 1031)
audit trail (p. 1024)
bonding (p. 1023)
bookkeeping (p. 1021)
carrier (p. 1036)
change fund (p. 1024)
check (p. 1033)
check register (p. 1033)
coordination of benefits (COB) (p. 1039)
Current Dental Terminology (CDT) (p. 1039)
customary fee (p. 1036)
deposit slip (p. 1027)
disbursements (p. 1031)
expenses (p. 1031)
fixed overhead (p. 1031)
gross income (p. 1031)

invoice (p. 1032)
ledger (p. 1022)
net income (p. 1031)
packing slip (p. 1032)
payee (p. 1033)
pegboard system (p. 1023)
petty cash (p. 1032)
posted (p. 1024)
provider (p. 1036)
reasonable fee (p. 1036)
responsible party (p. 1024)
statement (p. 1032)
transaction (p. 1022)
usual fee (p. 1036)
variable overhead (p. 1031)
walkout statement (p. 1024)

ADDITIONAL RESOURCES

PowerPoint slides (Evolve): 1-52

Legend

CTQ
Critical
Thinking
Question

DVD
Multimedia
Procedures
Videos and
Animations

ESLR
EVOLVE
Student
Learning
Resources

IDO
Interactive
Dental
Office
CD-ROM

SW
Student
Workbook

TB
Test Bank
on the
TEACH
CD-ROM

PPT
PowerPoint
Slides

Class Activities are indicated in ***bold italic***.

Torres and Ehrlich Modern Dental Assisting, 9th ed.
Bird/Robinson

LESSON 63.1

PRETEST

1. Accounting is
   a. recording of investment procedures.
   b. process of recording, classifying, and summarizing financial transactions.
   c. daily bookkeeping procedures.
   d. basic practice financial policies.

2. Pegboard accounting is also known as
   a. bookkeeping.
   b. accounts receivable.
   c. one-write system.
   d. integrated accounting.

3. What might the dental office obtain if staff members handle practice funds?
   a. bonding insurance
   b. consumer credit report
   c. employee policy manuals
   d. personal data

4. What is the most frequently used type of accounts receivable bookkeeping system?
   a. walk-out accounting
   b. integrated accounting
   c. charge slips
   d. pegboard system

5. Payments on any outstanding accounts payable are known as
   a. petty cash.
   b. disbursements.
   c. customary fees.
   d. usual fees.

6. Charge slips are used to
   a. audit.
   b. transmit financial information between the treatment area and the business office.
   c. record all checks issued on, and deposits made to, a specific account.
   d. coordinate insurance coverage between two insurance carriers.

7. The ledger is
   a. a written indication of any balance due on an account.
   b. the overhead costs of a business.
   c. a financial statement that maintains all account transactions.
   d. an itemized listing of shipped goods.

8. What is vital in the event of theft, fire, or disaster?
   a. backup records and files
   b. charge slips
   c. office equipment
   d. accounting records

9. The guarantor is the
   a. person who agreed to be responsible for payment.
   b. person providing the services.
   c. health insurance carrier.
   d. dental insurance carrier responsible for payment.

Bird/Robinson

10. An example of variable overhead is
    a. insurance premiums.
    b. salaries.
    c. electricity.
    d. office supplies.

Answers

1. b	3. a	5. b	7. c	9. a
2. c	4. d	6. b	8. a	10. d

BACKGROUND ASSESSMENT

Question: What is the Federal Income Contributions Act (FICA)?

Answer: FICA—or Social Security—requires that the employer deduct a certain percentage of the employee's gross pay. The employer is also required to match the contribution. These contributions are forwarded to the federal government to be credited to the employee's account. The employee receives a Statement of Earnings annually.

Question: What are the three most commonly used methods of calculating fee-for-service benefits?

Answer: The three most commonly used methods are usual, customary, and reasonable (UCR); schedule of benefits; and fixed fee schedule. Usual fee refers to a fee that the dentist charges private patients for a given service. A customary fee is one that is within the range of the usual fees charged for the same service by other dentists. A reasonable fee is one that is considered justified by special circumstances requiring extensive treatment. A schedule of benefits, also known as a schedule of allowances, is a list of fixed specific amounts that the carrier will pay toward the cost of covered services. A fixed fee schedule is an established fee for any treatment received by the patient.

CRITICAL THINKING QUESTION

A new patient visits the dental office, and the business assistant asks the patient to fill out a registration form. Then the dentist examines the patient and explains a plan of treatment. What information should the assistant make certain is on the registration form? What should happen before the treatment plan is implemented?

Guidelines: The registration form should gather all the basic financial information needed to manage the account history and complete the patient identification portion of an insurance claim form. The following information should be included on the form: name, address, telephone number, and place of employment of the person responsible for the account; information about patient coverage under a dental insurance plan; and identification information for all individuals included in the account. Before the treatment is implemented, a fee estimate must be prepared based on the treatment plan recommended by the dentist. The fee charged should represent a fair return to the dentist for professional services. After the dentist has completed the plan of treatment, the business assistant should present the fee information and make payment arrangements to the satisfaction of the patient and dentist.

OBJECTIVES	CONTENT	TEACHING RESOURCES
Pronounce, define, and spell the Key Terms.	■ Key terms (pp. 1020-1021)	▨ SW Fill in the Blank questions 1-20 (pp. 554-555) ℰ ESLR Electronic Flashcards ▸ Discuss each of the Key Terms, focusing on the definition, pronunciation, and spelling of each term. *Class Activity **Divide the class into groups, and give each group one-third of the key terms. Ask each group to develop a crossword puzzle using its assigned terms. They can use a Web site for crossword puzzles or make a puzzle on their own. Then have groups complete one another's puzzles until every group has considered each set of terms.***

OBJECTIVES	CONTENT	TEACHING RESOURCES
Demonstrate making financial arrangements with a patient.	■ Accounting (p. 1021) ■ Preventive account management (p. 1021) □ Gathering financial information (p. 1021) – Credit reports (p. 1022) – Fee presentation (p. 1022) – Making financial arrangements (p. 1022)	PPT 4-6 TB questions 1-3 SW Short-Answer Questions 2; Fill in the Blank questions 4, 11; Multiple Choice question 3 (pp. 553-555) Figure 63-1 Computerized registration form (p. 1022) Recall questions 1-3 (p. 1022) CTQ 3 (p. 1046) ▶ Discuss the difference between accounting and bookkeeping. Explain how managing accounts preventively can contribute to the financial health of a practice. ▶ Discuss the communication skills required when making financial arrangements with a patient. *Class Activity Divide the class into pairs, and present the following situation:* *A patient requires a root canal on one tooth and replacement of a crown on another tooth, both of which are expensive procedures. The patient's insurance will pay only part of the cost.* *Ask pairs of students to take turns role-playing a business assistant explaining the fees and office policy and making payment arrangements with the patient. Then ask volunteer pairs to make presentations to the class for discussion.*
Describe the function of computerized practice management systems and manual bookkeeping systems.	■ Accounts receivable (p. 1022) □ Types of accounts receivable systems (p. 1023) – Pegboard accounts receivable management (p. 1023) – Computerized accounts receivable management (p. 1023)	PPT 7-11 TB questions 4-5 SW Short-Answer Questions 1; Fill in the Blank questions 13, 20; Multiple Choice questions 1-2, 4-5 (pp. 553-555) Figure 63-2 Manual pegboard system (p. 1023) Figure 63-3 Computerized accounts receivable management system (p. 1023) ▶ Discuss types of accounts receivable systems. Outline the advantages and disadvantages of pegboard and computerized systems. ▶ Discuss the importance of confidentiality when maintaining accounts receivable. *Class Activity Divide the class into groups. Assign some of the groups computerized practice management systems and the other groups manual bookkeeping systems. Have groups discuss the function, benefits, and drawbacks of*

Torres and Ehrlich Modern Dental Assisting, 9th ed.

Bird/Robinson

OBJECTIVES	CONTENT	TEACHING RESOURCES
		their assigned systems. Then reconvene the class and lead a discussion in which students compare their findings.
Describe the importance and management of collections in the dental office.	☐ Accounts receivable management basics (p. 1023) – Charge slips (p. 1024) – Daily journal page (p. 1024) – Receipts and walkout statements (p. 1024) ☐ Recording payments (p. 1024) – Patient account records (p. 1024) ☐ Payment (p. 1024) – Payment at the time of treatment (p. 1024) – Cash (p. 1024) – Check (p. 1027) – Credit cards (p. 1027) – Professional courtesy and discounts (p. 1027) ☐ Daily proof of posting (p. 1027) ☐ Bank deposits (p. 1027) ☐ Monthly statement (p. 1027) – Cycle billing (p. 1027) – Divided payment plans (p. 1028) ■ Collections (p. 1028) ☐ Accounts receivable report (p. 1028) – Management of collection efforts (p. 1028)	⊠▤ PPT 12-28 ▦ TB questions 6-10 ▰ SW Short-Answer Questions 3; Fill in the Blank questions 1, 3, 6, 9-10, 12, 15, 17-19; Multiple Choice questions 6-14 (pp. 553-556) Figure 63-4 A computerized statement. A printout of this provides a walkout statement for the patient (p. 1025) Figure 63-5 A walkout statement if presented to the patient for his or her records (p. 1026) Figure 63-6 Deposit slip (p. 1028) Recall questions 4-8 (p. 1028) Collection Follow-Through (p. 1029) Box 63-1 Suggestions for Composing Collection Letters (p. 1029) Figure 63-7 An example of a collection letter (p. 1030) Recall questions 9-10 (p. 1031) Figure 63-8 Petty cash voucher (p. 1032) Recall questions 11-14 (p. 1033) ♀ CTQ 1-2 (p. 1045) ▸ Discuss the purpose and use of charge slips, the daily journal page, receipts, and walkout statements. ▸ Discuss the various forms of payment. Note the specific requirements of the business assistant when handling cash, checks, and credit cards. ▸ Discuss collection follow-through. Discuss the follow-through timetable and why such a timetable can help ensure the financial health of a dental practice. *Class Activity Invite the business manager of a dental office to speak to the class about the importance and management of collections. Ask the speaker to address various forms of payment, collection follow-through, and guidelines for communication strategies. Ask students to prepare questions in advance.*

OBJECTIVES	CONTENT	TEACHING RESOURCES
	– Collection letters (p. 1029)	
	– Collection telephone calls (p. 1029)	
	– Final collection options (p. 1031)	
	– Collection agency (p. 1031)	
	– Small claims court (p. 1031)	
	■ Accounts payable management (p. 1031)	
	☐ Dental office overhead (p. 1031)	
	– Fixed overhead (p. 1031)	
	– Variable overhead (p. 1031)	
	– Gross versus net income (p. 1031)	
	☐ Disbursements (p. 1031)	
	– Packing slips, invoices, and statements (p. 1032)	
	☐ Organizing expenditure records (p. 1032)	
	– Payment of accounts (p. 1032)	
	– Cash on delivery (p. 1032)	
	– Petty cash (p. 1032)	

ELSEVIER

Torres and Ehrlich Modern Dental Assisting, 9th ed.

Bird/Robinson

63.1 Homework/Assignments:

63.1 Instructor's Notes/Student Feedback:

LESSON 63.2

CRITICAL THINKING QUESTION

A new business assistant who has been hired for a dental practice will be responsible for handling payroll. Because the practice has not had a policy manual, the owner of the practice asks the new business assistant to develop a policy manual, which will be used to determine the type of payroll records the practice keeps. What records should the business assistant include in the policy manual?

Guidelines: Federal regulations require an employer to take certain deductions from an employee's pay and also to pay certain payroll taxes. The government requires each employer to keep records of the hours worked, the amount paid, and the amounts deducted for tax purposes. Employee records must be kept up to date at all times and must be complete and accurate. Separate payroll sheets should be kept for each employee, with the employee's full name, social security number, address, and number of exemptions.

OBJECTIVES	CONTENT	TEACHING RESOURCES
Describe check writing.	■ Writing checks (p. 1033) □ Check terminology (p. 1033) – Check endorsement (p. 1033) – Stop payment order (p. 1033) – Nonsufficient funds (p. 1033)	PPT 32-33 TB questions 11-13 SW Short-Answer Questions 4; Fill in the Blank question 2; Multiple Choice questions 15-16 (pp. 553-554, 556) Figure 63-9 Correct way to write a check (p. 1034) Recall questions 15-16 (p. 1034) ▶ Discuss check writing and check endorsement. Note the important elements that should be included in the check register entry. What is the difference between blanket endorsement and restrictive endorsement? ▶ Discuss nonsufficient funds. Explain the bookkeeping process that occurs when a check is returned. *Class Activity **Hand out sample blank checks to the class, and ask students to write a check correctly. Ask students to exchange checks and endorse them for payment. As a class, discuss errors and incorrect procedures. How should they be corrected?***
Explain the purpose of business summaries.	– Business summaries (p. 1034)	SW Short-Answer Questions 5 (p. 553) ▶ Discuss the business summaries that are used in the practice. Note the purpose of these summaries. *Class Activity **Lead a discussion in which students discuss business summaries used by a dental practice. What are the purposes? In what ways does the practice use the information?***
Identify common payroll withholding taxes and discuss the financial responsibility of	■ Payroll (p. 1035) □ Payroll deductions (p. 1035) – Income tax withholding	PPT 34-36 TB questions 14-17 SW Short-Answer Questions 6 (p. 553) Figure 63-10 Payroll report (p. 1035)

ELSEVIER

Torres and Ehrlich Modern Dental Assisting, 9th ed.

Bird/Robinson

OBJECTIVES	CONTENT	TEACHING RESOURCES
the employer.	(p. 1035) – Federal Insurance Contributions Act (p. 1035) – Other deductions (p. 1036) – Government remittance (p. 1036)	CTQ 4 (p. 1046) ▸ Discuss the items that must be recorded by each employer with regard to employees, including hours worked, amount paid, and amounts deducted for tax purposes. ▸ Discuss income tax withholding. Explain the three times when an employer must complete a W-2 form for each employee. *Class Activity Divide the class into groups, and assign each group a type of payroll deduction: federal income tax withholding; FICA; additional federal, state, and local taxes; or health insurance. Have each group discuss its assigned deduction and the financial responsibility of the employer. Then have each group share its information with the class for feedback and discussion.*
Discuss the purpose of dental insurance.	■ Dental insurance (p. 1036)	PPT 37 TB question 18 SW Short-Answer Questions 7 (p. 553) ▸ Discuss dental insurance and its purpose. Note the two ways in which people can obtain dental insurance. *Class Activity Lead a class discussion in which you propose each of the following as a possible purpose of dental insurance and ask the students to respond.* *– Pay for all dental costs* *– Reduce cost to patient* *– Increase payments to dentist* *– Decrease fraud* *Then discuss why it is important that claims are processed accurately and efficiently.*
Identify the parties involved with dental insurance.	☐ Parties involved in dental insurance (p. 1036)	PPT 38 TB question 19 SW Short-Answer Questions 9; Fill in the Blank questions 7, 14 (pp. 553-555) ▸ Discuss the parties involved in dental insurance. *Class Activity Divide the class into small groups, and assign each group one of the following parties involved in dental insurance:* *– Subscriber* *– Dependent*

Torres and Ehrlich Modern Dental Assisting, 9th ed.

Bird/Robinson

OBJECTIVES	CONTENT	TEACHING RESOURCES
		– *Group* – *Carrier* – *Provider* *Ask each group to discuss how its assigned party is involved with dental insurance and then discuss as a class.*
Identify the types of prepaid dental programs.	☐ Types of prepaid dental programs (p. 1036) – Usual, customary, and reasonable fees (p. 1036) – Schedule of benefits (p. 1037) – Fixed fee schedule (p. 1037) – Alternative payment plans (p. 1037)	⊠ PPT 39-42 TB question 20 SW Short-Answer Questions 10; Fill in the Blank questions 5, 16 (pp. 553-555) Recall question 17 (p. 1045) ▸ Discuss alternative payment plans, including capitation programs, direct reimbursement plans, individual practice associations, and preferred provider organizations. List the advantages and disadvantages of each to the patient and to the provider. *Class Activity Divide the class into three groups, and assign each group one of the types of prepaid dental programs: usual, customary, and reasonable fees; schedule of benefits; and fixed-fee schedule. Have each group discuss its assigned type of prepaid dental program, and then compare and contrast as a class.*

63.2 Homework/Assignments:

63.2 Instructor's Notes/Student Feedback:

Bird/Robinson

LESSON 63.3

CRITICAL THINKING QUESTION

A business assistant proposes simplifying the coding of dental procedures and reducing coding errors in a busy dental office. What kind of system could the assistant recommend that would simplify the coding process and reduce errors?

Guidelines: Each dental procedure has a specific code issued by the American Dental Association. One way to simplify and eliminate coding errors is to develop a standard preprinted form. The preprinted form can be attached to the patient's folder. After performing a procedure, the dentist can check off the box for services and charges along with any additional comments. Using this system can reduce the incidence of errors and unnecessary costs associated with the fees for procedures performed.

OBJECTIVES	CONTENT	TEACHING RESOURCES
Define managed care.	– Managed care (p. 1037)	PPT 37 TB question 21 SW Short-Answer Questions 11 (p. 553) ▸ Discuss the types of plans that are considered managed care plans. ***Class Activity** **Lead a discussion in which students describe managed health care. How does it differ from other forms of health care delivery? What are the pros and cons? Why should the dental assistant keep up to date on dental health care policies and procedures?***
Discuss and define basic dental terminology.	– Managed care (p. 1037) ☐ Determining eligibility (p. 1037)	TB question 22 SW Short-Answer Questions 12; Multiple Choice questions 17-20 (pp. 554-556) Table 63-1 Basic Dental Insurance Terminology (p. 1038) Recall questions 18-19 (p. 1045) CTQ 5 (p. 1046) ▸ Discuss determining eligibility. Note the proper types of identification the assistant should request of the patient to confirm eligibility. ***Class Activity** **Divide the class into pairs, and have them explain to each other basic dental insurance terminology using Table 63-1 for reference. Ask each pair to use the term correctly in a sentence. Then ask each pair to write its sentences on the board, leaving the term blank for the class to fill in correctly.***
Explain dual coverage.	☐ Determining benefits (p. 1039) – Limitations (p. 1039)	PPT 46 TB questions 23-24 SW Short-Answer Questions 13 (p. 554)

ELSEVIER

Torres and Ehrlich Modern Dental Assisting, 9th ed.

Bird/Robinson

OBJECTIVES	CONTENT	TEACHING RESOURCES
	– Nonduplication of benefits (p. 1039)	Recall question 20 (p. 1045) ▸ Discuss determining benefits. Note that the carrier is responsible for covering only the level of treatment that is included in the dental plan. ▸ Discuss the coverage provided in a least expensive alternative treatment plan (also known as an alternative benefit policy). ***Class Activity Lead a discussion in which students describe dual coverage. Why is it important to determine primary and secondary carriers? What is the birthday rule? What is the business assistant's role in coordination of benefits?***
Identify dental procedures and coding.	☐ Dental procedure codes (p. 1039)	TB question 25 SW Short-Answer Questions 14; Fill in the Blank question 8 (p. 554) Table 63-2 Dental Procedure Codes (p. 1040) Recall questions 22-25 (p. 1045) ▸ Discuss dental procedure codes. Note the purpose of these codes, and explain the legal and financial reasons for coding accurately and thoroughly. ***Class Activity Ask students to match the dental procedures listed below with the appropriate codes. Then ask students what practices are commonly followed in dental offices to reduce the possibility of coding errors.*** ***Dental procedures:*** ***1. Diagnostic*** ***2. Restorative*** ***3. Periodontics*** ***4. Implant Services*** ***5. Endodontics*** ***Procedure codes:*** ***a. D6000-D6199*** ***b. D4000-D4999*** ***c. D0100-D0999*** ***d. D3000-D3999*** ***e. D2000-D2999***

OBJECTIVES	CONTENT	TEACHING RESOURCES
Detail claim forms processing.	☐ Claim forms (p. 1040) – Claim form preparation (p. 1040) – Paper claim (p. 1040) – Electronic claim (p. 1040) ☐ HIPAA and electronic transactions (p. 1044)	☒▤ PPT 47-48 ▤ TB questions 26-27 ▤ SW Short-Answer Questions 15; Activity (pp. 554, 556-557) Figure 63-11 ADA standard claim form (pp. 1041-1042) Figure 63-12 Computerized claim form submitted for payment (p. 1043) HIPAA Electronic Transfers (p. 1044) Recall question 21 (p. 1045) ▸ Discuss paper claims and electronic claims. Note the advantages and disadvantages of each. ▸ Discuss HIPAA. Note how HIPAA regulations affect the submission of claims by a dental practice. *Class Activity **Divide the class into three groups, and give each of them a blank claim form. Describe a different patient clinical situation and treatment to each group, and have each group fill out the claim form. Then have each group share its form with the class for evaluation and feedback.***
Describe the procedure and purpose of claim forms follow-up.	☐ Claim form processing (p. 1044) – Tracking claims in process (p. 1044) ☐ Payments from insurance carriers (p. 1044) ☐ Handling overpayments (p. 1045)	☒▤ PPT 49-51 ▤ SW Short-Answer Questions 16 (p. 554) ▸ Discuss explanation of benefits. Explain its purpose and list the information contained in the explanation of benefits report. ▸ Discuss the procedure that must be followed in cases of overpayment. *Class Activity **Lead the class in a discussion in which students describe the purpose and procedures followed when following up claim forms. What common reports are generated by computerized programs that can help track claims. What is the business assistant's role?***
Identify insurance fraud.	☐ Insurance fraud (p. 1045)	☒▤ PPT 52 ▤ TB question 28 ▤ SW Short-Answer Questions 8 (p. 553) Patient Education (p. 1045) Legal and Ethical Implications (p. 1045) Eye to the Future (p. 1045)

Bird/Robinson

OBJECTIVES	CONTENT	TEACHING RESOURCES
		▸ Discuss insurance fraud. Offer examples of insurance fraud in a dental practice. *Class Activity **Present the following information and ask which could be considered insurance fraud, and why.*** – *Billing for services not provided* – *Not billing patient* – *Changing fees on a claim form to obtain a higher payment* – *Disregarding a copayment or deductible, accepting only the insurance payment, and writing off the difference* *As a class, develop a plan to prevent insurance fraud in a dental office. What are the dental assistant's responsibilities?*
Performance Evaluation		🖥️ TB 📘 SW questions (pp. 553-556) *e* ESLR Electronic Flashcards *e* ESLR Practice Quiz Recall questions (pp. 1022-1045) 💡 CTQ (pp. 1045-1046)

63.3 Homework/Assignments:

63.3 Instructor's Notes/Student Feedback:

Torres and Ehrlich Modern Dental Assisting, 9th ed.

Bird/Robinson

Slide 1

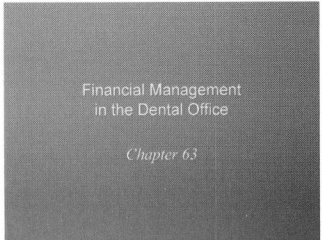

Slide 2

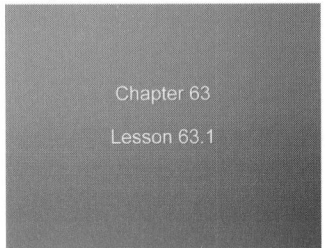

Slide 3

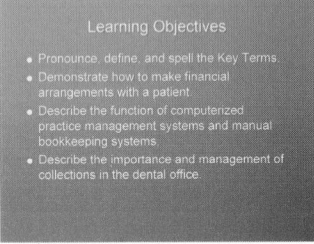

Slide 4

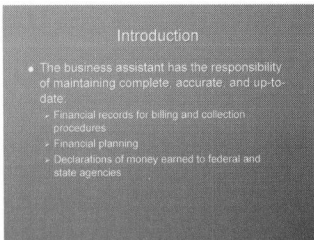

- What is the foundation for managing the financial transactions of a dental office? *(Business records.)*

Bird/Robinson

Slide 5

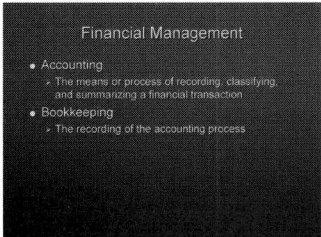

- What are two types of bookkeeping systems used in a dental practice? *(Accounts receivable and accounts payable systems.)*

Slide 6

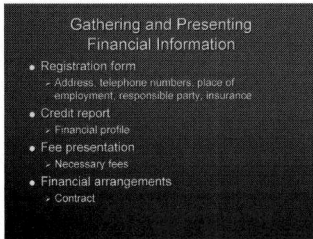

- What is the first step in preventive account management? *(Financial policies are established by the dentist and implemented by the business assistant. Fees will be paid in a more timely manner if the practice establishes financial guidelines.)*

Slide 7

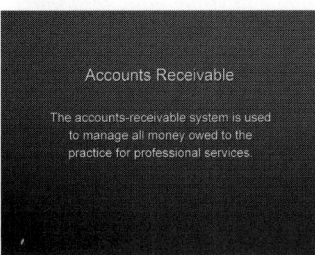

- The reimbursement process can be streamlined into an effective three-tier process. What are the three stages? *(Before the patient arrives, when the patient arrives, after the patient leaves.)*

Slide 8

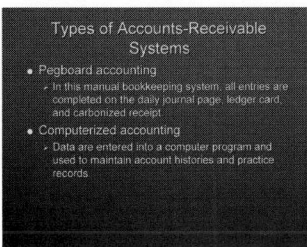

- What is the purpose of an accounts receivable management system? *(To record all transactions related to collecting fees for professional services provided.)*

- What can the dentist obtain on any staff members who handle practice funds? *(Bonding insurance.)*

Bird/Robinson

Slide 9

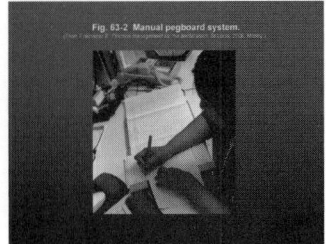

- In the average dental practice, what percentage of outstanding accounts are over 90 days past due? *(25% to 30%,: Advanced Dental Education Institute.)*

- What is a pegboard accounting system? *(A manual bookkeeping system in which all records are completed with a single entry.)*

Slide 10

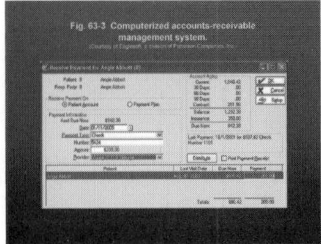

- What is a computerized accounts receivable management system? *(Data is entered into the system to maintain account histories and records of the practice.)*

- Why should an additional set of backup files be created and maintained? *(To avoid the loss of data contained in the files in the event of theft, fire, or another disaster.)*

Slide 11

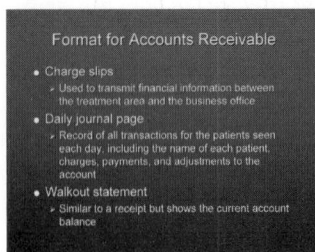

- How does the use of walkout statements improve cash flow? *(It speeds up payments and reduces the number of statements that must be prepared and mailed.)*

Slide 12

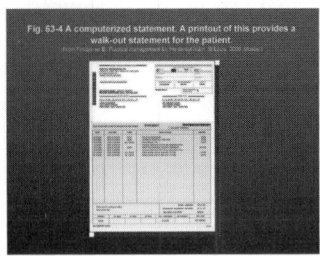

- A duplicate copy of the charge slip can be used as a receipt, a walkout statement, or both.

- In addition to maintaining patient accounts, all daily transactions posted to the bookkeeping system are used to generate the daily journal page.

Slide 13

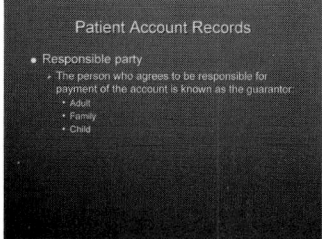

- The guarantor does not have to be in the same family as the patient, which makes divorce situations much easier.

Slide 14

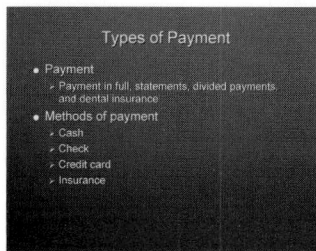

- What is the purpose of a pretreatment estimate form? *(It is submitted to the insurance carrier before treatment and provides information on what the insurance company will cover and what charges are the responsibility of the guarantor.)*

Slide 15

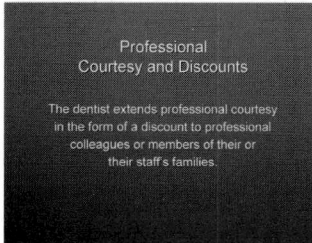

- What discount is generally extended to patients paying in full at the beginning of a planned treatment? *(5%.)*

Slide 16

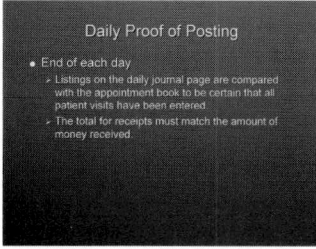

- What is the significance of the daily proof of posting? *(If the numbers do not match, the mistake can be caught early rather than further down the road.)*
- The total receipts collected should equal the payments in the cash drawer minus the change fund.

Bird/Robinson

Slide 17

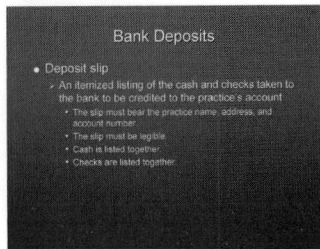

- How often should deposits be made? *(Once daily.)*
- What is one of the auditor's critical tests that involves the deposit ticket? *(The amount of the receipts should match the amount of the deposits.)*

Slide 18

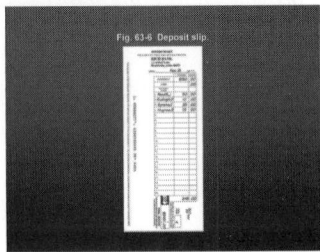

- What information must be imprinted on the deposit slip? *(Practice name, address, and account number.)*
- Checks are listed separately on the deposit ticket, usually by the last name of the person writing the check.

Slide 19

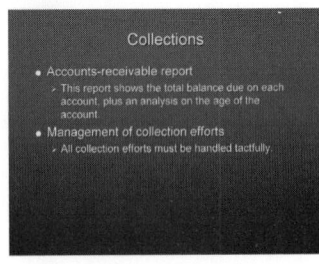

- The accounts receivable report shows how much of the balance is current; the noncurrent portion of the balance is categorized by age.
- Why should the business assistant ensure tactful collection procedures? *(To solicit cooperation and payment from patients.)*

Slide 20

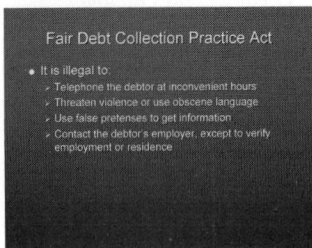

- Who regulates the Fair Debt Collection Practice Act? *(The Federal Trade Commission.)*

Torres and Ehrlich Modern Dental Assisting, 9th ed.

Bird/Robinson

Slide 21

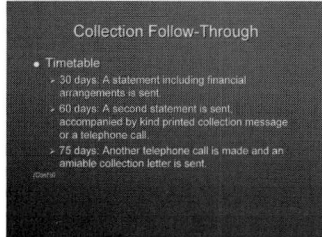

- Some statistics show that in-house debt collection efforts are only 70% effective on invoices more than 90-days outstanding.

Slide 22

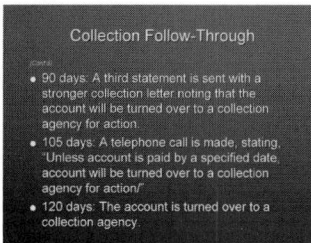

- Some companies offer outsourcing services on the collection of current accounts.

Slide 23

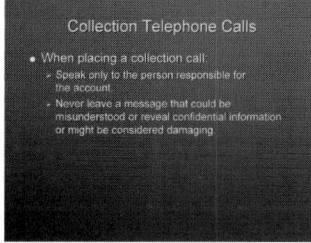

- Speak only to the person responsible for the account.
- Never leave a message that reveals confidential information.
- Do not become argumentative or defensive.

Slide 24

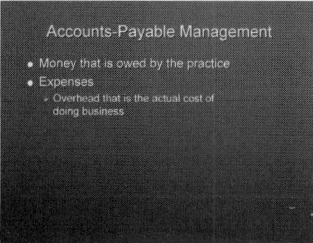

- What determines the cost of doing business in the dental office? *(Expenses and disbursements.)*

Torres and Ehrlich Modern Dental Assisting, 9th ed.

Bird/Robinson

Slide 25

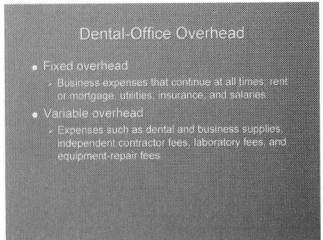

- Fee schedules must reflect both fixed and variable overhead expenses.

Slide 26

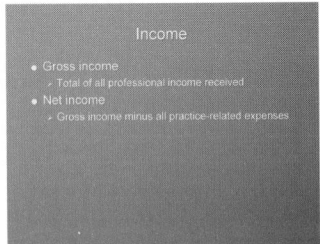

- Gross income minus practice-related expenses yields the dentist's net income from the practice.
- What is the business assistant's role with gross and net income? *(Usually responsible for management of day-to-day expenses and disbursements, provides records for accountant.)*

Slide 27

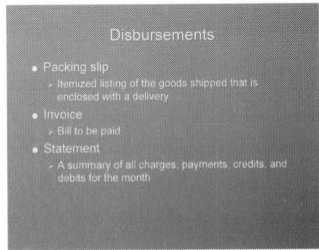

- What information is not found on a packing slip? *(Pricing information.)*
- When a delivery is received, what should be done with the packing slip? *(The contents should be checked against the packing list to identify any discrepancies.)*

Slide 28

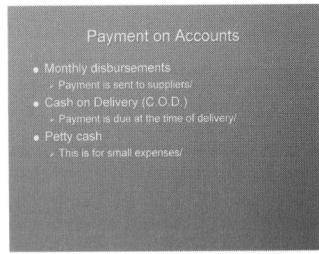

- What is the dentist's responsibility after a check is written but before it has been sent to the payee? *(To review and approve the bill.)*
- Besides the dentist, who is authorized to sign checks? *(Only an office manager who has been given limited power of attorney by the dentist based on appropriate papers on file at the bank.)*

Torres and Ehrlich Modern Dental Assisting, 9th ed.

Bird/Robinson

Slide 29

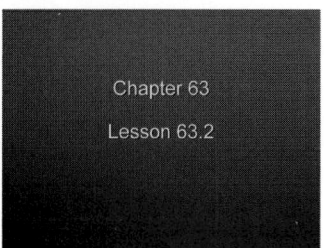

Chapter 63

Lesson 63.2

Slide 30

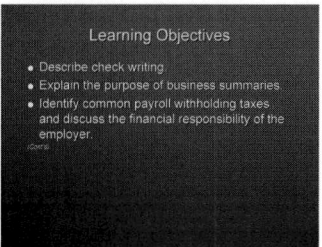

Learning Objectives

- Describe check writing
- Explain the purpose of business summaries
- Identify common payroll withholding taxes and discuss the financial responsibility of the employer.

Slide 31

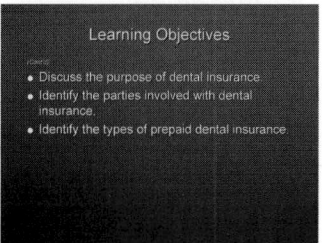

Learning Objectives

- Discuss the purpose of dental insurance
- Identify the parties involved with dental insurance.
- Identify the types of prepaid dental insurance

Slide 32

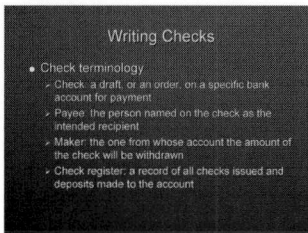

Writing Checks

- Check terminology
  - Check: a draft, or an order, on a specific bank account for payment
  - Payee: the person named on the check as the intended recipient
  - Maker: the one from whose account the amount of the check will be withdrawn
  - Check register: a record of all checks issued and deposits made to the account

- What are the advantages of computerized check writing? *(Savings in time, reduced possibility of error, ease of storage and retrieval of information.)*

- What is the difference between a blanket endorsement and a restrictive endorsement? *(Anyone can cash a check with a blanket endorsement; a check with a restrictive endorsement can be deposited only to the account of the payee.)*

ELSEVIER

Slide 33

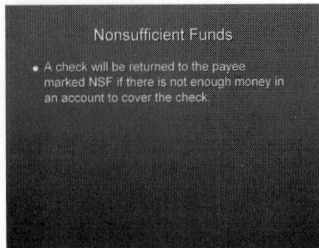

- Who is charged a fee for a returned item? *(The fee is charged to the account from which the check was written.)*
- Contacting the patient by telephone often resolves the issue and the check can be redeposited.

Slide 34

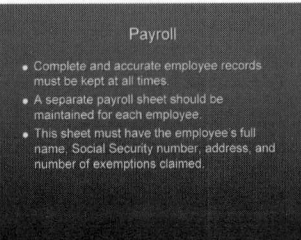

- Where can the business assistant find the federal requirements regarding issuing payroll? *(Circular E booklet issued by the IRS.)*

Slide 35

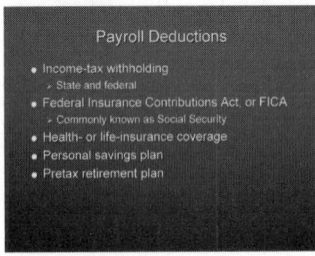

- Is the FICA withholding based on the number of exemptions that have been claimed on the W-4 form? *(No, FICA is a fixed amount regardless of the number of exemptions.)*
- The employer is required to match the employee's FICA contribution.

Slide 36

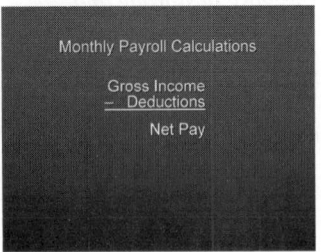

- Gross Income = pretax wages.

Slide 37

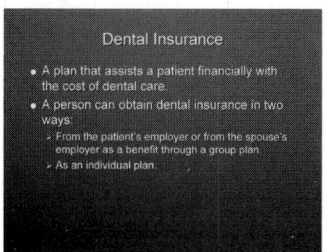

- The Surgeon General estimates that over 108 million children and adults do not have dental insurance.
- *Subscriber*: the person who carries the dental insurance plan.
- *Group*: the organization that has negotiated the dental insurance as part of its benefits package.
- *Carrier*: the party that pays the claims and collects the premiums.
- *Provider*: the dentist who renders treatment to the patient.

Slide 38

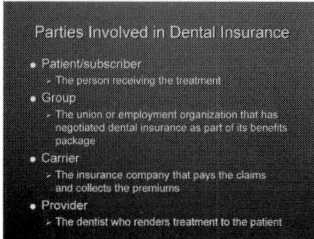

- Dental benefits are one of the most sought-after employee benefits.

Slide 39

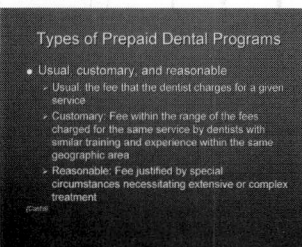

- These are the three most commonly used methods of calculating fee-for-service benefits.

Slide 40

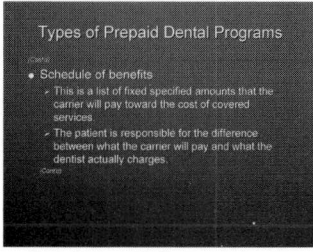

- The schedule of benefits is not related to the dentist's actual fee schedule. Generally the patient is responsible for paying the difference between the amount paid by the carrier under the schedule of benefits and the amount charged for the service based on the dentist's actual fee schedule.

ELSEVIER

Slide 41

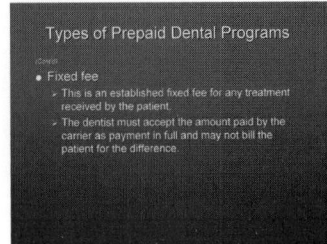

- Costs of dental health care account for approximately 30% of out-of-pocket expenditures for children's health care *(Surgeon General Report)*.

- According to the American Dental Hygienists' Association, about 75% of Americans have some form of periodontal disease.

Slide 42

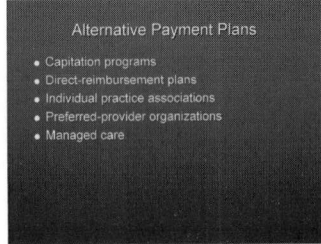

- In a capitation program payment to the dentist is based not on services rendered; instead, the dentist receives a fixed rate per covered member.

- Under a direct reimbursement plan, there is no insurance carrier involved - it is a self-funded program.

- An individual practice association is formed by a group of dentists for the purpose of collectively entering into a contract to provide dental services to an enrolled population.

Slide 43

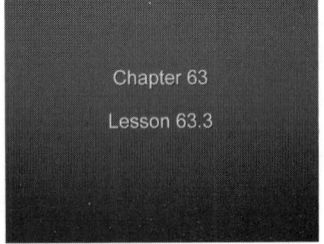

Slide 44

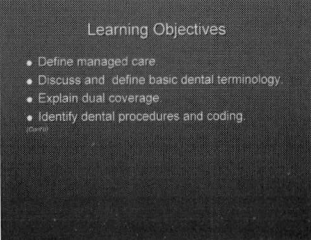

Torres and Ehrlich Modern Dental Assisting, 9th ed.

Bird/Robinson

Slide 45

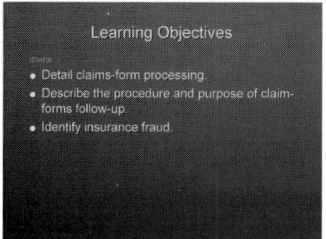

Slide 46

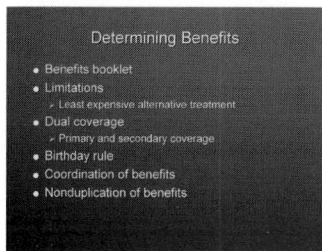

- For employees who receive coverage as a benefit from their employers, the two major factors that determine the amount to be paid by the carrier and the patient are the *method of payment* and the *limitations* within the plan.

- Under the nonduplication of benefits clause, if a patient is covered under two programs, then the patient may be reimbursed based on the higher of two allowed amounts but not for 100% of the fee.

- Tooth decay is the most chronic childhood disease. It is five times more common than asthma (*Oral Health in America: A Report of the Surgeon General, May 2000*).

Slide 47

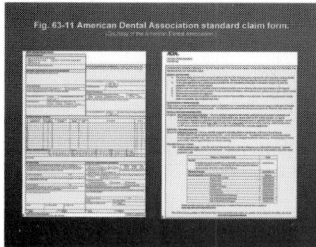

- Three primary areas of information required on the claim form: patient and subscriber identification, dentist identification, and details about the services provided.

- What percentage of children ages 2 to 17 have had a dental visit in the past year? *(74.3%.)*

- What percentage of adults ages 18 to 64 have had a dental visit in the past year? *(62.8%.)*

- What percentage of adults ages 65 and over have had a dental visit in the past year? *(55.4%.)*

Slide 48

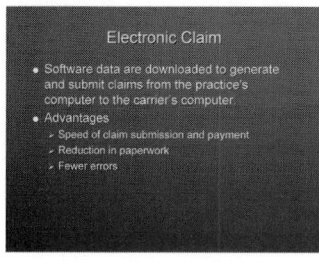

- Electronic claims lower the cost of processing claims.

- Electronic claim submission speeds the process and the payment, and reduces paperwork and errors.

- HIPAA specifies transaction standards to promote standardization of electronic claims submissions.

Torres and Ehrlich Modern Dental Assisting, 9th ed.

Bird/Robinson

Slide 49

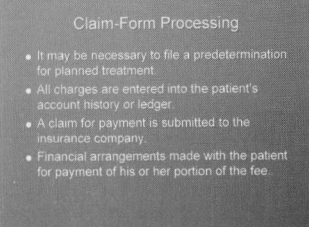

- Accurate information on a claim form helps speed the payment of claims.

Slide 50

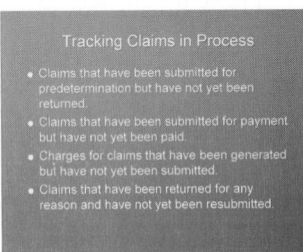

- Insurance claims are a form of accounts receivable.
- Developing a system to track claims in process will ensure that revenue is not lost.

Slide 51

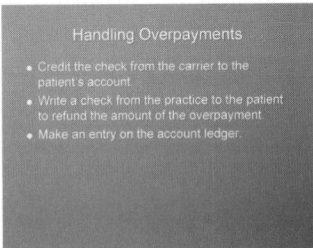

- Refunds should be issued to the patient for the amount of an overpayment.

Slide 52

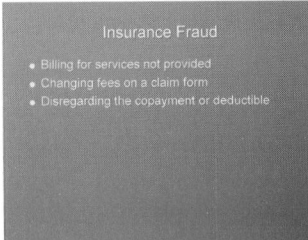

- Insurance companies are expanding their fraud investigation divisions to curb insurance fraud.
- According to the Coalition Against Insurance Fraud (CAIF), insurance companies lose approximately $26 billion a year because of fraud.

Torres and Ehrlich Modern Dental Assisting, 9th ed.

Bird/Robinson

TEACHING FOCUS

This chapter introduces students to topics related to marketing dental assistant skills. Students will have the opportunity to become acquainted with how to locate employment opportunities, prepare a resume and cover letter, seek employment, negotiate a salary, and meet career objectives.

MATERIALS AND RESOURCES

- ☐ computer and PowerPoint projector (Lesson 64.1)
- ☐ examples of employment agreements (Lesson 64.1)
- ☐ resume paper (Lesson 64.1)

LESSON CHECKLIST

Preparations for this lesson include:

- lecture
- guest speakers: representatives from a local dental society and an employment agency
- evaluation of student knowledge and skills needed to perform activities related to employment search, including:
  - o identifying career opportunities
  - o preparing for a job interview
  - o preparing a letter of application, resume, and job application form
  - o negotiating a salary
  - o understanding the elements of an employment agreement
  - o describing the steps for job termination
  - o achieving career objectives

KEY TERMS

career (p. 1048)   professional (p. 1050)
employment (p. 1049)   résumé (p. 1050)
interview (p. 1049)   termination (p. 1056)

ADDITIONAL RESOURCES

PowerPoint slides (Evolve): 1-20

Legend

CTQ
Critical
Thinking
Question

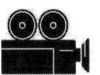

DVD
Multimedia
Procedures
Videos and
Animations

ESLR
EVOLVE
Student
Learning
Resources

IDO
Interactive
Dental
Office
CD-ROM

SW
Student
Workbook

TB
Test Bank
on the
TEACH
CD-ROM

PPT
PowerPoint
Slides

Class Activities are indicated in ***bold italic.***

Torres and Ehrlich Modern Dental Assisting, 9th ed.

LESSON 64.1

PRETEST

1. In general, what is the first contact with a prospective employer?
   - a. letter of application
   - b. resume
   - c. professional organization
   - d. telephone contact

2. The professional objective is part of the
   - a. resume.
   - b. cover letter.
   - c. letter of application.
   - d. newspaper advertisement.

3. Which of the following should not be stated on a resume?
   - a. professional objective
   - b. personal information
   - c. education
   - d. phone number

4. Which is the newest method of providing a resume?
   - a. sending it first class mail
   - b. faxing it with a cover letter
   - c. posting it on the Internet
   - d. hand delivery

5. Which of the following should be kept to a minimum at an interview?
   - a. jewelry and makeup
   - b. speaking
   - c. listening
   - d. smiling

6. What length should the resume be?
   - a. one-half page
   - b. one page
   - c. one legal-size page
   - d. two pages

7. How far in advance should you arrive for an interview appointment?
   - a. 5 minutes
   - b. 15 minutes
   - c. 30 minutes
   - d. 45 minutes

8. Which part of the interview is the most critical?
   - a. first 10 minutes
   - b. middle
   - c. last hour
   - d. conclusion

9. Title I of the ADA makes it illegal for an employer to
   - a. terminate an employee for disability.
   - b. require a uniform.
   - c. terminate an employee for stealing.
   - d. provide severance pay.

10. What is the single most important factor in achieving career goals?
    - a. education
    - b. networking ability
    - c. positive attitude
    - d. communication

Answers

1. d	3. b	5. a	7. b	9. a
2. a	4. c	6. b	8. a	10. c

Bird/Robinson

BACKGROUND ASSESSMENT

Question: What should a personal philosophy encompass?
Answer: The personal philosophy should reflect the individual's commitments, values, and concerns as they relate to future employment.

Question: What are the parts of a resume?
Answer: There are different styles of resumes, but overall the information provided in a resume is the same. The heading includes the applicant's name, address, and telephone number(s). Following the heading is a professional objective that describes the type of job being sought. The next section includes professional experience and lists each job held and duties performed. Education is included on the resume, with the most recent level completed listed first. Certifications and licensures relevant to the position should also be listed.

CRITICAL THINKING QUESTION

A recent graduate of an accredited dental assistant program has an appointment for a first job interview at a local dental office. The graduate knows a professional resume is important but has never prepared one. What key factors will ensure a resume that presents the applicant professionally? What should the applicant do after the interview, and why?

Guidelines: The applicant should limit the information on the resume to one page and make sure that it is neat and free of errors. Information should be concise, easy to read, and relevant to the job the applicant is applying for. All key elements should be present: name, address, and contact information; professional objective; education and training; certification and licensure; previous job experience; duties performed; and relevant skills. Within 48 hours after the interview, the applicant should send a thank-you letter to the interviewer. The thank-you letter helps the applicant stand out in the interviewer's memory, reaffirms the applicant's interest, and restates qualifications. The letter should be brief, thoughtful, and sincere.

OBJECTIVES	CONTENT	TEACHING RESOURCES
Pronounce, define, and spell the Key Terms.	■ Key terms (p. 1047)	SW Fill in the Blank questions 1-6 (pp. 559-560) ESLR Electronic Flashcards ▶ Discuss each of the Key Terms, focusing on the definition.

Determine career goals and develop a personal philosophy.	■ Your professional career (p. 1048)
	□ Goals and philosophy (p. 1048)
	□ Career opportunities (p. 1048)
	  – Private practice (p. 1048)
	  – Insurance (p. 1048)
	  – Sales (p. 1048)
	  – Research (p. 1048)
	  – Management consulting (p. 1048)
	  – Teaching (p. 1048)
	  – Dental schools (p. 1049)
	  – Hospitals (p. 1049)
		PPT 5-7
		
		TB questions 1-2
		
		SW Short-Answer Questions 1; Fill in the Blank questions 3-4, 6 (pp. 559-560)
		
		Factors to Remember When Seeking Employment (p. 1048)
		
		Recall question 1 (p. 1049)
		
		▶ Discuss goal setting. Offer suggestions for how students can think about their career goals and create a plan for achieving them.
		
		▶ Discuss career opportunities. Describe different employment choices and list advantages and disadvantages of each.
		
		▶ Discuss career goals. Make a list of career goals and describe the dental assisting careers that would offer opportunities to meet each goal.

Bird/Robinson

OBJECTIVES	CONTENT	TEACHING RESOURCES
	– Public health and government programs (p. 1049)	*Class Activity Divide the class into small groups. Have each group discuss career goals and develop personal philosophies to help meet the career goals. Have groups share their goals and philosophies with the class and invite feedback. What are some commonalities? Some differences?*
Identify potential career opportunities.	■ Locating employment opportunities (p. 1049) ☐ Newspaper advertisements (p. 1049) ☐ Campus placement (p. 1049) ☐ Employment agencies (p. 1049) ☐ Temporary agencies (p. 1049) ☐ Dental supply companies (p. 1049) ☐ Professional organizations (p. 1049) ☐ Internet (p. 1050)	PPT 8-9 TB question 3 SW Short-Answer Questions 2; Multiple Choice questions 1-2 (pp. 559-560) Recall question 2 (p. 1050) CTQ 1-2 (p. 1057) ▶ Discuss and describe employment sources and address the preparations necessary before pursuing each source. ▶ Discuss communication strategies for approaching sources at campus placement, employment agencies, temporary agencies, dental supply companies, and professional organizations. *Class Activity Invite representatives from a local dental society and an employment agency to speak to the class. Ask the speakers to identify and discuss potential career opportunities for dental assistants. What employment sources are appropriate for assistants just beginning their careers? Have students prepare questions in advance.*
Prepare a letter of application.	■ Seeking employment (p. 1050) ☐ Telephone contact (p. 1050) ☐ Cover letter (p. 1050)	PPT 10 TB question 4 SW Short-Answer Questions 3; Multiple Choice questions 3-4; Activities 1 (pp. 559- 560) Figure 64-1 Sample of a cover letter (p. 1051) Recall questions 3-4 (p. 1053) ▶ Discuss guidelines for telephone contact. Emphasize the importance of making a good first impression. ▶ Discuss the purpose of a letter of application. List general guidelines for composing a cover letter. *Class Activity Divide the class into small groups, and ask each group to develop a letter of application for a dental assistant position in one of the following job environments:*

Torres and Ehrlich Modern Dental Assisting, 9th ed.

Bird/Robinson

OBJECTIVES	CONTENT	TEACHING RESOURCES
		– Private local dental office *– Insurance* *– Research* *– Dental schools* *– Hospitals* *– Public health programs* ***Have each group share its letter of application with the class for feedback. How can each letter be improved?***
Prepare a professional resume.	☐ Résumé (p. 1050) – Electronic résumé (p. 1051) Procedure 64-1 Preparing a professional resume (p. 1052) (SW/ESLR Competency 64-1, p. 561)	PPT 11-13 TB questions 5-7 SW Short-Answer Questions 3; Fill in the Blank question 5; Multiple Choice questions 5-6; Activities 2 (pp. 559-560) SW/ESLR Competency 64-1 Preparing a Professional Résumé (p. 561) Figure 64-2 An example of a professional résumé (p. 1052) Recall questions 5-6 (p. 1053) CTQ 3 (p. 1057) ▸ Discuss the purpose of a résumé. Emphasize the importance of the appearance of the résumé. ▸ Discuss the elements of a résumé, using examples of different types. Describe the purpose of the heading, professional objective, professional experience, education, and certifications. Offer wording suggestions for each element. *Class Activity Ask students to prepare their own résumés or bring to class information that can be used to prepare a typical résumé for a dental assistant. Divide the class into small groups, and have the groups review the résumés. What was done appropriately? What might be improved?*
Describe the preparation and demeanor needed for a job interview.	☐ Completing a job application form (p. 1053) ☐ The interview (p. 1053) – Appearance (p. 1053) – Presenting yourself professionally (p. 1053)	PPT 14 TB question 8 SW Short-Answer Questions 4; Fill in the Blank question 1; Multiple Choice question 7 (pp. 559-560) Figure 64-3 Your first impression is very important (p. 1053) Recall question 7 (p. 1053)

OBJECTIVES	CONTENT	TEACHING RESOURCES
	– Interviewing professionally (p. 1053) – Concluding the interview (p. 1053)	▶ Discuss the job interview. Emphasize the importance of appearance and professional demeanor. Offer suggestions for making a positive impression. ▶ Discuss professional demeanor during the job interview. Note the importance of arriving early, sending positive nonverbal cues, answering questions honestly, and asking well-informed questions. ▶ Discuss appropriate interview questions. List questions that should not be asked by an interviewer, and offer suggestions for appropriate, polite responses by the applicant. ***Class Activity** Have student pairs take turns role-playing a dental assistant job applicant and interviewer. Ask volunteer pairs to present to the class for evaluation and feedback. Was the applicant prepared for the interview? Did the applicant present a professional demeanor? Were questions to the interviewer appropriate? Did the applicant answer the interviewer's questions clearly and in a positive manner?*
Prepare a follow-up letter.	– Follow-up letter (p. 1053)	🖥 PPT 15 💻 TB question 9 📖 SW Short-Answer Questions 5 (p. 559) Figure 64-4 An example of a follow-up letter (p. 1054) ▶ Discuss the purpose of the follow-up letter. Note the proper timing of the letter and offer suggestions for appropriate wording. ***Class Activity** Ask student pairs from the previous Class Activity to write a follow-up letter related to the interview. Have volunteer pairs present their letters to the class for review and feedback.*
Discuss factors to consider in salary negotiations.	■ Salary negotiations (p. 1053)	🖥 PPT 16 💻 TB question 10 📖 SW Short-Answer Questions 6 (p. 559) ▶ Discuss the factors that should be considered in determining a fair and equitable salary and benefits package. ▶ Discuss the specific benefits that should be addressed in addition to salary. ***Class Activity** Divide the class into groups, and present the following factors that an applicant should consider when negotiating compensation:*

ELSEVIER

Torres and Ehrlich Modern Dental Assisting, 9th ed.

   Bird/Robinson

OBJECTIVES	CONTENT	TEACHING RESOURCES
		– *Job duties/responsibilities*
		– *Work hours/schedule*
		– *Work environment/conditions*
		– *Advancement opportunities*
		– *Holidays/vacation*
		– *Health insurance/dental care*
		– *Retirement plan*
		Ask the groups to discuss (1) how each factor relates to an applicant's career goals and personal philosophy, as discussed in the first Class Activity, and (2) the role the factors play in negotiating salary. Then have groups share their conclusions with the class.
Discuss the elements of an employment agreement.	■ Employment agreement (p. 1054) ■ Americans with Disabilities Act (p. 1056)	PPT 17-18 TB question 11 SW Short-Answer Questions 7; Multiple Choice question 10 (pp. 559-560) Figure 64-5 An example of an employment agreement (p. 1055) Recall questions 8-9 (p. 1056) ▸ Discuss the employment agreement and how it offers protection to both employer and employee. ▸ Discuss the elements of an employment agreement. Describe the job description, work schedule, compensation, attire, termination, summary dismissal, and timeframe for giving notice. *Class Activity Present examples of employment agreements to the class, and lead a discussion in which students identify variations in job descriptions, duties, responsibilities, work schedules, compensation, performance reviews, attire, termination, summary dismissal, and time frame for giving notice. What can an employment agreement tell an applicant about the company?*
Describe the steps for job termination.	■ Job termination (p. 1056)	PPT 19 TB question 12 SW Short-Answer Questions 9; Fill in the Blank question 2; Multiple Choice question 8 (pp. 559-560) CTQ 4-5 (p. 1057)

Torres and Ehrlich Modern Dental Assisting, 9th ed.

Bird/Robinson

OBJECTIVES	CONTENT	TEACHING RESOURCES
		▸ Discuss job termination. Note that terms of the employment agreement should govern termination of employment. ▸ Discuss circumstances that might drive a dental assistant to terminate employment. Emphasize the need for perspective in evaluating a work situation. ▸ Discuss the professional way to give notice. Describe considerations in timing, phrasing, and demeanor. Emphasize the benefit of being able to use the employer as a reference when applying for future employment opportunities. *Class Activity Divide the class into three groups, and ask each group to discuss and develop a process for job termination. The groups should consider timing, phrasing, personal demeanor, and the ability to use the employer as a future reference. Then have each group share its process with the class for feedback.*
Describe the steps for achieving career objectives.	■ Achieving career objectives (p. 1056) ☐ Positive attitude (p. 1056) ☐ Professional responsibilities (p. 1056) ☐ Physical well-being (p. 1057)	PPT 20 TB questions 13-14 SW Short-Answer Questions 8; Multiple Choice question 9 (pp. 559-560) Recall question 10 (p. 1057) Patient Education (p. 1057) Legal and Ethical Implications (p. 1057) Eye to the Future (p. 1057) ▸ Discuss ways in which having a positive attitude can benefit the dental assistant on the job, in dealing with stress, and in attaining career goals. ▸ Discuss physical well-being. List the elements that are important in maintaining a healthy lifestyle. *Class Activity Present the following characteristics to the class. Ask the class to determine in what ways each contributes—positively or negatively—to achieving career objectives:* *– Positive attitude* *– Professional responsibility* *– Developing excuses* *– Physical well-being*

Bird/Robinson

OBJECTIVES	CONTENT	TEACHING RESOURCES
Performance Evaulation		TB SW questions (pp. 559- 560) SW/ESLR Competency 64-1 Preparing a Professional Resume (p. 561) ESLR Practice Quiz Recall questions (pp. 1049-1057) CTQ (p. 1057)

64.1 Homework/Assignments:

64.1 Instructor's Notes/Student Feedback:

Bird/Robinson

Slide 1

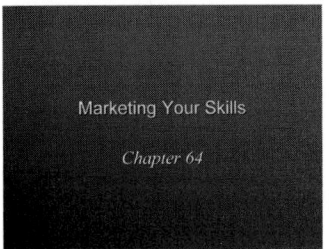

Slide 2

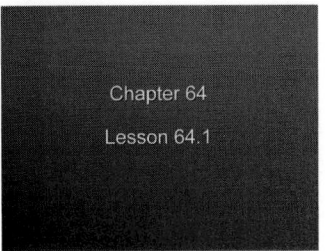

Slide 3

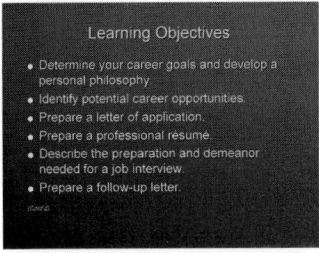

Slide 4

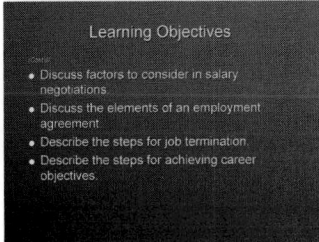

Slide 5

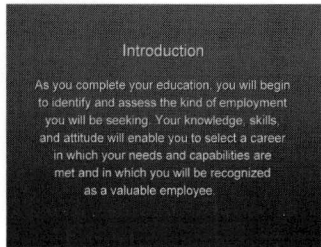

- Determining a career goal and personal philosophy can help focus the job search.

Slide 6

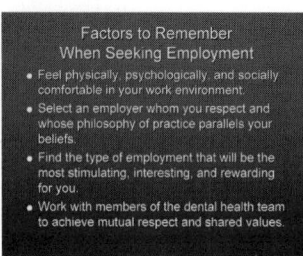

- The job of dental assistant is expected to be one of the fastest-growing occupations through the year 2012, according to the Bureau of Labor Statistics.

Slide 7

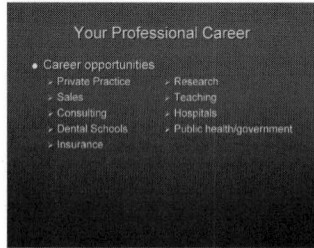

- Dental assistants have a range of choices once they complete training.

- Analyze your qualifications, interests, and goals to help choose a direction that will be rewarding for you.

Slide 8

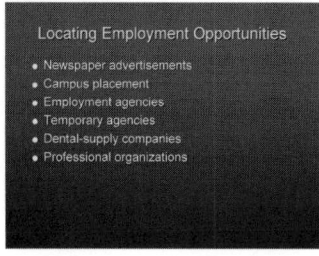

- In 2002, dental assistants held 266,000 jobs in the United States, according to the Bureau of Labor Statistics.

- A study by the University of Missouri showed that 48% of job openings were found through friends and family.

- How would a recent graduate go about contacting each of these job sources?

Torres and Ehrlich Modern Dental Assisting, 9th ed.

Bird/Robinson

Slide 9

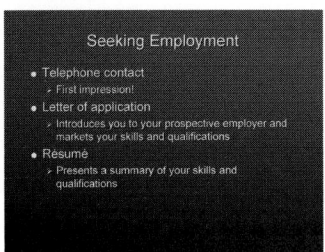

- How many hours a week should be spent job hunting? *(From 35 to 40 hours.)*

- Why is it important to do homework about yourself, that is, identify your skills, interests, and goals, in priority order?

- What information should a job applicant have in order to match qualifications with job function? Why is this matching important?

Slide 10

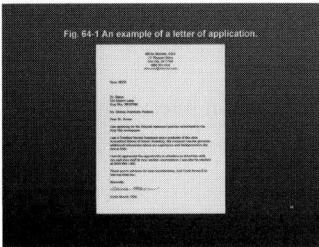

- What elements should be included in a letter of application?

- What are some additional guidelines to follow when writing a letter of application?

Slide 11

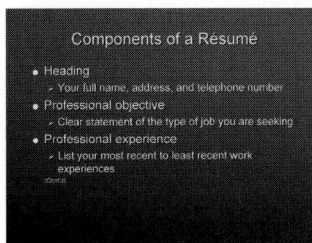

- Remember that the resume is a self-promotional piece and also a guide for the interviewer.

- What elements should be included on the resume?

- What elements should NOT be included on the resume?

Slide 12

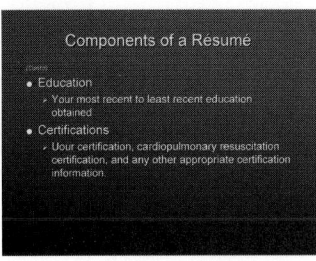

- What are the three different types of resumes?

- What type of resume is most appropriate for recent graduates of a technical program, such as dental assisting?

- How could different types of resumes be combined to present the applicant most effectively?

Bird/Robinson

Slide 13

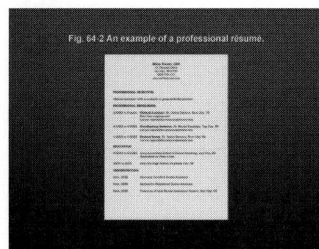

Fig. 64-2 An example of a professional resume.

- What elements in this resume make it look professional and thorough?
- Why is the appearance of a resume important?
- Visually, what should the resume NOT do?

Slide 14

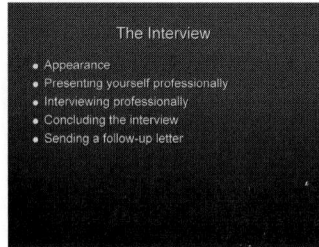

The Interview
- Appearance
- Presenting yourself professionally
- Interviewing professionally
- Concluding the interview
- Sending a follow-up letter

- Why is preparing emotionally for an interview as important as researching the company? *(The right mood brings the best performance.)*
- Initial answers to questions should be brief.
- Why is it important to write a thank-you note after an interview?

Slide 15

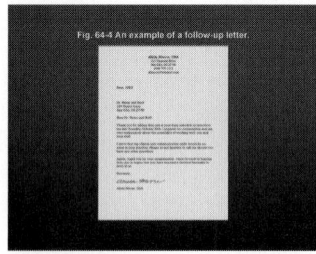

Fig. 64-4 An example of a follow-up letter.

- Why are follow-up letters often better than phone calls?
- What elements in this letter make it appropriate?
- If circumstances were different, what could be done differently in the thank-you note? Why?

Slide 16

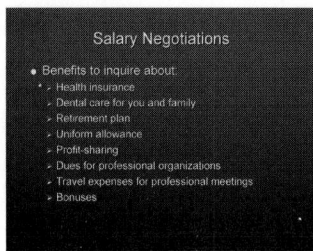

Salary Negotiations
- Benefits to inquire about:
  - Health insurance
  - Dental care for you and family
  - Retirement plan
  - Uniform allowance
  - Profit-sharing
  - Dues for professional organizations
  - Travel expenses for professional meetings
  - Bonuses

- Remember to look at the whole compensation picture.
- What factors should the job applicant consider relative to compensation?
- What is the best way to ask questions about benefits?

Slide 17

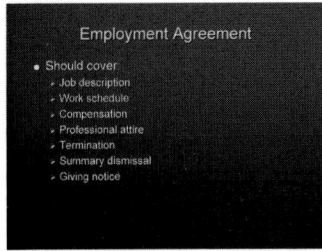

- A written employment agreement can eliminate misunderstandings in the future.
- In what ways does a written employment agreement protect both the employee and the company?
- If something is not covered in a written employment agreement, how should the job applicant proceed?

Slide 18

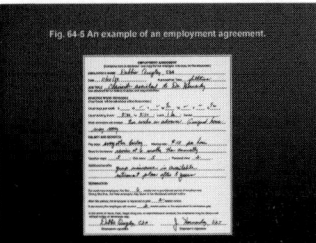

- What key elements are included in this agreement?
- Is anything missing?

Slide 19

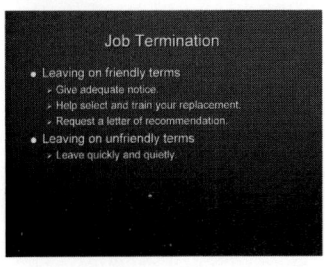

- A job termination handled successfully can lead to positive opportunities in the future.
- For what reasons might an employee want to terminate employment?
- For what reasons might an employer want to terminate an employee?
- How can both parties make the separation as positive as possible? Why is this important?

Slide 20

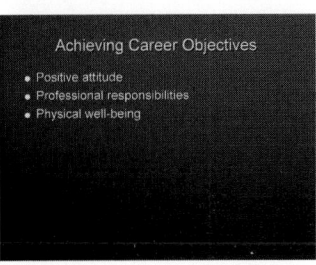

- Why is keeping a positive attitude helpful in attaining a career objective?
- How can a person relate positive attitude and professional responsibilities to career objectives and personal philosophy?
- What can a person do to maintain physical well-being?

1 Recall Questions and Answers

1. Who was Hesi-Re?
Hesi-Re was the earliest dentist whose name is known.

2. How long has dental disease existed?
Dental disease has always existed.

3. Who is the "Father of Medicine"?
The "Father of Medicine" was Hippocrates.

4. What is the Hippocratic Oath?
The Hippocratic Oath is an obligation to treat patients ethically, with confidentiality, and to the best of one's ability.

5. What dental procedures did the Romans practice?
The Romans performed oral hygiene, made gold crowns, and extracted teeth.

6. Were Western dentists the first to use silver amalgam as fillings?
No, the Chinese developed silver amalgam.

7. Which artist first distinguished molars and premolars?
The artist Leonardo da Vinci distinguished molars from premolars.

8. Who is the "Father of Modern Surgery"?
The "Father of Modern Surgery" is Ambroise Paré.

9. Who is the "Father of Modern Dentistry"?
The "Father of Modern Dentistry" is Pierre Fauchard.

10. Who was John Baker's famous patient?
John Baker's famous patient was George Washington.

11. Which famous colonial patriot first used forensic evidence?
Paul Revere was the first to use forensic evidence.

12. Who was Robert Woofendale?
Robert Woofendale was one of the first dentists to travel throughout the American colonies.

13. Who founded the first dental school in America?
Chapin and Harris founded the first dental school in America.

14. Who earned the title of "Grand Old Man of Dentistry"?
G.V. Black is known as the Grand Old Man of Dentistry.

15. Who was the first dentist to use nitrous oxide?
Horace Wells was the first dentist to use nitrous oxide.

16. Who discovered, and published the first paper on oral 'hairy' leukoplakia in male homosexuals?
Dr. Deborah Greenspan discovered, and published the first paper on, oral 'hairy' leukoplakia.

17. Who was the first dentist to use a dental assistant?
C. Edmund Kells was the first dentist to use a dental assistant.

18. Who founded dental hygiene education in America?
The founder of dental hygiene in America was Alfred C. Fones.

19. Who was the first woman in the world to graduate from dental school?
The first woman to graduate from dental school was Lucy Beaman Hobbs.

20. Who was the first African-American female dentist in the United States?
The first African-American woman to practice dentistry in the United States was Ida Gray Rollins.

21. Where is the Dr. Samuel D. Harris National Museum of Dentistry located?
The Dr. Samuel D. Harris National Museum of Dentistry is located in Baltimore, Maryland.

Torres and Ehrlich Modern Dental Assisting, 9th ed.

Bird/Robinson

2 ‖ Recall Questions and Answers

1. Name the three essential aspects of a professional appearance.

The essentials of a professional appearance are good health, good grooming, and appropriate dress.

2. How can you show that you are a responsible person?

You can demonstrate responsibility by arriving on time, staying for the full time, volunteering to help, learning additional skills, and showing initiative, among other actions.

3. What is the purpose of the ADAA?

The mission of the ADAA is to advance the careers of dental assistants, promote the dental-assisting profession, and enhance the delivery of quality dental healthcare to the public.

4. What credential is issued by the DANB?

The credential issued by the DANB is certified dental assistant.

5. Where can you obtain additional information about the DANB?

You may phone the DANB at 1-800-FOR-DANB or visit their website at http://www.danb.org.

Bird/Robinson

3   Recall Questions and Answers

1. What are the more common terms used for fixed prostheses?
Crowns and bridges are more common terms for fixed prostheses.

2. If a patient has poor dental hygiene habits, is fixed prosthodontics indicated?
No, fixed prosthodontics is not indicated for a patient with poor dental hygiene.

3. What type of indirect restoration is placed to improve the appearance of the facial surface of teeth?
A die is placed to improve the appearance of the facial surface of teeth.

4. What is the difference between an onlay and a three-quarter crown?
An onlay covers most of the occlusal and proximal surfaces; a three-quarter crown covers all but the facial or buccal surface.

5. How does a dentist convey to a laboratory technician what type of crown to make?
The dentist writes a laboratory prescription for the crown to be made.

6. What is the term for an exact replica of a tooth prepared by a laboratory technician?
A die is the exact replica of a prepared tooth.

7. What material does a laboratory technician use to create the pattern for a casting?
Wax is used to create the pattern for a casting.

8. How many appointments are required for a crown?
Two appointments are required for a crown.

9. What part of the tooth is covered by a full crown?
The anatomic portion is covered by a full crown.

10. What does the dentist use to reduce the height and contour of a tooth for a casting?
Rotary instruments are used to reduce the height and contour of a tooth.

11. If a tooth is non-vital, what is fabricated and placed into the pulp for better retention of a crown?
A post and core are placed into a non-vital tooth for better retention of a crown.

12. What is used during a crown and bridge preparation to displace gingival tissue?
Gingival retraction cord

13. What type of agent is applied to retraction cord to control bleeding?
A vasoconstrictor

14. What other terms are used for overgrown tissue?
Overgrown tissue is also called hypertrophied tissue or hyperplasia.

15. What types of impression are taken during crown preparation?
A preliminary impression and a final impression are taken during crown preparation.

16. What will the patient have on the prepared tooth while the laboratory is making a crown or bridge?
The patient has provisional coverage while the laboratory is making a crown or bridge.

Bird/Robinson

17. Who in the dental office is allowed to cement a crown or bridge permanently?
Only the dentist may permanently cement a crown or bridge.

18. How many appointments are required for a fixed bridge?
Two appointments are required for a fixed bridge.

19. What accessory is used to help in flossing a bridge?
A floss threader helps in flossing a bridge.

20. How is each unit of a bridge held together?
Each unit of a bridge is soldered.

Torres and Ehrlich Modern Dental Assisting, 9th ed.

Bird/Robinson

4   Recall Questions and Answers

1. What is the difference between ethics and law?
Legal issues are settled by using statutes and court decisions. Ethical issues are subject to individual interpretation as to the "right" or "wrong" of particular situations.

2. What are the four basic principles of ethics?
The four basic principles of ethics are autonomy, justice, do no harm, and promotion of well-being.

3. What establishes a guide to professional behavior?
The code of ethics is a profession's guide to professional behavior.

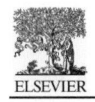   Bird/Robinson

5 Recall Questions and Answers

1. What are the two types of statutory law?
The two types of statutory law are criminal and civil.

2. What is the difference between an act of omission and an act of commission?
An act of omission is not doing something that should have been done, and an act of commission is doing something that should not have been done.

3. What is the difference between an expressed contract and an implied contract?
Expressed contracts are established through the written word or verbal agreement, and implied contracts are established by actions, not words.

4. What is the purpose of licensure?
Licensure is meant to protect the public from incompetent practitioners.

5. What authority does a state board of dentistry have?
The state board of dentistry has the authority not only to issue licenses, but also to revoke, suspend, or deny renewal of a license.

6. What is meant by reciprocity?
Reciprocity is when a state grants a license, usually without further testing, to an individual who is already licensed in another state.

7. What does *respondeat superior* mean?
Respondeat superior means that the employer is responsible for the actions of the employee.

8. What is the difference between direct supervision and general supervision?
Direct supervision is when a dentist is physically present when the dental auxiliary is performing an expanded function. Under general supervision, the dentist does not have to be physically present.

9. What is meant by abandonment?
Abandonment occurs when a dentist discontinues treatment of the patient without proper notice.

10. Can a dentist refuse to treat a patient because he or she has HIV infection?
A dentist cannot refuse to treat a patient with HIV, although, under specific conditions, the dentist may refer the patient to another dentist.

11. What are the "four Ds" necessary for a successful malpractice suit?
The "four Ds" necessary for a successful lawsuit are duty, dereliction, direct cause, and damages.

12. What does *res ipsa loquitur* mean?
Res ipsa loquitur means the act speaks for itself.

13. What are the best defenses against a malpractice suit?
Prevention and communication are the best defenses against malpractice lawsuits.

14. What is meant by *res gestae*?
Under *res gestae*, statements made by any person at the time of an alleged negligent act are admissible as evidence in a court of law.

15. What is the difference between implied consent and written consent?
An implied consent is demonstrated by actions, in contrast to a written consent, which is signed.

16. Why should broken appointments be noted on the patient's chart?
Broken appointments may be interpreted as contributory negligence on the part of the patient.

17. What is the primary purpose of reporting suspected cases of child abuse?
The purpose of reporting suspected cases of child abuse is to protect the child from further abuse.

18. What are mandated reporters?
Mandated reporters are professionals required by state law to report known or suspected cases of child abuse.

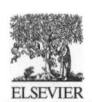

Bird/Robinson

6 Recall Questions and Answers

1. What is the difference between anatomy and physiology?
Anatomy is the study of the body's form and structure, and physiology is the study of the body's function.

2. What three imaginary lines are used to divide the body into sections?
The three imaginary lines used to divide the body into sections are the midsagittal, horizontal, and frontal planes.

3. What is the portion of the cell that carries genetic information?
The nucleus of the cell contains DNA and RNA, which carry genetic information.

4. What are the four types of tissues in the human body?
The four types of tissues are epithelial, muscle, connective, and nerve.

5. What are the four organizational levels of the human body, from simplest to most complex?
The four organizational levels of the human body are cells, tissues, organs, and body systems.

6. What are the two major body cavities?
The two major body cavities are the dorsal and the ventral cavities.

7. Which components make up the axial and appendicular regions of the human body?
The axial region consists of the head, neck, and trunk, and the appendicular region comprises the arms and legs.

ELSEVIER

7   Recall Questions and Answers

1. What are the two divisions of the skeleton?
The two divisions of the skeleton are the axial skeleton and the appendicular skeleton.

2. What is the connective tissue that covers all bones?
The periosteum is the connective tissue that covers all bones.

3. What are the two types of bone and their features?
The two types of bone are compact bone, which is dense and strong, and cancellous bone, which is light and spongy.

4. Where is cartilage found?
Cartilage is found where bones join together.

5. Articulation is another term for what structure?
Articulation is another term for joint.

6. What are the three types of muscle tissue?
The three types of muscle tissue are striated, smooth, and cardiac.

7. What distinguishes the appearance of each muscle type?
Striated muscle has dark and light bands, smooth muscle does not have bands, and cardiac muscle is striated in appearance but resembles smooth muscle in its action.

8. What are four disorders of the muscular system?
Disorders of the muscular system include sprains, strains, contusions, and progressive muscular dystrophy.

9. What are the two primary functions of the circulatory system?
The two primary functions of the circulatory system are to transport oxygen to cells and to regulate body temperature.

10. What are the upper and lower chambers of the heart?
The upper chambers of the heart are the atria, and the lower chambers are the ventricles.

11. What are the names and functions of the three main types of blood vessels?
The arteries carry blood away from the heart, the veins carry blood toward the heart, and the capillaries connect the arterial and venous systems.

12. What is a primary function of the lymphatic system?
The lymphatic system contributes to the immune system and destroys harmful organisms.

13. What tissues make up the lymphatic system?
The lymph tissues include lymph vessels, lymph nodes, lymph fluid, and lymphoid organs.

14. What two systems make up the nervous system?
The nervous system is made up of the central nervous system (CNS) and the peripheral nervous system (PNS).

15. What are the two divisions of the autonomic nervous system?
The autonomic nervous system is divided into the sympathetic and parasympathetic nervous systems.

16. What are the three types of neurons, according to their function?

The three types of neurons are sensory, motor, and associative.

17. What is the function of the respiratory system?

The respiratory system delivers oxygen to the cells and removes carbon dioxide from the body.

18. What is the role of the digestive system?

The digestive system provides the body with nutrients, water, and electrolytes.

19. What are the five actions of the digestive system?

The actions of the digestive system are ingestion, digestion, movement, absorption, and elimination.

20. What are the primary functions of the endocrine system?

The endocrine system regulates the body's activities through hormones.

21. What is the primary function of the urinary system?

The primary function of the urinary system is to maintain fluid volume and composition of the body fluids.

22. What are four functions of the skin?

The skin functions to regulate body temperature, provide a barrier against microorganisms, excrete salt and liquids, and provide sensitivity to touch.

23. What are the appendages to the skin?

The appendages to the skin include the hair, nails, and glands.

8   Recall Questions and Answers

1. What are the three periods of prenatal development?
The three periods of prenatal development are preimplantation, embryonic, and fetal.

2. Which period of prenatal development is the most critical, and why?
The embryonic period is the most critical because the major structures are being formed.

3. What are the three primary embryonic layers?
The three primary embryonic layers are the ectoderm, mesoderm, and endoderm.

4. Which branchial arch forms the bones, muscles, nerves of the face, and lower lip?
The first branchial arch forms the bones, muscles, nerves of the face, and the lower lip.

5. Which branchial arch forms the side and front of the neck?
The second branchial arch forms the side and front of the neck.

6. What are the three stages of palate formation?
The three stages of formation of the palate are primary, secondary, and fusion.

7. When does the development of the human face occur?
The development of the human face occurs between the fifth and eighth weeks.

8. When do the first signs of tooth development begin?
When the embryo is 5 to 6 weeks old, the first stages of tooth development are found.

9. What are the two major categories of factors that can adversely influence dental development?
The two categories of factors that can have an adverse influence on dental development are genetic and environmental.

10. What is the process of adding bone?
The process of bone deposit or addition is deposition.

11. What is the process of bone loss or removal?
The process of bone loss or removal is resorption.

12. What are the three primary periods in tooth formation?
The three primary periods in tooth formation are growth, calcification, and eruption.

13. What are the three stages in the growth period?
The three stages in the growth period are bud, cap, and bell.

14. When a tooth has several cusps, what structures are formed when the cusps join together?
When a tooth has several cusps, pits and fissures are formed as the cusps join together.

15. What is the name of the process by which teeth move into the oral cavity?
Eruption is the process by which teeth move into position in the oral cavity.

16. What is the difference between the anatomic crown and the clinical crown?
The anatomic crown is covered with enamel; the clinical crown is visible in the mouth.

Bird/Robinson

17. Where is the CEJ?

The cementoenamel junction is located at the neck of the tooth.

18. What is the hardest substance in the human body?

The hardest substance in the human body is enamel.

19. What is the most abundant mineral component in enamel?

The most abundant mineral component in enamel is hydroxyapatite, which consists primarily of calcium.

20. How does dentin transmit sensations of pain?

Sensations of pain are transmitted through the dentinal fibers.

21. What are the three types of dentin?

The three types of dentin are primary, secondary, and tertiary.

22. What are the two types of cementum?

The two types of cementum are primary and secondary.

23. What type of tissue makes up the pulp?

Blood vessels and nerves make up the pulp.

24. What cells form the intercellular substance of the pulp?

Fibroblasts form the intercellular substance of the pulp.

25. What are the functions of osteoblasts and osteoclasts?

The osteoblasts form bone; the osteoclasts resorb bone.

26. What is the primary function of the periodontal ligaments?

The primary function of the periodontal ligaments is to support, maintain, and retain the tooth in the jaw.

27. To which structures are the periodontal ligaments attached?

The periodontal ligaments attach to cementum and the alveolar bone, holding the tooth in place.

28. List the three types of oral mucosa, and provide an example of each.

Lining mucosa forms the inside of the cheeks, lips, and soft palate; masticatory mucosa covers the hard palate, attached gingiva, and dorsum of the tongue; specialized mucosa forms the papillae on the tongue.

9 | Recall Questions and Answers

1. What are the 11 regions of the head?
The 11 regions of the head are the frontal, parietal, occipital, temporal, orbital, nasal, infraorbital, zygomatic, buccal, oral, and mental.

2. What bone forms the forehead?
The frontal bone forms the forehead.

3. What bone forms the back and base of the cranium?
The occipital bone forms the back and base of the cranium.

4. What bones form the cheek?
The zygomatic bones form the cheek.

5. What bones form the upper jaw and hard palate?
The maxillary bones (maxillae) form the upper jaw and hard palate.

6. What is the only movable bone in the skull?
The only movable bone in the skull is the mandible.

7. Where is the mental foramen located?
The mental foramen is located on the left and right sides of the mandible between the apices of the first and second premolars.

8. What is the difference between the teeth of males and females?
Male teeth are larger and squared incisally, whereas female teeth are smaller with rounded incisal edges.

9. What are the two basic types of movement by the TMJ?
The two basic types of movement by the temporomandibular joint are hinge and glide.

10. What symptoms might a patient with a TMD have?
A patient with temporomandibular disorder may have symptoms of muscle spasms, pain, swelling, and difficulty opening the mouth.

11. Which cranial nerve innervates all muscles of mastication?
The mandibular division of the fifth cranial nerve innervates all muscles of mastication.

12. What is the name of the horseshoe-shaped bone where the muscles of the tongue and the floor of the mouth attach?
The hyoid is the horseshoe-shaped bone where the muscles of the tongue and the floor of the mouth attach.

13. Which of the major salivary glands is the largest?
The parotid gland is the largest salivary gland.

14. What is another name for the parotid duct?
Stensen's duct is another name for the parotid duct.

15. What artery is behind the ramus, and branches into five arteries?
The artery behind the ramus with five branches is the mandibular artery.

Torres and Ehrlich Modern Dental Assisting, 9th ed.

Bird/Robinson

16. What artery supplies the maxillary molars, premolars, and gingivae?

The posterior superior alveolar artery supplies the maxillary molars, premolars, and gingivae.

17. How many pairs of cranial nerves are connected to the brain?

Twelve pairs of cranial nerves are connected to the brain.

18. Which division of the trigeminal nerve subdivides into the buccal, lingual, and inferior alveolar nerves?

The mandibular division of the trigeminal nerve subdivides into the buccal, lingual, and inferior alveolar nerves.

19. During what type of dental examination are lymph nodes palpated?

Lymph nodes are palpated during an extraoral dental examination.

20. What is the term for enlarged or palpable lymph nodes?

Lymphadenopathy is the term for enlarged or palpable lymph nodes.

10   Recall Questions and Answers

1. What are the nine regions of the face?
The nine regions of the face are the forehead, temples, orbital area, external nose, zygomatic (malar) area, mouth and lips, cheeks, chin, and external ear.

2. What is the area of color change around the border of the lips?
The vermilion border is the area of color change around the lips.

3. What type of tissues cover the oral cavity?
Mucous membrane tissues cover the oral cavity.

4. What are the two regions of the oral cavity?
The vestibule and the oral cavity proper are the two regions of the oral cavity.

5. What is the name of the structure that passes from the oral mucosa to the facial midline of the mandibular arch?
The labial frenum is the structure from the oral mucosa to the facial midline of the mandibular arch.

6. What is the anatomic term for the gums?
The anatomic term for the gums is gingiva.

7. What is another term for unattached gingiva?
Marginal gingival or free gingival is another term for unattached gingiva.

8. What is another term for interdental gingiva?
Interdental papilla is another term for interdental gingiva.

9. What is the pear-shaped pad of tissue behind the maxillary incisors?
The incisive papilla is the pear-shaped pad of tissue behind the maxillary incisors.

10. What is the hanging projection of tissue at the border of the soft palate?
The uvula is the hanging projection of tissue at the border of the soft palate.

11. What is the term for the upper surface of the tongue?
The dorsum is the correct term for the upper surface of the tongue.

12. What is the thin fold of mucous membrane that extends from the floor of the mouth to the underside of the tongue?
The lingual frenum is the thin fold of mucous membrane that extends from the floor of the mouth to the underside of the tongue.

ELSEVIER

11   Recall Questions and Answers

1. What are the two sets of teeth that people have in their lifetime?
The two sets of teeth are primary and permanent.

2. How many teeth are in each dentition?
There are 20 teeth in the primary dentition and 32 in the permanent dentition.

3. What is the term for the four sections of the divided dental arches?
Quadrant is the term for the four sections of the divided dental arches.

4. What are the terms for the front teeth and for the back teeth?
Anterior is the term for the front teeth, and posterior is the term for the back teeth.

5. What are the four types of teeth?
The four types of teeth are incisors, canines, premolars, and molars.

6. Which tooth is referred to as the "cornerstone" of the dental arch?
The cornerstone of the dental arch is the canine.

7. What are the five surfaces of the teeth?
The five surfaces of the teeth are facial, lingual, mesial, distal, and occlusal or incisal.

8. What is the name for the space between adjacent teeth?
The space between adjacent teeth is called the interproximal space.

9. What is the name of the area where adjacent teeth physically touch?
The area where adjacent teeth physically touch is called the contact area.

10. What is the name of the triangular space toward the gingiva between adjacent teeth?
The triangular space toward the gingiva between adjacent teeth is the embrasure.

11. What is the term for the junction of two tooth surfaces?
The junction of two tooth surfaces is called an angle.

12. What is the name for the third of the tooth nearest the end of the root?
The third of the tooth nearest the end of the root is the apical third.

13. What is the name for the position of the teeth when they are in chewing movements?
The position of the teeth when they are chewing is called functional occlusion.

14. What is the term for teeth that are in poor occlusion?
Malocclusion is the term for teeth that are in poor occlusion.

15. What is the technical term for class III malocclusion?
The technical term for class III malocclusion is mesioclusion.

16. What classification is neutroclusion?
The classification for neut

17. What is the name for the curve of the occlusal plane?
The curve of the occlusal plane is called the Curve of Spee.

12   **Recall Questions and Answers**

1. How many anterior teeth are in the permanent dentition?
There are 12 anterior teeth in the permanent dentition.

2. What is the term for the permanent teeth that replace primary teeth?
Succedaneous is the term for the permanent teeth that replace primary teeth.

3. What is the term for the rounded, raised area on the cervical third of the lingual surface on anterior teeth?
Cingulum is the term for the rounded, raised area on the cervical third of the lingual surface on anterior teeth.

4. What feature do newly erupted central and lateral incisors have on the incisal ridge?
Newly erupted central and lateral incisors can have mamelons on the incisal ridge.

5. Which teeth are the longest ones in the permanent dentition?
The canines are the longest teeth in the permanent dentition.

6. Which teeth are the smallest ones in the permanent dentition?
The mandibular central incisors are the smallest teeth in the permanent dentition.

7. What is the name for the developmental horizontal lines on anterior teeth?
Imbrication lines are the developmental horizontal lines on anterior teeth.

8. What feature borders the occlusal table of a posterior tooth?
Marginal ridges border the occlusal table of a posterior tooth.

9. What are the pinpoint depressions where two or more grooves meet?
Occlusal developmental pits are the pinpoint depressions where two or more grooves meet.

10. Which teeth are frequently extracted as part of orthodontic treatment?
The first premolars are frequently extracted as part of orthodontic treatment.

11. What are the two forms of mandibular second premolars?
The two forms of mandibular second premolars are two-cusp and three-cusp forms.

12. What is the term for a tooth with three roots?
Trifurcated is the term for a tooth with three roots.

13. What is the term for a tooth that does not replace a primary tooth?
Nonsuccedaneous is the term for a tooth that does not replace a primary tooth.

14. What is the name of the fifth cusp on a maxillary first molar?
The cusp of Carabelli is the fifth cusp on a maxillary first molar.

15. How many roots do mandibular molars have?
Mandibular molars have two roots.

16. Which teeth are referred to as the "wisdom" teeth?
The third molars are often referred to as wisdom teeth.

17. How thick is the enamel covering on a primary tooth?
The enamel covering on a primary tooth is very thin.

18. What method of identification is used in the Universal/National System for the primary denti
Capital letters A to T are used to denote the teeth in the primary dentition using the Universal/National System.

19. Do primary anterior teeth have mamelons?
Primary anterior teeth do not have mamelons.

20. Which primary molar has an H-shaped groove pattern on the occlusal surface?
The primary maxillary molar has an H shaped groove pattern on the occlusal surface.

21. Which primary mandibular molar is the largest?
The second molar is the largest primary mandibular molar.

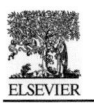

13   Recall Questions and Answers

1. What two types of bacteria primarily cause dental caries?
Mutans streptococci and lactobacilli cause dental caries.

2. Which of the above two types of bacteria is most responsible for dental caries?
Of the two types of bacteria, mutans streptococci cause the most dental caries.

3. What is the soft, sticky bacterial mass that adheres to the teeth?
Dental plaque is the bacterial mass that adheres to the teeth.

4. What is the mineral in the enamel that makes the crystal easier to dissolve?
Carbonated apatite is the mineral in the enamel that makes the crystal easier to dissolve.

5. What are the three factors necessary for the formation of dental caries?
The three factors necessary for the formation of dental caries are a susceptible tooth, bacteria, and fermentable carbohydrates.

6. What is the term for the dissolution of calcium and phosphate from the tooth?
Demineralization is the term for the dissolving of calcium and phosphate from the tooth.

7. What is the term for rapid and extensive formation of caries?
Rampant caries is the term for rapid and extensive formation of caries throughout the mouth.

8. What is the term for caries occurring under or adjacent to existing dental restorations?
Secondary caries, or recurrent caries, is the term for caries occurring under or around existing dental restorations.

9. What are the three protective mechanisms produced by saliva?
Saliva protects the teeth from dental caries through physical, chemical, and antibacterial actions.

14 Recall Questions and Answers

1. What is dental plaque?
Plaque is a soft mass of bacterial deposits that covers the tooth surfaces.

2. What is calculus?
Calculus is a hard, stone-like material that attaches to the tooth surface.

3. The term periodontal disease includes both_____ and _____.
The term periodontal disease includes both gingivitis and periodontitis.

4. What is the definition of periodontitis?
Periodontitis is inflammation of the supporting tissues of the teeth.

5. How many basic types of periodontal disease have been identified by the American Academy of Periodontology?
The American Academy of Periodontology has identified seven basic case types of periodontal disease.

6. How is the severity of periodontal disease determined?
The severity of the disease is determined by the amount of lost attachment.

15   Recall Questions and Answers

1. What is the goal of preventive dentistry?
The goal of preventive dentistry is to have a healthy mouth for a lifetime.

2. What are the two most common dental diseases?
Dental decay and periodontal disease are the two most common dental diseases.

3. What is the goal of a patient education program?
The goal of a patient education program is to enable patients to develop and maintain sound dental habits throughout their life.

4. What is the initial step in a patient education program?
The initial step in a patient education program is to listen carefully to the patient.

5. What is a dental sealant?
A dental sealant is a covering applied to the pits and fissures of the teeth.

6. What is the process by which fluoride prevents decay?
Demineralization and remineralization are the processes by which fluoride prevents decay.

7. What are the two routes or means by which the body receives fluoride?
Topical and systemic are the two routes by which the body receives fluoride.

8. What is the name of the dental condition that results from too much fluoride?
Fluorosis is the dental condition that results from too much fluoride.

9. What precautions are necessary for children using fluoridated toothpaste?
Precautions include adult supervision and reminders to not swallow the toothpaste.

10. What is the key dietary factor that relates to dental caries?
Sugar is the key dietary factor that relates to dental caries.

11. What information must a patient include in a food diary?
Food diaries must note the time the food was eaten, the quantity in household measures, and the amount of sugar that was added to any of the foods or beverages.

12. How do sugar-free sodas relate to dental caries?
Sugar-free sodas increase the acidity in the mouth.

13. What can patients do daily to remove plaque?
Patients can brush, floss, and use other aids daily to remove plaque.

14. Which type of toothbrush bristles is usually recommended?
A soft toothbrush with nylon bristles is usually recommended.

15. Which method of brushing teeth is generally recommended?
The modified Bass tooth brushing technique is most often recommended.

16. What is the difference between dental floss and dental tape?
Dental floss is round, and dental tape is flat.

Torres and Ehrlich Modern Dental Assisting, 9th ed.

Bird/Robinson

17. Which is more effective, waxed or unwaxed dental floss?
When used properly, waxed floss and unwaxed floss are equally effective.

18. What cleaners can be used to clean dentures?
A nonabrasive cleaner such as a commercial denture cleaner, mild soap, dishwashing liquid, or mild toothpaste can be used on the denture brush.

19. Will "tartar-control" toothpaste remove calculus?
"Tartar-control" toothpaste will not remove calculus but will help prevent re-formation after a professional cleaning.

20. If you cannot brush and floss after lunch, what should you do?
If you cannot brush and floss after lunch, you should rinse your mouth with water.

Torres and Ehrlich Modern Dental Assisting, 9th ed.

Bird/Robinson

16 Recall Questions and Answers

1. What are nutrients?
Nutrients are the components in food that provide energy, growth, and maintenance.

2. What are the three types of carbohydrates?
The three types of carbohydrates are simple sugars, complex carbohydrates, and fiber.

3. What is meant by cariogenicity?
Cariogenicity means a food is capable of causing tooth decay.

4. What is an amino acid?
An amino acid is part of a protein, used for building and repairing the human body.

5. How many of the amino acids are essential?
There are eight essential amino acids.

6. What is a complete protein?
A complete protein contains all eight essential amino acids.

7. Which systemic diseases are related to excess fat in the diet?
Cardiovascular disease, obesity, diabetes, and cancer are associated with excess fat in the diet.

8. Which cholesterol is "good," and which is "bad"?
HDL is the "good" and LDL is the "bad" cholesterol.

9. Which type of vitamin is stored in the body, and is not destroyed by cooking?
Fat-soluble vitamins are stored in the body and are not destroyed by cooking.

10. Which vitamins are referred to as the B-complex vitamins?
The water-soluble vitamins are referred to as the B-complex vitamins.

11. Which vitamins are fat-soluble?
Vitamins D, E, A, and K are fat-soluble.

12. Which minerals are present in the largest quantities?
Sodium, potassium, calcium, chlorine, phosphorus, and magnesium are present in the largest quantities.

13. What is often called "the forgotten nutrient"?
Water is often called "the forgotten nutrient."

14. Which governmental agency regulates the labeling of food products?
The U.S. Department of Agriculture (USDA) is the agency that regulates the labeling of food products.

15. What criteria are used to determine whether a product is "organic"?
Foods with the "organic" label must have been grown without the use of chemical pesticides herbicides, or fertilizers.

16. What are the two most serious eating disorders?
The two most serious eating disorders are anorexia nervosa and bulimia.

17 Recall Questions and Answers

1. Which lesions are below the mucosal surface?
Ulcers, cysts, and areas of erosion are lesions that occur below the mucosal surface.

2. Which lesions extend above the mucosal surface?
Blisters, pustules, and plaques are lesions that extend above the mucosal surface.

3. What lesion is even with the mucosal surface?
Ecchymosis (bruising) is a lesion that is even with the mucosal surface.

4. What condition appears as a white patch or area?
Leukoplakia appears as a white patch or area.

5. What condition is caused by a yeast-like fungal infection?
Candidiasis is caused by a yeast-like fungal infection.

6. What is another term for "canker sore"?
Aphthous ulcer is another term for "canker sore."

7. What is a condition in which inflammation causes severe pain and high fever?
Cellulitis is a condition in which inflammation causes severe pain and high fever.

8. What is the term for an inflammation of the tongue?
Glossitis is the term for an inflammation of the tongue.

9. What is the condition in which a pattern on the tongue changes?
Geographic tongue is the condition in which a pattern on the tongue changes.

10. What is the condition in which the body does not absorb vitamin B_{12}?
Pernicious anemia is the condition in which the body does not absorb vitamin B_{12}.

11. What type of cancer affects the blood-forming organs?
Leukemia is the cancer that affects the blood-forming organs.

12. What is a common precancerous lesion among users of smokeless tobacco?
Leukoplakia is a common precancerous lesion occurring among users of smokeless tobacco.

13. What is the term for a malignant lesion in the epithelial tissue of the oral cavity?
Carcinoma is the term for a malignant lesion in the epithelial tissue of the oral cavity.

14. What causes radiation caries?
The lack of saliva is the primary cause of radiation caries.

15. What is the term for a lack of saliva?
Xerostomia (also called "dry mouth") is the term for a lack of saliva.

16. What is the condition frequently seen on the lateral border of the tongue of patients with HIV/AIDS?
Hairy leukoplakia is the condition seen on the lateral border of the tongue of patients with HIV/AIDS.

17. Which opportunistic infection is seen as purplish lesions on the skin or oral mucosa of patients with HIV/AIDS?

Kaposi's sarcoma is seen as purplish lesions on the skin or oral mucosa of patients with HIV/AIDS.

18. What is the malignant condition that involves the lymph nodes of HIV/AIDS patients?

Lymphoma is the malignant condition that can involve the lymph nodes of HIV/AIDS patients.

19. What is the difference between developmental disorders and inherited disorders?

A developmental disorder is caused by a disruption of the cells during development, and an inherited disorder is caused by an abnormality in the gene.

20. What is a congenital disorder?

A congenital disorder is present at birth and may be developmental or inherited.

21. What is the term for abnormally large jaws?

Macrognathia is the term for abnormally large jaws.

22. What is the term for a bony growth in the palate?

Torus palatinus is the term for a bony growth in the palate.

23. What is a more common term for ankyloglossia?

Tongue-tie is a more common term for ankyloglossia.

24. What is the dental term for "tooth within a tooth"?

Dens in dente is the dental term for "tooth within a tooth."

25. What is the term used for abnormally small teeth?

Microdontia is the term for abnormally small teeth.

26. What term is used to describe two teeth joining together?

Fusion is the term used to describe two teeth joining together.

27. Which teeth are most often affected by ankylosis?

The deciduous molars are the teeth most often affected by ankylosis.

28. What is the hereditary condition that affects the dentin?

Dentinogenesis imperfecta is the hereditary condition that affects the formation of dentin.

29. What is the difference between attrition and abrasion?

Attrition is a normal process of tooth wear, and abrasion is caused by repetitive mechanical forces.

30. What is an oral indication of bulimia?

Erosion of the lingual surfaces of the teeth is an oral indication of bulimia.

31. What are three potential complications of orofacial piercing?

Three potential complications of orofacial piercing are infections, chipped teeth, and broken teeth.

ELSEVIER

Torres and Ehrlich Modern Dental Assisting, 9th ed.

      Bird/Robinson

18 Recall Questions and Answers

1. Why is microbiology important to the dental assistant?
Microbiology is important to the dental assistant for understanding infection-control protocol.

2. Who is referred to as the "Father of Microbiology"?
Louis Pasteur is known as the "Father of Microbiology."

3. Who recognized that airborne microorganisms were responsible for postsurgical infections?
Joseph Lister recognized that airborne microorganisms are responsible for postsurgical infections.

4. Who was responsible for discovering the rabies vaccine?
Louis Pasteur was responsible for discovering the rabies vaccine.

5. What are the three primary shapes of bacteria?
Cocci, bacilli, and spirochetes are the three primary shapes of bacteria.

6. What is the staining process for separating bacteria?
Gram's stain is the process for separating bacteria.

7. What is the term for bacteria that require oxygen to grow?
Aerobes are the type of bacteria that require oxygen to grow.

8. What is the most resistant form of bacterial life?
A spore is the most resistant form of bacterial life.

9. How are prions different from other microorganisms?
Prions contain only protein and no nucleic acids (DNA or RNA).

10. Which types of hepatitis are spread by exposure to blood?
HBV, HCV, and HDV are spread by contact with contaminated blood.

11. How is HIV spread?
HIV is spread by sexual contact with an infected person and by direct contact with infected blood (also) from infected mothers to their unborn children).

12. What tissues are affected by the West Nile virus?
West Nile virus affects a person's nervous system, causing inflammation of the brain and spinal cord.

13. How is the H5N1 influenza virus spread?
The H5N1 is spread by infected birds.

14. What microorganism is used as the benchmark for the effectiveness of a surface disinfectant?
The bacterium M. tuberculosis is the benchmark for the effectiveness of a surface disinfectant.

15. What disease is also known as lockjaw?
Tetanus is also known as lockjaw.

16. What is a sign of the first stage of syphilis?
The first stage of syphilis is a painless ulcerating sore known as a chancre.

17. What is a pandemic?
A pandemic is a global disease outbreak.

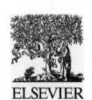

Torres and Ehrlich Modern Dental Assisting, 9th ed.

Bird/Robinson

19 Recall Questions and Answers

1. What is the most common route of contamination?
The most common route of contamination is through direct contact.

2. What is the term for acquiring an infection through mucosal tissues?
The term for acquiring an infection through mucosal tissues is droplet infection.

3. What infection-control measures help prevent disease transmission from the dental team to the patient?
The use of gloves, hand washing, masks, rubber dams, and patient mouth rinses helps prevent disease transmission from the dental team to the patient.

4. What is the purpose of the BBP?
The purpose of the Bloodborne Pathogens Standard is to protect healthcare employees.

5. How often should an exposure-control plan be reviewed and updated?
The exposure-control plan should be reviewed and updated at least annually.

6. What does the term Standard Precautions include?
Standard Precautions combine with Universal Precautions to include all body substances, regardless of whether or not they contain blood.

7. What information must be included in the employee training record?
The record of each training session must include the date of the session, name of the presenter, the topic, and names of all attendees.

8. What must an employee do if he or she does not want the hepatitis B vaccine?
The employee must sign an informed consent if he or she does not want the hepatitis B vaccine.

9. What is the most effective hand product on the market for use on clean hands?
An alcohol-based hand rub is the most effective hand product for use on clean hands.

10. Why should long or artificial nails and rings be avoided when working in a dental office?
Long or artificial nails and rings should be avoided when working in a dental office because they can harbor pathogens.

11. What are four examples of PPE?
Masks, gloves, protective eyewear, and protective clothing are examples of personal protective equipment.

12. What determines the type of PPE to be worn?
The anticipated risk of exposure determines the type of personal protective equipment to be worn.

13. What are the two types of protective eyewear?
Face shields and eyeglasses with side and bottom shields are types of protective eyewear.

14. What may be the most critical PPE?
Gloves may be the most critical personal protective equipment.

15. When should sterile gloves be worn?
Sterile gloves should be worn during procedures that involve cutting of bone or significant amounts of blood or saliva, such as oral surgery or periodontal treatment.

16. When should utility gloves be worn?
Utility gloves must be worn when the treatment room is cleaned and disinfected, while contaminated instruments are being cleaned or handled, and when surfaces are being cleaned and disinfected.

17. What type of glove should be worn to open drawers during a dental procedure?
Overgloves should be worn to open drawers during a dental procedure.

18. What type of response is irritant dermatitis?
Irritant dermatitis is a non-immunologic response.

19. What is the most common type of latex allergy?
The most common type of latex allergy is type IV sensitivity.

20. What is the most serious type of latex allergy?
Anaphylaxis is the most serious type of latex allergy.

21. What type of gloves should be used for a latex-sensitive patient?
Vinyl or nitrile gloves can be used for a latex-sensitive patient.

22. What are three examples of contaminated waste?
Surface barriers, patient bibs, and gloves are examples of contaminated waste.

23. What are three examples of general waste?
Paper towels, paper mixing pads, and empty food containers are examples of general waste.

24. What is another term for infectious waste?
Regulated waste is another term for infectious waste.

25. Which type of waste must be identified with the biohazard label?
Infectious or regulated waste must be identified with the biohazard label.

26. What is the BBP rule regarding refrigerators in dental offices?
Never store food or drink in refrigerators that contain potentially contaminated items.

27. What is the CDC guideline for using saliva ejectors?
Do not advise patients to close their lips tightly around the tip of the saliva ejector to evacuate oral fluids.

28. How does tuberculosis infection occur?
TB infection occurs when a susceptible person inhales bacteria, which then travel to the lungs.

29. What is the CDC recommendation on the use of pre-procedural mouth rinses?
The CDC does not make a recommendation on the use of pre-procedural mouth rinses.

30. Did the CDC make a recommendation on the effects of exposure to laser plumes on dental healthcare professionals? Why or why not?
The CDC has not made a recommendation because the effect on dental healthcare professionals from the use of lasers in dentistry has not been adequately evaluated.

20 Recall Questions and Answers

1. Why must surfaces in dental treatment rooms be disinfected or protected with barriers?
Surfaces in dental-treatment rooms should be disinfected or protected with barriers to prevent patient-to-patient transmission of microorganisms.

2. What are the two methods that deal with surface contamination?
Surface barriers and surface disinfection are methods of dealing with surface contamination.

3. What is the purpose of surface barriers?
The purpose of surface barriers is to prevent contamination of the surfaces beneath.

4. What should you do if the barrier becomes torn?
If the barrier becomes torn, the surface beneath must be cleaned and disinfected.

5. Which regulation requires the use of surface disinfection?
The OSHA Bloodborne Pathogens Standard requires the use of surface disinfection.

6. Why must surfaces be precleaned?
Surfaces must be precleaned because a thin film of bioburden can inactivate the disinfectant.

7. Which type of surfaces must have barriers placed?
Surfaces that are not easily cleaned and disinfected must have barriers placed.

8. How are antiseptics different from disinfectants?
Antiseptics are antimicrobial agents used on the skin. Disinfectants are chemicals intended to kill disease-causing microorganisms or inanimate surfaces such as countertops and dental equipment.

9. Which agency regulates disinfectants?
The Environmental Protection Agency regulates disinfectants.

10. What is the ideal disinfectant?
The ideal disinfectant is one that can rapidly kill a broad range of bacteria.

11. What disinfectant can leave a reddish or yellow stain?
Iodophors can leave a reddish or yellow stain.

12. What is a disadvantage of synthetic phenols?
Synthetic phenols can build up and leave a residue.

13. What is a more common term for sodium hypochlorite?
Household bleach is a more common term for sodium hypochlorite.

14. Are alcohol disinfectants effective when blood or saliva is present?
Alcohol disinfectants are not effective if blood or saliva is present.

15. What are two uses of chlorine dioxide?
Chlorine dioxide products may be used either as disinfectants or sterilants, depending on the duration of contact.

16. **How can you be sure that your general cleaning solutions are not contaminated?**
    To ensure that solutions are not contaminated, make fresh cleaning solution each day, discard any remaining solution, and let the container dry.

17. **What are the CDC's recommendations regarding carpeting and cloth furnishings in operatories, laboratories, and instrument-processing areas?**
    The CDC recommends avoiding the use of carpeting and cloth-upholstered furnishings in dental operatories, laboratories, and instrument-processing areas.

18. **With what should the majority of housekeeping surfaces be cleaned?**
    The majority of housekeeping surfaces need to be cleaned only with a detergent and water or an EPA-registered hospital disinfectant/detergent.

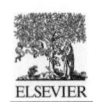

Bird/Robinson

21 Recall Questions and Answers

1. **What are the three instrument classifications used to determine the method of sterilization?**
   Critical, semicritical, and noncritical are the three instrument classifications used to determine the method of sterilization.

2. **What personal protective equipment is necessary when processing instruments?**
   Goggle-type eyewear, utility gloves, mask, and protective clothing are necessary when processing instruments.

3. **What is the basic rule of the workflow pattern in an instrument-processing area?**
   Linear or semicircular without "doubling back" is the basic rule of the workflow pattern in an instrument-processing area.

4. **If instruments cannot be processed immediately, what should be done with them?**
   If instruments cannot be processed immediately, they should be placed in a holding solution.

5. **Name the three methods of pre-cleaning instruments.**
   Hand scrubbing, ultrasonic cleaning, and thermal washing/disinfecting are three methods of pre-cleaning instruments.

6. **Which method of pre-cleaning instruments is the least desirable?**
   The hand-scrubbing method of precleaning instruments is the least desirable.

7. **How does an ultrasonic cleaner work?**
   The ultrasonic cleaner works by sound waves creating bubbles in the liquid.

8. **What prevents kitchen dishwashers from being used to pre-clean instruments?**
   Kitchen dishwashers cannot be used to preclean instruments because they are not FDA-approved.

9. **How can instrument rusting be prevented?**
   Lubrication can be used to prevent instrument rusting.

10. **Why should instruments be packaged before sterilization?**
    Instruments should be packaged before sterilization to maintain sterility.

11. **Why should you never use pins, staples, or paper clips on instrument packages?**
    Use of pins, staples, or paper clips on instrument packages can cause holes, and the instruments will no longer be sterile.

12. **What are the three forms of sterilization monitoring?**
    Physical, chemical, and biologic are the three forms of sterilization monitoring.

13. **What is a process indicator, and where is it placed?**
    A process indicator is placed on the outside of the pack to show that the pack has been exposed to heat.

14. **What is a process integrator, and where is it placed?**
    A process integrator is placed on the inside of the pack to show exposure to heat, temperature, and pressure.

15. Do process indicators and integrators ensure that an item is sterile?

Process indicators and integrators do not ensure that an item is sterile.

16. What is the best way to determine if sterilization has occurred?

Biologic monitoring is the best way to determine if sterilization has occurred.

17. What causes sterilization failure?

Failure occurs if the sterilizing agent does not come in contact with the item for the proper time.

18. What are the three most common forms of heat sterilization?

Steam, chemical vapor, and dry heat are the three most common forms of heat sterilization.

19. What is a primary disadvantage of flash sterilization?

The inability to wrap items is a primary disadvantage of flash sterilization.

20. What is a major advantage of chemical vapor sterilization?

No rusting of instruments is a major advantage of chemical vapor sterilization.

21. What are the two types of dry-heat sterilization?

Static air and forced air are two types of dry-heat sterilization.

22. What is the primary disadvantage of liquid chemical sterilization?

Inability to perform biologic monitoring is a primary disadvantage of liquid chemical sterilization.

23. How should instruments processed in a liquid chemical sterilant be rinsed?

Instruments processed in a liquid chemical sterilant should be rinsed with sterile water to maintain their sterility.

24. How should high-speed handpieces be processed before sterilization?

High-speed handpieces should be flushed before sterilization.

25. What types of heat sterilization are appropriate for high-speed handpieces?

Only steam and chemical vapor heat sterilization are appropriate for high-speed handpieces.

26. What does event-related packaging mean?

Event-related packaging means that unless some event occurs to contaminate the contents, it is assumed that the contents will remain sterile indefinitely.

27. How should clean supplies and instruments be stored?

Clean supplies and instruments should be stored in closed or covered cabinets, if possible.

Torres and Ehrlich Modern Dental Assisting, 9th ed.

Bird/Robinson

22   Recall Questions and Answers

1. What is the main difference between a recommendation and a regulation?
A recommendation is not enforceable, whereas a regulation is enforceable.

2. What is OSAP?a
OSAP is a not-for-profit organization dedicated to promoting dental asepsis and dental healthcare worker safety.

3. What is the primary role of the CDC in dentistry?
The primary role of the CDC in dentistry is to make recommendations for infection control.

4. What is the primary role of the FDA in dentistry?
The primary role of the FDA in dentistry is the regulation of dental devices.

5. What is the primary role of the EPA in dentistry?
The primary role of the EPA in dentistry is regulating and registering disinfectants.

6. What is the primary role of OSHA in dentistry?
The primary role of OSHA is to ensure a safe work environment.

7. What is the primary role of the NIH?
The primary role of the NIH is conducting and supporting medical research.

8. What is the primary role of NICDR?
The primary role of NIDCR is to promote the general health of the American people by improving their oral, dental, and craniofacial health.

Torres and Ehrlich Modern Dental Assisting, 9th ed.

Bird/Robinson

23   Recall Questions and Answers

1. **What types of health consequences could develop as a result of exposure to chemicals?**

    Heart, kidney, liver, and lung tissues could be damaged as a result of exposure to chemicals.

2. **Why is it important for the dental assistant to understand how to handle chemicals?**

    It is important for the dental assistant to understand how to handle chemicals so that he or she can avoid exposure.

3. **What are three primary methods of chemical exposure?**

    The three primary methods of chemical exposure are inhalation, ingestion, and skin absorption.

4. **What is the difference between acute and chronic chemical toxicity?**

    Acute chemical toxicity results from high levels of exposure over a short period; chronic chemical toxicity results from many repeated exposures, generally to lower levels, over a much longer time.

5. **What are four methods of personal protection against chemical exposure?**

    The four methods of personal protection against chemical exposure are hand protection, eye protection, protective clothing, and inhalation protection.

6. **What are the OSHA requirements regarding an eyewash unit?**

    OSHA requires an eyewash unit in areas where chemicals are used.

7. **What could be an effect of exposure to radiographic processing solutions kept in a poorly ventilated area?**

    Exposure to radiographic processing solutions in a poorly ventilated area may cause respiratory problems.

8. **In general, how should chemicals be stored?**

    In general, chemicals should be stored in a dry, cool, and dark place.

9. **In general, how are chemicals determined to be hazardous?**

    In general, chemicals are determined to be hazardous if they are ignitable, corrosive, reactive, or toxic.

10. **What is another name for the Hazard Communication Standard?**

    The "Employee Right-to-Know Law" is another name for the OSHA Hazard Communication Standard.

11. **What chemicals must be included in the chemical inventory?**

    All chemicals must be included in the chemical inventory.

12. **What is an MSDS?**

    An MSDS is a material safety data sheet.

13. **What materials are exempt from labeling requirements?**

    Tobacco and tobacco products, wood and wood products, food, drugs, cosmetics, and alcoholic beverages sold and packaged for consumer use are exempt from labeling requirements.

14. **Which employees must receive training about hazardous chemicals?**

    All employees who work around chemicals must receive training.

Torres and Ehrlich Modern Dental Assisting, 9th ed.

Bird/Robinson

15. **How long must training records be kept on file?**

    Employee training records must be kept on file for at least 5 years.

16. **What are three examples of regulated waste?**

    Used needles, contaminated broken glass, and endodontic reamers are examples of regulated waste.

17. **Why is x-ray (radiographic) fixer considered to be toxic?**

    X-ray fixer is considered to be toxic because of the high silver content.

24 Recall Questions and Answers

1. Are waterborne diseases limited to dentistry?

No, waterborne diseases are not limited to dentistry.

2. Is the presence of bacteria in dental unit waterlines a recent finding?

The presence of bacteria in dental unit waterlines was first reported more than 30 years ago.

3. Is there a widespread public health problem regarding contaminated dental water?

No, there is not a widespread public health problem regarding contaminated dental water.

4. What bacteria cause the disease legionellosis?

Legionella bacteria cause the disease legionellosis.

5. Where is biofilm found?

Biofilm is found on any solid surface that is wet or moist.

6. Is it appropriate to heat the water in dental units?

No, it is not appropriate to heat the water in dental units.

7. Is it possible to eliminate biofilm completely?

It is not possible to eliminate biofilms completely, but they can be reduced.

8. If sterile water is used in the self-contained reservoir, will the water that enters the patient's mouth be sterile?

If sterile water is used in the self-contained reservoir, it will not be sterile when it enters the patient's mouth because the traditional dental units are not capable of delivering sterile water.

9. How often should microfilters be changed?

Microfilters should be changed at least daily.

10. What precautions should you take when selecting a chemical for the dental unit?

You must check with the equipment manufacturer when selecting a chemical for the dental unit.

11. What type of water must be used as an irrigant for surgery involving bone?

Sterile water must be used as an irrigant for surgery involving bone.

12. Will flushing DUWLs remove biofilm?

Flushing DUWLs will not remove biofilm.

Torres and Ehrlich Modern Dental Assisting, 9th ed.

Bird/Robinson

13. When should the high-volume evacuator be used to minimize aerosol?

The high-volume evacuator should be used with the high-speed handpiece, ultrasonic scaler, and air-water syringe to minimize aerosol.

14. Will the use of a rubber dam totally eliminate exposure to microorganisms?

The use of a rubber dam will not totally eliminate exposure to microorganisms.

15. What methods are available to test the quality of dental unit water?

The quality of dental unit water can be tested by using a commercial service or by using in-office test kits.

Torres and Ehrlich Modern Dental Assisting, 9th ed.

Bird/Robinson

25 Recall Questions and Answers

1. What is meant by "ergonomics?"

Ergonomics is the adaptation of the work environment to the human body.

2. What is the goal of ergonomics?

The goal of ergonomics is to help people stay healthy while performing their work more effectively.

3. What types of disorders are considered to be MSDs?

Headaches, neck and shoulder pain, and carpal tunnel syndrome are types of MSDs.

4. What are the three categories of risk factors that contribute to MSDs?

The three categories of risk factors that contribute to MSDs are posture, repetition, and force.

5. What is the neutral position?

The neutral position is sitting upright with the weight evenly distributed.

6. What is meant by normal horizontal reach?

Normal horizontal reach is the reach created by the sweep of the forearm with the upper arm held at the side.

7. What type of glove is most likely to aggravate carpal tunnel syndrome?

Ambidextrous gloves are the most likely to aggravate carpal tunnel syndrome.

8. How can you reduce eyestrain?

You can reduce eyestrain by looking up from the task and focusing your eyes at a distance for about 20 seconds.

9. What exercise relieves neck strain?

Shoulder shrugging relieves neck strain.

10. What is one of the most important factors in preventing CTS?

Resting the hands is one of the most important factors in preventing CTS.

26 Recall Questions and Answers

1. **What forms must a business assistant hand to a patient to complete before any dental treatment can be provided?**
   The dentist must have a registration form, medical-dental health history form, medical alert, HIPAA, and consent forms.

2. **What term describes the collection of data by the dentist to make a correct diagnosis?**
   Assessment is the collection of data for a diagnosis.

3. **The patient record is a permanent document of whom?**
   The patient record is a permanent document of the dentist.

4. **Why is quality assurance so important in the maintenance of a dental practice?**
   Quality assurance defines the quality of care a patient is receiving.

5. **What does PHI represent?**
   PHI stands for protected health information.

6. **Where should the patient registration form be placed in a patient record?**
   The registration form should be placed at the front of the patient record.

7. **To verify that the information is accurate, what must a patient provide on the health history form?**
   The patient must provide a signature and date.

8. **What does the dental history section of the form provide for the dentist?**
   The dental history provides previous dental treatment and care.

9. **What is an example of a medical alert?**
   An allergy to medications is one example of a medical alert.

10. **What form in the patient record would inform the dental team of an existing restoration?**
    The clinical examination form would provide information about an existing restoration.

ELSEVIER

Torres and Ehrlich Modern Dental Assisting, 9th ed.
Bird/Robinson

27   Recall Questions and Answers

1. What are the four vital signs?

The four vital signs are temperature, pulse, respiration, and blood pressure.

2. What is the purpose of a thermometer?

The thermometer is used to measure body temperature.

3. What location on the body usually gives the highest temperature reading of the body?

The rectal area usually gives the highest temperature reading.

4. Where is the tympanic thermometer placed?

The tympanic thermometer is placed in the ear.

5. Which artery in the body has a pulse?

Every artery has a pulse.

6. Which artery would you normally palpate when taking a patient's pulse?

The radial artery is normally used to palpate a pulse.

7. What is the normal pulse rate for an adult?

An adult's normal pulse rate is 60 to 100 beats per minute.

8. Respiration is the process of doing what?

Respiration is the process of inhaling and exhaling, or breathing.

9. What is the term for excessively rapid breathing?

Tachypnea is excessively rapid breathing.

10. What is the normal rate of respiration for an adult?

An adult's normal respiratory rate is 10 to 20 breaths per minute.

11. Is the diastolic reading the first or last sound heard when taking a blood pressure?

The diastolic reading is the last sound heard.

12. What two instruments are used when taking a patient's blood pressure?

A sphygmomanometer and stethoscope are used for blood pressure readings.

13. What is the term for the small groove or fold on the inner arm?

The small fold on the inner arm is the antecubital space.

Bird/Robinson

14. Who first described a series of sounds (now named for him) heard during the taking of a blood pressure?

Korotkoff first described the series of sounds heard while taking blood pressure.

15. What is the range of a normal blood pressure reading for an adult?

Less than 130 systolic and less than 85 mm Hg diastolic is the normal adult blood pressure.

Torres and Ehrlich Modern Dental Assisting, 9th ed.

Bird/Robinson

28 Recall Questions and Answers

1. Identify four reasons why a patient seeks dental care.
The four reasons for a patient to seek dental care are examination (new patient), emergency, consultation, and review (returning patient).

2. What diagnostic techniques are used to evaluate a patient's oral condition?
Visual evaluation, instrumentation, radiography, and intraoral imaging are used to evaluate oral conditions.

3. What instrument is commonly used by the dentist to detect decay?
The explorer is used to detect decay.

4. Do you chart missing teeth? If so, how?
Yes. Place an X through the teeth on the chart.

5. Performing intraoral imaging is similar to what?
Intraoral imaging is similar to using a video camera.

6. What class(es) in Black's classification involves premolars and molars?
Classes I, II, V, and VI involve premolars and molars.

7. What class(es) in Black's classification system involves incisors?
Classes I, III, IV, and V involve incisors.

8. How would you chart an MOD amalgam on tooth 4?
Outline the mesial/occlusal/distal portion of the surface and color-code it with blue or black.

9. What members of the dental team can perform the periodontal examination for a patient?
The dental hygienist normally performs the periodontal examinations and charting.

29   Recall Questions and Answers

1. What role does the dental assistant have with the medically and physically compromised patient?
Aid the dentist in treatment, provide a source of information to the patient and family, make the patient more comfortable, and reduce anxiety.

2. What is the fastest-growing segment of the population?
Older people are the fastest-growing segment of the population.

3. What aging category would include a 76-year-old dental patient?
The "old" category would include a 76-year-old patient.

4. What is xerostomia?
Xerostomia results from certain disorders and medications and causes a decreased flow of saliva or a dry mouth.

5. What are four oral health conditions that affect the aging population?
Periodontal disease, tooth decay, dark and brittle teeth, and bone resorption are four oral conditions that affect the aging population.

6. What is dementia?
Dementia is the loss of memory, concentration, and judgment.

7. What common side effect occurs from taking phenytoin?
Hyperplasia occurs from taking phenytoin.

8. What is another term for cerebrovascular accident?
Stroke is another term for cerebrovascular accident.

9. What are two examples of neurologic disorders?
Alzheimer's disease and multiple sclerosis are examples of neurologic disorders.

10. What is the leading cause of death in the United States?
Heart disease is the leading cause of death in the United States.

11. Is epinephrine recommended for use in patients with heart disease?
Epinephrine and other vasoconstrictors can be administered, within limits, to patients with mild to moderate cardiovascular disease.

12. What is another term for hypertension?
High blood pressure is another term for hypertension.

13. What organs do pulmonary disorders affect in the body?
Pulmonary disorders affect the lungs.

14. What does the abbreviation COPD stand for?
COPD stands for chronic obstructive pulmonary disease.

ELSEVIER

Bird/Robinson

15. What disorder is associated with an overactive thyroid gland?

Graves' disease is associated with an overactive thyroid gland.

16. How is a patient with type 2 diabetes classified in relation to the need for insulin?

A patient with type 2 diabetes is classified as non-insulin-dependent.

Torres and Ehrlich Modern Dental Assisting, 9th ed.

Bird/Robinson

30 Recall Questions and Answers

1. Identify three sources of drugs.

Plants, animals, and the laboratory are three sources of drugs.

2. What type of drug name is Advil?

Advil is a brand name.

3. What agency regulates the sale of medicines?

The U.S. Food and Drug Administration (FDA) regulates the sale of medications.

4. Who is allowed to write prescriptions in the dental office?

The dentist writes prescriptions.

5. What part of the prescription includes the name and quantity of the drug?

The inscription includes the name and quantity of the drug.

6. What does the abbreviation b.i.d. stand for?

The abbreviation b.i.d. stands for twice a day.

7. Where is a sublingual drug administered?

A sublingual drug is administered (inserted) under the tongue.

8. Where is a subcutaneous drug administered?

A subcutaneous drug is administered (injected) under the skin.

9. What is the slowest route of absorption for a drug?

The oral route is the slowest route of absorption for a drug.

10. In which DEA drug schedule is Tylenol with codeine listed?

Tylenol with codeine is a Schedule III drug.

11. What is the term for the body's negative reaction to a drug?

The term for the body's negative reaction to a drug is adverse drug effect.

12. An analgesic is used for what action?

An analgesic is used for relief of pain.

13. What is an example of an antibiotic prescribed for plaque or gingivitis?

Chlorhexidine is prescribed for plaque or gingivitis.

14. What type of drug may be prescribed for high blood pressure?

Antihypertensive drugs, such as Lasix, are prescribed for high blood pressure.

15. Would a patient be taking a diuretic to treat a cold?

No, a patient might be taking an antihistamine to treat a cold.

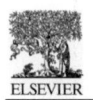

Torres and Ehrlich Modern Dental Assisting, 9th ed.

Bird/Robinson

31 Recall Questions and Answers

1. What is the best way to prevent an emergency?
The best way to prevent an emergency is to know your patient.

2. What is the cause of most medical emergencies in the dental office?
Stress causes most dental emergencies.

3. Who is responsible for a patient's safety in the dental office?
The dentist is responsible for the patient's safety.

4. Who in the dental office would most likely be in charge of calling the emergency medical services?
The front desk staff members, or business assistants, are most likely to call emergency medical services.

5. Where should emergency phone numbers be kept?
Emergency numbers should be kept next to each phone.

6. What minimum credentials must you have for emergency care standards as a dental assistant?
The minimum credentials are training in CPR, the Heimlich maneuver, and taking vital signs.

7. What does the abbreviation ABCD stand for in emergency care?
ABCD stands for airway, breathing, circulation, and defibrillation.

8. What is the proper ratio of chest compressions to breaths for an adult victim when doing CPR?
The proper ratio of chest compressions to breaths for an adult victim is 15:2.

9. What is the most frequently used "drug" in a medical emergency?
Oxygen is the most frequently used "drug" in a medical emergency.

10. What does the abbreviation AED stand for?
AED stands for automated external defibrillator.

11. What is the danger of ventricular fibrillation?
Ventricular fibrillation may cause cardiac arrest.

12. When patients tell you how they feel, what is the term for such a "feeling"?
The term for a patient's expressed "feeling" is symptom.

13. A patient who is unresponsive to sensory stimulation is in what state?
A patient unresponsive to sensory stimulation is unconscious.

14. What is the medical term for fainting?
Syncope is the medical term for fainting.

15. What is the medical term for chest pain caused by the heart muscle being deprived of oxygen?
Angina is the medical term for chest pain caused by the heart muscle being deprived of oxygen.

16. What is the medical term for a stroke?
Cerebrovascular accident is the medical term for a stroke.

17. A patient with asthma will usually carry what form of medication?
An asthmatic patient usually carries an inhaler.

ELSEVIER

Torres and Ehrlich Modern Dental Assisting, 9th ed.
 Bird/Robinson

18. What type of allergic reaction can be life-threatening?
Anaphylaxis can be life-threatening.

19. What condition results from an abnormal increase in blood glucose?
An abnormally increased blood glucose level is called hyperglycemia.

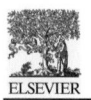

Torres and Ehrlich Modern Dental Assisting, 9th ed.

Bird/Robinson

32 Recall Questions and Answers

1. What is the ideal temperature for the reception area?

The ideal temperature of the reception area is 72° F.

2. What type of flooring should be placed in the clinical area?

Vinyl flooring should be placed in the clinical area.

3. What are the important features of the reception area?

The reception area should have good lighting, a comfortable temperature, reading material, and adequate seating.

4. Where in the dental office are dental procedures performed?

Dental procedures are performed in the treatment area.

5. What is another term for treatment area?

Operatory is another term for treatment area.

6. What patient chair position is used for most dental procedures?

The supine position is used for most dental procedures.

7. Which two features on the dental assistant's stool are not part of the operator's stool?

The dental assistant's stool has a foot platform or ring (footrest) and an abdominal bar.

8. What foot-controlled device is used to operate the dental handpiece?

A rheostat is used to operate the dental handpiece.

9. What does the abbreviation HVE represent?

HVE stands for high-volume evacuator.

10. Where should you place dental materials to be triturated?

You should place dental materials to be triturated in the amalgamator.

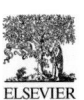
ELSEVIER

Torres and Ehrlich Modern Dental Assisting, 9th ed.
 Bird/Robinson

33 Recall Questions and Answers

1. **State two goals of the dental team that are intended to simplify dental treatment in the dental office.**
   The goals of the dental team are to increase patient comfort, minimize stress and fatigue, use appropriate moisture control, transfer instruments, and practice expanded functions.

2. **In relation to the operator, should the assistant be positioned lower or higher?**
   The assistant should be positioned higher than the operator.

3. **How should the operator maintain the forearms when working on a patient?**
   The operator should maintain the forearms parallel to the floor.

4. **When using the clock concept, where is the static zone for a right-handed operator?**
   The static zone for the right-handed operator is at the 12 o'clock to 2 o'clock position.

5. **Where are instruments exchanged during a procedure?**
   Instruments are exchanged in the transfer zone during a procedure.

6. **Besides the assistant, what may be located in the assistant's zone?**
   The mobile cabinet and countertop are also in the assistant's zone.

7. **Should the assistant use one hand or both hands to transfer instruments?**
   The assistant should use one-handed transfer.

8. **Which hand is primarily used to transfer instruments to a right-handed dentist?**
   The left hand is primarily used to hand instruments to a right-handed dentist.

9. **What is indirect vision?**
   Indirect vision is viewing an object through a mirror.

10. **What is another term for finger rest?**
    Fulcrum is another term for finger rest.

34 Recall Questions and Answers

1. **What type of dental instruments are more often referred to by a number than by name?**
   Pliers and forceps are more often referred to by number than by name.

2. **What part of the instrument is located between the handle and the working end?**
   The shank is between the handle and the working end.

3. **What classification of instruments is used to manually remove soft decay?**
   Hand (manual) cutting instruments are used to manually remove soft decay.

4. **What are the four uses of the mouth mirror?**
   Uses of the mouth mirror include indirect vision, light reflection, retraction, and tissue protection.

5. **What is the main feature of the working end of an explorer?**
   The working end has a sharp point.

6. **What instruments make up the basic setup?**
   The mouth mirror, explorer, and cotton pliers make up the basic setup.

7. **What instrument is used to measure the sulcus of a tooth?**
   The periodontal probe is used to measure the sulcus.

8. **What are the two most common excavators used in restorative dentistry?**
   The spoon excavator and black spoon are the most common excavators in restorative dentistry.

9. **What instrument would you transfer to the dentist to carve anatomy back into the interproximal portion of an amalgam restoration?**
   You would transfer a Hollenback carver for amalgam shaping.

10. **What instrument is used to pack amalgam?**
    An amalgam condenser is used to pack down amalgam.

11. **What type of instrument is discoid/cleoid?**
    A carver is discoid/cleoid.

12. **What type of scissors is placed on the restorative tray setup?**
    A crown and bridge scissors would be indicated in a restorative setup.

13. **What is another term for Howe pliers?**
    Howe pliers can also be referred to as #110 pliers.

14. **Where is the freshly mixed amalgam placed before transporting it in the amalgam carrier?**
    Freshly mixed amalgam is placed in the amalgam well.

Torres and Ehrlich Modern Dental Assisting, 9th ed.

Bird/Robinson

35 Recall Questions and Answers

1. How did the first dental handpiece operate?
The first dental handpiece was belt-driven.

2. What are the two most common types of dental handpiece?
Low-speed and high-speed handpieces are most often used in dentistry.

3. How fast does the low-speed handpiece rotate?
The low-speed handpiece can operate at 30,000 rpm.

4. Which attachment is used to hold a latch-type bur?
A contra angle is used to hold a latch-type bur.

5. How fast does the high-speed handpiece operate?
The high-speed handpiece can operate at 450,000 rpm.

6. How is the tooth kept cool and clean during the use of the high-speed handpiece?
A water coolant system keeps the tooth clean and cool during high-speed treatment.

7. What type of bur locking system is on the high-speed handpiece?
A high-speed handpiece holds a bur with a friction-grip device.

8. On the high-speed handpiece, what helps to illuminate the working field?
A fiberoptic system illuminates the working field.

9. What type of handpiece resembles a sandblaster?
An air abrasion handpiece resembles a sandblaster.

10. What type of shank fits into the contra-angle attachment?
The latch-type shank fits into the contra-angle attachment.

11. Restorative burs are made from what material?
Restorative burs are made of tungsten carbide.

12. What design of bur is a 33 ½?
A 33 ½ bur is an inverted cone.

13. What gives the diamond bur its advantage?
Cutting ability gives a diamond bur its advantage.

14. Finishing burs are used on what type of dental material?
Finishing burs are used on composite resin/esthetic materials.

15. What is used to hold a disc in the handpiece?
The mandrel is used to hold a disc in the handpiece.

Bird/Robinson

36 Recall Questions and Answers

1. What are the two types of evacuators used in operative dental procedures?
The two evacuators used in dental procedures are the saliva ejector and the high-volume evacuator.

2. What is the main function of the saliva ejector?
The main function of the saliva ejector is to remove saliva and water.

3. What are operative suction tips made from?
Disposable plastic, hard plastic, and stainless steel are used to make operative suction tips.

4. What type of rinsing technique is performed throughout a procedure?
A limited-area rinse is performed throughout a procedure.

5. What three means of isolation are most often used in dentistry?
Cotton rolls, dry angles, and dental dams are most often used to isolate teeth.

6. What type of isolation is commonly chosen for shorter procedures?
Cotton roll or dry-angle isolation is used in shorter procedures.

7. Why is it important to wet a cotton roll before removal?
If not wet, the rolls can pull on the lining of the mucosa.

8. What is the term for teeth that are visible through the dam?
Teeth visible through the dam are isolated or exposed.

9. What piece of equipment stabilizes and stretches the dam away from the tooth?
The frame stabilizes and stretches the dental dam.

10. If you are unable to slide the dam interproximally, what can be placed on the underside of the dam to help in the application?
Water-soluble lubricant can help in dam application.

11. The hole sizes on the rubber dam punch range from 1 to 5. Which is the smallest size?
Size 1 is the smallest hole size.

12. For what purposes would you use an anterior dental dam clamp?
You would use an anterior dental dam clamp for retraction of the gingiva, for class V restorations, and for endodontic treatment.

ELSEVIER

Torres and Ehrlich Modern Dental Assisting, 9th ed.

37   Recall Questions and Answers

1. Why are topical anesthetics used in dentistry?
Topical anesthetics are used in dentistry to numb the area where the injection is given.

2. What is the most frequently selected form of pain control used in dentistry?
Local anesthetics are most often used for pain control.

3. To create a numbing effect, where does a local anesthetic need to be injected?
Local anesthetics are injected near a nerve.

4. What is added to a local anesthetic to prolong its effect?
A vasoconstrictor is added to prolong an anesthetic's effect.

5. What type of injection technique does the dentist most frequently use for maxillary teeth?
Infiltration is most often used on maxillary teeth.

6. How many lengths of needles are used in dentistry, and for what are they used?
Two sizes of needle are used, long for block and short for infiltration.

7. Should a patient with an abscess receive local anesthesia? Why or why not?
No, a patient with an abscess should not receive local anesthesia because of the infection.

8. What is paresthesia?
Paresthesia refers to persistent numbness caused by damaged nerve endings.

9. Who was the first dentist to use nitrous oxide on his patients?
Horace Wells first used nitrous oxide.

10. What color code is used for nitrous oxide?
The nitrous oxide cylinder is blue.

11. How is the dental team at risk for overexposure to nitrous oxide?
The dental team may be at risk for N_2O overexposure from leakage around the mask and when a patient talks or breathes from the mouth.

12. What is given to the patient before and after N_2O/O_2 sedation?
Before and after N_2O/O_2 sedation, the patient is given 100 percent oxygen.

13. Is the patient conscious during intravenous sedation?
Yes, the patient is conscious during intravenous sedation.

14. Is the patient conscious during general anesthesia?
No, the patient is not conscious during general anesthesia.

15. In what environment is general anesthesia most often administered?
General anesthesia is most often administered in the hospital setting.

Torres and Ehrlich Modern Dental Assisting, 9th ed.

Bird/Robinson

38   Recall Questions and Answers

1. Who discovered x-rays?
Wilhelm Conrad Roentgen discovered x-rays.

2. Who was the first person to make practical use of x-rays in dentistry?
C. Edmund Kells was the first person to make practical use of x-rays in dentistry.

3. What is ionization?
Ionization is the process by which electrons are removed from electrically stable atoms through collisions with x-ray photons.

4. What are the primary components of a dental x-ray machine?
The primary components of a dental x-ray machine are the tubehead, the extension arm, and the control panel.

5. What is the negative electrode inside the x-ray tube?
The cathode is the negative electrode inside the x-ray tube.

6. What is the positive electrode inside the x-ray tube?
The anode is the positive electrode inside the x-ray tube.

7. What is usually found on a control panel?
The control panel of an x-ray unit contains the master switch and two indicator lights, exposure timer, milliamperage (mA) selector, and kilovoltage peak (kVp) selector.

8. During the production of x-rays, how much energy is lost as heat?
During the production of x-rays, 99% of the energy is lost as heat.

9. What are the three types of radiation?
The three types of radiation are primary, secondary, and scatter.

10. What does the term radiolucent mean?
Radiolucent refers to a dark appearance of a structure on a processed radiograph.

11. What does the term radiopaque mean?
Radiopaque refers to a white or light appearance of a structure on a processed radiograph.

12. What exposure factors control contrast?
Kilovoltage controls contrast.

13. What is meant by density?
Density is the overall darkness of a processed radiograph controlled by milliamperage and time.

14. What is the name of the process that results in the harmful effects of x-rays?
Ionization causes the harmful effects of x-rays.

15. What is the name of the time period between x-ray exposure and the appearance of symptoms?
The latent period is the time between x-ray exposure and the appearance of symptoms.

16. What is meant by genetic effects?
Genetic effects of radiation are those that are passed on to future generations.

17. What are the two systems of radiation measurement?
The traditional, or standard, system and the Systeme Internationale (SI) are used to measure radiation.

18. What is the maximum permissible dose of radiation for occupationally exposed persons?
The maximum permissible dose of radiation for occupationally exposed persons is 5.0 rem per year.

19. What is the purpose of the collimator?
The collimator is used to restrict the size of the primary beam.

20. What is the purpose of the aluminum filter?
The aluminum filter is used to remove the low-energy, long-wavelength rays.

21. What precautions should be taken when handling the lead apron?
Lead aprons and thyroid collars must not be folded when stored.

22. What is the most effective measure in reducing a patient's exposure to radiation?
The most effective measure in reducing patient exposure is the use of fast-speed film.

23. What is the purpose of personnel monitoring?
The purpose of personnel monitoring is to record the amount of occupational x-radiation that reaches the body.

24. What is the purpose of equipment monitoring?
Dental x-ray equipment should be monitored for leakage radiation.

25. What is the ALARA concept?
ALARA stands for "As Low As Reasonably Achievable."

39 Recall Questions and Answers

1. How does the use of film holders protect the patient from unnecessary radiation?
A film holder keeps the patient's hands and fingers from being exposed to x-radiation.

2. What makes up the basic type of film holder?
A basic-style film holder is a bite-block with a backing plate and a slot for film retention.

3. What is the purpose of a beam alignment device?
Beam alignment devices assist in the positioning of the position indicator device in relation to the tooth and film.

4. What are the five components of intraoral film?
Intraoral film consists of the (1) adhesive layer, (2) film emulsion, (3) gelatin, (4) silver halide crystals, and (5) protective layer.

5. What is a latent image?
The image on the film before processing is the latent image.

6. How can you tell which side of the film is placed toward the tube?
The white side of the film is placed toward the tube.

7. What number film is used for periapical radiographs?
Size #2 film is used for periapical radiographs.

8. What size film is used for occlusal radiographs?
Size #4 film is used for occlusal radiographs.

9. What are the two types of extraoral film cassettes?
Film cassettes may be either rigid or flexible.

10. What is an intensifying screen?
An intensifying screen converts radiographic energy into visible light.

11. How does extraoral film react differently from intraoral film?
The light from the screen exposes the extraoral film; the intraoral film is exposed directly by radiation.

12. When might it be necessary to duplicate x-rays?
It might be necessary to duplicate radiographs for the insurance company or for referral of patients to a specialist or another dental office.

13. What precautions should be taken when storing x-ray film?
Radiographic film should be stored away from light, heat, moisture, chemicals, and scatter radiation.

14. How can you find the expiration date of a package?
The expiration date of a package of radiographic film is on the outside of the box.

15. What are the five steps in processing dental radiographs?
Film processing involves (1) developing, (2) rinsing, (3) fixing, (4) washing, and (5) drying.

16. Which is the most widely used form of processing solution?
The liquid concentrate is the most widely used form of processing solution.

ELSEVIER

17. How often should processing solutions be replenished?

Processing solutions should be replenished daily.

18. What is a safelight?

A safelight is a low-intensity light composed of long wavelengths in the red-orange spectrum.

19. What is the minimum distance between the safelight and the working area?

The minimum distance between the safelight and the working area is 4 feet.

20. What is the optimum temperature for the water in the manual processing tanks?

The optimum temperature for the water in the manual processing tanks is 68° F.

21. What is the major advantage of automatic film processing?

Less time required for processing is the major advantage of automatic film processing.

22. How often should the levels of solution in the automatic processor be checked?

The levels of solution in the automatic processor are checked daily.

23. Are manual processing solutions and automatic processing solutions interchangeable?

Manual processing solutions and automatic processing solutions are not interchangeable.

Bird/Robinson

40 Recall Questions and Answers

1. What federal act requires persons who take radiographs to be trained and certified?
The Consumer-Patient Radiation Health and Safety Act requires persons who take radiographs to be trained and certified.

2. What type of consent is necessary before exposing a patient to x-rays?
Informed consent is necessary before exposing a patient to x-rays.

3. Under state laws, who is allowed to prescribe dental radiographs?
Under state laws, a dentist is allowed to prescribe dental radiographs.

4. Who legally owns a patient's dental radiographs?
The dentist legally owns a patient's dental radiographs.

5. What is meant by quality assurance?
Quality assurance is a way of ensuring that high-quality diagnostic radiographs are produced.

6. What are quality-control tests?
Quality-control tests are specific tests used to monitor dental radiographic equipment, supplies, and film processing.

7. When should you check a box of film for freshness?
You should check the film for freshness each time you open a box of new film.

8. Should you use a film cassette that has scratches?
No, you should not use a film cassette that has scratches.

9. What is one of the most critical areas in a quality-control program?
Film processing is one of the most critical areas in a quality-control program.

10. What is the purpose of the coin test?
The purpose of the coin test is to check the safelight.

11. How often should processing solutions be replenished?
Processing solutions should be replenished daily.

12. Why are the reference radiograph and stepwedge used?
A reference radiograph and stepwedge are used to check radiographic densities and contrast.

13. How can you tell when the fixer loses its strength?
When films take longer to "clear," the fixer is losing its strength.

14. What is the purpose of a quality administration program?
Quality administration deals with the management of the quality assurance program.

15. Which staff members need to be aware of the quality administration program?
All staff members need to be aware of the quality administration program.

Torres and Ehrlich Modern Dental Assisting, 9th ed.
Bird/Robinson

16. **What unique infection control problems occur in dental radiography?**
Constant movement by the operator—from the oral cavity to the exposure controls outside the operatory, to the darkroom, and finally to film mounting—increases the risk for exposing others to infectious diseases.

17. **What surfaces must be covered with barriers?**
Surfaces that are not easily cleaned and disinfected must be covered with barriers.

18. **What precautions should be taken when handling contaminated film?**
Saliva should be wiped off the film as soon as it is removed from the mouth.

19. **When should the packages containing the film-holding device be opened?**
The packages containing the film-holding device should be opened in front of the patient.

20. **What personal protective equipment (PPE) should the operator wear while exposing radiographs?**
The minimum PPE that the operator should wear while exposing radiographs is a gown and gloves. Masks and eyewear are optional.

21. **What type of gloves should be worn while disinfecting the radiography operatory?**
Utility gloves should be worn while disinfecting the radiography operatory.

22. **What precautions must be taken when transporting films to the darkroom?**
While taking the films to the darkroom, do not touch the inside of the cup or films.

Bird/Robinson

41 Recall Questions and Answers

1. What is the difference between a bite-wing and a periapical radiograph?
A bite-wing shows only the crowns, alveolar ridge, and a small portion of the root. The periapical shows the entire length of the tooth, including the apex and surrounding areas.

2. What are the two techniques for exposing radiographs?
The two techniques for exposing films are the paralleling and bisecting techniques.

3. Why is an exposure sequence important?
Using an exposure sequence is important so that areas of the mouth are not missed or repeated.

4. When exposing films, in which area of the mouth should you begin?
When exposing films, you should begin in the maxillary anterior area.

5. Which projection should be the first for posterior exposures?
For the patient's comfort, the premolar view is the first mandibular exposure.

6. Why is it not recommended to have the patient hold the film during exposure?
The patient's hand and finger receives unnecessary radiation when holding the film during exposure.

7. What type of film holders can be used in the bisecting technique?
BAI, EeZee-Grip, and Stabe are film holders that can be used in the bisecting technique.

8. What error occurs when the horizontal angulation is incorrect?
Overlapping of the contacts occurs when the horizontal angulation is incorrect.

9. What two errors occur when the vertical angulation is incorrect?
Elongation and foreshortening can occur when the vertical angulation is incorrect.

10. In the bisecting technique, how is the film placed in relation to the teeth?
In the bisecting technique, the film is placed close to the teeth.

11. What is the purpose of bite-wing radiographs?
Bite-wing radiographs are used to detect interproximal caries and evaluate crestal bone.

12. What horizontal angulation should be used for bite-wing radiographs?
The horizontal angulation should be +10 degrees for bite-wing radiographs.

13. What size film is used in the occlusal technique?
Size #4 film is used in the occlusal technique.

14. When are occlusal radiographs indicated?
Occlusal radiographs are indicated when a wide view of the arch is needed.

15. What physical disabilities may affect dental patients?
Patients may have vision, hearing, and mobility disabilities.

16. Under what circumstance would you hold a film for a patient?
Under no circumstances should you hold a film for a patient.

17. For partially edentulous patients, how can you modify the technique for using a bite-block?
For partially edentulous patients, you can modify the technique by placing cotton rolls where the bite-block would be placed.

18. When exposing films on a pediatric patient, how can you best describe the tubehead to the patient?
When exposing films on a pediatric patient, you can describe the tubehead as a "camera."

19. What changes must be made in the exposure factors when exposing radiographs on a pediatric patient?
The exposure factors must be reduced when exposing radiographs on a pediatric patient.

20. What size of film is recommended for a pediatric patient with all primary dentition?
Film size #0 is recommended for a pediatric patient with all primary dentition.

21. Why is the exposure sequence especially important when taking x-rays on a patient with a severe gag reflex?
Because patients are most likely to gag on posterior films, it is best to begin in the anterior areas.

22. What is the definition of a diagnostic-quality radiograph?
A diagnostic-quality endodontic radiograph is one in which the tooth is centered on the film, at least 5 mm of bone beyond the apex of the tooth is visible, and the image is as anatomically correct as possible.

23. When mounting radiographs, what is the recommendation concerning placement of the raised dot?
The ADA recommends mounting radiographs with the dot facing up.

24. Why is it important for the dental assistant to recognize anatomic landmarks?
It is important for the dental assistant to recognize anatomic landmarks because they are useful in mounting radiographs.

25. Why is it important to avoid retakes?
Retakes expose the patient to unnecessary radiation.

Torres and Ehrlich Modern Dental Assisting, 9th ed.

Bird/Robinson

42 | Recall Questions and Answers

1. When are extraoral radiographs needed?
Extraoral radiographs are taken when large areas of the skull or jaw must be examined.

2. What types of film are needed to supplement a panoramic radiograph? Why?
Bite-wing and selected periapicals are needed to supplement a panoramic radiograph because of the lack of detail in a panoramic film.

3. What is a focal trough?
A focal trough is an imaginary horseshoe-shaped area used for jaw placement during panoramic exposures.

4. What is the purpose of extraoral radiographs?
Extraoral radiographs are used to provide an overall image of the skull and jaws.

5. What is the name of the device that may be added to a panoramic unit to allow the operator to easily position the film and patient?
A cephalostat may be added on to a panoramic unit for this purpose.

6. What is the purpose of a grid?
A grid is a device used to reduce the amount of scatter radiation.

7. What type of imaging is best for soft tissues of the temporomandibular joint (TMJ)?
A computed tomography (CT) scan is the best type of imaging for soft tissues of the TMJ.

8. In digital radiography, what replaces the intraoral film?
In digital radiography the sensor replaces the intraoral film.

9. How are sensors sterilized?
Sensors cannot be sterilized; they must be protected with disposable plastic sleeves.

10. Which exposure technique is preferred when using digital radiography?
The paralleling exposure technique is preferred when using digital radiography.

ELSEVIER

43 Recall Questions and Answers

1. What professional organization evaluates a new dental material?
The American Dental Association (ADA) evaluates a new dental material.

2. What type of reaction does a dental material undergo when distortion occurs?
A dental material undergoes stress when distortion occurs.

3. What happens to a dental material when exposed to hot and cold?
A dental material undergoes contraction and expansion when exposed to hot or cold.

4. What is a source of galvanic action?
Saliva (salt conducting electrical currents) and two metals (acting as battery) are sources of galvanic action.

5. What are the four properties that must be considered in the application of a dental material?
Four properties that must be considered in applying dental materials are flow, adhesion, retention, and curing.

6. How does an auto-cured material harden or set?
An auto-cured material hardens, or sets, through a chemical reaction of the materials being mixed together.

7. What metals make up the alloy powder in amalgam?
The alloy powder in amalgam contains silver, tin, copper, and zinc.

8. Is dental amalgam placed in anterior teeth?
No, amalgam is not esthetically pleasing in the anterior teeth.

9. What does copper provide to amalgam restorations?
Copper provides strength and corrosion resistance to amalgam.

10. Where do you dispose of amalgam scraps?
Amalgam scraps are disposed of under water or under fixer solution.

11. How is the amalgam triturated?
Amalgam is triturated in an amalgamator.

12. How long do you triturate Sybraloy?
Sybraloy is triturated for 13 seconds.

13. What is the common term used for dimethacrylate?
The common term for dimethacrylate is Bis-GMA.

14. What filler type of composite resin is strongest and the one most often used for posterior restorations?
The macrofilled resin is strongest and used most often for posterior restorations.

15. When composite resins are being light-cured, what factors might require a longer curing time of the material?
Depth of restoration and color may require longer curing time.

16. What item is used to determine the color of composite for a procedure?
A shade guide is used to determine the color of composite.

17. What is the final step in finishing a composite resin?
The final step in finishing a composite resin is the use of a polishing paste.

18. What are some of the most common uses of glass ionomer materials?
Glass ionomer materials are commonly used as restorative materials, liners, bonding agents, and permanent cements.

19. What will contaminate the setting of glass ionomers?
Water will contaminate the setting of glass ionomers and should be avoided.

20. What does the abbreviation IRM stand for?
IRM stands for intermediate restorative material.

21. What temporary restorative material would be selected for a class II cavity preparation?
An IRM would be selected for a class II cavity preparation.

22. What material would you use to prepare for provisional coverage?
Acrylic resin or composite resin would be used to prepare for provisional coverage.

23. How many drops of monomer are recommended per tooth when mixing acrylic resin?
The recommended amount is 10 drops of monomer per tooth.

24. What are the three noble metals used in dentistry?
The three noble metals used in dentistry are gold, palladium, and platinum.

25. What type of restoration is made in the dental laboratory?
Indirect restorations are made in the dental laboratory.

44 Recall Questions and Answers

1. **What is the function of a dental liner?**
   A dental liner protects the pulp from irritation.

2. **On what tooth structure is a liner placed?**
   A liner, calcium hydroxide, is placed on dentin.

3. **What are the three unique qualities of calcium hydroxide?**
   Calcium hydroxide protects from chemical irritation, produces reparative dentin, and is compatible with all materials.

4. **What is the main ingredient in varnish?**
   Resin is the main ingredient in varnish.

5. **Can varnish be placed under all restorative materials? If not, which materials are contraindicated?**
   No, varnish cannot be placed under composite resins and glass ionomer restorations. Dentin sealers are contraindicated.

6. **What is the other name used for dentin sealer?**
   A dentin sealer is also known as a desensitizer.

7. **What does the dentin sealer seal?**
   The dentin sealer seals dentin tubules.

8. **What does an insulating base do for a tooth?**
   An insulating base protects the pulp from thermal shock.

9. **What effect does eugenol have on the pulp?**
   Eugenol has a soothing effect on the pulp.

10. **Where is a base applied in the preparation?**
    A base is applied on the pulpal floor.

11. **What dental instrument is used to adapt a base into place?**
    A condenser is used to adapt a base into place.

12. **What is the purpose of a dental bonding material?**
    A dental bonding material bonds restorative materials to tooth structure.

13. **What is an example of enamel bonding?**
    Examples of enamel bonding include placement of sealants, orthodontic brackets, bridges, and veneers.

14. **What must be removed from the tooth structure for bonding material to reach dentin?**
    The smear layer must be removed from the tooth for bonding material to reach the dentin.

15. **Which material is applied first: the bonding or etchant material?**
    The etchant is applied first.

45 | Recall Questions and Answers

1. What is another name used for permanent cement?
Another name for permanent cement is luting agent.

2. When is temporary cement used instead of permanent cement?
Temporary cement is used for provisional coverage or for cases in which there is concern about sensitivity or other symptoms.

3. What variable affects the addition or loss of water in a dental cement?
Humidity affects the addition or loss of water in a material.

4. Can glass ionomer cements be used for restorations?
Yes, class V glass ionomer cements may be used for restorations.

5. What ingredient in the powder of glass ionomer cement helps in inhibiting recurrent decay?
Calcium helps inhibit recurrent decay.

6. Can resin cements be used under metal castings?
Yes, resin cements may be used under metal castings.

7. What is important to complete in the composite resin cementation procedure before applying the composite resin cement?
Be free of all plaque and debris prior to acid etching.

8. What type of ZOE is used for permanent cementation?
Type II ZOE is used for permanent cementation.

9. On what mixing surface is ZOE mixed?
ZOE is mixed on an oil-resistant paper pad or a glass slab.

10. How is Tempbond supplied?
Tempbond is supplied in two tubes of paste.

11. In what two forms is the polycarboxylate cement liquid supplied?
Polycarboxylate cement liquid is supplied as powder or liquid.

12. How should polycarboxylate cement appear after the mixing process?
Polycarboxylate cement should appear glossy after mixing.

13. What is the main component in the liquid form of zinc phosphate cement?
The main component of the liquid form of zinc phosphate cement is phosphoric acid.

14. How do you dissipate the heat from zinc phosphate in the mixing process?
To dissipate the heat, spatulate over a large area of a cool glass slab.

15. What size of powder increment is first brought into the liquid of zinc phosphate when mixing?
The smallest increment of powder is first brought into the liquid when mixing.

16. Do you "fill" or "line" a crown with permanent cement?
You "line" a crown with permanent cement.

Torres and Ehrlich Modern Dental Assisting, 9th ed.

Bird/Robinson

46 Recall Questions and Answers

1. Is an impression a negative or positive reproduction?
An impression is a negative reproduction.

2. Of the three classifications of impressions, which one can the expanded-functions dental assistant legally take?
The EFDA can legally take a preliminary impression.

3. Which of the three classifications of impressions is used for occlusal relationship?
The bite registration is used for occlusal relationship.

4. Which type of impression tray covers half the arch?
A quadrant tray covers half the arch.

5. Which type of tray allows impression material to lock on mechanically?
A perforated tray allows the impression material to lock on mechanically.

6. Which type of impression tray is most often used for taking final impressions?
A custom tray is most often used for taking final impressions.

7. What is used to extend the length of a tray?
Utility wax is used to extend the length of a tray.

8. What is the organic substance of hydrocolloid materials?
The organic substance of hydrocolloid is seaweed.

9. Why would you select a fast-set alginate over a normal-set alginate?
You would select a fast-set alginate if the patient had a strong gag reflex.

10. What is the water-to-powder ratio for taking a maxillary impression?
The water-to-powder ratio for taking a maxillary impression is 3 measures to 3 measures.

11. What does the prefix "hydro-" mean?
"Hydro-" means water.

12. What is another name for irreversible hydrocolloid?
Another name for irreversible hydrocolloid is alginate.

13. Do you mix irreversible hydrocolloid on a paper pad or in a mixing bowl?
Irreversible hydrocolloid is mixed in a mixing bowl.

14. Before taking an impression with reversible hydrocolloid, where is the material kept?
Before taking a reversible-hydrocolloid impression, the material is kept in a conditioning bath.

15. Is an elastomeric material used for preliminary impressions or final impressions?
Elastomeric material is used for final impressions.

16. In which three ways are elastomeric materials supplied?
Elastomeric materials are supplied as pastes, cartridges, and putties.

ELSEVIER

17. What material does the dentist first apply to the teeth, the heavy-bodied or the light-bodied form?
The dentist first applies the light-bodied material to the teeth.

18. What is another term for polysulfide?
Another term for polysulfide is rubber base.

19. How is light-bodied material placed around a prepared tooth?
A syringe is used to place light-bodied material.

20. What system completes the mixing of final impression material for you?
An automix system completes the mixing of final impressions.

21. What material is most often used for a bite registration?
Baseplate wax is most often used for a bite registration.

22. What type of tray is used when using ZOE bite registration paste?
A gauze bite tray is used for ZOE bite registration paste.

23. Do you cool or warm the wax before placing the tray in the patient's mouth for a bite registration?
You warm the wax before placement in the patient's mouth.

47 Recall Questions and Answers

1. **Where would the dental laboratory be located in a dental office?**
   The dental laboratory would be a separate space or part of the sterilization center.

2. **What specialty practices might have a more extensive laboratory setup?**
   Specialty practices such as orthodontics, pediatric dentistry, and prosthodontics might have more extensive dental laboratories.

3. **What is an example of a contaminated item in the dental laboratory?**
   An impression or dental appliance would be a contaminated item in the dental laboratory.

4. **What piece of equipment is used to grind away plaster or stone?**
   A model trimmer is used to grind away plaster and stone.

5. **What piece of equipment does the dentist use to determine centric relation on a diagnostic model?**
   An articulator is used to determine centric relation.

6. **What is the most common number of wax spatula size used in the laboratory?**
   The #7 wax spatula is used most often in the laboratory.

7. **What is another term for a dental model?**
   Another term for a dental model is a study cast.

8. **What dental materials are used to make dental models?**
   Gypsum products are used to make dental models.

9. **What are the three forms of gypsum?**
   The three forms of gypsum are plaster, stone, and high-strength stone.

10. **What is the water/powder (g/ml) ratio of plaster?**
    The water/powder ratio of plaster is 100 g of powder to 45-50 ml of water.

11. **When mixing gypsum materials, do you add the powder to the water or the water to the powder?**
    When mixing gypsum materials, you add powder to water.

12. **What are gypsum materials mixed in?**
    Gypsum materials are mixed in a specialized rubber bowl.

13. **What are the two parts of a dental model?**
    A dental model consists of the anatomic and art portions.

14. **When pouring an impression, where do you begin placing the gypsum material in the maxillary impression?**
    The gypsum material is placed beginning in the palatal area and the last tooth.

15. **How long should you wait before you separate the model from the impression?**
    You should wait 40 to 60 minutes before separating the model.

16. **Which of the two models (maxillary or mandibular) do you begin measuring and trimming first?**
    The maxillary model is measured and trimmed first.

Torres and Ehrlich Modern Dental Assisting, 9th ed.

17. What area on the maxillary and mandibular model is trimmed differently?
The anterior portion of the maxillary and mandibular model is trimmed differently.

18. What should be placed between the two models when trimming them together?
A wax bite should be placed between two models when trimming.

19. Of the three types of custom trays discussed, which technique uses a more hazardous material?
A more hazardous material is used in acrylic resin trays.

20. Which type of custom tray is made for a vital bleaching procedure?
A vacuum-formed tray is made for a bleaching procedure.

21. In which two forms is acrylic resin supplied?
Acrylic resin is supplied as a powder and liquid.

22. Which type of material is used for a vacuum-formed custom tray?
Thermoplastic resin is used for a vacuum-formed tray.

23. What is the purpose of a spacer?
A spacer is used to create room in a tray.

24. How are undercuts corrected on a model when preparing a custom tray?
Undercuts are corrected by filling in with wax or molding material.

25. What type of wax is used to form a wall around a preliminary impression when pouring it up?
Boxing wax is used to form a wall around a preliminary impression.

26. To extend an impression tray, what type of wax would you use?
Utility wax is used to extend an impression tray.

27. What type of wax would you use to obtain a patient's bite impression?
Bite registration wax is used to obtain a patient's bite.

28. What is the most common wax used to create a pattern for an indirect restoration?
Inlay casting wax is most often used to create a pattern for an indirect restoration.

ELSEVIER

Bird/Robinson

48 Recall Questions and Answers

1. What is restorative and esthetic dentistry often referred to as?
Restorative dentistry is often called operative dentistry.

2. What is a common term used to describe decay?
Cavity is another term used to describe decayed teeth.

3. Which step in the initial preparation allows the dentist to determine the shape and placement of the cavity walls?
Cavity preparation, the process of removing decay, allows the dentist to determine the shape and placement of the cavity walls.

4. What wall of a cavity preparation is perpendicular to the long axis of the tooth?
The pulpal wall is perpendicular to the long axis of the tooth.

5. Where would you find a class I restoration in the mouth?
A class I restoration can be on the occlusal surface, occlusal two thirds of the facial surface of molars, and occlusal one third of lingual surfaces.

6. How many surfaces can be involved in a class II restoration?
A class II restoration can include two or more surfaces.

7. Would a class II restoration be located in anterior or posterior teeth?
A class II restoration is found in posterior teeth.

8. What restorative material would you set up for a class IV procedure?
Composite resin is used for a class IV restoration.

9. What kind of moisture control is recommended for class III and IV restorations?
The dental dam is used for moisture control in class III and IV restorations.

10. What population has a higher incidence of class V lesions?
The older population has a higher incidence of class V lesions.

11. What are three reasons for placing an intermediate restoration?
An intermediate restoration is placed for the health of the tooth, while waiting for permanent restoration, and for financial reasons.

12. Is the placement of an intermediate restoration an expanded function of the dental assistant?
Yes, placing an intermediate restoration is an expanded function.

13. What tooth surface would most often receive a veneer?
The facial tooth surface most often receives a veneer.

14. What is the difference between a direct and indirect veneer?
A direct veneer uses composite resin, whereas an indirect veneer uses porcelain.

15. What are the three primary indications for tooth whitening?
The three primary indications for tooth whitening are extrinsic stains, aged teeth, and intrinsic stains.

16. What is used to hold whitening gel to the teeth?
A thermoplastic resin tray holds gel to the teeth.

17. What is the main ingredient of whitening strip products?
Carbamide peroxide or hydrogen peroxide is the main ingredient of whitening products.

18. What side effects may a patient experience during tooth whitening?
The patient may experience hypersensitivity and gingival irritation during tooth whitening.

49 Recall Questions and Answers

1. What classification(s) of cavity preparation would use a posterior matrix system?
A class II cavity preparation uses a posterior matrix system.

2. What is the plural of matrix?
Matrices is the plural of matrix.

3. What is used to hold a posterior matrix band in position?
A universal (Tofflemire) retainer is used to hold a posterior matrix band in position.

4. When placing a matrix band, where is the smaller circumference of the band placed?
The smaller circumference of the band is placed toward the gingiva.

5. What instrument is commonly used to contour the matrix band?
A burnisher is used to contour the matrix band.

6. What additional item is used in the matrix system to re-establish a proper contact with an adjacent tooth?
A wedge is used to re-establish contact with an adjacent tooth

7. What can result from improper wedge placement?
Overhang or cupping can result from improper wedge placement.

8. Why can't a stainless steel matrix band be used with composites?
Metal bands scratch composites and interfere with the restoring process.

9. What is another term for a clear plastic matrix?
Another term for the clear plastic matrix is celluloid matrix or Mylar strip.

10. What matrix system is an alternative to the universal retainer?
The automatrix is an alternative to the universal retainer.

11. What type of matrix system uses a spot welder to fuse the ends together?
A spot-welded band uses a spot welder to fuse the ends together.

12. What is another term for a thin polished matrix band used for posterior composites?
A palodent is a thin polished matrix band used for posterior composites.

Bird/Robinson

50 Recall Questions and Answers

1. What are the more common terms used for fixed prostheses?
Crowns and bridges are more common terms for fixed prostheses.

2. If a patient has poor dental hygiene habits, is fixed prosthodontics indicated?
No, fixed prosthodontics is not indicated for a patient with poor dental hygiene.

3. What type of indirect restoration is placed to improve the appearance of the facial surface of teeth?
A die is placed to improve the appearance of the facial surface of teeth.

4. What is the difference between an onlay and a three-quarter crown?
An onlay covers most of the occlusal and proximal surfaces; a three-quarter crown covers all but the facial or buccal surface.

5. How does a dentist convey to a laboratory technician what type of crown to make?
The dentist writes a laboratory prescription for the crown to be made.

6. What is the term for an exact replica of a tooth prepared by a laboratory technician?
A die is the exact replica of a prepared tooth.

7. What material does a laboratory technician use to create the pattern for a casting?
Wax is used to create the pattern for a casting.

8. How many appointments are required for a crown?
Two appointments are required for a crown.

9. What part of the tooth is covered by a full crown?
The anatomic portion is covered by a full crown.

10. What does the dentist use to reduce the height and contour of a tooth for a casting?
Rotary instruments are used to reduce the height and contour of a tooth.

11. If a tooth is non-vital, what is fabricated and placed into the pulp for better retention of a crown?
A post and core are placed into a non-vital tooth for better retention of a crown.

12. What is used during a crown and bridge preparation to displace gingival tissue?
Gingival retraction cord

13. What type of agent is applied to retraction cord to control bleeding?
A vasoconstrictor

14. What other terms are used for overgrown tissue?
Overgrown tissue is also called hypertrophied tissue or hyperplasia.

15. What types of impression are taken during crown preparation?
A preliminary impression and a final impression are taken during crown preparation.

16. What will the patient have on the prepared tooth while the laboratory is making a crown or bridge?
The patient has provisional coverage while the laboratory is making a crown or bridge.

17. Who in the dental office is allowed to cement a crown or bridge permanently?
Only the dentist may permanently cement a crown or bridge.

18. How many appointments are required for a fixed bridge?
Two appointments are required for a fixed bridge.

19. What accessory is used to help in flossing a bridge?
A floss threader helps in flossing a bridge.

20. How is each unit of a bridge held together?
Each unit of a bridge is soldered.

Bird/Robinson

51 Recall Questions and Answers

1. What is the term for a temporary covering for a crown or bridge?
Provisional coverage is the term for a temporary covering for a crown or bridge.

2. How long does a patient normally wear provisional coverage?
A patient usually wears provisional coverage for two weeks to one month.

3. Why is it possible for the fabrication and cementation of provisional coverage to be an expanded function?
A provisional crown or bridge is not a permanent restoration, therefore it can be legal for an assistant to perform this function.

4. What type of provisional coverage provides the most natural-looking appearance?
Custom provisional coverage provides the most natural-looking appearance.

5. What types of provisional coverage can be used for anterior teeth?
Custom and polycarbonate provisional coverage can be used for anterior teeth.

6. What is required before tooth preparation in the making of custom provisional coverage?
A preliminary impression is required before tooth preparation in the making of custom provisional coverage.

7. What type of dental material is commonly used to fabricate custom provisional coverage?
Acrylic or composite resin is commonly used to fabricate custom provisional coverage.

8. After mixing the acrylic resin, where is it placed before seating it on the prepared tooth?
The acrylic resin is placed in an alginate impression or a thermoplastic tray before seating it on the prepared tooth.

9. When would an aluminum crown be selected for use?
An aluminum crown may be selected for cost factor or time constraints.

10. Does a polycarbonate crown remain on a prepared tooth, or is it just a mold for the provisional coverage?
A polycarbonate crown can be used either way.

ELSEVIER
Bird/Robinson

52 Recall Questions and Answers

1. **What type of removable prosthesis replaces one or more teeth?**
   A partial denture is a removable prosthesis that replaces one or more teeth.

2. **How does a person's occupation affect the choice of a removable prosthesis?**
   A person's occupation may call for a change in appearance.

3. **How does the addition of a prosthesis affect the flow of saliva?**
   The presence of a new prosthesis increases salivary flow.

4. **Why is it important that the alveolar ridge be evenly contoured for a removable prosthesis?**
   The alveolar ridge must be evenly contoured to fit properly and support mastication.

5. **What oral habits can affect the choice of a removable prosthesis?**
   Oral habits that affect prosthesis choice include clenching, grinding, and mouth breathing.

6. **What is the term for the metal skeleton on a partial denture?**
   The term for the metal skeleton on a partial denture is the framework.

7. **What is the term for the retainer on a partial denture?**
   The term for the retainer on a partial denture is the clasp.

8. **What component on a partial denture controls the way it is seated in the mouth?**
   The rest controls how a partial denture is seated in the mouth.

9. **What impression material is typically used when taking a final impression for a partial denture?**
   Elastomeric impression material is typically used when taking a final impression for a partial denture.

10. **What are the artificial teeth set in during the try-in appointment?**
    During the try-in appointment, the teeth are set in wax.

11. **What is the suction seal created between the denture and the mouth?**
    The suction seal between the denture and mouth is the post dam.

12. **How many teeth are in a full set of dentures?**
    A full set of dentures has 28 teeth.

13. **What technique does the dentist use to modify the borders of an impression?**
    The dentist uses border molding to modify the borders of an impression.

14. **What is a smile line?**
    The smile line represents the amount of teeth that show when smiling.

15. **What are the four jaw positions that the dentist measures when articulating a denture?**
    When articulating a denture, the dentist measures centric relation, protrusion, retrusion, and lateral excursion.

16. **When is an immediate denture used?**
    An immediate denture is used in extraction of anterior teeth.

17. What is the normal length of time an immediate denture is worn?

An immediate denture is usually worn for a few months.

18. How is an overdenture supported in the mouth?

The bony ridge, oral mucosa, natural teeth, and implants support an overdenture in the mouth.

19. What is the term for placing a new layer of resin over the tissue surface of a prosthesis?

The term for placing new resin over a prosthesis is relining.

20. Who can repair a denture?

The dentist and laboratory technician can repair a denture.

53 Recall Questions and Answers

1. Which dental specialists have training in dental implants?
The oral and maxillofacial surgeon, periodontist, prosthodontist, and implantologist have training in implants.

2. What is the success rate for dental implants?
The success rate for dental implants is 90%.

3. How long can dental implants last?
Dental implants can last a lifetime.

4. Is the financial investment for an implant greater or less than for a fixed prosthesis?
The financial investment for an implant is greater than for a fixed prosthesis.

5. How long can an implant procedure take to complete?
An implant procedure can take nine months to complete.

6. What are the three types of extraoral radiographs used by the dentist in evaluating the dental implant patient?
The dentist uses panoramic, cephalometric, and tomographic radiographs in evaluating a potential implant patient.

7. Why would a dentist use a surgical stent during implant surgery?
The dentist uses a surgical stent as a guide for placing the implant.

8. What material is commonly used to make an implant?
Titanium is used to make an implant.

9. What does osseo mean?
Osseo means "bone."

10. What component of the endosteal implant attaches to the artificial tooth or teeth?
The abutment post or cylinder of the endosteal implant attaches to the artificial tooth or teeth.

11. When would a subperiosteal implant be recommended to a patient?
A subperiosteal implant would be recommended as a mandibular full denture.

12. Why are plaque and calculus easier to remove from an implant than from a natural tooth?
Plaque and calculus are easier to remove from an implant than a natural tooth because the implant has a smooth surface.

13. What cleaning accessories are used to clean implants?
Toothbrushes, clasp brushes, interproximal brushes, and floss are used to clean implants.

Bird/Robinson

54 Recall Questions and Answers

1. What are periradicular tissues?
Periradicular tissues surround the root of a tooth.

2. What specialist performs root canal therapy?
An endodontist performs root canal therapy.

3. What will result if bacteria reach the nerves and blood vessels of a tooth?
An abscess will result if bacteria reach nerves and blood vessels of a tooth.

4. Is pain a subjective or objective component of a diagnosis?
Pain is a subjective component of a diagnosis.

5. Tooth #21 is being tested for possible endodontic treatment. What tooth would be used as a control tooth?
Tooth #28 would be used as the control tooth if #21 is being tested.

6. When the dentist taps on a tooth, what diagnostic test is being performed?
The dentist performs percussion when tapping on a tooth.

7. How many radiographs may be taken through the course of root canal therapy?
Five radiographs may be taken during the course of root canal therapy.

8. What diagnosis is given when pulpal tissues are inflamed?
The diagnosis is pulpitis when pulpal tissues are inflamed.

9. What is another term for necrotic or necrosis?
Non-vital is another term for necrotic or necrosis.

10. What dental material is used for pulp capping?
Calcium hydroxide is used for pulp capping.

11. How much of the pulp is removed in a pulpotomy?
Only the coronal portion is removed in a pulpotomy.

12. What dental instrument has tiny projections and is used to remove pulp tissue?
A broach has tiny projections and removes pulpal tissue.

13. Can endodontic files be placed in a handpiece for use?
Yes, endodontic files can be either hand-operated or placed in a high-torque handpiece.

14. What type of file is best suited for canal enlargement?
A Hedstrom file is best suited for canal enlargement.

15. Why is a rubber stop used on a file?
A rubber stop is used on a file to prevent perforation.

16. What does obturate mean?
Obturate means "to fill."

17. Which irrigation solution is most often used during root canal therapy?
Diluted sodium hypochlorite is most often used during root canal therapy.

18. What material is used for obturation of a canal?
Gutta-percha is used for obturation of a canal.

19. What type of moisture control is recommended for root canal therapy?
A dental dam is recommended for moisture control during root canal therapy.

20. What surface of an anterior tooth does the dentist enter when performing root canal therapy?
The dentist enters the lingual surface of an anterior tooth in root canal therapy.

21. What is the success rate of root canal therapy?
Root canal therapy has a 90 to 95% success rate.

22. What surgical procedure involves the removal of the apex of a root?
Apicoectomy removes the apex of a root.

55 Recall Questions and Answers

1. How do patients most often seek periodontal care?
A general dentist most often refers patients to a periodontist.

2. What information is included in the periodontal charting?
The periodontal charting includes pocket readings, furcations, tooth mobility, exudate (pus), and gingival recession.

3. Should teeth have any mobility?
All teeth have a slight degree of mobility.

4. What is the depth of a normal sulcus?
The depth of a normal sulcus is 1 to 3 mm.

5. What units of measurement are used on the periodontal probe?
Millimeters are the units of measurement on the periodontal probe.

6. What type of radiograph is especially useful in periodontics?
Bite-wing radiographs are especially useful in periodontics.

7. What instruments are used to remove calculus from supragingival surfaces?
Scalers are used to remove calculus from supragingival surfaces.

8. What instruments are used to remove calculus from subgingival surfaces?
Curettes are used to remove calculus from subgingival surfaces.

9. What is the purpose of explorers in periodontal treatment?
Explorers provide tactile information to the operator about the roughness or smoothness of the root surfaces.

10. What is the difference between a Universal curette and a Gracey curette?
A Universal curette has two cutting edges; a Gracey curette has only one edge.

11. What is the purpose of a periodontal pocket marker?
The periodontal pocket marker is used to make bleeding points as guides for surgical incisions.

12. How do ultrasonic scalers work?
Ultrasonic scalers work by converting very-high-frequency sound waves into mechanical energy in the form of very rapid vibrations.

13. What oral conditions would contraindicate the use of an ultrasonic scaler?
Use of an ultrasonic scaler would not be indicated for patients with demineralization, narrow periodontal pockets, titanium implants, or areas of exposed dentin.

14. Should an ultrasonic scaler be used on a patient with a communicable disease?
No, an ultrasonic scaler should not be used on a patient with a known communicable disease.

15. What are the more common terms for dental prophylaxis?
Dental cleaning or prophy are more common terms for dental prophylaxis.

16. Who can legally perform a dental prophylaxis procedure?

Only a dentist or dental hygienist can legally perform a dental prophylaxis procedure.

17. What are three nonsurgical periodontal treatments?

Scaling, root planing, and gingival curettage are three nonsurgical periodontal treatments.

18. How is tetracycline used in periodontal treatment?

Tetracycline is often used for the treatment of periodontitis, juvenile periodontitis, and rapidly destructive periodontitis.

19. What is the primary goal of periodontal surgery?

The primary goal of periodontal surgery is to gain access to the root surface for scaling and root planing.

20. From a patient's point of view, what are the primary disadvantages of periodontal surgery?

Esthetics, time, discomfort, and cost are the primary disadvantages of periodontal surgery from the patient's point of view.

21. What is a gingivectomy?

A gingivectomy is a type of excisional surgery performed to remove gingival tissue.

22. What is the purpose of osseous surgery?

The purpose of osseous surgery is to remove defects and to restore normal contours in the bone.

23. What is the function of a periodontal surgical dressing?

A periodontal surgical dressing protects the surgical site similar to a bandage.

24. What are the most common materials used for periodontal dressings?

The most common materials used for periodontal dressings are zinc oxide–eugenol dressings and noneugenol dressings.

25. Are there any training requirements for persons working with lasers?

Any person who operates a laser or assists during a laser operation must be thoroughly trained in use of the laser and all necessary safety precautions.

56 Recall Questions and Answers

1. Can a general dentist perform extractions?
Yes, a general dentist can perform simple extractions.

2. How can surgical assistants further their profession?
To further their profession, surgical assistants can continue their education, clinical training, and credentialing.

3. In which two settings can a patient receive oral surgery?
A patient can receive oral surgery in a private practice and a hospital operating room.

4. Are outpatient oral and maxillofacial surgical procedures considered major or minor surgeries?
Most outpatient oral and maxillofacial surgical procedures are minor surgeries.

5. What does the periosteal elevator reflect and retract?
The periosteal elevator retracts the periosteum.

6. What number is given to the universal forceps?
Universal forceps numbers are 150/151; these forceps allow the dentist to use the same instrument on both right and left sides of an arch.

7. What surgical instrument resembles a spoon excavator?
A surgical curette resembles a spoon excavator.

8. What surgical instrument is used to trim and shape bone?
A rongeur is used to trim and shape bone.

9. What is the difference between a hemostat and a needle holder?
The needle holder has crossed grooves to hold the needle.

10. When using the chisel, what additional surgical instrument must be used?
A mallet must be set out with a chisel.

11. What equipment is used when performing a surgical scrub?
Orange stick, antimicrobial soap, scrub brush, and sterile towel are used for a surgical scrub.

12. What does the term donning mean?
Donning is the act of placing on personal protective equipment, such as sterile gloves.

13. What procedure is completed after the removal of multiple teeth in the same quadrant or arch?
Alveoplasty is done after the removal of multiple teeth in the same quadrant or arch.

14. Which type of impaction occurs when a tooth is directly under the gingival tissue?
A tooth directly under the gingival tissue creates a soft tissue impaction.

15. Which type of biopsy is done when a surface lesion is scraped to attain cells?
Exfoliative cytology involves scraping cells from a lesion.

16. To what does the term suture refer?
Suture refers to stitching.

17. What are the three types of nonabsorbable suture material?
The three types of nonabsorbable suture material are silk, polyester, and nylon.

18. What is the approximate time frame for removing nonabsorbable sutures?
Nonabsorbable sutures are removed in about five to seven days.

19. How long should a pressure pack remain on a surgical site to control bleeding?
A pressure pack should remain on a surgical site for at least 30 minutes.

20. What analgesic may be prescribed for swelling?
Ibuprofen may be prescribed for swelling.

21. Would you instruct a patient to use a hot compress or cold compress for swelling?
You should instruct a patient to use a cold compress for swelling.

57 Recall Questions and Answers

1. **Would you expect to see a 17-year-old patient in a pediatric office?**
   No, it is not common to see a 17-year-old patient in a pediatric practice unless the patient has special needs.

2. **What is unique about the treatment areas of a pediatric practice?**
   Pediatric treatment rooms use an open bay concept.

3. **What types of patients are seen in a pediatric practice?**
   Infants through adolescents, as well as patients with special needs, are seen in a pediatric practice.

4. **Is it possible for a child to be 10 years old but to act like an 8-year-old? If so, what are you describing about this patient?**
   Yes, a patient with a chronologic age of 10 years can have the emotional age of an 8-year-old.

5. **At what developmental stage do children first want control and structure of their environment?**
   Children want control and structure at ages 3 through 5 years.

6. **How would Dr. Frankl describe a "positive" child?**
   Dr. Frankl would describe a "positive" child as one who accepts treatment, is willing to comply, follows directions, and is cooperative.

7. **When would a papoose board be used?**
   A papoose board is used with young children who are sedated.

8. **What types of skills are limited in a mentally challenged child?**
   IQ and adaptive skills are limited in a mentally challenged child.

9. **What is another term for Down syndrome?**
   Trisomy 21 is another term for Down syndrome.

10. **Is it possible for a 2-year-old child to have cerebral palsy?**
    Yes, a 2-year-old child can have cerebral palsy.

11. **When should a child first see a dentist?**
    A child should first see a dentist by 2 years of age.

12. **If a patient is at high risk for decay, how often should radiographs be taken?**
    Radiographs should be taken every 6 months in a patient at high risk for tooth decay.

13. **How is fluoride varnish used?**
    Fluoride varnish is used on patients with a high risk for carries.

14. **What procedure is recommended for children to protect the pits and fissures of posterior teeth?**
    Sealants are used to protect pits and fissures of teeth.

15. **Is an appliance that is placed to stop a patient from sucking the thumb considered interceptive or preventive orthodontics?**
    Using an appliance to stop thumb sucking would be considered preventive orthodontics.

16. **If you are a competitive swimmer, should you wear a mouth guard?**
    No, swimming does not require a mouth guard.

Bird/Robinson

17. What types of matrices are used on primary teeth?
T-band and spot-welded band matrices are used on primary teeth.

18. What endodontic procedure is commonly performed on primary teeth?
Pulpotomy is performed on primary teeth.

19. Would a child be referred to a prosthodontist for the placement of a stainless steel crown?
No, a child would not be referred to a prosthodontist for a stainless steel crown.

20. Which teeth are most frequently injured in the mouth?
Maxillary central incisors are most often injured.

21. What happens when a tooth is avulsed?
A tooth comes out when avulsed.

22. How would a dentist stabilize a tooth after an injury?
The dentist uses a temporary splint to stabilize an injured tooth.

23. Are you legally required to report child abuse?
No, a dental assistant is not legally required to report child abuse.

24. Could a fractured or broken nose be a result of child abuse?
Yes, a fractured nose could result from child abuse.

25. Who in the dental office should report child abuse?
The dentist reports child abuse.

Bird/Robinson

58 Recall Questions and Answers

1. What is a coronal polish?
A coronal polish is a procedure used to remove stains and plaque.

2. What is the difference between a coronal polish and an oral prophylaxis?
An oral prophylaxis is the complete removal of calculus and debris, as well as stain.

3. What is the purpose of selective polishing?
Selective polishing means that only the teeth with visible stain are polished.

4. What is an extrinsic stain?
An extrinsic stain is one that can be removed from the surfaces of the teeth.

5. What is an intrinsic stain?
An intrinsic stain occurs within the tooth and cannot be removed by polishing or scaling.

6. Which is the most common technique for stain removal?
Rubber cup coronal polishing is the most common technique for stain removal.

7. Which type of grasp is used to hold the handpiece?
The pen grasp is used to hold the handpiece.

8. What is the purpose of a fulcrum?
The purpose of a fulcrum is to provide stability for the operator.

9. What precaution should be taken when polishing esthetic type restorations?
Only very fine abrasives, such as diamond pastes or aluminum oxide pastes, should be used to avoid scratching the porcelain.

10. In which direction should the polishing stroke move?
The polishing stroke should be overlapping strokes from the gingival third toward the incisal (or occlusal) surface of the tooth.

11. What damage can result from using the prophy cup at a high speed?
Higher speeds produce frictional heat that can damage the tooth and burn the gingiva.

12. How should the patient's head be positioned for accessing the maxillary mandibular arch?
For access to the maxillary mandibular arch, the patient's head should be positioned with the chin tipped upward.

Bird/Robinson

59 Recall Questions and Answers

1. What is the purpose of dental sealants?
The purpose of dental sealants is to prevent dental caries in the pits and fissure areas.

2. Why are pits and fissures susceptible to caries?
Pits and fissures are susceptible to caries because bacteria cannot be removed from these areas.

3. Should sealants be the only preventive measure used?
Sealants should be used as part of a comprehensive preventive program.

4. What are the two types of polymerization?
The two types of polymerization are light-cured and self-cured.

5. Why is clear sealant material less desirable?
Clear sealant material is less desirable because it is difficult to see during placement and recalls.

6. Is there a difference in retention rates between filled and unfilled sealants?
There is no difference in retention rates between filled and unfilled sealants.

7. What is the reason for putting fluoride in dental sealant material?
In case the sealant is lost, it is thought that the fluoride will have already strengthened the base of the pit or fissure.

8. What is the range of shelf-life of sealant materials?
Sealant materials have a shelf-life between 18 and 36 months.

9. What are two patient safety precautions to keep in mind when using sealants?
Keeping the etchant off the soft tissue and patient eyewear are two patient safety precautions to remember when using sealants.

10. What determines the effectiveness of dental sealants?
Retention of the dental sealant determines the effectiveness of dental sealants.

60 Recall Questions and Answers

1. **What age groups seek orthodontic care?**
   All ages seek orthodontic care.

2. **What could be a genetic cause for malocclusion?**
   A genetic cause for malocclusion could be a smaller jaw size from one parent and a larger jaw size from the other.

3. **What term is used for abnormal occlusion?**
   Malocclusion is the term used for abnormal occlusion.

4. **What tooth determines a person's occlusion?**
   The maxillary first molar determines occlusion.

5. **If a tooth is not properly aligned with its opposing tooth, it is said to be in _____.**
   A tooth not properly aligned with its opposing tooth is in crossbite.

6. **If a person occludes and you cannot see the mandibular anteriors, what is that patient's diagnosis?**
   Overbite is the diagnosis.

7. **What two positions does the orthodontist evaluate for facial symmetry?**
   Frontal view and profile view are the two positions the orthodontist evaluates for facial symmetry.

8. **What type of radiograph is most commonly taken in orthodontics?**
   The cephalometric radiograph is most often taken in orthodontics.

9. **How many photographs are taken during the records appointment?**
   A total of five photographs are taken during the records appointment.

10. **What gypsum material is most commonly used for fabricating diagnostic models in an orthodontic office?**
    Plaster is the gypsum material used most commonly for fabricating diagnostic models in an orthodontic office.

11. **What instruments are used to seat a molar band?**
    Band pluggers and bite sticks are used to seat a molar band.

12. **Is the orthodontic scaler used for removing calculus from around the fixed appliance?**
    No, an orthodontic scaler, is not used to remove calculus from around the fixed appliance.

13. **What is another name for 110 pliers?**
    Another name for 110 pliers is Howe pliers.

14. **To ease in the placement of orthodontic bands, what procedure is completed to wedge teeth apart?**
    Separators are used to wedge teeth apart.

15. **When bands are being cemented, what can be used to prevent cement from getting into the buccal tubes or attachments?**
    Chapstick or utility wax can be used to prevent cement from getting into the buccal tubes or attachments.

16. Are brackets cemented or bonded to the tooth?
Brackets are bonded to the tooth.

17. Where would most auxiliary attachments be found on braces?
Most auxiliary attachments are found on the bands of braces.

18. What type of arch wire is indicated for correcting malaligned teeth?
A round wire is indicated for correcting malaligned teeth.

19. What two ways can you measure an arch wire without placing it in a patient's mouth?
You can use a diagnostic model or the arch wire that you are replacing.

20. Besides using ligature ties, what other technique is used to hold in an arch wire?
Elastomeric ties are used to hold in an arch wire.

21. What additional appliance might the orthodontist use to control growth and tooth movement?
Headgear might be used to control growth and tooth movement.

22. How can hard foods possibly harm braces?
Hard foods can loosen bands, pull out ligature ties, or bend arch wires.

23. How can a patient make flossing easier with braces?
A floss threader can be used to make flossing easier.

24. When a patient's braces come off, does that mean treatment is over?
No, it does not mean that treatment is over.

25. Give an example of a retention appliance.
Positioner, Hawley retainer, and lingual retainer are examples of retention appliances.

61 Recall Questions and Answers

1. **What psychologist believed that human beings are intrinsically good and friendly?**
   Carl Rogers believed that human beings are intrinsically good.

2. **What is the first basic need a person requires in Maslow's hierarchy of needs?**
   Psychologic needs are first in Maslow's hierarchy.

3. **What psychological term is used to describe the process by which society influences individuals?**
   Socialization is the process by which society influences individuals.

4. **What type of communication describes our body language?**
   Body language is nonverbal communication.

5. **What percentage of spoken words do we never hear?**
   It is estimated that 90% of spoken words are never heard.

6. **Can anxiety be communicated through facial expression?**
   Anxiety may be communicated through facial expression.

7. **Give a more effective word for "pulling" a tooth.**
   Removal and extraction are better terms for "pulling" a tooth.

8. **What is the key to a successful work environment?**
   Teamwork is the key to a successful work environment.

9. **Describe stressors in a dental office.**
   Stressors in the dental office include lack of staff, overbooking, multiple tasks, poor communication, and little job advancement.

10. **How can a patient be psychologically influenced by others' attitudes?**
    Others' negative or positive experiences can psychologically influence a person's attitude.

11. **Are objective fears acquired or learned?**
    Objective fears are learned.

12. **Describe a few of the techniques that can be used to calm an irate patient?**
    Careful listening, eye contact, and head nodding can be used to calm an irate patient.

13. **What is the most important piece of equipment used for public relations?**
    The phone is the most important piece of equipment for public relations.

14. **On which ring should you answer the phone?**
    It is best to answer the phone after the first ring.

15. **When the dental office is closed, how are messages obtained?**
    When an office is closed, messages are obtained by answering service or machine.

16. **What piece of equipment allows you to transmit hard-copy written messages?**
    The fax machine transmits written messages.

Torres and Ehrlich Modern Dental Assisting, 9th ed.
Bird/Robinson

17. What part of a letter includes the salutation?

The opening or introductory greeting includes the salutation.

18. In addition to patients, to who else might you send a business letter?

You may need to send business letters to dental colleagues and insurance carriers

19. Which members of the dental office should be involved in the marketing of the practice?

The dentist, dental assistant, business assistant, and dental hygienist should all be involved in the marketing of the practice.

20. What percentage of the office's gross revenue should be invested in marketing?

Between 3 and 5% of an office's gross revenue should be invested in marketing.

21. Give an example of an external marketing activity.

Health fairs, schools, senior citizens. Participating in a health fair, or visiting a school or senior citizen group are examples of external marketing activities.

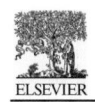

Torres and Ehrlich Modern Dental Assisting, 9th ed.

Bird/Robinson

62 Recall Questions and Answers

1. Is overseeing financial activities the responsibility of the clinical assistant or the business assistant?
Overseeing marketing activities is the responsibility of the business assistant.

2. What is the best way for a new employee to learn about office protocol?
Reading the operating procedure manual is the best way to learn about office protocol.

3. What continues to replace the "handwritten" operating procedures in the handling of business?
The computer continues to replace manual operating procedures.

4. What is another term used for a patient statement?
A ledger is another term for a patient statement.

5. How much free space should be left on each shelf of a filing cabinet?
At least four inches of free space should be left on each shelf.

6. What is used to mark a space from which a record has been taken?
An outguide is used to mark this space.

7. What is the easiest filing system to use?
Alphabetical order is the easiest filing system.

8. If a patient has not been seen within the last three years, would that patient be considered active or inactive?
This patient would be considered inactive.

9. What are the most common time lengths used for scheduling units of time in a dental practice?
Units of time are most commonly 10, 15, or 30 minutes each.

10. What four elements should be outlined in an appointment book?
Office hours, buffer time, meeting times, and holidays should be noted in an appointment book.

11. If a patient does not keep an appointment, where should this be recorded?
Missed appointments should be recorded in the patient record and on the appointment book.

12. What is the most common time period for recall?
The most common period of recall is six months.

13. If a patient was last seen in March, when would be his recall time?
A patient who was last seen in March would be recalled for September.

14. What two factors must be determined when a product needs to be reordered?
Rate of use and lead time determine when a product needs to be reordered.

15. How is an item marked for reorder?
A red flag reorder tag marks an item to be reordered.

16. Identify three ways that supplies can be ordered.
Supplies can be ordered through a sales representative, by catalog, or on the Internet.

17. If an item you ordered is not currently available from a supply company, the item is placed on _____ .

An item that is not available is placed on backorder.

18. Is a handpiece considered an expendable item? Why or why not?

No, a handpiece is not considered an expendable item, because of the cost of the item, and because, if properly cared for, it can last for years.

63 Recall Questions and Answers

1. **What two types of bookkeeping systems are used in dental practices?**
   Accounts receivable and accounts payable are two types of bookkeeping systems.

2. **What form in the patient record is used to gather financial information from a patient?**
   A registration form is used to gather financial information.

3. **Where should the business assistant discuss financial arrangements with a patient?**
   A private setting is ideal for discussing financial arrangements.

4. **Is money that is owed to the practice considered part of accounts payable?**
   No, it is considered accounts receivable.

5. **If a dental office does not have a computerized accounts receivable system, what type of system would be used?**
   A pegboard system is an alternative accounts receivable system.

6. **What form is used to transmit a patient's fee from the treatment area to the business office?**
   A charge slip is used to transmit a patient's fee.

7. **What methods of payment can a patient use to pay on an account?**
   Cash, check, credit card, and insurance are methods of payment.

8. **How often should bank deposits be made?**
   Bank deposits should be made daily.

9. **After how much time should an office begin collection efforts?**
   Collection efforts should begin after 30 days.

10. **Give four ways that a business can follow through on the collection of fees.**
    Letters, phone calls, collection agencies, and small claims court can be used to follow through on the collection of fees.

11. **Give an example of fixed overhead.**
    Mortgage, utilities, insurance, and salaries are all examples of fixed overhead.

12. **After a dental practice pays all practice-related expenses, what type of income is rendered?**
    The income represents a net income.

13. **What type of itemized listing of goods may be included in a shipment of supplies?**
    Packing slips are itemized listings of goods that may be included in a shipment.

14. **What does C.O.D. mean?**
    C.O.D. means that cash on delivery is required.

15. **Where in the checkbook do you record the checks written and deposits made on an account?**
    A check register is used to record checks issued and deposits.

16. **What term is used to indicate that an account does not have enough money in it to cover a check?**
    N.S.F (nonsufficient funds) is the term used to indicate that an account does not have enough money in it to cover a check.

ELSEVIER

Torres and Ehrlich Modern Dental Assisting, 9th ed.

Bird/Robinson

17. What are the three most commonly used methods of calculating fee-for-service benefits?
UCR (usual, customary, and reasonable) fees, schedule of benefits, and fixed fee schedule are three common methods.

18. _____ is a specified amount of money that an insured person must pay before the insurance goes into effect.
A deductible is the specified amount of money that the insured person must pay before insurance goes into effect.

19. A child or spouse of an insurance subscriber is considered to be a _____.
This person is considered a dependent.

20. Is it possible to be covered under two insurance policies?
Yes, a patient can be covered under two policies.

21. How is insurance submitted?
A claim form is used to submit insurance.

22. What category of service would include radiographs?
The category of service that includes radiographs is "diagnostic."

23. What category of service would include amalgam restorations?
The category of service that includes amalgam restorations is "restorative."

24. What category of service would include a full denture?
The category of service that includes a full denture is "prosthodontics, removable."

25. What category of service would include root planing and curettage?
The category of service that includes root planing and curettage is "periodontics."

64 Recall Questions and Answers

1. List the nine basic employment choices from which a dental assistant may choose.
Private practices, insurance, sales, research, consulting, teaching, dental school, hospital, and public health are nine employment choices.

2. Where might a dentist advertise for a job position?
A dentist might advertise in a newspaper, dental assisting program, or dental society newsletter.

3. What is the most common means of communication in your first contact made with a future employer?
The telephone is the most common means of communication.

4. What does a cover letter do?
A cover letter introduces you.

5. Should a resume list your gender, race, religion, and marital status?
No, your resume should not mention your gender, race, religion, or marital status.

6. How many pages should a resume be?
A resume should be one page long.

7. What time period is most critical in an interview?
The most critical part of an interview is the first 10 minutes.

8. What time frame is usually considered provisional employment?
The first several weeks to 90 days is usually considered provisional employment.

9. What is the term for termination without notice or severance pay?
Termination without notice or severance pay is called summary dismissal.

10. What is the most important factor in determining your professional success?
A positive attitude is the most important factor in determining your professional success.

Torres and Ehrlich Modern Dental Assisting, 9th ed.

Bird/Robinson

WORKBOOK ANSWERS

CHAPTER 1: HISTORY OF DENTISTRY

SHORT-ANSWER QUESTIONS

These questions reflect the Learning Outcomes listed at the beginning of this chapter in the textbook and can be used as class assignments. The answers can be found within the chapter and/or classroom discussion.

FILL IN THE BLANK

1. Irene Newman
2. preceptorship
3. forensic dentistry
4. periodontal disease
5. Commission on Dental Accreditation of the American Dental Association
6. Wilhelm Conrad Roentgen
7. Ida Gray-Rollins

MULTIPLE CHOICE

1. b	10. a
2. c	11. d
3. a	12. a
4. c	13. c
5. d	14. d
6. b	15. b
7. a	16. a
8. d	17. b
9. b	18. c

ACTIVITY

This activity is designed to open discussion and solicit varying opinions in the classroom. Several responses could be correct. The course director will determine whether a student's or a group's response is correct according to the factors presented and what is required.

CHAPTER 2: THE PROFESSIONAL DENTAL ASSISTANT

SHORT-ANSWER QUESTIONS

These questions reflect the Learning Outcomes listed at the beginning of this chapter in the textbook and can be used as class assignments. The answers can be found within the chapter and/or classroom discussion.

FILL IN THE BLANK

1. American Dental Assistants Association
2. Dental Assisting National Board
3. Certified Dental Assistant
4. HIPAA

Bird/Robinson

MULTIPLE CHOICE

1. d   4. b
2. d   5. d
3. d   6. b

ACTIVITIES

These activities are designed to open discussion and solicit varying opinions in the classroom. Several responses could be correct. The course director will determine whether a student's or a group's response is correct according to the factors presented and what is required.

CHAPTER 3: THE DENTAL HEALTHCARE TEAM

SHORT-ANSWER QUESTIONS

These questions reflect the Learning Outcomes listed at the beginning of this chapter in the textbook, and can be used as class assignments. The answers can be found within the chapter and/or classroom discussion.

FILL IN THE BLANK

1. dental assistant
2. periodontics
3. oral and maxillofacial radiology
4. dentist
5. dental laboratory technician
6. dental hygienist
7. dental public health
8. oral pathology
9. endodontist
10. oral and maxillofacial surgery
11. orthodontics
12. prosthodontics
13. pediatric dentistry

MULTIPLE CHOICE

1. b
2. b
3. a
4. b
5. c

CASE STUDY

This case study is designed to open discussion and to solicit varying opinions in the classroom. Several responses may be correct. The course director will determine whether a student's or a group's response is correct according to the factors presented and the course requirements.

ELSEVIER

Torres and Ehrlich Modern Dental Assisting, 9th ed.
Bird/Robinson

CHAPTER 4: DENTAL ETHICS

SHORT-ANSWER QUESTIONS

These questions reflect the Learning Outcomes listed at the beginning of this chapter in the textbook, and can be used as class assignments. The answers can be found within the chapter and/or classroom discussion.

FILL IN THE BLANK

1. laws
2. code of ethics
3. autonomy
4. ethics
5. nonmaleficence

MULTIPLE CHOICE

1. d
2. b
3. b
4. d

ACTIVITIES

These activities are designed to open discussion and to solicit varying opinions in the classroom. Several responses may be correct. The course director will determine whether a student's or a group's response is correct according to the factors presented and the course requirements.

CHAPTER 5: DENTISTRY AND THE LAW

SHORT-ANSWER QUESTIONS

These questions reflect the Learning Outcomes listed at the beginning of this chapter in the textbook, and can be used as class assignments. The answers can be found within the chapter and/or classroom discussion.

FILL IN THE BLANK

1. dental auxiliary
2. patient of record
3. direct supervision
4. expanded functions
5. respondeat superior
6. state dental practice act
7. board of dentistry
8. licensure
9. civil law
10. reciprocity
11. abandonment
12. due care
13. criminal law
14. general supervision
15. malpractice
16. implied consent
17. contract law
18. expressed contract
19. implied contract
20. written consent

Torres and Ehrlich Modern Dental Assisting, 9th ed.

Bird/Robinson

21. res gestae
22. mandated reporters
23. res ipsa loquitur

MULTIPLE CHOICE

1. b
2. d
3. c
4. b
5. a
6. c
7. c
8. b
9. d
10. d
11. b
12. d
13. b
14. a
15. c
16. c
17. a

ACTIVITIES

These activities are designed to open discussion and to solicit varying opinions in the classroom. Several responses may be correct. The course director will determine whether a student's or a group's response is correct according to the factors presented and the course requirements.

CHAPTER 6: GENERAL ANATOMY

SHORT-ANSWER QUESTIONS

These questions reflect the Learning Outcomes listed at the beginning of this chapter in the textbook, and can be used as class assignments. The answers can be found within the chapter and/or classroom discussion.

FILL IN THE BLANK

1. anatomy
2. physiology
3. anatomic position
4. midsagittal plane
5. horizontal plane
6. cytoplasm
7. organelle
8. nucleus
9. cranial cavity
10. epithelial
11. superior
12. anterior
13. medial
14. proximal
15. distal
16. superficial
17. visceral
18. parietal
19. axial
20. appendicular

ELSEVIER

Torres and Ehrlich Modern Dental Assisting, 9th ed.
Bird/Robinson

MULTIPLE CHOICE

1. b	7. b
2. a	8. d
3. c	9. d
4. b	10. d
5. d	11. d
6. c	

ACTIVITIES

These activities are designed to open discussion and to solicit varying opinions in the classroom. Several responses may be correct. The course director will determine whether a student's or a group's response is correct according to the factors presented and the course requirements.

CHAPTER 7: GENERAL PHYSIOLOGY

SHORT-ANSWER QUESTIONS

These questions reflect the Learning Outcomes listed at the beginning of this chapter in the textbook, and can be used as class assignments. The answers can be found within the chapter and/or classroom discussion.

FILL IN THE BLANK

1. axial skeleton
2. appendicular skeleton
3. periosteum
4. osteoblasts
5. Sharpey's fibers
6. compact bone
7. cancellous bone
8. cartilage
9. joints
10. articulations
11. involuntary muscles
12. muscle origin
13. muscle insertion
14. pericardium
15. arteries
16. veins
17. central nervous system
18. peripheral nervous system
19. neurons
20. peristalsis
21. integumentary system

MULTIPLE CHOICE

1. b	8. a	15. a	22. b
2. d	9. d	16. c	23. d
3. c	10. d	17. b	
4. b	11. d	18. a	
5. d	12. d	19. b	
6. e	13. d	20. d	
7. c	14. d	21. c	

ACTIVITIES

The result of this activity will vary depending on the individual.

CHAPTER 8: ORAL EMBRYOLOGY AND HISTOLOGY

SHORT-ANSWER QUESTIONS

These questions reflect the Learning Outcomes listed at the beginning of this chapter in the textbook, and can be used as class assignments. The answers can be found within the chapter and/or classroom discussion.

FILL IN THE BLANK

1. embryology
2. histology
3. prenatal development
4. embryonic period
5. conception
6. succedaneous
7. periodontium
8. ameloblasts
9. odontoblasts
10. cementoblasts
11. cementoclasts
12. osteoclasts
13. exfoliation
14. stratified squamous epithelium
15. masticatory mucosa

MULTIPLE CHOICE

1. c	14. d
2. a	15. a
3. c	16. d
4. a	17. d
5. b	18. b
6. c	19. a
7. c	20. b
8. d	21. c
9. d	22. d
10. a	23. b
11. c	24. d
12. b	25. c
13. c	

TOPICS FOR DISCUSSION

The topics presented are designed to open discussion and to solicit varying opinions and approaches to problems. The answers listed below are one set of possibilities, but several responses may be correct. The course director will determine whether a student's or a group's response is correct according to the factors presented and the course requirements

1. The first trimester is the most critical time, because during these weeks, development begins in all major structures of the body.
2. By the seventeenth week, all primary teeth are developed.
3. No, developmental disturbances can occur as a result of drug or alcohol consumption.

4. The overhanging forehead is the dominant feature of the embryo at one month after conception.

5. On average, birth occurs 38 weeks after conception.

CHAPTER 9: HEAD AND NECK ANATOMY

SHORT-ANSWER QUESTIONS

These questions reflect the Learning Outcomes listed at the beginning of this chapter in the textbook and can be used as class assignments. The answers can be found within the chapter and/or classroom discussion.

FILL IN THE BLANK

1. anterior jugular vein
2. cranium
3. greater palatine nerve
4. buccal
5. circumvallate lingual papillae
6. infraorbital region
7. lacrimal bones
8. masseter muscle
9. occipital region
10. salivary glands
11. sternocleidomastoid
12. articular space
13. abducens nerve
14. temporomandibular joint
15. temporomandibular disorder
16. trapezius
17. xerostomia
18. parotid duct

MULTIPLE CHOICE

1. c
2. b
3. c
4. b
5. d
6. c
7. c
8. b
9. d
10. c
11. a
12. c
13. d
14. c
15. b
16. d
17. a
18. c
19. a

TOPICS FOR DISCUSSION

The topics presented are designed to open discussion and to solicit varying opinions and approaches to problems. The answers listed below are one set of possibilities, but several responses may be correct. The course director will determine whether a student's or a group's response is correct according to the factors presented and the course requirements.

1. The patient's saliva can cause moisture contamination, as can water from the air-water syringe.
2. The salivary glands produce saliva.
3. Saliva is produced in the major and minor salivary glands, which are scattered in the tissues of the buccal, labial, and lingual mucosa, portions of the hard and soft palate, and under the tongue.
4. Cotton rolls, saliva ejectors, and use of a rubber dam can help control moisture.

CHAPTER 10: LANDMARKS OF THE FACE AND ORAL CAVITY

SHORT-ANSWER QUESTIONS

These questions reflect the Learning Outcomes listed at the beginning of this chapter in the textbook, and can be used as class assignments. The answers can be found within the chapter and/or classroom discussion.

FILL IN THE BLANK

1. canthus
2. ala of the nose
3. philtrum
4. tragus of the ear
5. nasion
6. glabella
7. septum
8. anterior naris
9. mental protuberance
10. vermilion border
11. commissure
12. vestibule
13. Fordyce's spots
14. labial frenum
15. gingiva

MULTIPLE CHOICE

1. c
2. b
3. a
4. d
5. b
6. d
7. c
8. a
9. b
10. c
11. b
12. c

ACTIVITIES

1. Refer to Figs. 10-1, 10-2, and 10-3 in the textbook for the features of the face.
2. Refer to Figs.10-4 through 10-12 for the major landmarks, structures, and normal tissues of the mouth.
3. 1. The vermilion border.
   2. The zygomatic arch.
   3. The eyes appear to be larger and more defined.

ELSEVIER

Torres and Ehrlich Modern Dental Assisting, 9th ed.

Bird/Robinson

CHAPTER 11: OVERVIEW OF THE DENTITIONS

SHORT-ANSWER QUESTIONS

These questions reflect the Learning Outcomes listed at the beginning of this chapter in the textbook, and can be used as class assignments. The answers can be found within the chapter and/or classroom discussion.

FILL IN THE BLANK

1. dentition
2. deciduous
3. occlusion
4. succedaneous teeth
5. anterior
6. maxilla
7. mandible
8. quadrant
9. sextant
10. mesial surface
11. distal surface
12. masticatory surface
13. interproximal space
14. embrasure
15. centric occlusion
16. functional occlusion
17. malocclusion
18. curve of Spee

MULTIPLE CHOICE

1. d	10. a
2. b	11. c
3. d	12. c
4. b	13. a
5. d	14. b
6. c	15. d
7. a	16. a
8. c	17. b
9. b	

ACTIVITIES

	Universal	Palmer Notation	ISO FDI
Maxillary right second molar	2	7⌋	17
Maxillary right first molar	3	6⌋	16
Maxillary right first premolar	5	4⌋	14

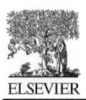

ELSEVIER

Torres and Ehrlich Modern Dental Assisting, 9th ed.

Bird/Robinson

Maxillary right canine	6	3⌋	13
Maxillary right lateral incisor	7	2⌋	12
Maxillary right central incisor	8	1⌋	11
Maxillary left central incisor	9	⌊1	21
Maxillary left canine	11	⌊3	23
Maxillary left second premolar	13	⌊5	25
Maxillary left first molar	14	⌊6	26
Maxillary left third molar	16	⌊8	28
Mandibular left second molar	18	⌈7	37
Mandibular left first molar	19	⌈6	36
Mandibular left canine	22	⌈3	33
Mandibular left lateral incisor	23	⌈2	32
Mandibular left central incisor	24	⌈1	31
Mandibular right central incisor	25	1⌉	41
Mandibular right canine	27	3⌉	43
Mandibular right second premolar	29	5⌉	45
Mandibular right second molar	31	7⌉	47

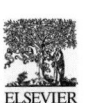
ELSEVIER

Torres and Ehrlich Modern Dental Assisting, 9th ed.
Bird/Robinson

CHAPTER 12: TOOTH MORPHOLOGY

SHORT-ANSWER QUESTIONS

These questions reflect the Learning Outcomes listed at the beginning of this chapter in the textbook, and can be used as class assignments. The answers can be found within the chapter and/or classroom discussion.

FILL IN THE BLANK

1. cusp
2. fossa
3. furcation
4. canine eminence
5. central groove
6. cingulum
7. imbrication lines
8. mamelon
9. marginal ridge
10. incisal edge
11. inclined cuspal planes
12. nonsuccedaneous
13. morphology

MULTIPLE CHOICE

1. b	11. d
2. c	12. c
3. a	13. b
4. b	14. d
5. d	15. b
6. d	16. d
7. a	17. a
8. c	18. c
9. d	19. d
10. b	20. b

ACTIVITIES

These activities are designed to open discussion and to solicit varying opinions in the classroom. Several responses may be correct. The course director will determine whether a student's or a group's response is correct according to the factors presented and the course requirements.

CHAPTER 13: DENTAL CARIES

SHORT-ANSWER QUESTIONS

These questions reflect the Learning Outcomes listed at the beginning of this chapter in the textbook, and can be used as class assignments. The answers can be found within the chapter and/or classroom discussion.

FILL IN THE BLANK

1. caries
2. demineralization
3. remineralization
4. mutans streptococci
5. lactobacillus
6. plaque

ELSEVIER

Torres and Ehrlich Modern Dental Assisting, 9th ed.

Bird/Robinson

7. cavitation
8. incipient caries
9. rampant caries
10. xerostomia
11. pellicle
12. fermentable carbohydrates

MULTIPLE CHOICE

1. b
2. c
3. a
4. c
5. a
6. c
7. d
8. d

CASE STUDY

This Case Study is designed to open discussion and to solicit varying opinions and approaches to problems. The answers listed below are one set of possibilities, but several responses may be correct. The course director will determine whether a student's or a group's response is correct according to the factors presented and the course requirements.

1. A 13-year-old should not have this many restorations.

2. Lack of home care, lack of fluoride, and a diet high in sweets could be responsible for the caries rate.

3. The chewing surface is referred to as the occlusal surface.

4. Provide fluoride treatments and dental sealants, if indicated, and teach him how to improve his diet.

5. Dietary analysis, home care instruction, and speaking with Jeremy's parents can help.

CHAPTER 14: PERIODONTAL DISEASE

SHORT-ANSWER QUESTIONS

These questions reflect the Learning Outcomes listed at the beginning of this chapter in the textbook, and can be used as class assignments. The answers can be found within the chapter and/or classroom discussion.

FILL IN THE BLANK

1. plaque
2. calculus
3. periodontium
4. periodontal diseases
5. supragingival
6. subgingival
7. gingivitis
8. periodontitis

ELSEVIER

MULTIPLE CHOICE

1. c
2. b
3. a
4. a
5. d

CASE STUDY

This Case Study is designed to open discussion and to solicit varying opinions and approaches to problems. The answers listed below are one set of possibilities, but several responses may be correct. The course director will determine whether a student's or a group's response is correct according to the factors presented and the course requirements.

1. It could be dental plaque or a variety of systemic factors.

2. Because of the orthodontic appliances, Sally may not be brushing thoroughly.

3. Notes of any changes should be made in the chart, so the dentist can evaluate whether a condition is im-proving or worsening.

4. Plaque-caused gingivitis is commonly seen in patients in orthodontic treatment. The orthodontist would make the diagnosis.

5. Assuming that gingivitis is caused by dental plaque, and that it is not a systemic disorder, Sally would benefit from some education on home care while undergoing orthodontic treatment.

CD-ROM Patient Case Exercise
1. Yes, Mrs. Van Doren's health history indicates that she has type 2 diabetes and osteoporosis.
2. Mrs. Van Doren's radiographs show generalized bone loss.

CHAPTER 15: PREVENTIVE DENTISTRY

SHORT-ANSWER QUESTIONS

These questions reflect the Learning Outcomes listed at the beginning of this chapter in the textbook, and can be used as class assignments. The answers can be found within the chapter and/or classroom discussion.

FILL IN THE BLANK

1. preventive dentistry
2. disclosing agent
3. dental sealants
4. systemic fluoride
5. topical fluoride

MULTIPLE CHOICE

1. c	11. d
2. b	12. c
3. a	13. d
4. c	14. a
5. d	15. b
6. d	16. b

ELSEVIER

7. b   17. d
8. c   18. d
9. a   19. c
10. d

TOPICS FOR DISCUSSION

These topics are designed to open discussion and to solicit varying opinions. Several responses may be correct. The course director will determine whether a student's or a group's response is correct according to the factors presented and the course requirements.

CHAPTER 16: NUTRITION

SHORT-ANSWER QUESTIONS

These questions reflect the Learning Outcomes listed at the beginning of this chapter in the textbook, and can be used as class assignments. The answers can be found within the chapter and/or classroom discussion.

FILL IN THE BLANK

1. amino acids
2. anorexia nervosa
3. bulimia
4. nutrients
5. organic

MULTIPLE CHOICE

1. d   9. c
2. c   10. b
3. b   11. c
4. d   12. b
5. c   13. d
6. b   14. b
7. a   15. a
8. a   16. a

TOPICS FOR DISCUSSION

These topics are designed to open discussion and to solicit varying opinions. Several responses may be correct. The course director will determine whether a student's or a group's response is correct according to the factors presented and the course requirements.

CHAPTER 17: ORAL PATHOLOGY

SHORT-ANSWER QUESTIONS

These questions reflect the Learning Outcomes listed at the beginning of this chapter in the textbook, and can be used as class assignments. The answers can be found within the chapter and/or classroom discussion.

FILL IN THE BLANK

1. pathology
2. lesion

3. erosion
4. cyst
5. abscess
6. hematoma
7. ecchymosis
8. granuloma
9. leukoplakia
10. lichen planus
11. candidiasis
12. cellulitis
13. glossitis
14. carcinoma
15. sarcoma
16. leukemia
17. xerostomia
18. congenital disorder
19. biopsy
20. metastasize

MULTIPLE CHOICE

1. a   14. d
2. c   15. a
3. d   16. b
4. c   17. c
5. d   18. a
6. a   19. d
7. b   20. c
8. c   21. b
9. d   22. b
10. a   23. d
11. c   24. c
12. b   25. d
13. c

CASE STUDY

This Case Study is designed to open discussion and to solicit varying opinions and approaches to problems. The answers listed below are one set of possibilities, but several responses may be correct. The course director will determine whether a student's or a group's response is correct according to the factors presented and the course requirements.

1. No, it is not from something you ate.

2. No, it is not caused by stress.

3. No, it is not harmful.

4. It is not uncommon for it to become suddenly noticeable.

CHAPTER 18: MICROBIOLOGY

SHORT-ANSWER QUESTIONS
These questions reflect the Learning Outcomes listed at the beginning of this chapter in the textbook and can be used as class assignments. The answers can be found within the chapter and/or classroom discussion.

FILL IN THE BLANK
1. microbiology
2. pathogenic
3. nonpathogenic
4. virulent
5. aerobes
6. anaerobes
7. facultative anaerobes
8. protozoa
9. provirus viruses
10. prions
11. spore
12. Creutzfeldt-Jakob disease
13. oral candidiasis
14. HBV
15. HAV
16. West Nile virus
17. H5N1

MULTIPLE CHOICE
1. b	9. b
2. c	10. d
3. b	11. d
4. c	12. b
5. b	13. d
6. d	14. c
7. a	15. a
8. c	

TOPICS FOR DISCUSSION
The topics presented are designed to open discussion and to solicit varying opinions and approaches to problems. The answers listed below are one set of possibilities, but several responses may be correct. The course director will determine whether a student's or a group's response is correct according to the factors presented and the course requirements.

1. Antibiotics cannot destroy viruses.

2. Viruses change to resist efforts to kill them.

3. It is difficult to develop a vaccine against viruses because they have the ability to change their genetic code.

4. Viruses may be transmitted through direct contact, or by inhalation of droplets spread by coughing or sneezing.

CHAPTER 19: : DISEASE TRANSMISSION AND INFECTION CONTROL

SHORT-ANSWER QUESTIONS

These questions reflect the Learning Outcomes listed at the beginning of this chapter in the textbook, and can be used as class assignments. The answers can be found within the chapter and/or classroom discussion.

FILL IN THE BLANK

1. latent infection
2. acute infection
3. chronic infection
4. OSHA Blood-borne Pathogens Standard
5. direct contact
6. indirect contact
7. droplet infection
8. percutaneous
9. permucosal
10. occupational exposure
11. standard precautions
12. personal protective equipment
13. hazardous waste
14. infectious waste
15. sharps
16. contaminated waste
17. anaphylaxis
18. communicable diseases
19. inherited immunity
20. acquired immunity
21. natural acquired immunity
22. artificially acquired immunity

MULTIPLE CHOICE

1. b	11. c
2. c	12. b
3. d	13. a
4. c	14. c
5. d	15. d
6. a	16. c
7. a	17. d
8. d	18. b
9. a	19. d
10. b	20. c

CASE STUDY

This Case Study is designed to open discussion and to solicit varying opinions and approaches to problems. The answers listed below are one set of possibilities, but several responses may be correct. The course director will determine whether a student's or a group's response is correct according to the factors presented and the course requirements.

1. Knowledge about disease transmission has increased over the years, and we now recognize hazards we did not recognize before.

Torres and Ehrlich Modern Dental Assisting, 9th ed.

Bird/Robinson

2. Dentistry has made every effort to keep abreast of scientific changes to keep dental patients and dental team members safe and healthy.

3. When working in the laboratory, you should wear utility gloves, a gown, protective eyewear, and a mask.

4. Protective clothing, mask, eyewear, and utility (chemical resistant) gloves should be worn.

5. The dentist should explain to Sheila why infection control is important both for her safety and for the safety of her teammates and patients.

CHAPTER 20: PRINCIPLES AND TECHNIQUES OF DISINFECTION

SHORT-ANSWER QUESTIONS

These questions reflect the Learning Outcomes listed at the beginning of this chapter in the textbook and can be used as class assignments. The answers can be found within the chapter and/or classroom discussion.

FILL IN THE BLANK

1. surface barrier
2. transfer surfaces
3. splash, spatter, and droplet surfaces
4. precleaning
5. disinfectant
6. residual activity
7. bioburden
8. tuberculocidal
9. broad-spectrum
10. iodophor
11. synthetic phenol compound
12. glutaraldehyde
13. chlorine dioxide
14. intermediate-level disinfectant
15. low-level disinfectant

MULTIPLE CHOICE

1. b   9. d
2. d   10. a
3. a   11. c
4. d   12. b
5. a   13. d
6. a   14. a
7. b   15. d
8. c

TOPICS FOR DISCUSSION

The topics presented are designed to open discussion and to solicit varying opinions and approaches to problems. The answers listed below are one set of possibilities, but several responses may be correct. The course director will determine whether a student's or a group's response is correct according to the factors presented and the course requirements.

Torres and Ehrlich Modern Dental Assisting, 9th ed.

Bird/Robinson

1. You should never get in the habit of cutting corners to save time.

2. Barriers can be changed more quickly. Remember that if the barrier is torn or dislodged, the undersurface must still be disinfected.

3. All surface barriers, the saliva ejector, and the air-water syringe tip will have to be replaced for the next patient on the dental-assisting unit.

4. All surface barriers, the dental handpiece, the air-water syringe tip, the patient's protective eyewear, and the evacuator tip will have to be replaced for the next patient on the dental unit.

5. The mask and gloves will have to be replaced. The gown need not be changed unless it is visibly soiled. The protective eyewear should be cleaned and disinfected between uses.

CHAPTER 21: PRINCIPLES AND TECHNIQUES OF STERILIZATION

SHORT-ANSWER QUESTIONS

These questions reflect the Learning Outcomes listed at the beginning of this chapter in the textbook, and can be used as class assignments. The answers can be found within the chapter and/or classroom discussion.

FILL IN THE BLANK

1. sterilization
2. sterilant
3. autoclave
4. biologic indicators
5. chemical vapor sterilizer
6. critical instrument
7. semicritical instruments
8. noncritical instruments
9. clean area
10. contaminated area
11. dry-heat sterilizer
12. use-life
13. biologic monitor
14. single-parameter indicator
15. endospore
16. ultrasonic cleaner
17. multiparameter indicator

MULTIPLE CHOICE

1. d	13. b
2. a	14. a
3. c	15. b
4. d	16. c
5. d	17. d
6. a	18. d
7. b	19. b
8. c	20. c
9. b	21. a
10. a	22. c
11. d	23. b
12. d	24. d

ELSEVIER

Bird/Robinson

TOPICS FOR DISCUSSION
The topics presented are designed to open discussion and to solicit varying opinions and approaches to problems. The answers listed below are one set of possibilities, but several responses may be correct. The course director will determine whether a student's or a group's response is correct according to the factors presented and the course requirements.

1. The addition of a sterilization assistant would be very helpful in such a busy practice.

2. Be certain that you have not overloaded the ultrasonic cleaner. If it is overloaded, the instruments will not be properly cleaned.

3. Placing the instruments in a holding solution would be helpful to prevent the debris from drying.

4. Perhaps the receptionist or the hygienist could lend a hand if his or her schedule permits. Remember that dentistry is a team effort.

5. Yes, you should discuss this with the dentist.

CHAPTER 22: REGULATORY AND ADVISORY AGENCIES

SHORT-ANSWER QUESTIONS
These questions reflect the Learning Outcomes listed at the beginning of this chapter in the textbook and can be used as class assignments. The answers can be found within the chapter and/or classroom discussion

FILL IN THE BLANK
1. FDA
2. CDC
3. ADA
4. OSHA
5. OSAP
6. NIOSH
7. EPA

MULTIPLE CHOICE
1. a
2. c
3. d
4. b

TOPICS FOR DISCUSSION
The topics presented are designed to open discussion and to solicit varying opinions and approaches to problems. The answers listed below are one set of possibilities, but several responses may be correct. The course director will determine whether a student's or a group's response is correct according to the factors presented and the course requirements.

1. You can check on the OSHA Web site, contact the local dental society, and contact OSAP.

2. You can check the CDC, OSAP, EPA, OSHA, and FDA Web sites.

CHAPTER 23: CHEMICAL AND WASTE MANAGEMENT

SHORT-ANSWER QUESTIONS
These questions reflect the Learning Outcomes listed at the beginning of this chapter in the textbook and can be used as class assignments. The answers can be found within the chapter and/or classroom discussion.

ELSEVIER

FILL IN THE BLANK
1. Hazard Communication Standard
2. material safety data sheet (MSDS)
3. chronic exposure
4. acute
5. hazardous waste
6. chemical inventory
7. Environmental Protection Agency
8. contaminated waste
9. infectious waste
10. regulated waste
11. toxic waste

MULTIPLE CHOICE
1. c	9. b
2. d	10. c
3. a	11. b
4. c	12. d
5. b	13. d
6. c	14. b
7. a	15. b
8. d	

CASE STUDY
This case study is designed to open discussion and to solicit varying opinions in the classroom. Several responses may be correct. The course director will determine whether a student's or a group's response is correct according to the factors presented and the course requirements.

1. Pamela will need to label all containers of chemicals that do not have a manufacturer's label and are not going to be used immediately.

2. 3

3. 4

4. 4

5. Pamela can obtain material safety data sheets from the manufacturer of the other products in the office.

CHAPTER 24: DENTAL UNIT WATERLINES

SHORT-ANSWER QUESTIONS
These questions reflect the Learning Outcomes listed at the beginning of this chapter in the textbook, and can be used as class assignments. The answers can be found within the chapter and/or classroom discussion.

FILL IN THE BLANK
1. biofilm
2. Legionella
3. microfiltration
4. colony-forming units
5. dental unit waterlines
6. self-contained water reservoir
7. retraction
8. planktonic bacteria

Torres and Ehrlich Modern Dental Assisting, 9th ed.

Bird/Robinson

MULTIPLE CHOICE

1. b	9. a
2. d	10. b
3. c	11. c
4. b	12. b
5. d	13. d
6. b	14. b
7. b	15. d
8. b	

CASE STUDY

This case study is designed to open discussion and to solicit varying opinions in the classroom. Several responses may be correct. The course director will determine whether a student's or a group's response is correct according to the factors presented and the course requirements.

1. No, HIV is not transmitted from dental unit water.

2. Describe your waterline protocol (e.g., filters, flushing, chemicals).

3. The practice uses sterile water for surgery.

4. Yes, it is safe to have dental treatment that requires water.

CHAPTER 25: ERGONOMICS

SHORT-ANSWER QUESTIONS

These questions reflect the Learning Outcomes listed at the beginning of this chapter in the textbook and can be used as class assignments. The answers can be found within the chapter and/or classroom discussion.

FILL IN THE BLANK

1. ergonomics
2. cumulative trauma disorders
3. musculoskeletal disorders
4. normal horizontal reach
5. maximum vertical reach
6. maximum horizontal reach
7. strains
8. sprains
9. thenar eminence
10. carpal tunnel syndrome
11. neutral position

MULTIPLE CHOICE

1. b	6. b
2. d	7. c
3. a	8. b
4. c	9. d
5. d	10. c

Torres and Ehrlich Modern Dental Assisting, 9th ed.
Bird/Robinson

TOPICS FOR DISCUSSION

The topics presented are designed to open discussion and to solicit varying opinions and approaches to problems. The answers listed below are one set of possibilities, but several responses may be correct. The course director will determine whether a student's or a group's response is correct according to the factors presented and the course requirements.

1. Sleeping in an awkward position may have caused your stiff neck, but you should consider other causes as well.

2. Sitting at chairside for several hours, in positions that may have been awkward, could have caused your pain.

3. To prevent the pain from getting worse, you can do some muscle-strengthening exercises and take rest periods between lengthy procedures.

4. You can have a meeting to discuss the problem, and suggest to the person who schedules patients that long appointments could be separated by shorter ones, or that assistants assigned to help on each procedure could be staggered. This will give each assistant an opportunity to move around and loosen the shoulder muscles.

5. To loosen your neck and shoulders, you can do head rotations, full back releases, and shoulder shrugs.

CHAPTER 26: THE PATIENT RECORD

SHORT-ANSWER QUESTIONS

These questions reflect the Learning Outcomes listed at the beginning of this chapter in the textbook, and can be used as class assignments. The answers can be found within the chapter and/or classroom discussion.

FILL IN THE BLANK

1. litigation
2. assessment
3. chronic
4. chronologic
5. demographics
6. alert
7. registration
8. forensics

MULTIPLE CHOICE

1. b	6. a
2. a	7. b
3. b	8. b
4. c	9. c
5. d	10. d

CASE STUDY

This case study is designed to open discussion and to solicit varying opinions in the classroom. Several responses may be correct. The course director will determine whether a student's or a group's response is correct according to the factors presented and the course requirements.

1. The patient registration form and the medical-dental health history form are completed in the reception area.

2. By reviewing the medical history, interviewing the patient, asking to see the medication, and having the dentist call the patient's doctor to learn more about the patient's health status

3. Yes, Ms. Stewart is allergic to several antibiotics. The names and allergy alerts should be noted on the inside cover of the patient record.

4. Charting should be completed on the clinical examination form.

5. Date: new patient visit, reviewed medical/dental history with patient. Vital signs: BP- Resp-Temp-Pulse. Extraoral/Intraoral exam. Schedule patient to return for prophylaxis and radiographs. Dental Assistant Initials/Dentist Initials.

CHAPTER 27: VITAL SIGNS

SHORT-ANSWER QUESTIONS
These questions reflect the Learning Outcomes listed at the beginning of this chapter in the textbook, and can be used as class assignments. The answers can be found within the chapter and/or classroom discussion.

FILL IN THE BLANK
1. diastolic
2. electrocardiogram
3. metabolism
4. arrhythmia
5. antecubital space
6. pulse
7. radial
8. respiration
9. sphygmomanometer
10. stethoscope
11. temperature
12. thermometer
13. rhythm
14. tympanic
15. volume

MULTIPLE CHOICE
1. d   9. c
2. b   10. b
3. c   11. d
4. d   12. b
5. d   13. a
6. b   14. c
7. c   15. c
8. b

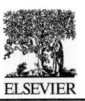
ELSEVIER

CASE STUDY

This case study is designed to open discussion and to solicit varying opinions in the classroom. Several responses may be correct. The course director will determine whether a student's or a group's response is correct according to the factors presented and the course requirements.

1. A dental prophylaxis is a procedure that is commonly performed by the dental hygienist. The procedure includes the complete removal of calculus, debris, stains, and plaque from the teeth.

2. A patient should be seated comfortably in an upright position when taking vital signs.

3. Besides noting a respiration rate, you should indicate the patient's breathing rhythm (breathing pattern) and depth (amount of air inhaled and exhaled during a breath).

4. The patient's blood pressure is high (systolic reading at stage 1 hypertension, and diastolic reading at stage 2 hypertension).

5. Allow the patient to rest for 10 minutes, and then retake the blood pressure. If the reading is still high, consult with the dentist before the procedure is begun.

CHAPTER 28: ORAL DIAGNOSIS AND TREATMENT PLANNING

SHORT-ANSWER QUESTIONS

These questions reflect the Learning Outcomes listed at the beginning of this chapter in the textbook, and can be used as class assignments. The answers can be found within the chapter and/or classroom discussion.

FILL IN THE BLANK

1. restoration
2. detection
3. furcation
4. mobility
5. morphology
6. palpation
7. extraoral
8. probing
9. recession
10. mucogingival
11. symmetric
12. intraoral

MULTIPLE CHOICE

1. b	9. d
2. d	10. d
3. c	11. d
4. d	12. d
5. a	13. a
6. d	14. b
7. d	15. c
8. b	

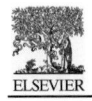

Torres and Ehrlich Modern Dental Assisting, 9th ed.

CHARTING

Descriptions of Charting Symbols

#1 Red circle around tooth

#2 Distal and occlusal surface outlined in blue/black and colored in

#3 Mesial, occlusal, and distal surfaces outlined in blue/black and colored in

#4 Coronal portion of tooth outlined in blue/black

#5 Coronal portions of teeth outlined in blue/black with diagonal lines. Tooth #6 root contains X and the three teeth with a line connecting each tooth.

#8 Coronal portions of teeth outlined in blue/black and a blue/black line down center of root

#9 Coronal portions of teeth outlined in blue/black and a blue/black line down center of root

#10 Small moon-shaped outline in blue/black on the gingival third

#11 Small moon shaped outline in red on the gingival third

#12 Mesial and occlusal surfaces outlined in blue/black

#13 Small red circle at tip of root

#14 Small blue/black dot on lingual pit and the abbreviation S in blue/black on the occlusal surface

#15 The abbreviation S in blue/black on the occlusal surface

#16 Red circle around tooth

#17 Red circle around tooth

#18-21 Coronal portions of teeth outlined in blue/black with diagonal lines. Roots of #19 and #20 contain an X, and a line connects the four teeth. #18 has a blue/black line down the center of the roots.

#24 Small half-moon shape outlined in blue/black on mesial surface

#25 Small half-moon shape outlined in blue/black on mesial surface

#26 Red zigzag line crossing over the mesial/incisal surface

#28 Mesial and occlusal surface outlined in blue/black and colored in

#29 Blue/black X through tooth and root

#30 Mesial, occlusal, distal surfaces outlined in red and colored in

#31 Occlusal pit colored in blue/black with a red line on outside

#32 Red circle around tooth

1. 6, 19, and 20
2. One to two appointments
3. Where tooth number 29 is missing
4. Esthetic reason. They may be visible when the patient smiles.
5. 1, 16, 17, and 32

CHAPTER 29: THE MEDICALLY AND PHYSICALLY COMPROMISED PATIENT

SHORT-ANSWER QUESTIONS

These questions reflect the Learning Outcomes listed at the beginning of this chapter in the textbook, and can be used as class assignments. The answers can be found within the chapter and/or classroom discussion.

FILL IN THE BLANK

1. anemia
2. atrophy
3. seizure
4. bacteremia

Torres and Ehrlich Modern Dental Assisting, 9th ed.

Bird/Robinson

5. xerostomia
6. angina
7. epilepsy
8. aging
9. Alzheimer's
10. hemophilia
11. hyperplasia
12. bronchitis
13. hyperthyroidism
14. leukemia
15. myocardial infarction
16. arthritis
17. asthma
18. hypothyroidism
19. stroke
20. diabetes

MULTIPLE CHOICE

1. d	9. c
2. c	10. b
3. d	11. a
4. d	12. c
5. b	13. d
6. a	14. b
7. b	15. d
8. d	

CASE STUDY

This case study is designed to open discussion and to solicit varying opinions in the classroom. Several responses may be correct. The course director will determine whether a student's or a group's response is correct according to the factors presented and the course requirements.

1. With multiple sclerosis, the time of day does not affect the patient's energy level. However, because Josh is wheelchair bound, it may take him longer in the morning to get ready for the appointment.

2. Josh may be taking adrenal suppressants such as prednisone, and muscle relaxants, such as diazepam, to help control muscle spasms during the appointment.

3. Josh would be transferred to the patient dental chair for the appointment.

4. When you are moving a patient from a wheelchair to a dental chair, clear all items from the pathway, position the patient the same way he or she would be seated, move the wheelchair as close to the dental chair as possible, lock the wheelchair, and raise the footrests.

5. To protect yourself from injury, have the patient remain on the edge of the chair before lifting, use your legs (not your back) to lift, pivot the patient's body to keep weight distributed, and lower the patient slowly to the chair.

CHAPTER 30: PRINCIPLES OF PHARMACOLOGY

SHORT-ANSWER QUESTIONS

These questions reflect the Learning Outcomes listed at the beginning of this chapter in the textbook, and can be used as class assignments. The answers can be found within the chapter and/or classroom discussion.

Torres and Ehrlich Modern Dental Assisting, 9th ed.

Bird/Robinson

FILL IN THE BLANK
1. excretion
2. absorption
3. superscription
4. systemic
5. dose
6. drug
7. distribution
8. signature
9. dosage
10. patent
11. pharmacology
12. prescription
13. antibiotic prophylaxis
14. subscription
15. generic

MULTIPLE CHOICE
1. d	8. d
2. b	9. c
3. c	10. a
4. d	11. d
5. d	12. c
6. b	13. c
7. c	14. c

CASE STUDY
This case study is designed to open discussion and to solicit varying opinions in the classroom. Several responses may be correct. The course director will determine whether a student's or a group's response is correct according to the factors presented and the course requirements.

1. An alert sticker provides immediate information on health conditions, allergies, and medications that must be taken.

2. Yes, because Mr. Miller has been diagnosed with mitral valve prolapse, it is important to ask the physician whether there have been any changes to his condition.

3. Mr. Miller is having a gingivectomy on the lower right quadrant.

4. No, the gingivectomy procedure is not considered a high-risk procedure for a patient with this medical condition.

5. It is necessary to know that Mr. Miller is allergic to penicillin so that this type of antibiotic is not prescribed for this patient.

6. No, the AHA and the ADA recommend that no antibiotic be prescribed before this appointment.

CHAPTER 31: ASSISTING IN A MEDICAL EMERGENCY

SHORT-ANSWER QUESTIONS
These questions reflect the Learning Outcomes listed at the beginning of this chapter in the textbook, and can be used as class assignments. The answers can be found within the chapter and/or classroom discussion.

FILL IN THE BLANK
1. convulsion
2. erythema
3. cardiopulmonary resuscitation
4. acute
5. allergy
6. allergen
7. syncope
8. gait
9. asthma
10. anaphylaxis
11. antibodies
12. antigen
13. aspiration
14. hypoglycemia
15. hypotension
16. myocardial infarction
17. hyperglycemia
18. hyperventilating

MULTIPLE CHOICE
1. b	11. b
2. c	12. d
3. d	13. b
4. b	14. c
5. a	15. b
6. b	16. a
7. c	17. c
8. c	18. b
9. d	19. d
10. a	20. b

CASE STUDY
This case study is designed to open discussion and to solicit varying opinions in the classroom. Several responses may be correct. The course director will determine whether a student's or a group's response is correct according to the factors presented and the course requirements.

1. Because Renee is in her third trimester, her pregnancy should not pose any problems for dental treatment. However, it is important to get approval from the patient's obstetrician before providing dental treatment.

2. Renee may feel faint as a result of pressure of the enlarged uterus on the abdominal veins, causing a lack of blood flow to the brain.

3. Renee is experiencing postural hypotension.

4. To respond to this emergency, turn the patient on her left side, or move her into an upright sitting position. The change of position should relieve the pressure on the involved blood vessels.

5. No drugs are indicated, but have the oxygen nearby.

Torres and Ehrlich Modern Dental Assisting, 9th ed.

Bird/Robinson

6. To prevent this emergency, keep appointments short for patients who are pregnant, and position the patient in a more upright position.

CHAPTER 32: THE DENTAL OFFICE

SHORT-ANSWER QUESTIONS

These questions reflect the Learning Outcomes listed at the beginning of this chapter in the textbook, and can be used as class assignments. The answers can be found within the chapter and/or classroom discussion.

FILL IN THE BLANK

1. subsupine
2. triturate
3. consultation
4. condensation
5. upright
6. dental operatory
7. rheostat
8. supine

MULTIPLE CHOICE

1. b	6. c
2. c	7. d
3. d	8. c
4. c	9. a
5. b	10. b

CASE STUDY

This Case Study is designed to open discussion and to solicit varying opinions and approaches to problems. The answers listed below are one set of possibilities, but several responses may be correct. The course director will determine whether a student's or a group's response is correct according to the factors presented and the course requirements.

1. When a new employee begins, a designated employee will review the office procedure manual, which will describe the areas of the office, how to operate and care for clinical equipment, and specific routines that are followed for clinical procedures.

2. In an office with four treatment areas, one is designated as an oral hygiene room, two for operative dentistry, and the fourth as a spillover for patient care. Each room should be designed for the dental team's comfort and mobility, and for the patient's privacy and comfort. Also, materials and instruments should be set up the same way in each room for easy access.

3. Personal items that may be added to a dental treatment area are certificates or diplomas from school and professional associations, a plant set at a distance from the dental treatment chair, a bird feeder or birdbath outside the window, hanging mobiles, or a poster on the ceiling to add visual enhancement for patients.

4. Always be open to a new employee with new ideas, but be sure that the dentist is involved, so as to ensure that everyone agrees with the changes, and that the changes are entered into the office procedure manual.

ELSEVIER

Torres and Ehrlich Modern Dental Assisting, 9th ed.
Bird/Robinson

CHAPTER 33: DELIVERING DENTAL CARE

SHORT-ANSWER QUESTIONS
These questions reflect the Learning Outcomes listed at the beginning of this chapter in the textbook, and can be used as class assignments. The answers can be found within the chapter and/or classroom discussion.

FILL IN THE BLANK
1. direct supervision
2. operating zones
3. indirect vision
4. expanded function
5. fulcrum
6. four-handed dentistry
7. grasp
8. indirect supervision
9. delegate

MULTIPLE CHOICE
1. d	9. d
2. a	10. c
3. c	11. d
4. c	12. b
5. b	14. d
7. b	15. c
8. a	

TOPICS FOR DISCUSSION
The topics presented are designed to open discussion and to solicit varying opinions and approaches to problems. The answers listed below are one set of possibilities, but several responses may be correct. The course director will determine whether a student's or a group's response is correct according to the factors presented and the course requirements.

1. Contact the state board of dental examiners in your state to find out what legal functions can be delegated to the certified dental assistant.

2. To become more proficient in expanded functions, you should understand dental anatomy, learn operator positioning, develop mirror skills, learn to use a fulcrum, understand cavity preparations, learn how to adapt instruments to areas of teeth, and learn to apply dental materials correctly.

3. Attain knowledge and skills by taking courses and by having open communication with the dentist that employs you, in order to maintain a competent level of performance.

4. Contact an accredited dental-assisting program and the Dental Assisting National Board to find out new procedures for the expanded-functions dental assistant, and take an approved course.

5. Depending on the "manpower" for the state in which you practice, preventive and restorative procedures may be performed by the expanded-functions dental assistant.

LABELING
12 o'clock to 2 o'clock	Static zone
2 o'clock to 4 o'clock	Assistant's zone
4 o'clock to 7 o'clock	Transfer zone
7 o'clock to 12 o'clock	Operator's zone

Torres and Ehrlich Modern Dental Assisting, 9th ed.
Bird/Robinson

CHAPTER 34: DENTAL HAND INSTRUMENTS

SHORT-ANSWER QUESTIONS

These questions reflect the Learning Outcomes listed at the beginning of this chapter in the textbook, and can be used as class assignments. The answers can be found within the chapter and/or classroom discussion

FILL IN THE BLANK

1. tactile
2. working end
3. handle
4. beveled
5. blade
6. nib
7. serrated
8. plane
9. shank
10. point

MULTIPLE CHOICE

1. c	9. d
2. b	10. c
3. b	11. a
4. c	12. c
5. d	13. b
6. b	14. d
7. d	15. c
8. b	

ACTIVITY

Tray setup for class II amalgam setup (left to right):

1. Mirror (for indirect vision, light reflection, retraction, tissue protection)
2. Explorer (to detect calculus and decay)
3. Cotton pliers (to carry, place, and retrieve small objects from the mouth)
4. Periodontal probe (to measure the sulcus or pocket depth of the periodontium)
5. Spoon excavator (to remove soft dentin, debris, and decay from the preparation)
6. Hoe (to prepare and plane walls and floors of the preparation)
7. Hatchet (to cut enamel and to smooth walls and floors of the preparation)
8. Chisel (to cut the enamel margin of the tooth preparation, form sharp lines and point angles, and place retention grooves)
9. Gingival margin trimmer (to cut enamel and place bevels along the gingival margins of the preparation)
10. Amalgam carrier (to carry mixed amalgam to the prepared tooth)
11. Condenser (to condense the placed amalgam into the preparation)
12. Burnisher (to smooth the surface of the freshly placed amalgam restoration)
13. Discoid/cleoid carvers (to carve the amalgam on occlusal surfaces)
14. Hollenback carver (to carve the amalgam on interproximal surfaces)
15. Amalgam knife (to remove excess restorative material along the margins)
16. Articulating paper holder/paper (to carry the paper to the mouth/to check the patient's bite)

Torres and Ehrlich Modern Dental Assisting, 9th ed.
Bird/Robinson

CHAPTER 35: DENTAL HANDPIECES AND ACCESSORIES

SHORT-ANSWER QUESTIONS

These questions reflect the Learning Outcomes listed at the beginning of this chapter in the textbook, and can be used as class assignments. The answers can be found within the chapter and/or classroom discussion.

FILL IN THE BLANK

1. friction grip
2. laser
3. rotary
4. flutes
5. console
6. tungsten carbide
7. shank
8. latch-type
9. fiberoptic
10. ultrasonic
11. torque
12. mandrel

MULTIPLE CHOICE

1. c	6. c	11. b
2. a	7. a	12. c
3. c	8. c	13. a
4. b	9. c	14. d
5. b	10. d	15. c

TOPICS FOR DISCUSSION

The topics presented are designed to open discussion and to solicit varying opinions and approaches to problems. The answers listed below are one set of possibilities, but several responses may be correct. The course director will determine whether a student's or a group's response is correct according to the factors presented and the course requirements.

1. On a high-speed handpiece, there are two portal entries (air/water). On a low-speed handpiece, there is only one (air).

2. You attach the contra-angle attachment to the low-speed handpiece.

3. You attach the #169L bur to the high-speed handpiece.

4. You attach the #4 round bur to the low-speed handpiece.

5. To prepare for the next procedure, you must wear PPE, remove handpieces from the hoses, remove burs from the handpieces, and follow the manufacturers' directions regarding how to clean debris from handpieces, clean internal components, dry and wrap, sterilize, and lubricate.

CHAPTER 36: MOISTURE CONTROL

SHORT-ANSWER QUESTIONS

These questions reflect the Learning Outcomes listed at the beginning of this chapter in the textbook, and can be used as class assignments. The answers can be found within the chapter and/or classroom discussion.

ELSEVIER

Torres and Ehrlich Modern Dental Assisting, 9th ed.

Bird/Robinson

FILL IN THE BLANK
1. bow
2. beveled
3. inverted
4. jaw
5. stylus
6. universal
7. malaligned
8. septum
9. exposed
10. aspirate

MULTIPLE CHOICE

1. b		11. d	
2. c		12. c	
3. d		13. d	
4. a		14. c	
5. b		15. a	
6. a		16. b	
7. c		17. b	
8. b		18. d	
9. a		19. d	
10. c		20. a	

TOPICS FOR DISCUSSION

The topics presented are designed to open discussion and to solicit varying opinions and approaches to problems. The answers listed below are one set of possibilities, but several responses may be correct. The course director will determine whether a student's or a group's response is correct according to the factors presented and the course requirements.

1. A saliva ejector or HVE tip can be used to rinse the patient's mouth after anesthesia.

2. Dental dam application takes place after the administration of anesthesia and after shade selection is completed.

3. The dental dam will be punched from canine to canine (tooth #6 to tooth #11). The hole sizes are #2.

4. Commonly, there would not be a clamp used for a class III restoration in the anterior application, but dental tape or a small cut of dam can be wedged interproximally between the canine and the first premolar on each side to secure it in place.

5. The dental dam will be removed once the restoration is completed, but before the patient's occlusion is checked, if needed.

ACTIVITY

The teeth to be exposed on the dental dam would include the following:

#22, hole size 2

#23, hole size 1

#24, hole size 1

#25, hole size 1

#26, hole size 1

#27, hole size 2

#28, hole size 3

#29, hole size 3

#30, hole size 5

CHAPTER 37: ANESTHESIA AND PAIN CONTROL

SHORT-ANSWER QUESTIONS

These questions reflect the Learning Outcomes listed at the beginning of this chapter in the textbook, and can be used as class assignments. The answers can be found within the chapter and/or classroom discussion.

FILL IN THE BLANK

1. anesthetic
2. oximetry
3. duration
4. gauge
5. tidal volume
6. anesthesia
7. vasoconstrictor
8. permeate
9. titration
10. porous
11. innervation
12. lumen
13. induction
14. analgesia

MULTIPLE CHOICE

1. c	11. b
2. b	12. a
3. c	13. c
4. d	14. c
5. b	15. d
6. d	16. b
7. a	17. c
8. c	18. a
9. b	19. c
10. d	20. b

CASE STUDY

This Case Study is designed to open discussion and to solicit varying opinions and approaches to problems. The answers listed below are one set of possibilities, but several responses may be correct. The course director will determine whether a student's or a group's response is correct according to the factors presented and the course requirements.

1. Topical anesthesia, local anesthesia, and N_2O/O_2 sedation most likely will be provided for Ms. Smith.

2. A history of a heart condition is a contraindication to the vasoconstrictor in a local anesthetic. The local anesthetic would be administered without a vasoconstrictor. The contraindications for N_2O/O_2 sedation are pregnancy, nasal obstruction, emphysema, multiple sclerosis, and emotional instability.

3. You would find these contraindications by viewing the patient's health history and asking specific questions.

Bird/Robinson

4. N_2O/O_2 sedation would be administered first, then topical anesthesia, and then local anesthesia.

5. You would need gauze, topical anesthetic ointment, a cotton-tipped applicator, a sterile syringe, a sealed disposable needle, a sterile local anesthetic cartridge, a sterile scavenger-type mask, and equipment for measuring vital signs.

CHAPTER 38: FOUNDATIONS OF RADIOGRAPHY, RADIOGRAPHIC EQUIPMENT, AND RADIOLOGIC SAFETY

SHORT-ANSWER QUESTIONS
These questions reflect the Learning Outcomes listed at the beginning of this chapter in the textbook, and can be used as class assignments. The answers can be found within the chapter and/or classroom discussion.

FILL IN THE BLANK
1. radiation
2. x-radiation
3. x-ray
4. radiology
5. radiograph
6. dental radiography
7. ionizing radiation
8. anode
9. cathode
10. primary beam
11. ion
12. peak kilovoltage
13. milliampere
14. electrons
15. tungsten target
16. contrast
17. density
18. dose
19. genetic effects
20. somatic effects
21. latent period
22. ALARA
23. photon
24. matter
25. energy
26. penumbra

MULTIPLE CHOICE
1. b		14. b
2. a		15. d
3. c		16. c
4. d		17. d
5. a		18. a
6. c		19. c
7. c		20. b
8. d		21. d
9. d		22. b
10. b		23. d

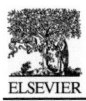

11. a   24. b
12. b   25. b
13. c

TOPICS FOR DISCUSSION
The topics presented are designed to open discussion and to solicit varying opinions and approaches to problems. The answers listed below are one set of possibilities, but several responses may be correct. The course director will determine whether a student's or a group's response is correct according to the factors presented and the course requirements.

1. Explain to your patient that many conditions that could be serious later can be detected early only with the use of radiographs.

2. Explain that the lead apron is another safety precaution taken for her protection.

3. Explain that you would be continually exposed to x-rays, unlike a patient who is exposed to only one series of radiographs.

4. Explain that you will take only the number of films the dentist has prescribed.

5. Explain the advantages of radiographs and the consequences of not having them. Then explain the safety precautions taken for her protection.

CD-ROM Patient Case Exercise

1. Exposure to radiation is cumulative, and under no circumstances should a dental assistant hold film for a patient.

CHAPTER 39: DENTAL FILM AND PROCESSING RADIOGRAPHS

SHORT-ANSWER QUESTIONS
These questions reflect the Learning Outcomes listed at the beginning of this chapter in the textbook and can be used as class assignments. The answers can be found within the chapter and/or classroom discussion.

FILL IN THE BLANK
1. latent image
2. film emulsion
3. tube side
4. label side
5. manual processing
6. automatic processing
7. film-holding devices
8. beam alignment devices
9. intraoral film
10. extraoral film
11. duplicating film
12. periapical radiograph
13. bitewing radiograph
14. occlusal radiograph
15. film cassette
16. film speed
17. intensifying screen
18. processing errors

Bird/Robinson

MULTIPLE CHOICE

1. b	5. c	9. c	13. c	17. d
2. d	6. c	10. d	14. b	18. b
3. a	7. c	11. a	15. a	19. b
4. b	8. d	12. b	16. b	20. b

ACTIVITY

Patient One: 28 years old

Maxillary right molar	#2
Maxillary left molar	#2
Maxillary central	#1
Mandibular right molar	#2
Mandibular left molar	#2
Mandibular central	#1
Right bitewing	#2
Left bitewing	#2

Patient Two: 8 years old

Maxillary right molar	#1
Maxillary left molar	#1
Maxillary central	#1
Mandibular right molar	#1
Mandibular left molar	#1
Mandibular central	#1
Right bitewing	#2
Left bitewing	#2

Patient Three: 4 years old

Maxillary occlusal	#4
Mandibular occlusal	#4

CD-ROM Patient Case Exercises

1. No, the dark area is a normal anatomic landmark.
2. Number 2 film was used for the molar and bitewing projections.
3. Because of missing teeth, only 13 films were necessary.
4. No processing errors occurred.
5. No, the dark area is not caused by a processing error.
6. The circle that appears at the bottom of the film is actually the raised dot on the film. The film should have been placed in the mouth with the raised dot on the occlusal surface.

CHAPTER 40: LEGAL ISSUES, QUALITY ASSURANCE, AND INFECTION CONTROL

SHORT-ANSWER QUESTIONS

These questions reflect the Learning Outcomes listed at the beginning of this chapter in the textbook, and can be used as class assignments. The answers can be found within the chapter and/or classroom discussion.

ELSEVIER

FILL IN THE BLANK
1. disclosure
2. informed consent
3. liable
4. quality assurance
5. quality control tests

MULTIPLE CHOICE

1. c	10. b
2. c	11. a
3. d	12. c
4. c	13. a
5. b	14. b
6. a	15. d
7. d	16. b
8. b	17. c
9. c	18. c

TOPICS FOR DISCUSSION
The topics presented are designed to open discussion and to solicit varying opinions and approaches to problems. The answers listed below are one set of possibilities, but several responses may be correct. The course director will determine whether a student's or a group's response is correct according to the factors presented and the course requirements.

Time: Leaving the film in the developer too long can cause films to be dark.

Solution strength Weak solution can make films lighter, although fresh solution cannot make films dark.

Temperature: Setting the developer temperature too high can cause films to be dark.

Light leaks: Exposure to white light can turn films black.

Improper fixation: Improper fixation cannot cause films to turn black.

Paper left on film: Leaving black paper on the film can result in loss of the image.

CHAPTER 41: INTRAORAL RADIOGRAPHY
SHORT-ANSWER QUESTIONS
These questions reflect the Learning Outcomes listed at the beginning of this chapter in the textbook, and can be used as class assignments. The answers can be found within the chapter and/or classroom discussion.

FILL IN THE BLANK
1. paralleling technique
2. bisection of the angle technique
3. diagnostic quality
4. interproximal
5. bitewing film
6. alveolar bone
7. crestal bone
8. contact area
9. open contacts
10. parallel
11. intersecting
12. perpendicular

Torres and Ehrlich Modern Dental Assisting, 9th ed.

Bird/Robinson

13. right angle
14. long axis of the tooth
15. central ray

MULTIPLE CHOICE

1. d	13. d
2. b	14. a
3. a	15. b
4. d	16. c
5. b	17. b
6. c	18. a
7. d	19. d
8. b	20. c
9. d	21. d
10. c	22. b
11. d	23. b
12. c	

CD-ROM PATIENT CASE EXERCISES

CHRISTOPHER BROOKS

1. Two bitewings and one maxillary occlusal projection were taken.
2. The bitewings were taken with #1 size film, and the occlusal was taken with #2 size film.

ANTONIO DEANGELIS

1. The technique error was incorrect horizontal angulation.
2. The film should have been placed farther back.
3. There is a cone cut. The cone should have been placed farther mesially.

CHAPTER 42: EXTRAORAL AND DIGITAL RADIOGRAPHY

SHORT-ANSWER QUESTIONS

These questions reflect the Learning Outcomes listed at the beginning of this chapter in the textbook, and can be used as class assignments. The answers can be found within the chapter and/or classroom discussion.

FILL IN THE BLANK

1. focal trough
2. Frankfort plane
3. midsagittal plane
4. tomography
5. charge-coupled device
6. digitize
7. sensor
8. digital radiography

MULTIPLE CHOICE

1. b	4. a	7. b	10. d
2. b	5. a	8. d	
3. a	6. d	9. b	

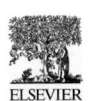

CASE STUDY

This case study is designed to open discussion and to solicit varying opinions in the classroom. Several responses may be correct. The course director will determine whether a student's or a group's response is correct according to the factors presented and the course requirements.

1. A cephalometric film would reveal a class III occlusion.
2. Bitewings or periapicals would reveal crowding.
3. Jeremy should be referred to an orthodontist.
4. Bitewings would reveal recurrent decay.
5. Radiographs are not capable of showing changes in soft tissues such as those that occur in gingivitis.

CD-ROM Patient Case Exercises

CINDY VALLADARES
1. Improper patient positioning caused the dark area.
2. The radiograph is not diagnostically acceptable because not all apices are visible.

INGRID PEDERSEN
1. The teeth on panoramic radiographs are frequently overlapped; this is not considered a positioning error. This is why bitewings are taken along with panoramic films.

TIFFANY COLE
1. Tiffany is 8 years old.
2. When the student clicks on #27, the screen will indicate a correct answer.

CHAPTER 43: RESTORATIVE AND ESTHETIC DENTAL MATERIALS

SHORT-ANSWER QUESTIONS

These questions reflect the Learning Outcomes listed at the beginning of this chapter in the textbook, and can be used as class assignments. The answers can be found within the chapter and/or classroom discussion.

FILL IN THE BLANK

1. galvanic
2. ceramic
3. cured
4. adhere
5. palladium
6. restorative
7. pestle
8. porcelain
9. esthetic
10. gold
11. viscosity
12. amalgam
13. auto-cure
14. microleakage
15. alloy
16. retention
17. spherical
18. strain
19. stress
20. trituration

MULTIPLE CHOICE

1. c	11. d
2. b	12. a
3. a	13. b
4. d	14. c
5. b	15. c
6. d	16. b
7. a	17. d
8. d	18. b
9. c	19. a
10. b	20. c

CASE STUDY

This Case Study is designed to open discussion and to solicit varying opinions and approaches to problems. The answers listed below are one set of possibilities, but several responses may be correct. The course director will determine whether a student's or a group's response is correct according to the factors presented and the course requirements.

1. This type of decay represents a class V restoration.

2. Composite resin would be selected for esthetics.

3. The dental dam is the best selection for maintaining moisture control. Moisture is of concern when teeth are restored, because of proximity to gingival tissues.

4. A composite or plastic instrument would be used to apply the material to the preparation.

5. The charting would include a small half-circle outlined in blue at the gingival third.

CHAPTER 44: DENTAL LINERS, BASES, AND BONDING SYSTEMS

SHORT-ANSWER QUESTIONS

These questions reflect the Learning Outcomes listed at the beginning of this chapter in the textbook, and can be used as class assignments. The answers can be found within the chapter and/or classroom discussion.

FILL IN THE BLANK

1. smear layer
2. thermal
3. hybrid
4. insulating
5. etching
6. polymerization
7. eugenol
8. desiccate
9.\micromechanical
10. obliterating
11. sedative
12. retention

Bird/Robinson

MULTIPLE CHOICE

1. b	9. b
2. c	10. d
3. d	11. c
4. a	12. b
5. d	13. d
6. b	14. c
7. c	15. a
8. a	

TOPICS FOR DISCUSSION

The topics presented are designed to open discussion and to solicit varying opinions and approaches to problems. The answers listed below are one set of possibilities, but several responses may be correct. The course director will determine whether a student's or a group's response is correct according to the factors presented and the course requirements.

1. Composite resin most likely would be selected for a class III restoration on tooth #7.

2. For a moderately deep restoration in an anterior tooth, you would set up a bonding system that includes an etchant and a bonding liquid.

3. It would take a minimum of two steps: a step for etching and another for application of the bonding material.

4. For best results in maintaining moisture control, a dental dam would be used.

5. Etching and bonding application may be legal in your state. Review your state's legal responsibilities.

CHAPTER 45: DENTAL CEMENTS

SHORT-ANSWER QUESTIONS

These questions reflect the Learning Outcomes listed at the beginning of this chapter in the textbook, and can be used as class assignments. The answers can be found within the chapter and/or classroom discussion.

FILL IN THE BLANK

1. spatulate
2. exothermic
3. provisional
4. cement
5. retard
6. luting agent

MULTIPLE CHOICE

1. b	9. a
2. d	10. c
3. c	11. d
4. b	12. b
5. a	13. a
6. c	14. d
7. d	15. a
8. b	

CASE STUDY

This Case Study is designed to open discussion and to solicit varying opinions and approaches to problems. The answers listed below are one set of possibilities, but several responses may be correct. The course director will determine whether a student's or a group's response is correct according to the factors presented and the course requirements.

1. A stainless steel crown is considered permanent when placed on primary teeth.

2. Duralon is a polycarboxylate.

3. You would set up a treated paper pad, a stainless steel spatula, polycarboxylate powder and dispenser, polycarboxylate liquid, and gauze.

4. To mix the cement, incorporate all powder quickly into the liquid at one time; the mixing should be completed within 30 seconds.

5. To clean the cement from around the crown (after it has completed its initial setting), use an explorer with a horizontal movement, and pull excess material away from the tooth. Once all pieces have been removed, tie a knot in dental floss and pass it through the contact on both sides of the tooth. Then rinse, dry, and examine the area.

CHAPTER 46: IMPRESSION MATERIALS

SHORT-ANSWER QUESTIONS

These questions reflect the Learning Outcomes listed at the beginning of this chapter in the textbook, and can be used as class assignments. The answers can be found within the chapter and/or classroom discussion.

FILL IN THE BLANK

1. colloid
2. border molding
3. elastomeric
4. base
5. centric
6. agar
7. syneresis
8. tempering
9. viscosity
10. alginate
11. extrude
12. hydro-
13. occlusal registration
14. catalyst
15. imbibition

MULTIPLE CHOICE

1. a	13. b
2. d	14. d
3. c	15. a
4. b	16. d
5. d	17. a
6. c	18. b
7. a	19. c
8. c	20. d

9. b	21. a
10. c	22. c
11. c	23. d
12. a	24. c
	25. b

CASE STUDY

This Case Study is designed to open discussion and to solicit varying opinions and approaches to problems. The answers listed below are one set of possibilities, but several responses may be correct. The course director will determine whether a student's or a group's response is correct according to the factors presented and the course requirements.

1. Alginate would be selected to take preliminary impressions.

2. You would set up alginate powder, an alginate measure scoop, a water measure, a rubber bowl, a wide-blade spatula, sterile impression trays, tray adhesive, utility wax, a saliva ejector, and a precaution bag.

3. Place water in a bowl, fluff alginate and sift powder into the water, and use a spatula to mix it with a stirring action until completely moistened. Firmly spread the alginate between the spatula and the side of the bowl. Mix until smooth and creamy.

4. The central and lateral incisors must be centered in the impression. A complete peripheral roll should be visible on both sides, and the tray must not be overseated. The impression should be free from tears or voids, with sharp anatomic detail of teeth and soft tissues. Specific areas for each impression are the retromolar reproduced on the mandibular impression and the hard palate on the maxillary impression.

5. Impressions are to be rinsed with cool water, sprayed with an approved disinfectant, wrapped in a moist paper towel, and placed in a precaution bag with the patient's name and date.

CHAPTER 47: LABORATORY MATERIALS AND PROCEDURES

SHORT-ANSWER QUESTIONS

These questions reflect the Learning Outcomes listed at the beginning of this chapter in the textbook, and can be used as class assignments. The answers can be found within the chapter and/or classroom discussion.

FILL IN THE BLANK

1. homogeneous
2. lathe
3. gypsum
4. volatile
5. dihydrate
6. dimensionally stable
7. facebow
8. polymer
9. crystallization
10. hemihydrate
11. model
12. anatomic
13. articulator
14. monomer
15. slurry

ELSEVIER

Torres and Ehrlich Modern Dental Assisting, 9th ed.

Bird/Robinson

MULTIPLE CHOICE

1. c	14. c
2. d	15. c
3. c	16. a
4. a	17. d
5. c	18. b
6. d	19. a
7. c	20. c
8. b	21. d
9. c	22. b
10. a	23. a
11. c	24. d
12. a	25. c
13. d	

CASE STUDY

This Case Study is designed to open discussion and to solicit varying opinions and approaches to problems. The answers listed below are one set of possibilities, but several responses may be correct. The course director will determine whether a student's or a group's response is correct according to the factors presented and the course requirements.

1. Preliminary impressions are gently rinsed under cold water, sprayed with an approved disinfectant, wrapped in a damp paper towel, and stored in the plastic precaution bag with the patient's name and date.

2. No, Alginate materials must be poured up within 1 hour. Because so much of the material is made from water, a slight change in its environment could distort the impression and cause dimensional change.

3. Plaster is commonly used for presentation purposes because it can be trimmed and polished for a more professional quality appearance.

4. The art portion of the cast would be trimmed on a model trimmer, then finished with a mix of slurry of gypsum to fill in any voids.

5. To polish the finished model, soak it in a soapy solution for 24 hours, allow it to dry, and then polish it with a soft cloth. You can also use a commercial model gloss spray.

CHAPTER 48: GENERAL DENTISTRY

SHORT-ANSWER QUESTIONS

These questions reflect the Learning Outcomes listed at the beginning of this chapter in the textbook, and can be used as class assignments. The answers can be found within the chapter and/or classroom discussion.

FILL IN THE BLANK

1. restoration
2. cavity wall
3. retention form
4. diastema
5. veneer
6. cavity
7. convenience form
8. pulpal wall

9. outline form
10. operative dentistry
11. line angle
12. axial wall

MULTIPLE CHOICE

1. b	11. d
2. d	12. b
3. a	13. d
4. b	14. d
5. d	15. a
6. d	16. c
7. b	17. c
8. a	18. b
9. c	19. a
10. d	20. d

CASE STUDY

This Case Study is designed to open discussion and to solicit varying opinions and approaches to problems. The answers listed below are one set of possibilities, but several responses may be correct. The course director will determine whether a student's or a group's response is correct according to the factors presented and the course requirements.

1. Commonly, you would see amalgam placed in this tooth for its strength and durability, but composite resin could be a choice for esthetics.

2. Tooth #18 would be the anchor tooth for the dental dam clamp and would continue to tooth #27.

3. Yes, because the mesial surface of tooth #19 is to be restored, and matrix will be required.

4. If amalgam is used, a base, a dentin sealer, and bonding system should be set out for the procedure.

5. The procedure would be charted as follows: mesial-occlusal surface outlined and colored in blue for amalgam.

CD-ROM Patient Case Exercise

CRYSTAL MALONE

1. I—1, II—7, III—0, IV—0
2. No, Crystal does not have any composite restorations in place.
3. Crystal should be scheduled for a posterior MO composite.
4. The dental team could advise her on over-the-counter whitening products and their use.
5. An endodontist and a fixed prosthodontist might have been involved.

CHAPTER 49: MATRIX SYSTEMS FOR RESTORATIVE DENTISTRY

SHORT-ANSWER QUESTIONS

These questions reflect the Learning Outcomes listed at the beginning of this chapter in the textbook, and can be used as class assignments. The answers can be found within the chapter and/or classroom discussion.

FILL IN THE BLANK
1. Mylar and celluloid strip
2. overhang
3. cupping
4. wedge
5. matrix
6. palodent
7. automatrix
8. universal retainer

MULTIPLE CHOICE

1. b	6. b
2. c	7. d
3. d	8. d
4. a	9. c
5. d	10. d

ACTIVITIES
This Case Study is designed to open discussion and to solicit varying opinions and approaches to problems. The answers listed below are one set of possibilities, but several responses could be correct. The course director will determine whether a student's or a group's response is correct according to the factors presented and the course requirements.

1. A universal retainer and a matrix band

2. You would need to select a molar extension band to adapt to the preparation that is being extended.

3. Using the crown and bridge scissors, you would remove the extension area for the distal side, leaving the remaining extension for the mesial facial surface.

4. You will need two wedges (one for mesial and one for distal contacts). The wedges would be inserted from the lingual.

5. Depending on the extension, an automatrix or a sectional matrix could be used.

CD-ROM Patient Case Exercise

MIGUEL RICARDO

1. Teeth #2, #3, #14, and #19 received a matrix in the restoration process.
2. No, Miguel does not have any composite restorations in place at this time.
3. Miguel should be scheduled for replacement of an amalgam restoration.
4. Tooth #3 will be restored.
5. A universal retainer and a matrix band will be prepared for the procedure.

CHAPTER 50: FIXED PROSTHODONTICS

SHORT-ANSWER QUESTIONS
These questions reflect the Learning Outcomes listed at the beginning of this chapter in the textbook, and can be used as class assignments. The answers can be found within the chapter and/or classroom discussion.

Torres and Ehrlich Modern Dental Assisting, 9th ed.

Bird/Robinson

FILL IN THE BLANK

1. cast post
2. core
3. die
4. abutment
5. articulator
6. fixed bridge
7. gingival retraction
8. crown
9. inlay
10. hypertrophied
11. master cast
12. investment material
13. pontic
14. porcelain-fused-to-metal
15. veneer
16. onlay
17. resin-bonded bridge
18. opaquer
19. three-quarter crown
20. unit

MULTIPLE CHOICE

1. b	9. c
2. c	10. b
3. d	11. b
4. a	12. a
5. c	13. d
6. b	14. c
7. d	15. d
8. b	

CASE STUDY

This Case Study is designed to open discussion and to solicit varying opinions and approaches to problems. The answers listed below are one set of possibilities, but several responses may be correct. The course director will determine whether a student's or a group's response is correct according to the factors presented and the course requirements.

1. If toothbrushing and flossing are done poorly, the gingival tissues will not be healthy enough to receive the prosthesis. This situation would have to be brought under control before the patient could receive a bridge.

2. Because of its location, a porcelain or porcelain-fused-to-metal bridge would be selected because of esthetics.

3. Teeth #11 and #13 serve as the abutment, and tooth #12 is the pontic or artificial tooth.

4. A custom temporary bridge would be fabricated during the crown and bridge preparation.

5. If a porcelain bridge was used, crowns for teeth #11 to #13 would be outlined in blue with each tooth connected by a crossbar, and the root of tooth #12 would be crossed out. If the bridge was porcelain-fused-to-metal, crowns for teeth #11 to #13 would be outlined in blue (with diagonal lines on

the lingual section representing the metal portion) with each tooth connected by a crossbar, and the root of tooth #12 would be crossed out

.

CD-ROM Patient Case Exercise

Jessica Brooks

1. No, Ms. Brooks does not have any crown and bridge work.
2. The tooth fractured, creating a larger surface area to be restored.
3. Ms. Brooks required a core buildup because the tooth was badly decayed.
4. Gold was prescribed for the preparation.
5. Ms. Brooks should be instructed to continue brushing and flossing as usual.

CHAPTER 51: PROVISIONAL COVERAGE

SHORT-ANSWER QUESTIONS

These questions reflect the Learning Outcomes listed at the beginning of this chapter in the textbook, and can be used as class assignments. The answers can be found within the chapter and/or classroom discussion.

FILL IN THE BLANK

1. custom provisional
2. provisional
3. preformed
4. stainless steel crown
5. polycarbonate crown

MULTIPLE CHOICE

1. b   6. a
2. a   7. c
3. d   8. b
4. d   9. c
5. c   10. d

CASE STUDY

This Case Study is designed to open discussion and to solicit varying opinions and approaches to problems. The answers listed below are one set of possibilities, but several responses may be correct. The course director will determine whether a student's or a group's response is correct according to the factors presented and the course requirements.

1. Yes, a preformed polymer or an aluminum crown could be used for a posterior provisional.

2. Two ways to make a provisional are to make a custom provisional from an impression or custom tray, and to use a preformed crown that is fitted for size.

3. You can add additional acrylic resin to the marginal area and reseat the provisional until the material sets, or you can refill with acrylic material and reseat if you are using a preformed crown.

4. Polish the provisional using a rag wheel and pumice on the lathe.

5. You will need to set up tempbond, a paper pad, basic setup, and floss. Once the cement has set, use the explorer to remove excess cement from around the margin. Using dental floss, tie a knot and pass it through the contact to remove any excess cement interproximally. Then rinse and dry and have the dentist evaluate the procedure.

ELSEVIER

Torres and Ehrlich Modern Dental Assisting, 9th ed.
Bird/Robinson

CD-ROM Patient Case Exercise
1. Teeth #2, #3, and #4 are involved in the three-unit bridge.
2. A custom provisional was selected for this case.
3. A thermoplastic vacuum-formed tray also could be used.
4. Tempbond (zinc oxide–eugenol) should be used for cementation of the provisional.
5. Instruct the patient to continue brushing. When flossing, do not "pop" the floss into and out of the contact. Contact the office immediately if the provisional becomes loose.

CHAPTER 52: REMOVABLE PROSTHODONTICS

SHORT-ANSWER QUESTIONS

These questions reflect the Learning Outcomes listed at the beginning of this chapter in the textbook, and can be used as class assignments. The answers can be found within the chapter and/or classroom discussion.

FILL IN THE BLANK

1. centric relation
2. connector
3. border molding
4. coping
5. edentulous
6. festooning
7. flange
8. framework
9. mastication
10. full denture
11. immediate denture
12. lateral excursion
13. occlusal rim
14. post dam
15. pressure points
16. protrusion
17. partial denture
18. relining
19. retainer
20. retrusion

MULTIPLE CHOICE

1. c	11. a
2. d	12. c
3. a	13. d
4. d	14. b
5. d	15. d
6. b	16. b
7. d	17. c
8. c	18. d
9. b	19. b
10. d	20. d

CASE STUDY

This Case Study is designed to open discussion and to solicit varying opinions and approaches to problems. The answers listed below are one set of possibilities, but several responses may be correct. The course director will determine whether a student's or a group's response is correct according to the factors presented and the course requirements.

1. You should welcome questions from friends and family about their dental health. You are now an advocate for the profession and will help people see the importance of healthy teeth.

2. A bridge would not be a good choice because there is no distal abutment for stability.

3. A dentist will want to keep as many natural teeth as possible in a dentition. Natural teeth are better for the patient's health, speech, and dental care.

4. There would be fewer appointments for the patient, the cost would be less, and good tooth structure would not be reduced.

5. Along with the final impression, the laboratory technician receives a prescription that describes the specific construction of the prosthesis.

CD-ROM Patient Case Exercise
1. Mr. Escobar has ten missing teeth.
2. An oral surgeon, periodontist, endodontist, and prosthodontist might be involved in the treatment plan.
3. Mr. Escobar will be receiving a full denture.
4. Implants were not discussed because of the patient's medical complications.
5. Because of the surgical alveoplasty, Mr. Escobar's supporting tissues will continue to heal and will change in shape.

CHAPTER 53: DENTAL IMPLANTS

SHORT-ANSWER QUESTIONS
These questions reflect the Learning Outcomes listed at the beginning of this chapter in the textbook, and can be used as class assignments. The answers can be found within the chapter and/or classroom discussion.

FILL IN THE BLANK
1. transosteal
2. endosteal
3. osseointegration
4. circumoral
5. subperiosteal
6. peri-implant tissue
7. surgical stent
8. implants
9. titanium

MULTIPLE CHOICE
1. d	9. d
2. c	10. d
3. d	11. b
4. a	12. c
5. c	13. d
6. d	14. b
7. b	15. d
8. c	

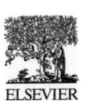

CASE STUDY

This Case Study is designed to open discussion and to solicit varying opinions and approaches to problems. The answers listed below are one set of possibilities, but several responses may be correct. The course director will determine whether a student's or a group's response is correct according to the factors presented and the course requirements.

1. Contraindications that should be reviewed are financial investment, length of treatment, risk of infection, bruxism, certain medical conditions, and the challenge for some patients.

2. After the first surgery, a healing period takes place, and the osseointegration period allows time for the fixture to bond with the bone.

3. Because implants are considered a surgical procedure, infection is the primary concern. The tissue and the bone are exposed for the implantation procedure. The patient's mouth is rinsed, the head is draped, and sterile gloves and a sterile setup are used to prevent disease transmission.

4. With this type of procedure, financial assistance may be available through dental insurance, installment payments, or credit card payments.

5. Several types of devices are essential in plaque removal for implant patients, such as manual or electric toothbrushes, single-tufted toothbrushes, denture clasp brushes, interproximal brushes, and floss.

CD-ROM Patient Case Exercise

1. Mr. Brooks has a crown on tooth #4 and a bridge on tooth #19.
2. Mr. Brooks decided to have an endosteal implant.
3. A fixed bridge would be the second choice of treatment.
4. Instruct the patient to remove plaque by using a manual or electric toothbrush, a denture clasp brush, an interproximal brush, and regular or implant floss.
5. After completion of the implant, Mr. Brooks will be scheduled for a recall appointment.

CHAPTER 54: ENDODONTICS

SHORT-ANSWER QUESTIONS

These questions reflect the Learning Outcomes listed at the beginning of this chapter in the textbook and can be used as class assignments. The answers can be found within the chapter and/or classroom discussion.

FILL IN THE BLANK

1. apical curettage

2. control tooth

3. abscess

4. percussion

5. gutta-percha

6. hemisection

7. indirect pulp cap

8. nonvital

9. debridement

10. palpation

11. root amputation

12. root canal therapy

13. pulp cap

14. perforation

15. periradicular

16. pulpotomy

17. pulpitis

18. retrograde restoration

19. endodontist

20. reversible pulpitis

MULTIPLE CHOICE

1. b	11. a
2. c	12. b
3. a	13. d
4. a	14. d
5. c	15. c
6. d	16. b
7. c	17. c
8. a	18. d
9. d	19. a
10. c	20. b

CASE STUDY

This Case Study is designed to open discussion and to solicit varying opinions and approaches to problems. The answers listed below are one set of possibilities, but several responses may be correct. The course director will determine whether a student's or a group's response is correct according to the factors presented and the course requirements.

1. Mr. Allen's general dentist would have referred him to the endodontist.

2. Tooth #20 is a mandibular left second premolar that has one root.

3. The dentist may choose from the following tests: percussion, palpation, thermal sensitivity, or electric pulp testing.

4. Tooth #29 would be used as a control tooth. A control tooth is used for comparison.

5. Local anesthetic and N_2O/O_2 could be used to alleviate pain and discomfort.

CD-ROM Patient Case Exercise

1. No, no existing root canals are charted for Mr. DeAngelis.
2. Tooth #7 was used as the control tooth for the testing.
3. To chart the tooth after completion of the root canal, a blue line is drawn through the root of tooth #10.
4. Mr. DeAngelis would be referred to a prosthodontist for the porcelain-fused-to-metal crown.
5. Yes, Mr. DeAngelis should be scheduled for a recall appointment.

CHAPTER 55: PERIODONTICS

SHORT-ANSWER QUESTIONS

These questions reflect the Learning Outcomes listed at the beginning of this chapter in the textbook, and can be used as class assignments. The answers can be found within the chapter and/or classroom discussion.

FILL IN THE BLANK
1. periodontics
2. periodontist
3. periodontal pocket
4. periodontal dressing
5. mobility
6. bleeding index
7. periodontal explorer
8. ultrasonic scaler
9. osseous surgery
10. gingivectomy
11. gingivoplasty
12. osteoplasty
13. ostectomy
14. laser beam

MULTIPLE CHOICE
1. b	10. a
2. d	11. b
3. c	12. c
4. a	13. d
5. b	14. b
6. c	15. a
7. b	16. d
8. d	17. c
9. b	18. b

TOPICS FOR DISCUSSION
The topics presented are designed to open discussion and to solicit varying opinions and approaches to problems. The answers listed below are one set of possibilities, but several responses could be correct. The course director will determine whether a student's or a group's response is correct according to the factors presented and the course requirements.
1. A periodontist would complete the procedure.
2. Flap surgery is another name for incisional periodontal surgery.
3. The surgeon would use sutures to close the flap.
4. To protect the surgical site and promote healing, you would prepare a periodontal pack to be placed over the surgical site.

CD-ROM Patient Case Exercises

LOUISA VAN DOREN

1. If Mrs. Van Doren's diabetes were not well-controlled, it would be a contraindication to the use of an ultrasonic scaler.
2. The gingivectomy is scheduled for the area of tooth #31.
3. Yes, Dr. Bowman will place a periodontal dressing.

JANET FOLKNER

4. Mrs. Folkner has a pacemaker. It would be wise to consult her cardiologist before using the ultrasonic scaler.
5. The radiographs indicate generalized bone loss.
    Curettes would be used to remove the subgingival calculus.

Bird/Robinson

CHAPTER 56: ORAL AND MAXILLOFACIAL SURGERY

SHORT-ANSWER QUESTIONS

These questions reflect the Learning Outcomes listed at the beginning of this chapter in the textbook, and can be used as class assignments. The answers can be found within the chapter and/or classroom discussion.

FILL IN THE BLANK

1. chisel
2. elevator
3. hard tissue impaction
4. hemostat
5. surgical curette
6. alveoplasty
7. bone file
8. soft tissue impaction
9. exfoliative biopsy
10. forceps
11. donning
12. impacted
13. incisional biopsy
14. mallet
15. scalpel
16. oral and maxillofacial surgeon
17. oral and maxillofacial surgery
18. outpatient
19. retractor
20. rongeur

MULTIPLE CHOICE

1. a	11. b
2. c	12. d
3. d	13. b
4. b	14. c
5. c	15. b
6. d	16. d
7. b	17. c
8. a	18. a
9. c	19. b
10. d	20. c

CASE STUDY

This Case Study is designed to open discussion and to solicit varying opinions and approaches to problems. The answers listed below are one set of possibilities, but several responses may be correct. The course director will determine whether a student's or a group's response is correct according to the factors presented and the course requirements.

1. Because Katie's teeth were impacted, an oral and maxillofacial surgeon would be the specialist of choice for the removal of impacted teeth.

2. Alveolitis, also referred to as dry socket, is the possible diagnosis for the pain.

Torres and Ehrlich Modern Dental Assisting, 9th ed.
Bird/Robinson

3. Specific causes include inadequate blood supply to the socket, trauma to the socket, infection within the socket, or dislodgment of the clot from the socket. For treatment of alveolitis, the socket is gently irrigated with warm saline solution, then a strip of iodoform gauze is dipped in medication and is packed into the socket.

4. The patient should come in immediately to have this process started.

CD-ROM Patient Case Exercise

1. The charting for tooth #30 indicates recurrent decay and an abscess.

2. N_2O/O_2 also could be used to calm the patient.

3. Sterile gloves, a mask, protective eyewear, and a sterile gown were worn during the procedure.

4. No, sutures were not placed after the extraction.

5. A strip of iodoform gauze is dipped in medication and is packed into the socket.

CHAPTER 57: PEDIATRIC DENTISTRY

SHORT-ANSWER QUESTIONS

These questions reflect the Learning Outcomes listed at the beginning of this chapter in the textbook, and can be used as class assignments. The answers can be found within the chapter and/or classroom discussion.

FILL IN THE BLANK

1. cerebral palsy
2. chronologic age
3. autonomy
4. avulsed
5. Down syndrome
6. athetosis
7. extrusion
8. intrusion
9. T-band
10. luxation
11. mental age
12. Frankl scale
13. pediatric dentistry
14. postnatal
15. mental retardation
16. neural
17. open bay
18. papoose board
19. pulpotomy
20. prenatal

MULTIPLE CHOICE

1. b	14. d
2. c	15. b
3. d	16. a
4. b	17. d
5. b	18. c
6. d	19. b
7. b	20. c

8. d	21. b
9. a	22. a
10. c	23. d
11. a	24. d
12. b	25. b
13. a	

CASE STUDY

This Case Study is designed to open discussion and to solicit varying opinions and approaches to problems. The answers listed below are one set of possibilities, but several responses may be correct. The course director will determine whether a student's or a group's response is correct according to the factors presented and the course requirements.

1. Ashley should be instructed to come in immediately.

2. A periapical radiograph should be taken for a diagnosis.

3. Traumatic intrusion results from an injury during which the tooth is forcibly driven into the alveolus.

4. Because Ashley is 12 years old, this would be her permanent central incisor.

5. Nothing would be completed at the emergency appointment. The teeth would be allowed to re-erupt naturally, but endodontic treatment likely will be required later.

CD-ROM Patient Case Exercise
1. Maxillary primary and permanent anteriors are visible on the occlusal film.
2. Probably not. Even though fluoride is important in the prevention of decay, the use of a bottle with sweetened liquid at bedtime would still affect this area.
3. At 5 to 7 years of age, the permanent first molars erupt.
4. No, this is not considered an expanded function because it is a permanent placement. If a stainless steel crown were used temporarily, this would be considered an expanded function.
5. The cement used for cementation of the stainless steel crown is permanent cement.

CHAPTER 58: CORONAL POLISHING

SHORT-ANSWER QUESTIONS

These questions reflect the Learning Outcomes listed at the beginning of this chapter in the textbook, and can be used as class assignments. The answers can be found within the chapter and/or classroom discussion.

FILL IN THE BLANK

1. calculus
2. oral prophylaxis
3. clinical crown
4. intrinsic stains
5. extrinsic stains
6. fulcrum
7. rubber cup polishing

MULTIPLE CHOICE

1. b	7. b
2. b	8. c
3. c	9. b
4. a	10. d
5. c	11. a
6. d	12. c

CASE STUDY

This Case Study is designed to open discussion and to solicit varying opinions and approaches to problems. The answers listed below are one set of possibilities, but several responses may be correct. The course director will determine whether a student's or a group's response is correct according to the factors presented and the course requirements.

1. While doing a coronal polish, you would be responsible for checking the patient's medical history, answering patient questions, inspecting the oral cavity for oral lesions, missing teeth, tori, etc., and polishing the surfaces of teeth.

2. Yes, in some pediatric offices, the dentist will remove any calculus and will instruct the educationally qualified dental assistant to perform the coronal polish.

3. Contraindications that would keep you from completing a coronal polish on a pediatric patient include the presence of calculus, stains that cannot be removed by polishing, and lack of parental permission.

4. If you notice calculus on the lingual surfaces of the lower anteriors, ask the dentist or the dental hygienist to remove the calculus before you begin polishing.

5. Remove calculus before performing coronal polishing.

CHAPTER 59: DENTAL SEALANTS

SHORT-ANSWER QUESTIONS

These questions reflect the Learning Outcomes listed at the beginning of this chapter in the textbook, and can be used as class assignments. The answers can be found within the chapter and/or classroom discussion.

FILL IN THE BLANK

1. dental sealant
2. polymerization
3. self-cured
4. light-cured
5. filled resin
6. unfilled resin
7. microleakage
8. acrylate
9. sealant retention

MULTIPLE CHOICE

1. b	6. a
2. e	7. a
3. b	8. c
4. d	9. d
5. b	10. b

CASE STUDY

This Case Study is designed to open discussion and to solicit varying opinions and approaches to problems. The answers listed below are one set of possibilities, but several responses may be correct. The course director will determine whether a student's or a group's response is correct according to the factors presented and the course requirements.

1. Before you begin the procedure, Dr. Allen must examine the teeth to ensure that there is no decay.

2. Sealants will be placed on her first four permanent molars.

3. You could use a rubber dam or cotton roll isolation.

4. Set out the necessary materials. Using a slurry of pumice and water, polish the occlusal surface of each tooth to be sealed. Establish moisture control in the area where the first sealant will be placed. Apply the etching agent for the appropriate length of time, then rinse thoroughly and dry the tooth. Maintain moisture control while applying the sealant to the occlusal surface. When the sealant has set, check the margins and the occusal surface for excess material. Follow this procedure for each of the remaining molars.

5. The sealant is a little too high. Using a stone mounted in the slow handpiece, carefully smooth off the excess. You should know and follow the requirements in the dental practice act of your state. Not all states allow a dental assistant to use the low-speed handpiece. In this case, Dr. Allen would remove the excess sealant material.

CD-ROM Patient Case Exercises

TODD LEDBETTER

1. Todd will have sealants on teeth #2, #4, #13, #15, #18, #19, #20, #29, and #31.
2. The lingual pits on the anterior teeth do not need sealants.
3. The setup would include polishing cup and pumice, cotton rolls, etchant material, sealant material, applicator and tip, and articulating paper.

CHRISTOPHER BROOKS

1. Christopher will have sealants on teeth #3, #14, #19, and #30.
2. A rubber dam or cotton rolls can be used for moisture control.
3. The teeth to receive sealants should first be polished with pumice and water.
4. Contaminated teeth must be reconditioned before sealant material is applied.

ELSEVIER

Torres and Ehrlich Modern Dental Assisting, 9th ed.
Bird/Robinson

CHAPTER 60: ORTHODONTICS

SHORT-ANSWER QUESTIONS

These questions reflect the Learning Outcomes listed at the beginning of this chapter in the textbook, and can be used as class assignments. The answers can be found within the chapter and/or classroom discussion.

FILL IN THE BLANK

1. band
2. braces
3. bracket
4. ligature tie
5. auxiliary
6. arch wire
7. separator
8. malocclusion
9. mesioclusion
10. cephalometric
11. distoclusion
12. headgear
13. retainer
14. overjet
15. open bite
16. orthodontics
17. occlusion
18. positioner
19. overbite
20. fetal molding

MULTIPLE CHOICE

1. d	14. d
2. a	15. d
3. c	16. c
4. d	17. c
5. b	18. a
6. d	19. d
7. d	20. b
8. b	21. d
9. c	22. d
10. a	23. a
11. b	24. b
12. d	25. d
13.b	

CASE STUDY

This Case Study is designed to open discussion and to solicit varying opinions and approaches to problems. The answers listed below are one set of possibilities, but several responses may be correct. The course director will determine whether a student's or a group's response is correct according to the factors presented and the course requirements.

Torres and Ehrlich Modern Dental Assisting, 9th ed.

Bird/Robinson

1. Photographs, radiographs (cephalometric), cephalometric tracing, and diagnostic models are used to evaluate Matt's case.

2. This meeting provides the patient and his parents a clear statement of the responsibility of the patient in helping to ensure successful completion of treatment.

3. Separators are placed interproximally on the teeth to be banded. The separator slightly separates the teeth to make seating of the bands easier.

4. You are responsible for laying out the correct setup, which includes the basic setup, preselected orthodontic bands, glass slab, spatula, gauze, band pusher, band seater, scaler, band remover, contouring pliers, alcohol, masking tape, lip balm or wax, and selected cement.

5. After banding, the patient is scheduled for the bonding of brackets.

CD-ROM Patient Case Exercise

1. The first molars are banded.
2. Elastomeric ties are the ligatures used for Kevin's orthodontic treatment.
3. The labial hooks are used for interarch elastics.
4. Kevin would be instructed to floss teeth using a floss threader, and to brush daily.
5. The sealant can be placed on tooth #19 because this tooth is not involved in the orthodontic treatment and would not interfere with it.

CHAPTER 61: COMMUNICATION IN THE DENTAL OFFICE

SHORT-ANSWER QUESTIONS

These questions reflect the Learning Outcomes listed at the beginning of this chapter in the textbook, and can be used as class assignments. The answers can be found within the chapter and/or classroom discussion.

FILL IN THE BLANK

1. salutation
2. verbal communication
3. word processing software
4. copier
5. FAX machine
6. nonverbal communication
7. letterhead
8. marketing

MULTIPLE CHOICE

1. c	11. b
2. c	12. c
3. d	13. d
4. c	14. c
5. a	15. b
6. b	16. b
7. d	17. b
8. c	18. a
9. a	19. c
10. d	20. b

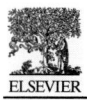

ACTIVITIES

This activity may be interpreted differently by each student. The course director will determine whether a student's or a group's response is acceptable.

CHAPTER 62: BUSINESS OPERATING SYSTEMS

SHORT-ANSWER QUESTIONS

These questions reflect the Learning Outcomes listed at the beginning of this chapter in the textbook, and can be used as class assignments. The answers can be found within the chapter and/or classroom discussion.

FILL IN THE BLANK

1. lead time
2. active
3. chronologic file
4. buffer time
5. inactive
6. cross-reference file
7. call list
8. daily schedule
9. filing
10. ledger
11. outguide
12. warranty
13. purchase order
14. patient of record
15. shelf life
16. units
17. want list
18. rate of use
19. requisition
20. reorder tags

MULTIPLE CHOICE

1. d	11. d
2. b	12. b
3. d	13. d
4. b	14. d
5. b	15. a
6. d	16. d
7. b	17. c
8. d	18. a
9. b	19. d
10. d	20. b

TOPICS FOR DISCUSSION

The topics presented are designed to open discussion and to solicit varying opinions and approaches to problems. The answers listed below are one set of possibilities, but several responses may be correct. The course director will determine whether a student's or a group's response is correct according to the factors presented and the course requirements.

ELSEVIER

Bird/Robinson

1. When there is a change in the number of patients or a change in revenue, this is a matter of concern for all staff.

2. A decrease in revenue could result in the loss of an employee, or a decrease in hours for an employee.

3. The following systems could increase the number of daily patients who are active patients of the practice:

Scheduling: Review the appointment book, and look for a discrepancy in scheduling. Examples could include late morning and early afternoon openings, longer appointments scheduled for morning, or follow-up on patient treatment plans.

Recall: Ensure that all active patients are placed on recall. Review patient records for patients who have not been seen in the past six months.

Broken appointments: Review the appointment book for broken appointments, and call these patients to reschedule.

Quality assurance: Send a letter to all patients asking for input on their dental care. This will help to better prepare the office for patient expansion.

4. To increase the number of new patients, the practice can publish a newsletter, develop promotional materials, and send thank-you notes to patients who refer a new patient.

CHAPTER 63: FINANCIAL MANAGEMENT IN THE DENTAL OFFICE

SHORT-ANSWER QUESTIONS

These questions reflect the Learning Outcomes listed at the beginning of this chapter in the textbook, and can be used as class assignments. The answers can be found within the chapter and/or classroom discussion.

FILL IN THE BLANK

1. accounts payable
2. check
3. expenses
4. accounting
5. customary
6. deposit slip
7. carrier
8. CDT
9. gross income
10. invoice
11. ledger
12. net income
13. posted
14. provider
15. walkout statement
16. reasonable
17. responsible party
18. petty cash

Torres and Ehrlich Modern Dental Assisting, 9th ed.

Bird/Robinson

19. statement
20. transaction

MULTIPLE CHOICE

1. d	11. c
2. c	12. b
3. d	13. d
4. c	14. c
5. c	15. b
6. d	16. a
7. d	17. d
8. a	18. b
9. b	19. c
10. d	20. c

CHAPTER 64: MARKETING YOUR SKILLS

SHORT-ANSWER QUESTIONS

These questions reflect the Learning Outcomes listed at the beginning of this chapter in the textbook, and can be used as class assignments. The answers can be found within the chapter and/or classroom discussion.

FILL IN THE BLANK

1. interview
2. termination
3. career
4. professional
5. resume
6. employment

MULTIPLE CHOICE

1. d	6. b
2. d	7. c
3. b	8. a
4. d	9. c
5. d	10. c

ACTIVITIES

These activities may be interpreted differently by each student. The course director will determine whether a student's or a group's response is acceptable.

Torres and Ehrlich Modern Dental Assisting, 9th ed.
Bird/Robinson